Filtration
IN THE
Biopharmaceutical Industry

Filtration IN THE Biopharmaceutical Industry

EDITED BY

Theodore H. Meltzer
Capitola Consulting Company
Bethesda, Maryland

Maik W. Jornitz
Sartorius AG
Göttingen, Germany

MARCEL DEKKER

MARCEL DEKKER, INC. NEW YORK • BASEL

ISBN: 0-8247-9896-1

The publisher offers discounts on this book when ordered in bulk quantities. For more information, write to Special Sales/Professional Marketing at the address below.

This book is printed on acid-free paper.

MARCEL DEKKER, INC.
270 Madison Avenue, New York, New York 10016
http://www.dekker.com

Current printing (last digit):
10 9 8 7

PRINTED IN THE UNITED STATES OF AMERICA

With love and respect
we dedicate this work to those who inspire us

To Wolfgang and Irene Jornitz, my parents –M.W.J.

To the memory of Xavier Magdalene Meltzer,
my wife and companion –T.H.M.

Foreword

In his Preface to *Filtration in the Pharmaceutical Industry* (Dekker, 1987), Theodore Meltzer addressed the subjects to be covered in this seminal opus. He noted that "Theoretical underpinnings are sought," but proceeded to plunge headlong into the real world by adding "but the approach is to the practical." And therein lies its value. That he achieved his objectives is a tribute to Dr. Meltzer's long and varied experience in the field and the body of practical knowledge residing with the myriad contributors he gathered to bring the book to fruition.

In the Foreword to that volume, Dr. K. H. Wallhäusser presents a lucid, concise history of filtration in the pharmaceutical industry up to the time of publication. This, in itself, should be required reading for anyone interested in the subject and perhaps points a way for some latter day author to pursue in much greater detail.

A decade has passed since publication of that work, yet much of its content is pertinent today. This may seem, at first consideration, to contraindicate the need for a reexamination of the subject, especially in an industry not noted for rapid change. On closer scrutiny, however, much has changed or evolved in the pharmaceutical industry, particularly in its biopharmaceutical areas, and in the filter industry, that clearly warrants an update. This second volume moves on from 1987 to cover the work that has been done since then in the manufacture of biopharmaceuticals and the filters that play a vital role in the processes that make it possible.

Some years ago a commentary appeared in print questioning the need for filters with removal ratings smaller than 0.2 μm, then, as now, considered to be the required rating for the sterile filtration of parenteral drugs. The need for smaller micron removal ratings was not generally recognized and, indeed, was considered by some as perhaps a marketing tool to expand the use of submicron filters. However, developments in the pharmaceutical industry were already underway that would dictate the need for such new products. The most notable, of course, was the development of biotechnology with its grounding in cell-derived protein drugs. Mycoplasma removal using 0.1 μm filters became a recognized need. Removal ratings in the nanometer range were needed for clearance of viruses not only in protein drug preparation but also in the production of human therapeutic blood fractions.

Validation of sterilizing filters used in aseptic processing grew from a need recognized by the filter industry to a regulatory requirement. The several techniques to accomplish validation have already filled volumes. Related to validation is the requirement for integrity. One does not need a long memory to recall that integrity testing in process used to be more or less optional. Over the past few years succeeding generations of sophisticated, computerized integrity test instruments have become available. They provide greater accuracy, for example, by measuring direct mass flow, or offer different approaches, such as water intrusion and multipoint testing. Other issues that have loomed larger in the past decade include protein binding, preservative binding, the need for certifying documentation and traceability of filters, and a stronger focus on filter extractables. The regulations for bulk pharmaceutical chemicals have dictated a need for filters designed specifically for this application. This past decade has also seen the emergence of a maturity of thought relative to the removal rating system of membrane filters. Legitimate questions have been asked regarding the numbers, and emphasis seems to be focusing more clearly on validated functionality.

Dr. Meltzer concludes his preface to the previous work by noting that a beginning has been made and hoping that it may serve the interests of filtration in the pharmaceutical field. It has, and if second beginnings are possible, that hope is reiterated for this volume dedicated to the biopharmaceutical field by Maik W. Jornitz and Theodore H. Meltzer.

David B. Pall
Founder/Chairman
Pall Corporation
East Hills, New York

Preface

In 1987 the book *Filtration in the Pharmaceutical Industry* was published and since this time it has served as the most complete reference on aspects of filtration in the pharmaceutical industry.

Most certainly within these last years filtration technology and all accompanying issues including regulatory topics have developed rapidly and changed. Filter systems and components have become more sophisticated and have achieved even higher quality, security, and economics, and production processes have improved dramatically. New filtration flow methods have been developed and optimized, and filter validation has become a firm part of every process and is now well understood within the industry. Integrity testing of filters has also experienced a high degree of positive changes, especially in respect to test sensitivity, automation, and easy of use. Nowadays most integrity tests are performed with automatic test machines, which again raises issues of computer validation requirements. Additionally, processes and theoretical hypotheses not fully understood in earlier years are now clearly defined and questions of the past have been answered.

Since 1987, biotechnology has taken its place alongside the traditional pharmaceutical industry and has brought the industry together as the biopharmaceutical industries. Thus, an up-to-date presentation was deemed to be necessary and is accomplished in *Filtration in the Biopharmaceutical Industry*.

This book elaborates on all the above-described points of filtration and their implications and discusses regulatory issues in detail in the most updated fashion. Not only are all different types of filters, their construction, and their retentive capabilities reviewed, but also specific issues such as extractables, endotoxins, unspecific adsorption, and filter validation are fully covered. Furthermore, the most common applications are thoroughly discussed and specific experiences are pointed out.

The authors did their best to create a compendium that will serve the biopharmaceutical industry in the most comprehensive and useful way. The intention of each individual author is to give answers to questions experienced in the industry, provide a prospective training tool, and document their expertise. We all hope we achieved our intention.

ACKNOWLEDGMENTS

There may be as many motives for editing or writing books as there are editors and authors. The unlimited wealth resulting from royalties may be one. Fame and enhanced personal reputation may be another. A search for knowledge may figure prominently, and for some the dissemination of knowledge may be the valued goal. There may be other reasons as well.

For the writers of life-influencing biopharmaceutical information there can be another motive of considerable merit. There is a tradition of some two thousand years or more that holds that the Good Lord undertook creation for the benefit of all humanity, but that each of us is so individual that in effect all of creation was manifest as if intended totally for each. From this it is concluded that one who preserves even a single life saves creation entire. The pharmaceutical and biotechnical industries being dedicated to mankind's well-being and longevity, the contributors to this book may have striven to attain this meritorious goal. We hope that their efforts and ours prove successful.

We acknowledge with thanks the collaborative efforts of our associates, the contributors to this work, its true authors. This book is of their making; it speaks of their professionalism and expertise. We are very grateful for their collegiality.

There are always enablers, individuals without whose hard work and devoted assistance very little would have been accomplished. In this instance, the hard work and Irish determination of Karen Storm were truly indispensable. The inspirational influences of Xavier Magdalene Meltzer, whom we dearly miss, are deeply avowed. We add our gratitude to Lila Harris and the others of the Marcel Dekker staff. We honor them all with sincere acknowledgment of our profound indebtedness to them.

Maik W. Jornitz
Theodore H. Meltzer

Contents

Part III Utilitarian Considerations

Part IV Applications

Contributors

Tony Alex Pall Corporation, Port Washington, New York

C. Thomas Badenhop Badenhop Engineering Services, Westport, Connecticut

Forest Badmington Millipore Corporation, Bedford, Massachusetts

Chris Bailey W. L. Gore and Associates, Elkton, Maryland

Daniel Brose Chemica Technologies, Inc., Bend, Oregon

Jeffrey R. Carter Millipore Corporation, Bedford, Massachusetts

Anthony C. Celeste AAC Consulting Group, Inc., Bethesda, Maryland

Michael Dosmar Sartorius Corporation, Edgewood, New York

Marilyn J. Gould Associates of Cape Cod, Inc., Falmouth, Massachusetts

Harwood Green Becton Dickinson and Company, Franklin Lakes, New Jersey

John Gulliford Pall Corporation, Pleasanton, California

Holly Haughney Pall Corporation, Port Washington, New York

Maik W. Jornitz Sartorius AG, Göttingen, Germany

Hyman B. Katz Pall Corporation, East Hills, New York

Julius Z. Knapp Research & Development Associates, Inc., Somerset, New Jersey

Rodney A. Knight Cuno, Inc., Meriden, Connecticut

Karen Lange W. L. Gore and Associates, Elkton, Maryland

Richard V. Levy Millipore Corporation, Bedford, Massachusetts

Alvin Lieberman Particle Measuring Systems, Fremont, California

Herbert Lutz Millipore Corporation, Bedford, Massachusetts

Theodore H. Meltzer Capitola Consulting Company, Bethesda, Maryland

Marc W. Mittelman Centre for Infection & Biomaterials Research, The Toronto Hospital, Toronto, Ontario, Canada

Wayne P. Olson Oldevco, Beecher, Illinois

Eugene A. Ostreicher Cuno, Inc., Meriden, Connecticut

Michael W. Phillips Millipore Corporation, Bedford, Massachusetts

Oscar W. Reif Sartorius AG, Göttingen, Germany

Juergen Rupp Sartorius AG, Göttingen, Germany

Larry A. Scheer Pall Corporation, Ann Arbor, Michigan

Anthony C. Shucosky Memtec Group, Timonium, Maryland

Gordon R. S. Smith Consultant, North East, Maryland

Peter Soelkner Sartorius AG, Göttingen, Germany

Srikanth Sundaram Pall Corporation, Port Washington, New York

Michael Sutsko W. L. Gore and Associates, Elkton, Maryland

Stanley W. Tarry Sartorius Corporation, Edgewood, New York

Karen Tronto W. L. Gore and Associates, Elkton, Maryland

A. Mark Trotter Sartorius Corporation, Edgewood, New York

Michael Wikol W. L. Gore and Associates, Elkton, Maryland

1

Filter Aid Filtration

GORDON R. S. SMITH
North East, Maryland

1 INTRODUCTION

1.1 Nonstructured Filter Media

The removal of particles from the fluids containing them can often be accomplished by contacting the suspension with finely divided solids onto whose surfaces the particles absorb or within whose layers they can become sieve removed (Fiore et al., 1980). Thus, deep-bed filters of sand (Ogedengloe, 1984), garnet, anthracite, coal, charcoal, etc., perform the particle-removal actions desired of them in water purification contexts. Particles are captured in such instances throughout the deep-bed filter, hence the term *depth filter* (as distinct from surface or screen filter) to describe the loci of particle removal. Such nonstructured depth filters are also devised by stirring finely divided solids such as diatomaceous earth, perlite, and/or various other filter aids, into the suspension, followed by the filtrative removal of both the purifying particle and the particles it has entrapped by adsorption.

Thus, in pharmaceutical manufacturing, filter aids find application in serum purification, antibiotic manufacture, and in vitro diagnostics preparation. Granulated activated carbon is used for color removal in the manufacture of large-volume parenterals (LVPs) and antibiotics. Fumed silica is used in the preparation of certain therapeutic blood fractions. Since these finely divided solids are often used in the form of layers supported on a septum or in the form of deep beds, they are defined as nonstructured filters or prefilters, the latter term stressing their customary usage. The prefilter in turn implies a filtrative action involving adsorptive removal (as well as sieve retention), especially for the particles of impurities small enough to enter the filter pores, the interstices among the solid granules, along with the permeating liquid.

There is a group of granulated solids among these materials that, because of their sizes, shapes, and mode of disposition, form layers whose filtrative action differs from that of the conventional unstructured depth filters such as sand or carbon. These nonstructured filtered materials are given the appellation of filter aids in the industrial filtration field where they are most widely used. Actually, however, they are not filter aids in the sense that flocculating agents may be said to assist in the filtrative removal of fine particles. Rather, they comprise the primary filter material. Their cakes, when properly composed, are tight enough to restrain particles chiefly by sieve retention. Because of the way they are used these nonstructured filter aids can provide a high particle loading capacity even while permitting high rates of flow. These materials are unique in that when used in the precoat body feed mode they provide what is, in effect, continuous surface filtration and thus combine the near positive separations of surface filtration with the dirt-holding properties of depth filters.

1.2 An Outline of Methods of Use

There are two basic ways in which filter aids are used: the precoat body feed method, which is almost always a pressure filtration, and the rotary drum precoat method, which is almost always under vacuum.

In the precoat body feed method (Fig. 1), a thin layer of filter aid, about $^1/_{16}$ in. thick, is first formed on a septum by recirculation of a filter aid slurry. After the precoat is in place, filtration is started as filter aid is continually added to the liquid being filtered. This produces a more permeable filter cake and lengthens the filter cycle. At the end of the filter cycle the precoat and cake are removed from the filter, and the process is repeated.

In the second method (Fig. 2), a layer of filter aid up to 6 in. thick is formed on a filter drum (usually under vacuum) as it rotates in a filter aid slurry. As filtration takes place, the filter cake that forms on the surface of the precoat is shaved off, along with a small amount of precoat, by a doctor blade. When the blade nears the drum, the remaining precoat is removed and the process is repeated.

1.3 Grades and Types

Filter aids come in a variety of materials and grades, each with various particle shapes, sizes, and distributions. Thus, it is possible to adjust the filter medium to meet changes in filtration needs and conditions by simply changing the grade, type, or amount of filter aid used.

1.4 Uses

Filter aids are useful industrially in the filtrative breaking of oil emulsions by the removal of stabilizing solids and in the removal of solids from aqueous streams even when the solids contents are too low for flocculation (i.e., below 5 ppm), reducing them to as low as 0.1 ppm. Filter aids in conjunction with a rotary vacuum drum have been used to remove particles too fine to be separated by most fixed media. An example is 6% or higher of solids from antibiotic fermentation broth filtration where the median particle range is only some 1–2 μm.

Filter aids are also used to filter a wide variety of liquids such as wine, beer, fruit juices, vegetable oils, corn, cane and beet sugars, various chemicals, and a wide variety of waste liquids and sludges. Because the filtered suspended solids emerge from the filter mixed with filter aids, this type of filtration is used primarily for clarification of liquids.

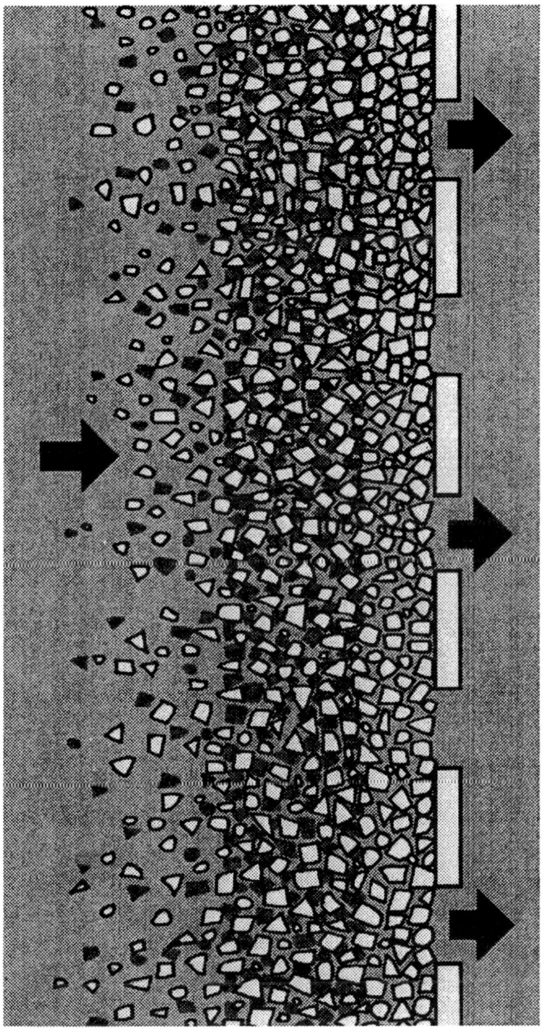

Figure 1 Schematic of filter cake and precoat. (Courtesy of Celite Co., Lompoc, CA.)

1.5 Typical Characteristics of Slurries Filtered

Typically the particles in the liquids filtered with the use of filter aids have a settling rate in water of from <0.02 to 0.2 feet per minute (fpm), particle sizes as low as 0.1 μm, and an undissolved solids content of a few parts per million to 4%. Flow volumes range from less than 30 gpm for sludges and viscous liquids to 10,000 gpm for water filtration. Unit flow rates will range from less than 0.1 gallon per square foot per minute (gsfm) to 1 gsfm. Solids can be recovered as a dry cake or as a thickened slurry (Ernst et al., 1991).

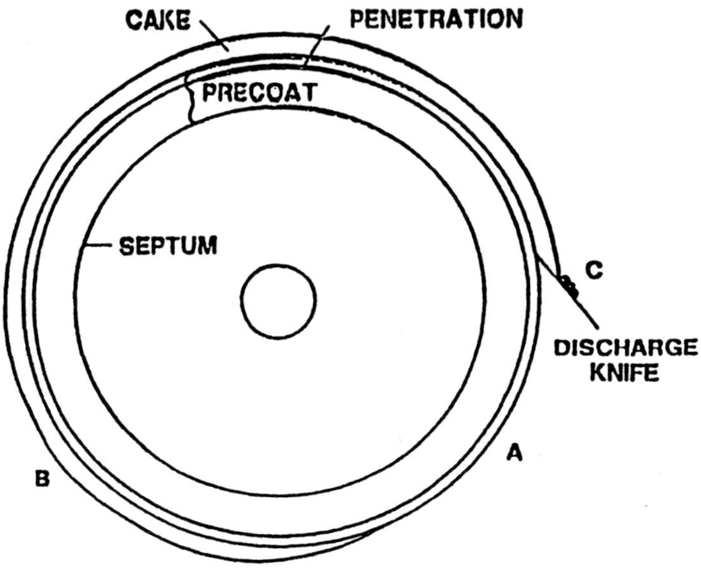

Figure 2 Cross section of a rotary vacuum precoat filter.

1.6 Clarification Properties of Filter Aids

There are so many factors affecting the clarification properties of filter aids that it is impossible to make any definitive statements as to what size particles will be removed by a specific grade of filter aid. These include, first, the particle shape, size and size distribution, charge, rigidity (or compressibility), and concentration. Next are operating conditions such as flow velocity, steadiness of pressure, and system vibration. Viscosity will tend to drag more fines through the cake, and the liquid may cause particles to either coagulate or peptize. Clarity may also increase as the filter cycle lengthens due to increased compaction of the filter cake with increased pressure (and whether the filter is run at constant pressure or constant rate or some combination of the two).

Considering these factors, the clarification abilities of filter aids can be described by means of examples and some studies. For example, the finer grades of diatomite filter aids have been shown to be able to remove, in laboratory tests, 100% of the coliform organism (Hunter et al., 1966). Numerous examples exist of the use of diatomite filter aids for the removal of amebic cysts and *Gardia lamblia* (Logsdon et al., 1981). The most stable filter cakes in terms of particle retention have been shown to be those in which the median particle size is matched by the median pore size of the filter aid (Cain, 1973).

1.7 Costs

Filter aid coats cost on the order of $0.10–0.30/lb with a dirt-holding capacity of 0.1–5 lb filter solids per pound of filter aid, making them one of the least expensive types of filter media available. The principal disadvantages of filter aid filtration are the capital costs of the equipment required to use a filter aid, contamination of the filtered solids with the filter aid, and additional cake disposal costs due to the presence of filter aids. Dust containment may also be a cost factor.

2 GENERAL PROPERTIES OF FILTER AIDS

2.1 Introduction

There are a number of properties of the filter cakes or layers built of the various nonstructured depth filters that determine their suitability for particular filter applications. The pore sizes of their interstices govern their sieve retentivity and influence their rate of flow. Flow rate is also dependent on the number of pores, but pore size is more important. The cake permeability to liquids is therefore dependent on the number of pores but more dependent on their size. The density of packing and the cake incompressibility in turn define the pore sizes, for it is the dimensional stability of the cake structure that governs the permanence of pore sizes, the retentivity, and the low rates achieved under the differential pressures over the duration of the filtration.

Table 1 illustrates the ranges of permeability, median pore sizes, and wet densities obtainable from the more common types of filter aids. The information in this table is useful in the preliminary evaluation of the physical properties of a material as a prospective filter aid.

The permeability of the filter aid cakes also defines the accessibility of the suspension being filtered to the filter cloth, pad, or septum on which the cake is constructed by deposition of the discrete filter aid particles. This is important when cleaning operations are involved. It is desired that the impurities not penetrate the filter cake to foul the septum. It is found that some 3% of larger particles, above 150 mesh in size, should be in the particle mix. This serves to bridge over the septum openings and therefore helps to form a stable precoat. Low cake densities make for good permeability. The densities should be on the order of 160–320 kg/m^3 (10–20 lb/ft^3), depending on the filter aid. Small and more regularly shaped particles have higher normal packing densities and lower permeability. This makes for the retention of finer particles by sieving but may unduly penalize the rate of flow. Generally speaking, the more narrow the particle size distribution, the more efficient the filter

Table 1 Properties of Filter Aids

Property	Filter aid		
	Diatomite	Perlite	Cellulose
Permeability (darcies)	0.06–30	0.4–6	0.4–12
Median cake pore size (μm)	1.1–30	7–16	—
Wet density			
(kg/m^3)	260–320	150–270	60–320
(lb/ft^3)	16–20	9–17	7–20
Compressibility	Low	Medium	High

aid cake because the more regular its degree of packing and the smaller its interstices. The median particle sizes of filter aids will range from 6 to 30 μm or more.

Filter aids come in many grades, but with the finest grades it is possible to remove more than 90% of 0.2 μm latex beads and other particles down in the colloidal range. Slightly coarser diatomite grades, of 0.3 darcy[1] permeability, have been shown capable of quantitative removal of coliform organisms (Hunter, 1966). It is possible to remove, with 1 lb of filter aid, anywhere from 0.1 to 5 lb (90 g to 2.2 kg) of suspended solids. In addition to the cake pore size, permeability, and compressibility, properties of interest in the screen analysis include the solubility and wet densities of the filter aid particles.

2.2 Types of Filter Aids

Diatomaceous Earth

Diatomaceous earth (Breese, 1989), called kieselguhr in Europe, is the most widely used type of filter aid. It consists of skeletal remains, millions of years old, of aquatic plants. It is mined from its natural deposits. As mined, dried, and sized by air classification, the diatomite particles are very fine (Fig. 3). Hence, they give filter cakes of high retentivity but low permeability. Calcining, with or without a flux, serves to adhere the very small particles to one another, making for larger aggregates. When a sodium carbonate flux is used in the calcining process, even coarser particles result. These yield filter aid cakes of greater permeability.

Most of the non-silica elements are bound up as silicates and are therefore relatively insoluble. For instance, solubility in dilute acids (except HF) is on the order of 0.1% for calcined filter aids and 0.2% for flux calcined filter aids. However, a 10% mixture of the soda ash flux calcined diatomite will have a pH of about 10. Its major soluble constituents will be calcium and iron. Smaller amounts of other ions will also be present. Acid-washed grades with substantially smaller amounts of such ingredients are also available. Diatomite is approximately 90% silica. It is therefore rather soluble, except in hot caustic (although it has been used to filter 50% sodium hydroxide solutions at room temperature).

Table 3 shows typical properties of various grades of diatomaceous earth. Filter-Cel is raw, uncalcined diatomite. It can be washed free of its iron and inorganic leachables by rinsing with several volumes of 2% salt solution (NaCl). When used in plasma/serum filtration, this is followed by a similar volume wash of ethanol in water of the same concentration and pH as the solution it is meant to precede. It is used in 2.5–5 g/L concentrations to form a precoat; a similar, or higher, quantity is mixed into the liquid to be filtered to serve as a body feed.

Because of its wider range of permeability and pore sizes, diatomaceous earth is used when high rates of flow are required (high permeability grades) or high degrees of clarification are being sought (low permeability grades). Its irregular shapes give highly porous beds of high flow rates.

Particle size analysis and typical physical and chemical properties are shown in Tables 2 and 3. In Table 3 note that the median pore size goes from approximately

---

[1]One darcy equals a flow through a geometric section 1 cm^2 in area and 1 cm thick of 1 mL/s of a liquid of 1 cP viscosity at 1 atm differential pressure.

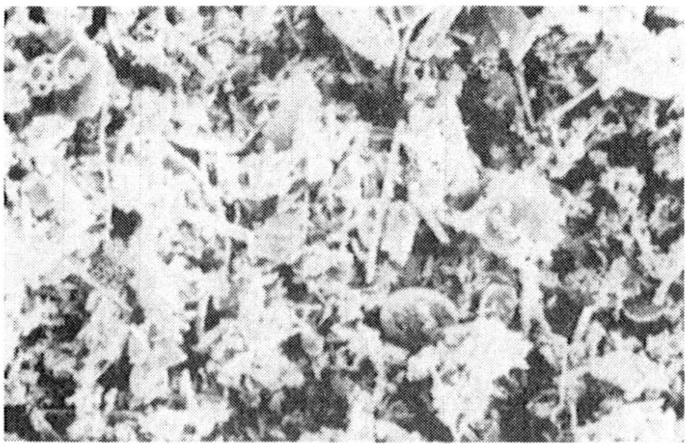

Figure 3 A midrange diatomite filter aid (200× scanning electron micrograph). (Courtesy of Celite Co.)

6 μm for the finest (lowest permeability) grade to approximately 120 μm for the highest permeability grade or a 20-fold increase whereas the permeability in darcies (Table 3) ranges from 0.09 to 30, over a 300-fold increase.

Perlite

Perlite is derived from volcanic rock and contains about two-thirds aluminum and one-third sodium silicate plus combined water (see Fig. 4). Thus, its solubility is essentially that of diatomite; its amounts of iron and calcium will be slightly lower. It is prepared by sizing the ore, expanding it with heat, milling, sizing, and packaging. As shown in Table 4, perlite filter aids yield filter cakes having permeability or flow rates equivalent to the middle of the diatomite range. The pore size of the smaller perlite particle cakes is significantly larger, however, than that of the smaller diatomite cakes. The smaller the particle size, the closer its degree of normal packing (at least to the extent permitted by the particle shape), and hence the smaller the spatial interstices of the resulting cake and the concomitant permeability and rates of flow. Therefore, where the removal of microorganisms or other fine particles is desired, diatomite filter cakes are preferred.

The perlite particles consist of large flat impermeable surfaces. This shape inclines perlite filter cakes to exhibit lower pore size-to-permeability ratios. Nevertheless, given diatomite and perlite filter aids of equal permeability, the perlite will have a higher median pore size and thus a higher pore size-to-permeability ratio. The wet densities of perlite cakes are, however, significantly lower than those of diatomite. Therefore, given the same weight of material, perlite cakes are thicker, giving them greater solids-holding capacity, and for cakes of equal thickness, less perlite on a weight basis will be needed. Perlite is somewhat more compressible than diatomaceous earth. (This property comes to bear in later discussions on vacuum filtration.)

Along with the particle size distributions there should be few if any unmilled particles, or "floaters."

Table 4 lists typical properties of Dicalite perlite filter aids. These properties are also similar to those of perlite filter aids made by Celite. Note that the pH of all grades is 7.0–7.5 as no flux is used in their manufacture.

Table 2 Typical Particle Size[a]

Filter	Weight % finer than micrometer size (lazer sizer) Micrometer size 1.0	1.5	2.0	3.0	4.0	6.0	8.0	12.0	16.0	24.0	32.0	48.0	64.0	96.0	128.0	196.0	Median particle size (μm)
Celite 500	2	2	4	6	10	19	27	41	54	69	78	90	93	97	100	100	14.7
Filter Cel	2	3	4	8	12	22	31	45	58	72	80	92	94	98	100	100	14.0
Celite 577	2	3	4	7	12	21	30	41	52	66	75	83	87	95	99	100	14.6
Std. Super-Cel	2	3	4	6	9	17	25	39	52	69	77	90	93	99	100	100	15.4
Celite 512	2	2	4	5	8	15	22	36	49	65	75	87	92	97	99	100	16.4
Hyflo Super-Cel	2	2	3	5	7	11	16	25	36	53	67	86	91	97	99	100	22.3
Hyflo RV	1.4	1.7	2.7	3.4	4.5	6.2	8.3	13.5	25.6	37.9	50.2	67.6	75.7	88.3	94.8	100	30
Celite 501	2	2	3	4	6	9	13	20	32	50	64	82	88	95	99	100	24.3
Celite 503	2	2	3	4	5	7	10	16	25	42	56	76	84	92	98	100	28.6
Celite 503 RV	1	1.4	2.2	2.7	3.9	4.8	6.1	9	14.4	26	37.1	56.2	63.7	76.1	81.1	100	40.0
Celite 535	1	2	3	4	5	7	10	16	23	36	49	70	79	91	98	100	34.3
Celite 545	1	2	2	3	4	5	6	9	14	26	40	55	78	92	99	100	36.2
Celite 580	1.3	1.5	2	2.6	3.3	4.6	5.9	8	12.1	20.6	32	53.2	65.5	82.4	95.6	100	45
Celite 560	1.3	1.6	2.3	3.2	4.5	6.9	9.5	13.9	19.2	26.2	34	47.8	55.8	70.1	92.5	100	55

[a]The coarsest particles of the coarser grades of filter aid exceed the dynamic range of a laser sizer, so data shown for those grades indicate a somewhat finer particle size distribution than actual.

Source: Celite Bulletin FA-84A, 1989, Celite Co., Lompoc, CA.

Table 3 Typical Physical Properties[a]

Grade	Color	Fibra-Cel–diatomite blend equiv.[b]	Median pore size (μm)	Approx. ΔP at 1 gsfm with 0.15 lb/ft^2 precoat	Estimated gsfh water; 6 in. precoat, 24 in. Hg ΔP	Permeability (Da)	Density lb/ft^3 Dry	Density lb/ft^3 Wet	150 mesh, % retained	% Moisture as shipped	pH	% Solubles
Celite 500	Gray	NA	1.5	3.2	NA	0.057	7.0	16	2	3.0	7.0	0.15
Filter Cel	Pink	1	2.5	2.6	NA	0.062	7.5	17	1	1.0	8.0	0.20
577	Pink	2	2.5	1.2	NA	0.16	8.0	18	2	0.5	7.0	0.10
Standard Super-Cel	Pink	5	3.5	0.7	10	0.28	8.0	18	4	0.5	7.0	0.10
512	Pink	6	5.0	0.4	20	0.53	8.0	19	7	0.5	7.0	0.10
Hyflo Super-Cel	White	7	7.0	0.1	50	1.2	9.0	18	6	0.1	10.0	0.15
Hyflo RV	White	NA	7.5	0.09	60	1.25	10.0	20	14	0.1	10.0	0.15
501	White	8	9.0	0.07	65	1.4	9.5	18	8	0.1	10.0	0.15
503	White	9	10.0	0.06	130	2.0	9.5	18	9	0.1	10.0	0.15
503 RV	White	NA	14.0	0.03	300	3.5	14.0	20.5	20	0.1	10.0	0.15
535	White	10	13.0	0.03	240	3.1	12.0	19	10	0.1	10.0	0.15
545	White	11	17.0	0.02	370	4.8	12.0	19	12	0.1	10.0	0.15
580	White	NA	17.0	0.02	370	5.8	18.0	21	30	0.1	10.0	0.15
560	White	13	22.0	0.005	1400	30.0	16.0	20	40	0.1	10.0	0.15

NA = Not applicable; gsfm = gallons per square foot per minute; gsfh = gallons per square foot per hour.

[a]As expressed, these are typical or estimated physical properties, not specifications, and should be used accordingly.

[b]Fibra-Cel grades are designated by a number plus a letter (i.e., Fibra-Cel 7F). The number refers to the equivalent grade of Celite filter aid and the letter to the percent cellulose in multiples of 2½%; i.e., A = 2½%, B = 5%, C = 7½%, etc.

Source: Celite Bulletin FA-84A, Celite Co., Lompoc, CA.

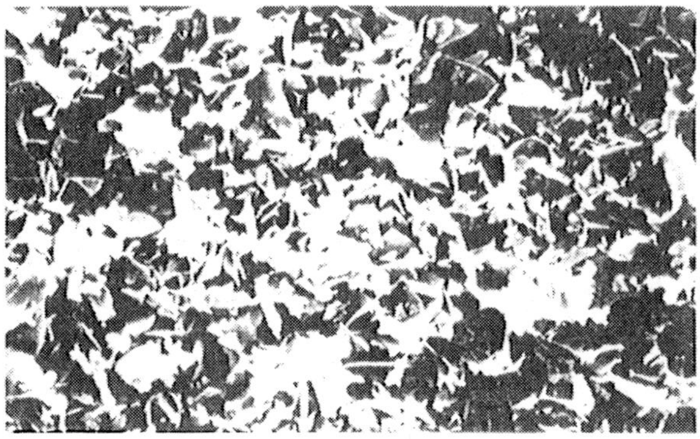

Figure 4 Perlite filter aid (200× scanning electron micrograph).

For a given type of filter aid with a particular basic particle structure, grades with lower cakes densities will have better clarification and dirt-holding efficiencies. Note that the relative flow rates of perlite filter aids range from 300 to 900, which puts them in the midrange of the filter aids shown in Table 5. It is in this flow rate range, therefore, that perlite filter aids are most likely to perform well.

Perlite filter aids made by Silbrico Corp. (Hodgkins, IL) have lower cake densities that also decrease steadily as flow rates increase (Table 5).

A comparison of diatomite and perlite filter aids is given in Table 6.

Cellulose Filter Aids

Cellulose filter aids (see Fig. 5 and Table 7) are used where a fibrous filter aid is needed to enhance filter aid performance or where their chemical resistance and combustibility are required. They are produced in two grades of cellulose: cellulose grades, which are highly purified, and the less purified and less costly brown grades.

The most common use of cellulose filter aids is in adding stability to diatomite or perlite precoats. Here they may be used as a pre-precoat to be followed by a diatomite or perlite precoat or, more commonly, blended with diatomite filter aids in amounts of 2.5–10% or higher as shown in the third column of Table 3.

Cellulose filter aids are also used where trace amounts of silica cannot be tolerated such as in the filtration of alkaline solutions and condensate in high pressure boilers. They can also be used as precoat on rotary vacuum precoat filters.

Specialty Filter Aids

Acid-washed diatomite filter aids, such as those made by the Celite Co. (Lompoc, CA) have reduced soluble iron and other impurities.

Celite analytical filter aids provide maximum acid washing for use in analytical filtrations.

Coating filter aids with such compounds as iron and aluminum hydrates as well as various surfactive agents greatly increases their effectiveness in removing turbidity, color, and coliform from water (Bell, 1961). Diatomite filter aids can be used with magnesite for iron removal (Bell, 1965b; Pittendreigh, 1966) and with potassium permanganate for manganese removal from potable water (Bell, 1965a; Coogan, 1962). Sorbo-Cel is an activated filter aid that can remove emulsified oil to 0.1 ppmw (Bell,

Table 4 Typical Properties of Dicalite Perlite Filter Aids[a]

Grade	Relative flow rate	Density (lb/ft^3) Loose wt.	Density (lb/ft^3) Filter cake	Density (kg/m^3) Loose wt.	Density (kg/m^3) Filter cake	% Retained, 150 mesh	Specific gravity	pH	Ignition loss[b] (%)	Color
416	130	5.5	21.0	88	336	—	2.3	7.0	3.0	White
426	175	5.0	20.0	80	320	—	2.3	7.0	3.0	White
436	300	6.0	15.0	96	240	3.0	2.3	7.0	3.0	White
476	650	7.0	15.0	112	240	4.0	2.3	7.0	3.0	White
CP-150	700	11.0	18.0	176	288	9.0	2.3	7.5	3.0	White
4106	900	9.0	15.5	144	248	13.0	2.3	7.5	3.0	White
CP-175	1000	12.0	18.0	192	288	20.0	2.3	7.5	3.0	White
4156	1325	11.0	18.0	176	288	17.0	2.3	7.5	3.0	White

[a]Based on U.S. produced perlite grades.
[b]4 h at 1700°F (927°C).
Source: Dicalite Technical Filtration Bulletin B-16, Grefco, Inc.

Table 5 Typical Properties of Silbrico Perlite Filter Aids

Grade	Weight of bags (lb/bag)	Cake permeability (Da)	Relative flow (mL)	Avg wet cake (lb/ft^3)
27-M	40	2	300	12.5
25-M	32	5	550	10.0
23-S	34	1.0	750	9.0
21-S	32	1.5	950	8.5
19-S	29	2.0	1100	8.0
17-S	25	3.0	1300	7.0
15-S	23	5.0	1700	6.0

Note: Tested with tap water under constant pressure.
Source: Silbrico Technical Bulletin, Silbrico Corporation, Hodgkins, IL.

1952). Diatomite filter aid filtration used in conjunction with cationic polyelectrolyte has been shown to be effective in removing viruses from water (Amirhor, 1952).

Celite AF is treated to prevent flocculation due to moisture in organic solvents.

3 FILTER AID FILTRATION WITH PRECOAT AND BODY FEED

3.1 Introduction

The essential parts of the pressure filter aid system are shown in Fig. 6.

There are three steps in pressure precoat filtration. The first step is the formation of the precoat layer. This is done by recirculating a mixture of the filter aid [equal, more commonly, to 0.1–0.15 lb/ft^2 (0.0488–0.0732 g/cm^2) of filter area] and clarified liquid or filtrate from the precoat tank through the filter and return. The precoat layer or filter aid cake is generally not in excess of $\frac{1}{16}$ in. (3 mm) in thickness. In the second step, filter aid as body feed is added to the liquid to be filtered. The addition of filter aid in this manner greatly increases cake permeability and decreases cake compressibility, resulting in much longer filtration cycles. Filtration is generally carried out at a constant or nearly constant rate and continues until a differential pressure of usually 30–50 psi (2.1–3.5 kg/cm^2) is reached or maximum cake is built, as defined by the cake space (the space available in the equipment for occupancy by the filter aid cake). Ideally, the maximum cake space and maximum pressure are reached at approximately the same time. The degree of clarification, cycle length, and filter aid consumption depend on the type grades of filter aid selected for precoat and body feed and the amount of filter aid added as body feed. The type and amount of body feel required to increase filter cycle length significantly depend on the compressibility and amount of undissolved solids, with the amount ranging from one-fourth the weight of incompressible solids to five or more times the weight of gelatinous compressible solids.

Used in the above manner, the precoat provides a surface filtration with the body feed continually renewing the filter surface. Separation is essentially positive and generally increases with cake thickness.

Table 6 Diatomite/Perlite Filter Aid Comparison Chart

Relative flow rate	Permeability (Da)	Celite	Grefco (Dicalite)[a]	Eagle-Picher (Celatom)	Celite Witco (Kenite)	Sil-Flo perlite	Silbrico (Sil-Kleer)	Femco perlite
100	0.09	Filter Cel	115	FW-2	100	—	—	—
135	0.2	Celite 577	Superaid	FP-2	—	—	27M	—
			215					
200	0.5	Std. Super-Cel	Speedflow	FP-4	200	—	32M	—
			416 (P)					
300	0.9	Celite 512	Sp. Speedflow	FP-6	300	—	23M	—
			426 (P)	FW-6				
			231					
500	2.0	Hyflow Super-Cel	Speedplus	FW-14	700	443	29M	505-S
			436 (P)	FW-12	720			HX-1
			476 (P)	FW-10	723			
750	2.5	Celite 501	—	FW-18	—	272	25M	—
900	3.5	Celite 503	Speedex	FW-20	1000	332	—	V-404
			4106 (P)	FW-14S	2500			V-505
			375	FWS	3000			
			CP-150 (P)					
			CP-175 (P)					
1350	5.5	Celite 535	4156 (P)	FW-50	—	—		—
			4200					
2200	8.5	Celite 545	—	FW-60	—	—		—
7500	30	Celite 560	6000	FW-80	5500	—		—

[a](P) after Dicalite grade indicates perlite.
Source: Eagle-Picher Industries, Inc., Cincinnati, OH.

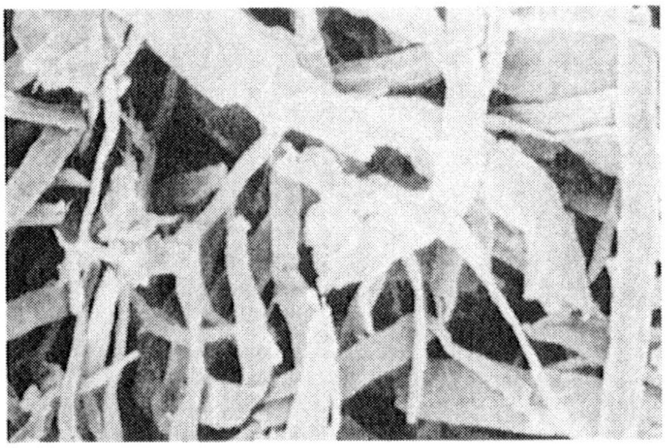

Figure 5 Cellulose filter aid (200× scanning electron micrograph). (Courtesy of Celite Co., Lompoc, CA.)

In those applications where body feed/solids ratios are roughly equal, it is not necessary to account for the density of the undissolved solids being removed, as these will fit into the interstices of the filter aid and will not increase cake volume.

3.2 Precoat

The precoat serves three purposes. First, it protects the septum from becoming fouled by the suspended impurities. Thus it is particularly important if the impurities are compressible and therefore likely to be sticky. Second, the precoat provides immediate filtrate clarity; and third, the precoat greatly facilitates cake removal from the septum at the end of the filter cycle.

In selecting the grade of filter aid for precoating, the coarsest grade that will prevent penetration by the impurities being removed, particularly where they may be slimy, should be selected. Tests can easily be run in a Buchner funnel. With the correct grade, a distinct line should be visible between the precoat and suspended solids. At this point, a slightly finer grade may be selected if filtrate clarity is still too poor.

Depending on the type of septum used and the need to minimize precoat bleed-through, a mixture of diatomite or perlite and cellulose may be used. Alternatively, a pre-precoat of 100% cellulose followed by a granular filter aid material may be used.

Septum Selection

Wire screens or cloths may be used as septa. In some applications such as those in the beverage industry, fibrous pads, felts, or paper may be used. Occasionally, the use of these materials will result in exceptionally high precoat pressures (they are ordinarily 1–2 psi) due to precoat/septum interface resistance. In these cases, a base, or pre-, precoat can be applied or the septum can be changed.

Screens are of higher capital cost but are more permanent, lasting up to 5 years. Cloths are cheaper to install and usually have lower corrosion resistance and, of course, lower temperature resistance. With both wire and cloth, the larger the fiber diameter, the more durable the material. Thus, a wire mesh with 0.011 in. wire may last longer than 0.007 in. wire, and a monofilament cloth may be more durable than a multifilament or staple. In each of these cases, the longer lasting material will have

Table 7 Typical Properties of Solka-Floc Cellulose Filter Aids

Grade	Color	Density (lb/ft^3) Loose wt.	Density (lb/ft^3) Filter cake	Density (kg/m^3) Loose wt.	Density (kg/m^3) Filter cake	Specific gravity	% Retention (U.S. std. screens) 40M	% Retention (U.S. std. screens) 100M	% Retention (U.S. std. screens) 325M	Fiber length (μm)	pH	Ignition loss (%)
KS-1016	White	3.2	10.5	50	170	1.5	16.0	52.0	87.0	290	7.0	99.8
SW-40	White	4.0	10.3	65	165	1.5	0.5	37.0	81.0	100–140	6.5	99.8
BW-20	White	6.5	13.5	105	215	1.5	9.0	33.0	68.0	80–120	6.0	99.8
BW-40	White	8.0	14.0	130	225	1.5	1.0	14.0	56.0	50–60	6.0	99.8
BW-100	White	12.5	19.0	200	305	1.5	tr.	6.0	31.0	35–45	6.0	99.8
BW-200	White	14.5	20.0	230	320	1.5	0	2.4	25.0	30–35	6.0	99.8

Source: Grefco, Inc.

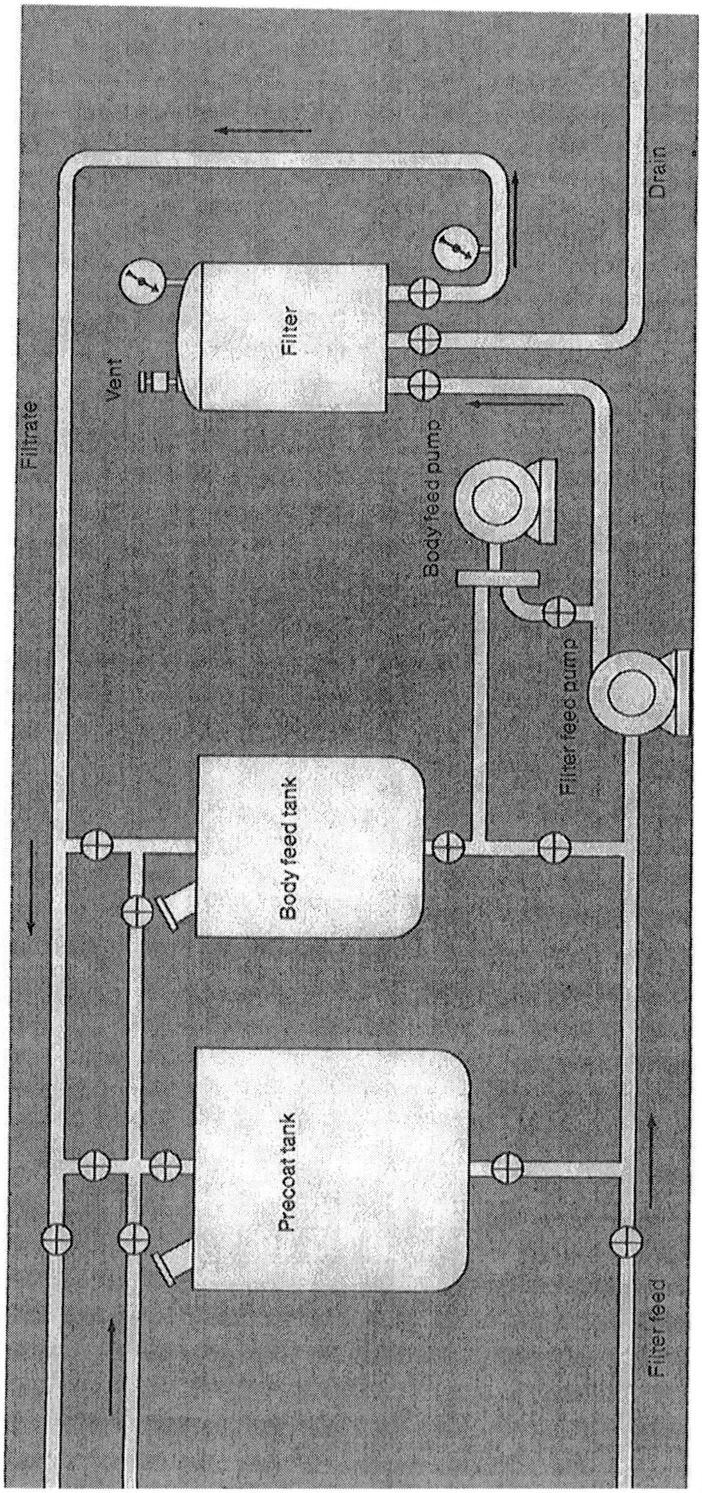

Figure 6 Typical filter aid filtration system. (Courtesy of Celite Co.)

larger openings and will therefore be harder to precoat and result in a less stable precoat. For wire screens, which may be woven, or well screen tubes, the maximum size opening that can be bridged by a precoat is 0.005 in.

Commonly used screen meshes are

24 × 110 Dutch weave (0.16 × 0.11 in. diameter wire)
70 × 80 mesh (0.007 in.)
60 mesh twilled (0.007–0.011 in.)

Precoat Formation

Precoat formation depends on the filter aid particle size, the septum opening size, the precoat slurry concentration, precoat slurry distribution within the filter, and recirculation rate. Filter aid particle size varies widely, of course, from grade to grade of filter aid. For good precoat formation on all but the tightest septa there should be at least 3% retained on a 150 mesh screen.

The septum opening sizes will depend on factors discussed above. The larger openings, up to 0.005 in., will require precoat concentrations on the order of 0.6–0.9% whereas a 0.3% concentration may be satisfactory for cloth septa.

The required precoat concentrations for commonly used filter aids are shown in Table 8. It should be noted here that the amounts shown are based on even precoat formation and are therefore about 2 lb lower than commonly recommended doses. This is indicative of possible precoat savings to be had with good internal filter hydraulics.

Table 9 shows the mean time for clarity for a wire septum at various flow rates. These times should be corrected for finer septa.

For a precoat to function properly, essentially all of it must be deposited on the septum. Table 10 shows the percent applied vs. tank volume circulated, assuming 100% retention.

It should be noted that even after four tank volumes, 2% of the precoat material remains in the slurry. This is extremely fine material, and if recirculation is allowed to continue when it should be delayed from going on stream, it will significantly increase the resistance of the precoat. This problem can be reduced by lowering the recirculation rate or, better still, adding body feed (discussed in the next section).

Table 8 Screen Precoat Amounts and Slurry Concentration Required

Material grade or equivalent	Wet density (lb/ft^3)	$lb/100\ ft^2$ (1/16 in. depth)	Slurry density (gal/lb)	PPM concn
All Solka Floc grades	12–16	8	20	6000
Perlites	12–14	8	20	6000
Standard Super-Cel	14–16	8	20	6000
Hyflo Super-Cel	17–19	10	17	7000
Celite 501	18–20	10	16	7500
Celite 503	20–21	11	15	8000
Celite 535	20–22	11	14	8600
Celite 545	21–23	12	14	8600

Source: Ulrich (1966).

Table 9 Pressure Leaf Clarity vs. Time at Various Precoat Rates

Precoat rate (gph/ft^2)	Mean time to clarify[a] (min)
10	10
15	7
20	5
30	3.5
40	2.5
50	2.0
60	1.6
75	1.3

[a]From when flow starts.

Precoat rates are generally on the order of 0.5 gal/(ft$^2 \cdot$min) for water and proportionately lower for higher viscosity liquids. The rate should be high enough to maintain an upward flow of 4 ft/min, which is required to keep the coarsest grades in suspension. Precoat pressures are shown in Table 3, column 4.

Precoat Troubleshooting

Precoat filtrate should clear up in 2–5 min or after a maximum of three turnovers. Poor, or delayed, clarity may be caused by

1. Improper venting of the filter preventing the slurry level from completely covering the filter elements.
2. Precoat erosion caused by high inlet velocities and poor baffling.
3. Blinded septum, resulting in unstable precoat formation.
4. Tears in the septum.
5. Wrinkles in the septum, causing enlarged openings.
6. Old screens with openings enlarged due to wear or corrosion (in the case of wire screens).
7. Poor circulation in the filter preventing even distribution of the precoat.
8. Low precoat rate failing to keep precoat in suspension.
9. Low precoat concentration. Precoat formation depends partly on a crowding effect of filter aid particles around the septum openings.

Table 10 Precoat Applied vs. Tank Volumes Circulated

Tank volume circulated	Precoat applied (%)
3/4	50
1	60
1 1/2	80
2	85
3	95
4	98

10. Worn gaskets between the filter elements and discharge manifold.
11. Negative discharge pressure, which may cause flashing of volatile liquids at the septum/precoat interface causing particles of filter aid to bleed through the septum.
12. Siphoning caused by precoat tank being lower than the filter.

3.3 Filtering with Body Feed

After the precoat is in place, body feed addition is started and the filter is switched from precoating to filtering. To quote the American Water Works Association,

> During filtration, cake permeability is maintained by adding small, predetermined amounts, of filter aid (body feed) to the unfiltered liquid before it enters the filter. The body feed mixes with solid particles in the filter feed and is deposited along with them on the precoat. As filtration proceeds, the cake deposited on the precoat is a mixture of suspended solids removed from the filter feed surrounded by filter aid. As the cake gradually increases in thickness, and although the cake remains permeable so that liquid passes through, the differential pressure across the cake gradually increases due to the increased thickness and resistance of the cake. Eventually, the differential pressure drop, or cake thickness reaches a maximum limit, and at that point the filter cycle is terminated (AWWA Manual M30, 1988).

The amount of body feed to be added is determined by the nature and amount of solids to be removed. Bench scale and/or pilot testing will generally indicate the type and range of solids that will be encountered and the amount and type of body feed necessary for efficient operation. As a rule of thumb, nondeformable solids require 1 part, or less, of body feed for each part of suspended solids. Deformable solids such as metal hydroxides and algae may require up to 10 parts or more of filter aid for each part of suspended solids.

> Proper control of the body-feed system and rate of application are the most important factors contributing to economic operation of a precoat-filtration plant. Accuracy of feed rate and continuity of feed are critical to the operation. Feeders should be designed to maintain accuracy over a wide range of feed rates so they can be closely matched to varying conditions. Plants may be equipped with instrumentation so that body-feed rates automatically adjust to changing turbidity. Interruptions in body feed should be avoided as much as possible to lessen the chances of cake blinding. Any sudden increase in pressure drop due to the blinding by turbidity that is associated with loss of body feed cannot be offset by subsequent higher body-feed rates. The net result is that the filter cycle will be shortened (AWWA Manual M30).

3.4 Spent Cake Removal

Introduction

Efficient and complete removal of the cake from the filter septum at the end of the filter cycle is essential to continued good filter performance. Poorly or incompletely cleaned septa result in higher filtration pressures, very thin precoats, or no precoat at all. The result is shortened filter cycles, lower quality filtrate, and higher operating costs.

Methods

Methods for cake removal vary according to the type of filter as described in more detail in Section 3.5. The three basic methods are (1) sluicing, (2) backwashing, and (3) dry cake discharge after blowing the cake with air.

Blowing Cake with Air

If the filter cake must be blown dry, the filter should be furnished with an air line (in addition to the pipelines already mentioned) and a filtrate return pipeline to either the body feed or filter feed tank (or, possibly, to still another tank). The filtrate must not be blown to the filtrate tank as the air will disrupt the cake and bleed solids into the filtrate. The flow of liquid from the filter must be controlled to maintain a differential pressure in the filter to prevent the cake from sloughing off the leaves.

3.5 Filter Equipment

Introduction

Following are descriptions of the major types of filters used in precoat filtration. As a practical matter, almost any type of filter, including some types of cartridges, can be precoated providing cake space exists and the filter has a suitable filter medium. The clarification properties of almost any filter medium (with the exception of membranes) can be improved by using a properly selected grade of filter aid.

Filter Press

The filter press has the lowest cost of all the pressure filters but the highest operating costs if operated manually (see Figs. 7–10).

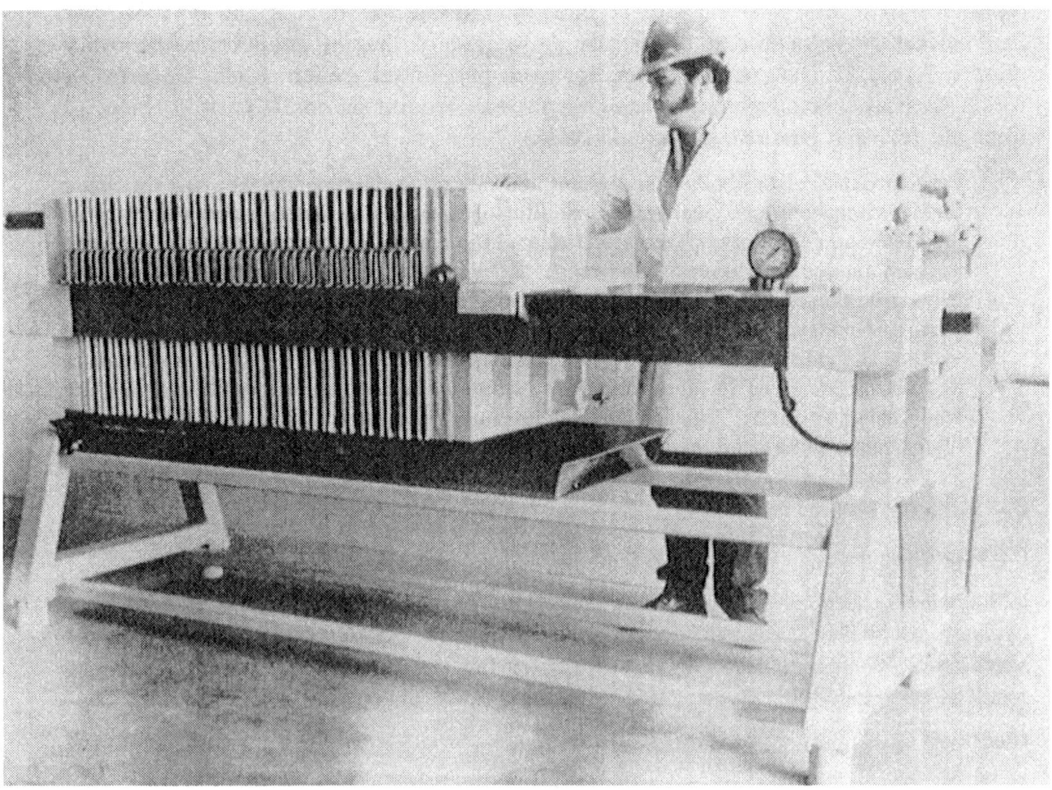

Figure 7 Plate-and-frame filter. Model 42-24A-SQ.

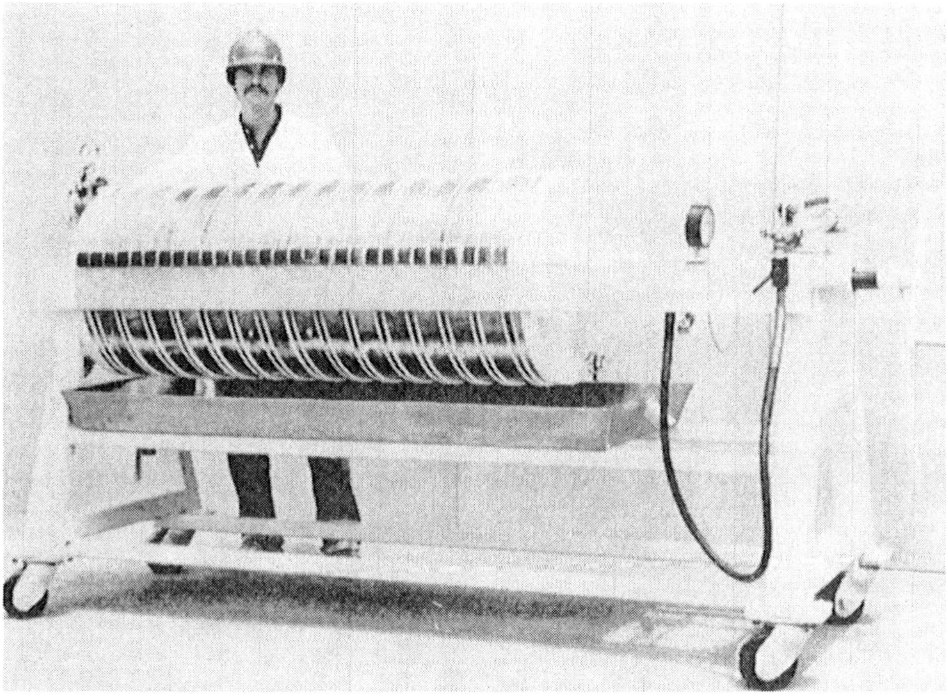

Figure 8 Plate-and-frame filters. Model 30-24D, 30 sheets, 24 in. (61 cm) diameter. Six to 50 round sheets, each 12–18 in. (30.5–45.7 cm) square; 6–42 sheets, 24 in. (61 cm) square. 1½ in. wide sludge frames. Sheets 6–30 in. (15.2–76.2 cm) square. (Courtesy of Star Systems Filtration Division, Timmonsville, SC.)

Filter presses are made as both plate-and-frame and recessed plate filters, with the latter being currently used almost exclusively. Recessed plate filters can be automated but must still be inspected after each cycle for complete cake release. Plate shifters can be provided for large filters. Recessed plate filters come in sizes of a few square feet to over 10,000 ft^2. They are used for everything from fine pharmaceuticals and beverages to large volumes of waste products. In the first of these applications, the septum may be woven or felt cloth, paper, or cellulose pads. If paper is used, filtration rates can be significantly increased by the use of a heavy wire screen backing. Even though the pads may be made of finely divided fibers and considered "tight," their clarification properties are still enhanced by a properly chosen filter aid.

These filters have the advantage of lower cost and near indestructibility. They provide good separation between unfiltered and filtered liquids and can easily be inspected. The large seal area around the plates, however, makes them unsuitable for hazardous liquids.

When properly sized, cake space is completely filled, with no liquid space remaining in the chamber. Membranes can be provided for maximum cake dewatering.

Although the great majority of these filters are used without precoat, they can be precoated. To obtain an even precoat, they should have a bottom inlet and a top

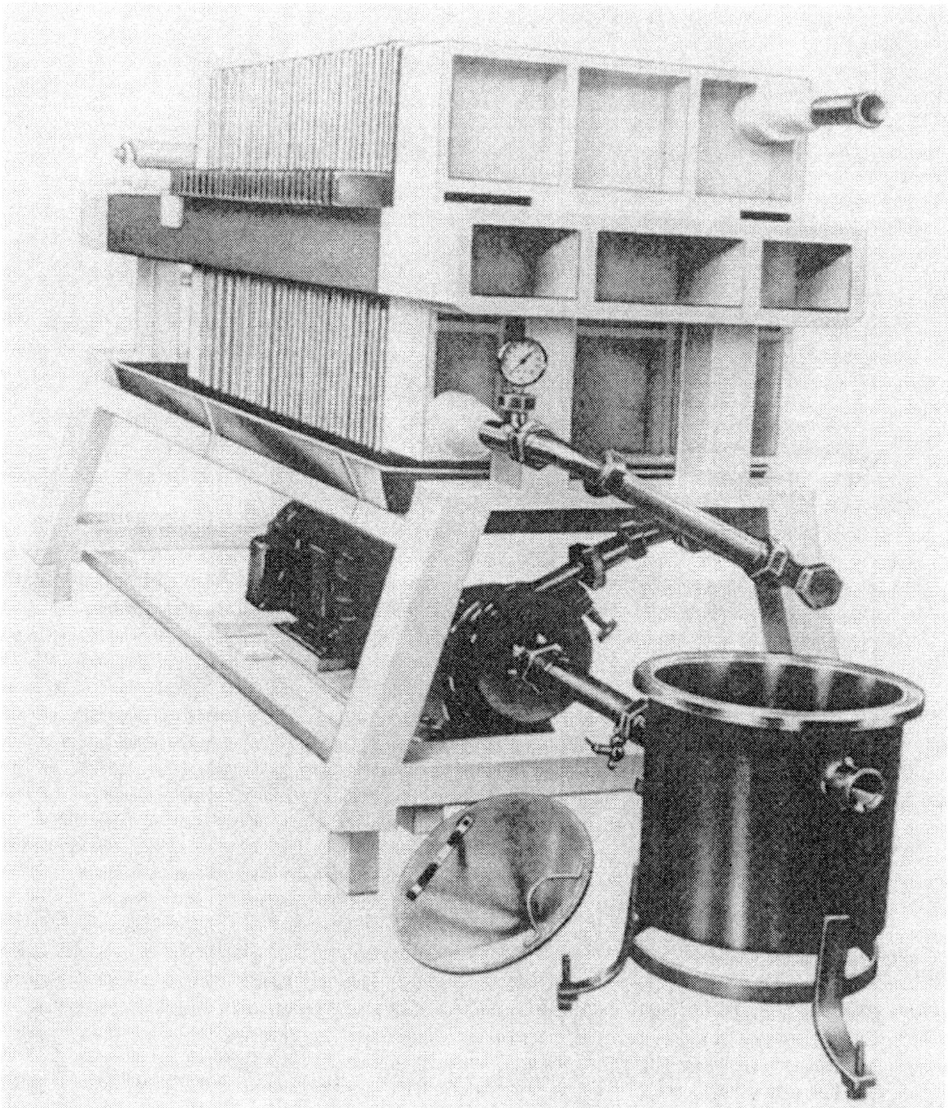

Figure 8 *Continued*

outlet. All air should be out of the filter before recirculation starts. Filters much larger than 300 ft^2 in area should have inlets and outlets at opposite ends of the filter.

Horizontal Plate Filters

Horizontal plate filters consist of a series of horizontal plates, usually covered with paper, separated by spacing rings (see Fig. 11). Flow is into the filter shell, through holes in the spacing rings, through the top of the leaves, and out the center shaft. Precoat is applied to the paper before filtration. Filtration takes place on the top of

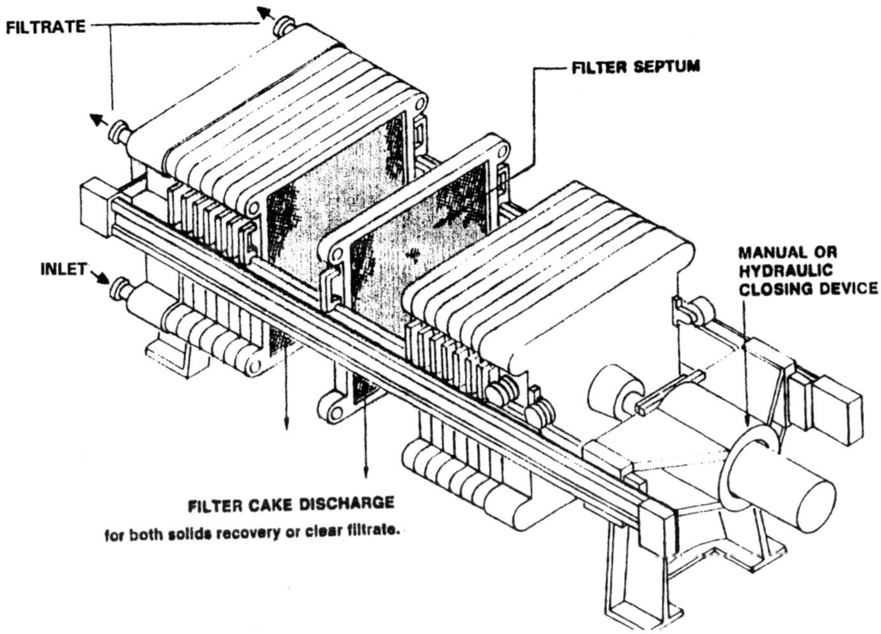

Figure 9 Recessed plate filter press. (Courtesy of Grefco, Inc., Los Angeles, CA).

the leaves only. For this reason, flow through the filter can be interrupted without disrupting the precoat.

Horizontal plate filters are also made in which the flow is into the center shaft through the plates and into the filter shell. This arrangement results in a smaller unfiltered heel at the end of the cycle.

For cleaning, the plates are removed from the shell as a bundle and disassembled. This is obviously a labor-intensive process, so these filters are used primarily as guard or polishing filters where filter cycles are usually 8 h or longer.

Tubular, or Candle, Filters

Tubular, or candle, filters consist of a series of up to (typically) 300–400 tubes (up to 600 ft^2) suspended from a tube sheet and enclosed in a filter vessel (see Fig. 12). They feature low cost construction and high flow rates. It is essential to use a high pressure "air bump" backwash when cleaning to keep tubes from becoming blinded.

These filters are of interest because of their low cost construction and high area-to-volume ratio. The cake is most commonly discharged as a slurry.

Leaf Filters

Leaf filters are essentially a series of leaves contained in a vessel or shell. Flow is into the filter shell through the leaves into a leaf manifold and out of the shell.

The cake is discharged either by blowing the cake dry and vibrating it off the leaves or by sluicing (or, in the last example, by leaf rotation). Sluices may be stationary, oscillating, or, in horizontal tank filters, moving. Sluicing typically takes about 2 gal liquid per square foot of filter area. Most of the cake is removed in the

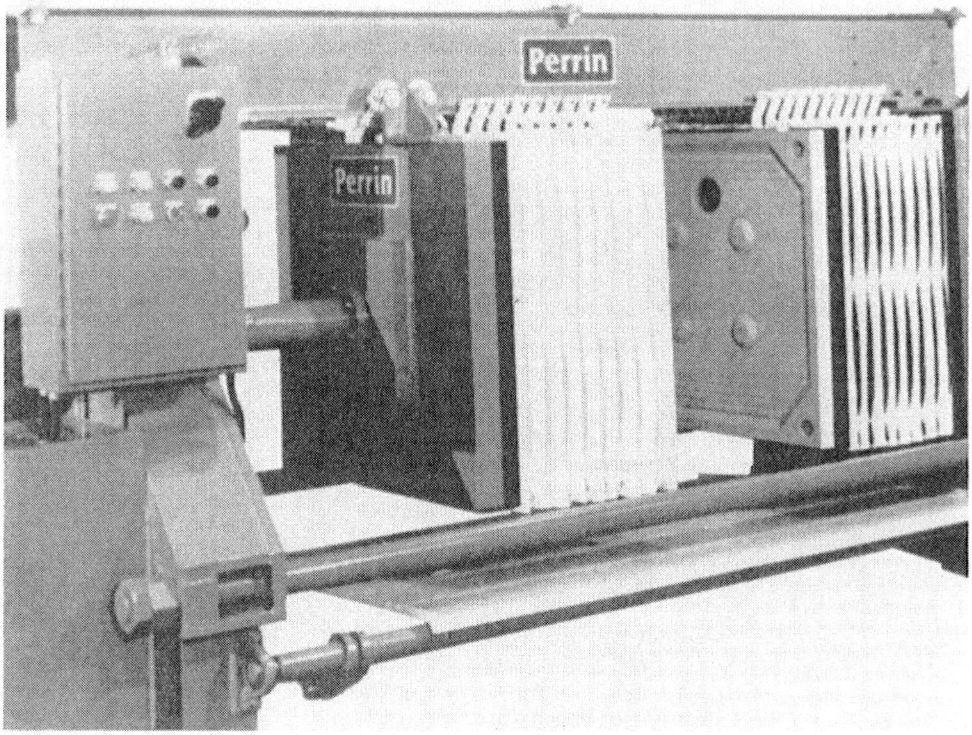

Figure 10 Automated recessed plate filter press. (Courtesy of Perrin Mfg. Co., Toronto, Canada.)

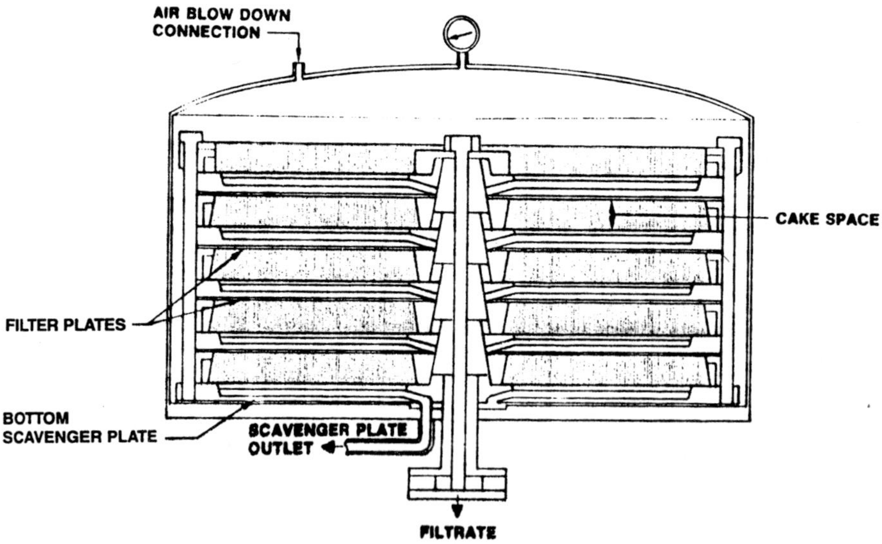

Figure 11 Horizontal plate filter. (Courtesy of Grefco, Inc.)

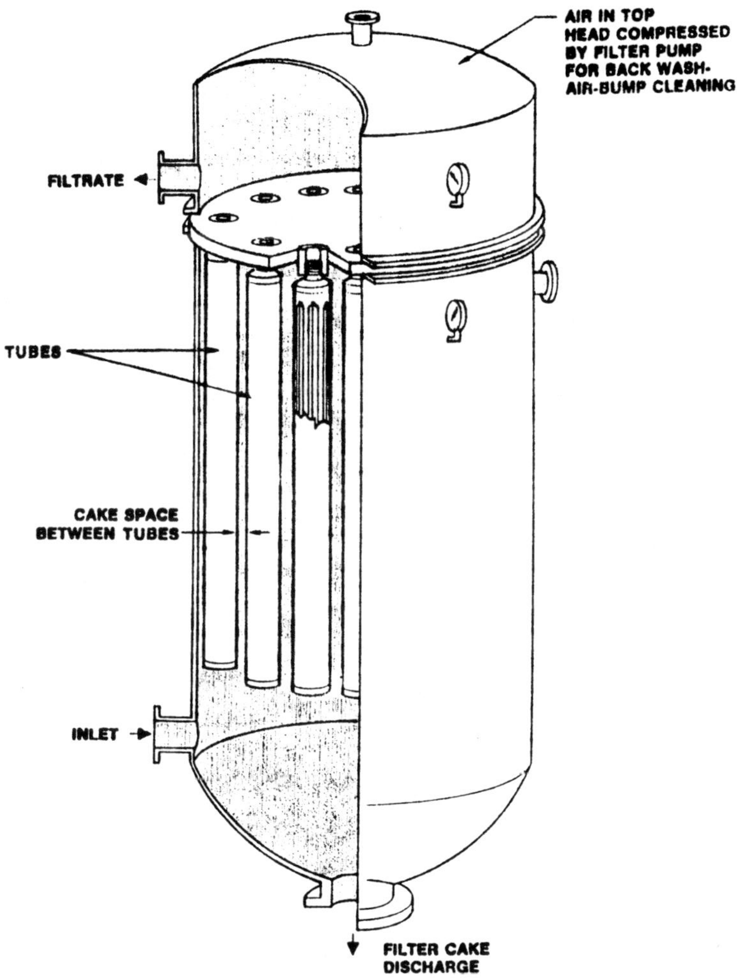

Figure 12 Tubular (candle) filter. (Courtesy of Grefco, Inc.)

first 0.5–1 gal of sluice liquid, so if it is important to minimize the volume of sluice slurry, the first portion can be separated for dewatering or other processing and the second portion, which will have relatively few suspended solids, added to the body feed tank. For good sluicing it is essential that the pumps and lines used for sluicing be of sufficient capacity to maintain sluice pressure (which is typically on the order of 50 psig) during sluicing.

Vertical Leaf, Vertical Tank Filters

Vertical leaf, vertical tank filters (see Fig. 13) are the least expensive and have the lowest volume-to-area ratio of the leaf-type filters. As with all filters, the inlet must be properly baffled for even precoat and cake formation. A disadvantage is the use of leaves of different sizes. Because the center leaves can be very large, these filters are limited in area to about 500 ft^2. For dry cake discharge, they can be supplied with wide-opening bottom doors.

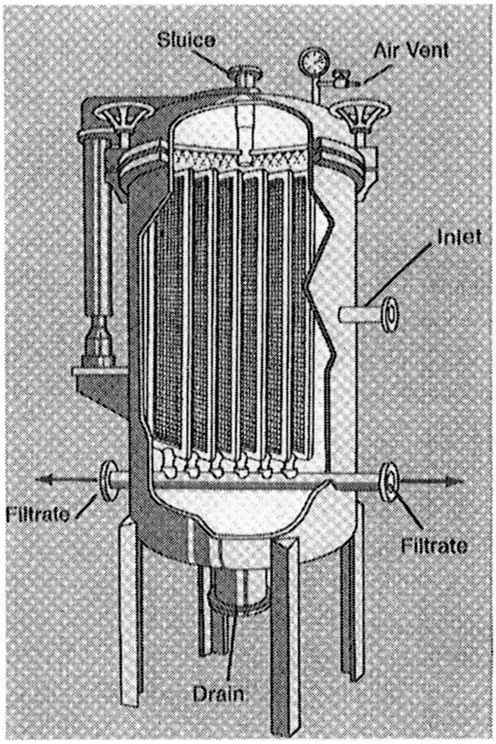

Figure 13 Vertical leaf, vertical tank filter. (Courtesy of Celite Co., Lompoc, CA.)

Vertical Leaf, Horizontal Tank Filters

Vertical leaf, horizontal tank filters (Fig. 14) can have areas of up to 2000 ft^2 or more. The leaves, which are all the same size, can be rolled out of the shell (or vice versa) for dry cake discharge or inspection. After dry cake discharge the leaves can be given a final sluice in the shell. Sluicing is done with either stationary, oscillating, or movable sluices.

These filters have a higher volume-to-area ratio than the vertical leaf, vertical tank filters, which is a disadvantage in batch operations.

Rotating Vertical Leaf, Horizontal Tank Filters

In rotating vertical leaf, horizontal tank filters the leaves are round and are mounted on a center shaft through which the filtrate flows out of the filter (see Fig. 15). The leaves are rotated during sluicing so that each part of the leaf receives the maximum force of the sluice. The leaves are stationary during filtration.

Some filters have two oscillating sluice headers running the length of the tube bundle at 180° to (opposite) each other.

Rotating Horizontal Leaf, Vertical Tank Filters

The construction of rotating horizontal leaf, vertical tank filters (Fig. 16) is similar to that of their horizontal tank counterparts just discussed except that the shaft is vertical. Filtration takes place on the tops of the leaves only. At the end of the filter

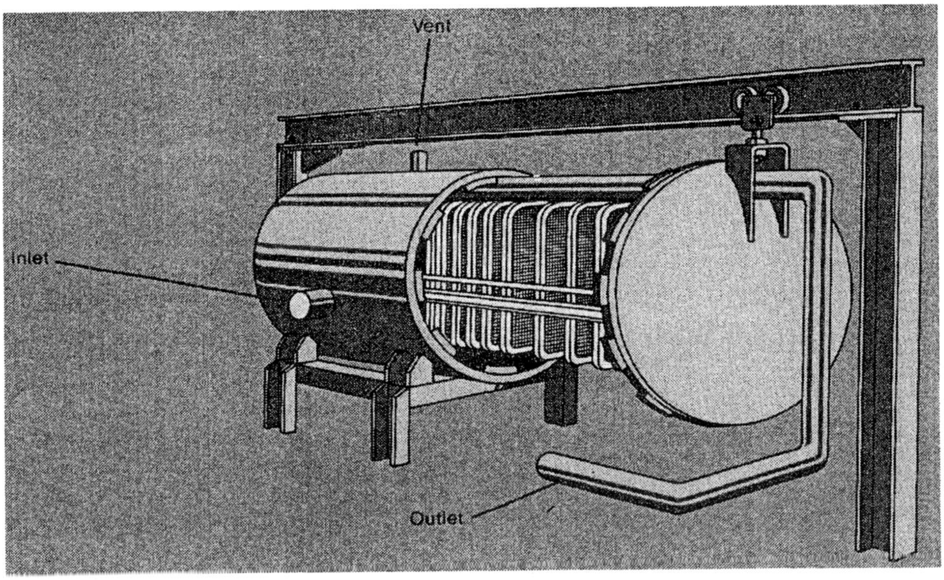

Figure 14 Vertical leaf, horizontal tank filter. (Courtesy of Celite Co., Lompoc, CA.)

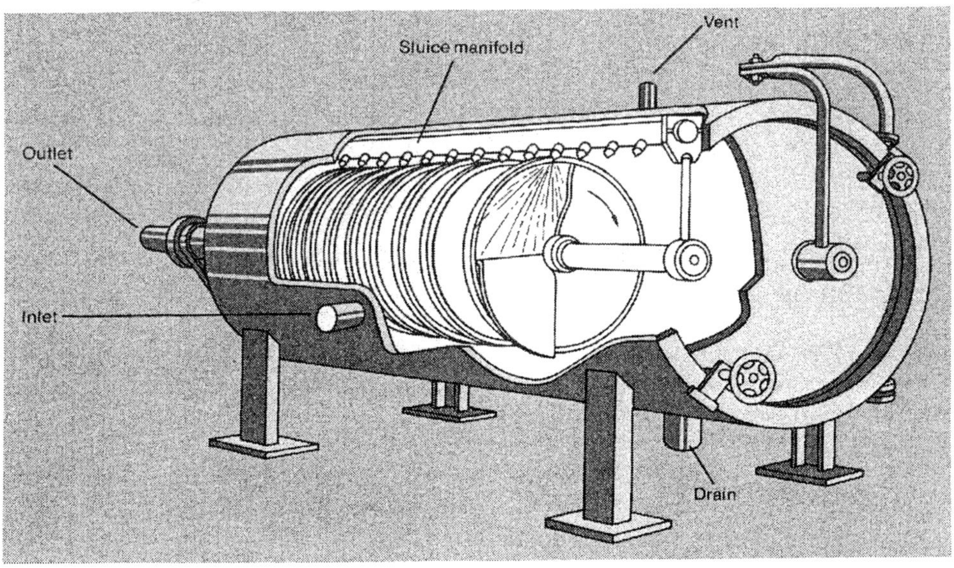

Figure 15 Rotating vertical leaf, horizontal tank filter. (Courtesy of Celite Co., Lompoc, CA.)

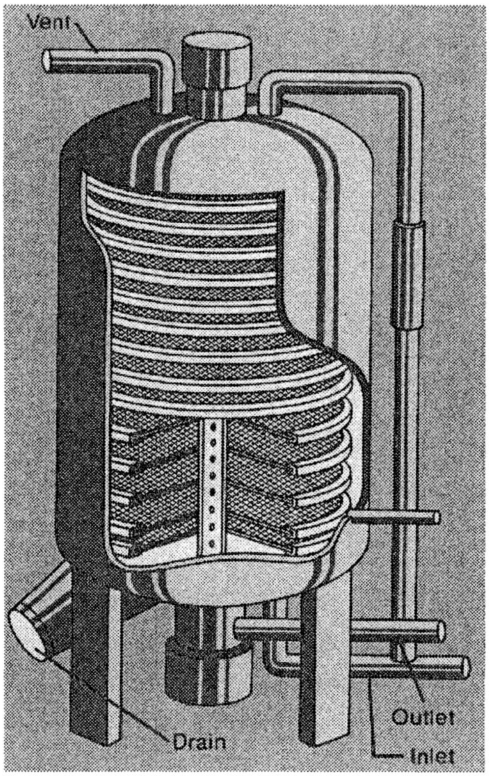

Figure 16 Rotating horizontal leaf, vertical tank filter. (Courtesy of Celite Co., Lompoc, CA.)

cycle the cake is removed by rotating the leaves at speeds of up to 400 rpm. Areas are also up to 400 ft^2.

Vacuum Leaf Filters

In a vacuum leaf filter (Fig. 17), liquid is drawn through the leaves by the filtrate pump. These filters are used mostly for large swimming pools and potable water. They are open tank, easily accessible, and relatively inexpensive.

3.6 Auxiliary Equipment

Introduction

Failures in filter aid filtration systems are probably caused more often by the poor design and malfunction of auxiliary equipment than by any faults of the filters themselves. For instance, filtrate clarity can be disrupted by air in the precoat tank or by an improperly designed precoat system causing an uneven precoat. An erratic body feed pump or uneven flow through the filter can shorten the filtration cycle. Often, even if the system works acceptably, better designed auxiliary equipment can improve the effectiveness of the filter aid, increase cycle length, and lower labor costs.

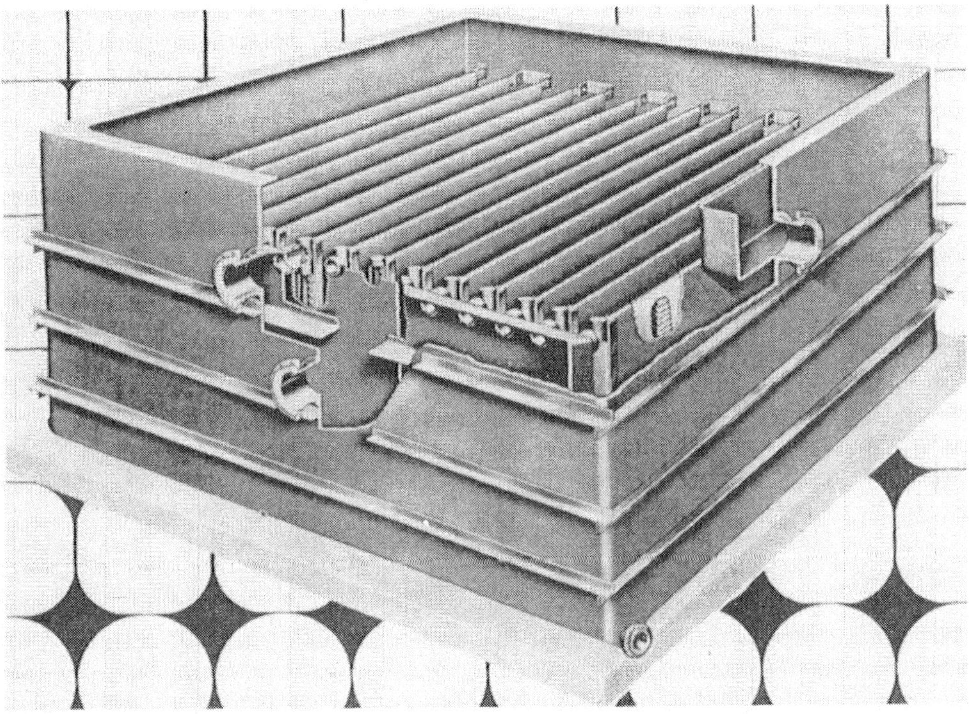

Figure 17 Vacuum leaf fiberglass filter. (Courtesy of Westfall Mfg. Co., Bristol, RI.)

Filter aid filtration systems consist mainly of precoat and body feed tanks, filter and body feed pumps, agitators, lines, valves, and instrumentation that includes pressure gauges, flowmeters, and clarity indicators. The system may also be automated.

One important requirement of a well-designed system is that it be as flexible as possible. Note, for example, the arrangement of the pipelines and valves shown in Fig. 6. For instance, the body feed tank can be filled with filtrate from either the filter or the filtrate tank or with unfiltered liquor through the filter feed pipeline. The precoat tank can be charged from either the filter or the filtrate tank.

Precoat and Body Feed Tanks

Both precoat and body feed tanks should have conical, dish-shaped, or sloped bottoms for good drainage and to maintain pump suction with a minimum amount of liquid. This is particularly important for precoat tanks, where a small heel greatly increases precoat slurry turnover.

Agitators may be sweep arm or propeller. If propeller, limit speed to between 40 and 60 rpm—this is easier on both the filter aid and the agitator. If there is any chance of power loss, design the agitator so it can be started after the filter aid has settled. This is particularly important for remote, unattended, automated systems.

Air must be kept out of the precoat pump and the filter. If the pump cavitates, flow will be disrupted, which will cause some or all of the filter aid on the filter leaves to fall off. Also, air may collect at the top of the filter if the filter is not vented and prevent complete formation of the precoat. There are automatic vent valves that will prevent this from happening.

Precoat System

If the precoat slurry is to be made up ahead of time, the capacity of the precoat tank should be 125% of the volume of the filter and connecting piping. This will allow a large enough heel in the tank to maintain suction after the slurry has been pumped to the filter and, along with proper tank baffling, prevent air from being drawn into the filter during recirculation. If the recommended amount of 10–15 lb per 100 ft^2 of filter area is used, a slurry concentration of 0.3–0.6% in the filter will result if the filter has the usual volume/area ratio.

The precoat return line should be extended below the heel level to minimize aeration and foaming (where that is a problem). If the precoat tank is located much below the level of the filter, the return line should be throttled to prevent liquid from siphoning from the filter back into the precoat tank. This can also be accomplished by installing an inverted U in the line with a vent valve at the top of the U.

If the filter is to be filled before precoating and filter aid added during recirculation, the tank need be only large enough to enable slurrying the filter aid during precoating while preventing air from getting into the system. It should be noted at this point, however, that to get an even precoat in a large filter, especially a leaf filter, the internal baffling must provide fast and good distribution of the incoming precoat material. This system is also not suitable for many fibrous filter aids as there is not enough agitation in the filter to get the fibers to separate and form an even precoat.

Body Feed Systems

Batch Addition

If the filtration is a batch operation, body feed can be added directly to the batch. This is the simplest method but has the disadvantage of wearing out the filter feed pump if filter aid concentrations are much above 0.01%.

Continuous Addition, Slurry

Proper design of body feed metering equipment is critical for good system performance. Inadequate design in this area has been the principal cause of difficulty with precoat filtration systems in the past. Any interruption or slowing of flow will cause a layer of high resistance in the filter cake that cannot be overcome by increasing the body feed rate. The result is an irreversible shortening of that particular filter cycle.

The size of the body feed tank depends on such factors as batch size (if the operation is not continuous), concentration of the slurry, and the desired time before refilling. To prevent large particles of filter aid from getting into the body feed pump and jamming or plugging the check valves, the suction pipeline should

1. Be located approximately 6 in. above the bottom of the body feed tank.
2. Be turned so that it faces in the direction of slurry rotation.

Filter media are relatively abrasive and settle out rapidly from slow-moving liquids. Certain designs are recommended to minimize problems in operation. Piston, diaphragm, or tubular diaphragm pumps can be used for body feed addition. Piston pumps can handle up to 18 wt % slurries. Pumps should be sized so that at least a 50% stroke is used. This will minimize filter aid settling in the lines. Flush-out connections should also be provided to clean filter aid out of the lines before shutting the system down.

> Ball check valves with hard steel balls and wear-resistant elastomeric seats are suggested. In addition, pumps should be equipped with flush connections so that they can be flushed periodically with clean liquid to minimize potential plugging, or they should be provided with clean-out fittings. The body-feed lines carrying the slurry from the feed pump to the raw-water feed line should be as short as possible and should have as few 90° elbows as possible. Flexible transparent tubing, process conditions permitting, instead of pipe will allow any clogging to be easily located and dislodged. Body-feed pipe or tubing should be sized to just maintain turbulent velocities to keep the media in suspension. Before extended shut-down periods, all slurry lines should be flushed (AWWA Manual M30).

A three-way valve should be placed in the line so that the slurry can be diverted back to the precoat tank during precoating.

Continuous Addition, Dry

Dry feeding of filter aid is frequently done in large installations, such as those employing rotary vacuum precoat filtration of fermentation broths (described in Section 4.2) and large water supply and waste plants. In pressure filtrations where filter aid is fed in at the suction side of the filter feed pump, dry feeding is limited to body feed addition rates of less than 0.01% to minimize pump abrasion. Filter aid can be fed downstream of the feed pump with an eductor and a booster pump (if necessary).

A major advantage of dry feeding is the reduction in the amount of space required for equipment and storage. Where filter aid is received in bulk, feeding can be done directly from the bulk storage tank.

In a dry feed system, an eductor takes slurry from a flooded funnel at a constant rate as long as the rate of the driving fluid through the eductor is constant. The level in the flooded funnel is kept constant by a float valve, while the body feed rate is maintained by controlling the rate at which the dry filter aid is fed into the flooded funnel. The eductor, which can be a standard liquid jet, should be capable of handling slurries at concentrations of 5–10% while operating at a discharge pressure slightly higher than that in the filter. Because the eductor will be run with process liquid, thus requiring no addition of liquid, it may be a high volume design that will result in less wear on the eductor. Because any holdup in the flooded funnel is small, it is important that feed be consistent.

Dry feeders come in two basic types. In one, the feed rate is changed by varying the speed of rotation of an auger or screw. The filter aid drops into the screw from a hopper located above it. If there is a tendency for the filter aid to bridge in the hopper, the hopper or the whole casing may be vibrated. The filter aid will be fed evenly through these feeders if the vibration is along the axis of the screw. The second type of dry feeder, which also has a screw and vibrator, is different from the first only in that changes in its feed rate are made by varying vibration frequency. These feeders, which are much less expensive than the first type, are generally accurate enough for regulating body feed if the slurrying tank is large enough to even out the intermittent feed.

Since all the dry feeders work volumetrically, the rates at which filter aid is fed will vary between grades due to their different flow characteristics. A higher density filter aid, for instance, will not only be fed at a greater rate on a weight basis at the same feed rate setting but will also flow with greater ease. For these reasons, volumetric dry feeders must be calibrated for each grade and type of filter aid used.

Dry feeders are usually supplied with a hopper that holds only about 50 lb of filter aid. For some installations, it may be necessary to substitute a larger hopper. Most manufacturers of dry feeders also make vibrating (“live bottom”) bins for supplying larger quantities of filter aid. These bins must be furnished with the correct vibrating devices and baffles to ensure that the filter aid will flow continuously. If vibration is too vigorous, the filter aid will become compacted and bridge over the opening at the bottom of the bin.

Filter Feed Pumps

Centrifugal pumps are usually used for filter feeders. To minimize particle degradation in the feed slurry they should have open impellers and operate at 1800 rpm maximum. If the precoat rate is substantially higher than the filter rate a second pump may be desirable.

3.7 Filter Aid Selection and Testing

Introduction

Once the decision has been made to investigate the effect of filter aids in enhancing a filtration it would be nice to have a filter aid very small amounts of which would remove essentially all the solids in the filter feed material at very high filtration rates. As this is not likely, priorities must be set and compromises made. Included in these compromises are not only the items mentioned above but also costs other than the purchase price of the filter aid. These costs include

1. Consequences of off-spec or imperfectly filtered materials.
2. Capital costs.
3. Filter aid storage and handling.
4. Filter aid disposal costs in addition to filtered solids disposal, especially for hazardous wastes.
5. Power. Pumping costs increase with higher filter pressures.
6. Maintenance. Shorter cycles may result in higher capacity but also in more wear on equipment.
7. Labor.
8. Heat, if needed to increase rates.
9. Product left in the filter cake. This may range (for vegetable oils) from 30% for steam blowing to 50% for hydraulically pressed cakes.

Precoat Selection

With all the grades and types of filter aids available one might well wonder where to start. If the median size of the suspended solids is known, a good place to start is with a filter aid with a similar median pore size (Cain, 1973). (The chances are that a midrange filter aid will be chosen, as these grades account for the bulk of filter aids used.)

The primary purpose of the precoat, as described above, is to keep solids, especially sticky ones, off the filter septum and to provide easy and as complete as possible removal of the filter cake. To do this, a certain minimum clarity, or solids removal efficiency, must be obtained. This minimum clarity can be observed as a clear line of demarcation between the precoat and the cake of solids removed by the precoat. The filtrate should be visually clear. The coarsest grade of filter aid that results in these conditions should be selected for initial testing. [There are many ways to measure clarity beyond ''just looking'' (although to a trained eye observing the Tyndall effect of a beam of light shining through a sample in a darkened room can match some very good optical instruments), and these are described elsewhere in this book.] If, based on other clarity measurements, the grade selected does not give the desired clarity, body feed should be added before the final precoat grade selection is made because although the primary purpose of body feed is to lower cake resistance, it is also a major contributor to clarity.

Büchner Funnel Tests

The simplest way to screen filter aids for precoat is, if the slurry permits, with a Büchner funnel. Otherwise, a pressure cell, as will be described later, can be used. In either case, the septum must be open enough not to retain any of the solids, and air must not be allowed to pass through the cake as it would drag particulate matter through the precoat and cake. Indeed, for the best results, air should be kept out altogether by following the precoat slurry with the sample before the filter is drawn dry.

Body Feed Selection

The primary purpose of body feeding is to lengthen filter cycles by decreasing cake resistance and compressibility. This is done by optimal selection of grade and type of filter aid. Having run the precoat tests, the search is narrowed down somewhat. The filtration operation will be simplest if the same filter aid can be used for both functions. If a coarser grade of body feed is used it should be limited to no more than two grades difference. Otherwise, particles will penetrate the body feed cake, coat out on the precoat, and increase the pressure drop. If a new installation is planned there will be no constraints on either cake thickness or flow rates. If an existing filter is to be used, however, cake thickness and flow rates will be determined by equipment and process demands (Tiller, 1988).

Most filter aid filtrations are run at a constant flow rate. Bench scale tests can also be run at constant pressure. Constant pressure tests are faster to run but are not as accurate. For instance, the greater hydraulic drag of the higher rates will cause fine particles to migrate through the cake, reducing its resistance as well as the clarity of the filtrate. Additional distortions occur if the cake is at all compressible. Other distortions are due to rearrangement, bending, and possible breaking of the particles in the cake. All that said, however, these tests can be useful for screening. If results are inconsistent, then a change to constant rate tests should be made.

Constant Rate Tests

A clear approach to constant pressure testing using vacuum is described in Cain (1990). (Higher pressure tests run in a pressure cell are described below.) In these tests filtration time is plotted versus volume as shown in Fig. 18. The results of these

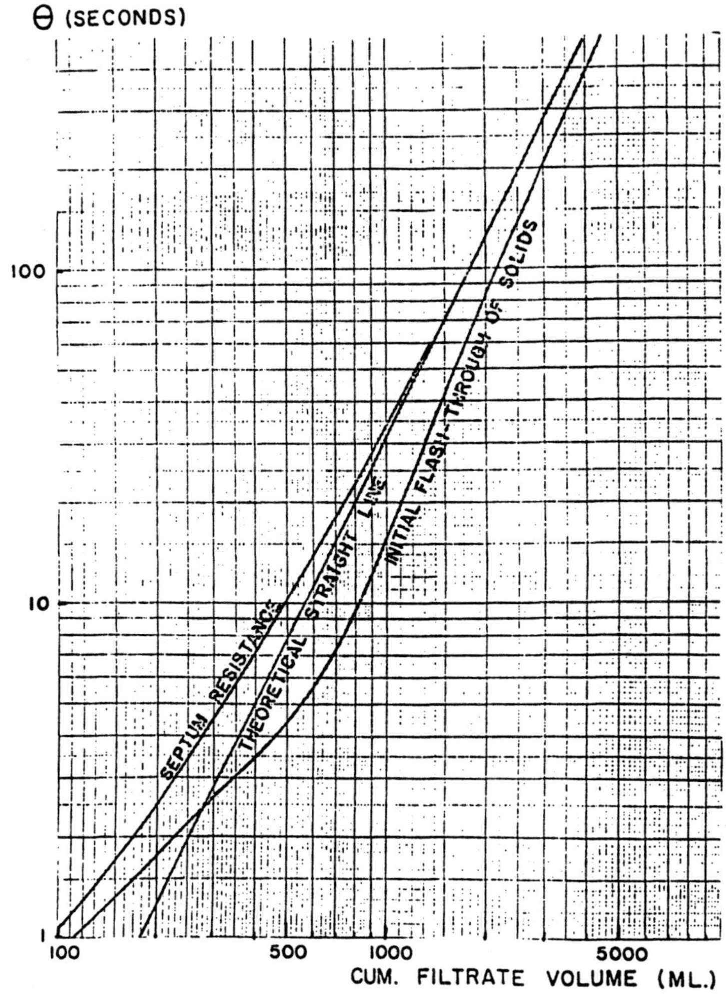

Figure 18 Constant pressure test data on log-log paper. (From Cain, 1990.)

plots should be a line that should either start out with a slope of 2 or approach that slope as the test progresses. Not doing so indicates either septum resistance or an unstable cake.

A different and more detailed treatment of constant pressure test data is described by Cook (1984), he also uses the data to estimate optimum costs. Both batch and continuous filtrations are discussed.

Constant Volume (Rate) Tests

The results of constant volume tests can be plotted arithmetically. Some of these plots are shown in Figs. 20 and 21. From these data and cake density figures from the tables on filter aid properties, the cake thickness can be calculated. In general,

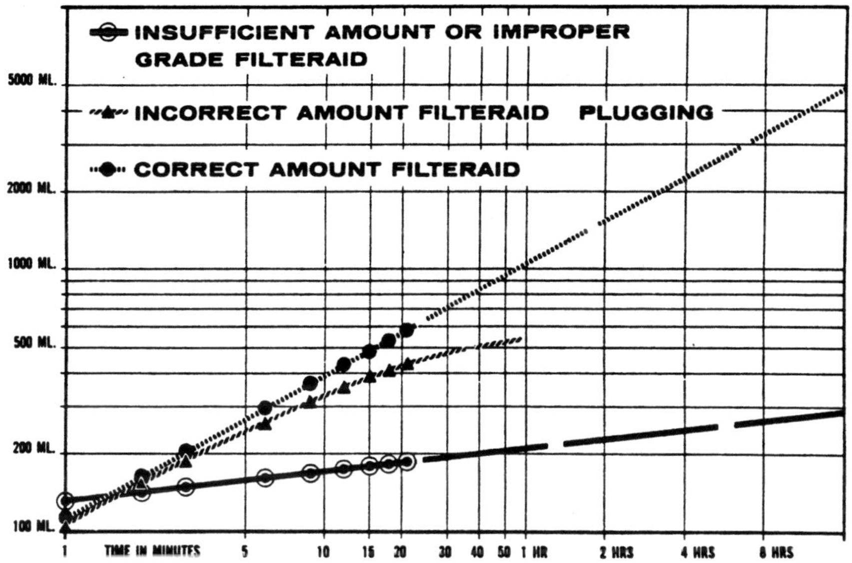

Figure 19 Test results showing correct and incorrect amounts of body feed. (Courtesy of Grefco, Inc., Los Angles, CA.)

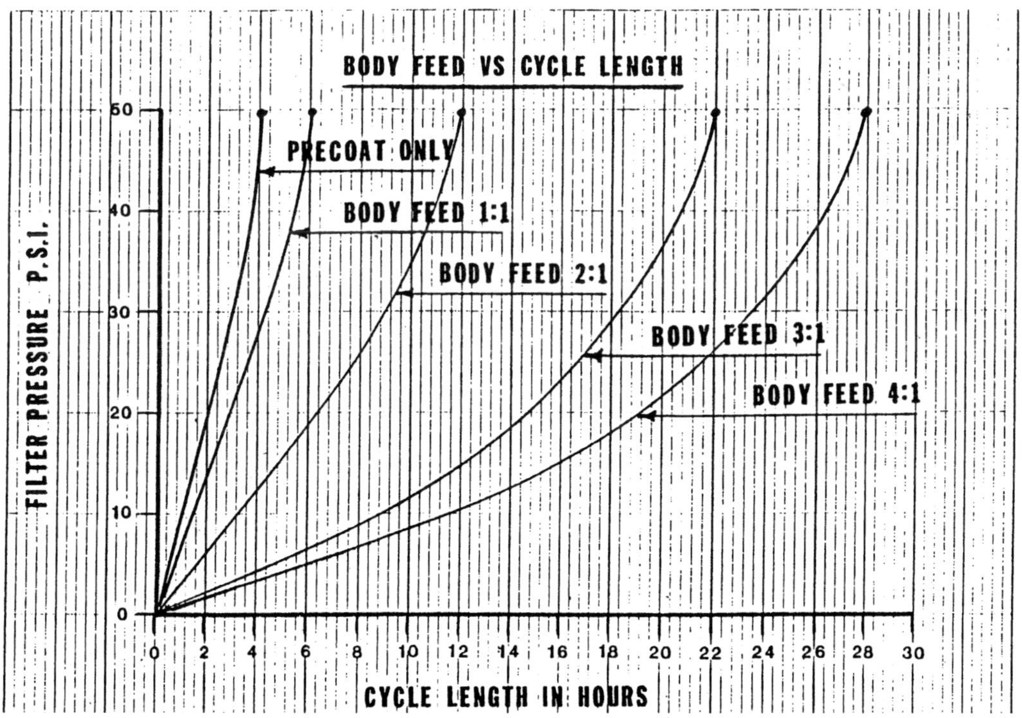

Figure 20 Effect of body feed amounts on cycle length. (Courtesy of Celite Co., Lompoc, CA.)

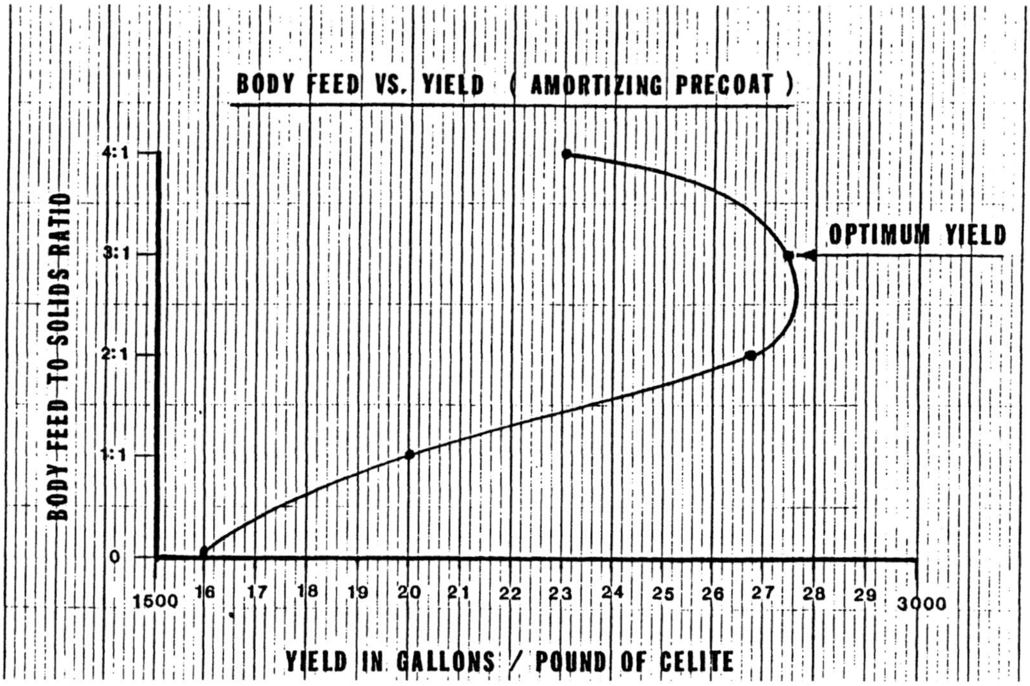

Figure 21 Body feed ratio vs. yield. (Courtesy of Celite Co., Lompoc, CA.)

the solids fit into the interstices of the filter aid (which is on the order of 90% void space) and therefore do not enter into these calculations.

Typically, for incompressible solids, body feed amounts to 0.25–1 times the weight of solids. For compressible solids, body feed may amount to as much as 6 times the weight of solids as in the case of yeast filtration.

Test Equipment

Constant Pressure

A constant pressure test cell is shown in Fig. 22. It is pressured by air. The filter element can be precoated outside the cell, the precoat held on by vacuum, and the element inserted into the cell for filtration. Results are plotted on log-log paper and extrapolated to desired cycle lengths (Fig. 19). Results can be considered fairly reliable if the resultant curve has a slope of ½. As stated earlier, this test method is subject to many disruptions that can distort or make the data useless. In these cases constant rate testing must be used. A yield curve similar to the one shown for the constant rate test can then be developed.

Constant Rate

The Walton test filter is a self-contained unit that is ideal for running bench-scale constant rate test. A unique and important feature is a variable chamber whereby volume can be adjusted to cake thickness. This overcomes one of the major imperfections of test equipment.

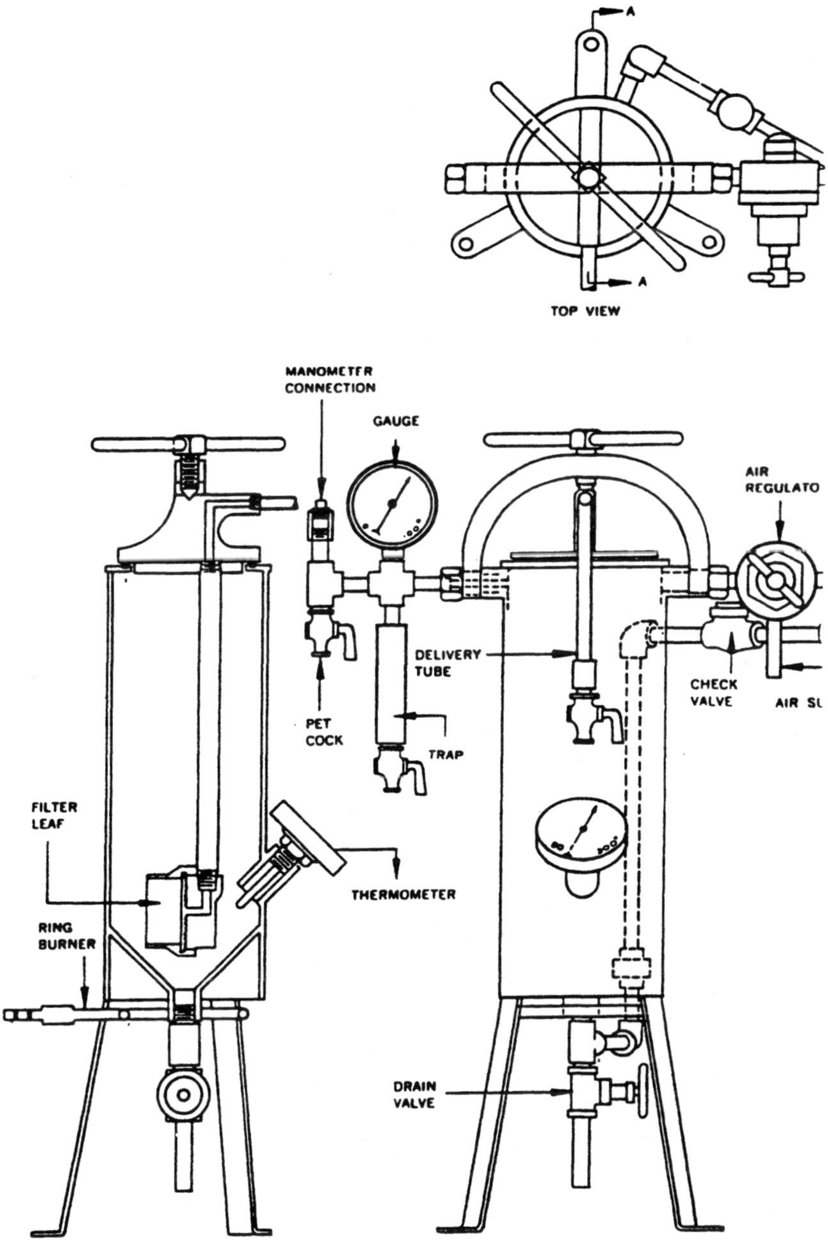

Figure 22 Laboratory pressure test filter. (Courtesy of Grefco, Inc., Los Angles, CA.)

4 ROTARY VACUUM PRECOAT FILTER

4.1 Introduction

The use of rotary drums constitutes the second mode of filter aid utilization. Some rotary drum equipment uses pressure as the means of generating the filtrative flow. Most usually, however, the rotary drums are vacuum operated (see Fig. 23).

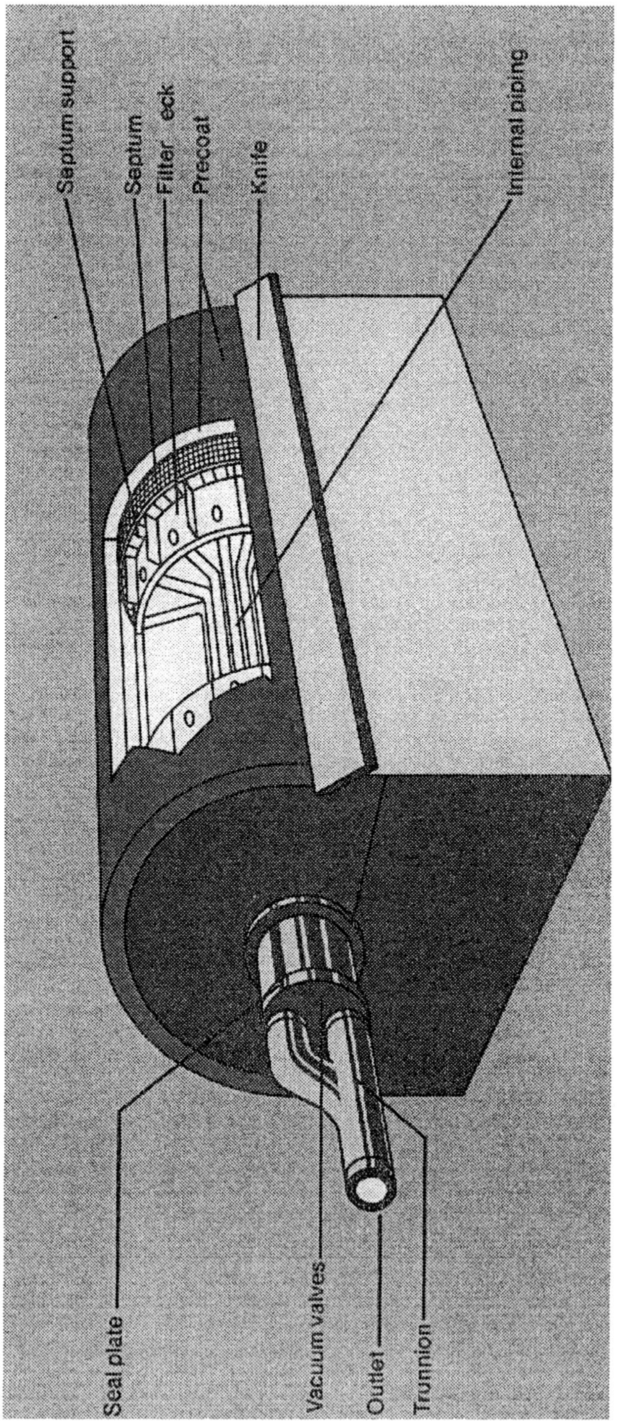

Figure 23 Rotary vacuum precoat filter.

This section emphasizes the mechanics of the rotary vacuum precoat filter with only brief references to theory. The reason for this is that, with the probable exception of smaller area packaged units now being sold mostly for waste filtration, the majority of filters, including many that have been operated for years on antibiotic broths, could be operated at significantly higher rates and at the same time lower precoat use. These improvements would come mostly from mechanical tune-up of the filter, different precoating and operating techniques, and precoat filter aid selection.

Sizes

Drum filters used for rotary vacuum precoat filtration have areas ranging from 3 to 1000 ft^2 (for a drum 12 ft in diameter by 24 ft long). The drum is covered with a highly permeable cloth (80–200 cfm air/ft^2 at 0.5 in. of water differential pressure) or wire. The drum may be simply a hollow cylinder with an internal "foot" extending from a center shaft to the bottom of the drum to pick up filtrate or, more conventionally, contain internal piping to convey the vacuum from a valve at the end of the drum to its surface. The largest area for the first type of drum is 500 ft^2.

Operation

Vacuum of 20–24 in. (51–61 cm) of mercury is applied to the drum from an outside vacuum source. The drum rotates at 0.5–3 rpm in a vat of liquid with submergence ranging from less than 10% to 30% (commonly) of the drum diameter. Before filtration takes place, a layer of filter aid is applied to the surface of the drum by adding a mixture of filter aid and water (or filtrate) to the bowl, whereupon the precoat forms on the drum as it rotates. This continues until the desired thickness of precoat is obtained (3–6 in; 7.6–15.2 cm), at which point the remaining slurry may be dropped or removed from the filter bowl and unfiltered liquid added. During filtration the filter cake that forms on the surface of the precoat is removed, along with a small amount of precoat, by means of a doctor blade running along the length of the drum and advancing toward the drum surface at a rate of 1–10 mils per drum revolution. This continues until the blade is approximately 3/8–1/2 in. (0.93–1.27 cm) from the drum surface, at which point the unfiltered liquid is removed from the drum, the remaining precoat is washed off the drum and bowl, and the drum is again dressed with a precoat. The efficiency of this piece of equipment depends on mechanical considerations, which are highly critical, the precoat filter aid type and grade and the method of application, and, during filtration, optimization of drum speed, knife advance, and drum submergence.

Applications

The rotary vacuum precoat filter is most useful in applications that deal with

- Blinding, compressible solids.
- Fine particle removal.
- Filtration of oil–water suspensions.

Rotary vacuum precoat filters are most commonly used in the pharmaceutical industry for the filtration of fermentation broths although they are being replaced by other separation methods. Currently, their largest areas of application are for the filtration of waste sludges such as those from air flotation units, clarifiers, wet scrubbers, chemical precipitation systems, de-inking processes, and for filtering various process liquors. Typically, filtrates contain from 50 to 1000 ppm suspended solids as compared to less than 0.1 ppm for pressure filtrations.

Advantages

The advantages of the rotary vacuum precoat filter are its thin cake discharge, which gives it the ability to filter highly compressible solids, and its filtration of relatively large amounts (5% to almost 100% apparent volume) of highly compressible solids such as fermentation broths, metal hydroxide sludges, corn syrups, oily wastes, and other materials. For very compressible solids, cakes may be drier than those from filter presses.

The use of filter aid precoat distinguishes this drum filtration operation from that of ordinary drum or belt-type filtrations.

Disadvantages

Disadvantages include

- High capital cost
- Cost of precoat
- Precoating downtime
- Cake contamination with precoat
- Poorer clarity than with pressure precoat filtration
- Inability to separate filtrate and wash liquids
- Odor from vacuum exhaust for certain types of liquids

4.2 Equipment Description

The conventional rotary vacuum precoat filter is shown in Fig. 23. The drum serves as a support for the precoat (a layer of filter powder), which is the actual filtration medium. This precoat is supported on a fabric or stainless steel wire cloth supported on top of a series of drainage grids approximately 3/4 in. thick. The drum surface is divided longitudinally into a series of panels (or sectors). Each sector has a drainage line, or lines, going from the sector toward the center of the filter drum and then out through the end of the drum into a valve arrangement. The filtrate with its entrained gas flows into a filtrate receiver, where the filter and gas are separated. The doctor blade for cake removal is mounted along the length of the drum.

Filter Operating Characteristics

The rotary vacuum precoat filter is a constant pressure filter with an element (drum) rotating at speeds up to 3 rpm. Each time the element rotates, the following functions are performed: filtration and cake formation, cake washing (when needed), cake drying, and cake removal. These operations may be carried out at drum speeds of up to 3 rpm so that each one is completed in a matter of seconds. For the filter to perform efficiently it must be precisely built and operated with great attention paid to detail.

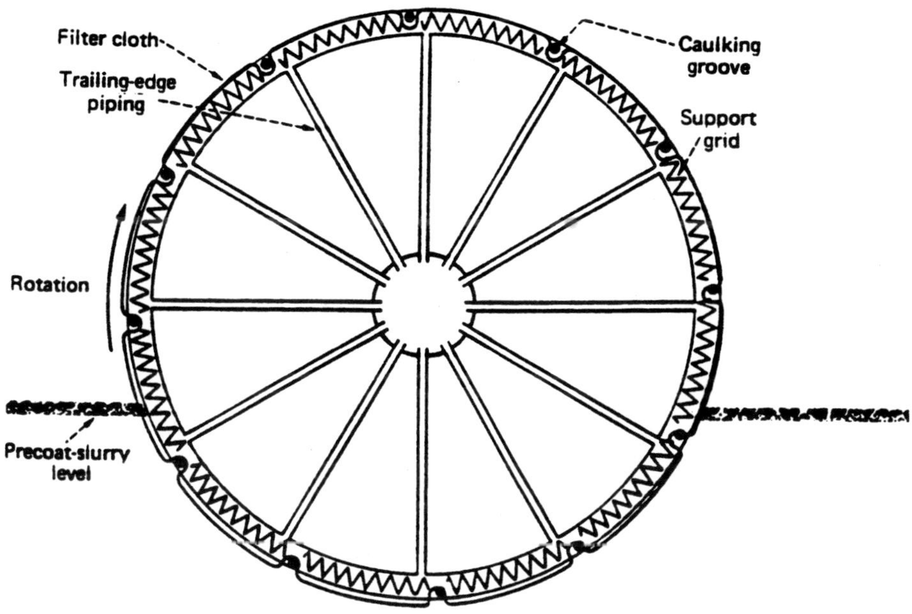

Figure 24 Cross section of a filter drum. (From Smith, 1976b.)

A cross section of a drum is shown in Fig. 24. Note that the vacuum is only on the surface of the drum, that the drum is divided into sectors, and that the drainage pipes are attached to the trailing edge of each sector in relation to drum rotation.

Pipeless Drum Rotary Vacuum Precoat Filters

Partly Submerged Drum

While the conventional drum filter contains internal piping, most filters being sold today are equipped with drums that have no internal piping. The entire inside of the drum is evacuated. Filtrate is withdrawn through a shaft that runs down the center of the drum. Areas of these filters range from 3 to 500 ft^2. The filters are sold as packaged units including auxiliary equipment (see Bulletin FP 3-91, Alar Engineering Co., Mokena, IL). This simplified construction results in much lower prices than for conventionally constructed filters.

For users of one of these packaged filters, this section should give a better understanding of operating principles and assist in optimizing the filtration.

Top Feed Precoating and Filtering

A new entrant in top feed precoating and filtering is the Nagaoka MJP filter drum (Nagaoka USA, Houston, TX) (Fig. 25). The filter is unique in that it is not submerged in slurry. Instead, precoat and unfiltered slurry are added to the drum at the 10–11 o'clock position and discharged at the 8–9 o'clock position. This, of course, eliminates the bowl, agitators, and level controls and results in less drum space being needed for cake discharge. Vacuum is provided by a water/air eductor also designed for the filter. A higher than usual vacuum (~24 in. Hg) is claimed. The filter can be fully enclosed.

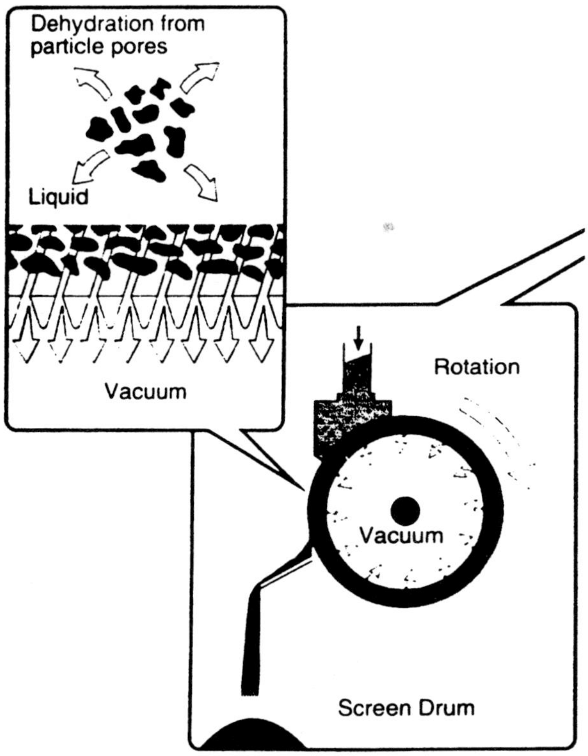

Figure 25 Nagaoka MJP filter drum. (Courtesy of Nagaoka USA, Houston, TX.)

4.3 Precoat Selection and Testing

Introduction

Filtration on the rotary vacuum precoat (RVP) filter (see Fig. 26) is best understood by reviewing the precoat selection process. The selection of the correct grade of precoat filter aid will have a dramatic effect on the operation in terms of both precoat consumption and throughput. If the grade is too coarse, unfiltered solids will penetrate into the precoat and filtration will stop. Too tight a grade will unnecessarily reduce the flow rate.

Filtering Factors

Filtering factors that govern filtration conditions include

1. Liquid viscosity
2. Liquid vapor pressure
3. Cake filterability and cohesiveness
4. Cake-drying time
5. Undissolved solids: particle size, distribution, and amount
6. Grade and type of precoat filter aid
7. Solids penetration into precoat
8. Knife advance rate

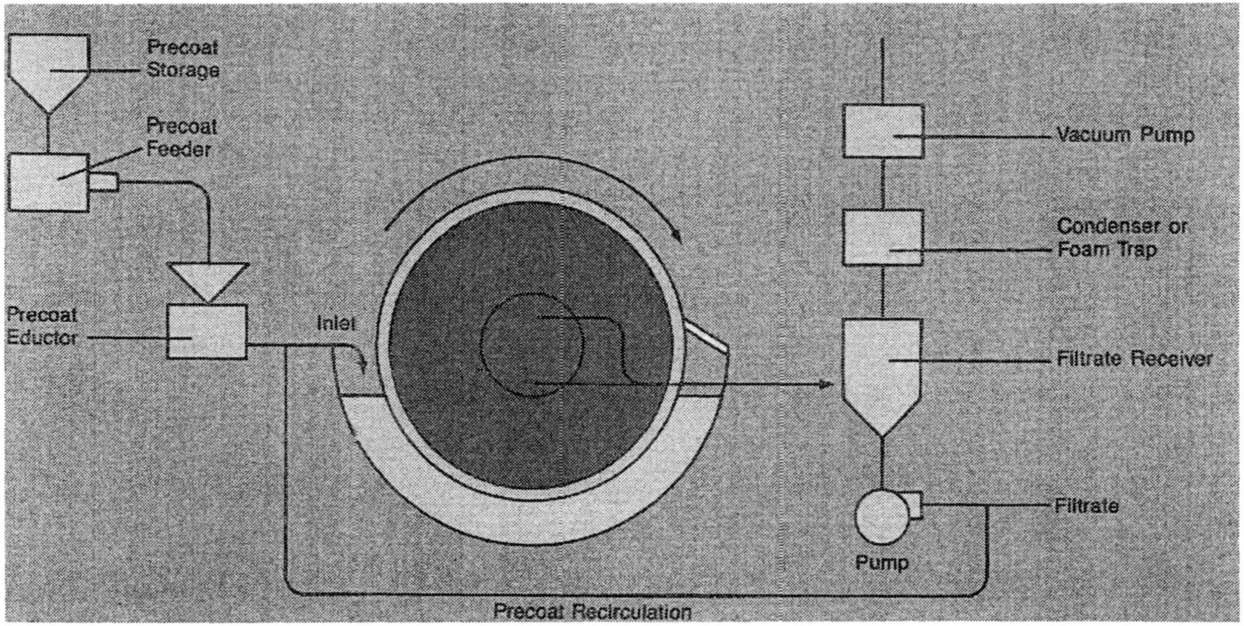

Figure 26 Schematic of a rotary vacuum precoat filter system showing dry precoat addition. Other precoat systems include concentrated slurry addition (discussed in Section 4.4) and slurry recirculation. All systems should be capable of maintaining a 10% slurry in the filter bowl.

9. Drum speed
10. Drum submergence
11. Precoat cutting efficiency
12. Vacuum
13. Precoat thickness
14. Continuous filter aid addition

The first five items are related to the nature of the slurry and determine the settings for the remaining items. Precoat thickness is usually a factor only with viscous liquids or with grades of less than 700 relative flow rate and high filtration rates (flow rates for 6 in. precoats are shown in Table 3).

The right combination of these factors for maximum throughput, minimum filter aid consumption, or a combination of the two can be determined with a test leaf or by plant observation. The results of changes in these factors may be much more dramatic than most changes that can be made on a pressure leaf filter.

Rotary Vacuum Precoat Filter Test Leaf

The effects of the factors just listed are best described by outlining test procedures. A test leaf designed by Celite is shown in Fig. 27. The leaf is a maximum of 2 in. deep and is attached to a clutch so that it can be left in any position without being

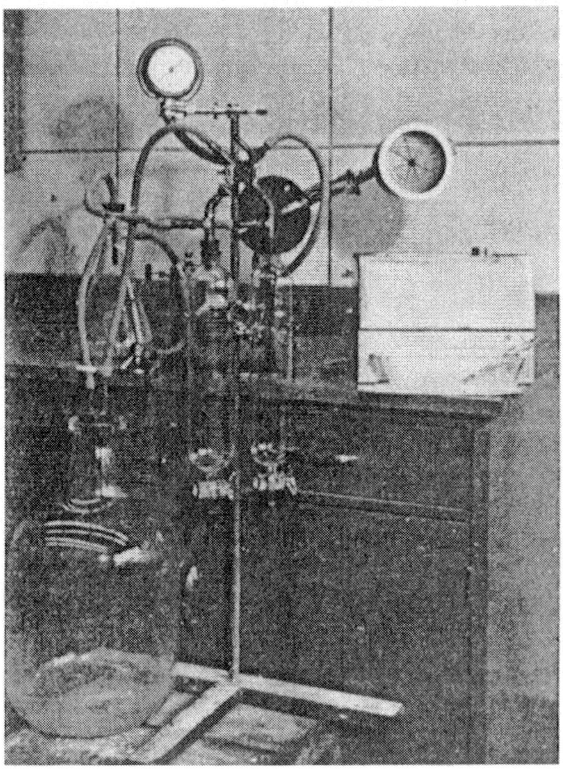

Figure 27 Rotary vacuum precoat filter test leaf with auxiliary equipment. (Courtesy of Celite Co.)

held by an operator. Crossover valves send filtrate to alternative receivers for draining and for venting unused receivers. An agitated temperature-controlled test liquid tank, vacuum gauge, and lines and receivers are shown.

In operation, a precoat is first formed on the leaf by alternately submerging and raising it to simulate a rotating drum. The leaf is then submerged in test liquid for the desired length of time, removed, and the cake and precoat extruded axially out the end of the leaf, which has a machined surface. The cake and precoat are then cut from the leaf, the precoat is allowed to dry, and the cycle is repeated as many times as needed. All of this is done in a rigid time sequence to simulate submergence drying and cutting time, based on a given drum speed, submergence time, and rate of knife advance. The quantity of the test liquid, the knife advance rate (i.e., mils per dip), and other items are recorded.

Screening Tests

A quick series of screening tests are first run to determine the fastest grade of precoat filter aid that, from visual observation, shows no penetration of solids into the precoat. A precoat approximately ½ in. thick is formed in the leaf and trimmed. A cake is formed on the leaf, and a 10 mil cut is taken. The remaining precoat should be clean. Faster (coarser) grades are tried until the remaining precoat is stained with unfiltered solids. These tests narrow down the grades of filter aid for further testing.

The second series of tests determine filtration rates versus submergence time of the drum in the filter feed. Because most solids for which the RVP filter is considered are very slimy, filtration rate frequently drops off rapidly in the first 2–8 s. Rates can best be estimated by applying a thin (about ½ in.) precoat to the filter test leaf and then submerging it for the desired length of time (i.e., 2, 4, 8 s). The filter leaf and lines are drained after each submergence, and the filtrate volume and time are recorded. Drying time is also recorded.

The results of one such series of tests are shown in Table 11, where a 0.1 ft^2 area leaf was used. Revolutions per hour were calculated based on the drying times required for the various submergences as well as on the position of the knife on the filter, which is very similar for all makes of filters. Thus, for a 4 s submergence (with the conventional knife), the filter cycle would be submergence, 4 s; drying time, 7¾ s; precoat cutting (distance between knife and slurry), 3¾ s or 15 s/rev. Based on these figures, the rate shown in the last column is 22 gal per square foot of filter area per hour. This is, of course, a much higher drum rotation than is conventionally used, but it is not beyond the range of practicality.

Table 11 Filtration Rates Versus Drum Submergence Time

Submergence time (s)	Filtrate volume (gal/ft^2)	Calculated drum speed (rev/h)	Calculated rate [$gal/(ft^2 \cdot h)$]
4	0.09	240	22
8	0.11	120	12
16	0.14	70	10
32	0.17	40	7

Submergence under these conditions is 27% of the filter area. There is a sharp drop in rate at 4 s submergence, which indicates an extremely high initial filtration rate. This may be due to two factors. First, the high rate occurs during cake formation on the precoat at a time when the resistance of the cake is at its lowest. Second, because the precoat entering the slurry is partly dewatered, its resistance to flow is at a minimum. Once the precoat is filled with liquid, its resistance increases to flow decreases.

Precoat Leaf Tests

The rest of the tests are run starting with the full 2 in. precoat in the test leaf as outlined above in the description of the leaf. It is important to adhere strictly to each part of the cycle time during these tests.

With these tests the optimum precoat grade and operating conditions can be determined for the grades of filter aid selected from the screening tests. The types of data that can be obtained are shown below.

EFFECT OF KNIFE ADVANCE ON FILTRATION RATE FOR DIFFERENT PRECOAT GRADES. This test, which measures penetration of solids into the precoat, is carried out with different grades of filter aids with relative flow rates of (for instance) 500, 750, and 900 at knife advance rates of 2–10 mil/rev. Typical results are shown in Fig. 28. When the knife advance rate is increased from 2 to 4 mil/rev, filtration rates for the two finer grades of precoat increase rapidly and then slow. The increase in filtration rate for the fastest grade is more gradual, indicating a greater degree of solids penetration into the precoat. The filtration rate obtained using the fastest grade at a knife advance of 10 mil/rev can be obtained with the slowest grade at a knife advance rate of 4 mil/rev. Very large savings in precoat cost can frequently be obtained by using a finer precoat grade.

DIATOMITE AND PERLITE AS PRECOAT MATERIALS. Figure 28, comparing different grades of diatomite, is also helpful in understanding the choice to be made between diatomite and perlite. Both are purchased on a weight basis but used on a volume basis. Perlite, having a higher volume, would seen to be the natural choice. For equal flow rates, however, perlite has larger pores that permit particles to pen-

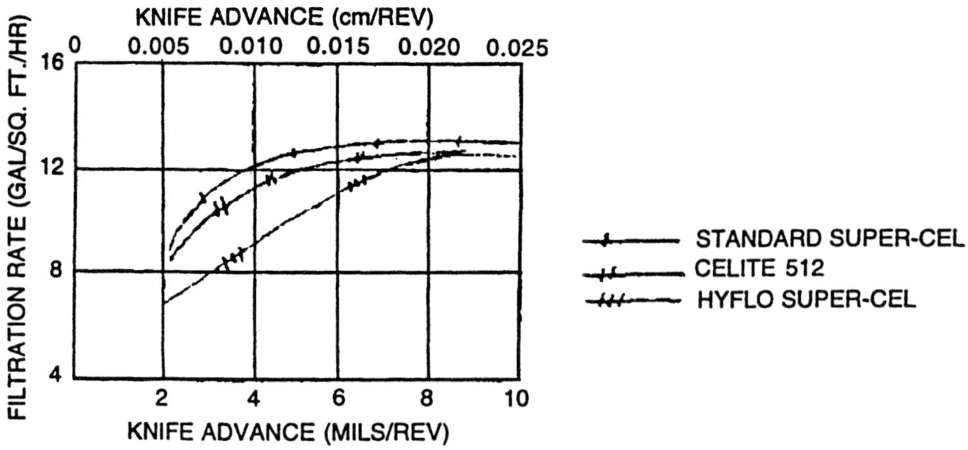

Figure 28 Knife advance rate versus filtration rate for various precoat grades.

etrate further into it as demonstrated below. As a result, a higher knife advance will be required for equal rates, thus negating the benefits of perlite's lower density. Of course, if the mechanical condition of the filter is such that the lowest knife advance that can be maintained is 4–6 mil/rev, then perlite may be the best choice.

As Fig. 29 shows, for equal permeabilities the penetration of particulate matter (in this case carbon) is much less for diatomite than for perlite. This means that knife advance rates required to remove solids from the surface of the precoat will be much lower for diatomite than for perlite for equal flow rates.

The diatomite and perlite in this demonstration have the same permeability. The diatomite is shown on the left in Fig. 29. A precoat of each material was formed. A mixture of powdered carbon and the corresponding type of filter aid was then filtered, forming a cake on each of the precoats. The degree of carbon penetration into each precoat was then measured. The following can be seen from the photographs. The penetration of carbon into the diatomite precoat is only about 25 μm, with a few particles reaching a depth of over 100 μm. Significant amounts of carbon particles penetrate 300 μm into the perlite precoat. The pore openings in the perlite

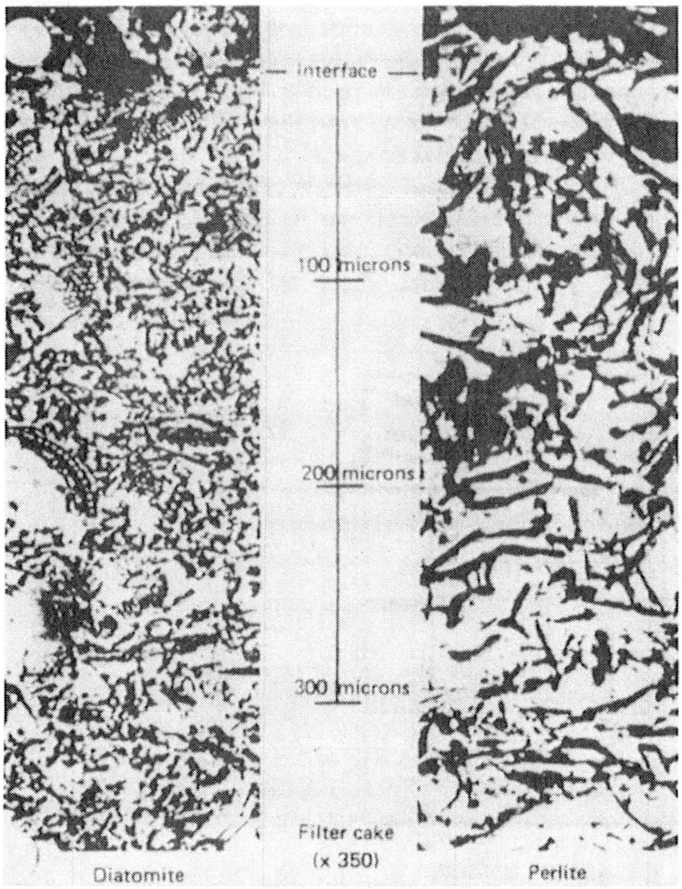

Figure 29 Penetration of powdered carbon into diatomite and perlite precoats—petrographic analysis. (Courtesy of Celite Co., Lompoc, CA.)

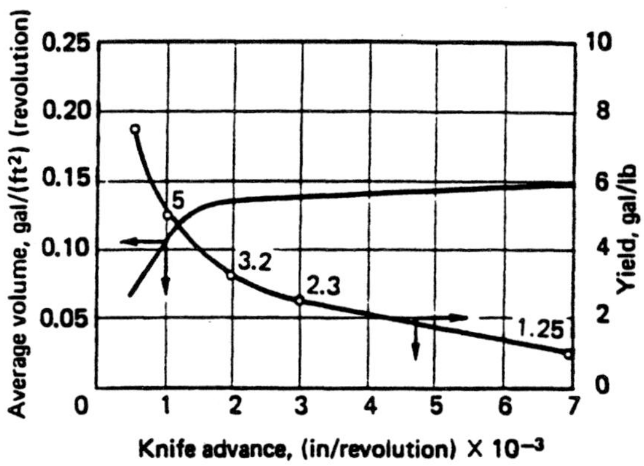

Figure 30 Knife advance vs. precoat usage and yield for a single grade of filter aid. (From Smith, 1976b.)

precoat are much larger than those in the diatomite precoat even though the precoat permeabilities are equal. The deeper penetration of solids into the perlite precoat will require a greater knife advance rate to remove these solids compared to the diatomite precoat, resulting in higher precoat consumption for perlite.

The data shown in Fig. 28 can be recalculated (see Fig. 30) to show the yield in terms of gallons throughput per pound of filter aid.

RATE VS. PRECOAT THICKNESS. As precoat thickness is reduced by the cutting of the knife, its resistance to flow decreases as shown in Fig. 31. Filtration rate, therefore, should increase as precoat thickness decreases provided penetration is not a factor. The 3 mil cut keeps up with penetration. The 1 mil cut does not.

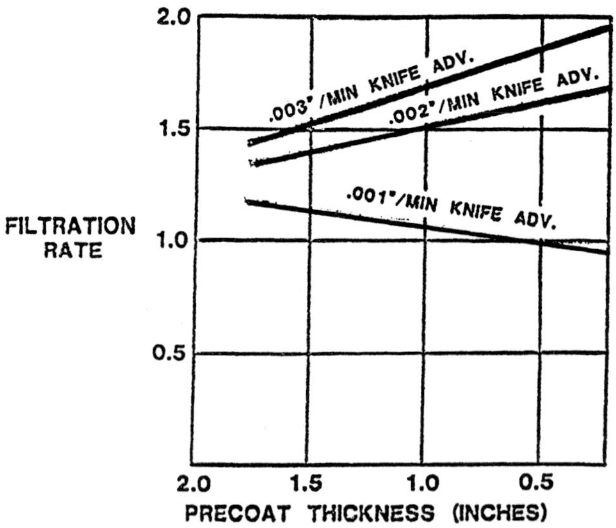

Figure 31 Filtration rate vs. precoat thickness relative to knife advance for 0.5% $Al(OH)_3$ at 90 s/rev. (From Bell, 1958.)

RATE VS. DRUM SPEED. Filtration rate versus drum speed is shown in Fig. 32 for three different knife advance rates. For example, when the drum speed is increased from 0.5 to 3 rpm and the knife advance rate is 4 mil/rev, the filtration rate increases from less than 4 to over 12 gsfh. At a drum speed of 1.5 rpm, the filtration rate increases from slightly under 6 to approximately 9 gsfh as the knife advance is increased from 2 to 4 mil/rev. The 4 mil/rev curve is shown leveling off at approximately 13 gsfh to illustrate the hydraulic limitations of the precoat–septum system.

Figure 32 also shows rates obtainable for different combinations of drum speed and knife advance. For instance, if a rate of 10 gsfh is desired, the filter may be operated in the following ways:

Knife advance (mil/rev)	Drum speed (rpm)
4	1¾
2	2¼
1	3

Some mechanisms advance the knife on a time basis rather than keeping the rate constant with drum speed. Increasing drum speed in this instance reduces knife advance per revolution. This has a negative effect on flow (see Fig. 33). Increasing drum speed, therefore, may increase the filtration rate up to the point at which the knife is too low to keep up with solids penetration into the precoat, and flow rate will decrease. Thus, a maximum rate is reached for a given knife advance versus time. To further increase rate, knife advance must be increased.

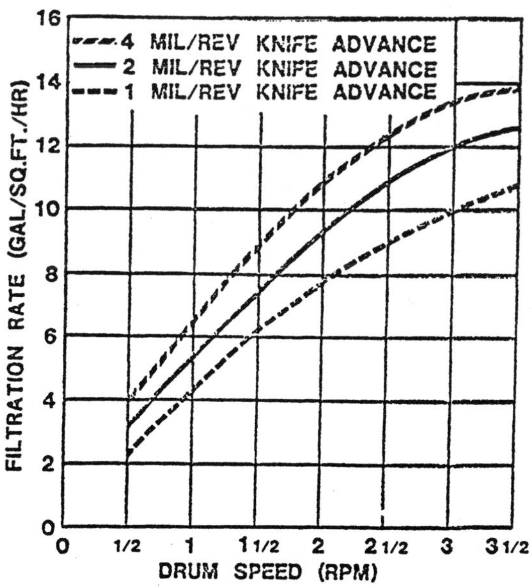

Figure 32 Filtration rate versus drum speed. (From Smith, 1977.)

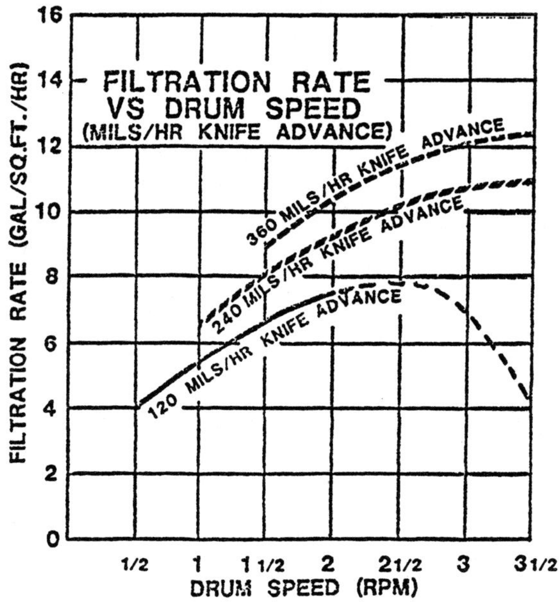

Figure 33 Rate versus drum speed when knife advance is constant with time.

PRECOAT USAGE VERSUS DRUM SPEED FOR DIFFERENT FLOW RATES AND KNIFE ADVANCE RATES. Figure 34 summarizes the information provided in this section. It shows knife advance rates and drum speeds for flow rates of 6, 8, 10, and 12 gsfh. For instance, if a 10 gsfh rate is needed, it can be obtained at a 4 mil/rev knife advance and a drum speed of 1¾ (with a precoat usage of 70 lb/1000 gal) or at a 1 mil/rev knife advance and a 3 rpm knife advance, in which case the precoat usage is only 30 lb/1000 gal. If an accurate knife advance rate of 1 mil/rev cannot be maintained, then a higher knife advance rate must be used, and filter aid costs will increase accordingly.

The following formulas were used in calculations for the graph in Fig. 34.

$$\frac{\text{Drum speed (rev/min)} \times 60\ \text{mil/hr} \times \text{knife advance (mil/rev)}}{1000\ \text{mil/in.} \times 12\ \text{in./ft} \times \text{precoat density (lb/ft}^3) \times \text{filtration rate (gal/(ft}^2 \cdot \text{h))}}$$

$$\times\ 1000 = \text{lb precoat/1000 gal filtrate}$$

The constants in the above equation can be combined to give

$$\frac{\text{Drum speed (rpm)} \times \text{knife advance (mils/rev)} \times \text{precoat density (lb/ft}^3)}{\text{filtration rate (gsfh)} \times 5}$$

$$= \text{lb precoat/1000 gal}$$

[A more theoretical approach has been taken by Hoflinger and Hackl (1990).]

The calculations show, for instance, that with the 4 mil knife advance condition, precoat consumption is doubled compared to that of the 1 mil knife advance. This

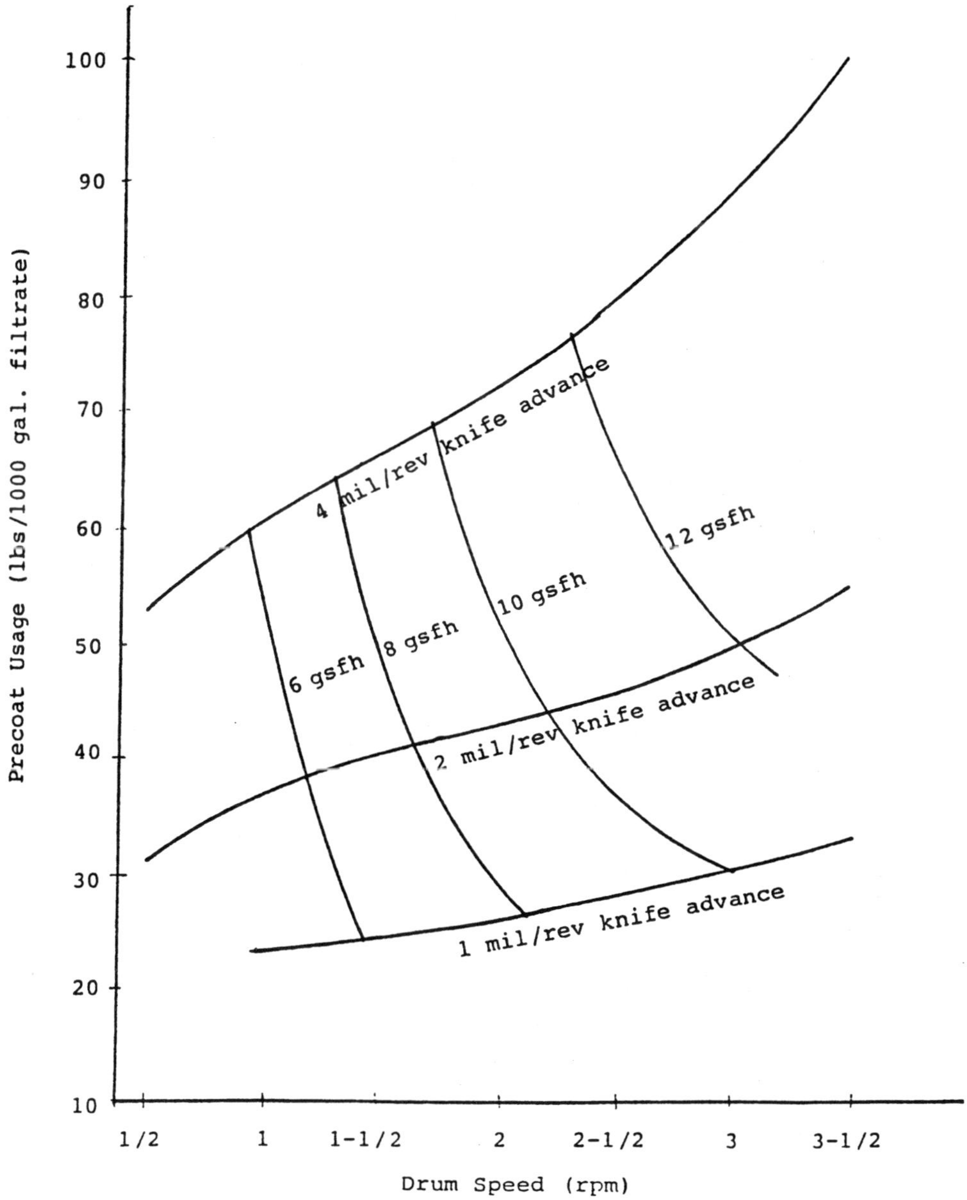

Figure 34 Precoat usages versus drum speed for different knife advance rates.

assumes that the cake is cut cleanly and evenly from the precoat under all conditions. If this is not the case, then the above assumptions are meaningless. Assuming good cake cutting, however, the conditions for minimum precoat consumption rate are those of higher drum speeds and lower knife advance rates, emphasizing the importance of good knife design and maintenance.

4.4 Precoating

Introduction

For a specific grade of precoat material, the way in which the precoat is applied will have a very significant effect on filtration efficiency. During filtration the knife may advance into the precoat at rates as low as 0.5 mm per drum revolution. It is necessary, therefore, to apply as firm a precoat as possible to minimize breathing of the precoat due to changes in vacuum and other operating factors.

The objectives of the precoat operation are to attain

A precoat thickness of up to 6 in.
An application time of 15–30 min
Maximum permeability
Maximum firmness (which translates into maximum density)
Uniformity on completion of ±¼ in.
No, or minimum, cracking

Precoat Laminations

As the filter drum rotates, the precoat alternately forms and is dewatered. Because the dewatered precoat entering the precoat slurry is mostly empty, at this point the flow of liquid into the precoat is at a maximum, and the precoat formed contains filter aid particle sizes typical of those of the filter aid in the precoat slurry. After the precoat fills with liquid, flow through it slows, and finer and finer particles of filter aid are drawn onto the precoat. This phenomenon results in the formation of a laminated precoat with laminations ranging from ⅛ to over ¼ in. in thickness, depending on precoat conditions. The slower the drum rotation, the higher the drum submergence; and the more dilute the precoat slurry, the greater the degree of lamination and the slower the flow through the precoat.

When precoating is carried out at maximum vacuum (4 standard cfm/ft^2 of filter area), maximum drum speed (preferably 30 s/rev), and minimum drum submergence, a greater amount of precoat formation occurs at maximum rates, while the precoat is filling with liquid, and laminations are thereby minimized. The precoat is firmer and more permeable and will give higher filtration rates and lower precoat consumption.

Precoating Systems

Metering into a Recirculation Line

After recirculation is established (making sure the liquid level in the filter tub is not touching the filter drum), a concentrated precoat slurry of up to 18% concentration is metered into the precoat recirculation line (see Fig. 35) at a rate such that the transfer is complete in 15–20 min, the desired precoating time. Excess liquid is removed (line not shown) from the precoat recirculation line to maintain a constant drum level of not more than 10% in the bowl. Precoat may also be metered in dry form into the recirculation line by means of an eductor. Again, the metering must be complete in 15–20 min.

After all precoat has been added, recirculation is continued until all precoat material is on the drum.

For smaller systems the "metering" may be a matter of dumping bags of filter powder into a tank during the precoat operation. If so, it is important to maintain a steady rate of addition.

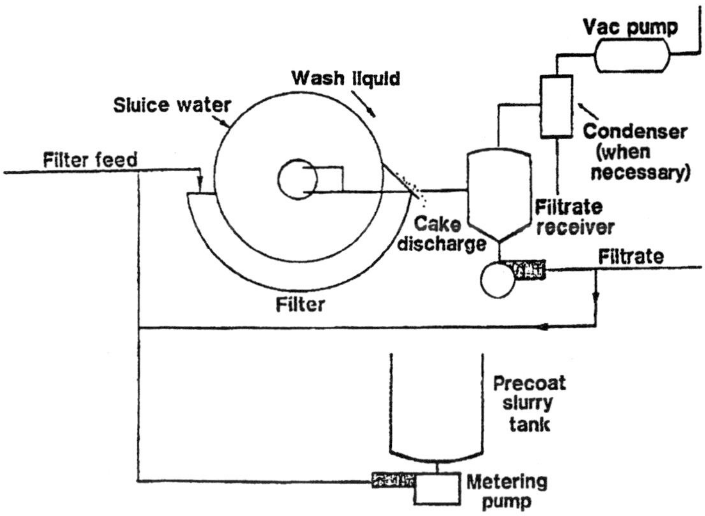

Figure 35 Rotary vacuum precoat filter system showing precoat addition by metering a concentrated slurry into the precoat recirculation line. (Courtesy of Celite Co., Lompoc, CA.)

In a variation of the above method, the precoat is added in dry form to an eductor in the recirculation line, as shown in Fig. 26. Other precoat systems are described in a Harborlite Corp. paper, Rotary vacuum precoat filter system design and operation, for the American Filtration Conference, May, 1992, Chicago. IL. This method is particularly suitable for large systems that use filter aid in bulk.

Precoat Losses

There are two major sources of filter aid losses in precoating:

1. The precoat remaining in the filter bowl at the end of the precoat operation. This material will be mixed in with feed slurry at the start of the filter cycle and cause a temporary increase in filter rates, but it is an inefficient use of filter aid.
2. Any excess amount of precoat trimmed from the drum as the precoat builds out beyond the knife. If this is a persistant problem, the precoat can be returned to the bowl by installing a movable plate under the knife.

The best solution to both the above situations is, of course, to add the correct amount of precoat.

Precoat Procedures

The following precoat procedures are recommended for diatomite and perlite filter aids.

1. Make up the precoat slurry. Adjust pH to approximately 2 if cracking is expected or to get the most stable precoat.
2. Start vacuum pumps at maximum (close all bleed valves between pump and filter).

3. Start drum at 30 s/rev.
4. Start precoat slurry to filter. Maintain a 10% slurry at all times.
5. Allow drum submergence to seek its own level throughout the precoat operation. If vacuum is adequate and the filter cloth is clean and not too tight (see below), the level should not rise much above 10%.
6. Start sprays when precoat first forms on drum if cracking is expected.
7. Continue above until precoat is within approximately $1/2$–$1/4$ in. of the knife.
8. Stop slurry feed to filter.
9. Continue precoating (applying precoat remaining in the bowl) until the precoat is cut evenly by the knife.
10. If it is desirable to separate the precoat from the precoat liquid, and if the precoat is free of cracks, the precoat liquid may be dropped from the bowl at this point. It may help to turn on wash sprays to keep the precoat moist. A vacuum of only 10 in. Hg, however, will hold on a 6 in. precoat.
11. Start feed to filter.
12. Manually advance the knife to maintain continuous cutting, then set the knife advance at a high rate until the precoat is stabilized.
13. Continue with normal filtration operation until the knife is a minimum distance from the drum (preferably not more than $1/4$–$1/2$ in.).

On occasion, a precoat of 100% cellulose is required either as a basecoat to reduce precoat bleed-through (in which case it may be only $1/8$–$1/4$ in. thick) or as the entire precoat where its chemical resistance is required. The high drum speeds, however, called for in the above procedures will cause the cellulose to form small rolls on the drum and prevent precoat formation. This can be avoided by using a drum speed of 1–2 min/rev instead of the higher speeds recommended above.

Precoat Removal and Filter Washdown

1. Drain the tub with the vacuum kept on to keep bare cloth from coming in contact with unfiltered slurry.
2. Fast advance the knife to the minimum distance from the drum to remove remaining precoat.
3. Stop the wash sprays if they are being used.
4. Stop the vacuum.
5. Turn high pressure wash sprays (if available) on to wash the septum.
6. Wash the tub and drum walls.
7. Purge all lines to be used for precoating of unfiltered material.

Cake should be removed from behind the knife at the end of each precoat cycle.

Use of a Basecoat Under a Precoat

In using a basecoat, the basecoat is first formed under the precoat using the coarsest grade of precoat filter aid available. For a 6 in. precoat the basecoat is usually 1 in. thick.

(Coarse grades of cellulose may also be used, in which case the precoat drum speed must be $1/2$–1 rpm rather than the 2 rpm recommended.)

The basecoat serves five functions:

1. It forms a renewable support layer for the precoat, permitting faster reprecoating.
2. It protects the septum from being blinded by unfiltered material during precoating.
3. It results in higher flow rates due to lower resistance.
4. The use of a coarser grade of precoat for the basecoat reduces blinding which frequently occurs when reprecoating over a heel of the same grade as was used for filtration.
5. It reduces precoat bleeding through the septum.

Precoat Troubleshooting

Precoat Formation Problems

If the vacuum pump is operating properly and has the specified capacity of 4 scfm per square foot of filter area and the filter cloth is clean and has a permeability of 80–200 cfm, the vacuum at the pump with a clean, bare cloth will be on the order of 3–5 in. Hg.

Inadequate vacuum on the surface of the drum causes the precoat to not pick up (or form) on the drum or to turn mushy when 1–2 in. thick, or even to fall off.

These problems, which may be indicated by a higher vacuum, may be caused by:

1. Blinding of the cloth (this is sometimes not readily seen with the naked eye).
2. Plugged internal piping either in the filter or between the filter and the receiver or the pump.
3. In new installations, an upward slope in the filtrate line between the filter and receiver, which causes liquid to flow back into the filter and out through the cloth, thus washing off the precoat at the bottom of each panel.

Precoat Cracking

Occasionally precoats crack despite all precautions and care taken in application. The following affords some understanding of the causes of and solutions to precoat cracking. Special noncracking filter aids exist, but familiarity with possible causes of cracking will enable almost any filter aid to be used as a precoat. Some of these causes of cracks are

1. The nature and origin of the precoat material.
2. The way in which the precoat is applied.
3. Partially blinded filter cloths, which set up stresses in the precoat.
4. Excessive compression of the precoat when the filter is first put on-stream caused by allowing solids to build up on the precoat before the knife is run in.
5. Flocculation of precoat material. Precoat materials tend to flocculate to different degrees in different types of liquids. The degree of flocculation can be measured by putting a 10% slurry or precoat and precoating liquid in a graduate and noting the degree of settling. Flocculation of diatomite filter aids can be reduced by lowering the pH (to as far as 2).

4.5 Filter Operation

Filtration Start-Up After Precoat Has Been Applied

1. Start wash sprays if they are not already on.
2. Start filter feed to filter. Knife advance may be left off at this point to compress and stabilize the precoat.
3. Fast advance the knife to start cutting.
4. Set the knife on slow advance.
5. Adjust the knife advance rate, drum speed, and submergence for optimum operation.
6. Continue until approximately 1/8 in. of precoat remains on the basecoat.
7. Stop the filter feed. Proceed as in Section 4.4.

Filter Adjustment for Blinding Solids and Maximum Rate

For maximum flow rate, the drum should be run at high speeds. If additional cake drying time is needed, drum submergence should be decreased instead of reducing the drum speed. Reducing the drum speed to get additional drying time (the most common reaction) will greatly reduce the flow rate, especially for blinding cakes. Thus, if the cake seals and reduces or stops the flow after 5–10 s of submergence, increasing the drying time by slowing the drum speed will result in little or no increase in the volume of filtrate for each drum revolution. Therefore, since there are fewer drum revolutions per hour, the filtration rate will decrease. For instance, I have run a 12 ft diameter by 24 ft long RVP filter on wine lees at 1 ft diameter submergence and at 20 s/rev. If the submergence were allowed to increase to 18 in., the cake at the knife would be too wet for proper discharge. Because this filter was specially designed, it was operated at knife advance rates of 0.005 in./rev, which made the filtration process very economical. Filtration rates were as high as 9 gsfh, compared to less than 3 gsfh running at the conventional rates of 1–2 mm/rev and higher submergences.

4.6 Troubleshooting Filtration Problems

Uneven Precoat

1. If precoat thickness is even around the circumference but varies in thickness along the length of the drum, the cause is poor feed distribution or inadequate agitation.
2. If thickness varies randomly throughout the precoat, the cause is septum, or cloth, blinding (see discussion of cloth cleaning in Section 4.8), or incomplete removal of all unfiltered material from the filter and lines before precoating.

Lost Precoats

Occasionally a precoat is lost during precoating due to excessive cracking. If the cracks are large and extensive and extend to cloth and the cloth is too open to seal quickly, vacuum will be lost and the precoat will fall off the drum. This may also happen during filtration. This situation can usually be avoided by using a cloth with a maximum Frazier rating of 200 cfm (see discussion of cloth selection in Section 4.8). (See Fig. 36.)

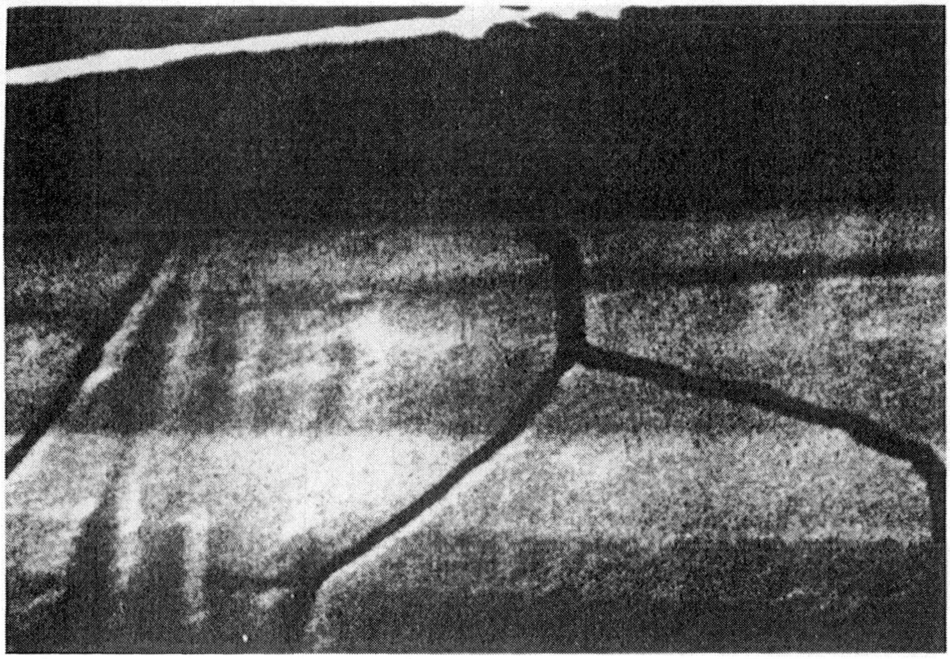

Figure 36 When the recommended cloths are used, even these cracks will not cause precoat to drop off the drum.

Precoat Patterns Caused by Too Open a Septum

Patterns can be produced by precoat bleeding through too open a septum (see Fig. 37).

Penetration of Solids into a Precoat

Filtration problems can result from solids being retained by layers of fine precoat material. (See Figs. 38 and 39.) They indicate use of too coarse a precoat material.

Uneven Knife Advance

Occasionally, it will be noticed that the surface of the precoat is alternately glossy (indicating that it is sealed and not filtering) and dull, with a dry cake. This situation may be the result of the following:

Dull or incorrectly mounted blades. Dull blades tend to smear the cake into the precoat, leaving the precoat partially blinded, especially at low knife advance rates. To overcome smearing, higher knife advance rates must be used.

Knife flexing. If the programmed rate of knife advance is 2 mil/rev (not an unreasonable goal for continuous operation) and the knife flexes ± 1 mil, there will be a 50% deviation in the advance rate. This can cause very significant increases in precoat consumption. Knife flexing can be a problem on all makes of filters of large area unless the knife has been specially constructed. This subject is discussed further in Section 4.7.

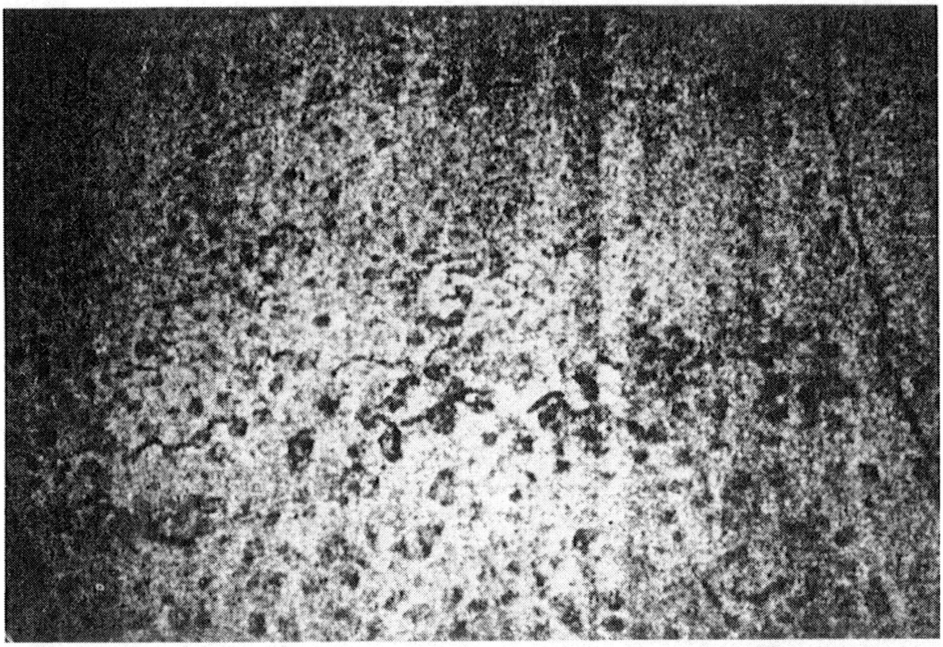

Figure 37 Pattern on a 1–2 in. thick precoat made by a continual bleed-through of filter aid through too open a septum.

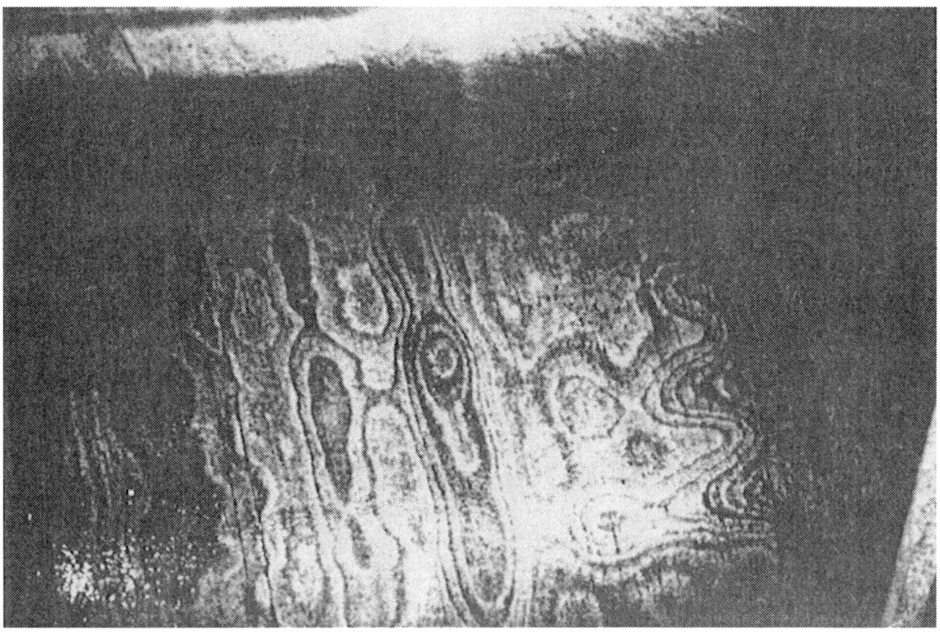

Figure 38 Wood grain patterns on precoat caused by excessive solids penetration due to too coarse a precoat.

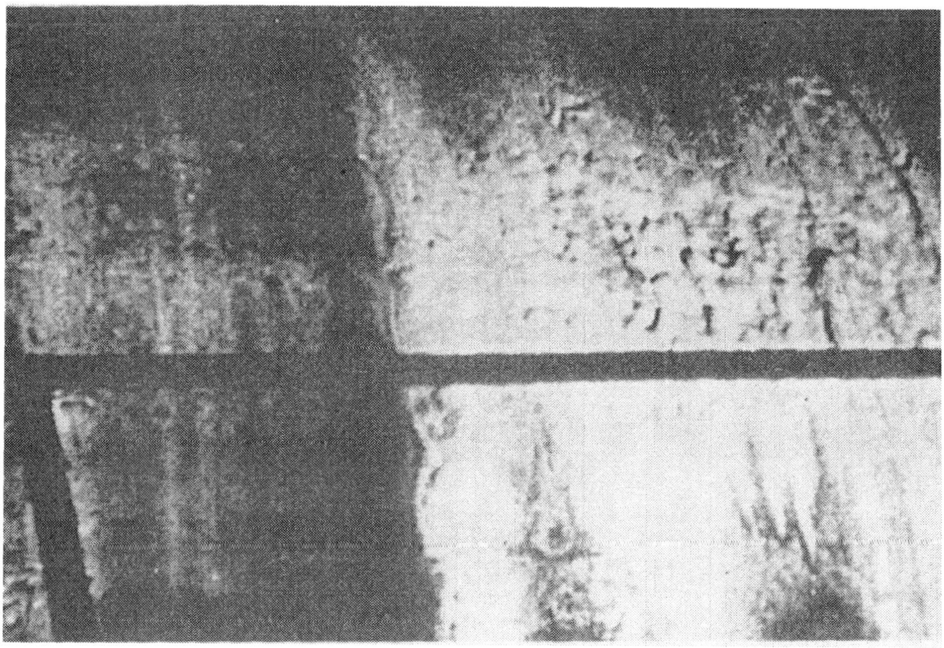

Figure 39 Precoat turns mushy and begins to wash off as solids penetrate into it, preventing vacuum from reaching its surface.

Solids buildup behind the knife. Buildup of solid material underneath the knife blade increases the contact area between the knife and the precoat, resulting in greater forces being required for an even knife cut. These increased forces in turn result in increased flexing of the knife and decreased cutting accuracy. This problem is difficult to overcome as the area involved is inaccessible during filtration and fairly inaccessible during the filter cleaning operation.

Precoat Gouging

Some cakes will be thick and heavy enough that they rise up ahead of the knife, removing a portion of precoat as they are cut. The depression left in the surface of the precoat is then filled with filtered solids and will not be removed by the knife for the next several drum revolutions. This area of precoat is then partially blinded. While these areas are continually changing they can account for up to 75% or more of the filter area and may result in filtration rates that are much lower than normal. This situation can be overcome by decreasing drum submergence and increasing drum rotation speed. The cake thus formed is too thin to cause gouging. Without gouging, filtration takes place over 100% of the precoat surface, so the filter area is increased severalfold and the cake, being thinner, has much less resistance to flow. It is possible, as was done with grape lees, to increase filtration rates threefold while at the same time reducing precoat use. Figure 40 shows a precoat surface before and after these adjustments were made.

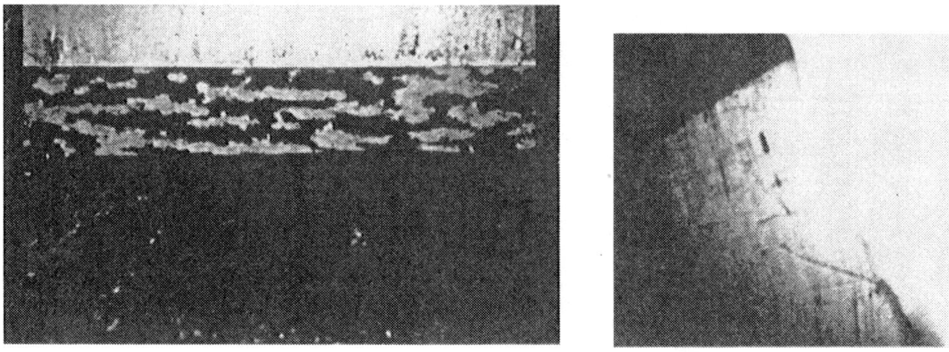

(a) (b)

Figure 40 (a) Precoat with gouging. (b) Precoat after operating adjustments.

Vibration

A vibrating blade and corresponding precoat pattern (Fig. 41) usually indicates too great an angle between the blade and the drum.

Intermittent Cutting

The pattern shown in Fig. 42 was due to the motion of the drum (due to loose trinion bearings) in concert with the oscillation of the agitator.

4.7 Equipment

Design aspects of the rotary vacuum precoat filter that are specific to this type of drum filter are summarized in this section.

The Filter Knife

The best-run laboratory and pilot tests are of little use if, at the plant, the cake is not removed from the precoat evenly and completely, leaving a smooth, clean precoat free of any unfiltered material. When a filter cake is being cut efficiently it will be removed continuously and evenly with only a small amount of precoat attached to it. (With the optimum grade of precoat, there will be almost no penetration of solids into the precoat beyond the precoat removed by the knife.) The cake may come off the knife in a continuous sheet (as in a wine lees filtration) or in varying degrees of dryness depending on its physical properties, but the precoat remaining on the drum should be smooth and free of any surface indentations or unfiltered solids. Poor removal of the cake will result in greater precoat consumption, lower flow rates, or both. Paying attention to the items outlined below can, in some instances, as much as double flow rates and at the same time halve precoat usage.

Knife Advance Mechanisms

Advance mechanisms fall into three general categories.

1. Time-controlled. The advance mechanism is independent of the drum and the advance rate is related to time. The advantage of this method is that

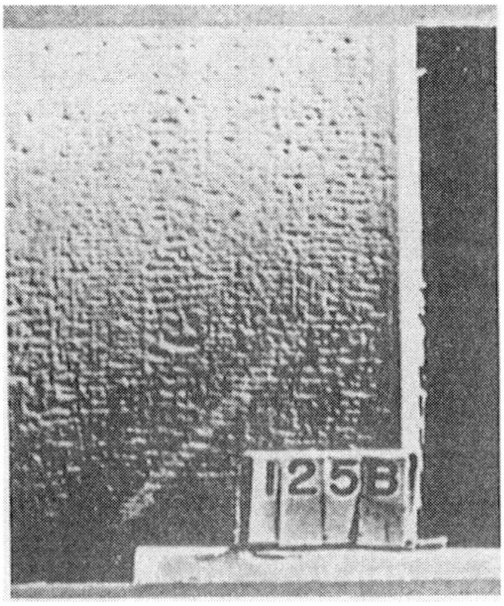

Figure 41 Pattern on precoat caused by vibration. (Courtesy of Celite Co., Lompoc, CA.)

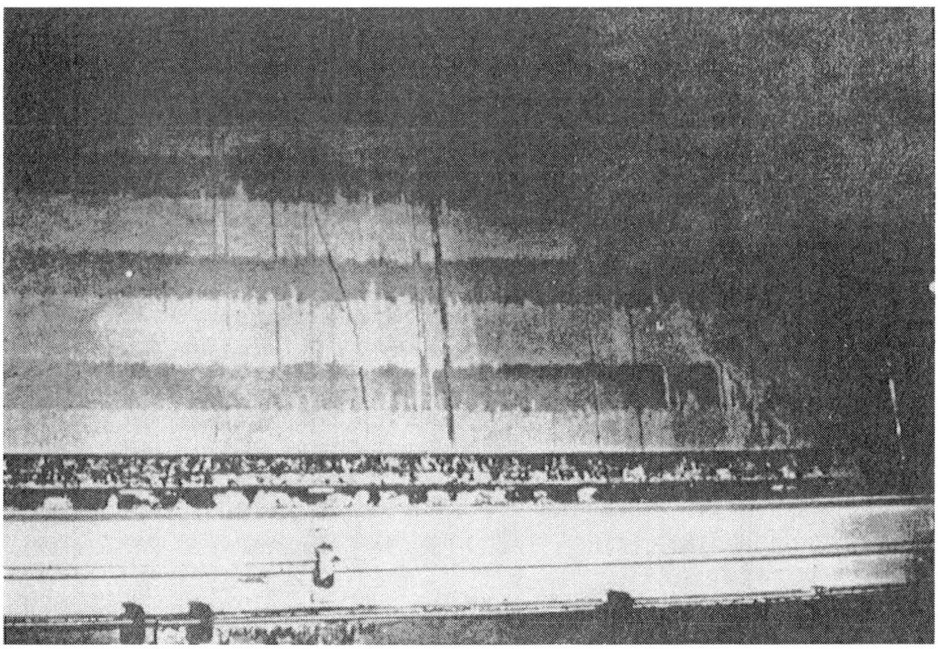

Figure 42 Striped pattern on precoat caused by excess agitation and loose trunion bearings.

once the optimum knife advance rate is determined, that rate is maintained for different drum speeds. The amount of precoat used per unit time is always known. To maintain a constant rate per revolution, however, an adjustment must be made each time the drum speed is changed.
2. Drum-controlled. In this case the advance rate is tied directly to drum rotation. The advance mechanism is run off the drum drive, and the knife advance rate is expressed as inches per drum revolution.
3. Process-controlled. In this case the knife advance rate is tied into tank levels or vacuum variations.

Knife Design

Knife flexing may be caused by any of the following:

1. Lack of overall rigidity of the knife structure
2. The angle of the knife to the precoat
3. Sharpness of the blade and the way it is mounted (bevel facing down)
4. Torque caused by the location of the blade on a radius originating from a line between the two end knife supports (on old knife designs)

The major cause of knife flexing is the angle of the knife to the precoat. There are two forces acting on the knife as it cuts cake from the drum. The first is the outward force on the knife exerted by the precoat and cake on the knife as they resist its advance into the precoat. This outward force is in turn dependent on the area of contact between the blade (and any solids buildup underneath it), the precoat, and the hardness, or resistance, of the cake. Minimizing this is the prime reason for mounting the knife with the bevel facing up, away from the precoat.

The second force is the downward force exerted by the rotation of the drum and the resistance of the cake and precoat to the cutting action of the knife. This force is related to drum speed, cake thickness, cake cohesiveness (in turn related to liquid viscosity), cake particle characteristics, degree of cake removal from the precoat on previous drum revolutions, knife sharpness, and area of contact between the knife and the precoat.

These outward and downward forces should be resolved by changing the angle of the knife to the precoat so that their resolution is along the plane of maximum knife assembly rigidity. This has been done in the past (on other types of knife assemblies) with very significant reductions in knife flexing.

The degree of knife flexing can be determined by use of an externally mounted dial indicator. Where it is necessary to take measurements on the knife itself, a portion of the blade (6 in. long) at the center of the knife is removed to prevent the cake from interfering with the dial indicator. The indicator is then placed on the knife below this point and time vs. knife position readings are taken. The data, when plotted, should give a straight line. If not, adjust the knife angle so that it gives a minimum of flexing.

An example of the results of some of these measurements showing the effects of knife flexing is given in Fig. 43. The line should, of course, be straight and the flow rates constant.

The Blade

The blade, which does the cutting, is mounted on the knife and is most commonly a 6 in. long piece of Stellite with a bevel along one side. It is essential that the blade

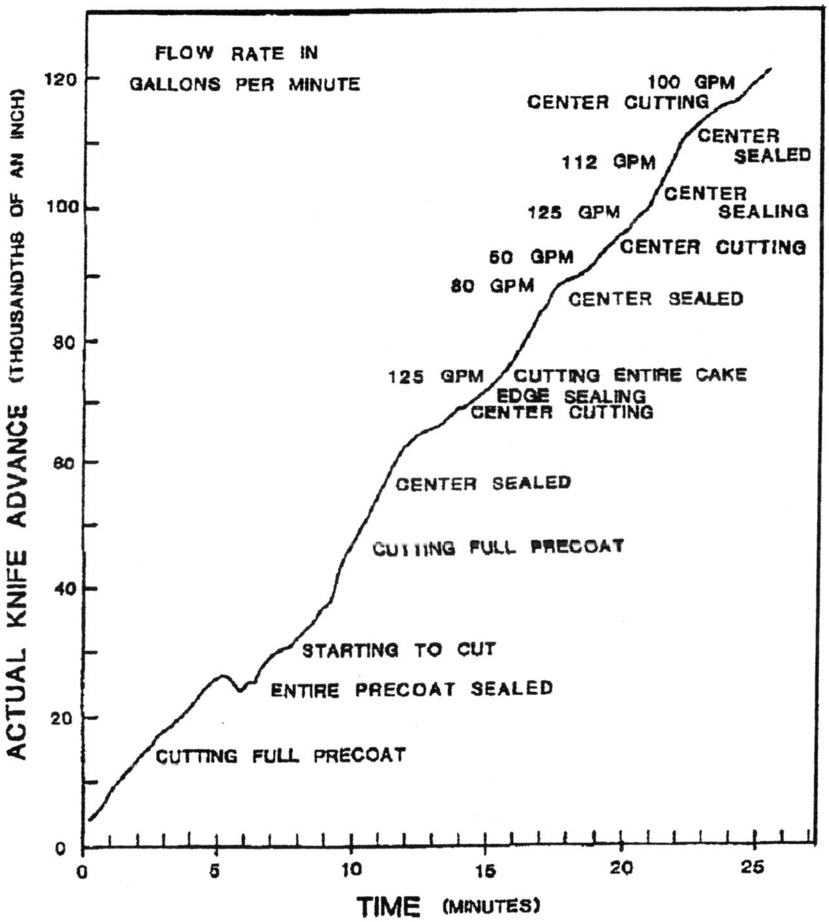

Figure 43 Effects of knife flexing on filter performance. (Courtesy of Celite Co., Lompoc, CA.)

be mounted with the bevel facing up to maximize cutting accuracy. Other materials such as Hastalloy may be used where corrosion is a problem.

It is possible to attach the blades to the knife with the bevel facing either up or down. Facing the precoat, the blade becomes self-sharpening. However, it also creates greater resistance to knife advance, accentuating any flexing problems. In addition, the bevel may tend to smear unfiltered solids into the precoat and lower filtration rates. Facing the bevel up provides minimum contact between the knife and precoat and minimizes flexing and cake smearing. This position will usually result in significantly higher precoat rates and lower precoat consumption and is worth the effort of keeping the knives sharp.

Aluminum oxide blades have greatly increased abrasion resistance and will last indefinitely where they are chemically compatible but are hard to use because of their brittleness. In tests, blades showed little or no wear after 18 months, whereas the Stellite blades were sharpened every 4–6 weeks. The aluminum oxide blades, however, are quite fragile and can easily break off if the knife angle is incorrect. A dimensional drawing of a filter blade is presented in Fig. 44 for those wishing to have such a blade made.

Cake Washing

For washing the filter cake, use flat, not conical, spray nozzles to get an even spray distribution.

The following suggestions are offered to reduce plugging of spray nozzles.

1. Install strainers at each spray header.
2. Mount nozzles on L's coming from the top of the header. This will allow any solids that either enter the header or form there to settle out rather than enter the nozzles.
3. Provide a connection at the opposite end of the header to be opened on a periodic basis to permit flushing out of accumulated solid material.

Should the plugging continue despite all the above, consider the use of Spraying Systems Company flat jet nozzles. These nozzles have a round opening (which will pass larger solids for equal capacity) and depend on a deflector to provide a flat spray pattern.

Wash Header

Despite the fact that unfiltered solids should never come in contact with the septum, the septum frequently becomes blinded over a period of time. Where this is the case, a wash header should be installed. Typically, Spraying Systems Corporation's Vee-Jet 9510 nozzles are mounted every 6 in. on a header, which is in turn mounted 6.5–7 in. from the drum. Pressures of up to 250 psig may be required to remove gelatinous substances. If these pressures are used, a baffle should be mounted behind the spray bar to prevent spray from bouncing off the drum into the operating area. The sluice is operated for several drum revolutions at the end of every precoat. Note that flat spray nozzles are used in place of the commonly supplied headers with drilled holes, as the latter are practically useless in maintaining a clean septum.

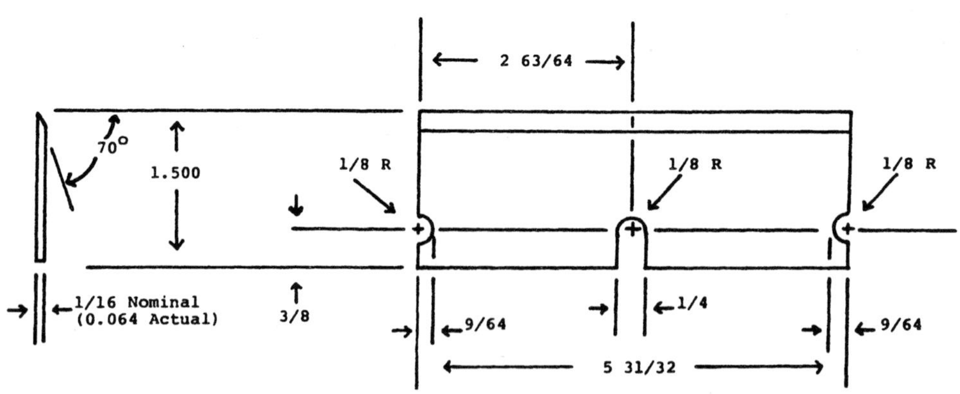

Figure 44 Rotary precoat filter blade.

Vacuum Pump Requirements

A vacuum pump capacity of 4 scfm is required per square foot of filter area for the formation of a good precoat. The vacuum required for filtration will depend on the permeability of the filter cake. It may be as low as 1 scfm per square foot of filter area. Where there is a significant difference between precoating and operating vacuums, it may be economical to have two vacuum pumps, using both for precoating and one for filtering.

4.8 Filter Cloths

Effects on Filter Performance

It should be possible with a rotary vacuum precoat filter to obtain a filtrate with solids of 0.1% or less. Some filters produce filtrates with a filtrate solids content of less than 10 ppm, and filtrate solids of less than 100 ppm are common. The cloth should be fine enough to prevent bleed-through of significant amounts of precoat and other suspended solids but be permeable enough to offer little or no resistance to liquid and gas flow (especially during precoating) in comparison to that of the precoat and filter cake. The cloth should be strong enough to support itself over the openings of the drum grid. If not, a support screen under the grid should be considered. In addition,

1. It should be resistant to abrasion.
2. It should be chemically resistant to the liquid being filtered.
3. It should have good dimensional stability.
4. It should not split when it is bent into a caulking groove.

A 10 × 10 mesh plastic screen between the cloth and the filter grid will greatly reduce cloth wear.

In selecting the cloth, the following characteristics should be considered:

The size of the cloth openings will increase as the cloth wears with use.
A cloth with thicker threads will be more resistant to abrasion.
The minimum size opening will depend on thread diameter and amount of calendering. Thus the thread thickness is limited.
A low thread count in one direction will result in a weaker cloth and one in which enlargement of openings due to thread shifting is more likely to occur.
Cloths made of monofilament fibers have the least tendency to blind compared to multifilament and staple fiber cloths.
Caulking the cloth at every one to three panels will minimize stretching and wrinkle formation, which in turn will reduce the distance within which the knife can be run to the drum without tearing the cloth (minimizes the precoat heel). It should be possible to reduce heel thickness to within $\frac{1}{4}$–$\frac{3}{8}$ in.

Considering the above, a cloth of the following characteristics is recommended.

Permeability: Air flow (Frazier rating) 100–200 cfm
Monofilament polypropylene
A maximum warp and fill count ratio of 2.5 (typical thread counts are 108 × 44 or 66 × 30)
Cloth weight: 8–10 oz/yd^2

Dutch-weave wire cloths (24 × 110) are also used in severe service.

4.9 Summary of Rotary Vacuum Precoat Filter Equipment Considerations

1. Internal piping must be on the trailing edge of the drum drainage panels or the precoat will not form on the drum.
2. Bridgeless valve construction. Vacuum has to be on 100% of the drum surface.
3. Minimum knife advance should be between 0.0005 and 0.001 in./rev.
4. The knife should be able to advance steadily during any one revolution of the drum and should not flex more than 0.0005 in. per revolution.
5. The knife should be able to advance within $\frac{1}{4}$–$\frac{3}{8}$ in. of the drum to minimize the amount of precoat left on the drum at the end of the filter cycle. Thus the drum should have a maximum runout of $\frac{1}{8}$ in.
6. The knife mounts should be such that the angle of the knife to the drum can be varied.
7. Filter must accept a 6 in. precoat.
8. After precoat is complete, the precoat should be uniform to within $\pm\frac{1}{8}$ in. over the face of the drum before trimming with the knife.
9. Tub level control: 10% drum diameter for precoat; as required for filtering.
10. The agitator in tub should have two speeds: high for precoating and slower for filtering. (Too high a speed can cause movement of the drum, resulting in uneven precoat cutting.)
11. The agitator should have extra large sealed bearings.
12. Cake wash sprays, if required, should be flat (not conical), and the spray header should be equipped with a cartridge to prevent sprays from plugging.
13. If solids are extremely blinding, the maximum drum speed should be 2–3 rpm.
14. If there is any tendency for the filter cloth to become blinded, a high pressure (up to 200 psig) flat-spray sluice header should be provided.
15. Vacuum: 4 cfm (mechanical) per square foot of area for precoating. Less capacity may be required for filtering, depending on the permeability of the filter cake. In some installations two pumps are used.
16. Precoat slurry entrance should be below the liquid level in the bowl to prevent foaming.
17. Sharp knives are critical for minimum precoat usage. An extra set of knife blades should be kept available.

BIBLIOGRAPHY

Alciatore, A. F., F. J. Bodman, and E. L. Neu. (1974). Advances in perlite and diatomite filter aid research, *Filtration Separ.*, Mar./April, pp. 121–124.

Amirhor, P., and R. S. Englebrecht. (1975). Virus removal by polyelectrolyte filtration, *J. Am. Water Works Assoc.*, April, pp. 187–192.

AWWA Manual M30. (1988). Precoat Filtration, Am. Water Works Assoc., Denver, CO.

Baumann, E., and R. L. LaFrenz. (1963). Optimal economic design for municipal diatomite filter plants, *J. AWWA*, *55*(1):48–58.

Bell, G. R. (1952). Removal of oil from condensate by diatomite filtration, Proceedings of the Thirteenth Annual Water Conf., Eng. Soc. Western PA, Oct. 22.

Bell, G. R. (1956). Comparison studies of diatomite and sand filtration, *J. Am. Water Works*, *48*(9):1103–1124.

Bell, G. R. (1961). Use of coagulant coated filter aids, Presented at Calif. Section, Am. Water Works, Oct. 27.

Bell, G. R. (1962). Design criteria for diatomite filters, *J. AWWA*, *54*(10):1241–1256.

Bell, G. R. (1965a). Removal of manganese by controlled precipitation and filtration, *J. AWWA*, *57*(5):655.

Bell, G. R. (1965b). Removal of soluble iron by filtration, *J. AWWA*, *57*(4):458–471.

Bell, G. R., and F. B. Hutto. (1958). Analysis of rotary precoat filter operation—new concepts, *Chem. Eng. Prog.*, *54*(12):69.

Bell, G. R., and F. B. Hutto. (1959). *Chem. Eng. Prog.*, *55*(1):75.

Breese, R. O. Y. (1989). Diatomite, occurrence and evaluation, Presented at Society of Mining Eng. Annual Mtg., Las Vegas, NV, Feb. 27–Mar. 2.

Bryant, E. A., and C. Yapijakis. (1977). Ozonation-diatomite filtration removes color and turbidity, Parts 1 and 2, Water Sewage Works (Sept. and Oct.).

Cain, C. W. (1973). Filter aid filtration, interaction of filter aid pore size and turbidity particle size, Presented at AIChE meeting, Vancouver, BC.

Cain, C. W. (1984). Filter aid use in filtration, in *Encyclopedia of Chemical Processing*, Marcel Dekker, New York, p. 348.

Cain, C. W. (1990). Filter cake filtration, putting the principles to work, *Chem. Eng.*, August.

Coogan, G. J. (1962). Diatomite filtration for removal of iron and manganese, *J. AWWA*, *54*(12):1507.

Cook, L. N. (1984). Laboratory approach optimizes filter aid addition, *Chem. Eng.*, July 23, pp. 45–50.

Cummins, A. B. (1942). Clarifying efficiency of diatomaceous filter aids, *Ind. Eng. Chem.*, *34*(4):403–414.

Cummins, A. B., and L. E. Weymouth. (1942). Filtration of sugar solutions, *Ind. Eng. Chem.*, *34*(4):392–398.

Dahlstrom, D. A. (1975). The 100% effective surface area continuous precoat filter, Presented at ACHEMA Meeting, June.

de Rijke, J. M., J. P. J. van Tilburg, B. Scarlett, J. A. Wesselingh, and A. H. Krap, Problems with filter aid in filtration equipment, *Filtr. Separ.*

Dillingham, J. I. I., J. L. Cleasby, and E. R. Baumann. (1967). Diatomite filtration equations for various septa, *J. Sanit. Eng. Div.*$_1$ 93:SAI:41 ASCE.

Dlouhy, P. E., and D. A. Dahlstrom. (1968). Continuous filtration in pharmaceutical production. *Chem. Eng. Prog.*, *64*(4):116–119.

Ernst, M., R. M. Talcott, H. C. Romans, and G. R. S. Smith. (1991). Tackle solid-liquid problems, *Chem. Eng. Prog.*, July, pp. 22–28, Vol. 87.

Fiore, J. V., W. P. Olson, and S. L. Holst. (1980). Depth Filtration, in J. Curling, ed., *Methods of Plasma Protein Fractionation*. Academic Press, New York, pp. 239–267.

Gregor, E. C. (1996). New and emerging filtration media, Presented at Assoc. of Nonwoven Fabrics Industry Conf. and Expo., Dec. 2–4.

Hofflinger, W., and A. Hackle. (1990). Evaluation of optimal knife advances for precoat filtration on rotary vacuum filters, *Filt. Separ.*, March/April:110–113.

Hunter, J. V., G. R. Bell, and C. N. Henderson. (1966). Coliform organisms removal by diatomite filtration, *J. AWWA*, *58*(9):1160–1169.

Hutto, F. B., Jr. (1957). Distribution of porosity in filter cakes, *Chem. Eng. Prog.*, *53*:7.

Kemper, E. A. (1984). Evaluating Walton filter data, *MBAA Tech. Quart.*, *21*(1):27–32.

Lange, K. P., W. D. Bellamy, and D. W. Hendricks. (1984). *Filtration of Giardia Cysts and Other Substances*, Vol. 1, *Diatomaceous Earth Filtration*, USEPA/600/52-84/1 14.

Lawrence, C. H. (1964). Design aspects of Lompoc water treatment plant, *J. Sanit. Eng. Div. ASCE*, *90*(SA6):81–113; Proc. Paper 4181.

Letterman, R. D., and G. S. Logsdon. (1976). Survey of direct filtration practice preliminary report, Proc. AWWA Annu. Conf., New Orleans, LA.

Logsdon, G. S., et al. (1981). Alternative filtration methods for removal of giardia cysts and cyst models, *J. AWWA*, *73*(2):111.

Mayer, E., and J. G. Wood. (1991). A new methodology for testing filter aids, *Fluid/Particle Separ. J.*, *4*(4):33–36.

Mefford, M. H., R. Lowder, and J. K. Coors. (1983). D.E. Filtration optimization and large scale filter systems start-up, *MBAA Tech. Quart.*, *20*(3):109–113.

O'Connor, J. T., and B. E. Benson. (1970). Iron removal using magnesium oxide, *J. Sanit. Eng. Div. ASCE*, December.

Ogedengbe, O. (1984). Characterization and specification of local sands for filters, *Filtr. Separ.*, *21*(4):331–333.

Pittendreigh, L. M. (1966). Recent experiences with diatomite filters for iron removal on potable water, Presented at Johns Manville Water Filtration Seminar, Boston, MA, April 14.

Purchos, D. B. (1977), Ed. *Solid-Liquid Separation Equipment and Scale-Up*, Uplands Press, Ltd., Crayden, England.

Prediction of diatomite filter cake resistance, *J. Sanit. Eng. Div. ASCE*, *93*(SA1):57.

Ris, J. I., I. A. Cooper, and W. R. Goddard. (1984). Pilot testing and predesign of two water treatment processes for removal of *Giardia lamblia* in Palisade, Colorado, Proc. AWWA Annu. Conf., Dallas, TX.

Silverblatt, C. E., H. Risbud, and F. M. Tiller. (1974). Batch, continuous processes for cake filtration, *Chem. Eng.*, *81*:127.

Smith, G. R. S. (1964). Standard liquor filtration, Presented at February Meeting of Am. Soc. Sugar Beet Technologists, San Francisco.

Smith, G. R. S. (1965). Prefiltration of beer before membrane filtration, *Brewers Dig.*

Smith, G. R. S. (1965). Improve your filter-aid filtration, *Chem. Eng.*, October 11, pp. 187–190.

Smith, G. R. S. (1966). Filter aid filtration, *Filtr. Eng.*, *1*(1):6–8.

Smith, G. R. S. (1971). The place of the rotary vacuum precoat filter in the winery, Presented at Am. Soc. Enologists 22nd Annu. Meeting, June.

Smith, G. R. S. (1972). Filter aid recovery and disposal, Presented at Am. Soc. Enologists 23rd Annu. Meeting.

Smith, G. R. S. (1973). Recovery of filter aid from spent filter cakes using liquid cyclones, Sugar Ind. Technicians Proc.

Smith, G. R. S. (1975). Filter aid regeneration and recovery, *Chem. Eng. Prog.* *71*(12).

Smith, G. R. S. (1976a). Filter aids—an overview, Sugar Industry Technician Proceedings, May.

Smith, G. R. S. (1976b). How to use rotary vacuum precoat filters, *Chem. Eng.*, Feb. 16.

Smith, G. R. S. (1990). Filter aids, in Ladislav Svarovsky, ed., *Solid Liquid Separation*, 3rd ed. Butterworths, Stoneham, MA.

Smith, G. R. S. (1978). Filtration equipment development for coal liquids, Electric Power Res. Inst., Res. Project 459-1, Phase 2, Final Report, November.

Smith, G. R. S. and Phillip C. Martin. (1977). Pressure filtration of liquified coal presented at the Fourth Annual International Conference on Coal Gasification, Liquefaction, and Conversion to Electricity, University of Pittsburgh, Aug. 2–4.

Syrotynski, S., and D. Stone. Microscreening and diatomite filtration, *J. AWWA*, *67*(10):545.

Task Group Report, Diatomite filters for municipal use, *J. AWWA*, *57*(2):157–180, and references therein.

Tiller, F. M. (1974). Bench-scale design of SLS systems, *Chem. Eng.*, Apr. 29, p. 117.

Tiller, F. M., J. R. Crump, W. Chen, and Y. L. Shen. (1988). *Cycle Optimization Involving the Use of Filter Aids*, Univ. Houston, Houston, TX.

Ulrich, E. A. (1966). Precoating Pressure Leaf Filters, Bull. SM-0025, Buffalo Filters, Inc.

Walton, H. G. (1977). Laboratory and filter for diatomite filtration test, Presented at the 43rd Annu. Am. Soc. Brewing Chemists Meeting, St. Louis, MO.

Walton, H. G. (1978). Laboratory procedure and filter for diatomite filtration tests, *Filtr. Separ.*, *1*:9–14.

Walton, H. G. (1982). Diatomite filtration—optimizing the body feed, *Filtr. Separ.*, *3*:237–238.

Walton, H. G. (1985). Filter septa, *Manville Filtration Manual*, Section IX, Manville Filtration and Minerals Group.

2

Expanded Polytetrafluoroethylene Membranes and Their Applications

MICHAEL WIKOL, CHRIS BAILEY, KAREN LANGE, MICHAEL SUTSKO and KAREN TRONTO

W. L. Gore and Associates, Elkton, Maryland

1 INTRODUCTION

The unique properties of expanded polytetrafluoroethylene (ePTFE) membrane make it a good choice for a number of pharmaceutical applications. Currently, ePTFE constructions are used for sterile filtration of fermentation feed air, process gases, and tank venting. The unique properties of ePTFE are also being exploited in a number of new innovative products and technologies. Lyophilization stoppers and bags, ultralow penetration air filters, and powder collectors are just a few of the new areas of interest to the pharmaceutical industry.

The purpose of this chapter is to

1. Discuss some pertinent properties of PTFE
2. Explain how PTFE is made into a microporous membrane
3. Describe the unique characteristics of ePTFE membranes
4. Discuss the benefits of the foregoing characteristics in pharmaceutical applications
5. Introduce a selection of emerging technologies based on ePTFE membranes

2 PROPERTIES OF PTFE

Polytetrafluoroethylene or PTFE $(CF_2—CF_2)_n$, commonly referred to by the DuPont trademark Teflon or the ICI trademark Fluon, is well known for its chemical resistance, thermal stability, and hydrophobicity. PTFE has these desirable characteristics because of its unique chemical structure.

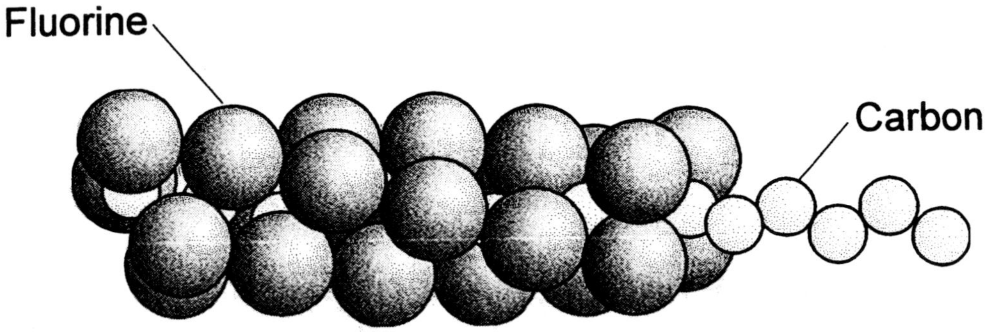

Figure 1 Chemical structure of PTFE molecule.

PTFE is a simple polymer because it is composed of only two elements: carbon and fluorine. PTFE has a long, straight carbon backbone to which the fluorine atoms are bonded (see Fig. 1). Both the C—C and C—F bonds are extremely strong. In addition, the electron cloud of the fluorine atoms forms a uniform helical sheath that protects the carbon backbone. The even distribution of fluorine atoms makes it nonpolar and nonreactive. The combination of strong bonds, protective sheath, and nonpolarity make PTFE extremely inert as well as thermally stable. This explains why PTFE is compatible with nearly all the processing and cleaning fluids that are typically used in the pharmaceutical industry including acids, bases, and solvents.

Because of the nonreactivity and nonpolarity of PTFE, it is difficult for anything to even bond to it. This is why PTFE (Teflon) is well-known as a nonsticking and easy-to-clean product.

Since fluorine is the most electronegative element in the periodic table, it does not want to share electrons with neighboring fluorine atoms. This results in a low surface free energy for PTFE. The lower the surface free energy of a material, the less likely it is to be wetted with higher surface energy fluids such as water. Table 1 summarizes some of the physical properties of PTFE.

In contrast, other polymeric membrane materials have some or all of the fluorine atoms replaced with hydrogen or other elements. This results in weaker bonds and a more polar and reactive molecule. The substitution also increases the surface free energy. Therefore, these polymers are less hydrophobic, less thermally stable, and more reactive than PTFE.

Figure 2 is a chemical compatibility and temperature map, which is a visual way to compare the chemical and thermal stability of various polymers.

Table 1 Physical Properties of PTFE

Structure	$—(CF_2CF_2)—_n$
Surface free energy	18.5 dyn/cm
Melt temperature	327°C
Continuous service temperature	288°C

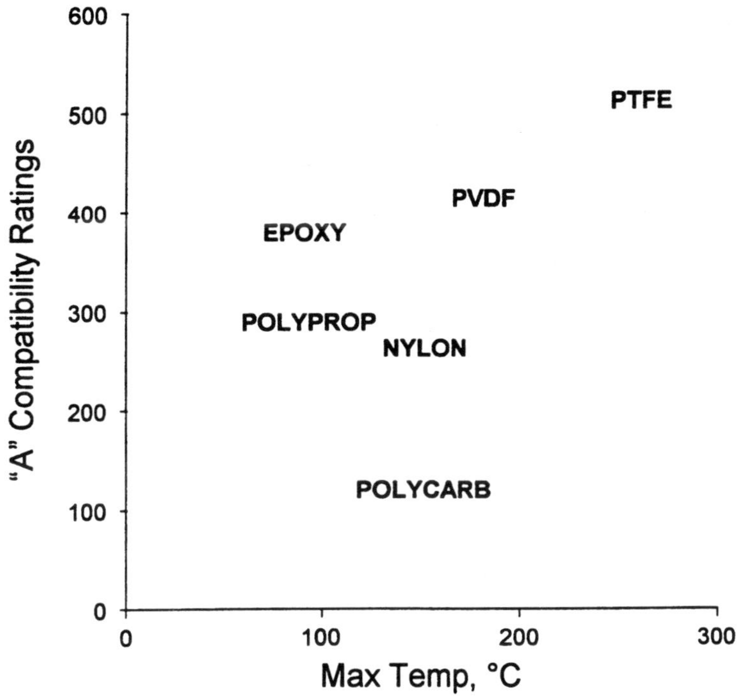

Figure 2 Chemical compatibility and temperature map.

3 MICROPOROUS PTFE

Since PTFE is chemically inert, thermally stable, and extremely hydrophobic, it is an ideal polymer for some applications in the pharmaceutical industry. As a microporous membrane, PTFE is a valuable air filter medium with high flow rates and filtration efficiency.

A schematic of how expanded PTFE membrane is made is shown in Fig. 3. In general, the process begins with pure PTFE fine powder resin. A lubricating agent is added so the powder forms a paste and can then be extruded in sheet form. This sheet is heated and expanded under the proper conditions to make a microporous sheet. The structure is stabilized in an amorphous locking step. Since the lubricating agent is extremely volatile, it is completely removed from the porous structure during processing. The resulting product is 100% PTFE. (It is interesting to note that expanding PTFE at extremely high rates actually increases the tensile strength of the polymer. This is unusual because most polymers fracture when subjected to a high rate of strain.)

Another method used to manufacture porous PTFE is by a replication process in which PTFE particles are mixed with burnable material such as paper fibers, then heated to remove the fibers. PTFE can also be made porous by the removal of a fugitive material such as a carbonate. Because these methods yield products that have lower flow rates and more contamination, they are of little commercial value

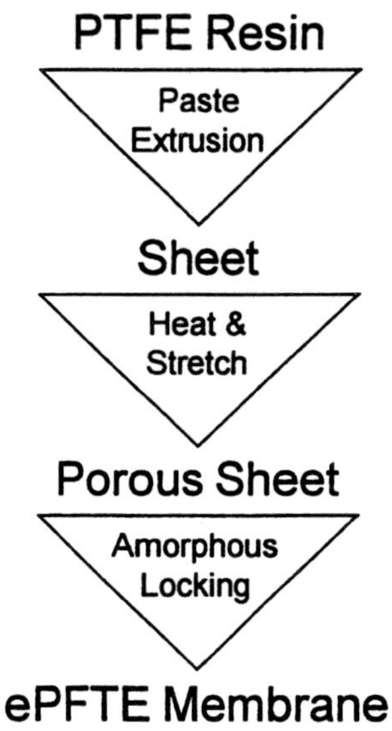

Figure 3 Expanded PTFE membrane process as described in a patent issued to R. W. Gore (Gore, 1980).

to the pharmaceutical industry. The balance of the discussion focuses on microporous expanded PTFE membranes.

Scanning electron micrographs (SEM) of an ePTFE structure that is commonly used in pharmaceutical microfiltration are shown in Fig. 4. The microstructure is characterized by nodes that are interconnected by fibrils. As you can see, this is a single, continuous structure where all the fibrils and nodes connect. There are no loose ends or particles to be shed or to contaminate a fluid stream. Even though there is a high density of thin fibrils, this structure is high flowing because it also has a high void volume (~85% porous).

As you can see from Table 2, ePTFE can have a broad range of physical properties including pore sizes, flow rates, and water breakthrough pressures. Membranes can be engineered and optimized to meet the needs of particular applications.

Because ePTFE membranes are extremely microporous and extremely hydrophobic, they will retain water droplets while allowing water vapor to readily pass through as illustrated in Fig. 5. Moisture vapor can flow through an ePTFE membrane by either bulk gas flow or diffusion. If there is a pressure differential across the membrane, gas will flow from the high pressure side to the low pressure side. Moisture vapor can also diffuse through the microporous structure if there is a humidity or temperature differential across the membrane.

ePTFE membranes are sometimes laminated to materials for additional structural reinforcement. They can be laminated to felts, wovens, and nonwovens made from a variety of materials including polypropylene, polyester, and PTFE. These support layers sometimes also function as a drainage layer in filters. Support materials should be selected according to the chemical, thermal, and mechanical requirements of the application.

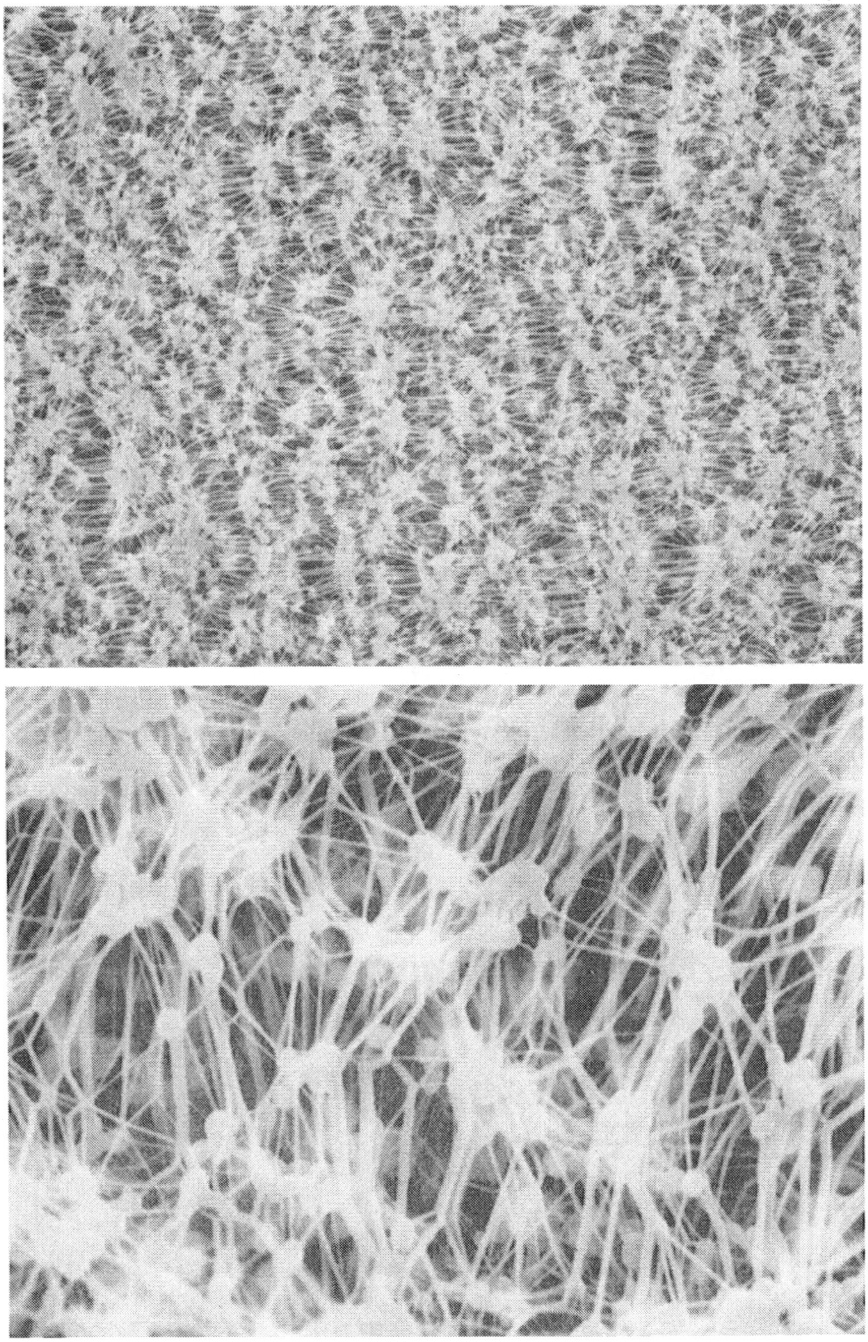

(a)

(b)

Figure 4 Scanning electron micrographs of expanded PTFE membrane. (a) 2000×; (b) 10,000×.

Table 2 Properties of ePTFE Membranes

Property	Range
Porosity	1–99%
Airflow	2.0–15,000 mL/cm[2a]
Methanol flow rate	1.0–10,000 mL/cm[2b]
Water entry pressure	0–350 psi
Isopropanol bubble point	0.1 to >50 psi
Pore size	0.02–40 μm[c]

[a]Airflow rate measured at 4.88 in. H_2O at 21°C.
[b]Methanol flow rate measured at 27.5 in. Hg at 21°C.
[c]Pore size as correlated to IPA bubble point.

4 "PORE SIZE" MEASUREMENT

As discussed elsewhere in this volume, pore size is a relative term, often depending on the application and the test method used to measure it. A common method for quantitatively determining the pore size of membranes including PTFE is the bubble point method. In this test, a membrane is wet out with an appropriate test fluid such as isopropyl alcohol and gas pressure is applied to one side of the membrane. The pressure at which the first steady stream of bubbles (or first measurable bulk gas flow) appears is said to be the bubble point. The inverse pressure–pore size relationship is given by the equation

$$D = \frac{C\delta}{P}$$

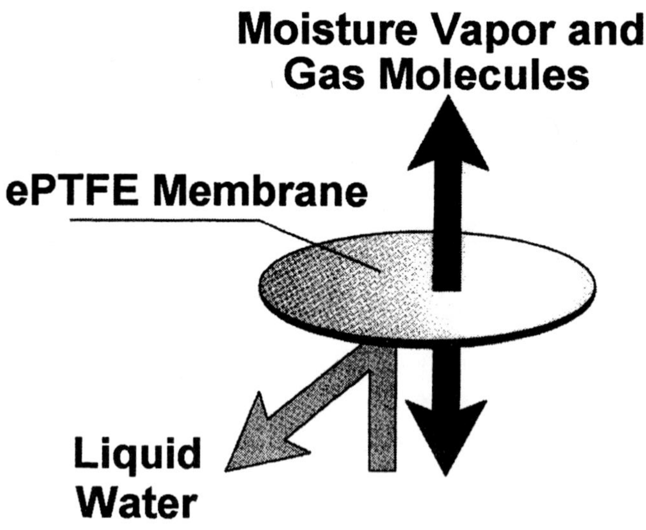

Figure 5 Illustration of how ePTFE membranes retain liquid water while allowing water vapor and other gases to be transmitted.

where

D = pore diameter
C = constant
δ = surface tension of wetting fluid
P = test pressure

For any pore structure other than a cylinder, modifying factors must be added to the equation. Since most membranes including ePTFE do not have a cylindrical pore structure, what is actually measured is a complex interaction of the wetting fluid, membrane, and test gas. Therefore, while the general inverse relationship holds that higher bubble point pressures indicate tighter membrane structures (smaller pore sizes), an actual pore diameter cannot be precisely determined from a bubble point measurement.

Water breakthrough or penetration pressure testing of hydrophobic membranes like ePTFE can also give a relative measure of the structure of a membrane.

Water breakthrough pressure is the minimum pressure required to force water through the largest pore of a dry hydrophobic membrane. Every hydrophobic membrane has a unique water breakthrough pressure that depends on the membrane's surface free energy, pore size, and shape. The inverse relationship between pressure and pore size also holds with this test in that tighter structures require higher pressures to force water through the membrane.

Filtration efficiency testing in both air and liquids can provide information about the pore structure of a membrane. In aerosol filtration, it can be difficult to determine the actual pore size of a membrane because adsorptive effects will allow the filter to capture particles that would otherwise pass easily through the structure. These tests can, however, be used as a comparative measure to determine the relative effectiveness of different filters in a given application.

5 AIR FILTRATION THEORY

5.1 Modes of Air Filtration

Air filtration occurs in two ways, surface filtration and depth filtration. Simply put, surface filtration occurs when particles are too large to fit into the pores of a filter and are trapped on the surface of the filter medium. Depth filtration occurs when particles are small enough to fit into the pores but are trapped during their journey through the depth of the filter medium. Therefore, the interaction between the particle size distribution and the pore size distribution determines whether surface or depth filtration occurs.

5.2 The Surface Filtration Mode

Air filters sometimes work by excluding large particles from the smaller pores in the filter, in the fashion of a sieve. This mechanism of particle capture is called sieving. In fact, most people are surprised to learn that this is not how air filters always work. In air filtration, this surface filtration mode is actually the less common of the two modes. It is only in this relatively uncommon mode of filtration that pore diameter is important. Particles that are larger than the pore diameter will not enter into the depth of the filter.

In one sense, there is no element of chance involved in surface filtration. If a particle is bigger than the pores, it is collected. But in another sense chance is still involved, because the pore sizes are not all equal but rather have some statistical distribution. If there is a tiny population of large pores, then some of the large particles will happen to be carried through those pores. If a particle enters the depth of a filter because it is not surface-filtered, depth filtration remains available to help capture it.

Expanded polytetrafluoroethylene is a highly porous material. Scanning electron micrographs (for example, those in Fig. 4) make it obvious that it resembles more a tangled forest than a neatly perforated plate; the fibers are well-defined units, but exactly how to define a unique pore between many of them at varying depths is hard to say. This is true of almost all porous materials.

The true pore size distribution of an air filter does not by itself determine the capture efficiency versus particle size curve, because most particles that can fit through the pores will still be captured by other mechanisms to be discussed later. Moreover, practical pore size measurement methods can only indirectly and imperfectly infer pore sizes. For example, many methods begin by assuming that the pores are cylindrical, but microscopy shows that this is far from true. Thus, it often happens that particles much smaller than the measured pore size of a filter are mostly surface-filtered. On the other hand, a pore size may be claimed for a filter on the basis that what is really meant is the size of the smallest particle that will be captured, which may vary tremendously depending on the details of how this is measured (for example, air velocity). Air filtration efficiency for an ePTFE membrane having a nominal pore size of 5.0 μm may be better than 99.99% at 0.1 μm. For these reasons, pore size can be a confusing specification for an air filter, and it is often more useful to specify to retention efficiency for the particle size and conditions of interest.

5.3 The Depth Filtration Mode

In depth filtration, particles small enough to enter the filter structure will be collected by chance interactions with the fibers of the filter. If the structure of the filter is the same at all depths, as it is in most filters, there is an exponential decay in the particle population as the air passes through the depth of the filter. This is consistent with a constant probability of collection within the next increment of depth for a particle that has survived the trip so far.

Depth filtration is sometimes wrongly considered the opposite of "absolute filtration." It is easy to demonstrate that the penetration through some depth filters must be 10^{-20} or 10^{-50} or less. A penetration of 10^{-20} cannot be measured, and a penetration of 10^{-50} has no physical significance at all (being about one atom's worth of the earth's mass). Thus such a depth filter at this efficiency level can be considered absolute.

Depth filtration works by several particle capture mechanisms, unlike surface filtration, which works only by sieving. These mechanisms are discussed in more detail elsewhere in this book and are thoroughly discussed in Hinds (1982). Briefly, all depth filtration mechanisms rely on van der Waals forces, electrostatic adhesion, or both to hold particles to filter fibers once the particles contact the fibers, but mechanisms differ in why particle–fiber contact occurs. In the "impaction" mechanism, large fast-moving particles hit fibers because their momentum overpowers the airflow deviating around the fibers. In the ''interception'' mechanism, relatively incompressible particles barely touch the fibers while airflow streamlines near them compress together around the particles to slip by the fibers. In the ''diffusion'' mechanism, small particles move more vigorously during collisions with individual air molecules, increasing the random contacts with fibers. Impaction and interception work better on larger particles, whereas diffusion favors the collection of small particles, so that extremely large or small particles are collected easily whereas an intermediate ''most penetrating'' size of particle is the most difficult to collect. Filters made of finer fibers have a smaller most penetrating particle size than filters made of coarser fibers.

The fibrils in ePTFE membranes designed for filtration are smaller in diameter than those in any other commonly used filtration medium. Many fibrils in ePTFE are as small as 0.01 or 0.02 μm, with a count median diameter on the order of 0.05 or 0.1 μm. In comparison, most fibers in microfiber glass paper are on the order of 1 μm, and fibers in filtration textiles on the order of 10 μm or more (other membranes may have ''fibers'' for which the diameter is hard to define, though numbers around 0.1–1 μm are plausible). From the viewpoint of the air filtration theorist, ePTFE is a nearly ideal random mesh of fine fibers distributed approximately perpendicularly to the airflow, with a high void fraction. The most penetrating particle size is around 0.07 μm, depending on air velocity. This makes ePTFE filters relatively efficient on the basis of total penetrating particle mass, as a 0.07 μm particle contains nearly 80 times less material than the 0.300 μm particle that is most penetrating for many typical filters such as HEPA filters (volume of a sphere varies as diameter cubed). Moreover, very fine fibers offer little resistance to passing air, and so good capture efficiency for ePTFE comes at little expense in air pressure drop.

5.4 Pressure Increase and Cleaning in the Two Modes

The most dramatic practical significance of surface versus depth filtration is that in surface filtration the particles accumulate in a thin dense layer right at the surface of the filter, whereas in depth filtration they accumulate gradually throughout some depth. The advantage of depositing the particles right on the surface is that they can more easily be removed and the filter can thus be cleaned and recover its initial airflow. The advantage of depositing the particles throughout the depth is that the particles are distributed throughout a diffuse and discontinuous region, which still has a large fraction of open space, and so airflow is more easily maintained without removing the particles than when there is a dense and impermeable particle layer right at the surface.

It is useful to consider three different cases in discussing the loading of a filter. In the lightest particulate loadings, such as those experienced by high purity point-of-use filters or recirculation filters sealed inside computer disk drives, the effect of particle loading is unimportant because there hardly is any. In this case, it is unimportant whether surface or depth filtration dominates, and filters are chosen on another basis.

At the opposite extreme, where particle loading is very heavy and rapid it is necessary to clean the filter many times, perhaps thousands of times or even more, during its lifetime. An example would be baghouse or cartridge collectors in an industrial process. In this case, surface filtration is very advantageous, making the thorough removal of particles easy for each cleaning ''cycle.'' ePTFE membrane filters are very useful in these applications because of their cleanability. An additional benefit of ePTFE is the minimal adhesion that exists specifically between polytetrafluoroethylene and particulate dirt (the same benefit that favors Teflon frying pans).

In the third case, intermediate between these two extremes, the particulate loading is low enough to make cleaning unnecessary but high enough to limit usable lifetime. In this case, surface filtration can be disadvantageous, especially if the particulate is oily and tends to wick into a continuous sheet. Membrane filters (including ePTFE membranes), if they are acting as surface filters, in this case require a prefiltering layer to perform depth filtration, especially for the larger particles that constitute the great majority of particulate mass. Such a prefilter layer with an efficiency of only 95% for all combined mass will extend the life of the membrane by around 20-fold, making this strategy a successful one. Interestingly, the classical DOP smoke efficiency test can fall into this class for ePTFE membranes if excessively high loadings are used, though, for example, the loadings used in the TSI Model AFT8160 filter tester do not cause a problem.

5.5 "Dust Cake" and Improved Efficiency During Cleaning

Filters used for extremely high particulate loadings must be cleaned repeatedly. Yet some such filters rely on particles bridging over openings in the filter to help capture other particles. During cleaning, these particle bridges are disrupted, and particle retention efficiency is reduced. Thus, it is common for a baghouse collector to exhibit a ''puff on pulse.'' Relative to most filters of this type, ePTFE filters have excellent retention efficiencies even during the cleaning cycle. The ePTFE membrane on the surface filter serves ''as a permanent dust cake,'' meaning that it replaces the particle bridges. However, this ''permanent dust cake'' is not an accumulation of permanently adhered dirt.

5.6 Summary of Air Filtration Theory

In comparison with most other air filtration media, ePTFE membranes are unusual in several ways.

1. Their high density of extremely fine fibrils provides better depth filtration efficiency.
2. High porosity and fine fibrils offer little resistance to airflow.
3. Small and consistent pores often provide surface filtration.
4. Cleaning of surface-filtered particles is very easy.
5. Filter efficiency is still high during and immediately after cleaning.
6. They have high air filtration efficiencies combined with low pressure drop.

6 STERILIZATION

Materials used in pharmaceutical manufacturing can be sterilized by numerous methods, including the use of dry heat, steam, ethylene oxide gas (ETO), or ionizing radiation. Because of PTFE's thermal stability, ePTFE can be repeatedly thermally sterilized under typical autoclave, steam in place, and dry heat oven conditions. Also, because PTFE is chemically inert, it is unaffected by ETO sterilization or cleaning solutions.

Steam and cleaning solutions could wet out the pores of a hydrophilic or less hydrophobic polymer. The liquid in the membrane pores can block gas flow as well as create an environment in which microorganisms can grow. Since PTFE is extremely hydrophobic, using ePTFE minimizes these risks.

Although microporous PTFE exhibits extraordinary resistance to chemical attack from a wide range of chemical species, it has only limited resistance to ionizing radiation. Ionizing radiation causes chain scission of the carbon bonds in the backbone of the helical PTFE molecule. This results in not only a reduction in molecular weight but also a reduction in the ultimate tensile strength and ultimate elongation. This decrease in physical properties is observed at relatively low levels of radiation; significant decreases are observed at less than 0.5 Mrad. Because of the decrease in physical properties, ionizing radiation is not a preferred method of sterilizing PTFE.

In some applications, it still may be desirable to sterilize components containing microporous PTFE with radiation. Properly designed and supported microporous laminates have been radiation sterilized and successfully used as hydrophobic vents and sterile barriers as transducer protectors, intravenous spike vents, and other medical components for a number of years. In these products, the support material(s) provide the proper dependable support to the PTFE to overcome the degradation of physical properties. The microstructure, physical dimensions, and performance of the laminate are not changed after radiation sterilization. Physical conditions that could cause a microporous PTFE membrane to fail after radiation sterilization include (1) excessive elongation, (2) puncture on sharp protrusions, and (3) concentration of stresses in limited areas. For example, since pleat peaks and valleys are areas of concentrated stresses, radiation sterilization is not recommended for pleated devices.

7 APPLICATIONS OF ePTFE MEMBRANES

7.1 Fermentation Feed Air and Exhaust Gas Filtration

Large volumes of sterile air and gases are required as a raw material in aerobic fermentation reactions. These gases require filtering for the removal of organisms and particulates. These exhaust gases are also filtered to prevent contamination from the fermentor into the environment as well as from the environment into the fermentor. During their service life (typically more than 1 year), these filters must undergo repeated steam sterilizations without binding or losing their integrity. Filter failure can be extremely costly in terms of product yield, product quality, maintenance, and downtime.

Historically, packed towers were used for these types of filtration. While they are better than no filtration, they have several disadvantages, including the fact that they are relatively inefficient, expensive to install and operate, wasteful of space, hydrophilic, and impossible to integrity test. Cartridges made of glass fiber and borosilicate glass fibers are more efficient than randomly packed towers, and they also save space. Significant improvements in filtration efficiency, pressure drop, hydrophobicity, and integrity testability are being realized by users of membrane filters containing ePTFE.

Because ePTFE membranes have a narrow pore size distribution, they are more efficient at retaining particles and organisms than nonwoven depth filtration media. Since PTFE is extremely hydrophobic, (1) it will remain hydrophobic through repeated sterilizations, (2) it will resume its presteam pressure drop with a minimal poststeaming blowdown, and (3) it is not susceptible to grow-through.

In addition to the benefits of improved reliability and efficiency, there are often significant economic benefits to using ePTFE membrane filters. The lower pressure drop of ePTFE filters results in significant energy savings in compressor operation. Capital and replacement costs can be further reduced because less filter may be required to obtain a desired flow rate and the filter will function through longer change-out cycles. Since ePTFE is extremely hydrophobic the time it takes to blow the filter dry is eliminated as well as the installation and capital cost of heat tracing filter housings. Studies have shown that contamination rates are 50% lower in fermentors with hydrophobic cartridge filters than in a control group of fermentors with packed towers. The contamination, energy, maintenance, and productivity cost savings realized by using ePTFE filters can be calculated to determine the total annual cost savings. The payback period for converting to hydrophobic filters is often less than 1 year.

7.2 Tank Vents

Tanks must be vented to allow gas to exit during filling and to enter during emptying. If a tank is not vented or a vent becomes blocked, the tank could either explode or implode. Even if the filter is only partially blocked, productivity could be reduced owing to slower tank drainage time. Therefore, a vent filter must allow for adequate flow of gas for pressure equalization while at the same time keeping the content of the tank free of contaminants.

Once again, filters made of ePTFE are ideal for this type of application. The filters allow for a high flow rate at a low pressure drop. These filters can be regularly tested to verify their integrity and their installation. Since they are hydrophobic, ePTFE filters will not "blind" from repeated steam sterilization or incidental aqueous solution contact.

7.3 Lyophilization

Many pharmaceutical products such as vaccines and anti-infectives are unstable in aqueous solution over time. Their shelf life could be enhanced by drying, but many of these substances are also unstable when exposed to heat. Lyophilization, or freeze-drying, allows these pharmaceutical products to be preserved with minimum degradation. During lyophilization, the product is frozen to −40 to −60°C. A very strong vacuum is then pulled, causing the moisture to be removed by sublimation. Lyophilization is a valuable pharmaceutical process because it allows long-term storage at room temperature for many otherwise unstable products.

Single-dose pharmaceutical products are typically freeze-dried in glass vials. The conventional method for freeze-drying in vials uses a split-bottom stopper. Drying is induced by leaving the split stopper in the "up" or open position throughout the cycle so that air and moisture vapor can escape through the physical openings in the stopper (see Fig. 6). Throughout this process the vial contents are exposed to

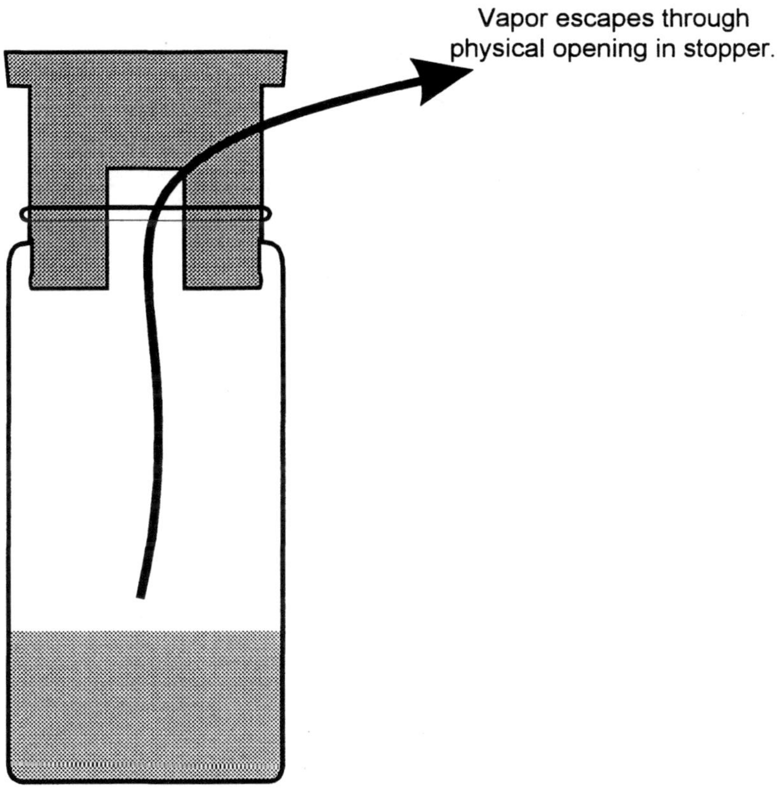

Figure 6 Configuration of conventional freeze-dry stopper.

the environment. This use of an open package to allow drying has several inherent risks:

1. Contamination of the product by the lyophilizer or surroundings
2. Cross contamination between containers in the lyophilizer
3. Product loss and difficult cleanup due to entrained powder
4. Worker exposure to toxic compounds being lyophilized

The unique microporous structure of the ePTFE membrane vent allows water vapor to escape from the package during lyophilization (see Fig. 7). The ePTFE membrane allows both bulk flow and diffusion of moisture vapor through it, ensuring that the sublimate has an exit path from the package throughout the freeze-dry cycle. At the same time, the filtration efficiency of the ePTFE vent not only contains the dried product within the package but also prevents the entrance of foreign particles into the package. Also, since ePTFE is extremely hydrophobic, it retains aqueous solutions during loading and drying.

The membrane is an effective sterile barrier that protects the product from bacteria, viruses, and other contaminants, allowing processors greater freedom in facility design. Since the product is in a closed, integral package after liquid filling, it can be transported between sterile areas or into nonsterile areas without risk of contamination. The thermal resistance of ePTFE allows it to withstand both freeze-

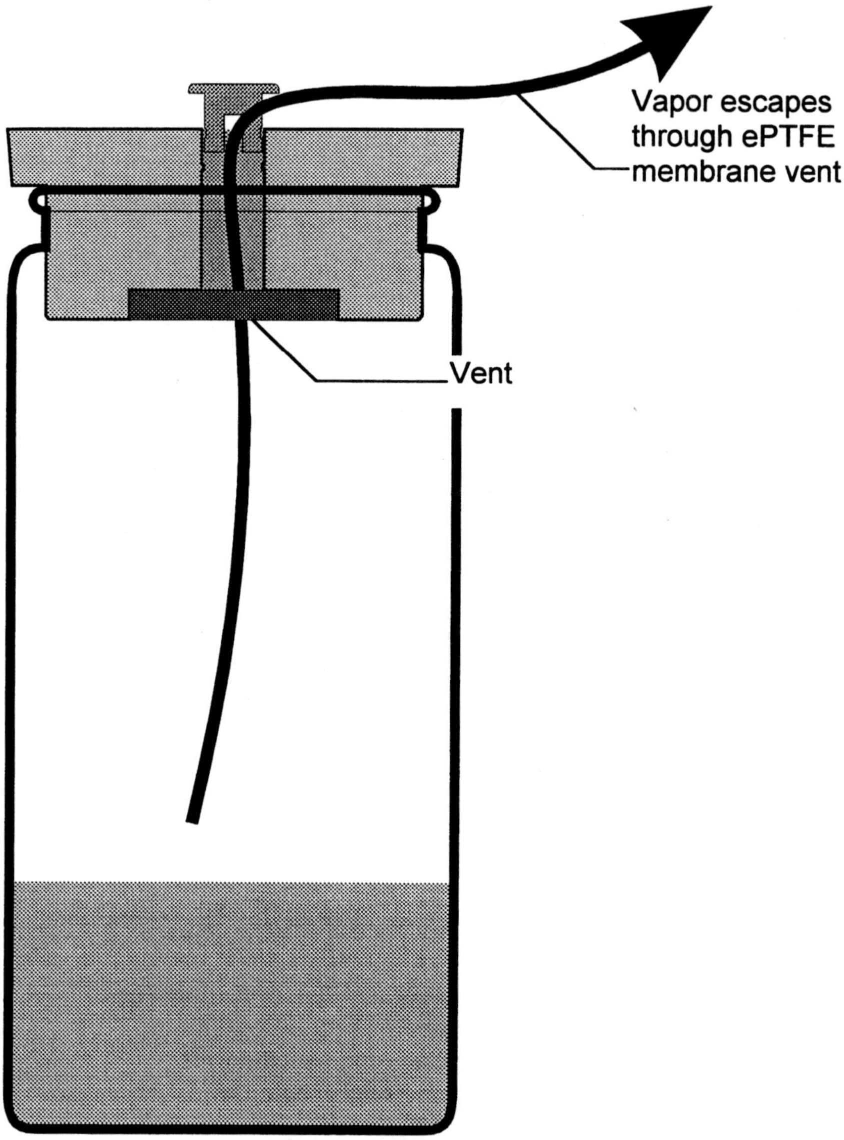

Figure 7 Configuration of freeze-dry stopper with ePTFE membrane vent.

drying and autoclave conditions. Likewise, ePTFE is chemically inert so it is not likely to react with the product throughout the packaged life of the product.

Barbaree and Sanchez (1982) investigated cross contamination rates from vial to vial in a freeze-dry run. Vials were filled with either of two bacteria, and the number of times these bacteria traveled from one vial to another during a standard freeze-dry run was counted. The study, using conventional split stoppers in glass vials, found cross contamination rates to be as high as 80% of vials per run. The Barbaree study was repeated and expanded upon by Lange et al. (1997). This study found cross contamination rates for conventionally stoppered vials to be as high as 91% of vials per run. The latter study also used two indicator organisms to track the path of cross contamination; however, it added a new component to the investigation. It compared the incidence of bacterial escape and cross contamination rates for conventional split stoppers to that for fully seated stoppers with an ePTFE vent.

The Lange et al. study found that in all cases the indicator organism that contaminated conventionally stoppered vials came from other conventionally stoppered vials. On the other hand, no bacteria were ever found to have either escaped from or entered the vials with the fully seated ePTFE vented stoppers. In each run, the incidence of cross contamination by indicator organisms in the vials with ePTFE vented stoppers was 0%. These results indicate that the ePTFE vented stoppers are an effective barrier to product contamination.

Such sterile barrier packages for freeze-drying can be designed in stopper form for single-dose applications or in bag form for bulk applications. Packages vented with ePTFE membranes or laminates are currently in use both in tissue banking and in the biotechnology industry. Bone grafts, which are often freeze-dried in large glass vials, use a rubber stopper fitted with an ePTFE vent. This bacteria-retentive vent allows the stoppers to be fully seated in the vial during the entire drying process. Freeze-drying of bulk products in both the tissue banking and biotechnology industries often uses flexible bags equipped with an ePTFE vent. The application of vented freeze-dry packaging takes advantage of several unique properties of ePTFE, including sterile barrier performance, temperature resistance, and permeability to moisture vapor. These same principles can simplify manufacturing for both single-dose and bulk pharmaceutical products.

7.4 Powder Collection and Containment

Many pharmaceutical products, whether they are antibiotics, buffers, antacids, vitamins, or other specialty products, at some point in time are in a powder form. In this section, we address filtration relative to the handling of these bulk powders. Typically, these powder forms are downstream in the purification stages or packaging operations. Separation of the powder from the gas stream requires filtration, which must satisfy two requirements:

1. It must prevent loss of product.
2. It must prevent exposure of product to the operators and to the environment.

Such areas requiring air filtration in the processing of pharmaceutical bulk powders are spray drying, fluid bed drying and granulating, tablet coating, milling and grinding, mechanical and pneumatic conveying, silos and bin vents, blending, packaging, and collection of nuisance dust (or local ventilation). The filtration units may actually be contained in the processing equipment or may be downstream from the processing equipment in the form of a dust collector. The filter elements used in these applications are typically filter bags or pleated filter cartridges (see Fig. 8).

Since ePTFE membranes are chemically inert, highly efficient, nonshedding, hydrophobic, and nonsticking, they are an ideal match for many of these applications. By laminating the ePTFE membrane to a backing textile substrate designed to give support and strength, a composite with synergistic properties is created. This backing

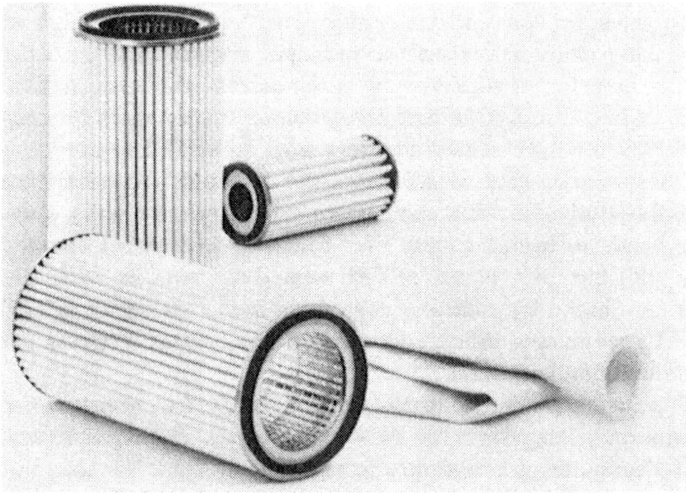

Figure 8 Examples of filter bags and filter cartridges used for powder collection and containment.

can be either woven or nonwoven and is chosen to suit the chemical and thermal conditions of the application.

In a dust collector, the "dirty" air is passed through a filter that retains particles and lets clean gas pass through. When the buildup on the filters becomes such that the flow through the system is restricted, the filters then go through a "cleaning cycle" during which the filters are pulsed with compressed air or mechanically shaken to release the dust, which then typically falls into a hopper where the solids are collected (see Fig. 9).

Conventional media for such applications typically consist of a felt or woven fabric such as polyester felt, Nomex felt, or woven nylon and rely on the presence of a primary dust layer or pre-coat to operate efficiently. Media composed of ePTFE membranes are considered to be the most efficient cleanable media in the fabric filtration industry. Collection efficiencies may exceed 99.97% at 0.3 μm right from the moment the system is started up. The fact that all the product being filtered is captured on the smooth membrane decreases product holdup and thus minimizes the potential for product degradation and carryover. It is often a concern with conventional fabric filters that fibers from the felts and fabrics will contaminate the product. Since product is collected on the membrane side of ePTFE membrane media, fibers from the support textile are prevented from contaminating the product. With the increase in demand these days for processing units with product containment systems (i.e., systems in which the filters are in the housing of the processing equipment, as opposed to a separate dust collector), there is an even greater need for an efficient nonlinting, FDA-acceptable material to be used as filters in these units. (Note: The PTFE used to produce Gore-Tex membrane filter medium complies with 21 CFR 177.1550 for perfluorocarbon resins that come in contact with foods.)

In addition to preventing fibers from contaminating the product, the ePTFE membrane has "nonstick" characteristics that allow the dust cake to release quite easily, with less frequent backpulsing (see Fig. 10). Since particulate matter is not

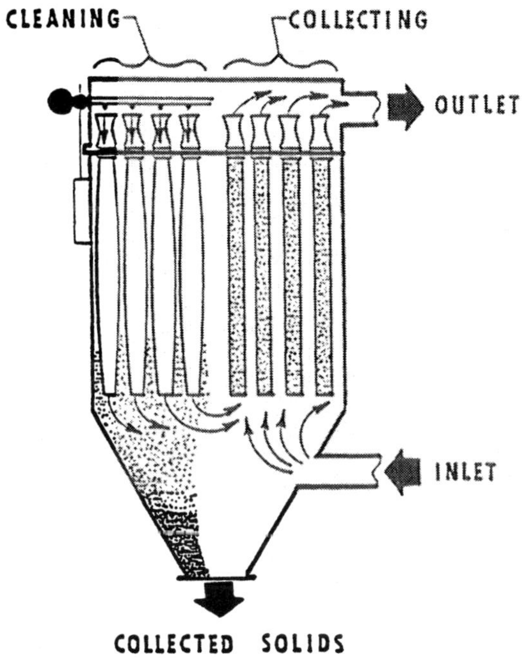

Figure 9 Schematic of powder collector.

held up within the medium, as with conventional media, valuable product is not lost when the filter must be cleaned or discarded. Rather, the powder can be recovered as useful product.

Table 3 shows the increase in yields obtained in a spray drying process handling aluminum-based powders when the filter medium in the dust collector following the dryer was changed from conventional Nomex felt to ePTFE membrane–laminated Nomex felt medium (see Fig. 11). In addition to the increase in yields, maintenance time during product changeover was reduced from 8 to 2 hours and cross contamination between products was minimized.

Since less frequent pulsing is required to release the dust cake, the differential pressure across the medium is kept to a minimum, allowing for higher airflows and greater production rates. The decrease in pulse frequency also helps extend the life of the filter. In air filtration, there is a compromise to be reached between differential pressure and filter life. The more frequent the pulsing, the greater the airflow. However, the violent motion of the pulse cycle on the filter eventually wears the fibers of the filter and decreases the strength and therefore the life of the medium. Therefore, when an ePTFE laminate filter is used, less frequent pulsing should extend the life of the filter.

Laminates composed of ePTFE membrane offer similar benefits in the pleated cartridge construction. Cartridges have more recently gained in popularity because of the ability to put more of the filter medium in a given space, which ultimately reduces capital costs. This in effect decreases the amount of time required for changeouts and thus decreases downtime. A typical medium for conventional filter cartridges is cellulose paper. The disadvantage of cellulose media is that cellulose has

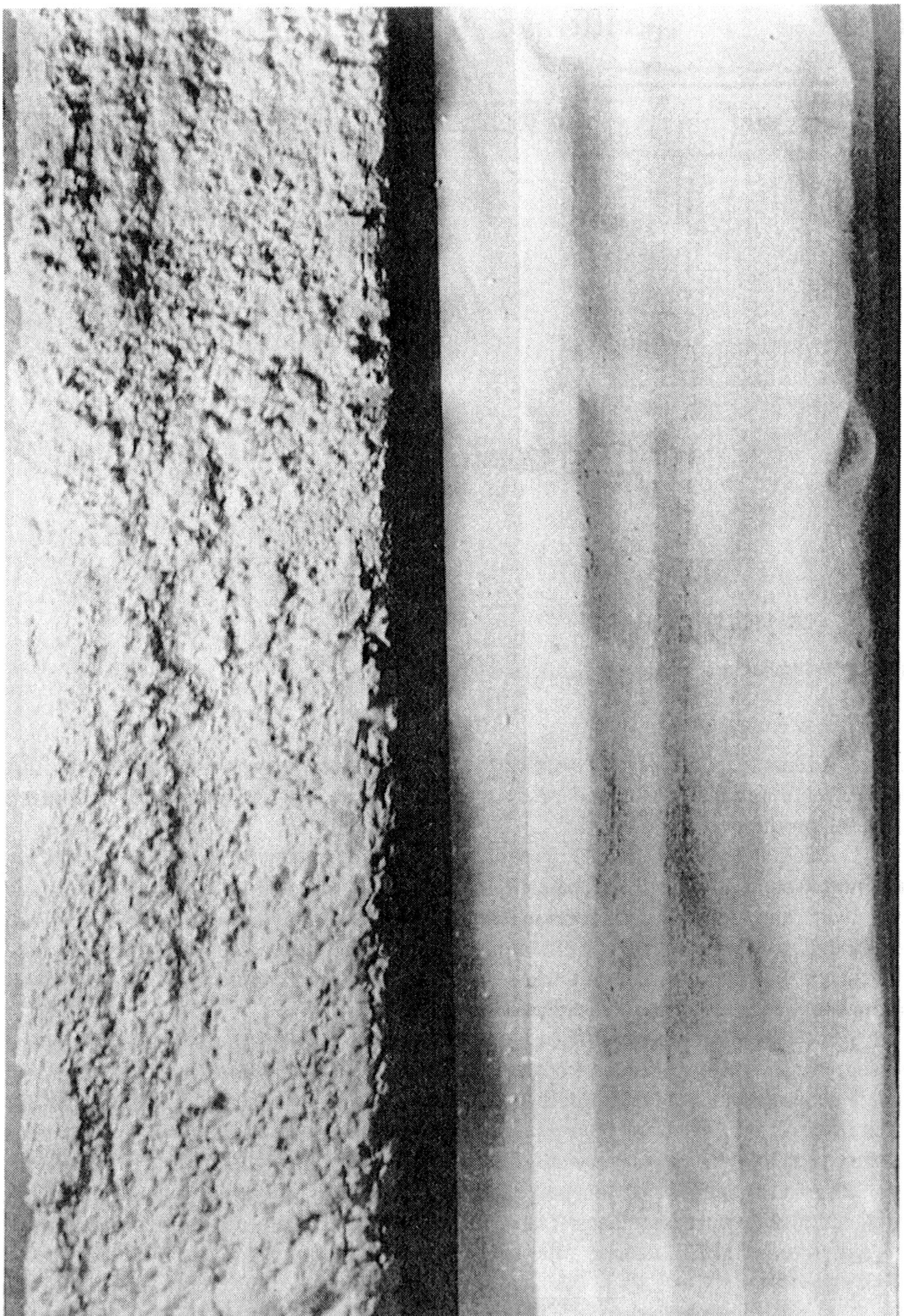

Figure 10 Illustration of the nonstick properties of ePTFE membrane. The powder cake sticks to the conventional filtration medium on the left. The powder does not stick to the ePTFE filtration medium on the right.

Table 3 Increase in Yield Obtained by Using ePTFE Membrane Laminated Nomex Felt Medium Instead of Conventional Nomex Felt

Product	Increase in yield
A	10.1%
B	8.0%
C	6.7%
D	15.2%

poor resistance to moisture and poor cake release on sticky dusts and is inefficient on very fine particulate unless precoated. Also, cellulose media often plug quickly (see Fig. 12). These filter cartridges are often limited to 180°F operating temperature.

Since PTFE is inherently hydrophobic, filters constructed with laminates consisting of an ePTFE membrane recover well from moisture upsets. After the moist cake is allowed to dry, the backpulsing should release the dust cake and continue to operate as it did prior to the moisture upset. This hydrophobic nature also allows these filters to be rinsed off with water for cleaning. As discussed previously, since PTFE is extremely inert and thermally stable, ePTFE is well suited for the processing and cleaning fluids that are typically used on the pharmaceutical industry, including acids, bases, and solvents. This ease of cleaning also decreases the potential for product cross contamination.

It is common to wash fabric filter bags to prevent contamination between product runs. Since the membranes used in ePTFE membrane filter bags are relatively thin, it is suggested that they not be laundered. Laundering may compromise the integrity of the membrane, thus decreasing the efficiency of the filter and potentially exposing fibers. Preferred ways to clean filters made of ePTFE laminates are to soak them in a bath or hose them down. Often, the good release characteristics of the ePTFE membrane enable its continued use without the need for laundering. Alternatively, it can be washed in place, thereby reducing the labor required to remove and launder it. The filters should always be thoroughly dried prior to baghouse startup.

An additional limitation of ePTFE laminates for dust collectors is that liquid hydrocarbons or oils may blind or plug the membrane, causing the air permeability to decrease.

Due to the unique properties of the ePTFE membrane, laminates made of it have gained wide acceptance not only in the pharmaceutical industry but also in the food, chemical processing, metals, boilers, incinerators, and minerals industries.

7.5 Ultralow Penetration Air and High Efficiency Particle Air

High efficiency particle air (HEPA) and ultralow penetration air (ULPA) filters represent a class of air filters that remove greater than 99.97% of airborne particles having a diameter in excess of 0.300 μm. Although the terms HEPA and ULPA have become standards with specific definitions, they originated as marketing terms for

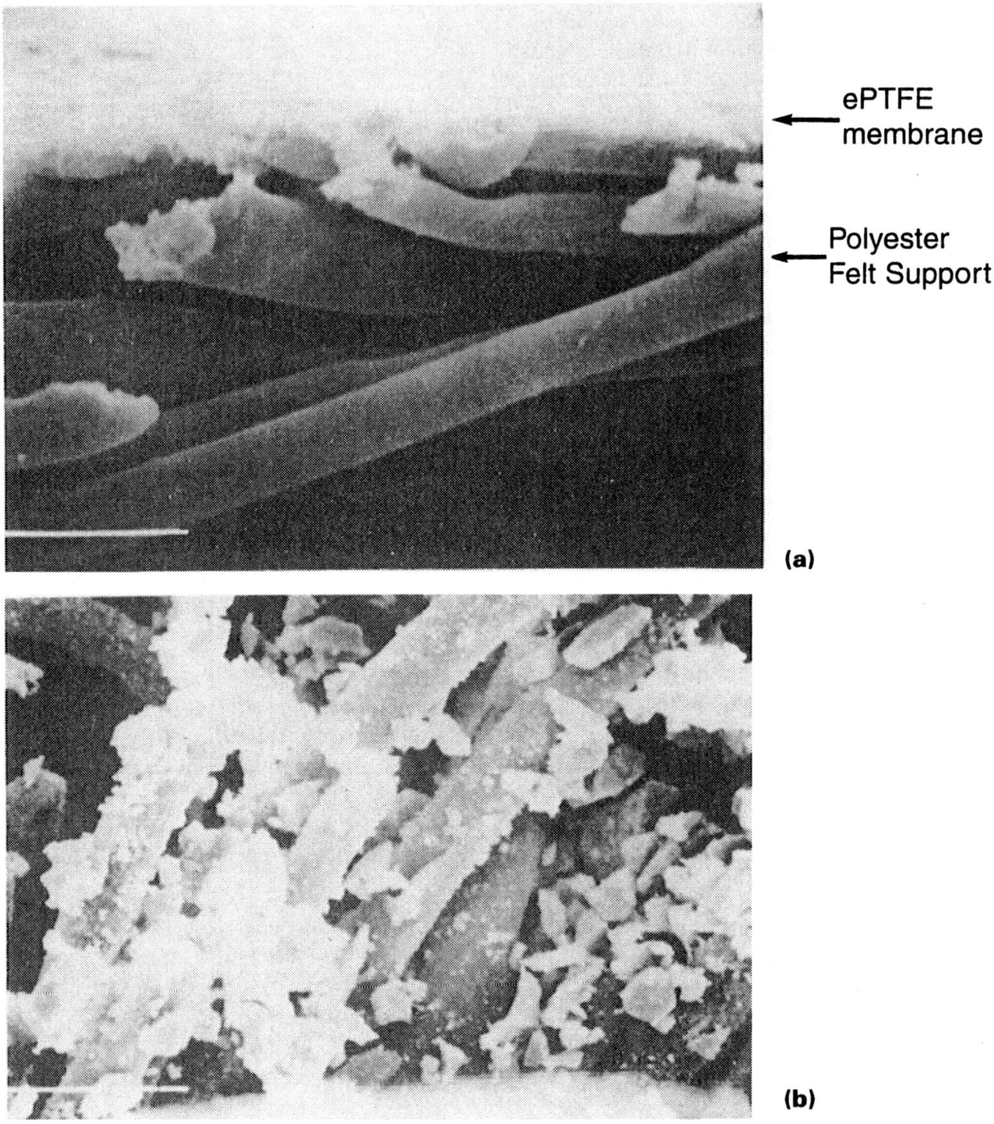

Figure 11 Cross section of (a) ePTFE polyester felt laminate and (b) conventional medium. Since the particulate is filtered at the surface of a ePTFE laminate (a), no product is held up in the depth of the medium. In the conventional filter (b), product is held up throughout the depth of the medium.

highly efficient, low resistance air filters. These filters were originally designed for use in nuclear HVAC systems but have since been adopted in the pharmaceutical industry as well as the food, electronics, and other industries. Use in the pharmaceutical industry has primarily been in heating, ventilating, and air conditioning (HVAC) and other air-handling systems like aseptic processing areas, clean benches, hazardous materials hoods, and, more recently, barrier isolation systems. Little has changed in the technology of these types of filters since their invention. They have

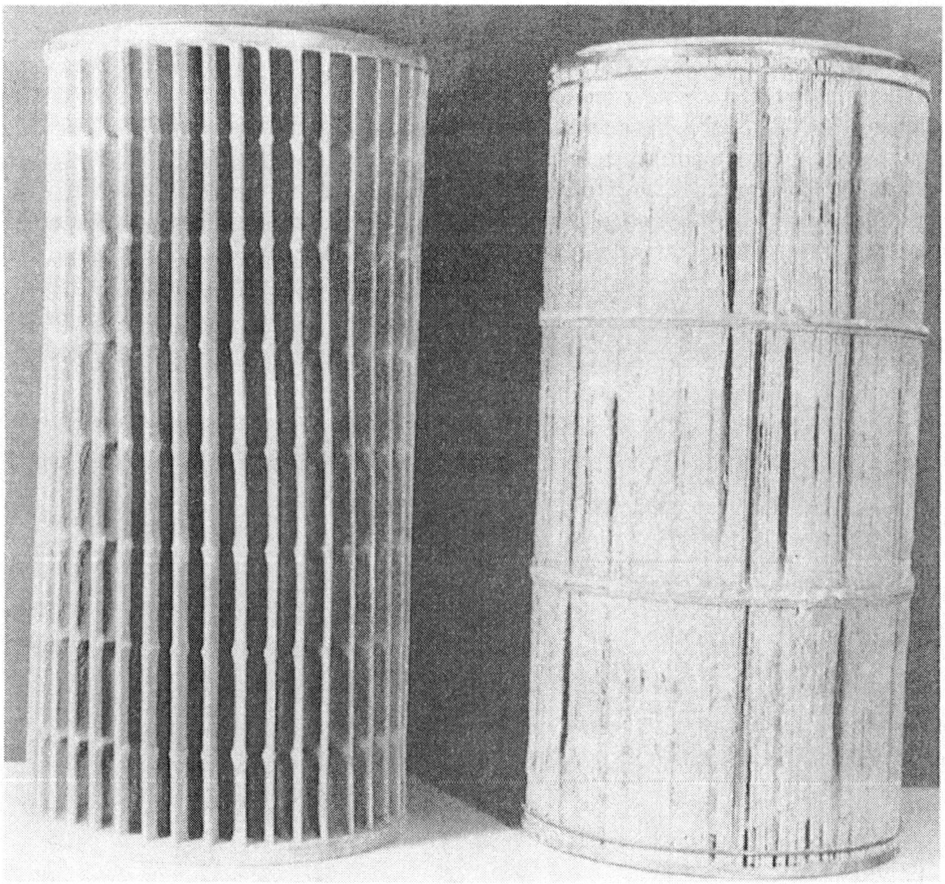

Figure 12 The cellulose cartridge (right) clogs more quickly than the ePTFE cartridge (left).

been basically pleated micro glass fiber paper filters adhered to a frame. Pleat depths range from less than 1 in. to 12 in. Frames are typically rectangular or circular and made of aluminum, stainless steel, or even wood.

The major problem with traditional micro glass fiber HEPA filters is that they have a relatively fragile filter medium. Not only are they easily damaged through normal handling and limited shelf life, but the rigors of many pharmaceutical applications can also harm them. The medium consists of many small glass fibers held together with an acrylic binder. Any breakdown of the binder or fiber can cause leaks or shedding. Agents of damage include handling; in-place contact; vibration; humid environments; exposure to chemicals such as cleaning agents, sterilizing agents, or process chemicals; elevated temperature; and age. Disposal of filters that are contaminated with hazardous materials also presents a problem. To circumvent these problems, zones between the clean space and the HEPA filter are usually covered and not subjected to full cleaning or sterilization. Also, filters must be checked for leaks, typically every 6 months, and are frequently replaced.

The newest innovation in HEPA and ULPA filtration is the use of an ePTFE membrane as the filter medium (see Fig. 13). These filters are inherently chemical-resistant, hydrophobic, easily cleaned, and very strong. They can have filtration efficiencies exceeding 99.99999% at a most penetrating particle size of 0.070 μm. The high strength of the medium, combined with the other properties, makes HEPA filters made of ePTFE an excellent choice for many applications including clean rooms, barrier isolators, aseptic processing and sterility testing areas, and anywhere else where cleanliness, sterility, and contamination control are needed. The filter medium can be exposed to cleaning and sterilizing agents, including water and steam, without breaking down. These filters can be subjected to handling and other physical stresses and still maintain their integrity. In some cases, the filters may be cleaned and reused.

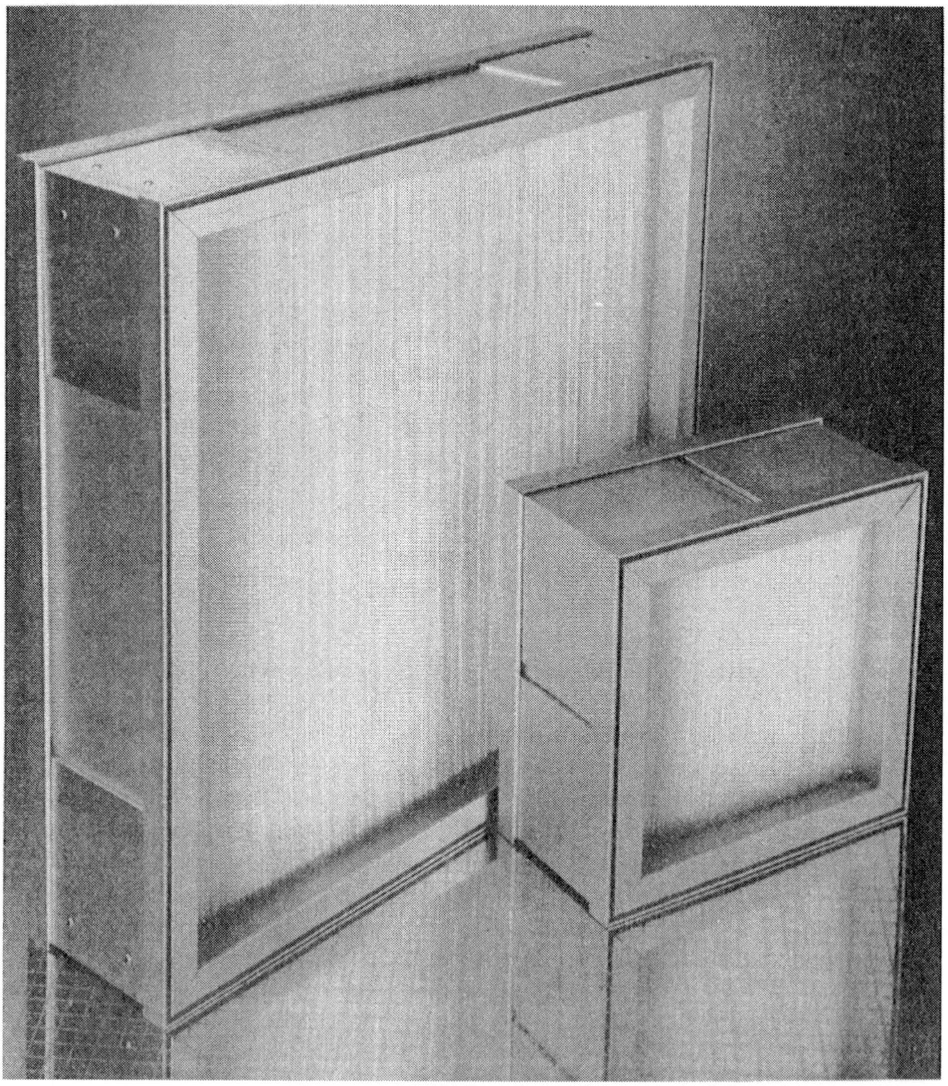

Figure 13 Examples of ULPA filters with ePTFE membranes.

HEPA filters are checked for leaks at the factory and in use. This is done by challenging the filter with particles and using a particle counter or photometer to detect areas of high penetration. One concern with the use of ePTFE membrane filters is the use of DOP, Emery 3004, or other oil-based particle challenges. As previously mentioned in this chapter, these oil smokes can wick into the filter medium and prematurely hinder airflow. Fortunately, there are many feasible solutions to this problem. As mentioned earlier, a 95% prefilter would remove enough mass of oil to prevent dampening of the airflow, leaving the HEPA filter to accomplish the fine, final filtration. Other particle challenges are acceptable and commonly used in the electronics industry. Polystyrene latex (PSL) spheres provide a solid challenge that will not overload the filter. Work has been done recently to demonstrate that leak location and sizing can be accomplished equally well using PSLs or DOP. DOP is a suspected carcinogen, and its use is diminishing for that and other reasons.

7.6 Filtering Liquids

Because of ePTFE membranes' chemical inertness and high flow rates, they are well suited for various liquid filtration applications. Low surface tension liquids such as methanol, isopropanol, and methyl ethyl ketone will readily wet ePTFE membranes. In these types of applications, no additional prewetting steps are required.

On the other hand, fluids with higher surface tensions such as water will not flow through hydrophobic membranes like ePTFE at normal operating pressures. If a hydrophobic membrane is to be used for an aqueous filtration, it must first be prewetted with a lower surface tension liquid such as isopropanol. Once properly wetted, aqueous solutions can be filtered through ePTFE membranes. Depending on the application, the prewetting solution can be flushed from the filter with water or with the aqueous solution to be filtered. Prewetting of ePTFE membranes is extensively practiced in the semiconductor industry.

Since prewetting can be inconvenient, a water-wettable or hydrophilic PTFE membrane would be desirable. The surfaces of PTFE membranes can be modified to render the membranes hydrophilic. Currently, hydrophilic PTFE membranes are suitable for room temperature filtration applications. These membranes often become unstable at elevated temperatures.

8 OTHER EMERGING MICROPOROUS PTFE MEMBRANE TECHNOLOGIES

An emerging technology worth mentioning is that of oleophobic ePTFE. As previously mentioned, the surface free energy of PTFE is 18.5 dyn/cm. There are some applications in which a lower surface free energy in an all-fluoropolymer membrane would be desirable. An oleophobic membrane is not wetted by lower surface tension fluids such as oils and solvents, whereas oils and solvents may wet out membranes that are merely hydrophobic. Characteristics of this type of membrane may be of interest in new processes and formulations.

9 CONCLUSION

As we have discussed, ePTFE membranes are valuable in a number of pharmaceutical filtration, separation, and venting applications. PTFE is inherently inert, thermally resistant, and extremely hyrophobic. PTFE can be engineered into a highly retentive and high-flowing microporous membrane. These characteristics are what makes ePTFE membranes the filtration media of choice in fermentation feed air and tank venting applications. These desirable characteristics of ePTFE are also being exploited in new pharmaceutical applications such as lyophilization stoppers and bags and ULPA filters. Because of the unique properties of ePTFE membranes they are a good choice for these as well as future challenging filtration, separation, and venting applications.

BIBLIOGRAPHY

American Type Culture Collection. (1992). *Catalogue of Bacteria & Bacteriophages*, Vol. 18.

Barbaree, J. M., and A. Sanchez. 1982. Cross contamination during lyophilization, *Cryobiology*, *19*:443–447.

Barbaree, J. M., A. Sanchez, and G. N. Sanden. (1985). Problems in freeze-drying: II. Cross contamination during lyophilization, *Dev. Ind. Microbiol.* *26*:407–409.

Bowser, J. J. (1991). U.S. Patent 5,019,140 (issued May 28).

Gore, R. W. (1980). U.S. Patent 4,187,390 (Feb. 5).

Hinds, W. C. 1982. *Aersol Technology*, Wiley-Interscience, New York.

Imbalzano, J. F., and J. R. Moody. 1985. Preliminary studies of the effects of semiconductor reagents on polymers containing fluorine and of trace metallic leachate from molded fluorocarbon resin, *J. Environ. Sci.*, July.

Lange, Zingle, Patten, and Franke. (1997). Bacterial cross contamination during lyophilization and its prevention, *Tissue Cell Rep.* (American Association of Tissue Bankers), August.

Pruett, K. M. (1983). *Compass Corrosion Guide II*, Compass Publications.

Rosenburger, Y., A. Siegman, M. Narkis, and S. Shkolnik. *J. Appl. Polym. Sci.* *45*:783–795.

Schubert, P. (1989). The Sterilization of Fermentation Inlet Air, Scientific and Technical Report, Pall Corporation, Glen Cove, NY.

Stein, C. D., and H. Rogers. (1950). Recovery of viable microorganisms and viruses from vapors removed from frozen suspensions of biological material during lyophilization, *Am. J. Vet. Res.* *11*:339–344.

3
Charge-Modified Filter Media

RODNEY A. KNIGHT and EUGENE A. OSTREICHER
Cuno, Inc., Meriden, Connecticut

1 INTRODUCTION

It has long been recognized that adsorptive effects can enhance the capture of particulate contaminants. Contaminant particles and a porous filter medium interact with two types of forces: van der Waals forces, which are short-range and always attractive, and the electrical double layer interactions, which may be attractive or repulsive depending on the surface charge of the contaminant particle and that of the pore surface. These interactions determine if a particle will be attracted to or repulsed by the pore surface. This chapter deals with the filtration process that is based on the control of these effects, namely, the electrokinetic interactions between suspended contaminants and porous filter media.

If the contaminant particle and the pore surface are of the same charge, and the double layers of the particle and the surface interact in a repulsive manner, then the capability of a filter medium to remove particles physically smaller than the pores of the medium is limited. On the other hand, if the contaminant particle and the pore surface are oppositely charged, and there is at least no repulsive interaction between the electrical double layers of the particle and the pore surface, then particles physically smaller than the pore size of the medium are capable of being removed by adsorption by the process called electrokinetic capture. Since most contaminants encountered in nature are electronegative, this mandates that the filter medium have a positive zeta potential.

Such a filter was developed over 100 years ago when chrysotile asbestos was first used as a filter medium. This naturally occurring mineral fiber carries an electropositive surface charge and has a positive zeta potential.

2 HISTORICAL OVERVIEW

The early history of fluid filtration revolves around the use of natural materials in the form of fine particulates or fibers to create porous media capable of removing contaminants from fluids. It is only in fairly recent times that filtration technology has taken upon itself the creation and use of synthetic materials specifically developed for the purpose of filtration. In many cases, these synthetic materials have been produced in an attempt to either imitate or improve upon the natural "prototype" material. So it was with the current technology of electrokinetic filtration. Any discussion of this technology must, as a basic premise, follow an understanding of its historical prototype, i.e., asbestos.

Commercial-scale mining of chrysotile asbestos was begun in Italy about 1866 (Kirk-Othmer, 1963). It did not take long for the potential suitability of this very fine inorganic fiber to be recognized for use in filter media. By the 1880s, the Seitz brothers had developed and commercialized the first asbestos-based filter sheets and founded the Seitz firm, which still exists today (Purchas, 1967). For nearly a century, chrysotile asbestos fiber filter media, primarily in the form of cellulose-asbestos filter sheets, were the filter media of choice for critical micrometric and submicrometric filtration applications. Asbestos filters were used extensively in the sterile filtration of many pharmaceutical products, particularly the biologicals. Even after the advent of sterilizing membrane filters in the early 1950s, cellulose-asbestos prefilters were found necessary to reduce the contaminant loading on the membranes. In the production of fractionated blood products, the use of asbestos filters was uniquely critical for the removal of lipids, denatured protein, and bacterial endotoxins (pyrogens). This use dates back to a paper by Cohn et al. (1946) on the fractionation of human blood, the basis for what is now a major health industry. In the alcoholic beverage industry, cellulose-asbestos sheet media or asbestos-based filter precoat mixtures were used for final polishing and sterilization (Neradt, 1971; Rose, 1977). In such applications, the asbestos was acid washed to reduce the calcium and magnesium extractables that produce haze in the finished product. Transformer and circuit breaker insulating oils were filtered with cellulose-asbestos sheet media to remove dissolved water and colloidal carbon particles to restore the dielectric strength of the oil.

By the late 1960s, cellulose-asbestos filter media were very mature, widely used, but no longer an exciting product. Under such conditions, there was little incentive for any investigation or development. There was limited recognition that the surface charge character of asbestos was somehow related to the unusual filtration capabilities exhibited by the material. In a patent for cellulose-asbestos filter pads (Seitz, 1939), George Seitz stated "I believe that the combination of two kinds of fiber in suitable proportions each having its special electrostatic qualities gives the filter sheet a special and unique adsorption power for germs." As best as can be determined, there was no serious attempt to define the nature of the surface charge and the functional filtration mechanism at work. As late as 1971, practitioners in the field were notably ambiguous in their description of the phenomenon. One expert covered his options by stating, "Asbestos fibers can hold the finest particles on their surface by adhesive, electrostatic and electrokinetic forces" (Neradt, 1971).

In the real world of the filtration industry, technical knowledge tends to be sought out only if it is clearly obvious that there will be an immediate and satisfying financial return. Had not history stepped in and rattled cages, our current knowledge of electrokinetic filtration probably would not have advanced beyond the level described above. However, in the late 1960s, chronic exposure to airborne asbestos was identified as a significant health hazard (Selikoff, 1968), with pulmonary fibrosis and a variety of neoplasms being linked to such exposures. Such reports aroused scientific interest in the possible health hazards associated with other forms of exposure. Asbestos contamination of fluids that had been filtered through cellulose-asbestos filter media was an obvious candidate for investigation, and soon reports were issued defining asbestos contamination of parenteral drugs (Nicholson et al., 1972), beer (Biles and Emerson, 1968), and a variety of alcoholic and nonalcoholic beverages (Cunningham and Pontefract, 1971).

The FDA proposed restrictions on the use of asbestos filters in the manufacture of parenteral drugs in 1973 (FDA, 1973) and issued appropriate regulations in 1975 (FDA, 1975) and 1976 (FDA, 1976). No regulations were ever proposed or issued governing the use of asbestos filters in food or beverage processing, but these industries were so sensitive to their public image and the threat of bad publicity that they needed no regulations to persuade them to seek a replacement for asbestos. Both the food and drug industries undertook programs to eliminate the use of asbestos filter media and challenged the filter industry to respond with safe and effective alternatives. Without exception, all of the "old line" cellulose-asbestos filter manufacturers initially responded either by ignoring the question or by attempting to persuade the government and customers that there really wasn't a problem.

3 DEVELOPMENT OF AN ASBESTOS SUBSTITUTE

The first step in the development of a substitute for asbestos in filter media was to develop a thorough understanding of what asbestos is and how it functions in the filtration process.

Asbestos-form minerals fall into two major categories identified as chrysotile and amphibole. It is the chrysotile that exhibits the classical fibrous morphology, and this was the asbestos used by the filter industry. The composition of the mineral on a unit cell basis is $Mg_6(OH)_8SIO_{10}$ (Pundsack, 1955). There is a size mismatch between the magnesium oxide-hydroxide octahedron and the silicon dioxide tetrahedral in the bonded layers that results in curvature of the sheet. This curvature is sufficient to roll the sheet into a spiral hollow fiber with the magnesium hydroxide on the outside (Speil and Leineweber 1969). Yada (1967) was able to produce a definitive scanning electron photomicrograph of the cross section of the basic asbestos fibril as shown in Fig. 1. This hollow fiber is the basic fibril and may in turn be bonded together with other basic fibrils to form larger fibers and bundles of fibers. This built-up structure explains the broad variation in Brumauer–Emmett–Teller (BET) nitrogen surface area measurements that have been reported for asbestos. The limiting upper surface area for highly fibrillated asbestos appears to be approximately 50 m^2/g.

As mentioned previously, the outer layer of the asbestos fibril, fiber, or bundle is composed of magnesium oxide-hydroxide. It is this layer that is responsible for the unique positive surface charge exhibited by asbestos. In water, the magnesium oxide-hydroxide will dissociate to give a chemically bonded magnesium ion at the fiber surface.

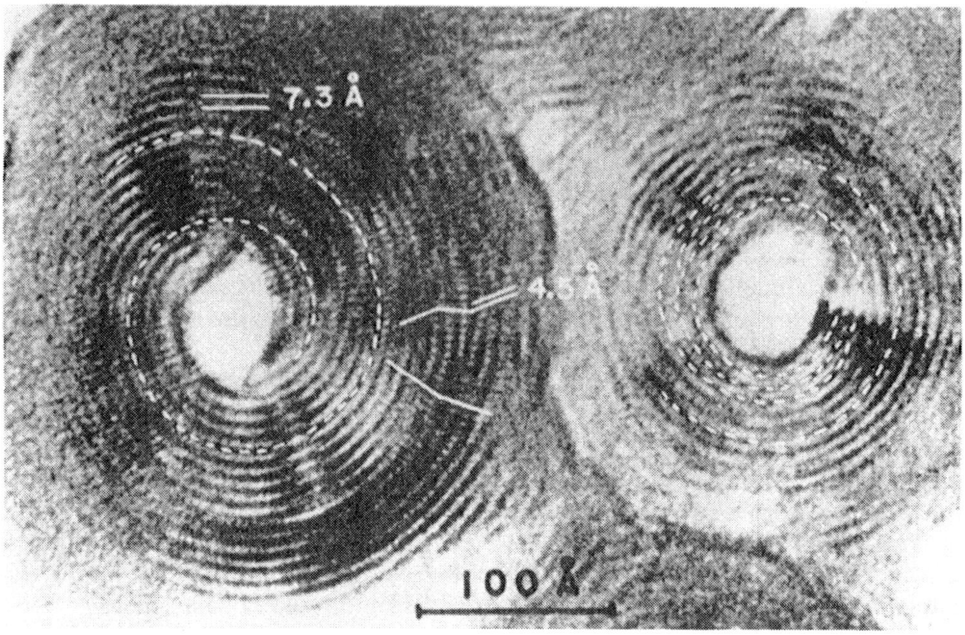

Figure 1 Electron photomicrograph of the fine chrysotile structure of asbestos. (Reproduced from Yada, 1967.)

If sufficient dissociation takes place, the net surface charge will be positive. Although it is impossible to measure surface charge directly, it can be indirectly measured by use of electrophoretic mobility or streaming potential measurements. These measurement techniques are described and discussed later in this chapter. Figure 2 shows the results of electrophoretic mobility measurements taken on unwashed and acid-washed fibers. The unwashed (standard) asbestos fibers demonstrated a positive surface charge at pH <8.3. This pH value is known as the isoelectric point, i.e., the point at which the net summation of positive (cationic) and negative (anionic) surface charge is zero.

The results achieved with the acid-washed asbestos were initially surprising. As mentioned earlier in the discussion of asbestos media applications, acid-washed asbestos was used in applications such as wine and beer filtration, where there was product sensitivity to calcium, magnesium, and iron extractions. The acid-washed asbestos exhibits a much lower isoelectric point and, in fact, behaves as a negatively charged material above pH 5.0. Given the fact that acid-washed asbestos media appeared to be giving adequate filtration performance, this finding brought into question the significance or necessity of a positive surface charge in an asbestos substitute.

Scanning electron microscopic evaluation of unwashed asbestos and acid-washed asbestos gave an answer to this seeming paradox. Acid washing stripped off the magnesium layer that produced the positive surface charge in unwashed asbestos. In doing so, it also "unglued" the asbestos bundles and fibers to produce a much higher level of fibrilization than could be achieved with unwashed asbestos.

The radically finer fibers of the acid-washed asbestos were capable of producing a filter medium with a much finer pore structure capable of very high mechanical

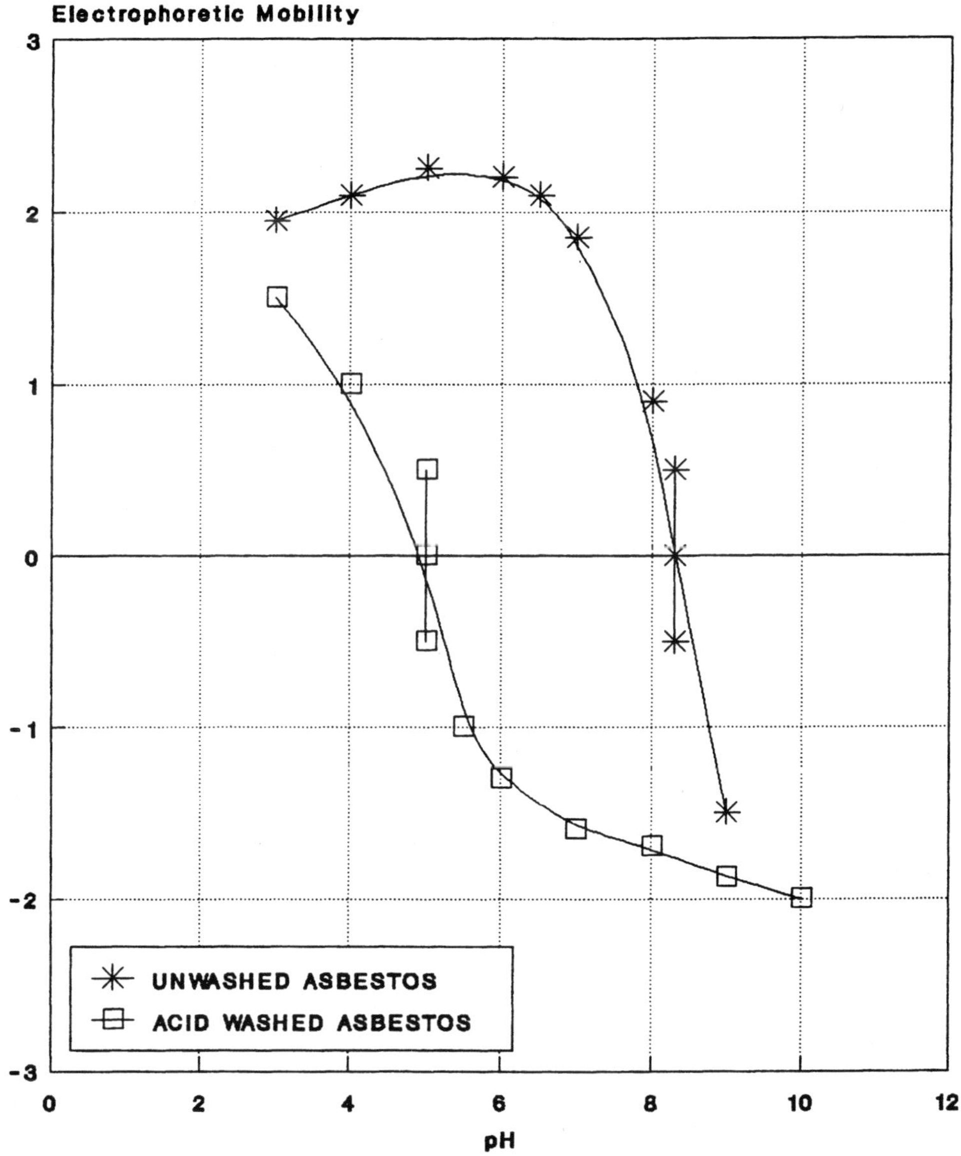

Figure 2 Electrophoretic mobility of chrysotile asbestos.

straining efficiencies. This appears to have compensated, to some degree, for the reduced capability of the medium to function via electrokinetic capture and adsorption. Wine and beer filtration concerns itself with the removal of yeast (≥2 μm) and lactobacilli (0.5 μm), and for such "giant" particles, mechanical straining is adequate. In the filtration of blood fractions, on the other hand, the user is concerned with the removal of certain colloidal and macromolecular materials of a size much smaller than the pore size of the filter medium. In this application, the users were forced to stay with unwashed asbestos media even though they would have preferred to use the cleaner acid-washed material. Finally, there was the actual test performance of the cellulose-asbestos medium itself. Figure 3 shows the performance of Seitz EK cellulose-asbestos filter medium when challenged with an anionic 0.109 μm monodisperse latex bead dispersion in water. The efficiency vs. throughput characteristics, showing high initial efficiency followed by breakthrough, are typical of electrokinetic capture and adsorption, not mechanical straining.

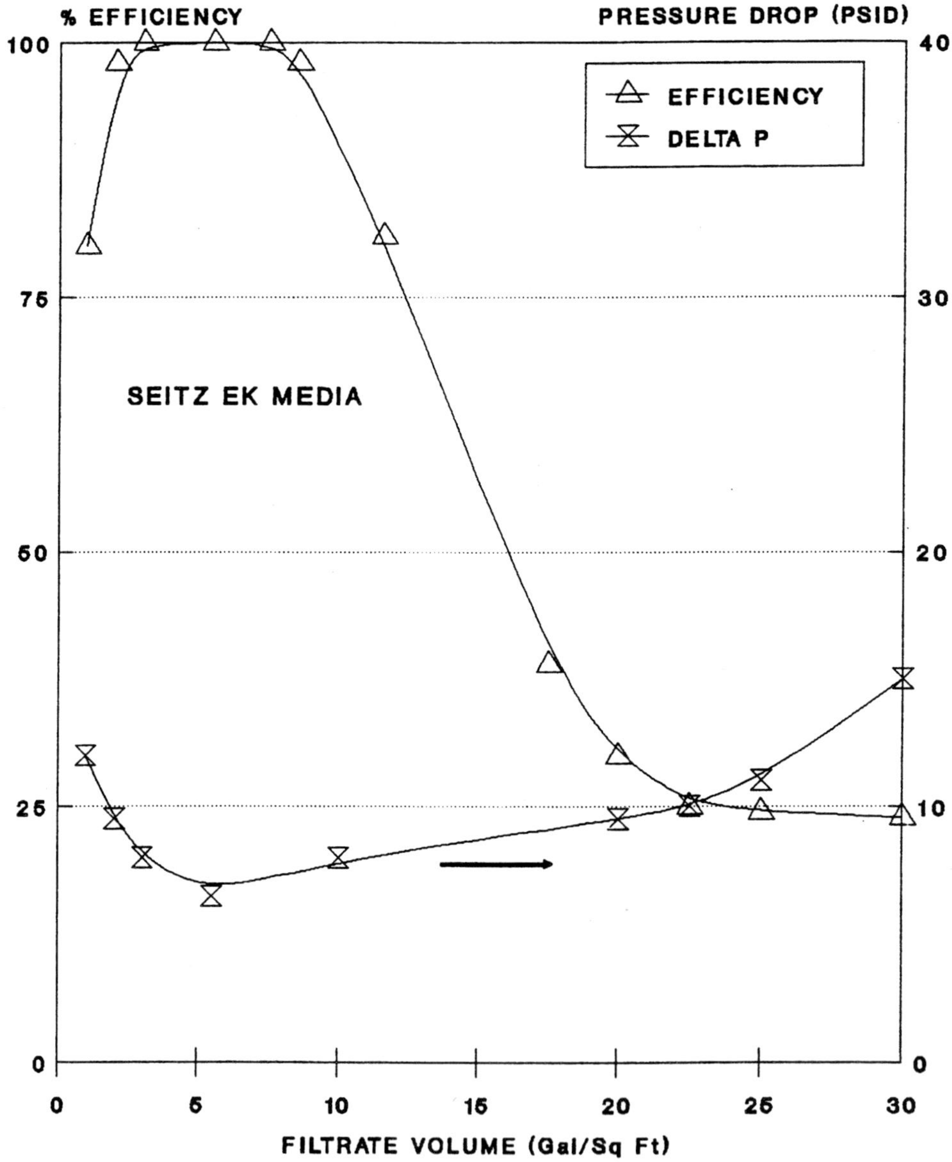

Figure 3 Filtration characteristics of cellulose-asbestos filter media.

4 SURFACE CHARGE MODIFICATION

As the situation stood in 1971, our evaluation of asbestos had given strong indication that the unique filtration properties of asbestos depended on its electropositive surface charge. It became obvious that if a substitute were to be developed, it would have to be possible to modify the surface charge characteristics of other types of fibers and/or particulate materials. A review of the technical and patent literature revealed that the concept of chemically modifying the surface of a filter medium to provide enhanced filtration characteristics was not a particularly new one. The earliest reference was a 1936 patent (Cummings, 1936) that described the treatment of diatomaceous earth to produce an electropositive, insoluble aluminum hydroxide coating. Such treated diatomaceous earth, when used as a filter aid, acted as a flocculant for colloidal contaminants. In 1938, another patent (Elliot and Elliott, 1938) was issued describing the treatment of filter sand with rosin. While there is nothing in the chemistry of rosin that would lead one to believe that it could function as a charge modifier, the inventors appeared to believe that there was such an effect, and their patent states, "Sometimes this coating carries an electrical charge; either positive or negative, and opposite to that of suspended colloid particles." In 1952, a patent (Rodman, 1952) was issued that described the use of a modified aliphatic amine to treat filter media intended for use in oil filtration. That patent attributed enhanced sludge removal to cellulose fiber filters so treated.

In the early 1960s, synthetic polyelectrolytes were developed for use in water treatment. These polyelectrolytes are water-soluble, high molecular weight synthetic organic polymers containing a series of repeating monomeric units. The monomeric units are characterized by having ionizable functional groups that dissociate in water to produce charged sites along the polymer chain. Initially, these polyelectrolytes were used as coagulants to improve the filterability of suspended solids. In such applications, they function by destabilizing colloid particles, through charge neutralization and/or bridging, so as to induce flocculation. In 1966 and 1967, Dow Chemical was issued patents (Guebert and Laman, 1966; Guebert and Jones, 1967) describing the use of cationic polyelectrolytes to charge-modify filter aids and the use of such charge-modified filter aids in removing microorganisms from water. In the early 1970s, Bauman and his coworkers at the University of Iowa did extensive work on the use of polyelectrolytes as a pretreatment to provide an adsorbed charge modifier coating on filter aids and filter media (Baumann et al., 1970; Burns et al., 1970; Oulman et al., 1971). Their work is particularly significant because they were the first experimenters to use electrokinetic (streaming potential) measurements to quantify the level of charge modification achieved (Oulman and Baumann, 1964).

5 DEVELOPMENTAL EFFORTS

The search for an asbestos substitute started, therefore, with a good understanding of both the filtration mechanism and the unique physical and chemical properties of chrysotile asbestos. Prior technology had demonstrated that it was feasible to charge-modify the surfaces of normally anionic filter materials so as to produce a cationic surface characteristic and that such charge modification did result in enhanced filtration properties. This knowledge allowed the definition of a set of basic requirements:

1. The basic filter material should be a fine, high surface area fiber or particulate with an ionic surface charge.
2. This material should be capable of being dispersed in a water slurry with cellulose fiber and being vacuum-formed into a thick (3/16 in.) sheet structure).
3. The chemical charge modifier should have a strong cationic functionality and should be capable of being chemically bonded to the anionic high surface area substrate.

This latter requirement was based on the needs of the pharmaceutical and food industries for a "clean" (low extraction) and "safe" (no toxicological problems) filter medium. Finding the appropriate charge modifier system to satisfy this requirement was the innovative step that moved us beyond all of the prior technology, which was based on the *adsorption* of a charge-modifying agent.

Unfortunately, adsorption is a reversible process, and such adsorbed charge modifiers exhibited high extraction levels. In practice, this meant that the charge-modifying agent must have an appropriate cross-linking functionality in addition to its cationic functionality. During the period 1972–1976, several basic types of "asbestos-free" filter media under the trademark Zeta Plus were developed and commercialized (Ostreicher, 1977a, 1977b, 1982; Hou and Ostreicher, 1991; Ostreicher and Hou, 1981).

Success in duplicating the performance of cellulose-asbestos filter media is most easily demonstrated by comparing the laboratory performance of a Zeta Plus media grade (Fig. 4a) with that of the corresponding Seitz cellulose-asbestos grade (Fig. 4b). These laboratory results were soon verified by the success of Zeta Plus in replacing cellulose-asbestos in a broad range of industrial filtration applications.

Because of the low wet strength of cellulose-asbestos, this medium had been limited to use as a sheet medium in filter presses, with all of the associated problems of leakage, sterilization, and lengthy changeout time and correspondingly high labor costs. In addition to having equivalent or superior filtration performance, Zeta Plus exhibited significantly better wet strength. This was a side benefit of the cross-linking characteristics of the charge modifier systems used, and it allowed the development of a new generation of radically improved disposable cartridges. In the intervening years, such cartridges have significantly displaced the use of filter presses.

The concept of charge modification of microporous membranes was first proposed, by Ostreicher, in the early 1970s. It was believed at that time that there was no advantage to trying to embellish the performance of an "absolute" filter that was already capable of achieving the level of performance demanded by the application. In the late 1970s, however, the reliability of such membrane filters came into question with several investigators reporting bacterial passage through such supposedly "absolute" membranes (Wallhäusser, 1979; Howard and Duberstein, 1980). In addition, the medical industry was coming to realize that other contaminants besides bacteria, namely viruses and bacterial endotoxins (pyrogens), had to be removed from parenteral drugs for patient safety (Brown, 1980). Significant success was achieved in removing both viruses and bacterial endotoxins (Sobsey and Jones, 1979; Gerba et al., 1980; Hou et al., 1980) by use of the charge-modified Zeta Plus filter medium, and it appeared that such enhanced performance could also be achieved with a charge-modified membrane. The new nylon membrane charge-modified filter media

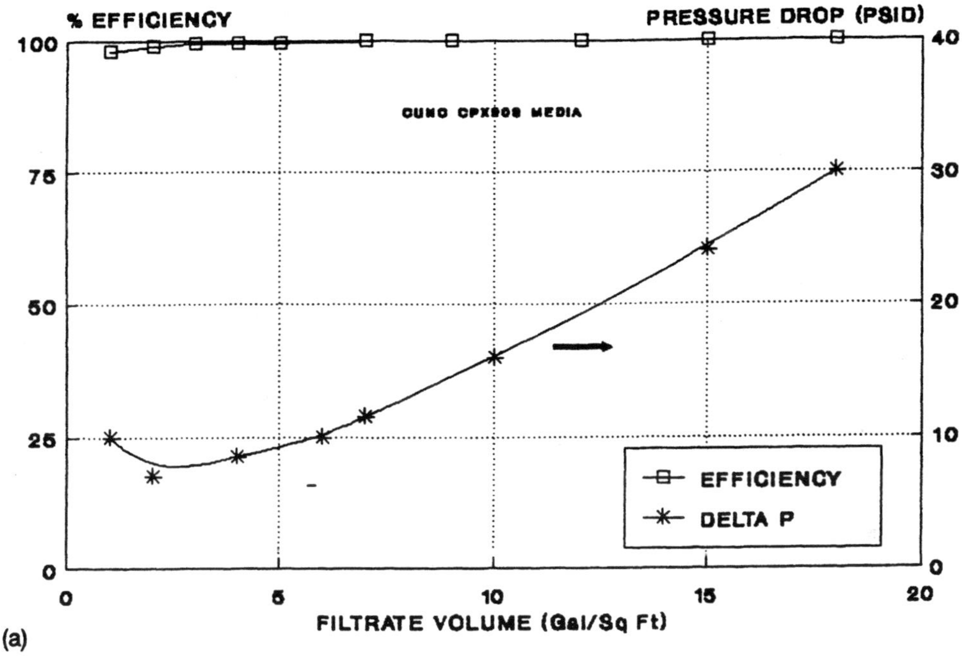

(a)

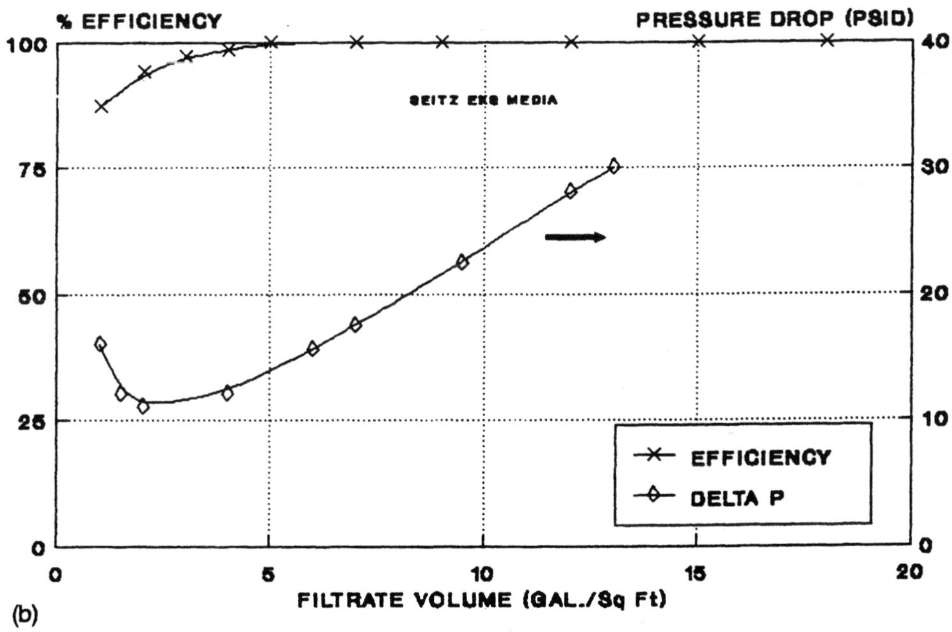

(b)

Figure 4 (a) Comparative filtration characteristics for Zeta Plus media. (b) Comparative filtration characteristics of cellulose-asbestos media.

were based on the unique morphology and surface chemistry of nylon (Ostreicher et al., 1984) and the very specialized requirements of the pharmaceutical industry (low organic extractions) and the semiconductor industry (low ionic extractions). This necessitated the development of two new two-component charge modifier systems (Ostreicher et al., 1984; Barnes et al., 1984).

The primary market, however, for such membranes was in the filtrative sterilization of pharmaceutical products. In this market, microporous polymeric membranes of 0.2 μm nominal rating have found widespread use in the sterilization of parenteral drugs. For this purpose, their performance was characterized in terms of the complete removal of the microorganism *Pseudomonas diminuta* (Pall, 1975).

The existence of the adsorptive phenomena in conventional microporous membranes is recognized (Tanny and Meltzer, 1976; Tanny et al., 1979). The effect of such adsorptive phenomena on the performance of "sterilizing" membranes was treated as a secondary and not very important attribute of the base polymer used to produce the membrane. Perhaps exaggeratedly, mechanical sieving was defined as the primary mode of filtration. All of the commonly accepted modes of membrane characterization concerned themselves with the determination of pore size distributions (especially maximum pore size) and the correlation of such physical parameters with the bacterial rejection characteristics exhibited by the membranes.

Historically, membranes were characterized as surface-type filters. In an SEM study, Knight et al. (1982) were able to rigorously demonstrate that a charge-modified nylon membrane functions as an adsorptive depth filter by virtue of the electrokinetic capture and adsorption function provided by the combination of charge modification and high internal membrane pore surface area. Figure 5 shows a cross section of such a charge-modified membrane after it was subjected to a 0.109 μm monodisperse latex bead challenge. This photograph demonstrates the reality of electrokinetic capture and adsorption with the monodisperse latex particles adhering to the surfaces of the relatively larger pore structure. That such removal is quantitative is shown graph-

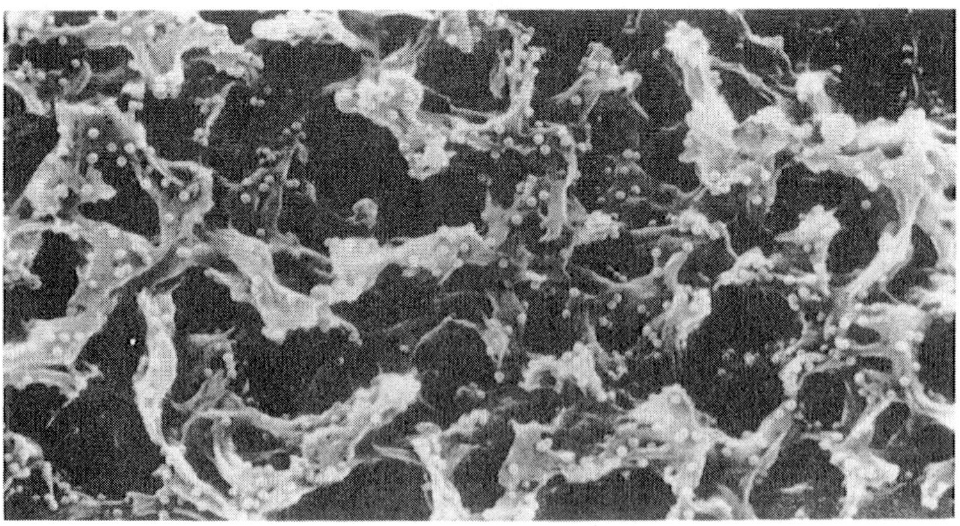

Figure 5 Electrokinetic capture of 0.109 μm particles on a charge-modified membrane.

ically in Fig. 6, which presents the particle removal efficiencies of a charge-modified 0.2 μm membrane and unmodified 0.1 μm and 0.2 μm membranes. The pressure drop characteristics for each of these membranes are shown superimposed on the efficiency curves in Fig. 7.

In addition to the sterilizing filtration of pharmaceuticals, the next most significant market segment for microporous membranes is the filtration of ultrahigh purity water used in the semiconductor industry. To be useful for such filtration, the

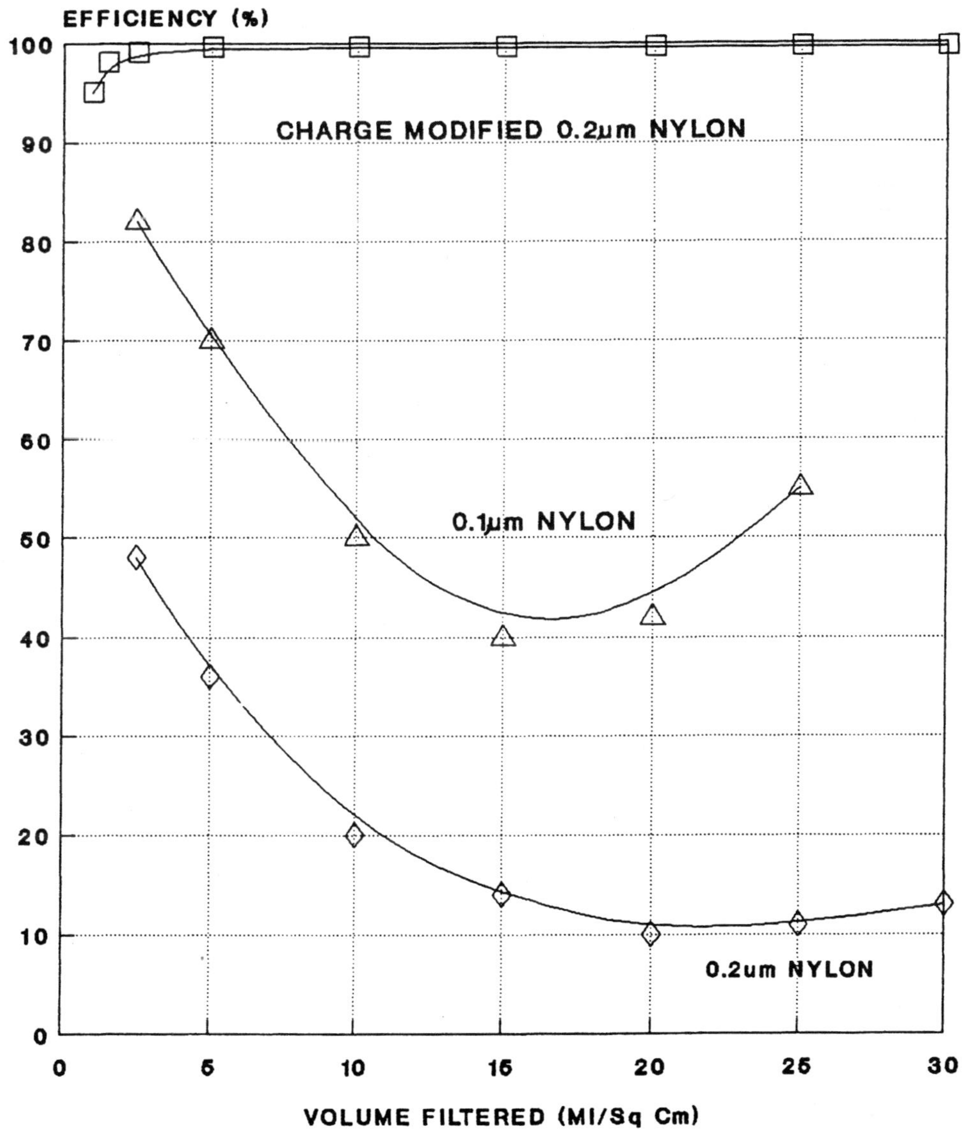

Figure 6 Filtration characteristics of modified and unmodified nylon 66 membranes, subjected to 0.109 μm MDL bead challenge.

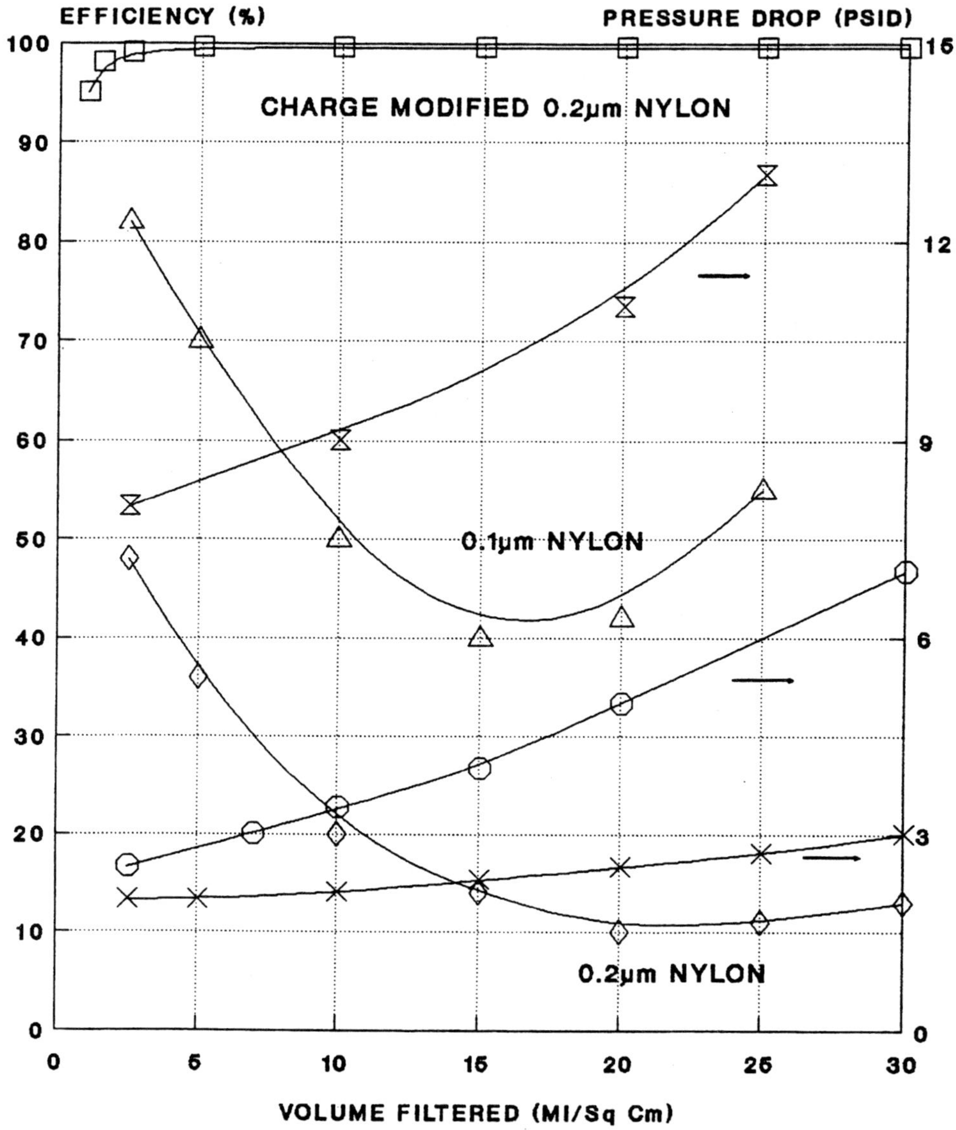

Figure 7 Filtration characteristics of modified and unmodified nylon 66 membranes subjected to 0.109 μm MDL bead challenge. ⧗, ΔP 0.1 μm nylon; ○, ΔP charge modified 0.2 μm nylon; ×, 0.2 μm nylon.

filter media must not contribute any ionic contamination to the 18 megohm·cm water. Given an appropriate charge-modified system (Barnes et al., 1984), it is possible to produce a charge-modified membrane that not only does not introduce ionic contamination but acts to remove ionic contaminants from solution and actually increase the resistivity of the water being filtered. Figure 8 demonstrates this type of performance.

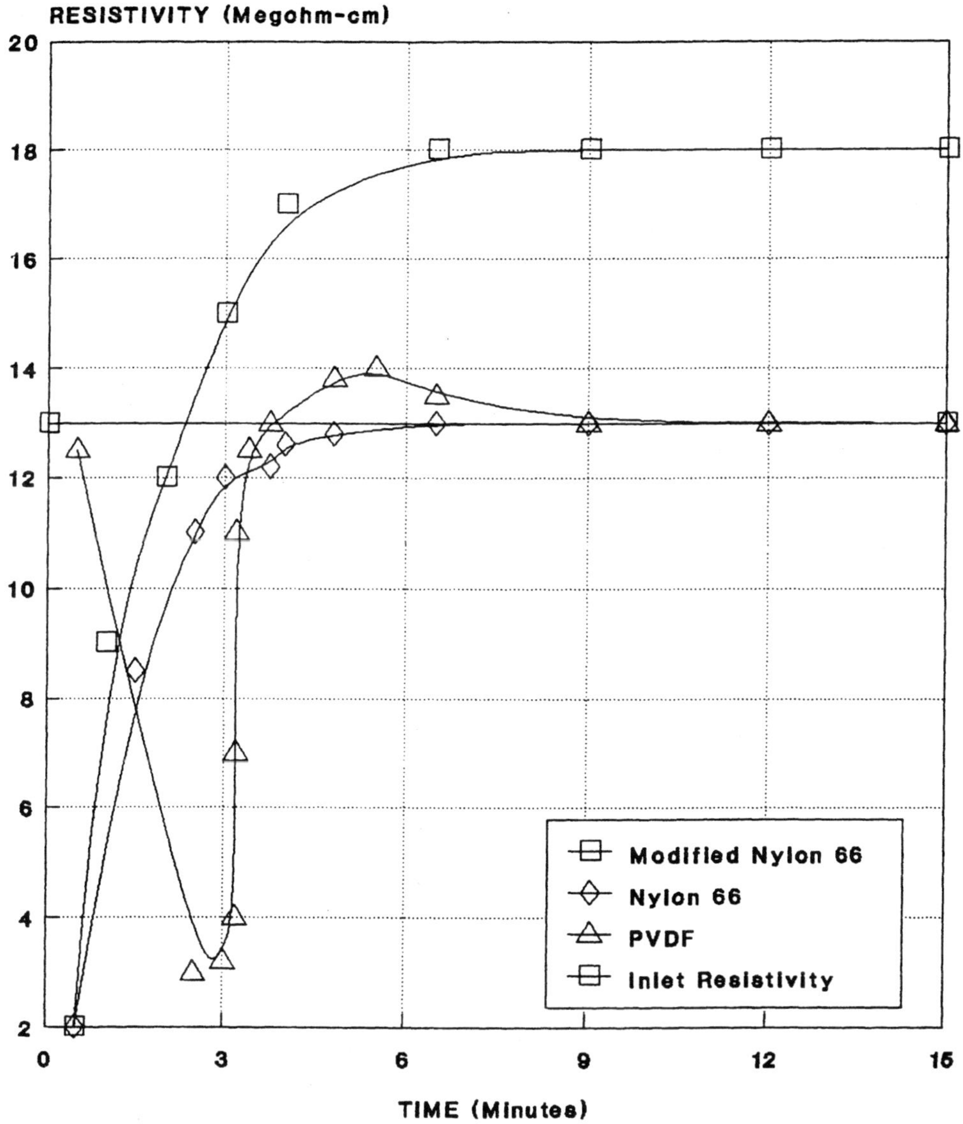

Figure 8 Behavior of modified and unmodified membrane cartridges in high purity water, inlet resistivity = 13 Megohm·cm.

6 OTHER DEVELOPMENTS

Charge modification techniques have been used to enhance the performance of micrometric rated resin-bonded (Kilty and Pernigott, 1980) and wound cotton (Hou and Kilty, 1981) industrial filter cartridges. Even on these coarser filtration ratings, electrokinetic capture and adsorption can produce a significant enhancement of the filtration performance as shown in Fig. 9.

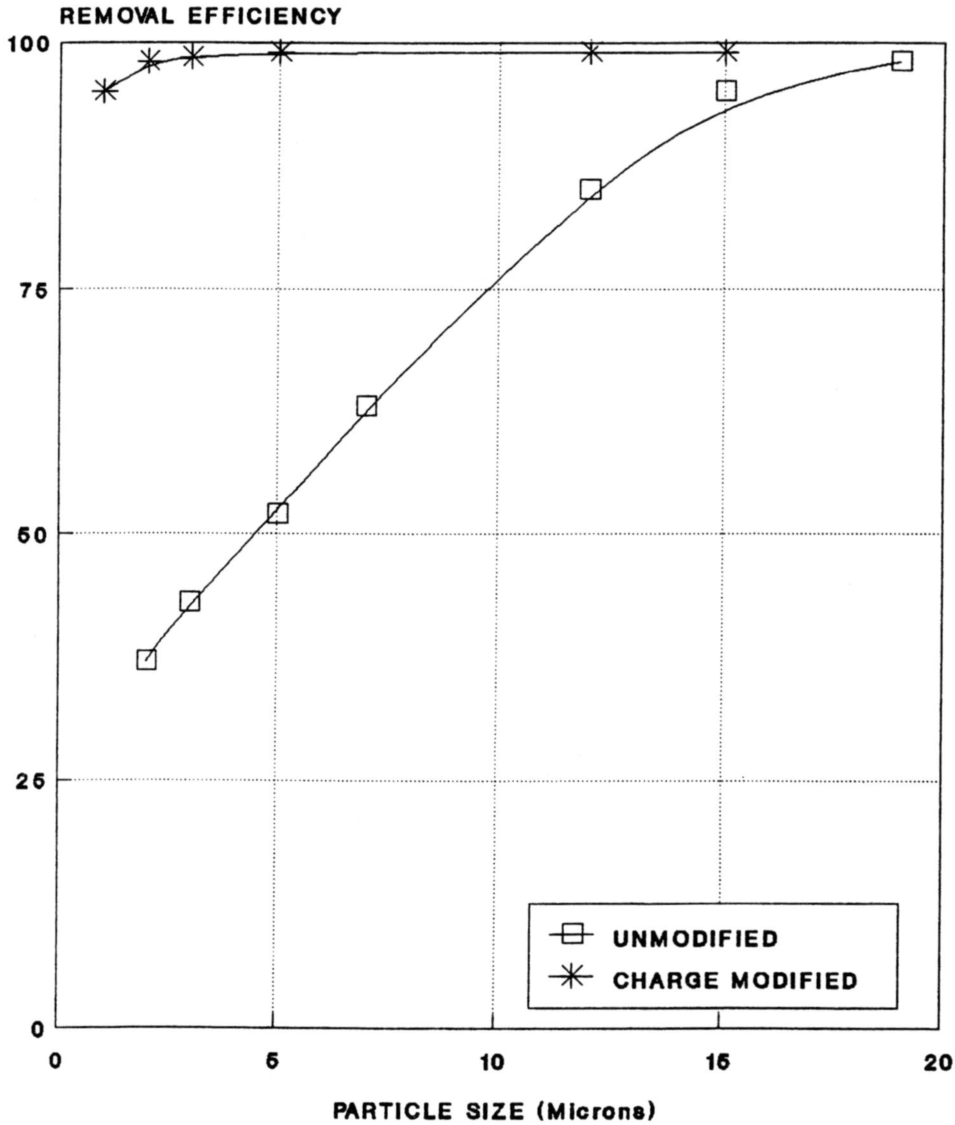

Figure 9 Effect of charge modification on cartridge performance of nominal 3 μm filter cartridge.

Initially, Cuno was the only filter manufacturer producing a charge-modified filter medium. Pall Corporation (nylon 66), Gelman, and Millipore have since joined in this technology. Gelman produces a positively charged polyethersulfone sulfate membrane, while Millipore produces a charge-modified poly(vinylidene difluoride) (PVDF) membrane.

7 TESTING CHARGE-MODIFIED FILTER MEDIA

New test methods had to be developed to evaluate and quantify the performance of candidate charge-modified media and, eventually, to provide process and quality control criteria for the final product. The primary performance characteristics for any filter medium are removal efficiency and capacity. The test techniques that had been developed to measure these characteristics in unmodified submicrometer filter media, such as bubble point, diffusion flow, and sterilization testing with specific microorganisms, dealt strictly with mechanical straining. They were not useful in measuring the efficiency and capacity of charge-modified media.

It was necessary that the contaminant particle size be smaller than the pore size of the medium being tested. In addition, it was necessary that the contaminants used have consistent and reproducible surface charge and particle size distribution characteristics. These requirements were necessary so that consistent and reproducible evaluation could be made of the electrokinetic capture and adsorption characteristics of the media independent of mechanical straining effects. The following test methods were developed to meet these requirements.

7.1 Monodisperse Latex Testing

Monodisperse latex testing, the "workhorse" of the developmental efforts, consists of challenging the filter medium sample, at a specified constant flow rate, with an aqueous dispersion of a single-size monodisperse polystyrene latex adjusted to a specified turbidity, pH, and resistivity. The effluent turbidity and medium pressure drop are measured and recorded as a function of the throughput. The particle removal efficiency of the media sample, for the specific particle size used, can be calculated directly from the inlet and effluent turbidity values (Knight and Ostreicher, 1981). These tests use relatively high contaminant challenge levels to reduce the time to breakthrough to an acceptable value for reasons of practicality as shown in Fig. 10. It is evident from the curves shown in this figure that at modest challenge concentrations, one is dealing with a billion particles per milliliter to evaluate filter media. It is also evident that to evaluate media with different sizes of monodisperse latex beads, a constant number of particles should be used rather than a constant concentration. These monodisperse latex particles are commercially available in a number of diameters ranging from 0.021 to >2.0 μm. The results shown in Figs. 3, 4, 6, 11, and 12 are based on the use of this particular monodisperse latex bead test technique.

7.2 Dye Testing

As developmental efforts led to the surface charge modification of ever finer pore size media, even the monodisperse latex test was impacted by interference from mechanical straining effects. To deal with this situation, a test technique was developed based on the use of metanil yellow, a water-soluble anionic dye with a molecular weight of approximately 375. The dimensions of this molecule are approximately 18 Å long by 9 Å wide (Graham, 1955), allowing it to be used as a test contaminant for almost any charge-modified media down into the microfiltration range without interference from mechanical straining effects. In this test method, the media sample is challenged, at a specified constant flow rate, with an aqueous dis-

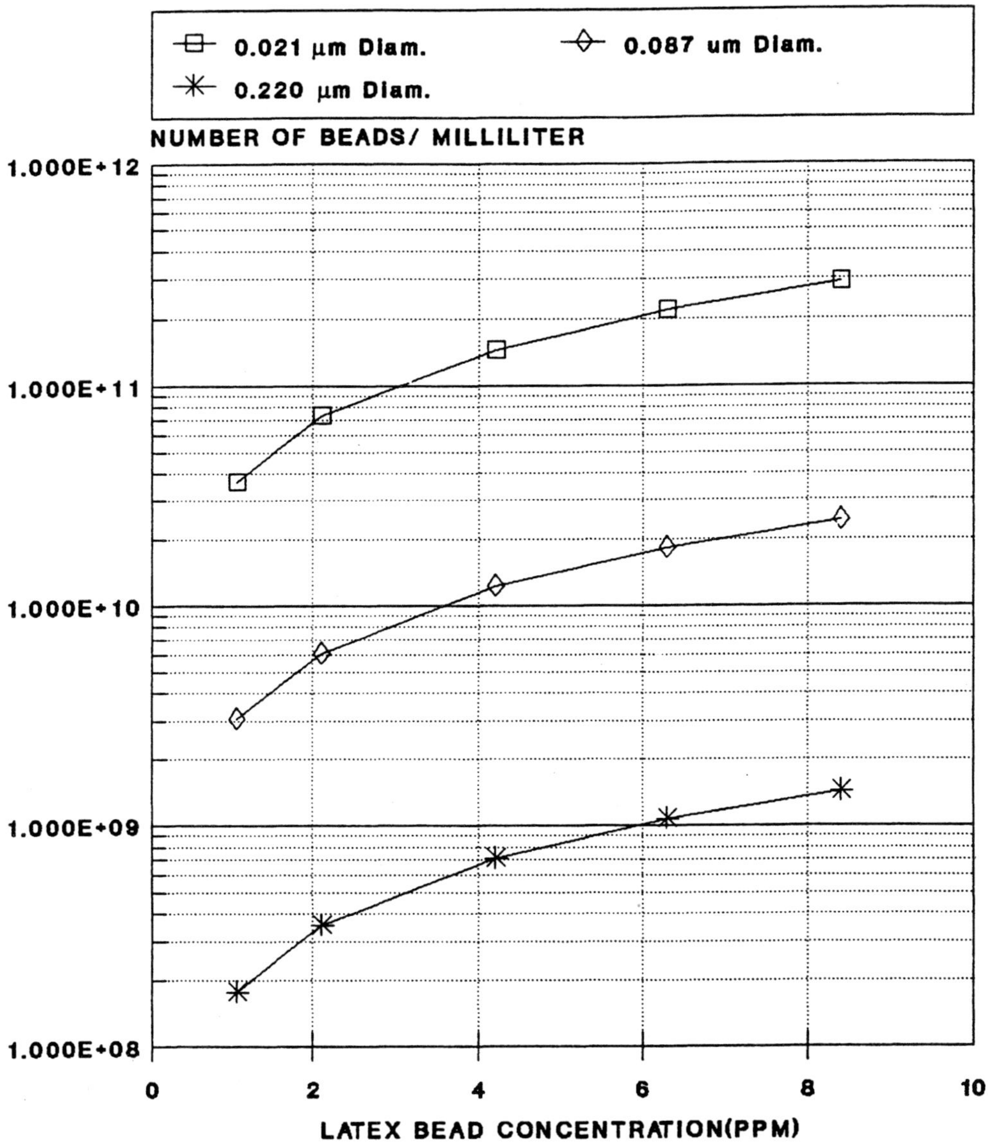

Figure 10 Number of latex per milliliter vs. latex bead concentration for beads of different diameters.

persion of metanil yellow adjusted to a specified pH and resistivity, and light transmittance is measured with a spectrophotometer. The light transmittance of the effluent is measured and recorded as a function of throughput.

7.3 Surface Charge Measurements

Surface charge cannot be measured directly or quantified by indirect techniques. Such indirect techniques as streaming potential (Knight and Ostreicher, 1981) for porous filter media allow the measurement of the potential at the hydrodynamic shear plane (zeta potential). The zeta potential is an important indicator of the electrokinetic status of a filter material and can be used to determine the capacity of a medium for contaminant and to determine its efficiency, as is shown later. Zeta potential is defined as the potential at the surface of shear between a liquid and a particle or a surface. It cannot be directly measured but can be calculated, for example, from streaming potential measurements, which is one of a series of four electrokinetic effects, the others being electrophoresis, electroosmosis, and sedimentation potential. All these effects are due to the disturbance of the static equilibrium conditions in the electrical double layer that exists at a solid/liquid interface.

The capillary pore model is used to demonstrate the concept of charge-modified membrane and is shown in Fig. 11. In this case, the capillary represents one pore of a network of pores. The wall of the capillary is shown as having a layer of positively charged ions attached to the capillary wall, with an equal number of ions of opposite charge loosely distributed in the second layer. The surface of shear, as indicated in Fig. 11, creates an imbalance in charge due to laminar flow of fluid through the capillary.

Streaming potential is the electric potential that is developed when a liquid is forced through a capillary or a network of capillaries such as a microporous membrane. It is due to the pressure drop across the end of a capillary or a porous plug such as a microporous membrane containing a liquid. The fluid flow created by the pressure drop across the capillary creates a disturbance in the electrical double layer, which sets up an electric potential across the ends of the capillary or porous medium. This potential can be measured directly by using a pair of inert electrodes in an external circuit of high impedance, so that all the current is forced to flow back through the system being measured, in this case a capillary. An apparatus for measuring streaming potential on a charged glass capillary is shown in Fig. 12. It should be obvious from Fig. 12 that a simple test apparatus can easily be assembled to evaluate the charge characteristics of filter material, whether it be microporous membrane, felted filter medium, or granular material.

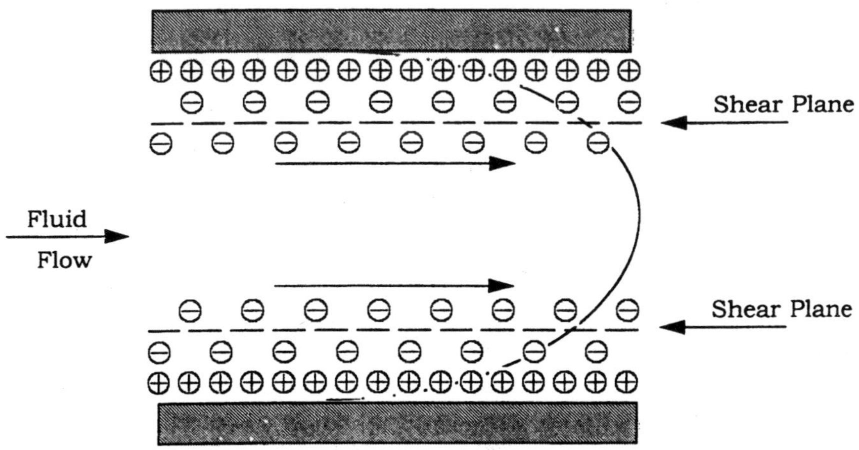

Figure 11 Ion distribution near the wall of a positively charged capillary.

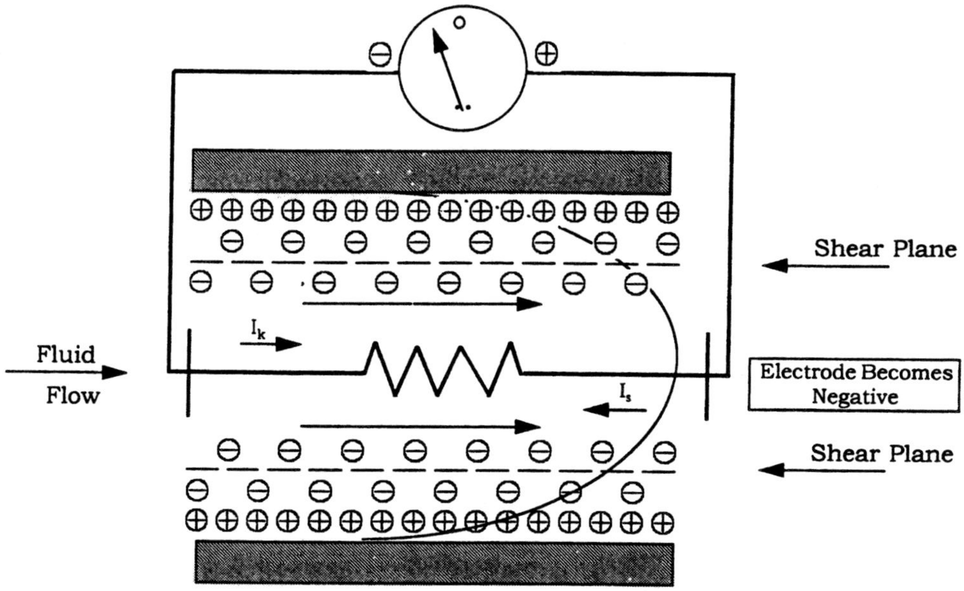

Figure 12 Ion distribution near the wall of a positively charged capillary with measuring circuit.

The relationship between the zeta potential and the surface potential is, however, a subjective one that depends on the ionic species and their concentrations in the test fluid. These test techniques are suitable for qualitative evaluations of the filtration mechanism and the effect of pH on both the charge modification process and the filtration process.

The monodisperse latex and dye tests are capable of providing a quantitative measure of the adsorptive capacity of a charge-modified filter medium. For reasons that are discussed later, the test results are sensitive to both the ionic content (species and concentration) and the pH of the test contaminant dispersion. Precise control of these two factors is critical to the reproducibility of the test results. Because of the abbreviated time frame, they are sensitive to the initial short-term pH shift and ionic extractions induced by the filter medium sample. Streaming potential measurements (Knight and Ostreicher, 1981) show that a potentially significant period of time is required for the media double layer to come into equilibrium with the bulk solution. Experimental precision requires that these factors be recognized and dealt with.

The electrokinetic behavior of colloidal particles, especially as it influences particle interactions and stability, has been the subject of a great deal of theoretical and experimental investigation, and there is an extensive literature available dealing with this aspect of electrokinetic phenomena. Unfortunately, no similar effort has been expended to investigate the electrokinetic interactions between colloidal particles and porous filter media. Cuno investigators were able to develop a "working" model of these interactions based on empirically derived understandings.

Wnek (1979), using the electrokinetic perspectives of colloidal chemistry, proposed that asbestos owed its unique filtration characteristics to the strong positive surface charge that it possessed at neutral and lower pH. He further proposed an operative filtration mechanism for such positively charged filter media that consisted of electrokinetic capture (via attractive double layer interaction) and adsorption of negatively charged particles, which in turn resulted in modification of the surface charge on the media from positive to negative. This, he further proposed, would eventually inhibit additional electrokinetic capture, allowing eventual breakthrough of the contaminant particles.

With the development of the previously described monodisperse latex bead test, it became possible to experimentally verify the breakthrough phenomena for cellulose-asbestos filter media (see Fig. 3) and, subsequently, for other forms of charge-modified filter media as shown, for example, in Figs. 4, 6, and 11.

Further testing combined the monodisperse latex bead test with streaming potential measurements (Knight and Ostreicher, 1981). This use of simultaneous streaming potential and particle removal efficiency measurements allowed the defining of the real-time relationship between the electrokinetic "status" of the media and the particle removal efficiency, as shown in Fig. 13. For a positive surface charge modified medium (Zeta Plus CPX-50S), the 0.109 μm negatively charged monodisperse latex particles are, initially, essentially quantitatively removed by electrokinetic capture and adsorption. The interaction between the constant-rate latex bead challenge and the medium gives a normalized streaming potential that decays linearly from a negative value (positive zeta potential) through zero and then asymptotically approaches a final positive normalized streaming potential (negative zeta potential). Only when the normalized streaming potential approaches and passes through zero does the particle removal efficiency, as measured by effluent turbidity, start to decrease. Finally, the particle removal efficiency asymptotically approaches zero (inlet turbidity = effluent turbidity) as the normalized streaming potential similarly approaches its final value. These results appear to verify the model proposed by Wnek, subject, perhaps, to some minor modifications. On the basis of Wnek's model, it was anticipated that the streaming potential would asymptotically approach zero with contaminant breakthrough starting at a low negative normalized streaming potential and going to zero filtration efficiency at zero streaming. These tests, however, showed that the filtration efficiency did not approach zero until the normalized steaming potential approached the high positive values exhibited by the unmodified filter medium. This actual performance appears to be indicative of a discrete, rather than uniform, positive charge deposition resulting in a grossly amphoteric surface, i.e., a surface possessing a heterogeneous distribution of anionic and cationic charge functionalities.

At first glance, it would appear that the adsorptive capacity of a medium might be predictable from the initial equilibrium value of the normalized streaming potential. To examine this question, a test series was run comparing the streaming potential and 0.109 μm monodisperse latex (MDL) capacity of single- vs. double-layer media samples. The results, shown in Fig. 14, demonstrated that although the adsorptive capacity is additive, the normalized streaming potentials for the single-layer and double-layer media samples were identical. At least in this case, therefore, the normalized streaming potential did not correlate with the adsorptive capacity. The correlation between effective medium thickness and adsorption capacity did appear to indicate that total charge-modified surface area might be the primary determinant of capacity.

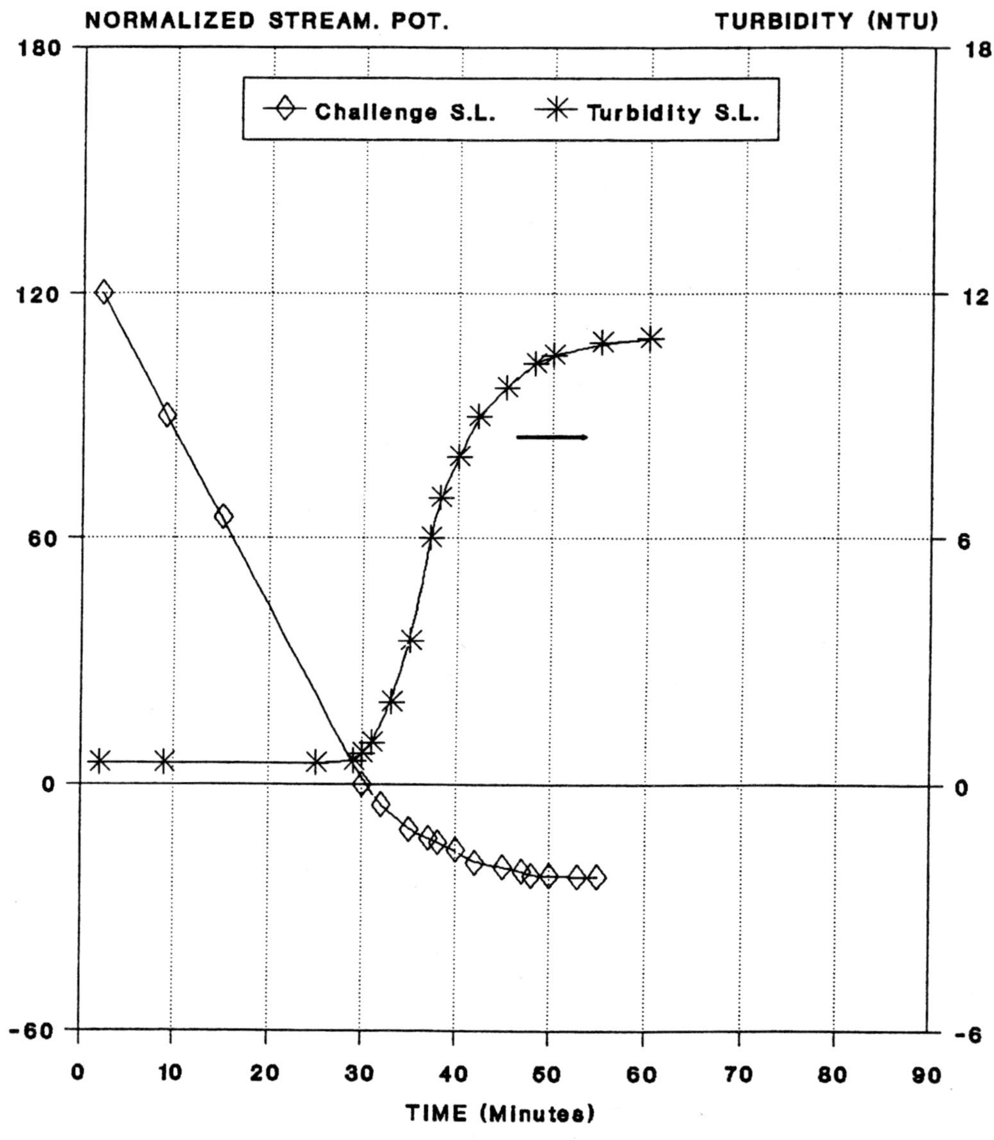

Figure 13 Results of 0.109 μm MDL bead challenge to single-layer type 50S Zeta Plus medium.

Early characterizations of the surface charge characteristics of asbestos (see Fig. 2) show a strong relationship between the electrokinetic characteristics and the pH of the water in which the asbestos fibers were dispersed. This relationship is the result of the effect of pH on the relative levels of dissociation of the various surface functional groups that, in a composite, determine the surface charge characteristics. More often than not, the surface chemistry of the systems with which we are dealing are amphoteric; i.e., both anionic and cationic functional groups exist at the surface.

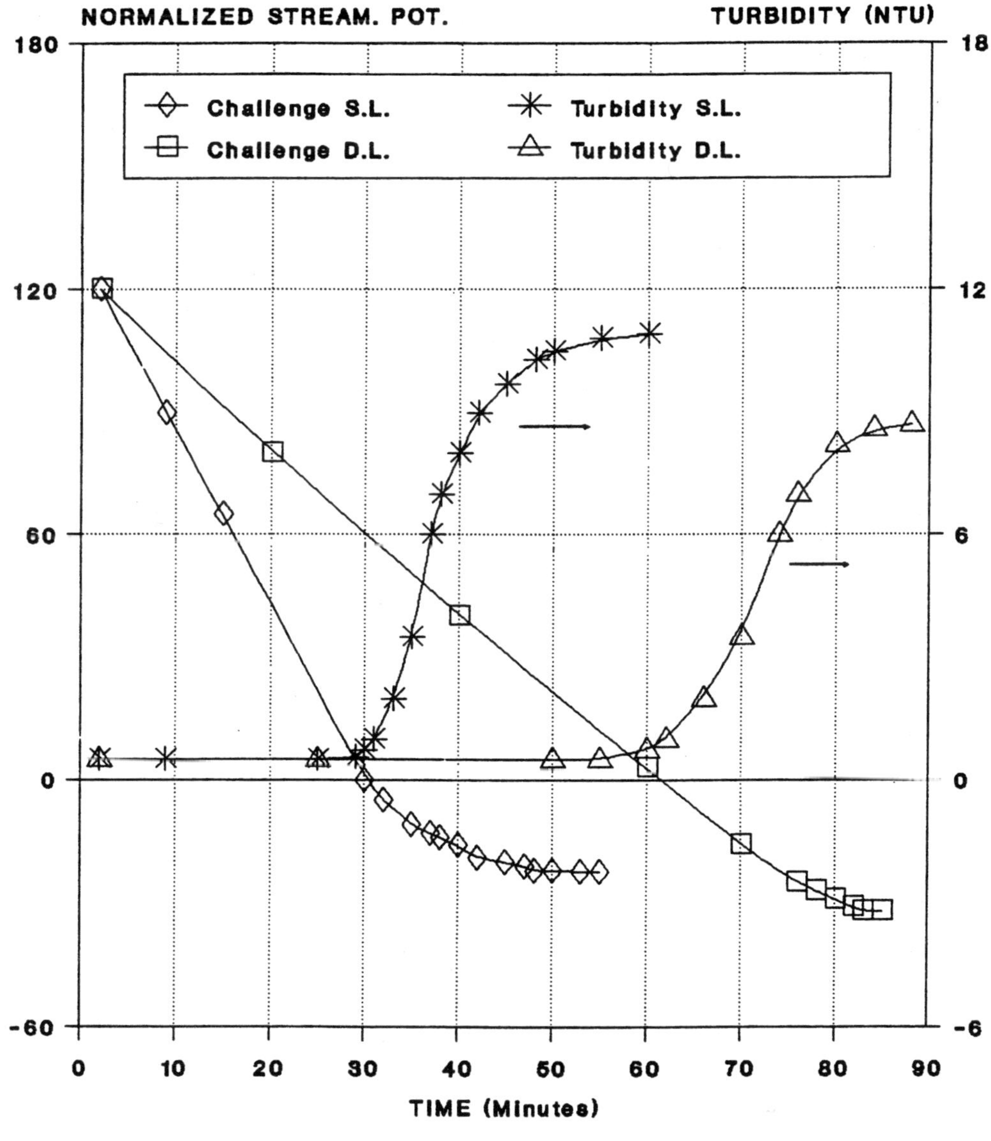

Figure 14 Results of 0.109 μm MDL bead challenge to single- and double-layer type 50S Zeta Plus medium. S.L. = single layer; D.L. = double layer.

Increasing the pH will suppress the dissociation of the cationic groups and increase the dissociation of the anionic groups, and vice versa.

Unmodified nylon 66 membrane, for example, has surface charge characteristics determined by the carboxyl and amine end groups of the nylon 66 molecule as shown conceptually in Fig. 15 and assumes that the carboxyl and amine end groups are uniformly distributed throughout the wetted pore surface.

In Fig. 16, it is seen that the unmodified nylon 66 membrane exhibits a negative surface charge at pH >6.0. Charge-modifying the nylon membrane surface with a

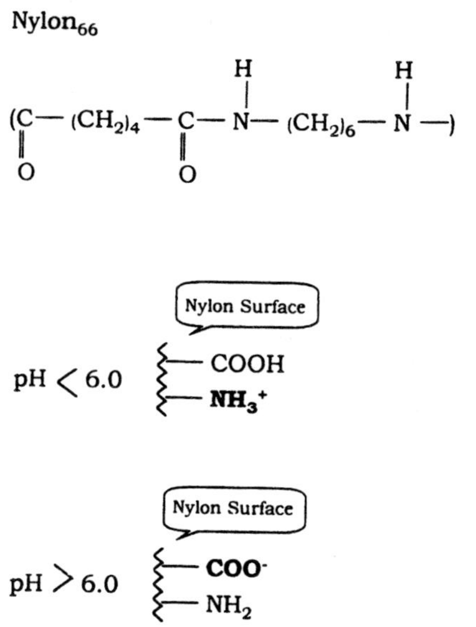

Figure 15 Surface charge characteristics of nylon 66.

strong quaternary amine charge modifier elicits a radical change in this characteristic, providing a positively charged surface up to pH 11.0.

One might expect that electrokinetic capture and adsorption performance would be impacted by pH, and in fact this is the case. The results of a metanil yellow dye challenge test on nylon microporous membrane are shown in Fig. 17. The effect of pH and type of charge modifier on membrane metanil yellow dye capacity is clearly shown.

Understanding the impact of pH on the electrokinetic capture and adsorption characteristics of a surface charge modified filter medium involves recognition that the surface charge characteristics of the medium and the contaminant change with pH. Given this combined effect, it becomes evident that pH can be adjusted to enhance and optimize the performance of charge-modified filter media, and, indeed, such techniques have been used in a number of applications.

The ionic environment plays an important role in the adsorptive capacity of charge-modified filter media. The size of the ionic double layer surrounding a charged particle or surface is controlled by the concentration and valence of the counterions in the solution. Riddick (1968) measured the electrophoretic mobility for a silica colloid in various concentrations of various electrolytes. The colloid concentration used was 100 ppm. Zeta potentials were calculated from the mobility values and were plotted against electrolyte concentration. The curves are shown in Fig. 18. Inorganic electrolytes can have a significant impact on the zeta potential. In this example, the zeta potential of a dilute solution of colloidal silica was modified by adding different electrolytes. The trivalent cation of aluminum chloride easily sends the zeta potential from a negative value toward a positive value, while the potassium sulfate, a monovalent cation, goes more negative until a plateau is reached. The zeta potential begins to rise because the high ionic concentration begins to compress the double layer.

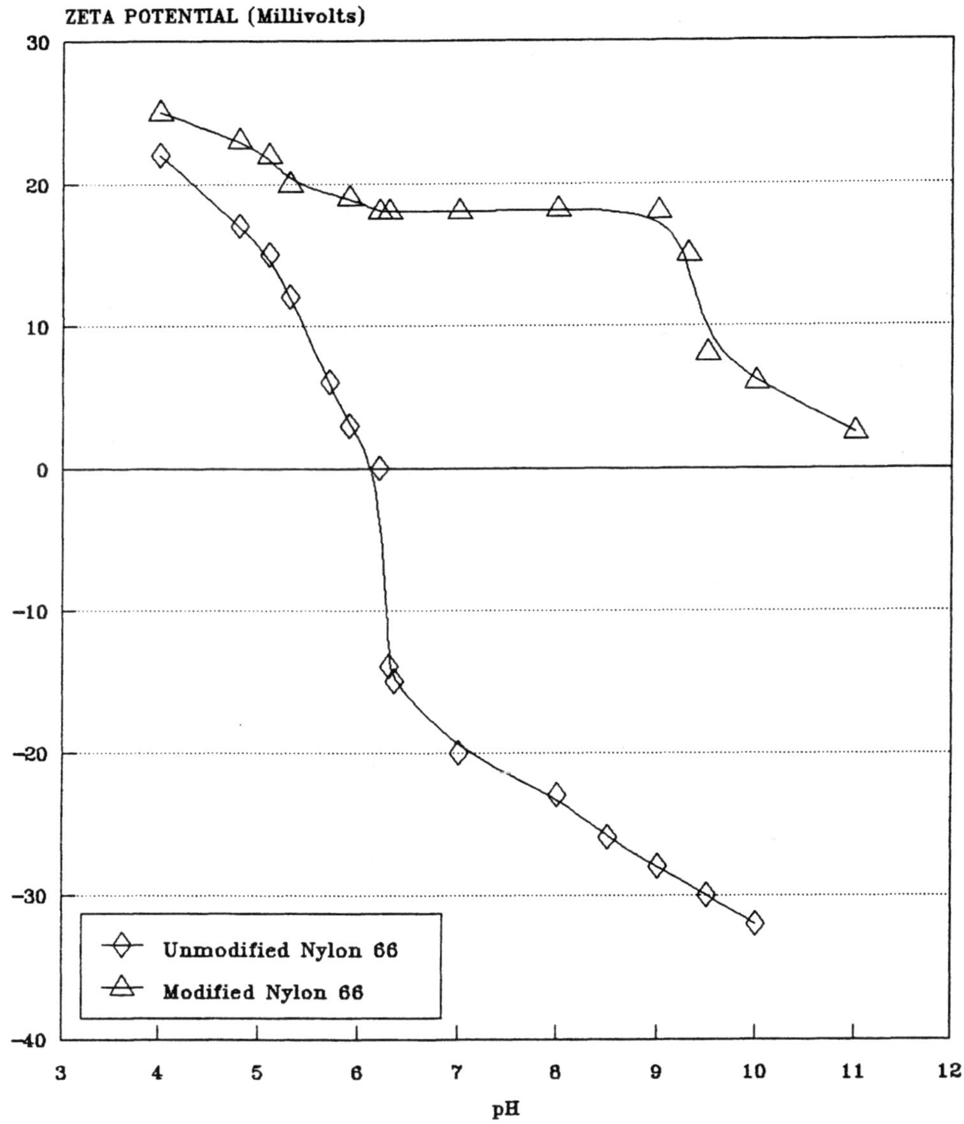

Figure 16 Electrokinetics of charge-modified and unmodified nylon 66—zeta potential vs. pH.

Increased ionic concentration and higher valence counterions reduce the thickness of the double layer, and vice versa. This has a significant impact on the repulsive or attractive interactions between particles and between a particle and the filter pore surface. The net effect of ionic concentration and valence can be, for evaluative purposes, quantified in terms of the resistivity of the solution. Decreasing the resistivity of the solution will increase the adsorptive capacity of a charge-modified filter medium. It does so, apparently, by reducing the thickness of the double layer surrounding the contaminant particles. Since there is a repulsive double-layer interaction

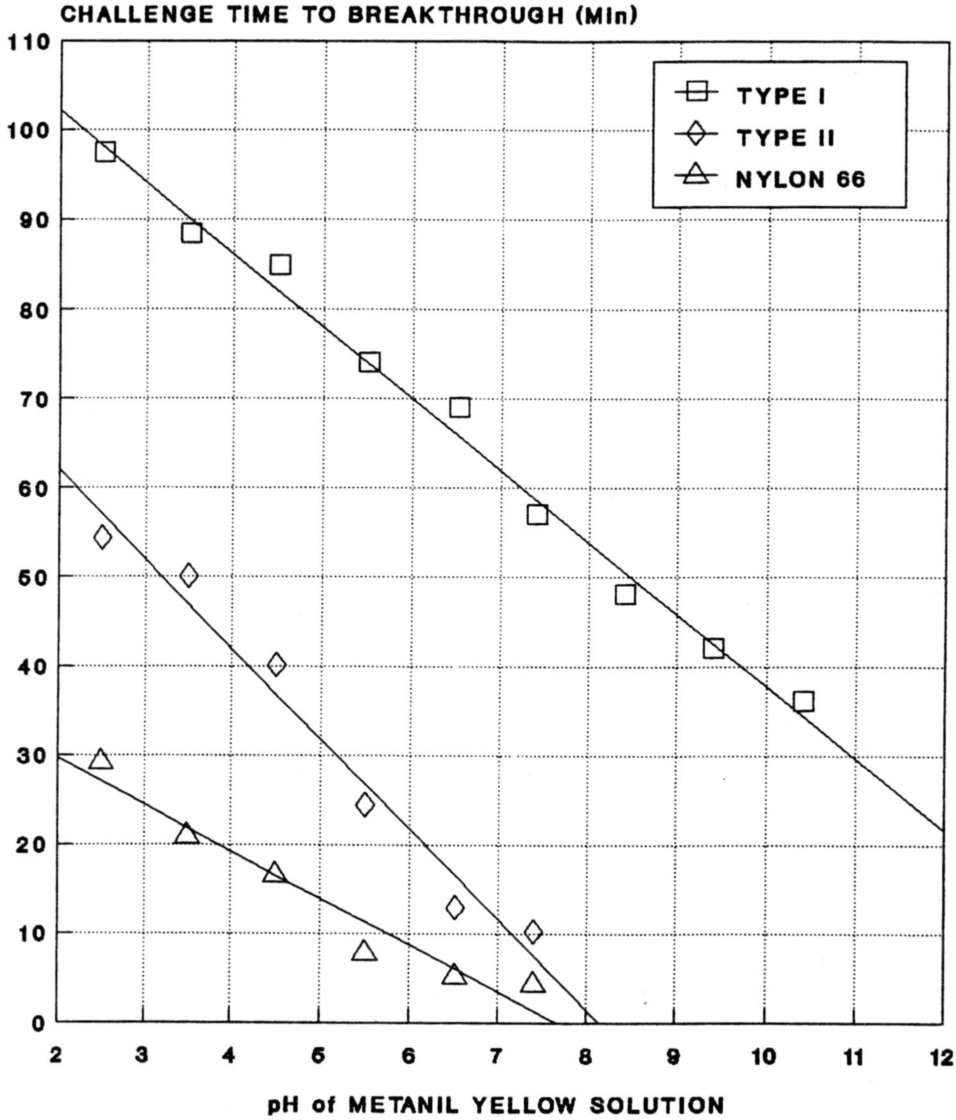

Figure 17 Effect of charge modification type on metanil yellow challenge capacity—pH vs. time to breakthrough.

between particles, this reduction allows the particles to approach each other more closely and decreases the amount of "space" taken up by an adsorbed particle on the oppositely charged filter medium pore surface. In one particularly interesting test, a Zeta Plus sample was subjected to a low conductivity 0.109 μm monodisperse latex bead challenge and run until breakthrough occurred. At that point, a salt was added to the contaminant dispersion to significantly increase the conductivity. As shown in Fig. 19, the effect of this salt addition was to restore the ability of the sample to adsorb contaminant particles.

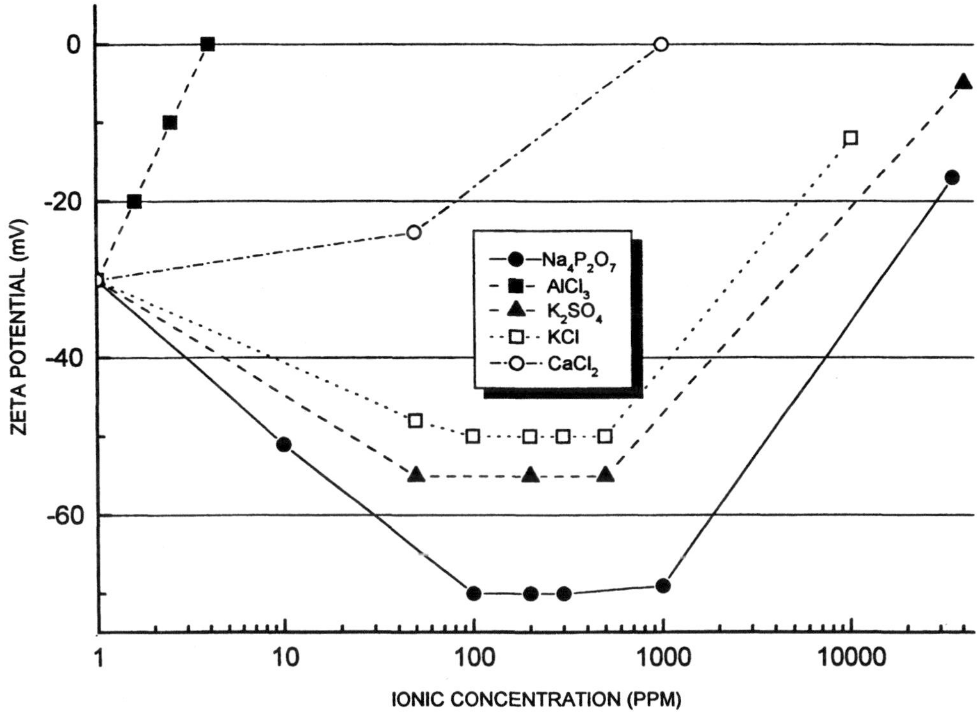

Figure 18 Zeta potential vs. concentration curves. (Reconstructed from Riddick, 1968.)

Charge-modified filter media are extremely effective in providing ultrapure water (UPW) systems. Charge-modified cartridges have demonstrated an exceptional ability to retain high concentrations of particles in semiconductor UPW systems.

The electropositive charge modification to the nylon microporous membrane enables such cartridges to remove particles much smaller than the rated pore size of the membrane. The electrokinetic adsorption and mechanical sieving have proven to be effective in removing contaminants such as colloidal silica and fragmented ion-exchange resin beads from UPW systems. The ability of such 0.04 μm membranes to adsorb 0.021 μm monodisperse latex beads is illustrated in Figs. 20 and 21.

Figure 20 shows the equilibrium flush-out of a 0.04 μm Zetapore microporous membrane subsequently challenged with a 4.2 ppm (1×10^{11} beads/mL) suspension of 0.21 μm monodisperse latex beads. Figure 21 is a scanning electron photomicrograph of the membrane challenged in Fig. 20.

8 APPLICATIONS

Charge-modified filter media are now widely used in the pharmaceutical industry for the removal or control of negatively charged contaminants such as endotoxins. Carazzone et al. (1985) investigated charge-modified filter media to determine if they were able to retain substances of opposite charge in solutions of different composi-

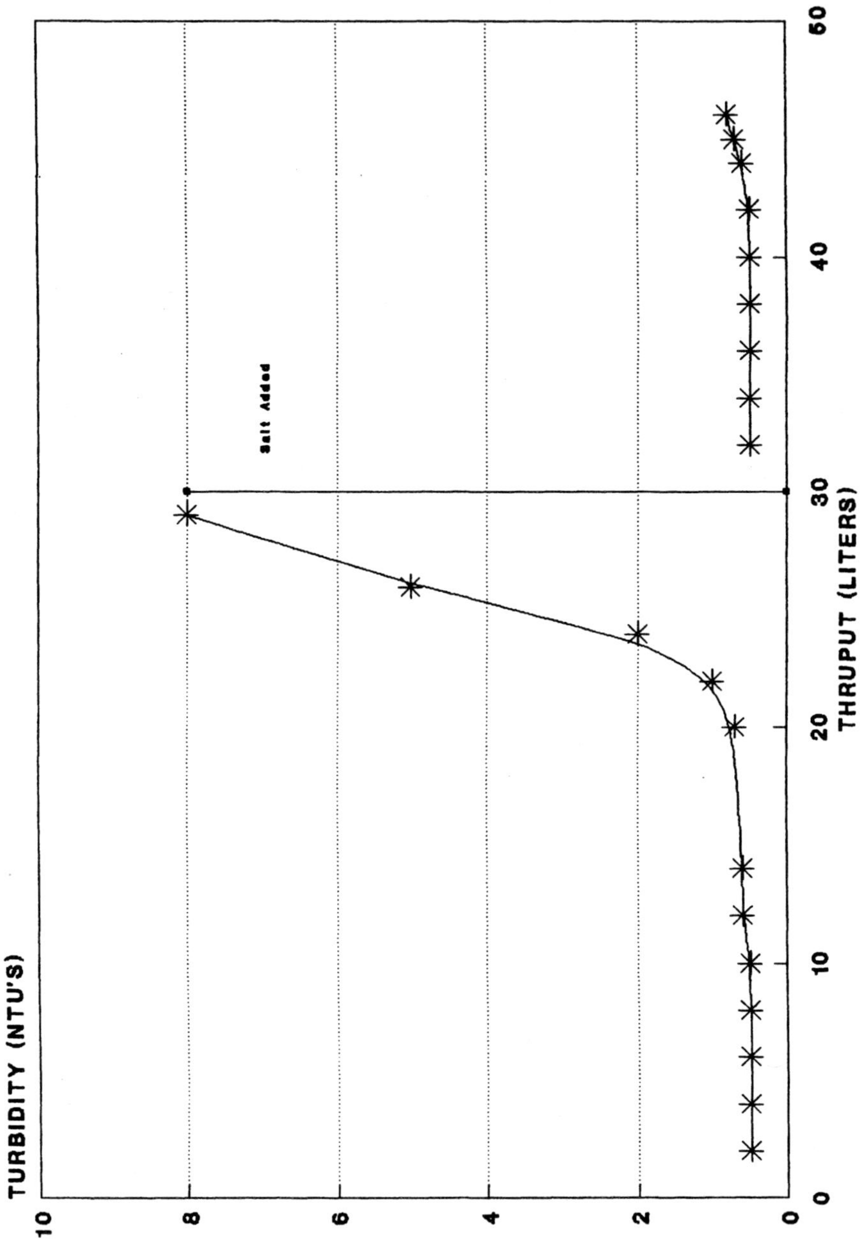

Figure 19 Effect of salt addition on adsorptive capacity.

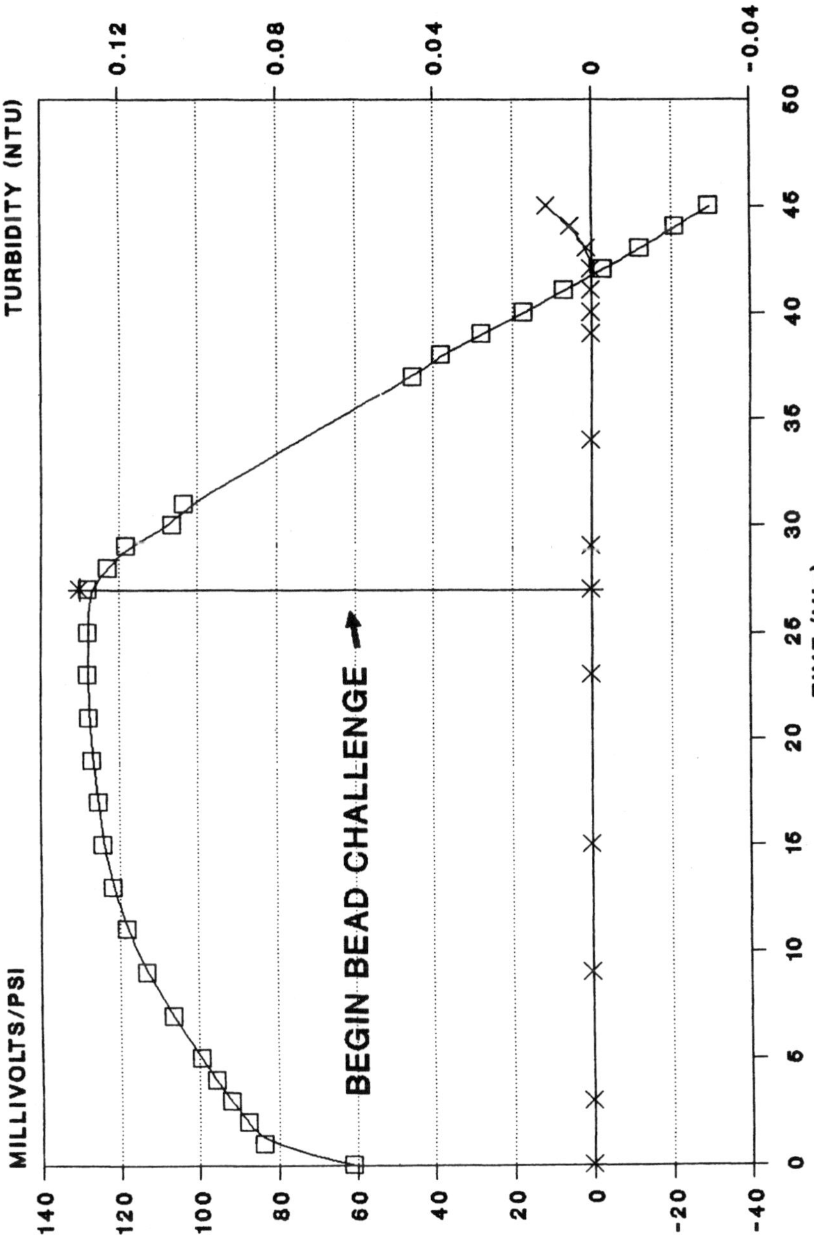

Figure 20 Streaming potential challenge curve. Challenged with 0.021 μm monodisperse latex beads (4.2 ppm).

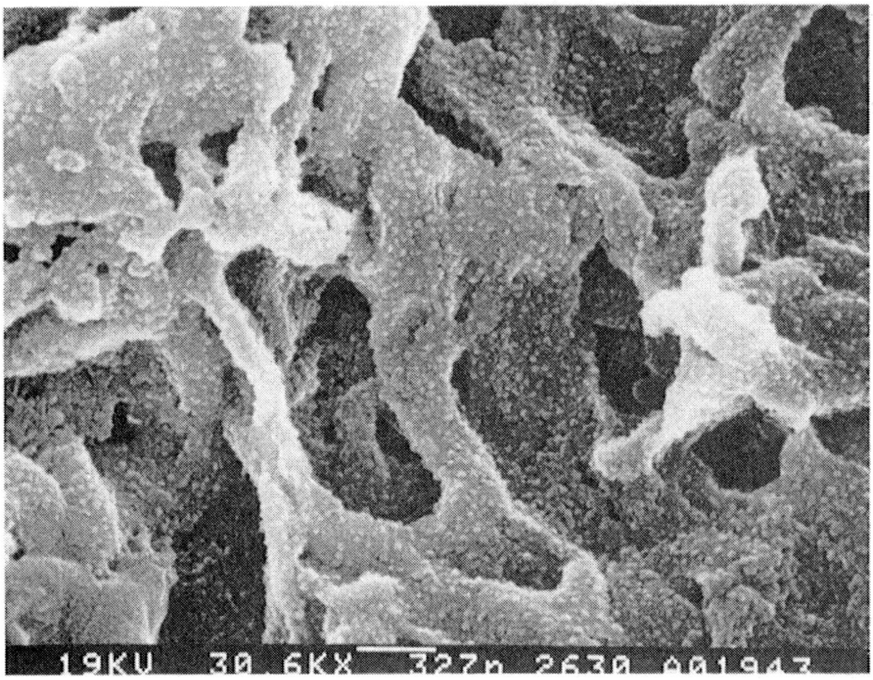

Figure 21 Micrograph of a 0.04 μm Zetapor membrane subjected to 0.021 μm monodisperse latex bead challenge.

tion, i.e., in both electrolytes and nonelectrolytes. The endotoxin used in this study was extracted from *E. coli* B5. Carazzone et al. found that (1) the removal of pyrogens to below detectable limits from distilled water is possible using both 0.2 and 1.2 μm charge-modified membranes, and (2) in the presence of 0.9% NaCl solution, neither the 0.2 or 1.2 μm membrane depyrogenated the challenge solution and, similarly, neither set of charge-modified membranes removed the endotoxin in a 2% peptone solution.

Evaluation of the same charge-modified filters with *Serratia marcescens* produced similar results in that organism retention was higher for charge-modified filters than for conventional membrane filters and the presence of electrolytes or peptone significantly reduces the efficiency of the charge-modified membrane.

Carazzone concluded that "the efficiency of positively charged filter media to remove pyrogenic substances and to improve microorganism removal from solutions vary with the composition of the solution to be filtered and with the pre-filter and final filter used."

Wickert (1993) reviewed the work of Barker and coworkers, who conducted a validation study to quantify the endotoxin removal capacity of charge-modified filters in water systems while evaluating the effect of flow rate, temperature, and steam sterilization conditions. The test system consisted of a 0.45 μm positively charged prefilter, a 0.2 μm positively charged filter to remove the endotoxin, and an additional 0.2 μm positively charged filter to retain endotoxin that might break through. All three filters were connected in series. The system was challenged with *E. coli* 0.55:

B5 purified endotoxin suspended in 0.5 mM EDTA at a challenge level of 8×10^7 EU. Variations in pH above 3 did not significantly affect the filter performance, but reducing the flow rate appeared to increase the filters' capacity for endotoxin. The effect of temperature and steam sterilization interval did not have an effect on endotoxin removal and therefore did not affect the stability of the charge modifier. Wickert concludes, "The information on the effect of varying process parameters also demonstrates the capability of this technology and confirms its flexibility."

Nagasaki (1988) evaluated nylon 66 charge-modified and unmodified filter cartridges after 5 months of identical service in a semiconductor high purity water system. He found that one of the key benefits of charge modification is that the membranes are much less susceptible to hydrolysis, speculating that the protection mechanism was the cross-linking of the charge modifier and the nylon. Hot water exposure testing was performed on both charge-modified and unmodified membranes. The result showed that the charge-modified membranes maintained elasticity, whereas the unmodified membranes became brittle after 2000 h of exposure. He concluded that "the added stability of the charge modified membrane is therefore another important factor to be taken into account in selecting a filtration system."

9 CONCLUSIONS

The current understanding of normal electrokinetic phenomena offers a particularly comprehensible or technically satisfying definition of why a given charge-modified medium functions at all, let alone so well. Understanding asbestos allowed us to create a significant new technology. We can only believe that further understanding of the mechanisms involved will lead to the creation of both new products and new applications.

Understanding of the mechanisms involved has been, for the most part, empirically derived. Much work remains to be done in terms of optimizing both the products and the applications. This, in turn, demands a more rigorous understanding of the chemical and electrokinetic phenomena involved both in producing a surface charge modified medium and in applying such media to both existing and new applications. It is known from practical experience that charge-modified filter media provide unique separation capabilities in systems where "normal" electrokinetic phenomena are probably not operative. The use of surface charge modified filter media to provide improved filtration performance has become an accepted technology.

REFERENCES

Barnes, R. G., C. Chu, G. T. Emond, and A. K. Roy. (1984). Charge modified microporous membrane process for charge modifying said membrane, and process for filtration of fluids, U.S. Patent 4,473,475.

Baumann, E. R. and C. S. Oulman. (1970). Polyelectrolyte coatings for filter media, *Filtr. Separ.* *7*(6):689.

Biles, B., and T. R. Emerson. (1968). Examination of fibers in beer, *Nature*, *219*:93.

Brown, D. G. (1980). Microbial contamination associated with hospital fluids, *CRC Crit. Rev. Environ. Control*, p. 279.

Burns, D. E., E. R. Baumann, and C. S. Oulman. (1970). Particulate removal on coated filter media, *J. AWWA 62*:121.

Carazzone, M., D. Arecco, M. Fava, and P. Sancin. (1985). A new type of positively charged filter: preliminary test results, *J. Parent. Sci. Technol.*, *39*(2):69–74.

Cohn, A. J., et al. (1946). A system for the separation into fractions of the protein and lipoprotein components of biological tissues and fluids, *J. Am. Chem. Soc.*, *69*:459–475.

Cummings, A. B. (1936). Electropositive composition and method of making the same, U.S. Patent 2,036,258.

Cunningham, H. M., and R. Pontefract. (1971). Asbestos fibers in beverages and drinking water, *Nature*, *232*:332.

Elliott, R. D., and M. J. Elliott. (1938). Filtering, U.S. Patent 2,106,318.

FDA. (1973). Asbestos Particles in Food and Drugs: Notice of Proposed Rulemaking, Food and Drug Admin., *Fed. Reg.* 38(188):27076.

FDA. (1975). Asbestos-form Particles in Drugs for Parenteral Injection, Food and Drug Admin. *Fed. Reg.* 40(51):11865.

FDA. (1976). Human and Veterinary Drugs, Food and Drug Admin., *Fed. Reg.* 41(31):6878.

Gerba, C. P., K. C. Hou, R. A. Babineau, and J. V. Fiore. (1980). Pyrogen control by depth filtration, *Pharm. Tech.*, *4*:83.

Graham, D. (1955). Characterization of physical adsorption systems. III. The separate effects of pore size and surface acidity upon the adsorbent capacities of activated carbon, *J. Phys. Chem.*, *59*.

Gsell, T. C., I. B. Joffee, and P. J. Degan. (1983). Polyamide membrane, Eur. Patent Appl. 0090483.

Guebert, K. W. and J. D. Laman. (1966). Removal of microorganisms from fluids, U.S. Patent 3,242,073.

Guebert, K. W., and I. C. Jones. (1967). Coated filter aids, U.S. Patent 3,352,424.

Hou, K. C., and M. Kilty. (1981). Wound cartridge filter, U.S. Patent 4,278,551.

Hou, K. C., and E. A. Ostreicher. (1981). Method for removing cationic contaminants from beverages, U.S. Patent 4,288,462.

Hou, K. C., and E. A. Ostreicher. (1982). Filter and method of making same, U.S. Patent 4,309,247.

Hou, K., C. P. Gerba, S. M. Goyal, and K. S. Zerda. (1980). Capture of latex beads, bacteria, endotoxin and viruses by charge modified filters, *Appl. Environ. Microbiol.*, *40*:892.

Howard, G., and R. Duberstein. A case of penetration of 0.2 μm rated membrane filters by bacteria, *J. Parenter. Drug Assoc.*, *34*(2):95.

Kilty, M., and A. Pernigotti. (1980). Cartridge filter and method of making same, U.S. Patent 4,230,573.

Kirk–Othmer Encyclopedia of Chemical Technology, 2nd ed. (1963). Wiley, New York, Vol. 2, p. 734.

Knight, R. A., and E. A. Ostreicher. (1981). Measuring the electrokinetic properties of charged filter media, *Filt. Separ.*, *18*(1):30.

Knight, R. A., J. V. Fiore, and J. V. Rossitto. (1982). Microporous membranes as depth filters, Presented at World Filtration Congress III (Filtration Society).

Marinaccio, P. J., and R. A. Knight. (1975). Process for producing microporous films and products, U.S. Patent 3,876,738.

Nagasaki, I. (1988). Charge-enhanced membranes for water filtration, *Solid State Technol.*

Neradt, F. (1971). Theoretical and practical aspects of sheet filtration in the wine and beverage industry, *Filt. Separ.*, *8*:263.

Nicholson, W. J., C. J. Maggiore, and I. J. Selikoff. (1972). Asbestos contamination of parenteral drugs, *Science*, *177*:171.

Ostreicher, E. A. (1977a). Particulate filter medium and process, U.S. Patent 4,007,113.

Ostreicher, E. A. (1977b). Fibrous filter medium and process, U.S. Patent 4,007,114.

Ostreicher, E. A. (1982). Process of making an improved filter media, U.S. Patent 4,321,288.

Ostreicher, E. A. (1991). Charge modified filter media, U.S. Patent 4,981,591.

Ostreicher, E. A., and K. C. Hou. (1981). Filter and method of making same, U.S. Patent 4,305,782.

Ostreicher, E. A., and K. C. Hou. (1982). Filter and method of making same, U.S. Patent 4,366,068.

Ostreicher, E. A., R. A. Knight, J. V. Fiore, G. T. Emond, and K. C. Hou. (1984). Charge modified microporous membrane, process for charge modifying same, and process for filtration of fluids, U.S. Patent 4,473,474.

Oulman, C. S., and E. R. Baumann. (1964). Streaming potentials in diatomite filtration of water, *J. AWWA*, *56*:915.

Oulman, C. S., and E. R. Baumann. (1971). Polyelectrolyte coatings for filter media, *Ind. Water Eng.* *8*(5):22.

Pall, D. B. (1975). Quality control of absolute bacteria removal filters, *Bull. Parenter. Drug Assoc.*, *29*:142.

Pundsack, F. L. (1955). The properties of asbestos. I: The colloidal and surface chemistry of chrysotile, *J. Phys. Chem.*, *60*:1218.

Purchas, D. B. (1967). *Industrial Filtration of Liquids*, Leonard Hill, London.

Riddick, T. M. (1968). Control of Colloid Stability Through Zeta Potential, Zeta-Meter Inc.

Rodman, C. A. (1952). Method of filtration by attracting sludge particles, U.S. Patent 2,613,813.

Rose, A. H. (1977). *Alcoholic Beverages*, Academic, London, p. 374.

Seitz, G. H. (1939). Filter pad and method of purifying liquids, U.S. Patent 2,144,781.

Selikoff, I. J., and D. H. K. Lee. (1968). *Asbestos and Disease*, Academic, New York.

Sobsey, M. D., and B. L. Jones. (1979). Concentration of poliovirus from tap water using positively charged microporous filters, *Appl. Environ. Microbiol.*, *37*:588.

Speil, S., and J. P. Leineweber. (1969). Asbestos minerals in modern technology, *Environ. Res.*, *2*:166.

Tanny, G. B., and T. H. Meltzer. (1976). The dominance of adsorptive effects in the filtrative purification of flu vaccine, *J. Parenter. Drug Assoc.*, *32*(6):258.

Tanny, G. B., D. K. Strong, W. G. Presswood, and T. H. Meltzer. (1979). Adsorptive removal of *Pseudomonas diminuta* by membrane filters, *J. Parenter. Drug Assoc.*, *33*(1):40.

Wallhäusser, K. H. (1979). Is the removal of microorganisms by filtration really a sterilization method, *J. Parenter. Drug Assoc.*, *33*(3):156.

Wickert, K. (1993). Validation of positively charged filters used for endotoxin control, *Pharm. Eng.*, *13*:41–45.

Wnek, W. (1979). Electrokinetic and chemical aspects of water filtration, *Filt. Separ.*, *11*(3): 237.

Yada, K. (1967). Study of chrysotile asbestos by a high resolution electron microscope, *Acta Cryst.*, *23*:704.

4
Prefilter Constructions

ANTHONY C. SHUCOSKY
Memtec Group, Timonium, Maryland

1 INTRODUCTION

The methods and materials employed in prefiltration are as many and as varied as the applications and the so-called final filters used. The notion of filtration and separation as an empirical science is reinforced when considering the unpredictability of the prefiltration event. Nonetheless, an understanding of the limitations as well as the advantages of prefiltration can greatly reduce the amount of trial and error needed to optimize a filtration and separation scheme. The idea behind prefiltration is to extend the life of more costly final filters by removing a portion of the injurious contaminants, primarily oversized, that would contribute to the premature plugging of the final filter. This classic concept and some of the various methods for applying it are covered elsewhere in the literature.

What is not covered, however, is an examination of cartridge prefilter devices in terms of their materials of construction, methods of assembly, and the importance of the materials selection and configuration design to the expected performance of the finished filter device. The prefilter can be a separate filter device in its own right, or it can be combined in some way as part of the final filter. The choice of materials and the methods of assembly obviously depend on the availability and state of the current relevant technologies at the disposal of the filter maker. Whereas the implication may be that only those interested in the actual design and manufacture of the device will benefit from such an examination, this is far from true. The filter user can benefit greatly from such information, including the simple treatment offered here. For example, a cursory understanding of the damage possible from using a woven mesh, instead of a nonwoven fabric as a membrane prefilter support layer can explain to a user why he is experiencing repeated failures in a pulsating or high viscosity fluid filtration process. Likewise, using a polypropylene fiber–based depth filter to remove nearly all particles greater than 1 μm may be doomed from the start by unreasonable expectations. Thus, understanding the inherent advantages and limitations of various prefilter constructs can help users minimize trial and error by allowing the proper placement of filters of various morphologies into the most appropriate filtration service for each design. Users can also select from among various filter designs as more informed consumers if they understand where each technology provides its optimal performance.

Because of the empirical nature of filtration already mentioned and the aura of misunderstanding that surrounds micrometric ratings, an understanding of the basics of fiber filtration technology and material selection provides users another tool that can help them quickly select from among an abundance of prefilter choices when trying to optimize a process.

The following discussion is in two sections. Section 2 addresses the relevance and impact that various construction material choices and manufacturing methods can have on a final filter microporous membrane cartridge device. Section 3 reviews the state of polypropylene fibrous depth filter design technology.

2 NONWOVEN FABRIC USE WITH MICROPOROUS MEMBRANE CARTRIDGES

Microporous membranes provide absolute levels of submicrometric particle removal from fluid streams. Applied properly, membranes can take a clean fluid and make it even cleaner to exacting and reproducible levels. This advanced technology permits the manufacture of megabite solid-state devices and injectable drugs with guaranteed sterility.

The membrane devices that routinely perform these modern miracles are able to do so only because of the use of nonwoven fabrics. These textile materials are vital to the proper functioning of the pleated membrane in a cartridge filter device. The nonwovens provide the dual function of membrane structural support and enhanced filtration performance.

The role of synthetic nonwoven fabrics in pleated cartridge membrane filters is examined here. Although many of the same concerns and guidelines apply to nonwovens used with other devices, the emphasis is on conventional pleated membrane cartridge filter devices.

2.1 Nonwoven Functions

Nonwovens provide physical protection and improve fluid dynamics and performance through prefiltration duty. Specific examples of these functions performed by nonwoven media in membrane cartridge devices include

- Protection during manufacture
- Protection and support during testing
- Pleat separation for fluid distribution
- Pleat separation for fluid egress
- Pleat support to prevent collapse
- Prefiltration

These functions are explored with the objective of familiarizing the novice to cartridge filter device fabrication with the important considerations of using nonwovens in this application. The various functions of the nonwoven for protecting the membrane are discussed on the basis of the location of the nonwoven relative to the membrane, i.e., on top of the membrane, below (under) the membrane in conventional outside-to-inside pleated cartridge design, or on both sides of the membrane.

Membrane Device Fabrication Protection

Protecting the membrane layer from damage while in use in a cartridge is an obvious role of nonwoven fabrics. Less obvious is the importance of nonwovens in protecting the fragile membrane from damage during cartridge device fabrication.

The polymeric microporous membranes available today come in a variety of robust materials. These include polysulfone, poly(vinylidene fluoride), and nylon. Most microporous membranes are made in a casting process that produces a homogeneous film. The film has discrete pore sizes, primarily in the submicrometric range. The membrane films are typically very thin, being on the order of 4–6 mils in thickness. While these modern polymer materials have broad chemical resistance and good tensile strength, they are still susceptible to physical puncture damage, damage from abrasion, or mechanical fatigue failure from overflexing.

The rigors of device fabrication (i.e., cutting, folding, stretching, melting, etc.) can weaken or damage the microporous film before the cartridge ever sees duty in filtration service. In fact, membrane cartridges will undergo the greatest stress and strain they are likely to experience when they are subjected to the intense pressures of integrity testing (an example is the bubble point test).

To protect the membrane film from damage during fabrication, it is generally sandwiched between two or more layers of support fabric. These supporting materials are typically made of polypropylene or polyester and may be nonwovens or extruded nets or meshes. Basis weights are usually low, 15–80 g/m^2. Thickness tends to be low also, on the order of 10–20 mils. (See Table 1.) Thin material is preferred to maximize the amount of membrane that can be folded or pleated into the cylindrical cartridge device.

A variety of melt-blown or spunbonded materials will work equally well as protectors of the membrane during device manufacture. The important point is that the web selected for this purpose must meet the requirements of being able to protect the membrane but not hinder the various process operations of cutting, pleating, and melting. In addition, the selected web must meet requirements for chemical compatibility and cleanliness.

Material compatibility and chemical purity must be matched with the membrane material and the intended filtration or separation application. Polypropylene is commonly used because of its broad chemical compatibility, low cost, and melting

Table 1 Web Requirements for Polypropylene or Polyester

Nonwoven type	Basis weight (g/cm^2)	Thickness (miles)
Melt-blown	15–80	5–30
Spunbonded	15–80	5–15
Extruded mesh	NA	5–20

characteristics. Polyester provides a better combination when used with nylon due to the higher melting temperatures of the two materials. Whether polypropylene or polyester is used, the polymer should be as chemically pure as possible. Virgin grades that have minimal additives are required. Heavy metals should not be used as antioxidants. FDA-listed material grades are almost always required, and the material must be nontoxic and nonpyrogenic. Testing such as USP Class V or VI and/or MEM elution may also be requested.

Some polymeric materials such as polypropylene are sensitive to UV light and atmospheric pollutant gases such as vehicle exhaust emissions. Exposure can cause discoloration over time, particularly in materials that are not stabilized. Some nylons or polyesters are susceptible to long-term hydrolysis. Such materials therefore require appropriate packaging that ensures protection from atmospheric gases, light, and moisture.

Material cleanliness must not be overlooked either. The degree of cleanliness required is dependent on the fragility of the membrane, the sensitivity of the fabrication process to damage, and the end use application. Manufacturing debris, shot, roping, or fly can damage fragile membranes or equipment such as calender rolls and thermal seamers. Needless to say, insects or carbonized polymer are not a welcome sight in the filter medium for any application from simply an aesthetics perspective. Insects, cellulose or cardboard fibers, or other debris from packaging and handling could wreak havoc in a sensitive electronic, pharmaceutical, beverage, or cosmetics application.

A vital concern in critical submicrometric filtration with cartridges is the issue of media shedding, sometimes called sloughing or media migration. The bottom nonwoven layer is the last surface contacted by the clean effluent; therefore the web must not contribute debris into the clean fluid.

As the fiber diameter of melt-blown webs decreases in size, a higher percentage of "fly" appears in the web. The fly consists of very small diameter branches off the main fibers and split fibers. These smaller fibrils are more likely to be entangled in the web than thermally fused. Pieces of these very small entangled fibrils may break or work loose and be dragged into the fluid. This is a limitation to currently available melt blowns.

Melt blowns are sometimes lightly calendered to reduce the probability of media shedding. The additional calendering step adds cost to the web and reduces permeability. Wet- or dry-laid webs and certain others rely on a chemical binder to hold fibers in place. Although some of these webs offer greater uniformity, the binder additive creates added chemical compatibility and chemical leaching concerns.

Downstream Layer

The downstream nonwoven layer adds structural support to the folded membrane in the face of the increasing differential pressure due to the fluid friction and buildup of contaminant. Selection requires a trade-off between thickness, permeability, and strength.

The downstream nonwoven layer must also promote fluid egress out of the pleat. This becomes more important as differential pressure increases due to contaminant buildup, increased fluid velocity, or increased fluid viscosity.

"Continuous-fiber" spunbonded webs of thermally fused polymeric polypropylene or polyester are frequently used as the downstream layer. The spunbonded webs are preferred over melt blowns because of their far superior strength. Spunbonded webs are stronger due to the greater molecular orientation of the individual fibers achieved by controlled drawing (during the manufacturing process) and the larger and more uniform fiber diameter.

Another choice is to use an extruded netting or mesh as the downstream support layer. Since the netting is homogeneous and "fiber free," it can be cleaner (less prone to shed) when used as the downstream layer. Nets or meshes are often made with different surfaces on either side, i.e., biplanar. If one side is raised and the other side is smooth, the orientation of the web in contact with the membrane may be important in preventing damage to the membrane or enhancing flow properties.

Extruded nets and meshes also tend to be thicker than nonwoven webs used for membrane support and may have less open area or porosity. The heavier netting may be an advantage when extra support is required or a hindrance when maximum area is required. The open spaces, windows, or "pores" of a net can create other problems in service.

Under certain conditions of high differential pressure across the membrane, the membrane can be forced tightly against the net surface. This can cause the area of membrane in contact with the solid structure of the net to essentially reduce or completely block fluid flow in those areas. Lateral flow out of the membrane can also be reduced. This increases the differential pressure even more, causing the filter to reach terminal or change-out pressure with some pores left unplugged with contaminant (i.e., with some unused life left).

The open areas of the net constitute unsupported areas of the membrane. Under increased differential pressure, some highly flexible polymeric membranes (like those made of PTFE) can stretch and deform such that the membrane "bulges" in these unsupported areas in response to the pressure gradient. The membrane pores are likewise altered. This may jeopardize the absolute retention of particles of certain sizes or shapes.

Upstream Layer

Maintaining proper fluid flow dynamics above the membrane is equally important. The upstream nonwoven layer must keep the flow channels open between adjacent pleats. Without proper support, adjacent pleats may "pinch" together and impede flow. Ideally, fluid will be transferred uniformly along the entire membrane surface from the apex of the fold to the trough. A textured or embossed surface may help in this regard.

The upstream layer has the yeoman's task of reducing the particle contaminant load on the final membrane filter. This prefiltration duty dramatically enhances the overall performance of the filtration scheme by reducing the total filtration cost and improving the filtration performance of the membrane filter. This can be accomplished by selecting appropriate media as part of the membrane device or as a separate stage filter for use in combination with the membrane final filter.

The major objective of the prefilter is to remove oversized particles so that the narrow-pore membrane layer is not prematurely plugged. Any layer placed on top of the membrane will provide some level of prefiltration. If a conscious design goal is to use the layer to optimize the life of the membrane, several guidelines should be followed.

The nonwoven layer must first be able to meet the requirements of physical protection and fluid dynamics addressed above. It is important that these protective layers not contribute significantly to fluid resistance. Thus, high permeability is a requirement. Frazier values of several hundred cubic feet per minute per square ft are common. Given this, attention can be focused on the filtration removal efficiency of the nonwoven. The easiest parameters to use as a measure of this are mean (flow) pore size, pore size distribution, and bubble point. The mean pore size correlates fairly well to the expected nominal retention efficiency of the nonwoven as filter medium. A narrow pore size distribution is generally preferable.

The conventional method for designing prefiltration relies on trial and error and is application-specific. The process begins by using a prefilter just slightly more open than the final filter. The combined prefilter and final filter system is run under actual operating conditions, and the increased (life and economic) benefit is measured. (A benchtop or small-scale test is often run first if a full-scale test is not practical.) If the prefilter plugs too quickly, a more open medium is tried. This can replace the first layer or be added to it in a staged or serial filtration approach. This procedure is repeated until the process is optimized in terms of the desired filtration and cost objectives.

It should be obvious that unless a filter is being designed for a specific application with fairly repeatable or consistent process conditions (i.e., contaminant load, particle size distribution, flow conditions, etc.), then what works in one application may not work in another. In addition, current nonwoven technology can produce webs with mean pore sizes down to about 1.0 μm that have reasonable permeability attributes when used alone. However, when a nonwoven this tight is used as a prefilter layer with a membrane, permeability may become a limiting factor in the performance of the membrane device. Consequently, the use of nonwovens pleated with membranes for precise prefiltration control is very limited at this time. A more reasonable approach is to use a separate filter device, or a series of staged pore size devices, composed of nonwoven filter media apart from the final membrane filter cartridge. The same method of trial-and-error optimization is used, but since the prefilter is now a separate device it can be sized on its own as a unit process.

In prefilters made entirely of nonwoven webs, several individual filter medium layers of increasing pore sizes can be combined into a single graded pore structure filter medium. The use of nonwoven prefilters can dramatically extend final filter life, thus improving the filtration economics. Historically, a separate prefilter usually extends the final filter life by 1.5–2 times. The novel use of multilayer designs can improve this manyfold. Figure 1 shows the results of using a multilayer nonwoven depth filter cartridge as a prefilter for a 0.45 μm membrane disk in a city water filtration system. The prefilter cartridge is made of layers of various pore sizes to create a graded cross section of large pores to small pores from the upstream side to the downstream side. The data document the increased service life of the final membrane and prefilter system. The benefits that can be derived from properly matched multilayered nonwoven webs are obvious.

The continuing challenge is the construction of better nonwoven webs that can be incorporated into these devices. By "better," it is meant that webs have high

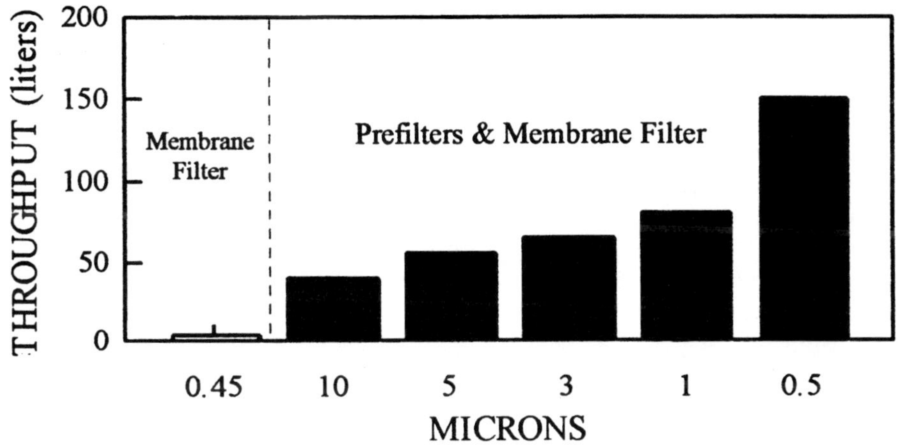

Figure 1 Prefiltration trials polypropylene nonwoven filters (Poly-Fine ARD). (Courtesy of Filterite, Memtec Corporation, Timonium, MD.)

permeability, uniform construction, and very fine retention properties. This can be achieved by making webs from the smallest diameter fibers possible.

There are, of course, many exceptions and many reasons to use different basis weights and thicknesses in conjunction with membranes based on the design of the membrane and its target application. For example, if the filter is destined for use in a slightly viscous fluid or to remove gels or deformable particles, a thicker nonwoven layer, or a combination of several thin layers, may be used to sequester the deformable or shear-sensitive particles. Left unrestrained, the deformable particles can spread across the membrane surface and prematurely blind the microporous sieve layer.

2.2 Summary

The proper design, selection, and application of nonwovens with membrane devices are critical to achieving the desired filtration objectives of performance and cost. The use of all types of nonwovens as part of fine filter and membrane filter devices continues to expand. Performance and low price are twin requirements, but performance takes precedence in this typically high end application.

To properly service this application it is important for nonwoven suppliers to learn more about the requirements of their customers. To the extent that a user understands the influence that the material construction can have on filter performance, he can select from among a variety of offerings or specify his requirements to a filter supplier.

The availability of nonwovens with ever finer fiber diameters, greater web cleanliness and uniformity, and in more engineered polymer materials will permit continued improvement in the performance of membrane filter systems and in their economic use in expanded application opportunities.

3 DEPTH PREFILTER CONSTRUCTION TECHNOLOGY

3.1 Introduction

The polypropylene depth filter cartridge offers a unique combination of performance and low cost characteristics that make it a logical and almost unbeatable choice for many industrial, food and beverage, electronic, coating, and general-purpose filtration uses [1]. In recent years, improvements in depth filter designs have increased the advantages of using depth filter cartridges in more and more applications. The characteristics of depth filtration that make it a universally accepted first choice for fine filtration are described below as well as the technological advances that have led to the current offerings. A new approach in melt blowing technology is described that produces a significantly improved design that combines a variety of desirable features into a single prefilter construction.

Depth vs Surface Filtration

In the accepted way of viewing the primary methods of how filters work, it is often stated that a fibrous filter medium will capture a particle from a fluid stream by either stopping the particle as it impinges upon the filter/fluid/particle interface, i.e., at the filter surface, or by trapping the particle somewhere within the internal body of the fiber matrix itself, i.e., within the depth of the filter medium. The events are not mutually exclusive; however, one or the other mechanism does tend to be the dominant one in a given application. Whether the particles are primarily captured on top of the filter medium layer or inside the filter medium simply depends on the relative size of the particles and the size of the openings in the filter that the particle encounters (actually the relationship between the entire particle and pore size distributions). If the particle is faced with a preponderance of openings that are too small for it to pass through unencumbered, then it will likely be arrested at that initial interface of particle, fluid, and filter contact. This is the traditional, fly on the window screen, or "sieve" filtration model. If, however, the particle is introduced to an array of openings that in general are larger than the diameter it presents to the openings, then chances are good that it will pass through one of the oversized entryways. Once inside the fibrous filter matrix, the particle will find itself in every-increasing proximity to the surface of one or more of the filter fibers or "pore" walls. As the particle is carried along in the fluid stream it may be forced to change direction, slow down, or find the random pore opening that is sufficiently small to capture and hold it.

Thus depth filtration uses the internal empty space, or voids volume, to hold particles. This very "open" design of a depth filter has at least two filtrative advantages over a filter designed to capture particles on the surface where the fluid, particles, and filter meet. First, the open design may be less restrictive to fluid flow. The fluids can move through the large openings with greater ease than through smaller ones. Second, these same openings can contain a larger quantity of contaminant before becoming so restrictive that the plugged filter must be replaced with a new one. The long service life and relatively low unit price contribute to the economic advantage of using disposable cartridge depth filters.

From a particle removal perspective, the depth filter, with its tortuous pathways and layer after layer of randomly intermingled fibers, presents the particle with a broad distribution of pore sizes. This feature makes depth filters an excellent choice for prefiltration, particularly where the particle size distribution and concentration are somewhat variable. This "forgiving" nature of depth filters contributes to their versatility of use and helps explain their widespread acceptance. Since particle capture may rely to a large extent on the chance of particle–fiber contact, the number of particles of any given size that are removed is somewhat unpredictable. The likelihood of fiber–particle contact can be increased if the particle moves more slowly or follows a longer path through a filter medium [2]. This can be accomplished by using a greater filter area (more filter cartridges) or a lower, steadier (nonpulsed) flow rate. Particle release under pulsing conditions or in response to increasing differential pressure is a drawback of classical depth filters [3].

Improving Depth Filter Cartridge Performance

Depth filters have traditionally been a lower cost alternative to filtration than surface filters that have a more precisely engineered pore size distribution. Removal of "most" of the contaminating particles from a liquid stream is all that is required in many applications. This is exactly what depth filters are designed to do. However, the trend for prefiltration continues to be a need for longer service life, finer levels of filtration, and more efficient particle removal. Finer filtration and longer life are by convention a mutually exclusive trade-off. Fortunately, there have been technological advances in depth filter design that have addressed the increasing demand for lower cost and higher performance.

Fiber Filter Efficiency

There are several ways to improve the filtration efficiency of fibrous depth filters. Given a certain minimum fiber diameter, fibers can be packed more closely together to make the openings smaller. The fibers can be stacked higher (thicker), thus increasing the chances of particle–fiber contact. Stacking fibers generally creates a number of smaller openings by virtue of layering fibers over previously unoccluded openings. These two techniques reflect what has traditionally been done in the design of yarn-wound depth filter cartridges since the 1950s.

Yarn-wound filters are manufactured from "staple" fibers that are typically between 20 and 30 μm in diameter and 1–2 in. (2.5–5 cm) in length. The short fibers are twisted into a yarn that is then "wound" in a selected "pattern" that essentially packs the fiber tightly together to achieve a certain "density." A number of layers are then built up to achieve a prescribed thickness. This combination of fiber diameter, yarn-wound packing density, and thickness produces the desired filtration level [4].

This technology produces a filter that is quite good at clarifying liquids. It should be remembered that the human eye can only resolve individual particles at or larger than about 40 μm. Thus, if using a visual interpretation of "clean," a yarn-wound depth filter proves to be an effective device in this size range. Aside from a "clean"-looking liquid, an increasing number of industrial and other more critical processes require quantitative removal of particles in the 10 μm range and below. They also require the removal of larger particles with a higher level of assurance. Although yarn-wound filters are available from the 1–100 μm size range, the fiber diameter is the same irrespective of the micrometer rating. Therefore, although the filters perform adequately, the best performance for this diameter fiber and packing technology is generally in the 20–40 μm range.

Fiber Filter Dirt-Holding Capacity

Packing the relatively large fibers together to effect removal of particles less than 20 μm in diameter requires a high density. Stated another way, the porosity or percentage of voids volume in these filters is very low (≈0.6). The result is a highly restrictive design that may plug quickly. A "graded density" approach is used to increase the dirt-holding capacity. In this approach, the smallest pores (area of high density) are near the center support core only. The pore size increases as the density decreases from the inside to the outside of the filter. The larger openings of the outer wraps offer less fluid flow resistance and create a tapered pore design to hold larger particles near the outside of the filter. The larger openings on the outside also help prevent blinding or fouling by deformable particles. The smaller particles in a given fluid stream will penetrate farther into the filter media (or wraps), where they can be captured by the more closely packed fibers.

The graded density approach helps to increase the dirt-holding capacity but becomes less effective as the filter becomes finer (<20 μm). This is because the thickness of the tightly packed (high density) zone increases to achieve the finer levels of filtration. A yarn-wound filter in the 1–5 μm range is so tightly packed throughout its total thickness that pore gradation is minimized. This highly restrictive tight packing is required to obtain a mean pore size that is smaller than the diameter of the fibers being used. The result is a low dirt-holding capacity in spite of the graded density design. Conversely, on very open grades (>50 μm) it is difficult to space the relatively small diameter fibers far enough apart to achieve the desired mean pore size and still maintain the strength of the yarn (due to the twisting together of the short staple fibers) needed for it to be processed on the winding equipment without breaking.

3.2 Depth Filter Advances

The first major advance in depth filter design technology was made in the 1970s. The advancement was centered on the development of a "melt spinning" process that produces depth filters by extruding melted polypropylene through a series of nozzles [5]. The nozzles are surrounded by an air stream that stretches the polymer stream into a fiber mass that collects on a rotating mandrel. A compactor roller packs the fibers more tightly around the core at the beginning of the process and less so as the fibers build to the desired outside filter diameter. This filter manufacturing process thus uses the "graded density" approach to extend the dirt-holding capacity like that used in yarn-wound filters. In addition, the longer melt-spun fibers coupled with some thermal fusion that occurs in the process all but eliminate concerns about fibers coming loose and passing into the filtered effluent. Fiber "migration" can occur with the staple fiber yarn-wound filter design.

The melt-spun filter design offers several other advantages over traditional textile winding technology. First, the process produces a filter free of lubricants or finishing agents. These are additives that are processing aids necessary to process the fiber and yarn used to make yarn-wound filters. Second, the extrusion process produces a distribution of fiber diameter sizes. Although this distribution is relatively uncontrolled in this process, the mean fiber size can be smaller than the traditional staple fiber diameters. The smaller mean fiber diameter coupled with the graded density method can produce filters in the 10–20 μm range that show enhanced efficiency and life performance over typical yarn-wound products. However, filters finer than 10 μm and coarser than 40 μm still lie outside the range of optimum application for the melt spinning process.

In addition, the melt spinning process does not use a center core in the filter. Instead, the fibers are packed together on the innermost layer to form a rigid structural support layer that allows the cartridge to be used at ambient temperatures and low pressures without a separate support core. For these applications, the lack of a center core reduces the cost of the filter. The absence of a center core also simplifies disposal considerations. However, the densely packed fiber material that is acting as a "core" can become the flow restriction point for the filter. This in turn can lead to less than optimum utilization of the fiber matrix for enhanced filtration performance, particularly in filters rated at 10 μm or less. In other words, a portion of the filter matrix is replaced by a zone of highly packed fibers for structural strength purposes. This zone can become the most flow-restricting part of the filter. Its composition can therefore dramatically affect the dirt-holding capacity as well as the retention efficiency of the filter. In addition, the formation of this critical inner "core-like structure" is difficult to control and contributes to variation in filter performance.

Melt-Blown Depth Filter Design

The next advance in depth filter technology occurred in the 1980s with the advent of the first melt-blown type of cartridge that incorporated various fiber diameters as the filter was manufactured to achieve a graded pore design by means other than varying the fiber packing density. This design is based on using a variation of standard melt blowing equipment. In this process, polypropylene is extruded through a multihole die and the polymer stream is stretched and attenuated by a high velocity heated air stream. The fibers are collected on a central core mounted on a rotating mandrel that reciprocates in front of the extruder. The mean fiber diameter is changed as the filter is being made by adjusting the air velocity or one of the other variables that contribute to the formation of the fiber sizes, e.g., temperature or polymer pumping rate.

The concept of using a graded or changing pore size to enhance filtration performance is a desirable one. This technique involves nothing more than incorporating a series of prefilters into a single stage to maximize the use of the entire filter and extend filter life (dirt-holding capacity). This same concept is used in a patented microporous membrane filter design referred to as a highly asymmetric pore structure [6]. Thus, varying the mean fiber size to change the mean pore size while keeping the (packing) density relatively constant throughout provides several advantages. First, the use of smaller diameter fibers that are a result of the melt blowing process (diameters as small as 3 μm mean size) permits efficient, repeatable removal of particles from a fluid stream down to 1 μm in size. Second, the smaller fiber diameters require a smaller zone (thickness) to achieve the small particle size removal desired compared to other previous technologies. Finally, the filter is less-flow-restrictive and allows for more prefiltration zones that enhance dirt-holding capacity.

The improvement in removal efficiency from the use of multiple layers of filter media made from fiber diameters similar to or smaller than the particle size to be removed (<10 μm) brought about the notion of "absolute" removal efficiency in a depth filter design. The concept of absolute removal efficiency had previously been applied to surface "sieve-type" filter designs only. "Absolute" in the context of depth filters is based on removal efficiency values of 99% or greater of particles of the rated micrometer size. Results are obviously test-dependent.

Another advantage of relying on a graded pore size structure made from decreasing mean fiber diameters instead of tighter packing (increased density) of one fiber size diameter (or limited fiber size diameter range) is the increase in filter porosity it grants. Theoretically, an increase in porosity (to 0.7–0.8) means less flow restriction and potentially more void volume for greater dirt-holding capacity [7].

The efficiency improvements in this technology, particularly down to the 1 μm level, are significant, but limitations still exist. Unfortunately, the same small diameter fibers that enhance removal efficiency are somewhat malleable in the face of increasing differential pressure. This is particularly true when the porosity is kept high (packing density is low). The result can be a change in the shape of the filter matrix as differential pressure across the filter cartridge increases. Such a change can cause the porosity of the filter element to decrease rapidly and, in certain conditions, cause the release of particles previously captured. Applications involving the filtration of viscous fluids or variable process flow conditions are very susceptible to this "unloading" phenomenon.

The use of a small fiber diameter melt-blown matrix also produces relatively "soft" cartridge ends. These soft ends make it difficult to effectively seal a cartridge in a housing if the vessel uses the traditional knife edge sealing system found on many industrial pressure vessels. Improper sealing of the filter cartridge into the filter housing can quickly negate the advantages of any filter cartridge because contaminants can readily bypass the filter [8].

Another drawback of this technology relates to the variability that is part of the melt blowing process used to manufacture this type of filter. The manufacturing method requires that the variables responsible for changing the mean fiber diameter of the polymer stream be changed in real time as each filter is produced. Even with advanced processor controls, there is variation from filter to filter due to the randomness of the changing fiber matrix structure from the nonequilibrium conditions maintained in the melt blowing equipment.

Finally, the melt blowing process uses a standard melt blowing die that consists of a series of uniform hole sizes along the die. Melt-blown fibers are typically smaller than melt-spun, spunbonded, staple, or other fibers used to make depth filter cartridges. This enables the formation of filter media capable of fine levels of particle size retention down to the 1 μm level. Unfortunately, the process conditions typically used are not conducive to making pore size grades ≥20 μm with optimum properties. The filters produced are typically much finer than their rating would indicate. The result is often premature plugging and shorter than expected life cycles. In addition, in critical classifying applications, particles of desired sizes may be removed.

Spiral-Wound Staple Fiber Felt Cartridges

A third technology was also introduced in the 1980s that can be described as a lateral approach to optimizing the use of staple fibers to make a depth filter cartridge. In this technology, staple fibers (of a monosize diameter or narrow size distribution) made of a bicomponent structure are laid onto a web that forms a felt. The fibers are typically made of a polypropylene core surrounded by a lower melting point polyethylene outer sheath. The web of fibers is then rolled under heat and pressure to make a rigid cartridge. The process optimizes the use of staple fibers to produce a depth filter that can have less variation in performance and some higher levels of filtration efficiency in the 5–10 μm range compared to yarn-wound filters. Mechanical strength is also good; however, the same limitations of staple fiber–based technology discussed apply here. These include a graded density design, textile lubricants, limited fiber diameter range, and fine filter efficiency limits.

Absolute Rated Depth Filter Cartridges

The next noteworthy improvement in depth filter technology was introduced in 1992. The spiral wrapped (absolute rated depth) filter design optimized the use of melt-blown web technology [9]. The advantages of the melt-blown cartridge are maintained and optimized while the shortcomings of variation and unloading are eliminated. The filter media pore size gradient is accomplished through the use of the preferred method of changing fiber diameters rather than increasing media density. A depth filter structure is produced by combining separately made web layers of melt-blown media in a spiral rolled configuration. This technique allows for the widest possible range of optimized absolute rated filtration grades.

By making discrete layers separately, the filtration properties of each layer can be optimized and checked in advance of making the filter. Variation in filter performance is eliminated. A rigid support mesh is spiral wound throughout the filter. This prevents compression or change of shape of the filter medium in viscous fluids or at high differential operating pressures. The ends of the cartridge are thermally sealed with a rigid cap of polypropylene. The use of gaskets and O-rings for cartridge-to-vessel sealing eliminates bypass concerns. This design approach requires several more manufacturing steps than the methods previously described. This extra manufacturing nonetheless produces a depth filter cartridge that has high repeatability of performance for a depth filter.

3.3 Melt Blowing Advancement

The next generation advance was introduced in 1995. It incorporates the features of the available technologies combined with several new process innovations. The result is a new technology dedicated to the production of advanced melt-blown filtration media. The depth filter cartridge design is manufactured by the patented CoLD MELT process [10] or advanced melt blowing (AMB) process.

This melt-blown depth filter uses the preferred methods of varying the mean fiber diameter to achieve the desired level of particle retention and a graded pore structure to increase contaminant-holding capacity but with some unique differences. For example, the conventional method of changing the mean fiber diameter uses a single extruder machine with a fixed die. Selected operating conditions, such as air velocity, are constantly changed to effect changes in the fiber diameters. As previously described, the melt blowing process is very sensitive to small changes in operating conditions. For a highly repeatable process, the melt blowing process requires a certain period of time to produce a balance or equilibrium under each new set of conditions. The speed of the melt-blown filter manufacturing process required to make it economically feasible does not allow sufficient stabilization time. The result is a notable variation in the performance of the filters produced. The new process eliminates this limitation.

Process Features

The AMB process apportions multiple extruding machines to produce the fiber structure of each depth filtration "zone." By using an array of extruding machines to create a single filter cartridge, each machine can be optimized to operate under conditions that will consistently produce the desired fiber structure for each zone. Each machine can also use its own specially designed die and be located in a position relative to the fiber collecting point that will optimize formation of the desired fiber matrix morphology. This new approach to melt blowing technology produces a high degree of process control and repeatability that is an improvement over conventional melt blowing techniques adapted to making depth filter cartridges. The control afforded by the use of more than one extruder means that a finer graduation of fiber diameters can be transitioned from one zone to the other if desired. The greater degree of control can increase dirt-holding capacity in general, but the opportunities for tailoring the filter structure for specific application conditions are obvious.

For example, the conventional melt blowing process uses a single die to produce the entire range of retention from 1 to 100 μm. Many variables can be adjusted (as previously noted) to modify the ultimate mean fiber size. However, there is a practical limit to the effective range of fiber sizes possible given a certain starting diameter. This means that, according to basic fiber filtration principles, there is a practical limit to the effective range of optimum removal and high dirt-holding capacity for certain particle size ranges (see Fig. 2). A positive point of melt blowing is the production of very fine fibers smaller than 10 μm. While this is viewed as an advance in the state of the art of achieving "absolute" retention of particles in the 1–10 μm range, it does a disservice to processes that need high performance removal of only the particles of 20 μm or larger. An example of this is fine coating appli-

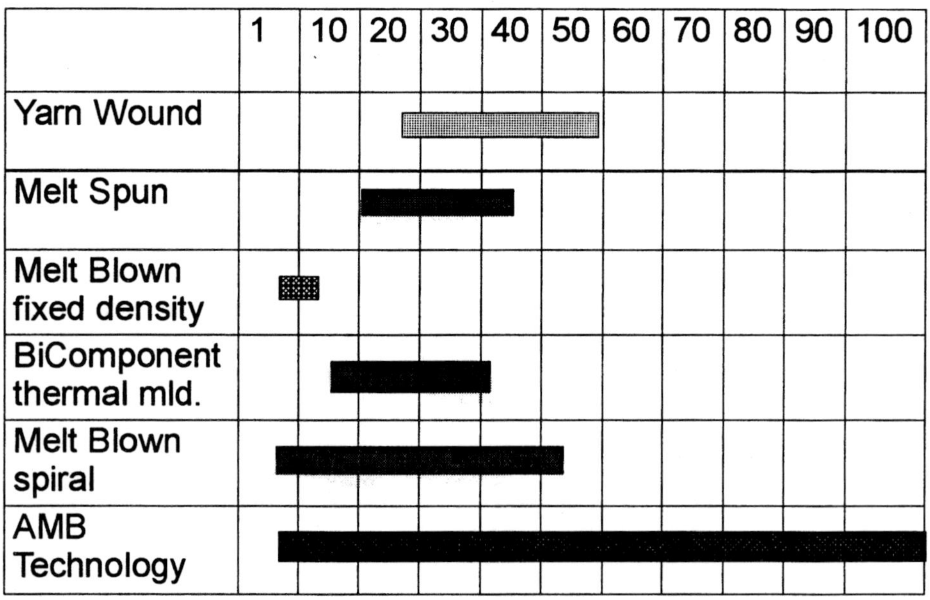

Figure 2 Optimum depth prefiltration range by technology.

cations where the classifying properties of the filter medium are paramount. Removal of desired small particles can be anything from an economic concern due to rapid filter plugging to a process disaster if the filtered product particle mix is out of specification.

The flexibility of the AMB process allows the multiple die designs to be in operation simultaneously. Thus, the filter-making process is not limited to a single fiber diameter (as in staple fiber–based processes) or a limited range of fiber diameters (as in conventional single-die melt blowing). The new patented process can produce any fiber diameter size, or combination of fiber diameter sizes, necessary to effect optimum filtration performance over the entire filtration range from below 1 μm to above 100 μm.

Another innovation of the AMB design is the addition of very large diameter fibers to the matrix of small diameter fibers that are optimized for a specified particle retention level. This is the root of the reference name CoLD, which refers to the "*co*located *l*arge *d*iameter fibers." Recall that one of the failings of using very small diameter melt-blown fibers (<5 μm) in a matrix of intermingled fibers is that the fibrous mass can change shape in response to increasing differential pressure. One consequence of this is a compression or partial collapse of the structure that can lead to increased flow resistance, variable particle removal efficiency, and reduced on-stream life cycles. Another concern is that the movement of the filter medium will release previously retained contaminant (unloading) [3] or the changed pore structure will alter the filtration characteristics of the filter.

The patented filter design selectively inserts very large diameter support fibers as a part of the fine filter matrix where they provide a rigid internal network. The added large diameter fibers perform a function similar to that of the support and drainage layers used in pleated surface media designs. These large diameter fibers allow the depth filter medium to maintain its shape in viscous fluid flow and as differential pressure increases. They also enhance the fluid transport properties of the matrix. The depth filter medium does not compress with increasing differential pressure because of the more rigid large diameter fibers. Thus flow passages and pore voids are maintained for further particle collection. This can significantly increase the dirt-holding capacity of all grades, in particular those at the fine end of the spectrum. The added strength imparted by the larger fibers also ensures positive sealing on knife edge, or "crush seal," sealing systems.

Tables 2 and Figs. 3 and 4 show comparative test results of a conventional melt-blown (CMB) depth filter tested head to head with the advanced melt-blown

Table 2 Conventional Versus AMB Technology Initial Particle Removal Efficiency

Beta ratio	Conventional melt blowing	AMB
10	5.5	7
20	6.1	7.8
50	7	8.9
100	7.7	9.9
1000	12	13

Conclusion: Efficiency unaffected by addition of CoLD fibers.

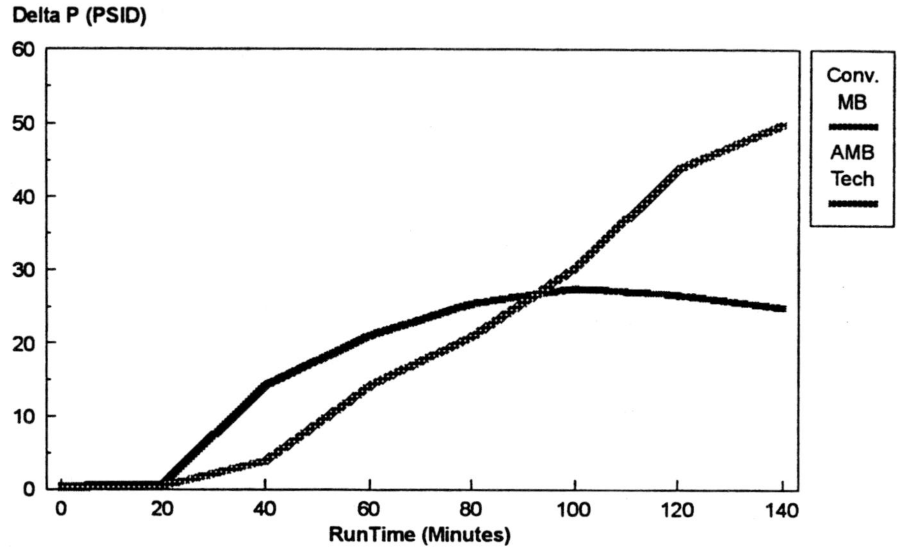

Figure 3 Conventional versus AMB technology plugging charts.

(AMB) fiber design depth filter cartridge. Table 2 shows the equivalent initial retention efficiency of the two filters. Figure 3 shows that the AMB fiber filter demonstrates a normal plugging curve over time, retaining its structural integrity. The flattening of the CMB (conventional melt-blown) filter plugging curve at about 20 psid suggests an unloading of particles. (The differential pressure does not increase because particles are passing through the filter.) This is confirmed in Fig. 4, which

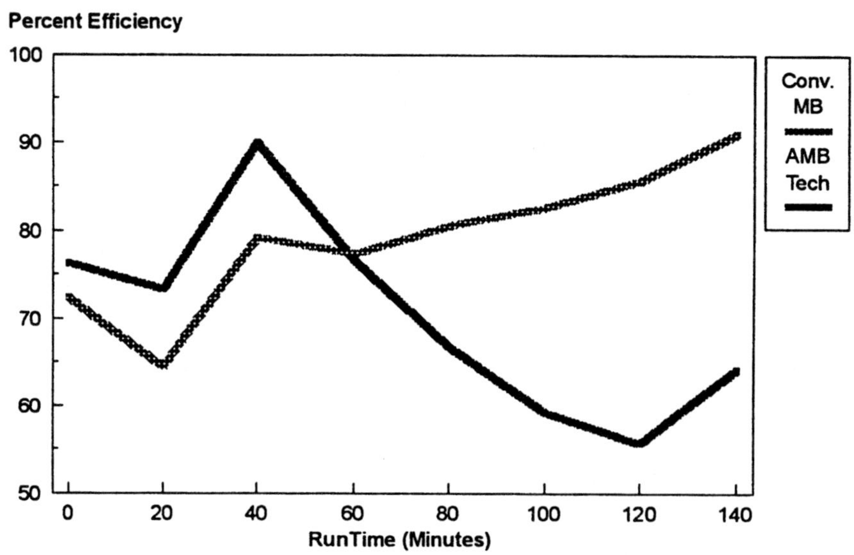

Figure 4 Conventional versus AMB technology—turbidimetric efficiency.

clearly shows the drop in turbidimetric efficiency of the CMB filter due to continuing unloading of contaminant into the filtrate.

4 SUMMARY

At least six approaches to making and combining fibers into a matrix or mass to create a depth filter cartridge design have been identified (see Fig. 2). Each technique produces a depth filter that performs best in a certain particle size range. The area of optimum performance appears to be related to several factors common to the fabrication technique chosen. The most important is fiber diameter. Yarn-wound depth filters use a fixed fiber diameter with mechanical packing differences to modify slightly the mean pore size. Advancements have sought to use smaller fiber diameters and fiber diameter distributions to increase removal efficiency and in some cases increase dirt-holding capacity. These advances have still been limited to a narrow optimum performance range because of the limited range of fiber diameters that can be made by simply combining conventional melt blowing and related technologies. Stated another way, most of the depth filter advances were made possible by marginally modifying available technology originally designed to make other products.

The recent technological advances promise a new generation of prefilter products to improve the filtration and separation performance of many filter design schemes. As those knowledgeable in the arts of filtration and melt blowing continue to combine their expertise, one can expect to see continued advances in the state of prefilter construction and a continued extension of prefilter applications into territory previously the sole domain of membrane technology.

REFERENCES

1. A. C. Shucosky, Select the right filter cartridge, *Chem. Eng.*, 1988, *95*:72–77.
2. J. J. Janas, and S. G. Meenan, Guidelines for choosing the optimum process filter, *Chem. Process*, January 1991, pp. 38–40.
3. C. J. Williams, Testing the performance of spool-wound cartridge filters, *Filtr. Separ.*, March/April 1992, pp. 162–168.
4. C. S. Hoffman, An empirical model for the design of fibrous filter media, INDA Filtration Workshop, November 1983.
5. C. M. Vogt, J. W. Soehngen, and J. C. Polise, Varying density cartridge filters, U.S. Patent 3,801,400 (to Celanese Corp) (issued April 2, 1974).
6. W. Wrasidlo, and K. J. Mysels, The structure and some properties of graded highly asymmetric porous membranes, *J. Parenter. Sci. Technol.*, January/February 1984.
7. L. C. Wadsworth, and S. B. Barboza, Relationships among melt blown web structure, air permeability and filtration, *INDA J. Nonwovens Res.*, *2*(1):43–48.
8. C. J. Williams, and R. G. J. Edyvean, Testing cartridge filters in aqueous media: interpreting the results—the pitfalls and problems. Part 2: The problems and pitfalls of cartridge filter performance evaluation, *Filtr. Separ.*, March 1995, pp. 255–259.
9. A. C. Shucosky, Absolute efficiency depth filter cartridge advances, *Filtr. Separ.*, January/February 1993.
10. A. C. Shucosky, Enhancing membrane performance with media, Proceedings of the Thirteenth Annual Membrane Technology/Separations Planning Conference, Business Communications Co., Inc., & Filtrex Inc., Newton, MA, October 1995.

5

Cartridge Filters

PETER SOELKNER and JUERGEN RUPP
Sartorius AG, Göttingen, Germany

1 INTRODUCTION

The configuration and construction of cartridge filters give them a large variety of advantages in comparison to common filter systems (flat or disk filters, etc.). Cartridges with a filter medium consisting of pleated membranes or fleeces constitute an increase in filter area in a confined and defined volume. That form of construction leads to higher flow rates, shorter process times, a lower differential pressure level, and less plant space compared to other types of filter units. These economic aspects are emphasized by a higher total throughput before the clogged filter elements have to be replaced. On the one hand this leads to lower production costs, and the reliability of the filter system is increased.

Progress in cartridge filter development has focused on mechanical and thermal stability with respect to applications in process filtration and a low extractable level afforded by the materials used for the cartridge filter. Legislation such as USP 23 of the U.S. Pharmacopeia, the U.S. Food and Drug Administration (FDA) guidelines for materials, and extractable testing under worst-case conditions developed by cartridge filter producers themselves have influenced the optimization of cartridge filters.

Cartridge filters are used in a variety of fluid and gas filtration applications in the pharmaceutical industry. Examples of applications in liquid filtration include

Prefiltration of suspensions
Final product clarification
Fractionation of suspensions
Bioburden reduction
Sterile filtration

and in gas filtration,

Retention of particles
Sterile filtration

These filter devices are used mainly in the field of microfiltration with retention rates and pore sizes of 0.05–50 μm. An application may require a combination of prefilter and endfilter cartridges to ensure both the product quality and the economy of the filtration process.

Cartridge filters and capsules for pharmaceutical process filtration are available from approximately 0.05 to 36 m^2 effective filter area in one filter device. Static filtration by cartridge filters is adaptable to processes of all sizes. A full scale-up is possible by using cartridge filters of the appropriate size and effective filter area (see Fig. 1) or their combination in multiple cartridge housings.

In general, cartridge filters are divided into two basic groups: prefilters and membrane end filters.

1.1 Prefilter Cartridges

Filter media for prefilter cartridges include a multitude of materials: fleeces of polypropylene, polyester, polyamide, resin-bonded or binder-free fibers, and other synthetics (woven and nonwoven fleece structures); sintered materials like polyolefins, metals, and ceramics; yarns; special filter papers (e.g., mixtures of fibers, cellulose, polyolefins, and binders); polymer membranes; and others. Prefilter cartridges have an effective filter area ranging from 0.05 to 36 m^2.

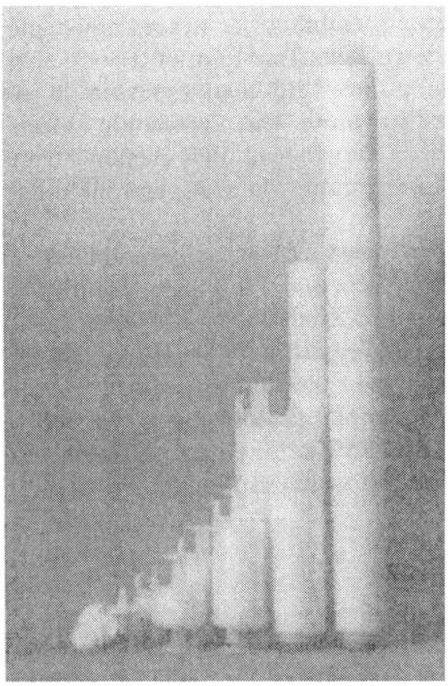

Figure 1 Cartridge filter scale-up line. (Courtesy of Sartorius AG.)

1.2 Membrane Endfilter Cartridges

Membrane endfilter cartridges incorporate testable polymer membranes based on polymer materials such as cellulose acetate (CA), polysulfone (PSU), polyethersulfone (PESU), polyamide (PA), poly(vinylidene fluoride) (PVDF), polytetrafluoroethylene (PTFE), polycarbonate (PC), and polypropylene (PP). (See Section 2.1.5.)

2 CONSTRUCTION OF CARTRIDGE FILTERS AND CAPSULES

2.1 Typical Components of Cartridge Filters

Modern pharmaceutical process filtration places high demands on the quality of cartridge filters. Due to the application requirements, cartridge filters have been optimized in their mechanical and thermal stability and the configuration and implementation of components and details (e.g., connectors) to meet the demands of sterile technology. Special attention has been paid to the selection of materials, with a focus on high performance and low extractable levels. As a result of developmental work over the past decade, the basic construction parts of cartridge filters, especially membrane sterile filter cartridges (Fig. 2) have a unique dimension and functionality.

Connector

To accommodate filter cartridges in housings, three basic types of fittings are in use: knife edges, flat gaskets, and O-rings. To ensure reliability of the seal with respect to safety against bypass, as determined by integrity testing by diffusion or pressure holding tests, and the microbiological safety of membrane sterile filter cartridges, connectors with external double O-rings are state-of-the-art integral components of the cartridge construction.

Knife-edge and flat gasket end fittings are not suitable for pharmaceutical applications. For example, the function of these types of end fittings depends on the exertion of considerable compressive force by the metal knife edges or pressure plates. According to the properties of the most common polymeric construction parts, with their tendency to expand or to shrink under thermal stress conditions [e.g., sterilization of the filter unit by in-line steaming (in situ steaming)], these adaptation techniques cannot avoid cross-contamination due to bypass of parts of the unfiltered liquid or gas stream.

Integral connectors with external double O-rings afford the best kind of cartridge sealing in accordance with the principles of sanitary design. To avoid having users replace their cartridges with competitors' cartridges, cartridge filter manufacturers at first designed their own forms of connectors. Nowadays, the manufacturers offer cartridges with the types of connectors established in the pharmaceutical industry.

The two connectors illustrated in Fig. 3 are examples of single- open-end cartridge connectors. In comparison to connector B, connector A has locking ears. These locking ears are more suitable for process filtration applications where backpressure caused by backflushing during the regeneration procedure or by an abrupt closing of valves in the downstream processing may unseat the cartridge filter or provide the opportunity for bypass. Usually multicartridge housings have plates installed to fix the cartridges in the correct position to avoid bypass and the unseating of the filter devices. There is no guarantee that under thermal stress (e.g., different expan-

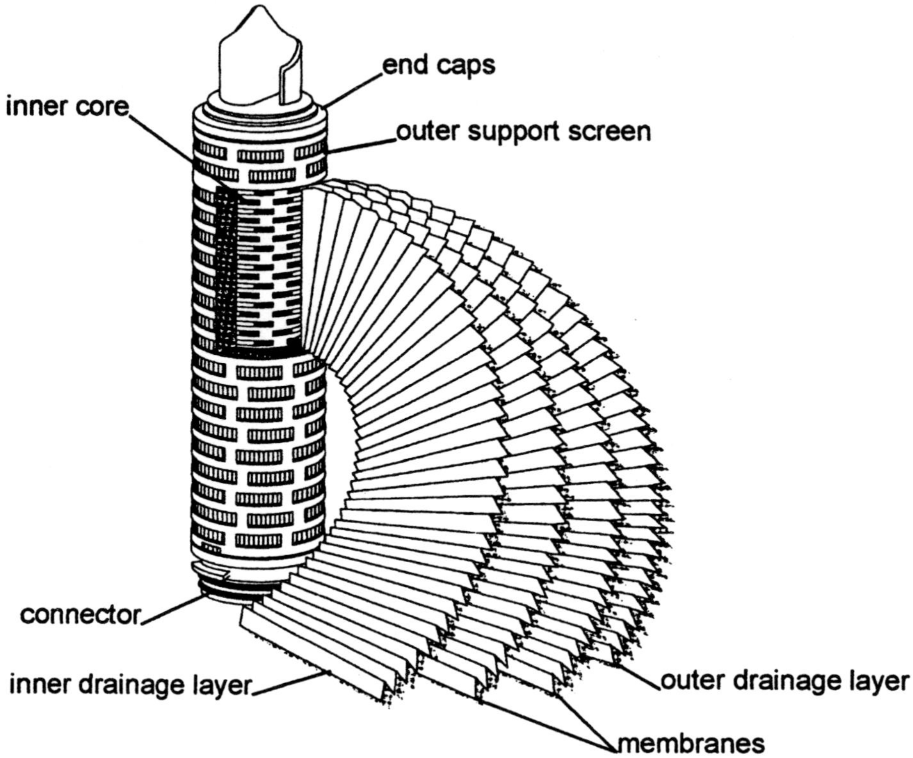

Figure 2 Typical components of a pleated cartridge filter. (Courtesy of Sartorius AG.)

sion or shrinking features of steel and polymeric materials) and extreme process conditions (e.g., pressure shocks) bypass or damage of the cartridge construction (e.g., deformation of the outer support screen or inner core) can be prevented with connector B.

To avoid shrinking of the adapter and resultant leakage or bypass, all connectors encapsulate a stainless steel ring or a ring consisting of polymeric material with a lower tendency to vary dimensionally under thermal stress conditions. This adapter design offers the advantage that repeated sterilization of the cartridges by steaming or autoclaving does not affect the safety of the connection between the housing and the filter device.

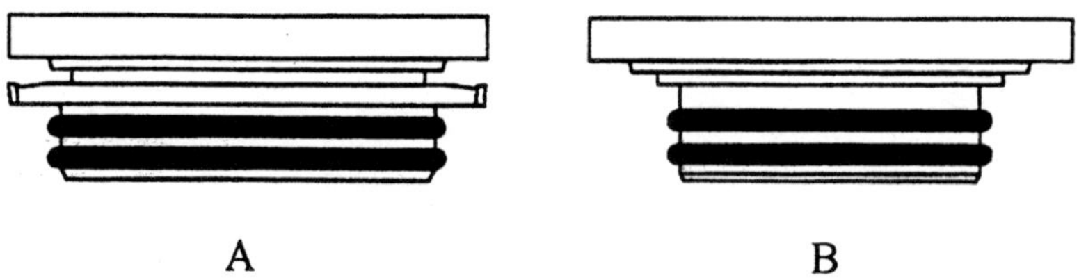

Figure 3 Common cartridge connectors with external double O-rings. (Courtesy of Sartorius AG.)

End Caps

The filter medium and other parts of the cartridge (inner core, outer support screen, connector, fin or flat cap, etc.) are assembled and bonded to a functional filter device by the end caps. To create a connection between the end caps, the filter medium, and the other constituents, hardening fluid binder [e.g., resins (epoxide resins or polyurethane)], additional polymeric melts (e.g., polypropylene, polyethylene, polysulfone, polyester) or a direct thermal welding of the cartridge components can be used. Every end-capping technique has to comply with the essential requirement that a leakproof filter element be produced that separates the unfiltered material from the filtrate side.

Direct thermal welding is the most advantageous technique. With respect to the extractables of a cartridge filter, the number of different construction materials should be limited. Resin binders especially significantly increase the extractable level.

Another consideration is that additional sealing compounds can damage the filter material. The differences in hydrodynamic resistance between the pleats caused by small differential distances between the pleats in the pleat pack are responsible for an uneven distribution of the fluid, polymeric melt, or fluid binder rising in the pleats. After cooling down or hardening of the sealing compounds in the pleats, little spears of compound can remain. The points of those spears threaten the integrity of the filter medium by changing the pressure demands due to motion of the pleat packs caused by the alternating forces.

Outer Support Screen

A basic requirement of the outer support screen is that it increase the mechanical and thermal stability of the cartridge, especially if it has a pleated filter medium, without limiting the flow rate and that it minimize the resultant decrease of the effective filter area. This screen prevents the deformation of the pleat pack by backpressure. It forms the cylindrical shape of the cartridge filter and facilitates handling of the filter device during installation and replacement.

The outer support screen and the inner core should consist of a material that has heat expansion coefficient comparable to that of the filter medium or pleat pack. Otherwise, the filter device may be destroyed by the thermal demands of autoclaving or steam sterilization.

Inner Core

The two basic functions of the inner core are to support the pleat pack to withstand pressure forces in the filtration direction and to draw off the filtrate through the perforations to the outlet of the cartridge. The design of the inner core has to be optimized to support the cartridge construction mechanically, which is best accomplished by a massive cylindrical tube, while at the same time avoiding limitation of the flow rate by construction parts.

The final assembly length of the cartridge is determined by the length of the inner core. In most cases the core consists of a thermoplastic polymeric material that tends to shrink or expand under thermal treatment. Due to that fact a 10 in. cartridge element has a tolerance in length of up to ± 1 mm. This has to be well suited to the properties of the pleat pack under thermal stress to avoid rips in the filter material.

The theoretical method used to calculate the behavior of the different materials regarding exposure of the cartridge to varying temperatures has to be tested during product validation by running autoclaving or in-line steam sterilization cycles.

Filter Media

Membranes

Microfiltration membranes assembled in cartridge filters consist of a variety of polymeric materials surrounding porous voids, thus building up the pores. These include for example, cellulose acetate (CA), polysulfone (PSU), polyethersulfone (PESU), polyamide (PA), poly(vinylidene fluoride) (PVDF), polytetrafluoroethylene (PTFE), polycarbonate (PC), and polypropylene (PP).

Pore sizes of microfiltration membranes for cartridges range between approximately 0.05 and 5 μm depending on the requirements of the application. The thickness of the membranes range from about 15 μm (track-etched polycarbonate membranes) to about 250 μm (reinforced polymeric membranes). The thickness of microfiltration membranes used in cartridge filters, with or without reinforcement, generally ranges between 130 and 190 μm.

Testable membrane endfilter cartridges are available in a pore size range from about 0.05 to 1.0 μm. Typical pore sizes for pharmaceutical applications range between 0.1 and 0.65 μm, mainly 0.2–0.45 μm.

Membrane endfilter cartridges are the only filter system with a defined and validated microbiological safety. The retention of these microporous layers can be correlated to nondestructive integrity test methods (e.g., pressure-holding test, diffusion test, and bubble point test). Special microorganisms in a defined concentration are used in bacteria challenge tests to determine or validate the microbiological retention rate (LRV = log reduction value). The only external test independent of filter manufacturers' bacteria challenge test procedures and parameters is the bacteria challenge test under the regulations of Health Industrial Manufacturer Association (HIMA), defined for a pore size of 0.2 μm (LRV = 7 cm^{-2}; test microorganism = *Brevundimonas diminuta*). Cartridge filters passing this test are considered sterile. For a pore size of 0.45 μm, the test method is not defined. To validate 0.45 μm cartridge filters for pharmaceutical applications, *Serratia marcescens* is often used. The microbiological retention rate varies from LRV 5 to LRV 7 cm^{-2}.

Particle retention tests, e.g., with monodisperse polystyrene particles, are not used to characterize the sterilize filtration capacity of microfiltration membranes. Particle retention is a function of several parameters, including the pH value because of its influence on the outer charge of the polymeric membrane material and its functional groups. Polyamide, for example, has a positive outer charge if the pH value is under the isoelectric point of the membrane. If the particle suspension possesses a pH value higher than the isoelectric point, the outer charge of the membrane is negative. In dependence on the outer charge of the used particles, adsorptive effects are able to influence the assessing of the real mechanical retention capacity of the membrane and the correlation to its sterile filtration capacity.

Other parameters influencing that kind of particle test are the ionic concentration of the suspension and the purity of the suspension. Surface-active substances (e.g., tensides) have an influence on the outer charge of the membrane and the particles. On the other hand, a particle retention test is limited to a maximum concentration of the unfiltered suspension. Modern particle counter systems are only able to detect approximately 10^6 particles, correlating the concentrations of the monodisperse particles on the up- and downstream sides at the same time. At higher concentrations, so-called coincident failures cannot be avoided. In the bacteria challenge test, bacterial concentrations of up to 10^{12} bacteria per 10 in. cartridge are used to verify LRV 7 cm^{-2}.

There is no defined particle retention test that can be used to validate the sterile filtration capacity of membrane cartridge filters. The bacteria challenge test is the only method of characterization for this purpose that delivers reliable results.

To meet the mechanical and thermal demands of process filtration and production of the pleat pack and cartridge assembly, robust membranes with a low tendency to brittleness or a pleat pack construction that prevents membrane damage have to be used. To meet the requirements of an integer membrane cartridge filter, several solutions are possible. On the other hand, the membrane material was improved over the past decade by the development of special reinforcement techniques and new polymeric materials (e.g., PSU, PESU, PVDF, PTFE) that can be pleated as a single-layer membrane without reinforcement. On the other hand, the pleat pack construction, the use of single- or double-layer membranes in combination with inner and outer drainage fleece, is decisive for the absolute function of a membrane filter cartridge. Figure 4 shows the three main membrane reinforcement configurations.

Apart from the improvement of the membrane reinforcements and the use of polymeric materials, special know-how before and during production of a membrane cartridge filter is irreplaceable. The main parameters for the pleating procedure are

1. Conditioning of the membrane before pleating (relative dampness of the membrane)
2. Steaming of the membrane during the pleating process
3. Use of special pleating knifes in correlation with the construction of the pleat pack
4. Velocity of the pleating process (pleats per minute)

(a)
(b)
(c)
(d)

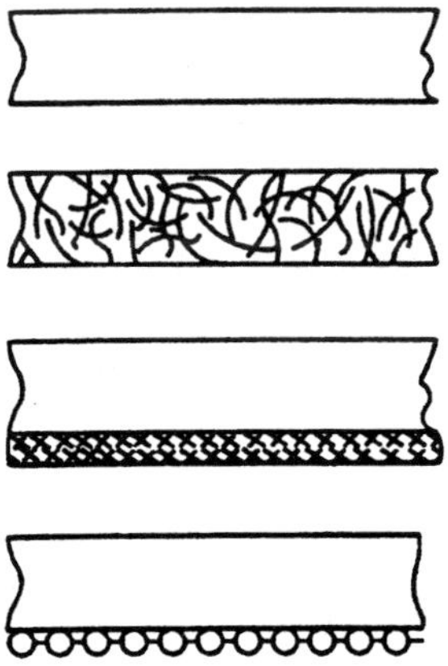

Figure 4 Types of membrane reinforcements used in cartridge filters: (a) No reinforcement; (b) integral fleece reinforcement; (c) sandwich-construction reinforcement; (d) laminated fleece reinforcement (one side).

Various pleated membrane cartridge filters with unsupported or reinforced membranes, single or double (homogeneous or heterogeneous) layer construction, and constructed of a variety of polymeric materials, as mentioned before, are available.

Inner and Outer Drainage Fleece

The inner and outer drainage fleeces preserve the pleated structure, forming the void between the pleats to ensure the passage of the liquid or gas through the entire filtration area during processing. The number of pleats in relation to the thickness of the drainage layers and the permeability of the pleat pack influences the performance of the cartridge with respect to flow rate and total throughput. In addition, the drainage layers protect the filter medium during the manufacturing process, that is, during pleating and the assembly of the pleat pack into the outer support screen.

The inner and outer drainage layers are usually nonwovens or extruded nets chosen with respect to functionality, filter specifications, and cost effectiveness. The heating of the polymeric fleeces during the pleating and exposure to room temperature after the pleating, the "thermofixing" of the pleat pack, fixes the shape of the pleats.

Prefilter Materials

In most cases prefilter cartridges are based on a vertical pleat pack construction, and multilayer cartridges are composed of wound filter media. Not so common are the horizontal pleated designs and the hybrid versions of wound and pleated constructions combined in one cartridge. (Figure 7, presented in Section 3.1, illustrates a number of these constructions.) Nowadays spiral-wound filter cartridges are not state-of-the-art for pharmaceutical applications; they commonly have knife-edge connectors, which present a danger of bypass, whereas wound fibers do not have a defined retention rate.

The following paragraphs give a brief overview of the most commonly used prefilter materials.

POLYPROPYLENE. Polypropylene (PP) nonwovens are mostly produced by melt blowing. The PP fibers are manufactured with two-way jets. The fluid PP melt passes the inner jet, and air blown through the outer jet cools the fibers. The fibers accumulate on a belt, building up a nonwoven fleece structure.

The performance of the nonwoven can be determined by the mass flow of the PP melt, mass flow of the air (fixing the diameter of the fiber), the distance from the jet to the belt, and a further processing step called calendering. In the calender the nonwovens are pressed between heated rolls to obtain a thinner and more compact fleece structure. Multiple polypropylene layers, with similar or progressively finer retention ratings, can be used to meet the demands of the filter device performance such as reliable, good total throughput and/or a fractionated, defined retention of particles.

Typical criteria for the selection of polypropylene nonwovens for cartridge designs are the following mechanical features and performance data.

Physical features. The price of nonwovens is based on their weight. Therefore, consideration of nonwovens is focused on the most effective performance of the fleece, but at the lowest suitable weight (calender nonwovens).

The thickness of nonwovens determines the maximum number of pleats (see Section 3.4, Table 1) and the resultant effective filter area.

Porometer values indicate the retention rate of the multiple polypropylene layers. This method is used to assess individual types of fleece and combinations of them.

Typical data on polypropylene nonwovens pleated in filter cartridges are listed below.

Retention rate (μm)	Weight (g/m^2)	Thickness (μm)	Porometer mean value (μm)
0–5	40–100	80–300	1–8
5–10	20–60	90–200	4–20
10–50	20–50	100–250	8–40

Performance data. For the evaluation of performance data such as total throughput, flow rate and the protection of subsequent separation units, especially sterilizing grade membrane cartridges, are the main focus in selecting a fleece. Chemical compatibility of the additives in the polymeric fibers are important criteria in meeting the requirements of pharmaceutical applications.

GLASS FIBER. Glass fibers have a high adsorptive capacity according to the positive or negative outer charge of the material. Glass fiber fleeces can be classified into two basic types: layers with binder and binder-free materials. Concerning mechanical stability and glass fiber shedding, fleeces with binder are advantageous, but extractables have to be evaluated separately. To increase its mechanical stability, glass fiber fleece can be laminated with a thin polymeric nonwoven (e.g., PP), which functions as a reinforcement.

Performance data. Due to the high adsorptive capacity, particles and colloids are retained by glass fiber fleeces, although the particles are even smaller than the effective mechanical retention based on a sieve effect. The total throughput combined with the protection of subsequent separation units has an impact on the cost effectiveness of the application. High yields of a cartridge filter line consisting of a prefilter and endfilter system are related to the performance of the prefilter cartridge.

Physical features. Additional physical features, e.g., flow rate, thickness, and porometer values, are issues in the selection of glass fiber fleeces.

Typical glass fiber fleece data are

Weight (g/m^2)	Thickness (μm)	Porometer mean value (μm)
70–200	150–500	1–4

2.2 Typical Components of Capsule Filters

Capsules are closing the gap between process scales in the laboratory, pilot plant, or full-scale filtration process. They are available in different sizes, leading to an effective filter area of $\approx$0.03–0.5 m^2. In most cases capsules are used in liquid filtration applications or gas filtration on a laboratory scale. The incorporated construction components of a capsule are based on cartridge technology (see Section 2.1). The capsule housing usually accommodates a minicartridge with an inner core, an outer support screen, and end caps. The filter medium is assembled as a pleat pack or wound around the inner core. To reach a full scale-up level, in most cases cartridge manufacturers use the same filter media combinations as in their process filtration devices.

Owing to their disposability, capsules represent a simple but complete and separate filter unit. They are often prepared as "ready to use right from the box." This implies, for pharmaceutical applications, a sterile product or a product that can be sterilized safely and easily with typical available sources in the associated area of the process (e.g., autoclaving with pure water steam at 121 or 134°C). On the other hand, presterilized filter devices, especially for the laboratory scale, help to save time during processing and are therefore more and more frequently requested. Three methods for the presterilization of capsules are well known: gamma irradiation, steam sterilization, and gas sterilization by ethylene oxide (ETO). None of the indicated sterilization methods can be favored generally.

Gamma irradiation is a safe method of sterilizing, depending on the radiation dose. On the other hand, not every material withstands the demands of gamma sterilization because of a post-irradiation aging phenomenon. Pure polypropylene, for example, continues to degrade after irradiation. Efforts to stabilize polypropylene fibers (e.g., inner and outer drainage layers) or solid PP (e.g., housing material) against this phenomenon have to be proved and validated in each case, because additives can cause unwelcome extractables that are not in accordance with the FDA guidelines or other application demands arising from USP 23 (water for injection) or USP plastic class VI tests (short-term toxicity test).

Gas sterilization by ETO is suspected to leave residues of the toxic gas. To ensure that after the sterilization proceedings the capsule filter is completely degassed, it must be kept for about 100–150 h in a special degassing chamber. This increases production time, which increases the production costs and decreases the flexibility of a manufacturing plant to produce just in time to meet incoming orders. On the other hand, ETO gas sterilization is well known as a safe method for obtaining a sterile product.

Steam sterilization does not have an impact on the quality of the filter device. In most cases capsules for pharmaceutical applications are constructed of materials that resist autoclaving at 121 or 134°C. The basic problem with that method of ensuring sterility, because the polymeric materials of the capsule housing work against the heat transfer of the steam. Because of their low heat conductivity they tend to insulate the inner parts of the capsule.

To guarantee the sterility of the filter device and ensure that each sterilization method has no impact on the quality of the product, the product and the process must be validated.

Figure 5 shows a capsule filter scale-up line together with three so-called minicartridges depicted in front of the capsules. These types of minicartridges are assem-

Figure 5 Capsule filter scale-up line. (Courtesy of Sartorius AG.)

bled into the capsule housing or are available as an original filter device in combination with a minicartridge housing.

Capsule Connectors

Common types of connectors for capsules are sanitary flanges, hose barbs, and NPT threads (Fig. 6). These standardized capsule connectors facilitate installation of the capsule filter and make possible the combination of capsules in series, for example, a prefilter and endfilter.

Capsule Housing

The combination of a housing and a cartridge filter as a matched design creates a complete, ready-to-use separation unit. For the operation of a cartridge or capsule filter, a driving differential pressure is indispensable. As a consequence the housing has to be designed as a container that resists inner pressure forces. In correlation to the pressure load, the shape and thickness of the housing material, which affect its mechanical stability, are defined. Common capsule housings resist inner pressure forces up to a level of 6 bar. In this respect, the welding of the cylindrical jacket with the cover and the bottom, which are in most cases connected directly with the capsule connectors as one plastic part produced in an injection molding process, is of special significance. Exceptional welding stability depends on a thermal bonding of these capsule parts, which consist of thermoplastic polymeric materials. These

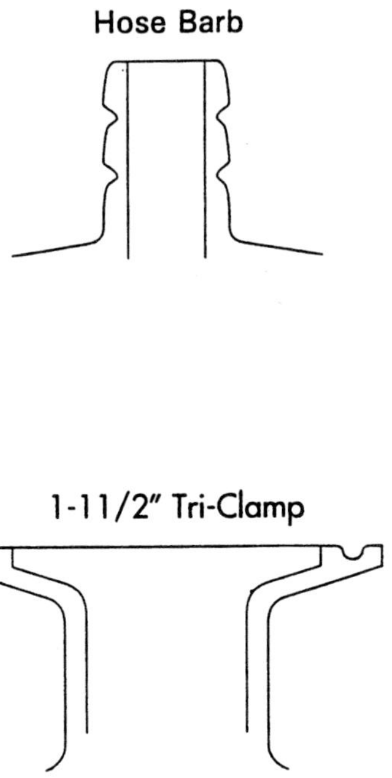

Figure 6 Common capsule filter connectors. (Courtesy of Sartorius AG.)

items concerning mechanical stability refer to room temperature conditions. In-line steam sterilization at 121 or 134°C may give rise to an impact on the mechanical stability of the housing or the dimensions of the connectors under thermal stress, caused by a maximum pressure of 2 bar in the housing (at 134°C) and a decreasing tensile strength of the polymeric material. Therefore, capsules should be sterilized by autoclaving. During autoclaving also, the filter device is exposed to a temperature to 121 or 134°C but without additional pressure forces on either side of the housing.

A significant feature of the construction of each capsule filter are the two venting valves on the up- and downstream sides. The valves are directly connected with the jacket and are fixed on both sides of the capsule (bottom and top). They serve the basic function of venting the housing before processing to ensure that the entire filter area is used during filtration. Otherwise the enclosed gas in the void between the encapsulated cartridge and the housing has to be pressed through the filter medium during the separation process. This can cause problems, especially with sterilizing grade filters where the filter medium consists of a single- or double-layered membrane. In this case the driving differential pressure must be higher than the bubble point of the utilized membranes [from ≈2.0 bar (the minimum bubble point for 0.45 μm) to ≈6.0 bar which implies a pore size of ca. 0.05 μm]. The positions (bottom and top side) and number (two) of valves are related to the different installation directions of the capsule to ensure easy handling and functional safety.

3 CARTRIDGE DESIGN

3.1 Construction and Design of the Pleat Pack

Pleating or rolling up a rectangular, track-shaped filter material is the most important and obvious form of processing a cartridge filter element, with regard to optimizing utilization of the filter material roll. Circular shapes, e.g., stamped out flat filter material or filter disks, require a logical division of the original dimension of the filter roll, which is based on a continuous manufacturing process such as casting membranes or producing melt-blown PP filter fleeces. The pleating method of processing filter material is more economical as it allows the complete use of the produced filter material and maximizes the filter area in a compact form.

Because of the diversity of filter applications and the cartridge filter manufacturers' philosophy, a number of different pleat pack constructions have been established on the market. Figure 7 gives a rough impression of the kinds of pleat pack constructions or configurations of the filter media, that are used in pre- and endfilter cartridges.

The pleat pack shown in Fig. 7a is the most common type for pleated cartridge filters. The folded edges of all pleats are oriented to the center of the inner core, orthogonal to its central axis. This form of construction can be handled safely due to the adaptation of pleat packs with end caps. The symmetric shape and configuration of the pleats is submerged in the hot melt of the end caps with a constant hydrodynamic resistance of the voids in the pleat pack, leading to a unique and safe welding of the materials. On the other hand, the shape of the voids, influenced by the relationship between the inner drainage layer and the outer protective layer, has a direct effect on the application or the performance of the cartridge filter in specific applications. For the filtration of liquids with low solids contents (e.g., sterile filtration of aqueous solutions), a ratio of the thickness of the outer to the inner drainage and support layers of 1–1.5:1 and a large number of pleats (high surface area) based on this construction guarantee high flow rates and a good total throughput with appropriate filter media.

The ratio of the thickness of the drainage fleeces and the number of pleats determine the angle between the folded filter media. Therefore the pleat pack of cartridge filters used in applications for the retention of high solids (e.g., particles) contents out of suspensions must be modified accordingly. The performance of the cartridge in retaining particles by surface filtration is most effective if the outer void between the pleats is able to cover the retained solids and maximizes the outer surface that can be reached by the solids of the suspension. Otherwise the retained solids build up a filter-active filter cake, blocking the space between the pleats in the first third or half of their depth and preventing the passage of the suspension into the deeper regions of the pleat pack. The effective filter area is limited by the construction of the pleats. The loss of pleats as a result of the assembly of a thicker outer drainage fleece (500–1000 μm thickness) with ratio of the thickness of outer to inner drainage fleece of up to 8 induces better performance of the cartridge according to requirements of the application. Comparison of surface areas is not sufficient for assessing the comparative merits of cartridge filters.

An additional advantage of a pleat pack is the resultant effectiveness of backflushing during the regeneration of the filter. Retained particles, for example, can be

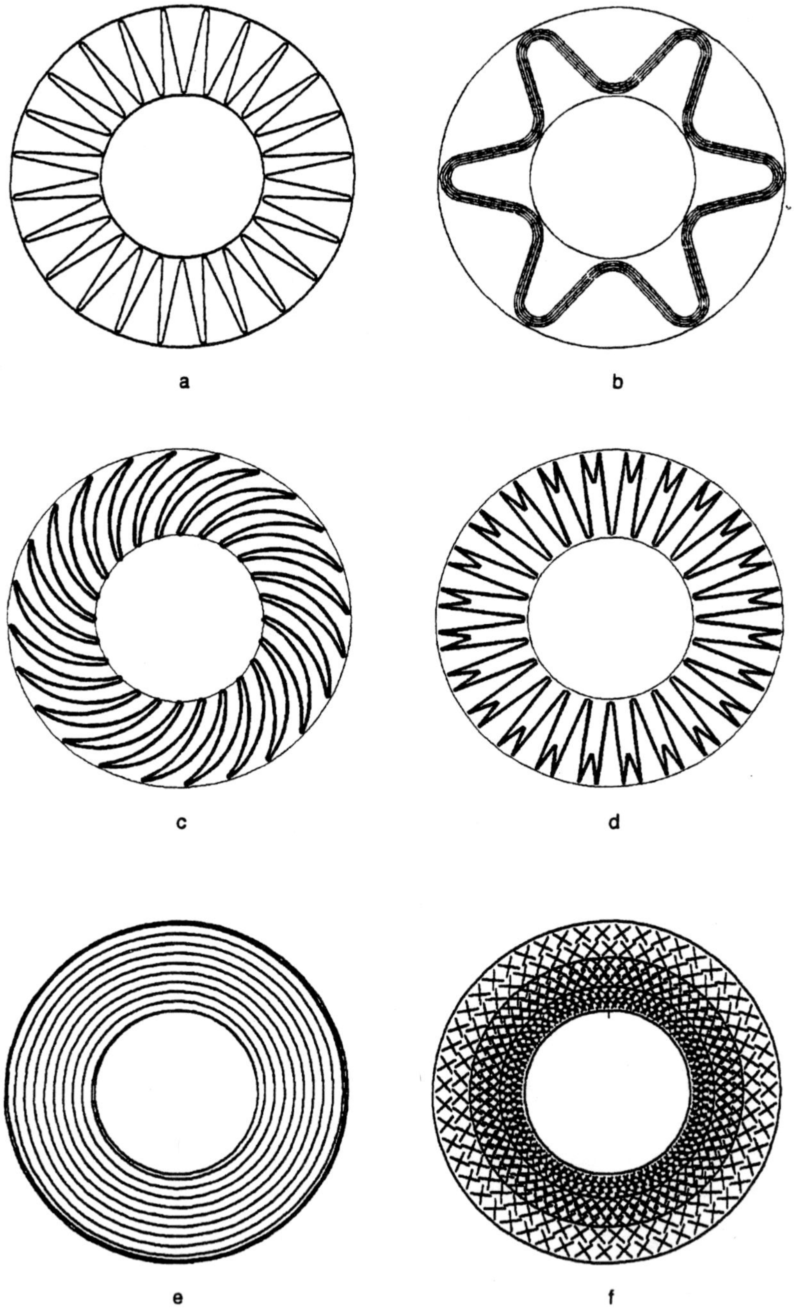

Figure 7 Pleat pack and filter media configurations of cartridge filters. (a) Pleat pack. (b) Pleat pack with thick multilayers. (c,d) Pleat pack with increased surface area. (e,f) Prefilter cartridges using fractionated depth filtration. (g) Pleat pack fixed on inner core and surrounded by nonwoven filter media. (h) Cross section showing hollow-fiber filter construction. (i) Multipleat construction. (j) Lampion, or Chinese lantern, filter.

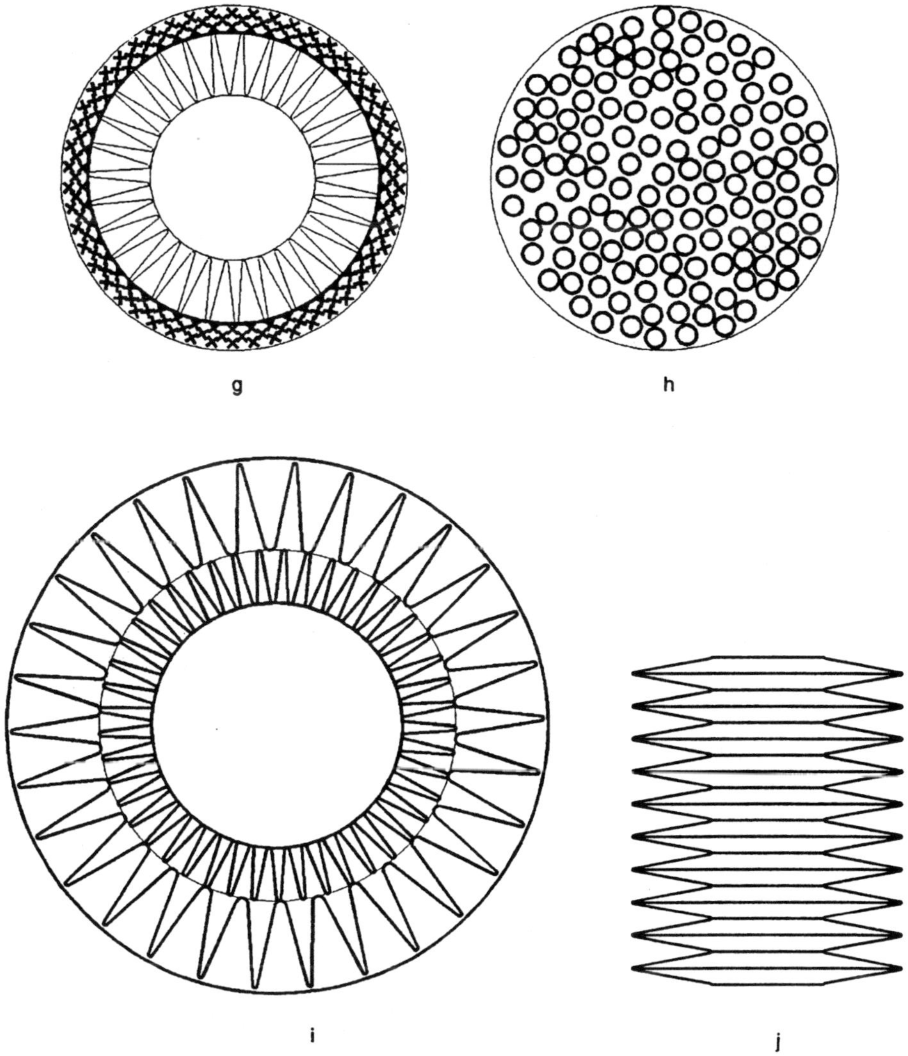

Figure 7 *Continued*

flushed out of the surface of the filter medium. This optimization of the pleat pack for highly loaded suspensions is mostly relevant for prefilter cartridges.

Figure 7b shows a way to pleat multilayers ($\approx 1-5$ mm) for the retention of particles and colloids by fractionated depth filtration. This configuration does not damage the thick filter medium in the critical area of the sharp folded edges of a common pleating by compressing the material on the inside and stressing it on the outside. Furthermore, this configuration offers good performance for the fractionated clarification of highly loaded suspensions with a wide range of particle sizes. This shape and the use of thick filter material are only appropriate in the field of prefiltration.

Figures 7c and 7d show how the surface area of a filter can be increased by up to 50%. Figure 7c is based on longer pleats that are wound tangentially to the core. This construction creates an antiproportional relation between the increase in surface area and the increase in flow rate and total throughput. The performance of the cartridge with respect to increased surface area is limited by the diversion of the liquid streamlines (which affect the flow rate) and the accessory buildup of a blocking filter cake between the pleats, especially in the clarification of suspensions. Figure 7d is based on the idea of using the void between the pleats in the vicinity of the outer support screen. The number of pleats in a cartridge filter, and therefore the surface area, is limited by the thickness of the pleated filter medium and the diameter of the inner core. The surface area in a confined volume can be increased by using alternating pleat heights. Like that of Fig. 7, this pleat pack configuration can be useful for filtering liquids with a very low solids content (<0.1 wt%), where a moderate flow rate and a good total throughput are desired. On the other hand, the endcapping of these pleat pack constructions can cause problems in attaining microbiologically safe bonding due to the hydrodynamic resistance gradient between the pleats upon submersion in the bonding material.

Figures 7e and 7f show typical forms of prefilter cartridges for the retention of particles by fractionated depth filtration. The filter in Fig. 7e is composed of a wound nonwoven multilayer, building up progressively finer filter zones from the nonfiltrate to the filtrate side. The filter in Fig. 7f is created by e.g., spraying the nonwovens in a kind of melt blowing procedure onto the inner core. It remains one layer with a graded density. The thickness of the multilayer or graded density layer usually varies between 0.45 and 0.6 in. The cartridge design of Fig. 7b can be used as an advanced construction of the types shown in Figs. 7e and 7f for special applications, where only a part of the depth of the multilayer is responsible for the performance of the cartridge. That means that the particle size spectrum of the unfiltered suspension is even smaller, with a tendency to give a monodisperse particle size distribution. Under these conditions the increase of the surface area due to the use of a pleated shape combined with the thinning of the multilayer lead to better performance of the cartridge filter with respect to flow rate and total throughput.

The cartridge filter shown in Fig. 7g is a combination of those in Fig. 7a and 7e or 7f. The pleat pack fixed on the inner core is surrounded by a nonwoven filter medium. The outer filter medium belt is filter-active with the function of protecting the pleat pack. On the other hand, this additional layer on the nonfiltrate side decreases the flow rate of the filter device, and because of the small surface area in comparison with that of the pleat pack it is difficult to find a balance between the two filter media to guarantee an increasing total throughput in different applications. If the outer layer shows good protection, it tends to block before the large surface area of the pleat pack is blocked. If the outer layer has a sufficient total throughput, the protection of the following pleat pack is questionable.

Figure 7h shows a cross section through a bundle of hollow fibers bonded by the end cap(s) of the filter device. The hollow fibers themselves represent the filter medium (membrane or nonwoven layer) dividing the nonfiltrate and filtrate sides. In most cases, hollow fibers are used in crossflow modules. This type of cartridge filter for static filtration is a kind of crossflow module without the typical retentate outlet for tangential flow. It is possible to accommodate a surface area of up to 1.5 m^2 in the confined volume of the 10 in. cartridge with a diameter of 2.5 in. In comparison with pleated membranes (e.g., Fig. 7a), the cost effectiveness of the hollow fiber construction as a cartridge filter is questionable, because the membrane material in the form of hollow fibers is three or four times as expensive as the same area of a flat filter material.

The construction illustrated in Fig. 7i allows a combination of two or three pleat packs in one cartridge, a multipleat construction. This can have major impacts on the performance regarding the filter medium employed:

1. The inner pleat pack contains a coarse filter medium that functions as a drainage layer and a mechanical support for the outer pleat pack. As a result the effective filter area increases as the number of pleats of the outer pleat pack, which contains the real filter medium, increases. The numbers of pleats are determined by the thickness of the filter medium and the outer diameter of the inner core or in this case the inner pleat pack.
2. A combined multipleat construction in which all pleat packs are filter-active facilitates fractionated retention with a high total throughput. The areas of the utilized filter media can be well suited to each other by the number and height of the pleats in the different pleat packs, due to the performance (flow rate, total throughput, and support of the inner filter medium) of each filter-active layer. To use the total filter capacity, all filter media should be plugged simultaneously, and on the other hand the endfilter system should be protected as efficiently as possible. To meet these demands of the cartridge design, special application know-how is necessary.

The largest cartridges with a multipleat construction have a height of 40 in., an outer diameter of 10 in., and an inner core diameter of 4 in. The resultant effective filter area amounts to at most 40 m^2. These cartridges are most efficient in prefilter applications with large volumes.

Figure 7j shows a Lampion or Chinese lantern filter. This configuration is an alternative to conventional pleat packs, changing the orientation of the pleats to an angle of 90°. This cartridge construction uses pleatable filter media tubes, mostly PP fleeces. It is claimed that this construction offers greater filter area in the same volume. The calculation illustrated in Fig. 8 and in the appendix on p. 168 was made on the assumption that the constructions of both Figs. 7a and 7j are based on the same geometrical dimensions (length of cartridge, diameter of inner core and outer support screen, thickness of filter media, etc.) to prove this theory.

Due to the conditions of this calculation, the Lampion filter element has 150% as much effective filter area as a conventional pleated cartridge filter. On the other hand, the filter area of the Lampion pleat pack configuration cannot be used completely owing to ineffective drainage, which draws off the fluid between the pleats. If the distance between the pleats is equal to the thickness of a single pleat ($\lambda = \tau$) (see Fig. 8), the equation for the number of pleats in the Lampion filter element is converted to

$$N_{\mathrm{lamp}} = \frac{L}{2\tau}$$

Under these conditions the drainage effect is comparable to that of the configuration of a ''conventional'' cartridge filter, and the Lampion filter element provides only 75% as much effective filter area as a conventional cartridge filter. The optimized

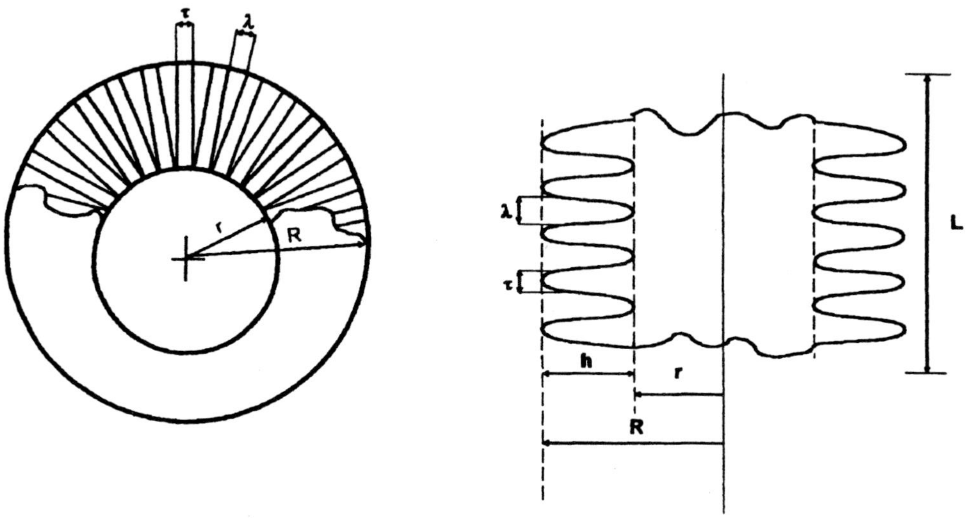

Figure 8 Comparative filter area calculation. (See Appendix on p. 168 for calculation.)

filter area with respect to performance data (total throughput and flow rate) is in between the two configurations (75 and 150%). Therefore there is no significant difference between construction-related parameters (effective filter area) and performance data (total throughput, flow rate) of the two designs.

An increase in the effective filter area of the Lampion filter element is related to an expansion of the diameter of the outer support screen. The utilization of the complete filter area of the resulting higher pleats, which are stacked on top of each other, is based on efficient drainage layers. Elements of this kind are available for prefilter applications.

3.4 Construction Data and Some Basic Thoughts on Fluid Dynamics of a Typical Standard Cartridge

Construction Data

The typical form and design of a cartridge filter used in pharmaceutical process filtration applications are based on a cylindrical filter element with the geometric data shown in Table 1.

Estimation of the Fluid Velocity and Differential Pressure in a Membrane Filter Cartridge

For the flow through small capillary pores, the law of laminar motion is valid. Therefore the pressure drop, according to the Hagen–Poiseuille law, is proportional to the velocity (Eck, 1988). The Hagen–Poiseuille law for laminar flow in tubes can be stated as

$$Q = \frac{\pi r^4 \Delta p}{8\eta \Delta l} \tag{1}$$

With Eq. (1), the water flow Q_{pore} through an ideal single pore can be estimated.

Table 1 Geometric Data for a Typical Cartridge (Scale-up) Filter Line

Dimension	10 in. standard	Minicartridge designs 1	2	3	4
Effective filter area (m^2)					
Membrane	0.6–0.8	0.2	0.1	0.05	0.03
PP Nonwoven	0.4–0.9				
GF Nonwoven	0.4–0.6				
Length (in.)	10	5.0–6.0	2.8–3.8	1.5–2	1.0
Outer diameter (outer support screen) (in.)	2.4–2.8	2.0–2.3	2.0–2.3	2.0–2.3	2.5
Inner diameter (inner core)	1.2–1.6	0.8–1.0	0.8–1.0	0.8–1.0	0.8–1.0
Number of pleats					
Membrane	100–160	50–80	50–80	50–80	60
PP Nonwoven	70–180				
GF Nonwoven	50–90				
Pleating height	10–13 mm (0.4–0.51 in.)	10–13 mm (0.4–0.51 in.)	10–13 mm (0.4–0.51 in.)	10–13 mm (0.4–0.51 in.)	10–13 mm (0.4–0.51 in.)
Weight (dry condition) (g)	280–320	105–130	75–85	45–55	45

As an example, the data for a sterilizing grade 10 filter cartridge, based on a PESU membrane, are given as

Mean pore radius (porometer mean value)	$r_{pore} = 2 \times 10^{-7}$ m
Pore sectional area	$A_{pore} = 1.256 \times 10^{-13}$ m^2
Length of pore (thickness of membrane)	$\Delta l = 1.4 \times 10^{-4}$ m

The calculation is based on the following process parameters:

Pressure drop	$\Delta_p = 5 \times 10^4$ Pa
Viscosity of water at 0°C	$\eta_0 = 1.79 \times 10^{-3}$ Pa·s
Viscosity of water at 20°C	$\eta_{20} = 1.01 \times 10^{-3}$ Pa·s
Viscosity of water at 50°C	$\eta_{50} = 0.55 \times 10^{-3}$ Pa·s

The flow rate of pure water at 20°C through a single pore, Q_{pore}, is then

$$Q_{pore}^{20°C} = 22.218 \times 10^{-17} \text{ m}^3\text{/s} = 1.333 \times 10^{-11} \text{ L/min}$$

To calculate the flow rate through a filter cartridge, the number of pores has to be determined.

The effective filter area of a sterilizing grade cartridge is $A_{cart} = 0.7$ m^2. The free volume or porosity of a typical microfiltration membrane is 70% (free pore area $\varepsilon = 0.7$).

The number of pores N can be described as

$$N = \frac{A_{cart}\varepsilon}{A_{pore}} \tag{2}$$

or in this case,

$$N = 3.901 \times 10^{12}$$

The theoretical flow rate through a 10 in. cartridge filter is

$$Q_m = NQ_{pore} \tag{3}$$

or for this example

$$Q_m = 52.0 \text{ L/min}$$

The actual water flow rate Q_r at $\Delta p = 0.5$ bar is 50 L/min. The deviation between model and reality is 4%,

$$\frac{Q_m - Q_r}{Q_r} = 0.04$$

The average fluid velocity in a single pore can be described as

$$\bar{v}_{pore} = \frac{Q_{pore}}{A_{pore}} \tag{4}$$

$$\bar{v}_{pore} = 1.769 \times 10^{-3} \text{ m/s}$$

The Reynolds number (Re) in a pore is given as

$$\mathrm{Re}_{\mathrm{pore}} = \frac{\rho v d_{\mathrm{pore}}}{\eta_{20}}$$

Based on an average porometer diameter of $d_{\mathrm{pore}} = 4 \times 10^{-7}$ m, the Reynolds number is

$$\mathrm{Re}_{\mathrm{pore}} = 7.006 \times 10^{-1}$$

Therefore it can be stated that the flow in a single pore is laminar!

Table 2 shows the influence of the temperature on the flow rate $Q(T)$, as an example for a 10 in. filter cartridge, for which the differential pressure is $\Delta p = 0.5$ bar = constant.

The pressure drop caused by the flux through the inner core is

$$\Delta p = \lambda \frac{\Delta l}{d_c} \left(\frac{\rho}{2}\right) c^2 \tag{5}$$

With the fluid velocity c in the core based on $Q_r = 50$ L/min,

$$c = Q_r/A_c \qquad \text{or} \qquad c = 1.18 \text{ m/s}$$

The difference between the mean velocity in the core c and that in the pore v_{pore} is 10^3 (factor of 1000!).

The Reynolds number of the fluid in the core is 3.54×10^4; the flow in the core is turbulent.

The resistance number λ is

$$\lambda = 0.316\ \mathrm{Re}^{-1/4} \qquad \text{(Blasius)}$$

so for the core,

$$\lambda = 0.024$$

and the pressure drop in the core is

$$\Delta p = 139.3 \text{ Pa} = 1.39 \text{ mbar}$$

The pressure drop caused by the inner core is negligibly small.

With $\lambda = 64/\mathrm{Re}_{\mathrm{pore}} = 91.35$ and Eq. (5), the pressure drop Δp_{pore} in a single pore is estimated as

$$\Delta p_{\mathrm{pore}} = 2.828 \times 10^{-2} \text{ mbar}$$

The actual pressure drop is 500 mbar, so that the ratio $\Delta p/\Delta p_{\mathrm{pore}}$ is ≈ 100. Therefore the pressure drop is the sum of the inlet losses in the pleat pack (Δp_i), push losses to the membrane (Δp_p), outlet losses (Δp_o) out of the membrane, and the dissipation in the core Δp_d:

Table 2 Water Flow Rate at $\Delta p = 0.5$ Bar

Temperature	0°C	20°C	50°C
Flow rate	29.3 L/min	52.0 L/min	95.4 L/min

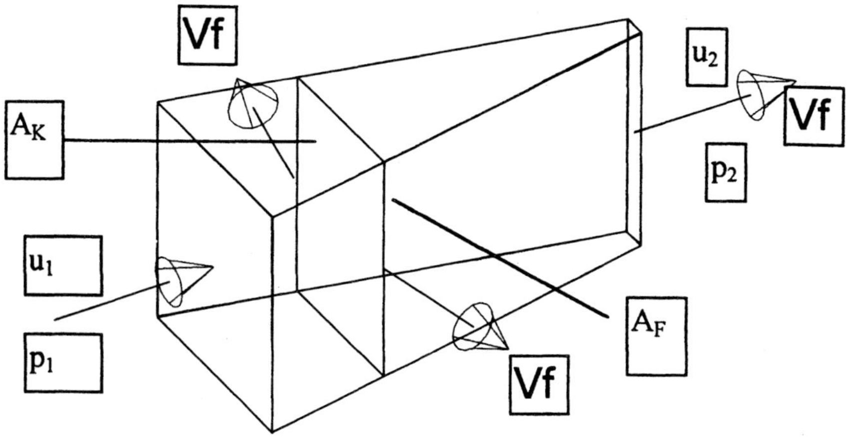

Figure 9 Infinite description of the volume of a pleat.

$$\Delta p = \Delta p_i + \Delta p_p + \Delta p_o + \Delta p_d$$

A common estimation to describe the pressure drop Δp_p in a pleat is to use the expression for impulse in an infinitesimal balance space (see Fig. 9).

$$\iint \Delta p_i \, dx \, d\phi = p_1 - p_2 = \rho(u_2^2 - u_1^2) + \Delta p_v + p \iint v_f \frac{V_f}{A_K} \, dx \, d\phi$$

The various terms have the following fluid dynamical meaning:

$\rho(u_2^2 - u_1^2)$ = increase in the pressure drop due to slowing down the volume stream

Δp_v = increase in the pressure drop due to friction

$\rho \iint v_f V_f / A_K \, dx \, d\phi$ = increase in the pressure drop due to a change in the impulse in the main flow direction caused by the volume stream leaving the balance space through the permeable membrane.

If the single pressure drops are an unknown quantity, the model of parallel connected tubes is valid (Eck, 1988). Between the inlet and the outlet, the streamline splits into several parallel connected tubes (see Fig. 10).

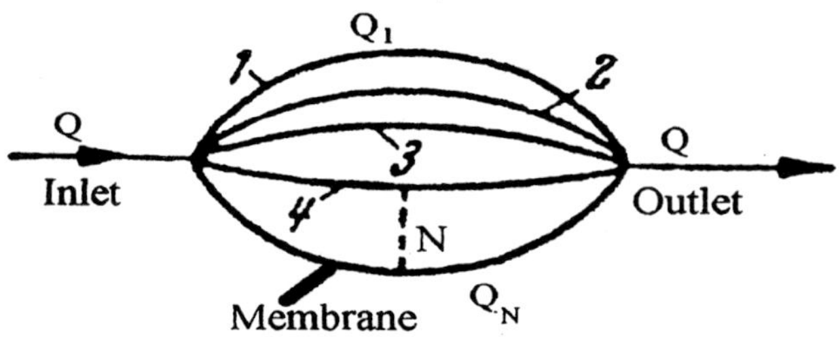

Figure 10 The parallel connected tube model. (From Eck, 1991.)

Table 3 Total Resistance Values for Different Cartridge Constructions

Cartridge construction	Total resistance R
Pleated	7.2×10^{10} kg/m^7
Wound	6.6×10^{12} kg/m^7

Equation (5) is now

$$\Delta p = \lambda \left(\frac{1}{d}\right)\left(\frac{\rho}{2}\right)\left(\frac{1}{A^2}\right) Q^2 = RQ^2$$

where R is the total resistance value, $R = (1/N^2)R_i$, the continuity equation is $Q = \Sigma_{i=1}^{N} Q_i$, and $\Delta p = RQ^2$.

For example, the total resistance value for this 10 in. cartridge example is $R = 4.5 \times 10^{10}$ kg/m^7. If we draw a comparison between this cartridge construction (see Fig. 7a) and a wound cartridge construction (Fig. 7e or 7f) with a similar filter material with respect to retention rate, a tremendous difference between the total resistance values of the two constructions is obvious (see Table 3).

These theoretical contemplations cannot substitute for the empirical testing of cartridge filters to meet the requirements of an application. Every construction has to be optimized with respect to the demands and conditions of the pharmaceutical process.

BIBLIOGRAPHY

Dickenson, C. (1994). *Filters and Filtration Handbook*, 3rd ed., Elsevier Science, New York.

Dubbel. (1987). *Taschenbuch für den Maschinenbau*, 16th ed., Springer-Verlag, Berlin.

Eck, B. (1988). *Technische Strömungslehre*, Bol. 1, Guwindlager, 9th ed., Springer-Verlag, Berlin.

Eck, B. (1991). *Technische Strömungslehre*, Bol. 2, Anwendlingen, 9th ed., Springer-Verlag, Berlin.

Gupta, R. K., R. J. Legare, and R. E. Kozulla (eds.). (1996). Index 96 Congress: *Applications and Properties of Nonwoven Fabric Containing Polyethylene Based Fibres*, European Disposbles and Nonwovens Association (EDANA), Brussels.

Matteson, M. J., and C. Orr. (1987). *Filtration Principles and Practices*, 2nd ed., Marcel Dekker, New York.

Meltzer, T. H. (1987). *Filtration in the Pharmaceutical Industry*, Marcel Dekker, New York.

APPENDIX (see Fig. 8)

COMPARATIVE FILTER AREA CALCULATION

Conditions: h = const. ; L = const. r = const. ; R = const. for both configurations

$$r = \frac{R}{2} \qquad h = (R - r)$$

with:
h = height of a pleat
L = length of the filter element
r = outer radius of the inner core
R = inner radius of the outer support screen
λ = free distance between the pleatings
τ = thickness of a pleat in the final configuration

Rem.: τ as a part of the effective filter area is neglectably small.

Conventional cartridge filter | **"Lampion"-filter element**

Maximum numbers of pleats:

$$N_{max}^{pleat} = \frac{2 \cdot \pi \cdot r}{\tau} \quad [-] \qquad\qquad N_{max}^{lamp} = \frac{L}{\tau} \quad [-]$$

Resultant effective filter area:

$$A_{pleat} = 2 \cdot h \cdot L \cdot N_{max}^{pleat} \quad [m^2] \qquad\qquad A_{lamp} = 2 \cdot \pi \cdot \left(R^2 - r^2\right) \cdot N_{max}^{lamp} \quad [m^2]$$

$$A_{pleat} = \frac{4 \cdot h \cdot L \cdot \pi \cdot r}{\tau} \quad [m^2] \qquad\qquad A_{lamp} = 2 \cdot \pi \cdot \left(R^2 - r^2\right) \cdot \frac{L}{\tau} \quad [m^2]$$

Comparison of the resultant, effective filter area:

$$\frac{A_{pleat}}{A_{lamp}} = \frac{2 \cdot \pi \cdot \left(R^2 - r^2\right) \cdot \frac{l}{\tau}}{4 \cdot \pi \cdot (R - r) \cdot r \cdot \frac{L}{\tau}} \quad [-]$$

<=>

$$= \frac{R^2 - r^2}{2 \cdot r \cdot (R - r)} = \frac{4r^2 - r^2}{4r^2 - 2r^2}$$

$$\frac{A_{lamp}}{A_{pleat}} = \frac{3}{2}$$

6

Quality Assurance of Filters for Fluid Clarification

HYMAN B. KATZ
Pall Corporation, East Hills, New York

1 INTRODUCTION

Quality has been defined as "the totality of characteristics of an entity that bear on its ability to satisfy stated and implied needs" (ISO, 1992). In the filter industry these stated and implied needs require a manufacturer to recognize the conditions of use of its products and handle its operations as an extension of its customers' manufacturing and testing facilities. This is being accomplished in part by implementing the ISO 9001 international standard for quality management (ISO, 1994) in each of the operations of a total quality system including those that encompass product development, manufacturing, performance testing, and technical support.

2 PRODUCT DEVELOPMENT

In product development, there should be close coordination between quality assurance and research and development on matters such as material selection, testing programs, and prototype production. All stages of product development also benefit from close interaction with design engineering, manufacturing engineering, and production. This is depicted schematically in Fig. 1. The engineering groups, for example, might be responsible for translating initial material selections into purchasing specifications. They might also draft packaging requirements and dimensional drawings. The quality assurance staff would be involved in surveys of materials vendors and in developing or structuring various specifications into a quality control manual. Periodic audits, including samples taken for performance testing, would help ensure that a filter manufactured at one location is comparable to a similar filter made at another site by the same manufacturer. In production, manufacturing and quality

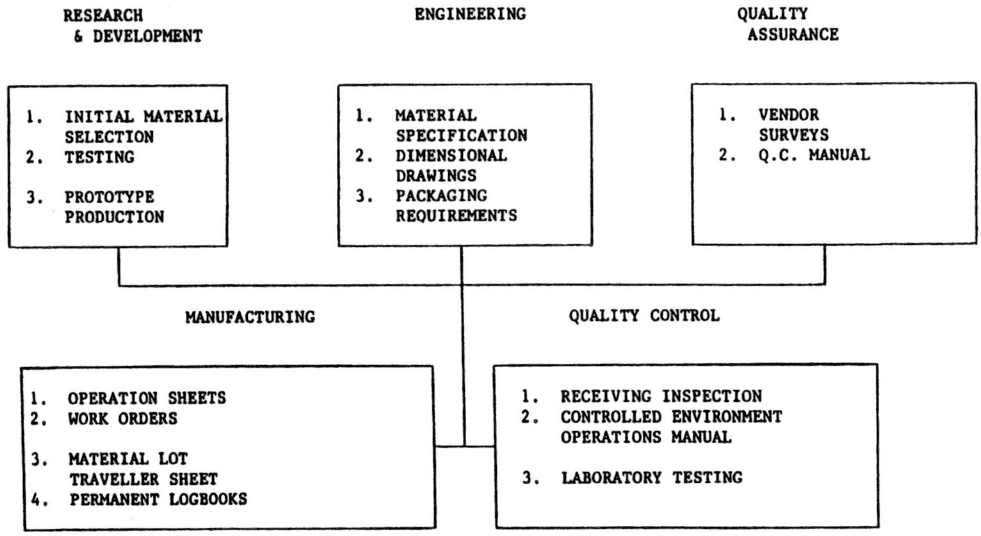

Figure 1 Coordination of quality control with various company departments.

control personnel would be closely involved in providing feedback to plant management and corporate staff. For example, manufacturing would involve drawing up operation sheets, work orders, and material lot traveler sheets.

3 MANUFACTURING

3.1 Lots

Material lot traveler sheets provide traceability for individual lots. They accompany materials staged for production of a given lot from their inspection through each manufacturing operation to final testing and release. Although the definition of a lot varies from manufacturer to manufacturer and from product to product, a lot may be defined as all filters produced from common vendor material lots in a single work shift. The definition of lot size should be considered by engineering and quality assurance, jointly with marketing, during product development. It will depend on material specifications, process variability, and intended use.

3.2 Control Stations

Control stations must also be considered during product development. Operations may be classified (Sender, 1962) as machine-dominant, operator-dominant, materials-dominant, or setup-dominant. Critical operations require in-process controls, and permanent log books or data entry terminals are maintained at various control stations in the manufacturing sequence. These log books are used by quality control personnel, individual operators, and/or production foremen to record various product/process characteristics. The quality control group, for example, will record measured dimensions and review certificates of analysis during receiving inspection. Similarly, they will conduct testing and inspection functions in the manufacturing area where first-piece production samples are taken to qualify machine setup in accordance with narrow-limit gauging (Ott, 1975) or other forms of statistical process control. Operators are charged with recording machine settings, product measurements, and yields at their workstations.

A generalized schematic flow diagram for the manufacture of cartridge filters is depicted in Fig. 2. Each box represents a workstation, the majority of which are monitored by quality control personnel (denoted by QC in Fig. 2). The dashed line denotes a controlled environment area. The extent of controls varies with the end use of the product. Pharmaceutical filters, for example, may be manufactured in a clean-room environment, an isolated portion of which would be maintained as a Class 100 area with the use of high efficiency particulate air (HEPA) filters.

Materials staged for production of a filter cartridge lot are brought into the controlled environment area and delivered to three distinct workstations. Filter media, for example, are corrugated, cut to size, and formed into a cylindrical configuration by joining two ends with a side seal. Setup personnel adjust equipment settings to optimize physical properties within product specifications. Operators continuously maintain and monitor these settings and product properties, while quality control inspectors periodically verify them. For example, at corrugation, the heights of individual pleats and the number of pleats per unit length are controlled. Corrugation increases the filter area per unit volume, allowing greater flow rates and longer service life than afforded by the corresponding flat sheet media, but requires careful precontrol.

An outer cage and inner support core are assembled around the filter material to provide greater ruggedness and ease of handling while simplifying installation and reducing labor time. End caps are then attached, completing the filter element by sealing both ends.

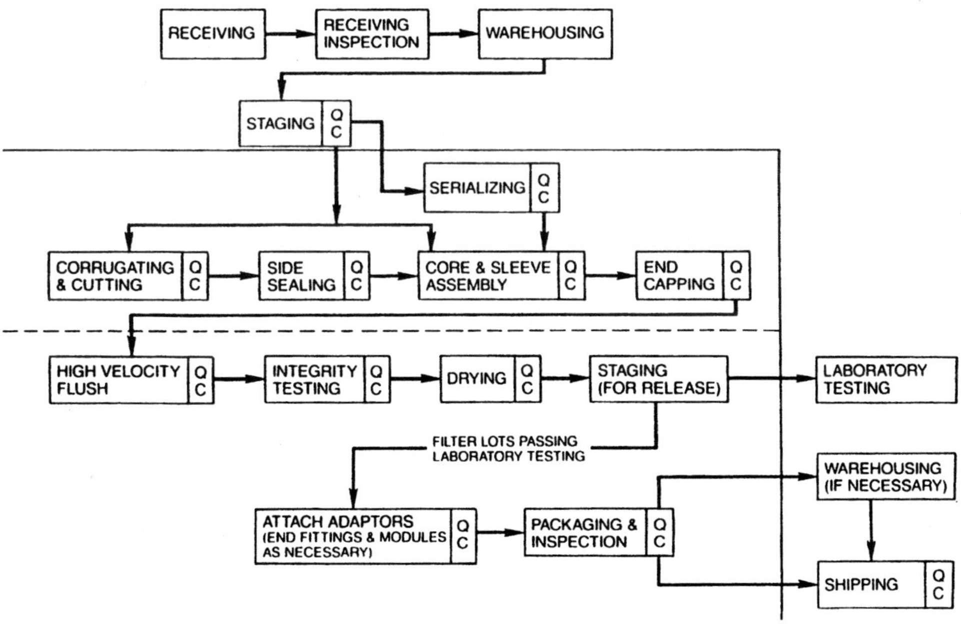

Figure 2 Generalized manufacturing flowsheet for cartridge filters.

A number of techniques are available for side sealing and end capping. Potting resins and adhesives may be used, but these introduce new and increased levels of extractables. Proprietary heat melt processes are often preferred in critical applications sensitive to extractables. These use specialized manufacturing equipment and novel thermocouples to provide greater control over heating time, temperature, and location. This has decreased the variability and improved the tensile strength of plastic welding. In addition, advanced tool design and molding techniques have allowed some plastic components to be formed as a single piece rather than as multiple pieces requiring subsequent heat treatment to achieve the robustness capable of withstanding extreme process conditions. Autoclaving stresses all such bonds and seals, serving as a useful, albeit destructive, qualification test on an acceptance sampling basis as well as an important part of validation for new filter constructions. Heat treatment has also been used to improve traceability. Outer cages or plastic sleeves have been sequentially heat stamped to provide unique serial numbers for individual filter elements.

4 CONTAMINATION CONTROL

All the operations up to and including end capping generate debris. They are performed in a controlled environment area that is separated from a second controlled environment area by a set of double-lock doors forming an air lock (denoted by a dashed line in Fig. 2). The second area does not contain any debris-generating operations but is restricted to flushing, integrity testing, drying, and packaging operations. This second controlled environment area is maintained in a Class 100 room and is so certified periodically by outside testing laboratories. It contains walls of HEPA filter banks to provide horizontal laminar air flow.

The process controls and inspections discussed above are essential to building quality into the product. Coupled with 100% integrity testing during production, they ensure the reproducibility of the removal capabilities of the filter.

Sampling for tests performed outside the controlled environment area, on the other hand, is useful in verifying the quality characteristics of the product. These tests are sometimes considered "destructive" inasmuch as the filters are handled differently from the remainder of the lot. They are performance tests intended to qualify the fitness for use of the product for selected applications. For example, effluent cleanliness testing is applicable to all process industries, while resistivity recovery testing is applicable to the electronics industry, and tests for oxidizable substances, pH shift, and pyrogenicity would be directed toward the pharmaceutical industry.

Effluent cleanliness testing is a good example of why filter manufacture may be considered an extension of a filter user's own manufacturing facilities. Filters are an essential component of a total contamination control program and require their own contamination control programs to ensure the proper degree of cleanliness. There are four basic steps in any contamination control program (NASA, 1966): design; implement; maintain; and verify.

First, one has to design with the proper degree of contamination control in mind. Then one has to implement those controls necessary to achieve this level of contamination control. Next, that level of cleanliness has to be maintained. Finally, one has to verify that those levels of cleanliness are being achieved.

In order to design with the proper degree of contamination control for the pharmaceutical industry, for example, the debris-generating operations are separated from the cleaning operations (which are performed in a Class 100 room). To implement a contamination control program, operators are required to wear caps and gowns, use captive footwear, and have restricted access into the controlled environment area. To maintain product cleanliness levels, filters are flushed provided they do not contain any wetting agents or desired adjuvants and they can be properly dried. A high velocity flush, providing a pressure differential of about 60 psid (4 bar) will produce consistent levels of cleanliness. Flushing at a lower pressure, near the flow rate commonly used in routine service, will not be adequate to ensure such levels of cleanliness. Flushing at about 60 psid (or 15 L/min) for about 3 min is adequate to achieve the levels of cleanliness specified in even the most restrictive current industry standards, provided the filter is nonshedding. This is generally true of filters with integral seals, bonded media, and a stable pore structure. Media shedding or migration typically results in a high level of contaminants that does not significantly improve with flush volume. This is reflected in the regulatory definition of a non-fiber-releasing filter given by the Food and Drug Administration (FDA) in Title 21, Part 210.3(b)(6) of the *Code of Federal Regulations* (CFR, 1995) as "any filter, which after any appropriate pretreatment such as washing or flushing, will not release fibers into the component or drug product that is being filtered." This definition allows for removal of manufacturing debris that is generated during all assembly operations and of particulate matter present in the ambient environment.

5 CLEANLINESS LEVELS

To verify that desired levels of cleanliness are being achieved, effluent cleanliness tests must be performed. Such a test (shown schematically in Fig. 3) uses a membrane to collect effluent from a test filter. These tests involve particle counting by an automated instrument or a manual optical microscopic method. Each has its advantages and disadvantages, and the data obtained from one type of measurement have no relationship to the data obtained from another method. Although automated particle counters with light-obscuration sensors allow real-time, continuous monitoring, they usually cannot differentiate between particles and air bubbles, and their sensors may be susceptible to cell blockage and contamination. While manual microscopic particle counting is labor-intensive and can be operator-dependent, it allows identification of particles and unusual contaminants. The *United States Pharmacopeia* (USP, 1995) permits either method for enumeration of particulate matter in injections (see Table 1), but individual monographs specify only the microscopic particle count test for any product that is not a pure solution with the clarity and viscosity of water (USP, 1996).

The apparatus and procedure for a manual microscopic counting method are presented below.

The test (shown schematically in Fig. 3) uses a membrane to collect effluent from a test filter. The analysis membrane is dried in a laminar flow hood, and particulates are counted microscopically. A disk or cartridge filter is used as a prefilter to isolate the system so that no extraneous particulates are introduced, and the whole system is flushed each day prior to testing in order to clean up the system to achieve an acceptable blank count. To obtain the system blank, an analysis membrane is

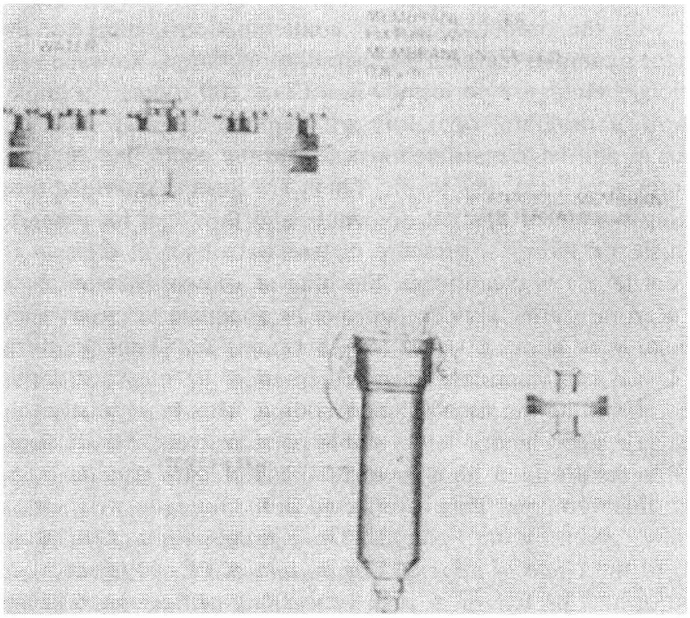

Figure 3 Schematic of effluent cleanliness test.

installed downstream without installing a test filter in the housing. Flow is initiated at 4 L/min for 5 min, and then the analysis membrane is removed, dried under a laminar flow hood, and counted microscopically. For the test count, a new analysis membrane is installed downstream and the test filter is installed in its housing. A test is run for 5 min at 4 L/min, using a total effluent of 20 L. Additional data for higher volumes can be obtained by installing another analysis membrane downstream, leaving the same filter in the test filter housing, and resuming flow.

Table 1 Particulate Matter in Injections, USP ⟨788⟩

	Size ranges and limits	
Particle count test method	≥10 μm	≥25 μm
Light obscuration		
Blank count (10 mL)	10	0.2 per mL
Large-volume injections	25	3 per mL
Small-volume injections	6000	600 per container
Microscopic		
Blank count (50 mL)	20	0.1 per mL
Large-volume injections	12	2 per mL
Small-volume injections	3000	300 per container

Source: Based on USP (1995).

Average initial particulate counts and ranges are given in Table 2 for 0.2 μm rated nylon membrane filters. For comparison purposes, unit effluent counts are given, reported per liter of water that was run through the filter per square foot of filter area. Particles 5 μm in diameter or larger are counted using an optical microscope at 100× magnification. The practical limit of this microscopic technique is about 1–2 μm, but counts at that limit are not as reproducible. Filter membrane manufacturing debris having an aspect ratio of 3:1 or larger is counted separately as fibers, in accordance with the regulatory definition of a fiber given by the Food and Drug Administration (FDA) in Title 21, Part 210.3(b) (5) of the *Code of Federal Regulations* (CFR, 1995). This has the advantage of providing a bivariate characterization of the manufacturing debris and improves operator recognition of anomalous contaminants, if any.

Cleanliness levels of filter cartridges are strongly influenced by type of construction and methods of production. Even in Class 100 areas, the use of a chemical adhesive in side sealing may increase initial unit particle counts by an order of magnitude over filters that do not require such additional handling.

Initial particulate counts are reduced with further flushing. Extending an effluent cleanliness test for an additional 30 min at 4 L/min, for example, decreases particle counts to about 3, and fiber counts drop down to about 0.4 fiber on average for the filters reported in Table 2. Running an additional 30 min (or 120 L) further reduces the particle count down to 1 and the fiber count down to 0.2 on average. These are the same values as are typically found for a 20 L blank extrapolated to 260 L, so that the net count would be zero if the blank count were subtracted.

The blank count cannot be completely eliminated. It arises from the test system itself, i.e., the piping and the filter housing. There is wear and fatigue of surfaces in the system as well. Another significant source for the blank count is the analysis membrane itself. Particle and fiber counts for particular lots for analysis membranes are often listed on the product container. Although prerinsing minimizes these, it does not eliminate them. Indeed, the very act of installing one of these analysis membranes in a test system by clamping it in place generates particles and fibers.

Once cleanliness levels are known, they may be compared with industry standards. In the pharmaceutical industry, one such comparison is with the *United States Pharmacopoeia* (USP) procedure in general chapter < 788 > where particulate matter limits are given for small- and large-volume parenterals for single-dose infusion (USP, 1995). This standard requires a valid blank for the test environment whether

Table 2 Initial Effluent Particulate Counts

Initial 20 liters	Particles larger than 5 μm	Fibers, 3:1 aspect ratio
Average	10	0.6
Range	0.8–21	0.1–0.9

Counts per liter per square foot of filter area for 5 ft^2 nylon membrane production elements; blank counts not subtracted. (Note that subsequent effluent counts are within the range of blank counts and are essentially zero.)

the testing is performed microscopically or by a light obscuration particle count test instrument. Once this background particle level is sufficiently low, an aliquot of a test preparation for a large-volume injection meets the requirements of the test with particle counts determined microscopically if the average number of particles present in the units tested does not exceed 12 particles that are 10 μm in diameter or larger per milliliter, with no more than two of these 12 particles/mL being allowed to be as large as 25 μm in diameter or larger.

In making a comparison with levels of cleanliness for filters, differences in test protocols should be understood. For example, only a 25 mL test aliquot may be taken in the USP procedure, whereas 20 L samples are taken in the filter effluent cleanliness test described above. In addition, the USP procedure counts only particles 10 μm in diameter or larger, while the filter effluent cleanliness test method counts particles down to 5 μm. Nevertheless, comparing that particle count given in Table 2 as the upper limit of the range observed in the initial 20 L results in a value of 0.1 particle/mL, whereas the USP particulate matter limit is 12 particles/mL. Therefore, the pharmaceutical grade filters reported in Table 2 are two orders of magnitude cleaner than that required for large-volume parenteral products. Of course, large-volume parenteral manufacturers have other contamination control problems to contend with, such as the cleanliness of container/closure systems. Nevertheless, having information on the cleanliness of their system components is important. Knowing the amount of debris to be expected if the filter has been properly flushed and maintained allows the development of meaningful internal operating procedures.

For filters not flushed during their manufacture, initial counts will be greater and the ranges more variable. On the other hand, extended flushing after installation in a process stream will reduce counts to acceptable levels (except in the case of media migration). Filter validation programs often require such testing to determine the amount of flushing to be performed after filter installation, based on company standards for finished-product cleanliness and product sensitivity to the flush fluid.

6 PERFORMANCE TESTING

Other tests intended to qualify fitness for use deal with effluent qualities closely related to performance in specific applications. For electronics applications, for example, a resistivity recovery test is performed to measure the "rinse-up" time required to flush a filter with deionized water so that the effluent is free of conducting ions as measured by the absence of any loss of resistivity. For pharmaceutical applications. a test of organic oxidizable substances mentioned in the *United States Pharmacopoeia* for purified water has been performed (USP, 1995). This test for oxidizable substances monitors the presence of certain organic impurities to ensure that none have come in contact with the filter materials of construction. While a high velocity flush is ineffective in reducing extractables, because migration within plastic materials is dependent on polymer bulk phase diffusion, it can serve to remove surface contaminants and leachable monomers. Purified water flushed through a test filter is treated with sulfuric acid, heated to boiling, and reacted with potassium permanganate, which is a powerful oxidizing agent with a pinkish coloration. The presence of most organic oxidizables will react with the potassium permanganate, and the pink color will disappear. If the pink color remains, there are no detectable organic oxidizables, and the test is passed. Some filters may require a preflush to remove trace organics and pass this test.

A test for total organic carbon (TOC) was introduced as USP ⟨ 643 ⟩ to serve as an alternative to, and eventually replace, the test for oxidizable substances in the USP water monographs (USP, 1996). As an indirect measure of organic molecules, TOC test methods are more sensitive than the colorimetric potassium permanganate assay used for oxidizable substances and can be performed either on-line or as an off-line laboratory test sample. Analytical technologies used to measure TOC must have a limit of detection of 0.05 ppm of carbon or lower, which is one order of magnitude below the 500 ppb maximum allowable. Water conductivity, USP ⟨ 645 ⟩, was also introduced to limit the allowed water impurity level and thus serves as a useful test of filter effluents.

The limulus amebocyte lysate (LAL) assay for endotoxins is another test used to ensure effluent quality in the pharmaceutical industry. Limulus test reagents vary in sensitivity from lot to lot and require a positive water control to establish a minimum sensitivity (e.g., 0.125 EU/mL). A positive sample control is also used to establish that nothing in the sample inhibits gel formation. A negative water control is used to determine whether any contamination invalidates the test. The test filter itself may be autoclaved at 121°C for 30 min or less in order to render the normal bioburden pyrogenic without depyrogenating the test sample and thereby maximize the test challenge. The test filter is then soaked for 1 h in the minimum volume of nonpyrogenic water necessary to cover all filter surfaces. A test soak aliquot is then incubated at 37°C for 1 h. Absence of gel formation indicates an acceptable test.

Filter integrity tests measure fitness for use not only by detecting leaks but also by verifying removal ratings. As nondestructive physical test methods, they can be performed 100% during production of filter cartridges used in critical applications. Filter integrity tests are typically liquid displacement tests consisting of measurement of air flow through a prewetted filter at defined test pressures (Pall, 1975). Empirical correlation of integrity test values with particulate or bacterial challenges is then used to verify removal ratings. The validity of the correlation rests on the reproducibility of the filter manufacturing process and the representativeness of the filter samples and the test challenge protocol. Further, the limiting integrity test value on which the removal rating is based may be combined with a safety factor to maximize the probability of absolute removal.

Since pore size distributions vary from one type of filter medium to another, each filter medium must be independently studied to correlate its integrity test parameters with particulate or bacterial challenges to validate removal ratings. It is important that a statistically significant number of specimen filters be evaluated in order to select suitable test parameters. The test pressure chosen for the integrity test must be high enough to produce a measurable flow and low enough to distinguish between bulk flow through open pores and diffusive flow through a liquid film that wets the filter medium. This allows detection of atypical pore size distributions and minor defects. Automated integrity test instruments create a pressure ramp and measure gas flow directly or indirectly through pressure decay. As a result of differences in instrument sensitivity and the algorithms used in the computer software to increase the applied pressure and define the inflection point, variation in measured integrity test values will occur between instruments of different manufacturers. Therefore, detailed test protocols must be performed in a consistent manner to obtain reproducible integrity test values that are to be correlated to bacterial retention. Offsetting this, from a practical viewpoint, a variety of pore size distributions are known to be microbially retentive because of the much greater number of smaller diameter pores present in most filter media.

In addition to such performance tests on finished products, performance testing during product development is an important part of a total quality program. Such qualification or prototype testing is essential, for example, in material selection. Engineering plastics tailored to individual process conditions are available, and membrane resins also can be chosen to optimize certain performance characteristics such as minimizing extractables. Materials for pharmaceutical use, for example, are often selected on the basis of having a listing in Title 21, parts 170–199, of the *Code of Federal Regulations* (CFR, 1995) as materials that may be processed for uses involving contact with human food. These materials are then also tested for biological reactivity, in vitro, as specified in the USP general chapter < 88 >. These USP biological safety tests for plastics list various options, including implantation and extraction in up to four solutions meant to simulate body fluids (USP, 1995). While the implantation test is often omitted, it provides an additional safety factor and is an important consideration for filter materials to be used in drug delivery systems. The extraction tests contain an additional option in that one of several time–temperature conditions may be chosen. This is significant because the higher temperatures, even at shorter times, can cause degradation of certain plastics and should be used with autoclavable filters. Other biocompatibility and toxicological tests have been advocated (HIMA 1978, 1980) and applied to evaluating the safety of materials used in filters. Such tests have been standardized (ISO, 1994) and modified by the FDA to replace the 1986 United States/United Kingdom/Canada Tripartite Biocompatibility Guidance.

7 TECHNICAL SUPPORT

Performance testing is conducted not only in regard to filter manufacture but also for filter use, where it is referred to as applications testing. Such technical support is a major feature of a total quality program because it is a service that often determines the ability of the product to satisfy user needs. It also constitutes a key factor in the product development spiral (Juran, 1974), frequently providing the field experience that leads to new research and development as well as redesign and corrective action. As a result, the movement toward separation systems is foretold in the development of those types of technical support capabilities for fluid clarification customers.

Technical support encompasses scientific and laboratory services, becoming an extension of user capabilities. Demand for these technical support services has increased as innovative technology, increasing specialization, and regulatory complexities have heightened user expectations. In the pharmaceutical industry, for example, customer–supplier partnerships have been fostered by regulatory guidance: "The agency recognizes that some of the more complex filter validation tests may be beyond the capabilities of some filter users. In such cases, it is acceptable to have the tests conducted by outside laboratories or by filter manufacturers" (FDA, 1987). This has led to the separation of specialized filter validation laboratories from other performance testing laboratories. Pharmaceutical filter validation laboratories perform services that include bacterial challenge testing with actual process fluids, filter extractables in drug product solvents, and preparation of documentation for in-plant validation of filter processes. Other performance testing laboratories carry out industrial applications testing including filterability determination of fluids, contamination analysis, effects of processing conditions on filter efficiency, and filter integrity testing. As an extension of user capabilities these laboratory services are frequently audited by customers, and some technical support departments in the United States, Europe, and Japan have completed third-party audits to attain supplier quality system certification to ISO 9001.

Fluid clarification may therefore be seen as a specialized discipline within a diverse range of process industries. The synergism provided by cooperative programs between manufacturer and user has led to many advances in filter product quality and fluid process technology.

REFERENCES

CFR. (1995). Code of Federal Regulations, U.S. Government Printing Office, Washington, DC.

FDA. (1987). *Guideline on Sterile Drug Products Produced by Aseptic Processing*, Division of Manufacturing and Product Quality (HFN-320), Center for Drugs and Biologics, Food and Drug Administration, Rockville, MD.

HIMA. (1978). Report 78-7, Guideline for the Safety of Materials Used in Medical Devices, Health Industry Manufacturers Association, Washington, DC.

HIMA. (1980). Report 80-1, Biocompatibility, Health Industry Manufacturers Association, Washington, DC.

ISO. (1994). *Quality systems—Model for quality assurance in design/development, production, installation and servicing*, ISO 9001: 1994, International Organization for Standardization, Geneva, Switzerland.

ISO. (1994). *Biological Evaluation of Medical Devices, Part 1: Evaluation and Testing*, ISO 10993-1, International Standards Organization, Geneva, Switzerland.

ISO. (1992). *Quality Management and Quality Assurance—Vocabulary*, ISO 8402, International Organization for Standardization, Geneva, Switzerland.

Juran, J.M. (Ed.) (1974). *Quality Control Handbook*, 3rd ed., McGraw-Hill, New York.

NASA (1966). *Handbook for Contamination Control on the Apollo Program*, Apollo Reliability and Quality Assurance Office, National Aeronautics and Space Administration, Washington, DC.

Ott, E.R. (1975). *Process Quality Control*. McGraw-Hill, New York, Chap. 7.

Pall, D.B. (1975). Quality control of absolute bacteria removal filters, *Bull. Parenteral Drug Assoc.*, *29*(4):192–204.

Sender, L.A., In *Quality Control Handbook*, 2nd ed. (J.M. Juran, Ed.) (1962). McGraw-Hill, New York, Sec. 26.

USP. (1995). *United States Pharmacopeia*, 23rd revision, United States Pharmacopeial Convention, Inc., Rockville, MD.

USP. (1996). USP 23, Supplement 5, *United States Pharmacopeia*, 23rd Revision, United States Pharmacopeial Convention, Inc., Rockville, MD. (Official Nov. 15, 1996).

7

Pore Sizes and Distributions

C. THOMAS BADENHOP
Badenhop Engineering Services, Westport, Connecticut

1 THE DETERMINATION OF THE PORE SIZE OF FINE FILTRATION MEDIA

Filters are used to separate particles from the fluid in which they are entrained for the following reasons or applications:

1. To separate large from smaller particles
2. To recover solids from fluid streams as a product
3. To recover solids from a fluid stream where the fluid is the product and the solid is a contaminant
4. Special applications such as growth of bacteria

The first of these processes is one of classification. Applications that involve the separation of aggregates into size classes, as by the use of Taylor sieves, are examples of classification processes. Of great commercial importance is the classification of fine particles used in the manufacture of magnetic devices such as tapes and computer drives. Here the particle separation must be made with very fine filters. The retention size range of these filters is very important to the process. Reverse osmosis (RO) and ultrafiltration are other instances of classification filtration.

When the removal of solids from a fluid stream is performed to recover the solid, as in filtering pigments or salts from a chemical process, total removal may not be needed. Here the medium may have a retention capability just sufficient to begin the formation of a filter cake. The cake then acts as the filter medium for the removal of the remaining solids in the stream. It is this cake that will be recovered as the product. The fluid may be disposed of or recovered and recycled in the process.

The third process is the removal of solids from a fluid stream so that the stream will be made clear, and the fluid is the product of the filtration. Beverage filtration represents this type of filtration, which is generally regarded as clarification filtration.

Membranes are generally regarded as classifying filter media. This is particularly true of uncharged media. In gas streams membranes remove particulates much smaller than their *mean flow pore size* (MFS) (Spurny, 1977) (Fig. 1), whereas in liquid filtration particles smaller than the MFS is retained less as the particle size decreases (Fig. 2).

Membranes that have been surface modified to produce a positive zeta potential during filtration will remove particles much smaller than the MFS. With such filters the residence time of filtration has an effect on the retention of particles smaller than the MFS. These membranes can act as clarifying filters.

Filter media which are constructed of a random distribution of small particles and fibers and generally called filter sheets are typically known to be clarifying filters. Their removal capacity is limited by the interactions with particulates and the internal surface area of the medium through zeta potential, hydrophobic and hydrophilic interactions. These materials are called depth filtration media.

Filter sheets, a specific type of depth filtration medium with barely measurable bubble points, have demonstrated virtually quantitative removal of virus particles. It is almost impossible to define a pore size or particle removal size for these filter materials. Pore size measurement of these materials is irrelevant; surface area measurement, however, is of significance in establishing retention characteristics.

The measurement of the particle-retaining capacity of a filter medium should be predictable from the characteristics of the medium itself. This is more likely for classifying media, than for clarifying media. The typical Taylor sieve size can be directly measured by examining the spacing between the wires of the sieve. It is obvious that particles larger than the openings of the sieve will be retained and also obvious that particles smaller than the sieve hole size will pass through the sieve. Particles just about the same size as the holes will sometimes pass through and sometimes be trapped in the holes. These sieves have a rather sharp particle separation characteristic. With these sieves there is only one layer of sieving action to retain particles, and the hole size is very narrowly distributed. Track-etched membranes from Nuclepore also have a very narrow distribution range of pore sizes with some overlapping of holes. These filters have essentially one pore size. Separation

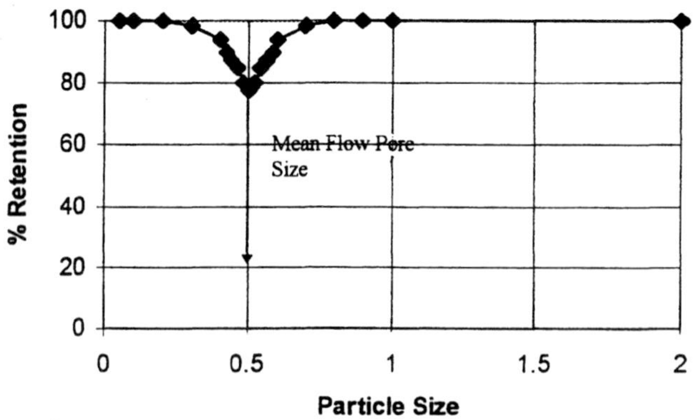

Figure 1 Retention in gas streams.

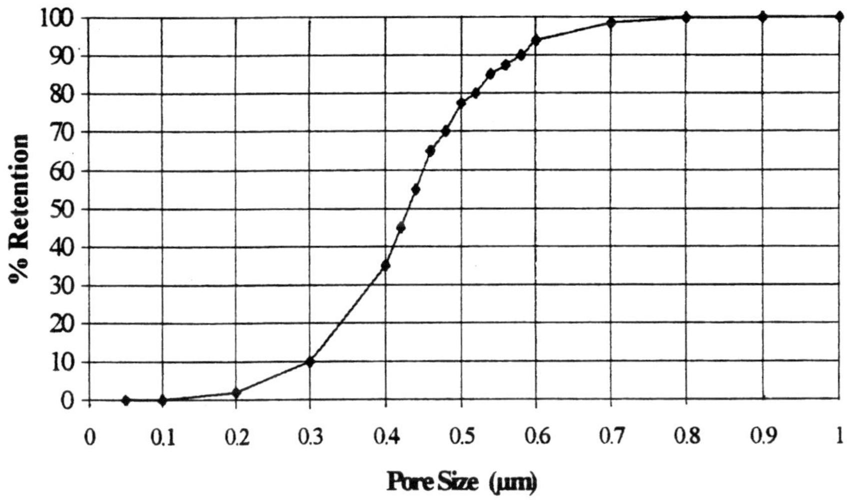

Figure 2 Membrane retention in liquids (noncharged media).

is extremely sharp. With these filters microphotographs can be used to exactly measure the pore size.

Filter media such as membranes formed from a phase inversion process produce a distribution of pore sizes, as is the case with most media other than woven sieves. Track-etched membranes have a narrower distribution than phase inversion membranes, but pore doubling and the etching process still result in some variation from the mean size of he filter.

With any medium there is the possibility of measuring the maximum pore size of the material by means of the bubble point. Assuming the maximum hole to be circular, the Canter equation [Eq. (1)] can be solved for the maximum-sized pore. The maximum pore is proportional to the pressure required to force air through the largest capillary or hole. With good wetting, the cosine of the wetting angle can be considered to be 1. The value of the maximum pore size obtained by using this test method has been shown to be reliable.

As the name implies, there can be only one pore of maximum size. All other pores must be smaller and not only smaller but greater in number. Finding the distribution of the pores according to their size is useful in establishing the retention and flow characteristics of the filter. Liquids flow through fine porous bodies in laminar flow (Brown, 1950) as opposed to turbulent flow. This means that the bulk flow through the capillary of the filter is inversely proportional to the viscosity of the liquid, directly proportional to the pressure differential across the filter, inversely proportional to the capillary length, and inversely proportional to the fourth power of the diameter of the capillary [Eq. (4)].

This results in the largest capillaries having the greatest proportion of total flow. Figure 3 demonstrates the amount of fluid flowing through the pores of the filter in relation to their size. The flow through the larger pores is so much greater that a numerical pore distribution is of little interest in characterizing membranes.

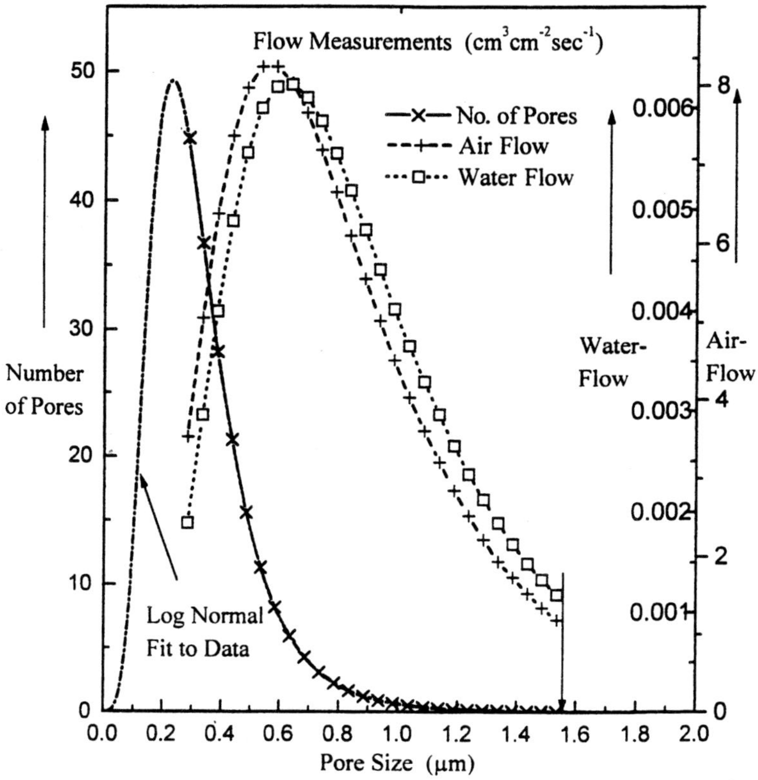

Figure 3 Distribution of a 0.65-μm mean flow pore filter as compared to the numerical distribution.

The flow distribution of the filter as shown in this figure (i.e., the percentage of the flow passing through each pore diameter) is significant. The pore size distribution of filters as represented by the flow distribution is what is usually meant when the "flow pore distribution" of a medium is discussed.

The distribution of flow through a filter of fine pore size (i.e., less than 1 μm) is different for liquids and gases. This is because the size of the capillaries of the filter produces a flow close to the mean free path of the gas molecules. Below 1 μm, gases flow proportionately more through a finer pore more than is predicted by the laminar flow equation. Below 0.5 μm this error is rather large. Thus, the mean flow pore size of a filter measured using gases is smaller than that which would be expected for liquids. The gas measurement gives a disproportionately higher contribution to the fine capillaries of the medium. This means that the pore size distribution of the filter should be calculated from gas flow first, and the distribution for liquids calculated from this result.

The current ASTM method does not take this factor into consideration. Media smaller than 0.2 μm will result in a considerable error in the flow distribution for liquids.

2 STANDARD TESTS TO CHARACTERIZE FILTER MEMBRANE MEDIA

2.1 Bubble Point

The bubble point is the measure of the maximum pore size of any filter or porous material. This is expressed by the *Cantor equation*, which may be derived through the analysis of the balance of forces in a capillary.

Let

ΔP = the pressure differential across the filter
D = the diameter of the capillary
θ = the wetting angle between the fluid and the surface of the filter
γ = the surface tension between the liquid and the solid interface material

then

$$D = \frac{4\gamma \cos \theta}{\Delta P} \tag{1}$$

It has been demonstrated (Knight et al.) that for fluids that wet porous material well, the contact angle θ is 0°. This eliminates the cosine term in the equation. If the wetting fluid is water and the pressure differential is measured in bar and the pore size in micrometers, the equations reduces to

$$D = \frac{3}{\Delta P} \tag{2}$$

The bubble point is a very important test as it indicates the *maximum pore size* of the filter. It will indicate if there is an outlier pore that is larger than an expected maximum pore size. It also indicates leaks or improper sealing of a filter, be it a cartridge or "O" ring seal of a flat membrane. In combination with other tests methods the bubble point can be used to establish the average pore size (nominal pore size) of filter media.

2.2 Water Flow Rate of Filter Media

The rate of water flow through a filter medium (Fig. 4), when determined without any pressure restrictions other than the media itself, can yield important information about the average or *hydrodynamic* pore size of the medium. With all fine pore size media the Reynolds number, Re, is usually very small, indicating laminar flow

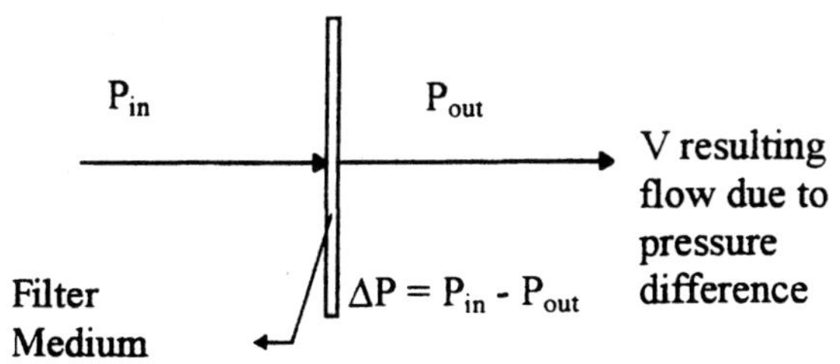

Figure 4 Flow of fluid through a membrane.

through the medium (Brown 1950). With laminar flow, the Hagen-Poiseuille equation may be applied directly.

Assuming circular cross sections of the capillaries:

L = the capillary length, in cm
V = the volume flow, in cm^3 sec^{-1}
η = the viscosity, in poise
N = number of capillaries in diameter D

then

$$\mathrm{Re} = \frac{DV\rho}{\eta} \tag{3}$$

and if the Re is less than 600, the flow is entirely laminar (Fig. 5). The flow of fluids follow streamlines ignoring the roughness and will flow around obstructions. If a particle touches the wall of a capillary, it will remain there. The layer of fluid immediately next to the capillary wall is stationary.

$$V = \frac{\pi D^4 \Delta P}{128 L \eta} N \tag{4}$$

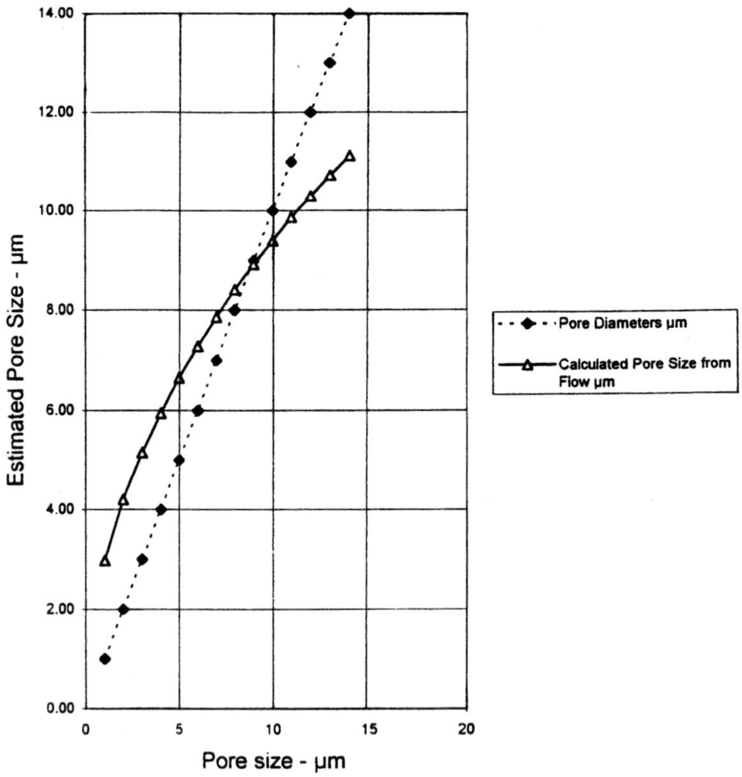

Figure 5 Hydrodynamic pore size estimate.

2.3 Void Volume

The water flow rate of a filter is insufficient for a determination of the average or hydrodynamic pore size of a filter medium. It is necessary to establish the area that represents the capillaries in the medium. This is determined by the void volume of the material.

Void volume V_v can be calculated from the density of the polymer or component of the medium ρ_m, the volume of the medium V_m, and the weight of the medium W_m:

$$V_v = \frac{W_m}{\rho_m V_m} \tag{5}$$

of the volume of an imbibed liquid V_{liq} divided by the volume of the media:

$$V_v = V_{\text{liq}} \div V_m \tag{6}$$

The diameter D cannot be directly determined from Eq. (4); however, the product D^4N can be determined, as L can be assumed to be the thickness of the medium. It is usually possible to determine the void volume of the medium from density determinations. With this information, the number of pores can be calculated as a function of pore size.

If V_v is the void volume of the medium and A is the area of the filter in square centimeters, then

$$N = \frac{4A}{\pi D^2} V_v \tag{7}$$

Solving Eqs. (4) and (7) simultaneously (which can be done graphically), the hydrodynamic pore size of the medium is determined. A medium that has a skin as the ultrafilter medium requires that the thickness of the skin be used in this determination instead of the thickness of the structure. If this is not done, the pore size can be calculated as being larger than the maximum pore size. The following example illustrates the procedure.

The medium is a porous carbon block filter, as represented in Fig. 6. An estimate of the average pore size was needed to see whether this material could retain a particular particle size. First, the bubble point of the carbon block was measured using water. The value of pressure at the bubble point was 3.61 psi or 0.25 bar. This, from Eq. (2), gives a maximum pore size of 12.05 μm. Second, the axial water flow rate of the block was measured. Next, the void volume of the block was determined. The volume of this block is 64 cm^2. Carbon's specific gravity is 1.68 g cm^3, which yields a carbon volume of 23.6 cm^3. When the carbon block was completely filled with water, which was accomplished by immersing the block in water in a vacuum, a water volume of 40.4 cm^3 was measured. This calculates to a void volume of 63.2%.

This means that if this block were composed of capillaries uniformly distributed throughout the block, the area of these capillaries must equal 8 cm^2. From the flow test, a flow of 6.67 cm^3 sec^{-1} was found with a capillary length (block length) of 4.9 cm at a pressure differential of 1.66 bar. The simultaneous solution of Eqs. (3) and (5), which is graphically solved in Fig. 5, is about 8.5 μm. The calculated hydrodynamic pore size of this filter is smaller than the maximum pore size, as

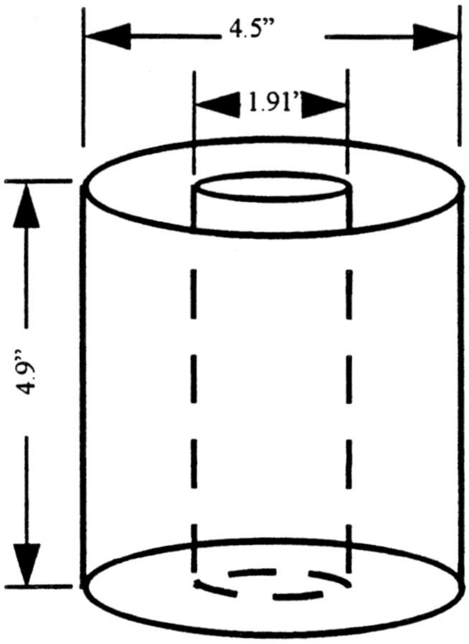

Figure 6 Carbon block filter dimensions.

determined by bubble point measurement. If this was reversed, it would indicate that the block had a nonuniform structure such as that produced by a dense surface skin. This means that the assumption that the capillary length is equal to the thickness of the medium is incorrect. In this block the flow radially through the filter resulted in the same pore size being calculated. There was obviously no skin or surface densification. When there is surface densification, there can be a discrepancy between the maximum pore size and the calculated hydrodynamic pore size. The value of L must be adjusted to take the densification into account. Sometimes it is difficult to make a conclusion that can be supported by data in the determination of L for a dense surface.

In membrane filters this can be very important in the determination of pore size and retention characteristics. It is possible to measure the pore size distribution independently of surface densification. A rigorous analysis of this process requires the solution of the flow equation for a wetted filter medium. For membrane filters in the pore size range of about 0.1 to 3 μm, the following equation has been developed:

$$PV = \frac{\pi D^4 \Delta P \bar{P}}{128 \eta L} = nRT \tag{8}$$

This represents the viscous portion of the gas flow. An additional term must be added to this equation when the Knudsen number, Kn, is greater than zero. The flow equation for small capillaries is (Carman, 1956):

$$PV = \frac{pD^4 DP\bar{P}}{128hL}\left[1 + 4\ \mathrm{Kn}\left(\frac{2}{f} - 1\right)\right] \tag{9}$$

Kn is the Knudsen number, the ratio of the mean free path of the gas molecules to

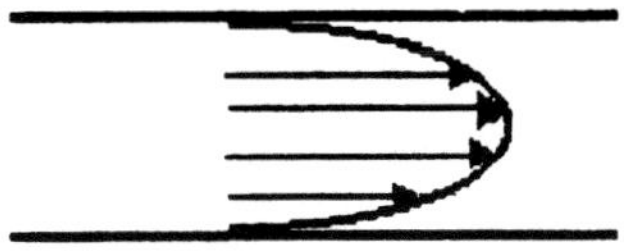

Figure 7 Vector representation of laminar flow in a capillary.

the diameter of the capillary. In membrane filters the value of Kn cannot be ignored. In this equation f is a reflection factor. This factor is absent from the viscous flow equation because the molecules never reach the surface of the capillary, because a layer of motionless fluid lies on this surface. The profile of the velocity within the capillary will have the shape shown in Fig. 7. The arrows are the varying velocity vectors and the curve is the profile of these vectors. When the Kn number becomes significant, the velocity at the surface of the capillary becomes greater than zero and the molecules can interact with this surface. Thus, there can be some reflection from rough spots in the surface.

Membrane filters are not capillaries but are composed of cells and openings in the cells, and thus there will be ample opportunity for reflection from the internal surfaces of the membrane. Streamlines will no longer completely surround the surfaces of the membrane structure preventing any reflection. The higher the Kn number, the greater is the proportion of reflected molecules (see Fig. 8) of the fluid stream (Tsien, 1946; Carman, 1956).

The value of f for a porous body is usually constant over a wide range of flows and pressures. This has been demonstrated in direct measurements of the flow of gases through membrane filters (Badenhop, 1983).

Substituting the specific gas characteristics for the value of the Kn number into Eq. (7) (Badenhop, 1983, pp. 41–55):

$$\text{Kn} = \frac{\text{Kn}}{\Delta PP} \tag{10}$$

and rearranging terms and dividing through the ΔP:

$$\frac{PV}{\Delta P} = \bar{P}\,\frac{\pi D^4}{128\ \mu L} + \frac{\pi D^3 4\ \text{Kn}}{128\ \mu L}\left(\frac{2}{f} - 1\right) \tag{11}$$

If the value of f is constant, the preceding equation is linear when $PV/\Delta P$ is plotted against $\bar{P}$. The graph of the flow of hydrogen and nitrogen through a 0.1 μm filter (Fig. 9) shows the linearity of the relation between $PV/\Delta P$ vs. $\bar{P}$, which proves that the value of f is constant through this membrane (under the conditions of the test).

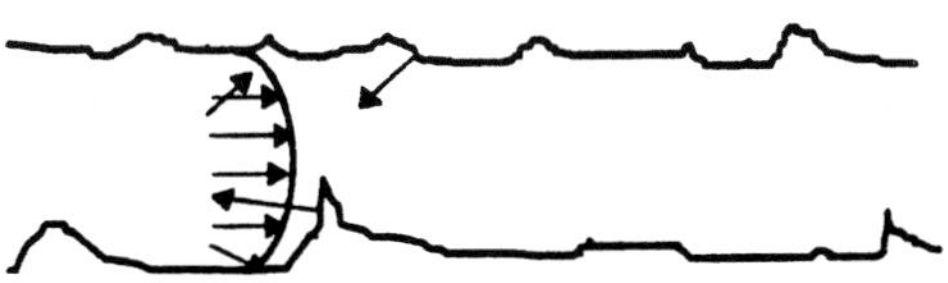

Figure 8 Partial molecular flow in a small capillary flow extends to wall of capillary, causing reflection due to roughness.

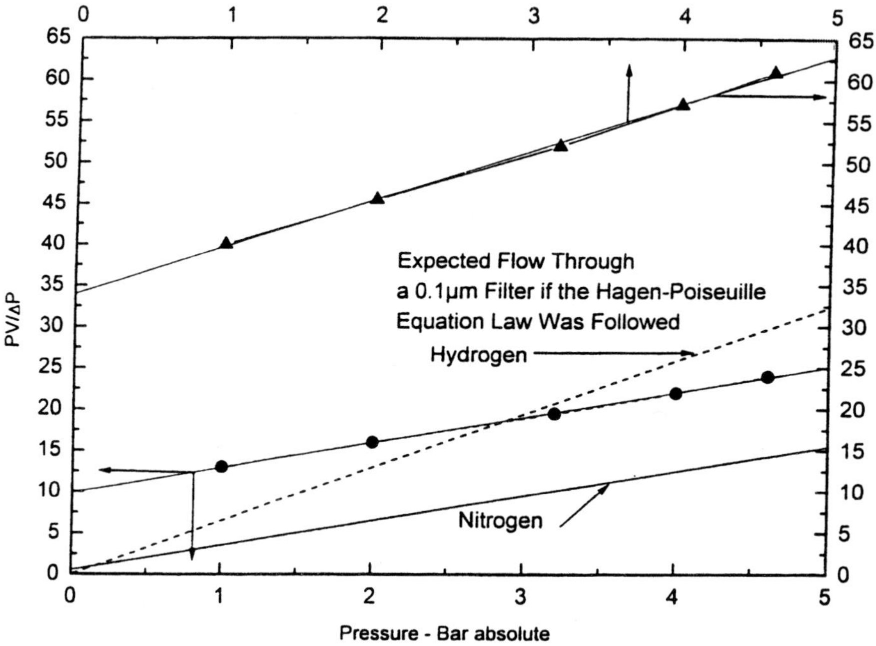

Figure 9 The reflection factor f is constant over the test range.

In addition, the intercept of this function does not pass through the origin as it would if the Hagen-Poiseuille law were followed.

Thus, a significant increase in the expected flow occurs through the gas slip effect. If the calculations used to determine a pore distribution of hydrodynamic pore size uses the Hagen-Poiseuille law, in this calculation, without the consideration of gas slip, errors occur. The smaller the capillaries, the greater the error. Note also that this linearity verifies Eq. (11). It correctly represents the flow of gases through membrane filters.

$$PV_{\text{wet}_i} = \frac{\pi \Delta P_i}{128\ \eta L} \left\{ \bar{P}_i \int_{D_i}^{D_{\text{BP}}} f(D) D^4 dD + 4\ \text{Kn} \int_{D_i}^{D_{\text{BP}}} f(D) D^3 dD \right\} \tag{12}$$

where

$f(D)$ = the pore distribution function
D_{BP} = the maximum pore size (bubble point)
D_i = a point on the wet flow curve between the bubble point and the smallest possible pore size

Each point D_i on the wet flow curve is represented by Eq. (12). From this equation the value of the distribution function $f(D)$ can be determined. Note that integrating this equation (assuming the distribution function $f(D)$ were known) would yield the dry flow of the membrane.

The procedure for development of the distribution function is one of careful measurement of the wet flow versus pore size at ever-increasing pressure in steps of constant pore size. At each step, beginning with the bubble point, where the flow is just >0, a step size is chosen small enough to generate a reasonable function but large enough to control pressure differentials exactly. It is also of critical importance that the wetting fluid be nonvolatile so that the only increase in flow, with each increase in pressure, is due to pores previously open flowing at a higher ΔP—and new pores being opened as the bubble point of these small capillaries are exceeded. The flow must be measured after sufficient time to assure the flow through the newly open capillaries has reached the maximum. The wetting fluid must have time to be blown out of the capillary. It sometimes requires up to 5 min to achieve constant flow. The number of pores is then calculated from the effect of the increase in pressure after taking into consideration the added flow from pressure increase from the previous step using Eq. (13), the general equation of flow (Badenhop, 1983, pp. 63–77):

$$PV = \frac{\pi D^4 \bar{P} \Delta P}{128\ \eta L} \left\{1 + \frac{4\ \mathrm{Kn}}{DP} \left(\frac{2}{f} - 1\right)\right\} N \tag{13}$$

For the normal pore distribution, as shown in Fig. 10, the flow pore distribution has been calculated using the preceding equation. Figure 10 is the normal distribution about a numerical mean pore of 0.6 μm and a maximum pore size of 1.2 μm. The resulting calculation of the flow pore distribution is shown in Fig. 11. Real membrane filters tend to be log normally distributed. An actual example of the pore distribution from measured data is shown in Fig. 12. Note that the distribution for air is slightly different from the distribution for water.

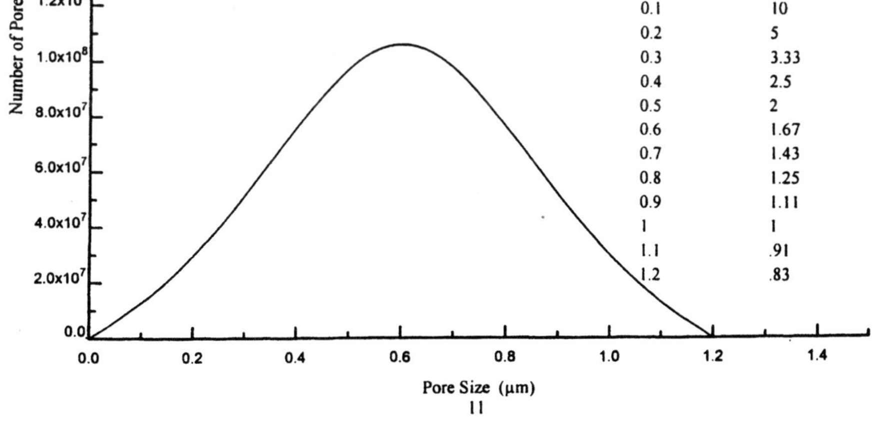

Figure 10 Numerical pore distribution, normally distributed.

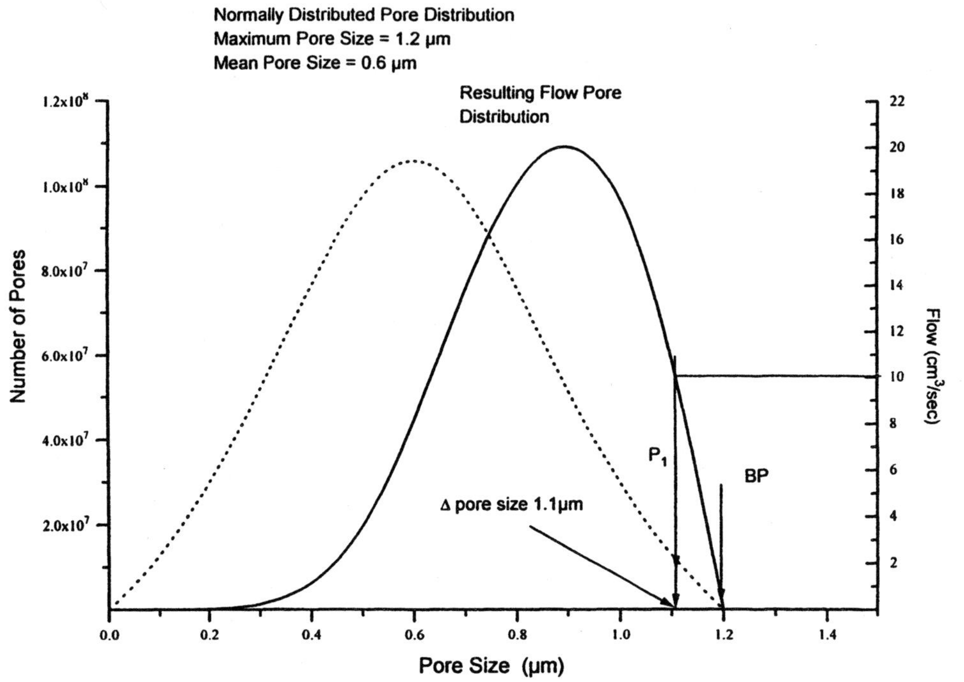

Figure 11 Normally distributed numerical pore distribution showing the resulting flow pore distribution.

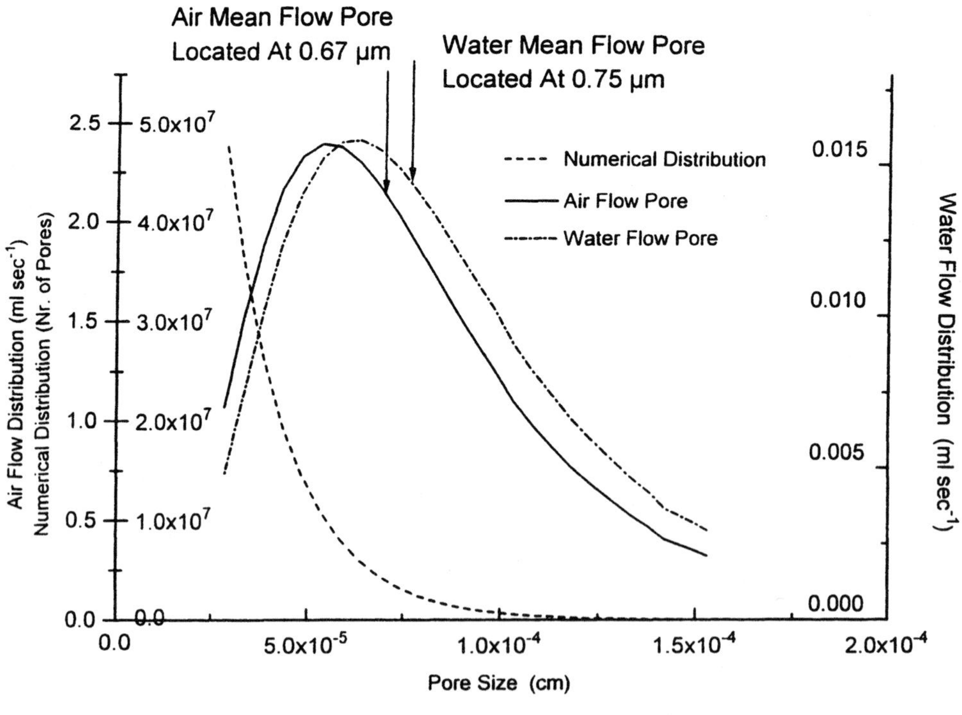

Figure 12 Distribution of a 0.65-µm membrane.

3 EVALUATION OF THE INTEGRITY OF LARGE-MEMBRANE FORMATS

The measurement of the bubble point of membranes in small formats presents no difficult as the initiation of flow may be either directly observed or measured with sensitive instruments. As the area of the membrane increases, the difficulty of determining the bubble point increases because of the parallel flow of gas from diffusion through the wet membrane. With small formats this diffusion is almost immeasurable. With larger formats diffusion flow becomes significant, especially at the high pressures needed to assure integrity of cartridges with very small pore size membranes.

The diffusion of gas through the membrane is not at all influenced by its pore size. Fick's law, which describes the diffusion of gases, states that the diffusion is proportional to the pressure across the membrane and inversely proportional to the thickness of the wetted film of the membrane. The rate of diffusion is also related to the solubility of the gas in the testing fluid. CO_2, for example, has a higher diffusivity through water wet membranes than does air. SF_6 has a lower diffusivity through water wet membrane than does air.

Membrane cartridges are normally tested with air, and the diffusion rate at a fixed pressure is used to indicate the integrity of the membrane composite. As this test measures the diffusion of gas through a wet film, it is not measuring the pore size of the membrane. For this reason the test pressure used in establishing the integrity of composites is usually set some point below the bubble point of the media (to avoid exceeding the bubble point, which would result in very high flow values), and high enough not to be below the bubble point of the next larger grade of membrane. Thus, the test is performed, for example, for a 0.2-μm cartridge at a pressure higher than a 0.45-μm membrane's bubble point and lower than the 0.2-μm bubble point. It is generally set at 80% of the bubble point of the medium used to produce the composite.

The level of diffusion flow will increase as the pressure increases and finer pore sizes are evaluated. It is, however, very difficult to distinguish between a level of diffusion flow and small defects in the cartridge. This is of critical importance when determining the integrity of pharmaceutical membrane cartridges, as a single defect can result in bacteria passing through the structure (11).

Attempts at developing testing procedures that would distinguish between diffusion and bulk flow have been undertaken since 1980 at AMF laboratories (12), using a procedure that utilizes the time delay in the establishment of diffusion of SF_6 gas from the almost instantaneous development of bulk flow.

Companies other than the membrane producers have begun developing testing equipment for the measurement of porous bodies. (These are well known in the industry and include Sartochek from Sartorius, Pall's Palltronic, etc.) Coulter has marketed a porometer for the measurement of pore size distribution, as has PMI (Porous Materials Incorporated). PMI has been developing integrity testing devices utilizing mass flow meters in their design. In addition, they have been able to build very repeatable equipment by using oversampling measurement techniques which hold pressure constant until flow has stabilized. This oversampling is of particular help in establishing the true diffusion/bulk flow characteristics of membrane cartridges. The PMI system is capable of establishing the distribution of the pore structure at the bubble point of cartridges because of the accuracy of the instrumentation.

In order to refine the measurement of cartridges, an improvement in the signal-to-noise ratio of the measurements is of considerable advantage in generating definitive data. This is critical in producing truly meaningful results that distinguish between bulk flow and diffusion. It is possible to develop such a system.

The foundation of the mechanical requirements of a highly precise system for reliable integrity testing is already available in the PMI equipment and software. The second step in the development of a high-sensitivity measurement system is the incorporation of gases other than air in the diffusion testing. With the use of other gases, the sensitivity of the mass flow meters improves significantly. Using SF_6, as an example, increases the sensitivity of the meters by a factor of 4.

Of particular interest are gases that are nontoxic, less soluble in water, and lower in viscosity than air. The Freons have this characteristic but are expensive and environmentally unsound. SF_6 is a nontoxic gas that we have studied in the past. It is nontoxic, the mass flow meters are four times more sensitive to SF_6 than to air, and it is lower in viscosity than air. The viscosity of air is 0.00186 cps and SF_6 is 0.00152 cps, an improvement of 22.37%. This has the net effect of enhancing the differentiation between bulk and diffusion flow measurements. SF_6 also is one-fourth less soluble in water than air. Thus, there is a bulk flow-to-diffusion improvement of almost 5 times that of air.

This difference is particularly noticeable when the output voltage off the mass flow meters using SF_6 are plotted against the output voltage of the mass flow meters flowing air (see Fig. 13).

The flow of gas through small pores (larger than 1 μm) is approximated by the viscous flow equation:

$$V = \frac{\pi D^4 \Delta P}{128\ \mu L} N \tag{4}$$

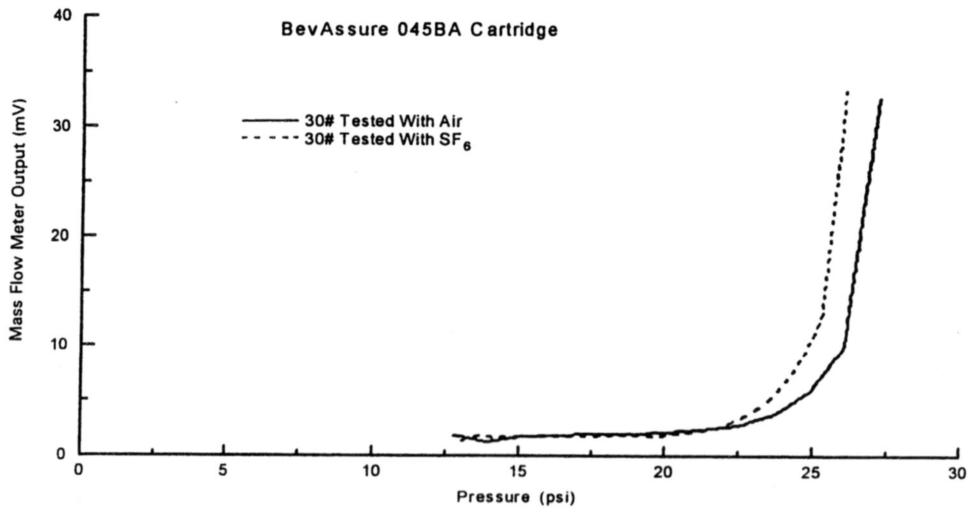

Figure 13 Output voltage off mass flow meters using SF_6 versus air.

From the Cantor equation, which relates the bubble point of the membrane to the pore size, the relation between bubble point and maximum pore size is given:

$$D = \frac{4\gamma \cos \theta}{\Delta P} \tag{1}$$

Since the wetting angle has been shown to be 0° (Knight et al.) this reduces for water and when the pressure difference (in bar) and diameter (in μm) to

$$D = \frac{2.88}{\Delta P}$$

With the pressure in psi the relation is

$$D = \frac{41.76}{\Delta P}$$

Using these relationships the number of pores in bulk flow can be calculated from the total of diffusion flow and bulk flow by measuring the flow above the linear Fick's law values.

The viscous flow equation holds for gases only when the velocity of flow is less than Mach number (Ma) 0.5. For membrane-sized pores this is not a consideration; however for defects, which are much larger than the membrane pore sizes, the effect of the Ma should be evaluated. The gas flow values for assumed defect sizes shown in Tables 1 and 2 have taken the compressibility of the gases into consideration. Note that once Ma = 1 no increase in flow through the pore is possible with a decrease in downstream pressure. Increasing upstream pressure increases flow due to density change only. This further complicates the flow calculations.

For SF_6 the molecular weight is 146 and the higher density results in a much lower speed of sound, which limits the flow at higher pressures. This, in effect, makes the use of the SF_6 more sensitive in the lower pore size areas for defects in the bubble point range. The Ma number exceeds 0.5 even at 0.5 bar pressure, indicating compressible flow.

Table 1 Gas Flow Values for Flow of Air Through Defects of Various Sizes

Test pressure bar gauge	Flow of air through defect size (ml/min)				
	10 μm	8 μm	6 μm	4 μm	2 μm
1	0.52308	0.22302	0.07200	0.01433	
1.5	0.85020	0.37626	0.12444	0.02503	0.00157
2	1.18560	0.54702	0.18630	0.03799	0.00239
2.5	1.53960	0.72900	0.25626	0.05315	0.00336
3	*1.61700*	0.91980	0.33282	0.07044	0.00448
3.5		*1.03500*	0.41478	0.08982	0.00575
4			0.50058	0.11088	0.00716
4.5			*0.58200*	0.13386	0.00872
5				0.15858	0.01044
5.5					

Italic numbers indicate choke flow.

Table 2 Gas Flow Values for Flow of SF_6 Through Defects of Various Sizes

Test pressure bar	Flow of SF_6 through indicated defect size (ml/min)				
	10 μm	8 μm	6 μm	4 μm	2 μm
1	0.00791	0.00380	0.00134	0.00028	
1.5	0.01199	0.00600	0.00223	0.00048	3.07E-05
2	*0.01384*	0.00843	0.00325	0.00072	4.68E-05
2.5		0.00957	0.00437	0.00100	6.58E-05
3		*0.01023*	0.00561	0.00132	8.76E-05
3.5			0.00167	0.00167	1.12E-04
4			*0.0064*	0.0021	1.40E-04
4.5				0.0024	1.70E-04
5				0.0029	2.04E-04
5.5				*0.0033*	2.40E-04

Italic numbers indicate choke flow.

The apparent accuracy of the measurements made with the PMI equipment is in the range of ±0.0125 ml of SF_6. Assuming that it is possible to read to ±0.02 ml of SF_6, with careful testing, the character of the defects can be discernible. This level of accuracy is not possible with air and is due to the enhanced sensitivity of the meters using SF_6.

The accuracy of the PMI equipment is largely due to the oversampling methods of developing the data. The equipment raises the pressure to a desired value and waits until the flow gauges give a constant reading. This allows time for pores to open because their bubble point are exceeded and to reach a steady flow rate. Once the steady flow is established and the measurement is recorded, the pressure is increased to the next level.

This oversampling is particularly critical in determining the bubble point and mean pore of the filter. Failure to wait for the flow to come to a constant rate will result in inaccurate and nonrepeatable test results. There can be a substantial time delay in the establishment of the mean pore that will require the instrument to wait for 5 min or longer at the pressure near the mean. The PMI equipment is capable of adjusting for this effect.

The incorporation of a halogen-containing gas, such as SF_6, in the testing allows the use of ECD detectors that can significantly increase sensitivity in determining the point at which bulk flow begins (detection of the bubble point).

Using a mixture of SF_6 and air in diffusion testing will take advantage of the wet membrane's gas separation capability. The mixture will have a different composition when passing through the filter by a diffusion mechanism than when passing through the filter by bulk flow. The difference in the solubility of air and SF_6 is about 4 to 1; thus most of the SF_6 will be retained as the mixture diffuses through the filter. The ECD detector is extremely sensitive to halogen-containing gases and the change in composition because of:

Bulk flow containing four times the SF_6 from bulk flow rather than diffusion

The lower viscosity of SF_6, which further enhances the sensitivity of the measurement

There is a considerable cost advantage in using a mixture of SF_6 rather than pure SF_6, and the detectors will be able to sample the total gas mixture when the correct composition is chosen. This latter point was a significant problem in the earlier work at AMF, complicating the sampling of the gases.

A definitive single-point measurement is possible with this system. It is only necessary to measure the composition of the gas to indicate whether bulk flow existed at the test pressure. As bulk flow occurs, there is an increase in the flow of the gas through the cartridge. This composition change of the mixture of the gases will be identified by the ECD detector. This is a far more sensitive measurement than a flow measurement made by mass flow meters.

In addition, when pressure is applied quickly, bulk flow occurs almost instantaneously, whereas diffusion flow requires saturating the water film with the gas mixture. This phenomenon has been described by Brown (1950). This time delay allows for true detection of leaks in a large filter system.

REFERENCES

Badenhop, C. Thomas. (1983). The determination of the pore distribution and consideration of methods leading to the prediction of retention characteristics of membrane filters. Doctoral thesis, Universität Dortmund, Dortmund, Germany, pp. 53–59.

Badenhop, C. T. (1990). *The Validation of Membrane Filtration Devices for Pharmaceutical Uses*. Cuno, Inc.

Brown, G. G. (1950). *Unit Operations*. John Wiley & Sons, Inc., New York, pp. 138–139.

Carman, P. C. (1956). *Flow of Gases Through Porous Media*. Butterworth's Scientific Publications, London, pp. 62–78.

Knight, Rodney A., and Badenhop, C. T. (1990). *New Integrity Test Method*. Cuno, Inc.

Knight, Rodney A., C. Gryte, and T. Hazlett. (1992). Effect of high temperature annealing on the capillary of polyamide microporous membranes. Polymer Solution, Blends and Interfaces; (I. Noda and D. N. Rubingh, Eds.). Elsevier Science Publishers, B.V.

Spurny, K. (1977). Nucleopore Sieve Filter Membrane: Ten years usage for dust and aerosol measurement. *Dust, Purity Air 37*(9):328–334.

Tsien, H. S. (1946). Superaerodynamics: Mechanics of rarefied gases. *J. Aeronaut. Sci. 12*: 653–664.

8

Extractables and Compatibilities of Filters

OSCAR W. REIF
Sartorius AG, Göttingen, Germany

1 INTRODUCTION

One important issue in the filtration of pharmaceutical formulations is the fundamental question about the interactions between the filter and the fluid to be filtered. The chemical and structural compatibility between a filter and the processing liquid are very important and are functions of various physical and chemical parameters of the filter and the fluid. Incompatibility can lead to ineffective filtration and process failure. Another consequence of fluid–filter interactions is the potential contamination of the filtrate by extractables and particle shedding of the filter. Such contamination would lead to an obsolete product, costly abortion of the production process, or a health risk to the consumer of the filtered pharmaceutical matter. In this chapter, consideration is given to extractables and the compatibilities of filters in the pharmaceutical industry and the relationship between the two.

2 EXTRACTABLES

The issue of extractables, both in type and in amount, is of growing concern to all filter users. The ability to evaluate extractables is vitally important for all applications, especially when the filtered solution is intended for therapeutic use. Pharmaceutical products such as solid drugs, injectable and infusion solutions, or preparations used to treat open wounds must comply exactly with defined quality standards. To ensure the quality of their products, the pharmaceutical industry subjects them to extensive testing for potential contaminants both during the initial development of the manufacturing process and as part of a continuing quality and process control. The improvement in analytical methods with regard to the sensitivity of detection, selectivity, and reproducibility has led to an increased awareness of the problem of impurities and contaminants in pharmaceutical formulations.

Consequently, the chemical nature and origin of extraneous contaminants are of growing concern to all pharmaceutical manufacturers. In general, all materials such as storage tanks, tubing, pipes, valves, packaging, and purification devices employed in the manufacturing process are a potential source of impurities and should be tested as such. The final steps in the downstream process on a pharmaceutical production line are especially critical with regard to substances that can be extracted from the equipment by the process conditions applied and have a direct impact on the quality of the formulation.

Filters and filtration equipment are an integral part of downstream processing, used primarily during prefiltration to reduce the bioburden and for sterile filtration of the pharmaceutical solution. As the final step in drug processing before packaging or formulation, sterilization of the product by membrane filtration, is especially critical because extractables from these downstream processing devices can directly contaminate the product. Not only are such extractables particularly detrimental in the manufacture of small batches where their concentrations can be greater than in large-volume filtrations (because the extracted contaminants are diluted), but they can also be of concern in the processing of large batches if the filtered solutions are concentrated by evaporation of the solvent or by lyophilization. Such methods concentrate the impurities together with the product and can shift the concentration of a specific contaminant from the nontoxic range to the toxic.

This chapter is devoted to extractables, particulates, and the soluble entities leached from filters by the liquids being filtered. The origin of the extractables of prefilter and sterile filter cartridges is discussed as well as current practices, development, and the results of extractables studies and flush protocols.

3 THE ORIGIN OF EXTRACTABLES

In the pharmaceutical industry, sterilizing filters are used in numerous device configurations. Cartridge filters are the most widely used in the industry and are produced in a wide variety of models constructed of many different materials. They are often designed as disposable components to be replaced when they clog but are sometimes also sold as cleanable and reusable. Filter media constitute various polymeric membranes, yarns, binder-free and binder-containing fibers (wovens and nonwovens), felts and other synthetics, woven wire cloths, and sintered metallic and ceramic structures. In the pharmaceutical industry, the filters used for sterile filtration are mainly made of colloidal film membranes containing cellulose acetate (CA) and other cellulose esters, polyamides (PA), polysulfone (PSU) and polyether sulfone (PESU), fluorocarbons like polytetrafluoroethylene (PTFE) or poly(vinylidene fluoride) (PVDF), polycarbonate (PC), polyetherimide (PEI), or polypropylene (PP). Several other polymers including olefins, polystyrene, and polyacrylics are also used but are less important in the downstream processing of pharmaceutical formulations. The membranes are manufactured with or without supporting webs made of polypropylene, polyethylene, or polyesters. These membranes and supporting materials are potential sources of extractables or particle shedding and can contribute to decomposition or degradation of the material resulting from thermal or mechanical stress during the sterilization process (such as autoclaving, steam sterilization, or gamma radiation). Moreover, fluid–filter interactions or even chemical reactions between aggressive solutions and the polymeric materials can produce various compounds that contaminate the filtrate. A detailed discussion of these compatibilities of filters is given in the following sections of this chapter. Before a membrane is selected for a specific application, its material should possess an inherent chemical and mechanical compatibility consistent with its intended use.

All polymeric membranes are produced from specific monomers or monomer blends that contain various additives to stabilize both the monomers and the membrane. These additives range from antioxidizing and antiaging agents to softeners, light-protecting compounds, and plasticizers and contain a large number of chemical substances such as polycyclic aromatic compounds, phenols and cresols, silicones, fatty acids, and esters. Each of these substances has a specific solubility in the individual solvents and can contribute to impurities in the filtrate. Even though the concentration of these additives is low compared to the amount of polymer in the membrane, it is impossible to exclude the possibility of extractables by ensuring the chemical resistance of the membrane polymer alone.

The production of microporous membranes is another source of extractables. In addition to monomers and their additives, pore formers and solvent residues may also be present. Solid particles may additionally be created by blushing, or dust particles that adhere to the membrane surface can also be present in the filtrate. Moreover, wetting agents are often added to the filter during or after membrane production. The casting formulas and the individual methods are usually known only to the manufacturers of the specific membranes.

A wide range of solvents to dissolve the polymers are used as swelling, gel-forming, or precipitation agents. Some combinations rely on acetone, formic acid, dioxane, alcohols, dimethylformamide, pyrrolidone, methylene chloride, hexane, or butanone as solvents, to mention a few. Because most membranes are washed after casting and during cartridge production, the contribution of the solvents or pore formers to the extractables in the filtrate is kept at a minimum. Furthermore, the solvents and pore formers often completely evaporate after initiating gel formation.

A more important issue regarding the origin of extractables is that of wetting agents. These agents are added to make a membrane water-wettable when hydrophobic membrane polymers are involved. Of the numerous wetting agents available, membrane manufacturers use those verified as acceptable for pharmaceutical applications or foodstuffs.

The wetting agents are either adsorbed or chemically bonded to the membrane. If the adsorption method is used, the agent can still be readily absorbed in the appropriate solvent, thus contributing to the amount of extractables. If the agent is chemically bonded to the membrane, it is more stable, but it can also be extracted if the chemical bond is dissolved when exposed to appropriate temperature or solvents. For example, PVDF membrane is made hydrophilic by chemical modification in which the fluorocarbon polymer is reacted with an organic amine (polyhydroxypropylacrylate) compound. Triton X-100 was a widely used adsorbing wetting agent until tissue culture experiments proved it to be cytotoxic. More important today is the application of pyrrolidones, especially polyvinylpyrrolidones, hydroxypropyl cellulose, and, to a lesser degree, glycerol. Some membranes made of materials such as nylon or some cellulosics are water-wettable even without a wetting agent thanks to the hydrophilic nature of the polymers.

Other sources of extractable particulates and impurities in the membrane or the cartridge that result from the membrane and cartridge production process include people, clothing, containers, packaging, transport, storage, and processing equipment. Casting equipment, which is often constructed of stainless steel, can pose particular problems as a potential source of extractables. Many polymeric membrane materials adhere to the steel with great tenacity. To impede this attraction, the steel is washed with various chemicals or coated with silicones or comparable agents; residues of this treatment may then be present as extractables in the finished membrane. Silicones are not only imported to the membrane by casting but can also result from the milling of the resin or polymer blends. Another factor attributable to production is that the membrane becomes electrically charged by the friction created between the membrane and the steel rolls, even if the whole system is continuously discharged. The electrically charged membrane attracts all sorts of airborne dust and particles.

Despite these problems, contaminants resulting from membrane production are often overestimated because, as mentioned above, the finished membranes are customarily washed during manufacture and the final filter is then also rinsed as part of intensive cartridge testing procedures.

The inner and outer supports, end caps, and adapters are constructed primarily of polypropylene because of its high chemical resistance, good temperature stability, and low production costs. Polypropylene, a polymeric compound, can naturally contribute to extractables in the same way as polymeric membranes. Consequently, degradation products of the polymers and their specific additives may be present in the filtered solution along with impurities resulting from the production process. A similar situation applies to the fleece materials used as drainage or membrane supports. These fleeces are mostly made of nonwoven polypropylene or polyester fibers. The adapters or cartridge-to-housing connections are also made of polypropylene or sometimes of stainless steel. More important are the O-rings: Although their contact area is relatively small, they can contaminate the filtrate. Chemical or physical degradation can extract silicones, particularly from O-rings made of the same polymer.

Prefilters are constructed of various materials. Polypropylene, for example, is used in pleated or wound fleece, wound fiber, bonded, or sintered filter cartridges. Other prefilters use membranes made of different polymers with large pore sizes. The potential extractables of these filter modules are comparable to those in final membrane cartridges.

Contaminants on glass fiber filters should also be mentioned, as such filters are commonly used (as prefilters) in conjunction with or sometimes to replace the membrane filters. Glass fiber filters are completely devoid of wetting agents but do contain significant amounts of inorganic material. The silicate they are made of contains most of all fairly water-soluble cations. Furthermore, the glass fiber fleeces primarily used in the pharmaceutical industry contain glues or binders that prevent the glass fibers from shedding from the filter. These binders or glues are soluble in several specific solvents at elevated temperatures and are a potential source of extractables.

Charge-modified depth (CMD) filters are produced by adsorption or chemical binding of the charged compound to the surface of the membrane, fiber, or resin. The charge modifiers are generally cross-linked or thermoset and are therefore very stable against most solvents. Nevertheless, like wetting agents, they may be absorbed or chemically altered under specific conditions.

The contribution of other prefilters based on charcoal cloth, carbon fibers, silica hydrogels, diatomaceous earth, perlite, and so on to the contaminants in the filtrate is similar to that of glass fiber filters. Inorganic ions as well as binders or glues can be extracted. An increased particle shedding of the nonbonded materials is observed if the prefilter materials are used to a filter bed. However, since these filtration media are not common in the downstream processing of pharmaceutical solutions, the extractables of these devices are not specifically discussed in this chapter.

In conclusion, virtually all prefilters and membrane filters yield some level of extractables. The sources of the extractables are as numerous as the various compounds of the potential contaminants. In light of the fact that extractables differ strongly in their concentration and represent the whole range of chemical compounds, analysis of filtrate impurities is a difficult task. Obviously, there is no single all-encompassing analytical method for determining extractables. However, a reasonable approach to the extractable analysis should be possible if the aspects presented above are considered.

4 PRELIMINARY STUDIES ON EXTRACTABLES

The qualitative and quantitative study of extractables from microporous membranes is linked to the development of the analytical method itself. The more analytical techniques have improved, the more aware filter manufacturers and customers have become that pharmaceutical solutions can be contaminated with filter extractables. Early investigations conducted by Saad and Higouchi (1965) showed that significant quantities of ultraviolet-adsorbing entities were extracted from cellulose ester filters. Interferences resulted from the determination of cholesterol by spectrophotometry at 205 nm. Chiou and Smith (1970) quantified this problem using chemical and spectrophotometric analytical methods and showed that absorbances as large as 0.406 could arise from such extractables in the range of 205–320 nm.

Furthermore, Cahn (1967) reported on the cytotoxic effects of the wetting agent Triton X-100, which can leach from microporous membranes. Remberg et al. (1971), Gandrud and Lazerus (1972), and Marvin et al. (1972) also proved the existence of extractables from filters using chemical and spectrophotometric analytical techniques. Both Cahn (1967) and Rosenbluth and Cribbs (1969) investigated the influence of temperature and the number and volume of water flushes needed to remove essentially all offending surfactants from membrane filters. They additionally recommended that the extraction solution be kept at a temperature of 90–100°C.

The ASTM Standard D3861 (ASTM, 1984) established a method for determining total extractables that was also adopted by the U.S. Environmental Protection Agency. In this test, water extractables are determined by weight loss arising after the filter is extracted with boiling water. Because this method involves measuring small differences in weight between the same filters before and after the extraction, it has a high potential for error if only a single filter is tested. Care must be taken to avoid weight changes in the filter resulting from the absorption of particles or moisture, or reactions between the membrane and the solvent.

Bordner et al. (1978) proposed a test in which the filter is immersed in high quality distilled water for 24 h and the extract is assayed for the compounds of interest such as metal ions, total organic carbon, phosphorus, and ammonia. Erroneous results were caused by bacterial growth inhibiting or promoting materials leaching out of a membrane filter used for bacterial water analysis (Bower and Kilham, 1978). Previously, Geldreich (1975) had reported that different types of extractable tests must be performed to evaluate membrane filters for growth-promoting and -inhibiting extractables. The release of extractables from polycarbonate and various cellulose ester membranes by ultraviolet (UV) absorption techniques was investigated by Cooney (1980), who showed that the measured level of contaminants in the extraction solution was strongly affected by the applied wavelength. He also showed that ionic extractables interfered with the determination of wetting agents by UV spectrophotometry. The report also confirmed that diffusion affects the extractive flushing of membranes. The removal of extractables from membranes by aqueous leaching appears to be concentration-dependent. Cooney showed that the thoroughness of such purification depends on the flow rate of water in a dynamic flow system and not just on volume. In static liquid/solid soak tests, the extracting liquid should be periodically replaced, and a large volume is preferable to a smaller one. Because elution of the extractables is concentration-dependent, the rate of extraction decreases with time and flush volume. Even though complete removal was found to be impracticable, compliance with USP regulations on total nonvolatile residuals in water for injection is possible. Olson et al. (1980) stated that water with a resistance of 750,000 Ω will usually be related to a total nonvolatile content of 10 ppm and that extensive washing of the filter leads to an extractable level below 10 ppm, thereby meeting the water for injection standard. The influence of temperature was also demonstrated in this study, which showed that an initial water wash at 5°C removes more extractables than a warm water flush at 45°C. This result is contrary to recently published data, which indicate a higher extractables level with increasing temperatures. A detailed evaluation of this impasse is discussed in the following sections of this chapter.

In their study, Olson et al. (1980) used high performance liquid chromatography (HPLC) and reversed-phase thin-layer chromatography (RP-TLC) to analyze wetting agents. The extracts were additionally tested with regard to their UV-active content and the use of methanol, water acetonitrile, and tetrahydrofuran as solvents. The extracts were quantitatively analyzed by reversed-phase HPLC based on the total peak areas measured with a UV detector at 454 nm. No attempt was made to identify the compounds. The results must be considered and interpreted carefully because the ultraviolet adsorption method exclusively detects UV-active substances containing unsaturated bonds or aromatic groups. This method does not detect compounds with saturated bonds or low UV activity. Furthermore, the substances have different UV-adsorbing capacities related to their class and the amount of UV-adsorbing functional groups in their chemical structure. As a result, compounds with identical concentrations but different chemical structures can produce different UV absorbance values. Olson (1979) also estimated that the amount of extractables from an untreated solvent-case filter is 900 mg/m^2. Later studies found this figure to be suitable for raw membranes but too high for the finished product by a factor of 10–50.

5 CURRENT PRACTICES

Filter manufacturers currently validate filter cartridges in compliance with USP 23 (USP, 1995). The validation guides contain information about extractables like construction materials, USP 23 extractables, USP 23 particle testing, LAL pyrogen testing, USP 23 Class VI plastics test, and chemical compatibility. Current extractables testing can be divided into two categories: toxicological and analytical.

In toxicological testing, the manufacturers select thermoplastic components that have passed the USP Class VI test, a well-established test for plastic materials. The USP Class IV test specifies not only the solvents to be tested but also the specific temperature and times of extraction. In this test, exhaustive extraction is performed in a closed vessel or under reflux using saline, ethanol in saline, polyethylene glycol, or vegetable oil as solvents. The specific solution to be filtered can also be tested. The solutions are chosen to represent a broad range of solvents, provide biocompatibility, and prevent any interference with the subsequent animal testing. The extraction is performed either at 121°C of 1 h, 70°C for 24 h, or 50°C for 72 h and thereby takes into account the worst-case conditions based on extreme extraction.

Additionally, a mutagenicity (Ames) test and the USP general mouse test are performed to provide clearance certification for all filter components. These toxicological tests show that the filter and cartridge materials have no biological reactivity, but none of the tests determines the amount of eluted substances or identifies specific extractables. Furthermore, the possibility of accumulating effects of a very low concentrated toxic compound cannot be excluded by these tests.

The analytical methods applied to validate a filter cartridge are also based on the extraction of filter cartridge components under extreme conditions. The complete filter cartridges are treated by a static soak method for an extended period of time and at medium-range temperatures. Rinse volumes are analyzed to obtain a flush protocol and to ensure that a minimum of extractables are obtained from the filter under application conditions. The extraction solvents of pure water, ethanol, or a mixture of the two are applied as model solutions. Both techniques are designed to exhaustively elute all extractable components from the filter or the cartridge. This approach does account for the process conditions of the end user, such as specific solvents, temperature, or time protocols. The applied extractions also provide general information about the extractables and cover most pharmaceutical applications. Several quantitative and qualitative analytical methods are applied to analyze the extracts.

Gravimetric determination of the nonvolatile residue (NVR) is a classic quantitative method and is used as a standard technique for extractables from most pharmaceutical process devices such as containers, packaging materials, tubing, and purification devices. According to USP 23, Requirements for Sterile Water for Injection, three cartridges from three different lots are wetted by soaking, autoclaved, and extracted in reverse-osmosis (RO) water and 20% and 70% ethanol for 3 h at 25°C under shaking. The solvent is then evaporated, and the weight of the nonvolatile residue is determined. For a flush protocol, the cartridge is rinsed after the autoclaving and 200 mL samples are taken from 1, 2.5, 5, and 10 L flush volumes. The solvent is also evaporated at 105°C for 60 min and the NVR measured. The maximum NVR limits described in USP 23 relate to the volume of the vessel (<30 mL, <0.004%; 30–100 mL, <0.003%; >100 mL, <0.002%).

The total organic carbon (TOC) test is a quantitative method of measuring the total oxidizable organic content of an aqueous solution. According to the old USP 22 (Sterile Water for Injection), 10 mL of 2 N sulfuric acid and 0.4 mL of 0.1 N permanganate solution are added to a 50 mL sample and heated to 100°C for 10 min. If the solution retains its color, the sample has met the requirements. Extraction and sampling are performed as described for the NVR test. Since ethanol is an organic solvent and would interfere with this method, RO water is the only extraction solvent tested. Another, now more important, means for measuring the oxidizable organic carbon content besides chemical TOC determination is to use a TOC analyzer. The sensitivity and precision of this instrumental TOC technique are superior to those of the chemical method, and the TOC determination protocol of the USP 23 is based on this method.

The extract solutions obtained by static extraction and flushing method are also assayed for the content of total heavy metal ions, sulfate, chloride, and ammonia using individual chemical tests for each ionic compound. The maximum concentration of the ions is also specified by USP 22. In the USP 23 test, the determinations of the calcium, sulfate, chloride, ammonia, and carbon dioxide are replaced by conductivity/resistivity measurements, and the recommended changes will be published in the USP 23 supplement in 1995.

The pH and conductivity/resistivity of the solutions are also measured. USP 23 for purified water sets the limits and the relationship between the pH and the maximum allowable conductivity. If both pH and conductivity are within the limits of this relationship, the USP requirements are met. Depending on the pH level, the proposal of USP 23 is that the filtered water should meet a standard of 4.7 and 5.8 microsiemens per centimeter (μS/cm). However, these recommended changes in USP 23 are still under discussion.

Particle shedding from the filters is determined according to USP 23 for "large volume parenterals for single dose infusion." Using the method "Light Obscuration Test Particle Count," the limits for a maximum number of particles per milliliter of product (in this case, large-volume injections for single-dose infusion) is set at 25 particles/mL >10 μm and 3 particles/mL >25 μm. The revisions of the old USP 22 that led to the USP 23 regarding the general test chapter. "Particulate Matter in Injections" are sill under discussion, and new recommendations are anticipated to be published in 1995. The British Pharmacopoeia has set the limits for particles in the LVP injections at 500 particles/mL 2–5 μm and 80 particles/mL >5 μm. Particle release from filters is determined as follows. The autoclaved and integrity-tested filters are statically soaked and rinsed with RO water. Samples (75 mL) are taken from 1, 2.5, 5, and 10 L flush volume for analysis. The particles in the solution are tested with regard to their size and number by a particle sensor at a constant flow rate of the sample through the sensor.

Although current practices for extractable analysis include various methods for quantifying the total amount of nonvolatile or organic elutable compounds, none of these techniques identifies or quantifies a specific compound in the "extractable cocktail." For example, it is not possible to rule out a low concentration extractable toxic compound capable of accumulating in an organism. This substance might not be detected by the toxicological test because of its low concentration and would not be identified by extractable analysis recommended by either the USP or BP. Moreover, the model solutions used in the extraction tests may have little effect on a specific compound in the filter that might well be soluble under actual process conditions. Recently, the trend has been to evaluate filtration devices under conditions of actual use. Several studies on extractables have been devoted to this problem.

6 METHODOLOGIES IN EXTRACTABLE TESTING

The different extractables were investigated using various approaches. A guide to extractables published by Pall Inc. presents a test method based on extraction of an autoclaved filter cartridge in 1500 mL of solvent at room temperature (Pall Inc., 1994). The NVR was determined for a large number of solvents and showed that the values of the nonvolatile residue fall in a range of roughly 20–400 mg per 10 in. cartridge. It was stated that neither longer exposure nor repeat extraction increases these NVR values appreciably. Thus, these NVR values approximate the total material that can be extracted from the cartridge into each solvent regardless of volume or contact time. The extraction procedure represented worst-case conditions based on autoclaving, although the definition of worst-case conditions for extractables and the exposure time should be the object of scrutiny. The publication reported that further testing yielded low percentages of a variety of other volatile components (such as benzyl alcohol, chlorobutanol, and cholesterol), substances that are not covered by the NVR test because, due to their low boiling points, they are evaporated with the solvents. No method described how this testing was performed. The nonvolatile residue was further analyzed to identify the components using Fourier transform infrared spectroscopy (FTIR), a powerful method for identifying functional groups and specific chemical bonds of the analyzed molecules. Because each molecule has its own specific infrared spectrum, it is possible to identify an unknown substance by matching the absorption spectra of unknown samples with characteristic absorption wavelengths of the relevant functional groups and bonds or by matching the spectra with those of known compounds. For this purpose, most FTIR instruments are supported by a large spectral library. Nevertheless, FTIR analysis has its limitations in analyzing unknown samples (Robinson, 1995). FTIR analysis of mixtures produces an overlaid spectrum of the characteristic absorption wavelengths of each compound in the mixture. The more substances in the mixture, the more complex are the resulting spectrum and its interpretation. Besides, substances with identical functional groups but different positions or sums of functional groups in the chemical structure can hardly be detected within one spectrum. Low concentration compounds are similarly hard to identify in a sample with a high concentration substance, because the spectrum of the high concentration overlie that of the low concentration one.

Despite these shortcomings, FTIR is an excellent method for identifying a purified unknown compound or even a mixture of a few substances. FTIR analysis of the NVR of the Ultipore N_{66} showed a spectrum of primarily nylon 66 and poly(ethylene terephthalate) (PET). Spectra of related or low concentration substances could not be identified because of the strong signals of polyamide and terephthalate. Spectra of extracts from 0.1, 0.2, and 1.2/0.45 micrometer-rated double-layer cartridges were examined and yielded essentially identical results. In this report, the same compounds were identified in the ethanol extract. Furthermore, our experience has shown that neither the amounts nor the identities of the extractables change significantly with filter pore size.

A method for analyzing filter extractables based on a model stream approach was presented by Stone et al. (1994a) in a pilot study. The extraction solvents were selected after reviewing the chemical classes of the solvents used in pharmaceutical formulations. More than 80% of all formulations were found to be primarily aqueous with various salt contents and different pH values. Also present were organic solvents (mainly ethanol) and solvating agents or surfactants. In this overview, worst-case extraction was performed using water, ethanol, 20% NaCl, 0.1% Tween 80, pH 2.0 HCl, and pH 12.5 NaOH as solvents. The cartridges were autoclaved twice at 126°C for 30 min, conditions that an earlier study found suitable to achieve a high extractable level (Stone et al., 1994b). After a static soak for 8.5 h at ambient temperature, the TOC and the NVR of the extracts were determined, followed by FTIR analysis of the nonvolatile residue. Additionally, the eluted compounds were investigated by reversed-phase high performance liquid chromatography (RP-HPLC or RPC). RPC is a powerful analytical tool that separates the substances according to their hydrophobicity and allows the detection of each substance. Analysis can be performed directly on the extraction solution for both nonvolatile and volatile components. Detection in RPC is generally performed by a UV detector and represents a very sensitive method. The disadvantage of UV detection is that only UV-active chemicals, particularly unsaturated or aromatic compounds, are detected. Chemicals with low UV absorbance might pass this analysis undetected. Moreover, even the detected chemicals cannot be identified by their UV absorbance. Stone et al. (1995) overcame the problem of RPC by identifying the separated and purified fractions of the RPC by FTIR analysis. The combination of RPC and FTIR is an excellent separating/analyzing system. Using this method, one signal peak was detected in the ethanol extract that had been isolated and identified by FTIR as oligomeric poly(vinylidene fluoride). In the ethanolic and water solution, FTIR analysis of the NVR additionally showed polyacrylate from the membrane and highly aliphatic components of the polypropylene membrane supports, cartridge core, and end caps. RPC was unable to detect any other compounds in the other extraction solutions. Stone et al. (1994b) also showed that sodium chloride, Tween, NaOH, and HCl solutions interfered with the FTIR and that reliable results with the NVR test can be achieved only with the water, ethanol, and HCl extract. High salt concentrations cause a very high background level that interferes with the method. The same problems arose in the TOC test when it was performed with ethanol, saline, or Tween-containing solutions.

Stone et al. (1995) also stated that the relatively high concentrations of organic components in pharmaceutical formulations make it impossible to detect or analyze very low levels of extractables. As an example, the RPC chromatogram of a pharmaceutical formulation versus those of filter extracts and water controls is presented in Fig. 1. Based on the results of the pilot studies, Stone proposed a model stream approach and suggested that extractables testing should approximate the actual process conditions as closely as possible. The approach can be defined in five basic steps: classifying the formulation components, selecting the analogous model streams, characterizing the process variables, selecting the extraction protocols, and selecting the appropriate analytical tools. Furthermore, worst-case process conditions should be selected in order to obtain results that reflect the effect of the actual pharmaceutical process on the filter material. This worst-case scenario can be included in the model stream approach, especially in the static extraction, yielding data that reflect the extractables of the specific process as closely as possible.

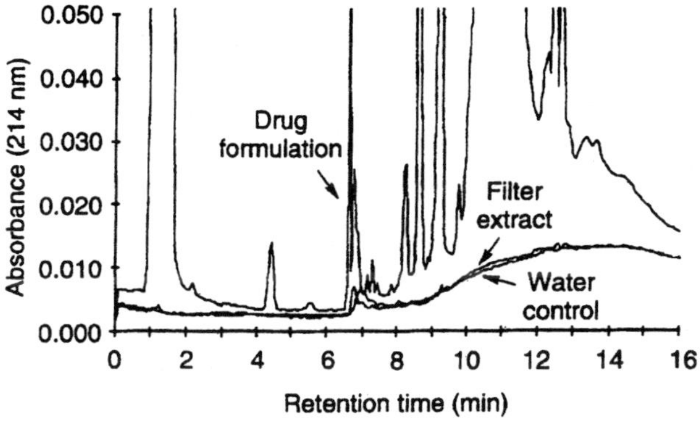

Figure 1 RP-HPLC chromatogram of pharmaceutical formulation versus filter extract. The relatively high concentration of organic components in the pharmaceutical formulation, indicated by the high number and intensity of peaks, makes it impossible to detect very low levels of extractables. (From Stone et al., 1995.)

7 ANALYSIS AND EVALUATION OF FILTER CARTRIDGE EXTRACTABLES

Making use of the results of previous investigations, a standard protocol for the analysis of extractables was developed (Fig. 2) and tested on 10 in. cartridges used for prefiltration and sterile filtration. The protocol includes an extensive extraction procedure followed by separation of the concentrated and unconcentrated extracts with various complementary methods and is combined with methods for identification of the compounds (Reif et al., 1995a).

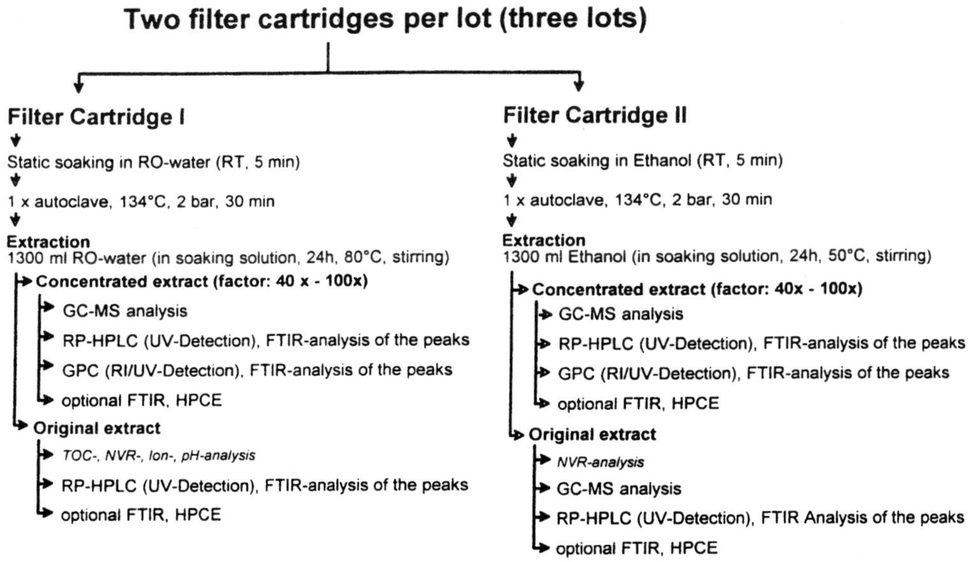

Figure 2 Standard scheme for extractables analysis. (From Reif et al., 1995a).

The following describes and discusses the analytical methodology as well as the extractable data of prefilter and sterile filter cartridges. The prefilter cartridges from various manufacturers included filter units with PP and GF nonwoven fleeces as well as large-pore prefilter membranes. The sterile filter cartridge study evaluated the 0.2 μm cartridges from various manufacturers with different membrane materials (CA, PA, PTFE, PVDF, PESU).

In an initial step, the sterile or prefilter cartridge was wetted in the extraction solution and then autoclaved. This procedure ensures worst-case extraction conditions because the extracting liquid boils in the prewetted cartridge and comes in direct contact with the polymers and the fleece or membrane pores. If a dry filter cartridge is used, the steam has to diffuse into the pores and condense on the polymers during autoclaving. This is a comparatively slow process that reduces the extraction strength.

In the method presented here, the autoclaved cartridge was placed back in the original extraction solution to prevent any extractables from being lost by the initial wetting. Preliminary studies had shown that a small amount of less than 12 μg NVR/cartridge was already eluted during the wetting process.

The extraction was performed with optimized equipment, which consisted of a glass cylinder with a ground glass cover and a reflux condenser on top. The bottom of the cylinder had a glass insert that facilitated the insertion of a magnetic stirring rod below the cartridge. The temperature of the extraction solution was controlled by means of a heating/cooling jacket around the cylinder. This construction had the advantage that a small extraction volume could be used to completely soak a 10 in. cartridge and allowed dynamic stirring to prevent temperature and concentration gradients. The solvent could be heated to 100°C under precise temperature control (±5°C). No loss of any highly volatile compounds was observed thanks to the large reflux cooler.

Distilled water and analytical grade ethanol were chosen as standard extraction media since most of pharmaceutical production and purification processes are based on these two solvents or a mixture of the two. Hence, the results of this study would support extractables analysis or evaluation of most pharmaceutical solutions based on water or ethanol. The pure solvents used here did not take into account the effect of additives such as salts and stabilizers on the pharmaceutical formulations. If possible, extractables should always be tested using the specific pharmaceutical solution as the extracting solvent.

To estimate the amount of the high and low concentration extractables, the eluates were analyzed in both original and concentrated form. Investigation of low concentration contaminants also provides data on pharmaceutical processes, particularly where the final product is packaged in concentrated form, e.g., lyophilized. In such cases, the extractables would also be concentrated, and any contaminating compound that may be nontoxic in diluted form but toxic in a concentrated state would pose a severe threat to the quality of the pharmaceutical product.

The concentrating procedure must be performed carefully to prevent the loss of highly volatile substances. Prior to this study, the potential loss of compounds in the concentration step had been determined. After solid-phase extraction to concentrate the water eluate and careful evaporation of the ethanol, no degradation of the sample was observed. If necessary, the ethanolic extract can also be analyzed for potentially highly volatile contaminants using headspace GC-MS, a technique that can analyze these compounds even in a concentrated form without any pretreatment.

Common analytical methods described in the guidelines of the FDA or the USP, such as the analysis of the nonvolatile residue (NVR), pH measurement, conductivity, and heavy metal ion concentration test or total organic carbon (TOC) assay, can be performed on the unconcentrated extracts prior to extractables analysis. Since these well-known methods are already referred to in an earlier section of this chapter and furnish no additional information about the chemical nature of the extractables, they are not discussed further here.

As mentioned above, some reports described the use of Fourier transform infrared spectroscopy (FTIR) to identify extractables. Infrared spectroscopy is probably the most versatile and flexible of the molecular spectroscopic techniques as it can be applied to a broad range of both organic or inorganic materials in all three physical states: solid, liquid, and gas. The information contained in the spectrum originates from molecular vibrations that are specific to the molecular bonds. Functional groups of the molecule can be determined, and a molecule can be identified by its unique spectrum, which represents a characteristic fingerprint of that molecular species.

The disadvantage of FTIR is that the spectra of the different compounds overlap and it is difficult to identify individual species in complex mixtures and to precisely quantify a single compound. FTIR is therefore not always the most accurate method for extractables testing. However, in the context of this study and for identifying an isolated and purified substance or as a fundamental analytical technique, FTIR can be considered a powerful tool and was used for these purposes.

The main problem in identifying the species in the extract is that there is no method for determining a single compound in a sample mixture that contains several equally concentrated substances. Therefore, appropriate methods must be applied to separate the mixture into its individual species and to identify isolated fractions. Several different separation techniques, such as gas chromatography (GC), liquid chromatography (LC), capillary electrophoresis (CE), and supercritical fluid extraction (SFE), can be used to solve this problem. These techniques stand for various modifications and several separation modes and are based on the same general principle, namely that the species are separated first and then detected by appropriate detectors. For standard extractables analysis, two of the most common and powerful separation techniques that combine high resolution with precise reproducibility were selected: GC and reversed-phase high performance liquid chromatography (RP-HPLC).

The first analytical method applied to each extraction sample should be GC, for it offers a unique combination of maximum resolution, detectability, and simplicity. The only major limitations GC faces involve three factors: the volatilities of the actual analytes, their thermal stabilities at the temperatures required for volatilization, and, less important for our protocol, the thermal stability of the column coatings and stationary phases. GC is thus limited to analytes with a molecular weight less than 300–500 g/mol and temperature-stable compounds. The column type selected must be appropriate for the sample.

Gas chromatographic detection of the separated compounds is mainly performed in a nonselective thermal conductivity detector (TCD). The disadvantage of this type of detector is that the separated compounds cannot be characterized. Better information about the nature of the analytes can be gathered using more selective instruments such as a flame ionization detector (FID), which shows a specific response to hydrocarbons, or the nitrogen photometric detector (NPD), which gives a selective response to nitrogen-containing compounds. Although the sensitivity of these detectors is very high, the problem of identifying single analytes in complex samples like extracts remains unsolved.

Preliminary studies showed that GC analysis of the extracts by flame ionization or nitrogen photometric detection resulted in a large number of peaks, but no substance was identified. Apart from the fact that the analytes contained nitrogen or carbon, the analysis provided no further data. The coupling of GC to mass spectrometry (MS) combines the resolution power of the gas chromatograph with the swiftness and reliability of identifying the separated analytes by their mass spectra. GC-MS is the method of choice for extractable analysis.

Figure 3 shows the chromatograms of the GC-MS analysis of the concentrated water extract. A few small peaks were observed in the chromatograms of each cartridge. The peaks were mainly identified as degradation products or as additives. Specifically, certain amounts of DOP were found in all cartridges. An exception is cartridge H, in which higher concentrations of caprolactam and some of its derivatives were identified. GC-MS analysis of the unconcentrated ethanol extract showed virtually no peaks (not shown here), whereas analysis of the concentrated eluate (Fig. 4) resulted in a large number of signals. Most of the peaks were identified as homologs of siloxanes from the O-rings or hydrocarbons from the polypropylene materials of the cartridge cores, caps, and supporting fleeces. Minor components were found to be various stabilizers and additives of the original polymer production that are necessary to ensure the quality of the polymeric product.

Considering the low detection limits of the MS detector, 1–0.1 ppm, and that the samples are concentrated 100-fold, all investigated cartridges can be said to have an extractable level of $\lesssim 1$ ppm per cartridge in approximately 1.3 L RO water. However, this applies only to contaminants that can be analyzed by GC-MS.

Although most extractables can be identified by GC-MS, compounds with a molecular mass above 500 g/mol such as polymers or temperature-sensitive analytes cannot be analyzed by GC as described above. RP-HPLC is used to fill this gap in the analytical protocol for extractable testing. RP-HPLC is a powerful analytical tool that separates substances according to their hydrophobicity and allows the detection of each individual compound. The compounds can be separated either under isocratic conditions or by gradient elution with increasing solvent strength. The advantage of gradient elution is that analysis time is reduced and both nonpolar and polar solutes can be separated in a single run. To achieve similarly optimal separation conditions for polar and nonpolar compounds, two runs with different solvents must be performed.

For better resolution and lab-to-lab reproducibility, two isocratic gradients were run for each sample—one using methanol/water and the other acetonitrile/water to achieve optimal separation conditions for both strong and weak hydrophobic compounds. The analysis was performed directly on the extraction solution and comprised both nonvolatile and volatile components. RP-HPLC detection is usually performed in a UV detector, a highly sensitive device. As mentioned earlier, the disadvantage of UV detection is that only UV-active chemicals, specifically unsaturated or aromatic compounds, are detectable, and chemicals with a low UV absorbance may go undetected. Besides, even chemicals that are detected are then not identifiable by their UV absorbance. As discussed in Section 6, this shortcoming of RP-HPLC can be overcome by subjecting the fractions separated and purified by RP-HPLC to FTIR analysis. The combination of the RPC and FTIR is an excellent separating and analyzing system.

Figure 5 presents the chromatograms of RP-HPLC of the original water extract, showing only a few, mostly minor, peaks. Some of the peaks are due to the system or the sample preparation methodology and could also be detected in the analysis of the blank. Figure 6 depicts chromatograms of the analysis of the ethanol extract, showing several peaks in the chromatograms of each cartridge with a strong UV response, which could be identified as additives or decomposition products of the specific membrane polymers. Most of the substances were already known from the initial GC-MS analysis. The strong UV response was mainly due to aromatic functional groups in the chemical structure of the individual compounds, e.g., terephthalates, benzoic acid derivatives, phthalates, or phenyl sulfones. In general, due to the different UV activities of the individual compounds, the concentrations of the substances cannot be estimated from the height of the single peaks or their specific areas. The concentration of the compounds cannot be evaluated by UV detection without taking into consideration the UV activity of the detected compounds. The analysis of the 40-fold concentrated ethanol and water extracts (now shown here) revealed some minor contaminants in addition to those identified in the original eluates, although the concentrations of these extractables were too low to be fractionated and identified by FTIR (<1 ppb).

As mentioned before, RP-HPLC, a method that relies on UV detection, is only capable of analyzing compounds that are UV active. Compounds with a molecular weight greater than 500 g/mol cannot be identified by GC-MS. To compensate for this deficiency in the analytical protocol, all concentrated extracts were analyzed by GPC with refractive index (RI) detection. GPC separates the solutes by size, while the RI detector is capable of detecting all substances in the solvent based on changes in the refractive index. The detected substances were further analyzed by FTIR. Although the resolution of the GPC is relatively low and the detection limits of the RI detector are high compared to UV detection, this method can detect the presence of high molecular weight compounds that are not identifiable by RP-HPLC. Nevertheless, in this study no contaminants were found in the extracts that had not already been identified by GC-MS or RP-HPLC.

The compounds identified in the water and ethanol extracts are listed in Table 1. The extractables originated from the decomposition products of either the polypropylene or the cartridge (oligomeric aliphates) or specific membrane. The nature of the decomposition product strongly depends on the extraction conditions applied. A solvent that reacts with or dissolves the membrane polymer or extreme temperatures will increase the concentration of the extractables and the amounts of the different contaminants. Therefore, the chemical compatibility of the membrane should be tested before starting extractables analysis under process conditions. This issue is discussed in the next section of this chapter.

Furthermore, all cartridges contain a certain amount of additives or starting materials from the initial polymerization. Specifically, the major softeners or plasticizers such as dibutylphthalate (DOP) or fatty acids can be found in each extract. Antioxidizers like 2,6-dibutylcresol or benzoic acid derivatives can also be found in each extract. These additives are necessary for the production and stability of the

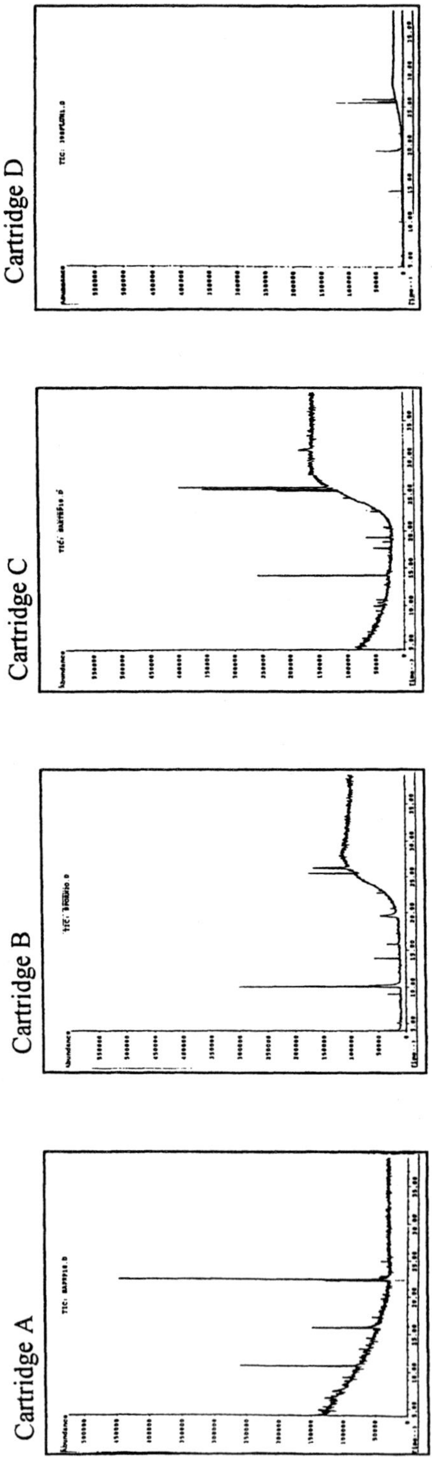
Cartridge D
Cartridge C
Cartridge B
Cartridge A

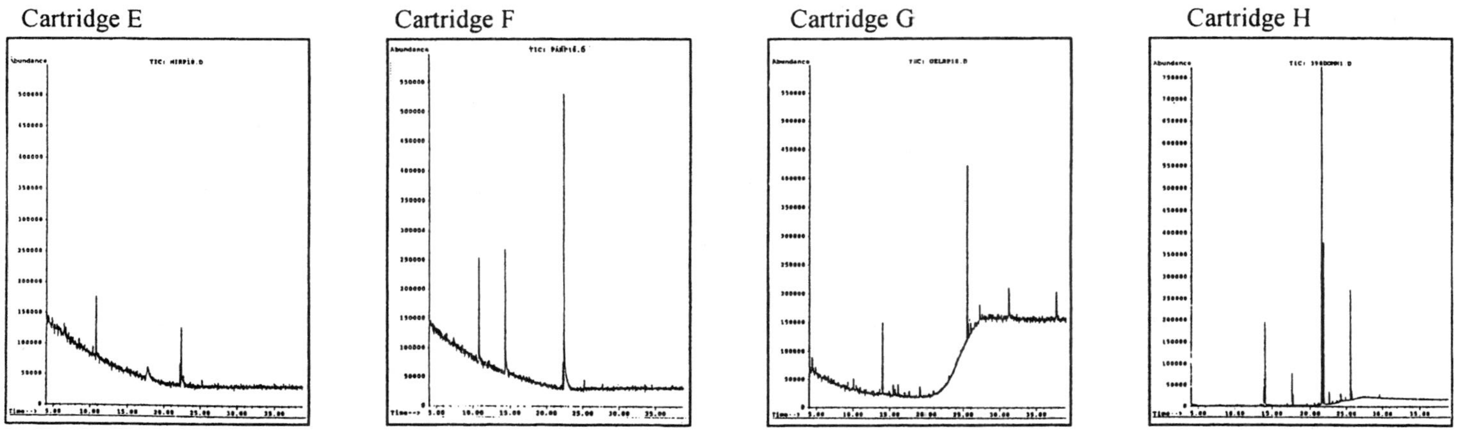

Figure 3 Chromatograms of GC-MS analysis of concentrated water extract using 0.2 μm sterile filter cartridges with different membrane materials (various manufacturers). (From Reif et al., 1995a.)

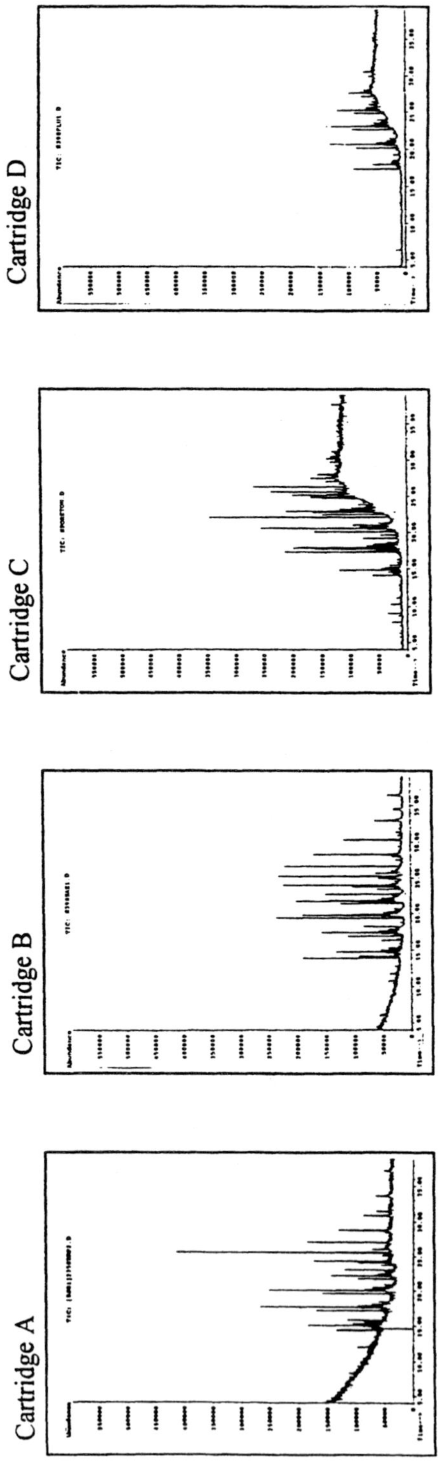
Cartridge A
Cartridge B
Cartridge C
Cartridge D

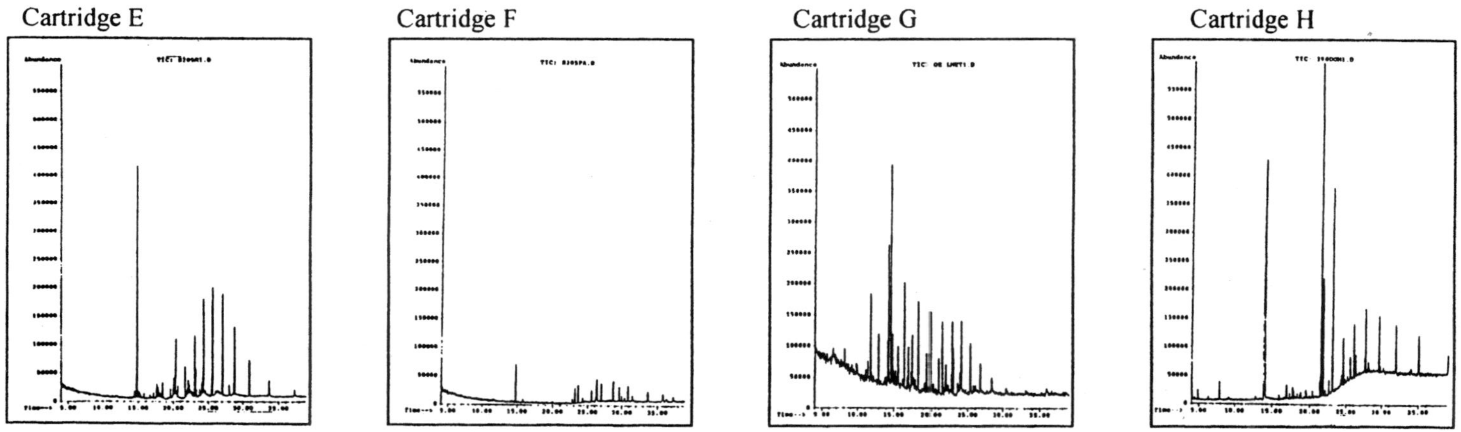

Figure 4 Chromatograms of GC-MS analysis of concentrated ethanol using 0.2 μm sterile filter cartridges with different membrane materials (various manufacturers). (From Reif et al., 1995a.)

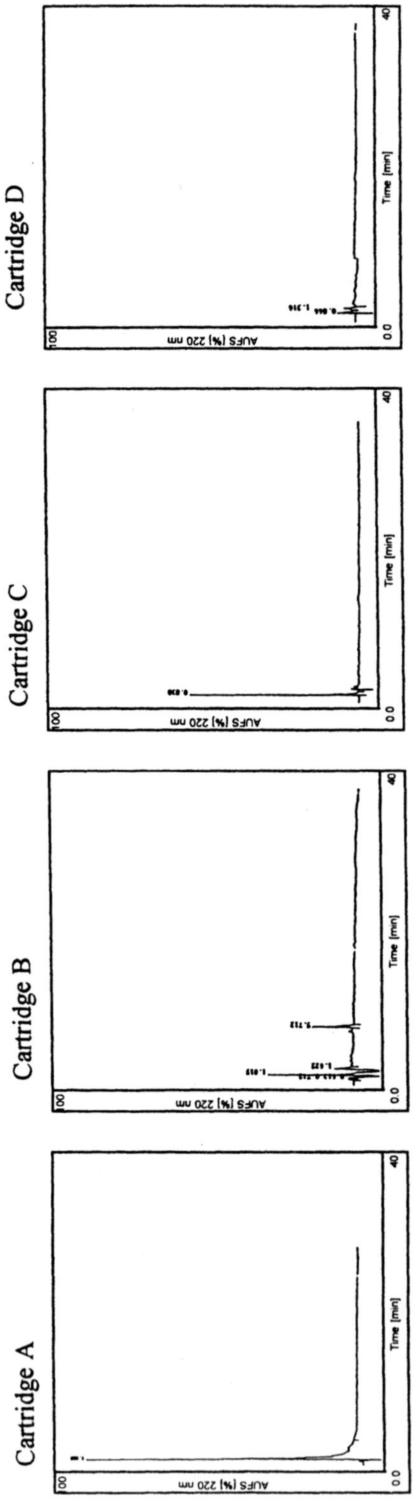
Cartridge D
Cartridge C
Cartridge B
Cartridge A
AUFS [%] 220 nm
Time [min]
100
0.0
40

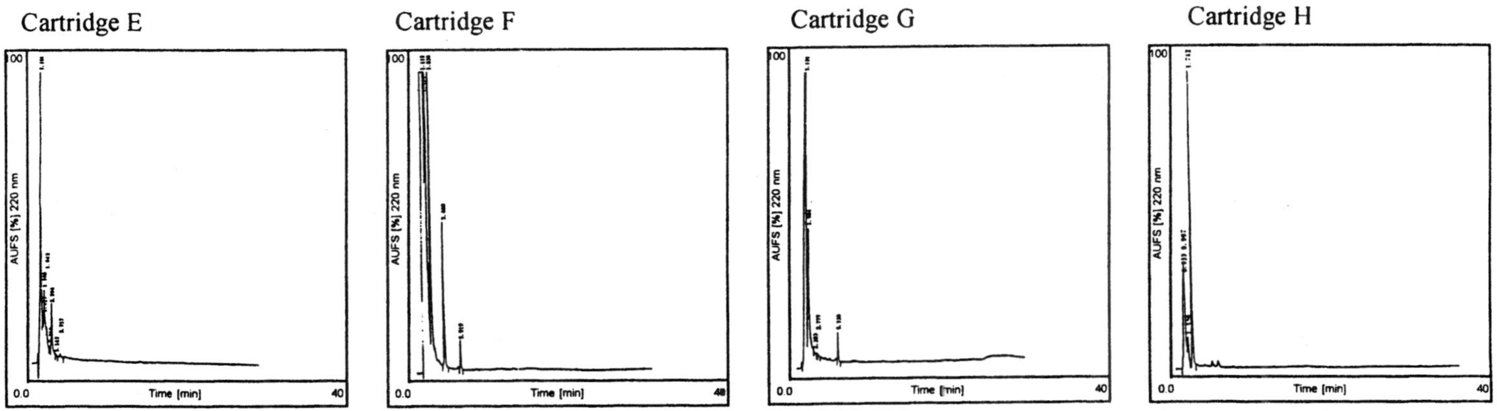

Figure 5 Chromatograms obtained by RP-HPLC analysis of original water extract using 0.2 μm sterile filter cartridges with different membrane materials (various manufacturers).

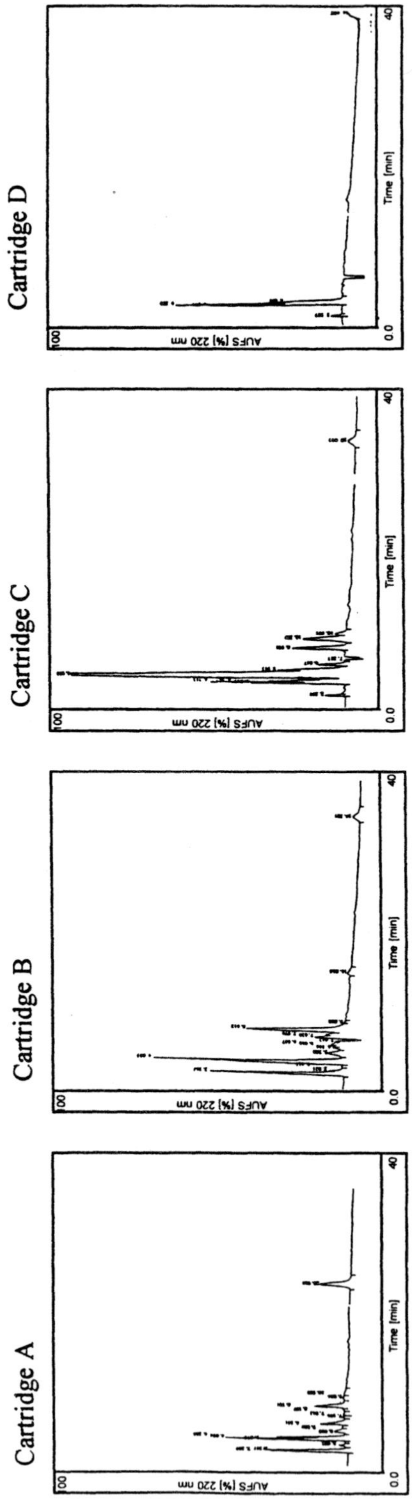
Cartridge A
Cartridge B
Cartridge C
Cartridge D
AUFS [%] 220 nm
Time [min]
100
0.0
40

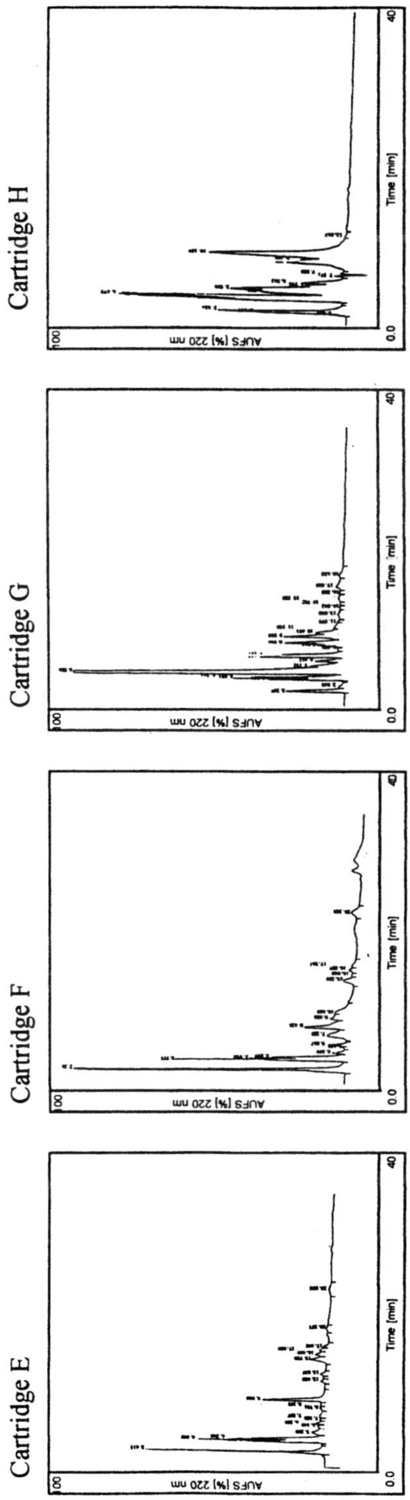

Figure 6 Chromatograms obtained by RP-HPLC analysis of original ethanol extract using 0.2 μm sterile filter cartridges with different membrane materials (various manufacturers). (From Reif et al., 1995a.)

Table 1 Extractables of 0.2 μm Sterile Filter Cartridges with Different Membrane Materials from Various Manufacturers

Cartridge A	Cartridge B	Cartridge C	Cartridge D	Cartridge E[a]	Cartridge F[a]	Cartridge G[a]	Cartridge H[a]
Diethylphthalate	Cyclohexan	Propionic acid	Dibutylphthalate	Acrylic acid	Dimethylbenzene	Etherthioether	Caprolactam
Stearic acid	Ethoxybenzoic acid	Diphenyl ether	12-Oligoaliphates	2-Phenolic oligomers	Etherthioether	Propionic acid	Butyrolactone
2,6-Di-*tert*-butylcresol	2,6-Di-*tert*-butylcresol	2,6-Di-*tert*-butylcresol	Hydroxybenzoic acid	2,6-Di-*tert*-butylcresol	2,6-Di-*tert*-butylcresol	2,6-Di-*tert*-butylcresol	Laurinlactam
2,2-Methylene-bis-4-ethyl-6-*tert*-butylphenol	Cyclohexadiene-1,4-dione	4-Methyl-2,5-cyclohexa-diene-1-one	*tert*-Butyl-methyl-2,5-cyclohexa-diene-1-one	3 oligo. Benzyldi-phenylmethane	3,5-Di-*tert*-butyl-4-hydroxy-phenyl propionate	2,6-Di-*tert*-butylmethyl-2,5-cyclohexa-diene-1-one	Laurinlactam derivative
Hydroxybenzoic acid	Phenylisocyanate	Hydroxybenzoic acid	2,4-Bis(1,1-di-methylethyl)-phenol	Triphenylphos-phite	2 N-containing high MW compounds	4,4-Dichloro-diphenylsulfone	4-Methoxy-4-chlordiphenyl-sulfone
7-Oligosiloxanes	Palmitic acid	Palmitic acid	Succinic acid	Stearic acid	Acetamide	Benzothiazolone	Adipinic acid
Bis-(2-ethyl-hexyl)-phthalate	Stearic acid	Dimethoxydi-phenyl sulfone	3-Oligosiloxanes	Bis-(2-ethyl-hexyl)-phthalate	N-containing aromatic high MW comp.	4-Hydroxypropyl benzoate	Dibutylphthalate
12-Oligoaliphates	12-Oligoaliphates	11-Oligoaliphates	Polyether	Polyacrylate	3-Oligoamides	6-Oligoaliphates	Ethylhexylphthal-ate

4-Methyl-2,5-cyclohexadiene-1-one	11-Oligosiloxanes	Methoxy-4-chlorodiphenylsulfone		Ethylacrylate	Bis-(2-ethylhexyl)-phthalate	Hydroxyphenyl acetamide	Dihydroethylphthalate
	Methyl-4-hydroxybenzoate	Bis-(2-ethylhexyl)phthalate		Diphenylphthalate	10-Oligosiloxanes	Methoxy-4-chlorodiphenylsulfone	2,6-Di-*tert*-butylcresol
	Etherthioether	Polyether		9-Oligosiloxanes	2-Oligoaliphates	7-Oligosiloxanes	Diisobutylphthalate
		7-Oligosiloxanes		6-Oligoaliphates		Cyclohexane	Diacetylbenzene
		2,4-Bis(1,1-dimethyl ethyl)-phenol				Methoxy-4-chlorodiphenylsulfone	Cyclotridecanone
							4,4-Dichlordiphenylsulfone
							Propionic acid
							4-Oligosiloxanes
							3-Oligoaliphates

[a]Identification of the RP-HPLC peaks by FTIR is still in progress; extractables list may be incomplete.
Source: Reif et al. (1995a).

polymers and can be found in nearly all polymeric products. Since solvents tend to diffuse into the polymer structure, virtually all polymeric materials undergo a certain extraction of these additives.

The amount of extractables was evaluated with regard to detection limits and the sample volumes. The extractables of all sterile filter cartridges were found to be equal to or less than 1 ppm in an extraction volume of approximately 1300 mL. None of the identified compounds were considered to be chemically toxic at the determined concentrations. Moreover, these results were obtained under worst-case extraction conditions, whereas in most applications the membrane cartridge has already been rinsed or the extractables diluted during filtration.

This study also examined the extractables of prefilters by including cartridges with polypropylene (PP) fleeces or glass fiber (GF) fleeces as filtration media as well as large-pore membranes (Reif et al., 1995b). RP-HPLC analysis of the original water and GC-MS and RP-HPLC analysis of the original ethanol extract resulted in no peaks in the chromatograms of the PP fleece prefilter cartridges except for those also present in the blank. Only minor peaks were shown for the GF fleece cartridges. The extractables obtained from the membrane prefilter cartridges were comparable with the results obtained with membrane sterile filter cartridges. GC-MS and RP-HPLC analysis of the concentrated water showed a few major peaks of the high concentration compounds and several minor fractions (Fig. 7). GC-MS analysis of the concentrated ethanol resulted in several peaks that chiefly resulted from oligomers of the aliphates and the siloxanes (Fig. 8). These extractables were caused by degradation of the cartridge core, supporting materials, or silicone O-rings. The results of extractables from the prefilter materials were comparable with those obtained from sterile filter cartridges. The components used in sterile membrane filter and prefilter cartridges are often identical.

A small amount of a solid residue was found in the ethanol and water extracts of the glass fiber cartridges and was examined using FTIR and thermogravimetric analysis (TGA). FTIR analysis showed typical absorbance signals for silica and small peaks indicating an aliphatic compound. The results of TGA showed that the solid residue was composed of 14% crystal water, 16% carbonic compound, and 65% silica, e.g., glass fibers. Further tests revealed no glass fibers in the filtrate of a rinsed cartridge as a result of the downstream supports and fleeces of the prefilter cartridges. The glass fiber testing is still in progress.

The extractables determined in the prefilter cartridges are listed in Table 2. The extractables were identified as by-products of the PP and GF fleeces, membranes, and cartridge materials or additives of the specific polymers (antioxidizers, stabilizers, softeners, UV light protectors, etc.). The concentration ranges of the extractables under worst-case conditions were parts per billion per 10 in. prefilter cartridge for the low concentration contaminants and parts per million per 10 in. cartridge for a few high concentration contaminants in approximately 1300 mL of solvent. In particular, the PP fleece prefilter units showed a very low level of extractables, whereas the results of the membrane prefilter cartridge were comparable with those of the sterile filters. None of the identified extractables were toxic at the determined concentrations, although this aspect must be considered separately for each individual formulation process. Similar to the sterile filter units, brief rinsing of the prefilter cartridges reduces the amount of extractables to negligible concentrations.

8 PREFLUSH EFFECT ON EXTRACTABLES

The evaluations of the extractables as discussed above were all based on a worst-case scenario to achieve the highest possible amount of extractables. In real pharmaceutical applications all process variables such as process temperature, contact time of the filter material with the solvent, sterilization methods, and flush procedures prior to the process application have a direct impact on the extractables level. The use of flush procedures especially reduces the amount of extractables in the process. Most manufacturers publish the extractable concentrations—determined by NVR or TOC methods—in the flush volumes of the individual filter cartridges, showing that the filter units meet USP 22 and USP 23 requirements. Figure 9 shows the capillary electrophoresis chromatograms of an on-line extractables analysis of a filtrate after different flush volumes. After a volume of 500 mL the extractables are below the detection limits (0.1–1 ppm) of the UV detector of the capillary electrophoresis system.

Of course, the reduction of the extractables during the flushing procedure depends on the solubility of the extractables in the applied flush solution. Therefore, the flush solvent should be as identical as possible to the pharmaceutical solution to prevent any additional extraction process with a change in the solvents between the flushing and filtration process.

9 PARTICLE SHEDDING OF FILTERS

Particle shedding of filter units is an extractables-related issue in the pharmaceutical issue, for both extracted compound and particles contaminate the filtrate. Therefore, particle shedding should be given special consideration in the field of sterile filtration of LVP injection products. Even though the particle matter in parenterals is at best controversial regarding health significance, injectable drugs should not contain particulates that could be introduced into the bloodstream. Clothing, containers, and processing equipment (pumps, valves, piping systems, etc.) are major sources of particulates as well as the individual drug or the specific solvent itself. Cleaning and preparation of containers and closures, aseptic processing, and isolation technologies have improved the particulate quality of the pharmaceutical products (Winston Ho and Sirkar, 1992). Yet the sterilizing filter itself may contribute to particle contamination. Prefilters and some final filters shed particles from their matrices, for particle shedding is related to the polymers used and the mode of construction. Woven and nonwoven filters or membrane support fleeces in particular are sources of particulate contamination of the filtrate. Most membrane cartridges are tested by the filter manufacturers in the cartridge validation process with respect to particle shedding under static soaking flushing procedures. The validation data ensure that the filter will generate only the lowest amount of particles even under intermittent flow conditions, where particle generation is a major point of concern. Figure 10 shows the size-dependent determination of particles in the filtrate volumes after 1, 2.5, 5, and 10 L according to USP 23 for large volume parenterals for single-dose infusion (Sartorius AG, 1995). The tested 10 in. sterile filter cartridge meets the requirements of USP 23 limits for a maximum number of particles per milliliter of product of 25 particles/mL >10 μm and 3 particles/mL >25 μm as well as the limits of the British Pharmacopoeia (500 particles/mL 2–5 μm and 80 particles/mL >5 μm). These data are

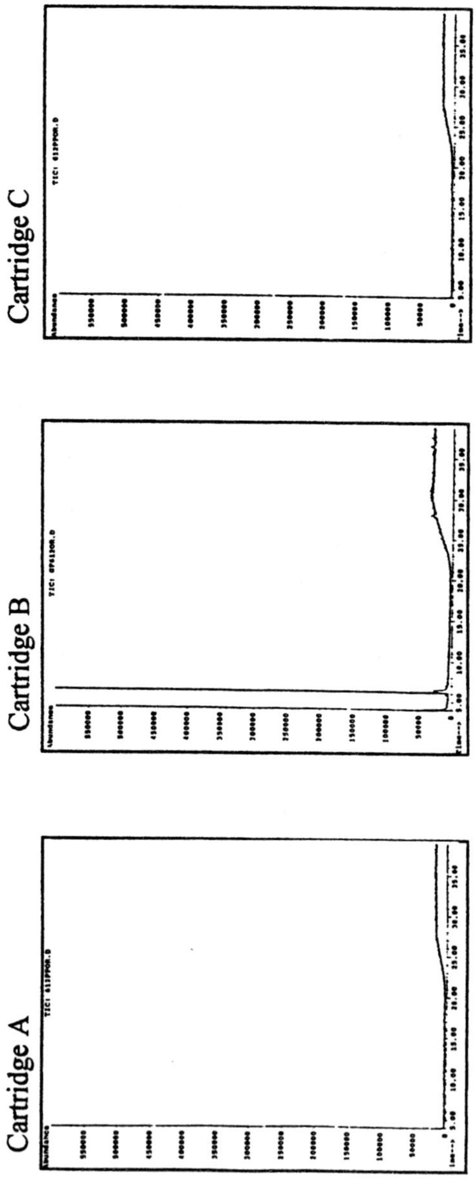

Cartridge A
Cartridge B
Cartridge C

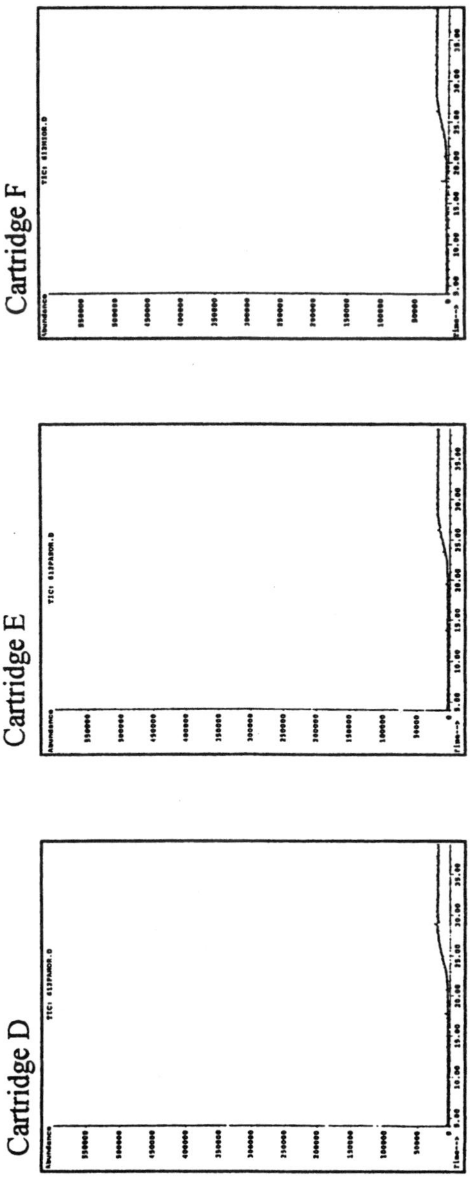

Figure 7 Chromatograms from GC-MS analysis of concentrated water using prefilter cartridges with different filter materials (various manufacturers). (From Reif et al., 1995b.)

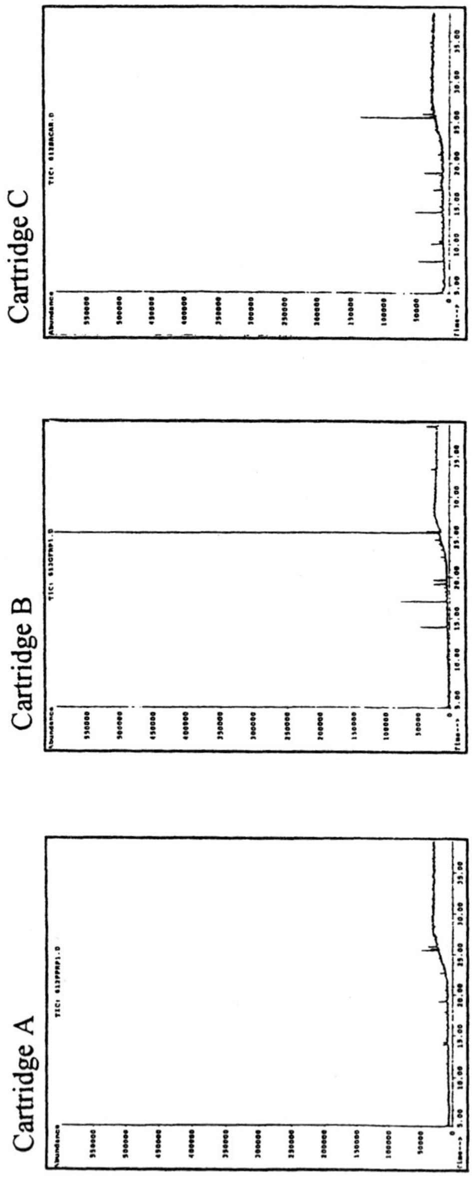
Cartridge C
Cartridge B
Cartridge A

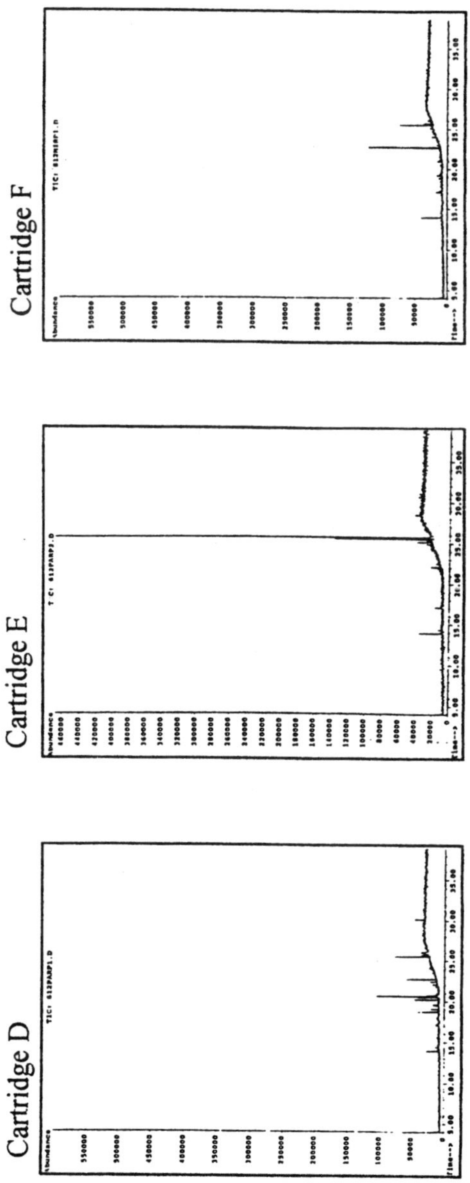

Figure 8 Chromatograms from GC-MS analysis of concentrated ethanol extract using prefilter cartridges with different filter materials (various manufacturers). (From Reif et al., 1995b.)

Table 2 Extractables of Prefilter Cartridges with Different Filter Materials from Various Manufacturers

Cartridge G (PP fleece prefilter)	Cartridge B (GF fleece prefilter)	Cartridge C (Membrane prefilter)	Cartridge D[a] (PP fleece prefilter)	Cartridge E[a] (GF fleece prefilter)	Cartridge F[a] (PP fleece prefilter)
Cyclohexane	Succinic acid	Methyl-2,4-pentadiol	Caprolactam	Caprolactam	Propionic acid
2,6-Di-*tert*-butylphenol	8-Oligoaliphates	Glycerol	Propionic acid	Dodecanol	Butyl-1-methoxybenzene
Hydroxybenzoic acid	2,4-Bis(1,1-dimethylethylphenol	2,4-Bis(1,1-dimethylethyl)phenol	4-(1-Methyl-1-phenylethyl)phenol	High MW N-containing compound	Naphthalenic compound
2,6-Di-*tert*-butylcresol	Ethoxyethyl benzoate	Butylphenoxyacetic acid	2,6-Di-*tert*-butylcresol	2,6-Di-*tert*-butylcresol	Polyether
Stearic acid	Diethyl terephthalate	Ethoxybenzoic acid	Benzoic acid	High MW aromatic	2,6-Di-*tert*-butylcresol
8-Oligoaliphates	Myristic acid	4-Oligosiloxanes	Dibutylphthalate	High MW aromatic	Dibutylphthalate
4-Oligosiloxanes	Palmitic acid	6-Oligoaliphates	2,2-Dimethoxy-1,2-diphenylethanone	Cyclododecane	High MW N-containing compound
Polyalkylic ether	Octadecene	Diethylphthalate	Butylmethoxybenzene	Butyl-4-methoxyphenol	Hexadecene
3-Oligosiloxanes	Stearic acid	Polyalkylic ether	5-Oligosiloxanes	3,3-Thiobispropionic acid	
	Polyalkylic ether		7-Oligoaliphates	7-Oligoaliphates	
	2-Oligosiloxanes		Caprolactam derivative	6-Oligosiloxanes	
	Glass fibers		Triphenylphosphine oxide	Polyether	
				Glass fibers	

[a]Identification of the RP-HPLC peaks by FTIR is still in progress; extractables list may be incomplete.
Source: Reif et al. (1995b).

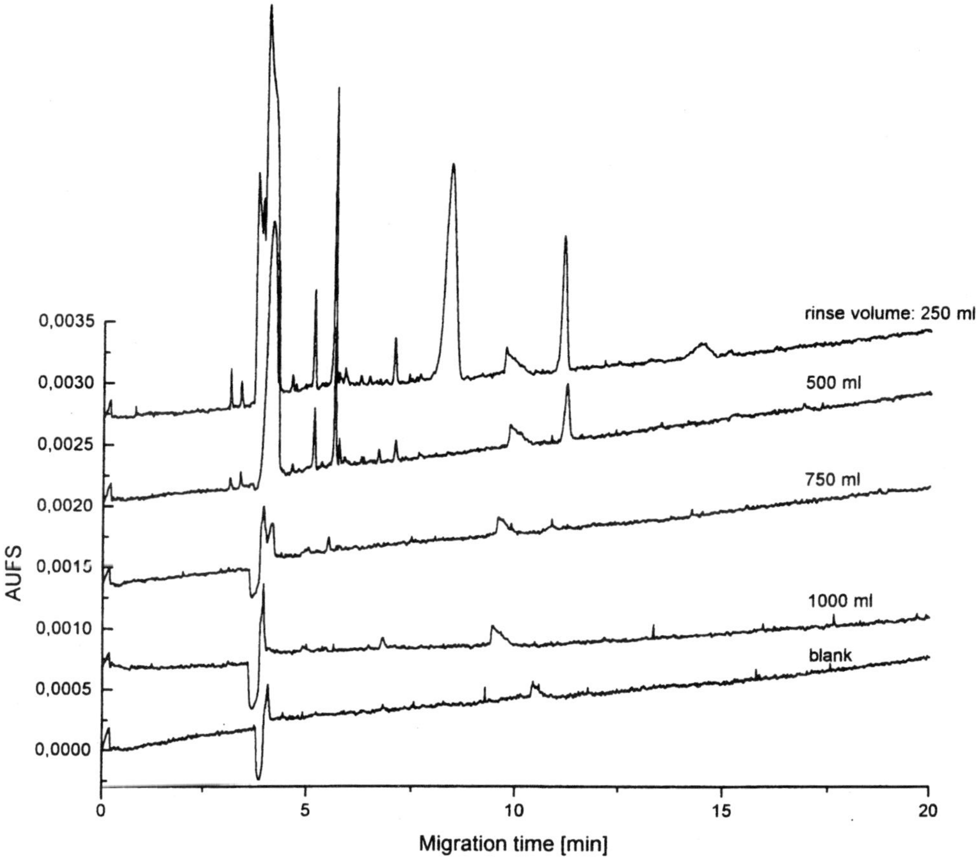

Figure 9 On-line analysis of reverse osmosis water flush volumes of 0.2 μm sterile filter cartridge with a cellulose acetate membrane by capillary electrophoresis. (From Reif, 1995.)

generally determined by the manufacturers and published in the individual validation guides.

10 CHEMICAL COMPATIBILITIES AND EXTRACTABLES

The extractables studies showed a significant difference of extractable concentrations between the various solvents, indicating a relationship of the extractables and the extracting liquid. If a membrane, a prefilter fleece, or the filter cartridge construction materials are incompatible with the solvent, the highest amount of extractables and particles could be observed. In a theoretically worst case, the filter polymers are dissolved in the liquid, resulting in the highest possible contamination of the "filtrate." Special consideration should therefore be given to the chemical compatibilities of the filter materials.

As mentioned earlier, the majority of the polymers are based not only on the polymer itself but also on various additives with different functions in the polymeric structure. Most of the additives stabilize the polymer (antioxidizers, aging and UV

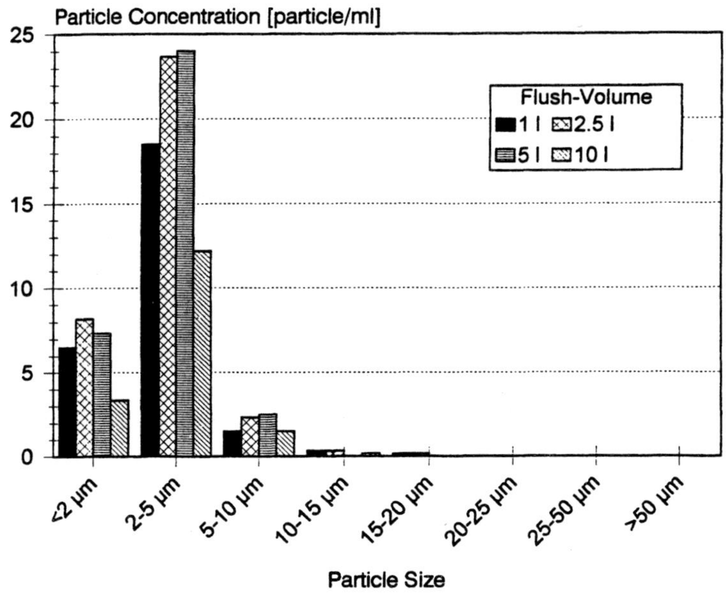

Figure 10 Particle content in the filtrate of a 0.2 μm sterile filter cartridge.

protectors, etc.) or enhance the polymer processing characteristics (lubricants, softeners, polymerization starters, etc.). The liquid additives are mainly molecularly dissolved in the polymer matrix whereas the solid additives are physically dispersed (Elias, 1993). Therefore, the additives do not influence the constitution or the configuration of the polymeric macromolecules, but they have a strong impact on polymer stability, conformation, morphology, and surface structure. Decreasing the additives in a membrane polymer would cause changes not only in the membrane structure but also in the chemical stability of the filter. The additives are often in unstable thermodynamical equilibrium with the surrounding polymer matrix and tend to dissociate. This self-dissociation process depends on various effects such as the type of additive–polymer interaction, additive concentration gradients, the viscosity of the system, and the temperature. The migration of an additive in a surrounding liquid is generally called bleeding (solid additives) or extraction (softeners). Bleeding or extraction can occur even in thermodynamically stable polymer–additive systems because of the attracting force of the differences in chemical potential between the additive in the polymer system and the contacting liquid. The velocity of the migration is mainly governed by the diffusional processes in the polymer matrix, and kinetic factors can slow down the extraction but are not able to impede the process. If the surrounding liquid is an optimal thermodynamical solvent with respect to the additives, all compounds incorporated in the polymer matrix will be extracted over a prolonged time. With the increasing loss of stabilizing additives, the polymer itself may show a decrease in chemical and physical stability as well as a changing morphology and surface structure. The diffusional controlled migration of the additive into the surrounding liquid will last until concentration equilibrium is achieved between the polymer matrix and the liquid. Because the volume of the solvent is often much greater than that of polymer matrix of the filter, the state of equilibrium cannot be reached, and the migration of the additives will continue until the polymer matrix is free of the extractable compounds.

Another factor that governs the loss of the stabilizing additives in the filter polymer and influences the matrix stability is the diffusion of the surrounding liquid into the polymer. The penetration of the solvent into the polymer matrix is also a diffusion-controlled process and is regulated by the glass temperature and the swelling rate of the polymer (Osada and Nakagawa, 1992). If a solvent migrates into the polymer matrix, the additives incorporated in the matrix can be dissolved and extracted. These penetrated and extracted areas of the solid polymer are weakened in their physical and chemical resistance, and if the polymer is exposed repeatedly to the solvent, even the deeper layers of the polymer matrix are destabilized. Furthermore, the penetration of the solvent into the matrix causes a swelling of the polymer, which may result in a relaxation of the polymers segments and thereby in a decrease of physical strength.

The migration, bleeding, and extraction of the additives result directly in extractables in the filtrates and additionally increase the degradation products of the polymer owing to the degradation of the additive-loss-based polymer matrix. The presented results of the extractable study showed various extracted chemical compounds that were identified either as decomposition products of the cartridge construction and membrane polymers or as additives of the individual polymers. An investigation of the time and temperature dependence of the extraction proved that not all extractables concentrations increase with higher temperature or prolonged extraction times. If the polymer is compatible with the solvent, the extraction of the additives increases with prolonged extraction times, but the contaminant concentrations based on polymer decomposition do not increase. If the solvent is capable of dissolving the weakened polymer matrix, both the additive and decomposition product of the polymer increase. Furthermore, due to the temperature dependence of the decomposition and the additive extraction, rising extraction temperatures enhance the extraction level of the additives and the polymer decomposition products. As an example, Fig. 11 shows the investigation of the time- and temperature-dependent extraction of an additive (softening agent di(2-ethylhexyl)phthalate (DOP) and a decomposition product (polyacrylate) of a polyamide membrane.

Regarding the wide variation in the susceptibility of membrane filters to attack by various solvents other than water (alcohols, hydrocarbons, esters, ketones, acids, alkalies, etc.), it is essential to investigate the solvent–polymer matrix interactions prior to the application of the filter. In particular, the preliminary step of an extractable validation of a filter unit should always be consideration of the compatibility of the filter with the specific solvent under process conditions. Furthermore, the effect of autoclaving or steam or gamma-radiation sterilization and CIP solutions may have a devastating impact on the integrity of the polymer matrix of the filter and could cause extremely high extractable levels. The specific process conditions should always be considered for extractable evaluation during filter validation processes.

11 STRUCTURAL AND CHEMICAL COMPATIBILITIES OF FILTERS

To be structurally or chemically suitable for the filtration of a liquid, a filter must be compatible with that liquid. That means that the filter must not undergo chemical attack and there should be no change or adverse alteration of its porous structure.

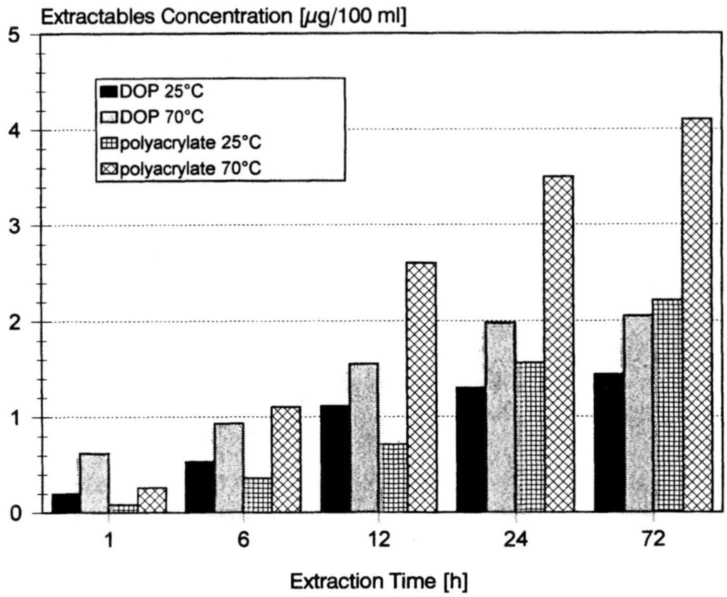

Figure 11 Time- and temperature-dependent extraction of an additive (softening agent di(2-ethylhexyl)phthalate, DOP) and a decomposition product (polyacrylate) of a polyamide membrane filter cartridge. (From Reif, 1995.)

Filter manufacturers commonly make available compatibility charts concerning their filters. Of necessity, these charts usually list only the actions of pure liquids. The assessment of the compatibilities of more complex fluids is left to those who formulate them or the filter manufacturer in a customer-oriented validation service.

Common methods for compatibility evaluation are visual observation of the appearance of the filter and determination of changes in filter dimensions or flow rates. Furthermore, integrity testing, especially with the bubble point method, and spectroscopic techniques such as scanning electron microscopy are common methods for investigating the impact of a liquid on the filter structure. Generally, four responses of a filter to a liquid can be recognized: no chemical effect, slight swelling or distortion of the filter, extended swelling and partial filter dissolution, and finally complete disintegration of the filter.

The compatibility of a filter depends not only on the filter–liquid interaction but also on the temperature and the applied pressure. If a mixture is to be filtered, all compounds of the liquid should be considered separately, although there is a chance that the detrimental impact of a minor component on a filter may diminish in the mixture. On the other hand, the influence of the aggressive compound on the filter stability even as a minor component in a fluid mixture cannot be predicted, and not all offensive action of a compound is muted by dilution. Furthermore, filters may be attacked by aggressive mixtures of compounds that may individually be harmless to the filter.

The compatibility of a filter with a given solvent will depend on the chemical composition of the filter. Certain rules can be given for the chemical resistance of various filter types (Brock, 1983):

Cellulose nitrate filters are susceptible to most solvents except aliphatic hydrocarbons and to most acids and alkalies.

Cellulose acetate filters are similar to the cellulose nitrate, except that they are more resistant to alcohols.

Regenerated cellulose filters are resistant to most solvents but show more sensitivity to alkalis and acids.

Vinyl filters are resistant to alcohols and alkalies, but they are not resistant to most other solvents or acids.

Poly(vinyl chloride) filters are resistant to most solvents but are sensitive to acids, ketones, and dioxane.

Acrylic filters are sensitive to acids and ketones but are resistant to most other liquids.

Nylon filters are resistant to most solvents but not to acids.

Polycarbonate filters are resistant to most acids and most organic solvents except halogenated hydrocarbons and strong alkalies.

Poly(vinylidene fluoride) filters are resistant to most solutions; exceptions include some specific solvents like acetone, dimethylformamide, and sulfuric acid.

Polytetrafluoroethylene filters are resistant to almost anything.

This estimation of filter compatibilities includes sterile filter membranes as well as prefilter media composed of materials mentioned about. Other prefilter media used in the pharmaceutical industry such as polypropylene or glass fleece and steel or ceramic prefilters show compatibilities that correspond to the technical data published for the raw materials. As our major concern regarding compatibilities is related to the sterile filtration media, the compatibilities of these specific prefilter materials are not discussed in this chapter.

12 COMPATIBILITY STUDIES OF MEMBRANE FILTERS

The following discussion is based mainly on the investigation of Lukaszewicz and Meltzer (1980), and portions are direct citations of their work. In this study, they examined three different types of membranes in each of several liquids, e.g., sesame seed oil, tri-*tert*-butylphosphate, and aqueous benzyl alcohol of varying strength. The compatibility results were described in terms of tensile and elongation properties, bubble point, flow, and dimensional changes in the filter. Furthermore, morphological changes were investigated using scanning electron microscopy. The impact of the structural changes of the filter in a specific solvent on organism retention were studied in a bacterial challenge test. The findings argue that compatibility complexities and subtleties require very specific assessments involving, comparable to the results of the extractable studies, the particular filter type and the precise challenging solutions.

As stated earlier, the migration of the liquid into the polymer matrix of the filter results in a softening and swelling of the membrane. Therefore, dimensional changes can be determined. Meanwhile, several manufacturers list alterations in the thickness and diameter of the membrane disks subjected to contact with liquids. The dimensional changes are so small, however, that their measurement, particularly of the thickness, is often difficult and somewhat imprecise. The application of stereomicroscopy with an integrated length-measuring system overcomes this problem, but owing to the high rate of deviation from filter to filter, the experimental compatibility assessment is unsuitable for reliable results or routine analysis. Typical values of measured change in the diameter of a 47 mm disk were found to be in the range of 0.05–2 mm (Reif, unpublished results, 1995). The thickness changes are proportionally far smaller.

Tensile and elongation studies can be used to study the softening or plasticizing effect. Normally, the tensile strength of a solid would be expected to decrease as the insinuating liquid molecules separate the polymeric segments from one another, thereby decreasing the aggregate strength contributions of the forces that bind the polymeric segments to one another in the bulk state. Similarly, while the percent elongation would increase due to the reduced binding forces, the elongation to break could be expected to decrease with the declining tensile strength. It was found that incompatibility effects result in lower tensile strength as well as in lower membrane elongation to break. As stated, this may be related to the migration of the liquid into the polymer matrix, which increases the space between the polymer chains and reduces the intramolecular forces between the individual polymers. It was found that the normal variability common to membranes, exaggerated by sensitivities of the highly porous state to tensile and elongation studies, would necessitate too large a sample replication to conveniently secure statistically meaningful results (Lukaszewicz and Meltzer, 1980). Therefore, tensile and elongation studies are not suitable for compatibility investigation, at least not in routine integrity testing.

Experiments concerning the swelling and flow rate showed that the swelling of a microporous membrane results in a decrease in flow rates. Thus, the increase in the diameter of a filter due to liquid contact and the migration of the liquid molecules into the polymer matrix is accompanied by a decrease in flow rate (Table 3). In Fig. 12, scanning electron micrographs (SEM) of cellulose triacetate before and after equilibrium with 10% benzyl alcohol in sesame seed oil are presented. The disruptive effect of the solution on the porous structure of the membrane is evident. Figure 13 shows the mutagenic effect of tri-*tert*-butyl phosphate on the 0.45 μm rated cellulose triacetate after 48 h of soaking. Swelling in nonporous films such as ultrafilters, at least when the weaker compressive resistance of the membrane is not overcome by the applied differential pressure, would be expected to result in enhanced throughput rates. This greater permeability, accompanied by reduced permselectivity, would be the consequences of the larger intersegmental space dimensions caused by plasticization of the ultrafilter. Liquid passage through the porous membranes depends, however, on the artificial voids that are the pores. It does not derive from the intersegmental spacings within the polymer. When a porous membrane becomes plasticized, its concomitant swelling occurs not only in its outer dimension but also internally, at the expense of its void volume. Decreased flow results. Lukaszewicz and Melter (1980) showed, furthermore, that a diminution in flow rate is not necessarily paralleled by a discernible increase in the filter's diameter of a nylon-supported vinyl chloride-acrylonitrile copolymer membrane (Table 3). It may be that the nylon supporting fleece serves to resist and to mask the swelling tendency to dimensional change. This indicates that fleece-supported membranes are superior to unsupported membranes with respect to the swelling rate–related changes in the porous structures. However, with an aqueous solution of less aggressive nature, flow

Table 3 Membrane Equilibration with Plasticizing Liquids of Cellulose Acetate and Vinyl Chloride-Acrylontrile Copolymer Membrane[a]

	Cellulose triacetate		Vinyl chloride-acrylonitrile copolymer	
	Disk diameter (mm)	Flow rate (mL/min)	Disk diameter (mm)	Flow rate (mL/min)
3% Aqueous benzyl alcohol				
Before	47	345	47	300
After	48	285	47	178
Difference	1	60	0	122
Sesame oil				
Before	47	410	47	295
After	48	150	47	105
Difference	1	260	0	190
10% Benzyl alcohol in sesame oil				
Before	47	385	47	303
After	48	170	47	120
Difference	1	215	0	183
Tri-*tert*-butyl phosphate				
Before	47	385	47	295
After	48	165	47	195
Difference	1	220	0	100

[a]Water flow rates: mL/min at 15 psi, 0.45 μm, filter diameter 47 mm, static equilibration for 48 h.
Source: Lukaszewicz and Meltzer (1980).

rate diminution without dimensional change is also observed for the unsupported membranes.

The lack of correlation between flow rate decrease and dimensional change remained significant. The effect may be only an apparent one, mirroring a relatively greater sensitivity of flow rates to differences in the membrane structure and hence to normal membrane variability than is indicated by dimensional changes (or bubble point values). Higher benzyl alcohol concentrations in contact with the same polysulfone membranes affect both the flow rate and the dimensional changes in the expected manner. However, scanning electron micrographs reveal no apparent changes in the 0.45 μm rated polysulfone membrane as a result of a 2-day equilibration with either 2% or 3% aqueous benzyl alcohol (Table 4).

Lukaszewicz and Meltzer (1980) stated that whatever the relationship between flow rate diminution and measurable increase in the diameter of a membrane disk, the large variability in the commercial filter's normal flow rate makes this parameter gives only a hint on the membrane–liquid compatibilities. Besides, a strong decrease in flow rate will always indicate a compatibility or filtration problem, and a substitution of the filter material would be advantageous.

Determination of the flow rate of deionized water before and after exposure of the filter to the specific solvent is an easy and reproducible way to quickly investigate the general chemical or structural compatibilities of membranes. Nevertheless, the

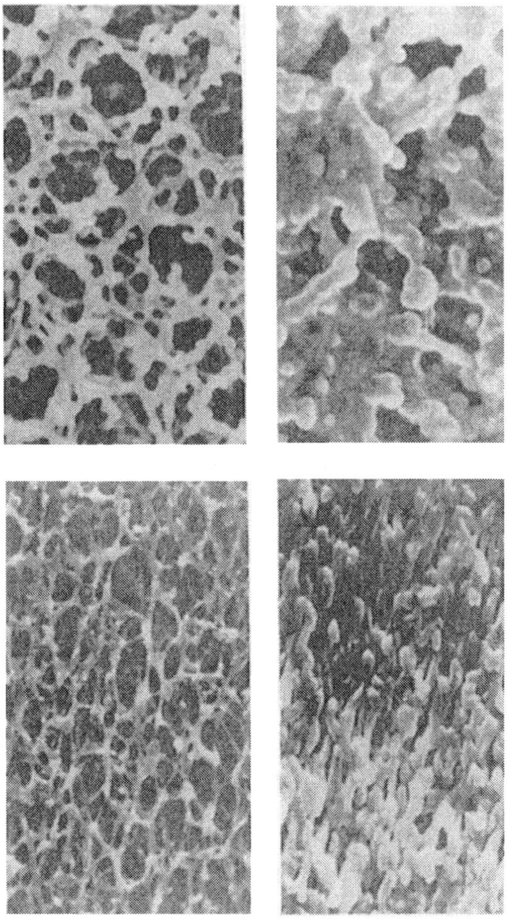

Figure 12 Scanning electron micrographs. Cellulose triacetate, 0.45 μm, 7000×, top left: dry control, top right: 10% benzyl alcohol in sesame seed oil; cellulose triacetate, 0.45 μm, 2000×, bottom left: dry control, bottom right: tri-*tert*-butyl phosphate. (From Lukaszewicz and Meltzer, 1980.)

results of the swelling and flow rate testing should always be considered at least in the integrity test context.

The diminution of water flow through the swollen membranes is presumably the consequence of pore-size restrictions caused by internal swelling, and variations in the bubble point would be expected. Lukaszewicz and Meltzer (1980) found that when a 0.2 μm rated cellulose triacetate membrane is exposed to aqueous 70% poly(propylene glycol) solution the bubble point increases with the swelling of the membrane (Table 5). Apparently an increase in bubble point is not an invariable accompaniment to decrease in flow rate, as shown by the effect of this same solution on 0.2 μm rated polysulfone filters. Here, the bubble point value seems unchanged, lying within the 10% accuracy commonly accorded to this test. The phenomenon can be rationalized on the grounds that flow rate is a more sensitive index to pore structure than is the bubble point. In either case, the particle retention capabilities,

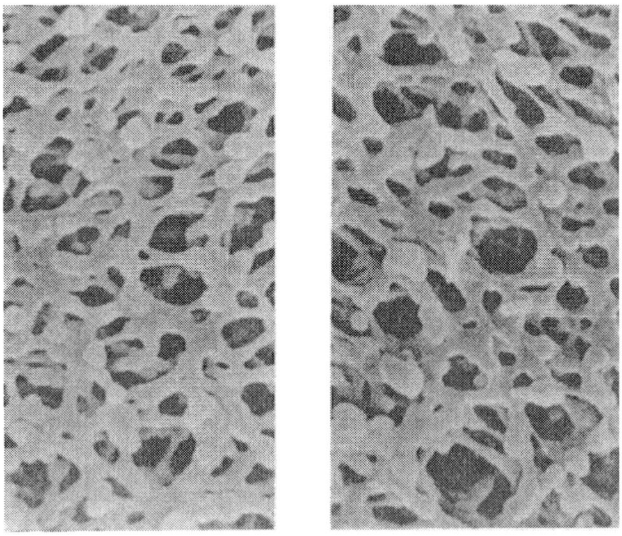

Figure 13 Scanning electron micrograph. Polysulfone, 0.45 μm, 7000×. Left: dry control. Right: 3% benzyl alcohol. (From Lukaszewicz and Meltzer, 1980.)

Table 4 Membrane Equilibration with Plasticizing Liquids of a Polysulfone Membrane[a]

	Disk diameter (mm)	Flow rate (mL/min)
0.5% Aq. benzyl alcohol		
Before	47	350
After	48	210
Difference	1	140
1.0% Aq. benzyl alcohol		
Before	47	350
After	47	195
Difference	0	155
2.0% Aq. benzyl alcohol		
Before	47	375
After	48	240
Difference	1	135
3.0% Aq. benzyl alcohol		
Before	47	350
After	48	168
Difference	1	182

[a]Water flow rates: mL/min at 15 psi, 0.45 μm, filter diameter 47 mm, static equilibration for 48 h.
Source: Lukaszewicz and Meltzer (1980).

Table 5 Membrane Equilibration with Plasticizing Liquids—Effect on Bubble Point[a]

Equilibration time (h)	Flow rate (mL/min)	Bubble point (psi)
Cellulose triacetate		
0	174	30
48	34	37
96	33	42
Polysulfone		
0	82	40
48	58	36
96	52	36

[a]0.2 μm rated, 48 h equilibration with 70% polypropylene glycol, filter diameter 47 mm.

assuming sieve-type capture, would indicate unimpairment; in fact, the cellulose triacetate membrane has become tighter.

However, the use of more aggressive swelling agents, such as varying strengths of water or benzyl alcohol in sesame seed oil or of tri-*tert*-butyl phosphate, yields situations where the bubble point values diminish and the aqueous flow rates decrease. This phenomenon merits elucidation and can be explained only by disturbing impacts of the test fluid or test procedure on the bubble point tests.

Lukaszewicż and Meltzer (1980) also considered the possibility of false bubble point readings. In the experimental design, the 47 mm filter disks, after equilibration with test solution, were each flushed with 1 L of water prior to having their flow rates and bubble points redetermined with water. It is conceivable that despite the presumably ample water flush, swelling agent remained on and/or in the filter pore walls. Also, especially in the case of the oil preparations, imperfect water wetting could result. This could lead to more easily evacuated pores in the bubble point test, with correspondingly lower bubble point values.

The surface tension of the test fluid also appears as a term in the bubble point equation. The fluid in the pores at the time of the bubble point testing need not be of the same purity or of the surface tension as the water that filled them after the flush. The pure water may acquire wetting agent that diffuses from within the pore walls at some finite rate in response to the drive of the concentration gradient. Conceivably the pore "water" surface tension is different. This could lead to lower bubble point values. It is possible that the depressed bubble point values genuinely indicate larger pores, whose presence can be rationalized. In the membrane casting operations, stresses are inevitably created that in some degree become locked into the finished filter. These are released when plasticization of the test membranes reduces the solid-state viscosity to the point where polymeric segmental motion (and subsequent swelling) can occur. Such stress release for extended polymer segments would result in membrane shrinkage. In general it is said that the "membrane remembers its original orientation during production." In the complex of antagonistic swelling and shrinking forces, it is conceivable that individual pores may become larger even as most are diminished by internal swelling.

In general, bubble point values decrease where marginal compatibilities are involved. A test of organism retention capabilities was performed in such a case by Lukaszewicz and Meltzer (1980) who used *B. subtilis* spore challenges against membranes whose bubble point values decreased following filter exposure to swelling liquids. The results, summarized in Table 6, reveal a failure to retain the challenge. The subjected membranes, previously determined to be 100% retentive for *Brevundimonas diminuta* (former *Pseudomonas diminuta*), were challenged with spores of *B. subtilis* suspended in the test solution. As shown in Table 6, 0.2 μm rated cellulose triacetate membranes exposed to sesame seed oil compositions containing 0.5% phenol showed sterility failures. These failures assume that a lowering of a membrane's bubble point subsequent to liquid contact may indicate an increase in the largest pore size characterizing that filter. It may not be assumed, however, that an artificial or anomalous reading has been obtained, although such cases may be encountered when product is the wetting liquid.

Another integrity test method is the diffusion test, in which the diffusion of air through a wetted membrane at a constant pressure is measured. The diffusion can be correlated to a pore size–specific organism retention value and is regarded as a very sensible test method for membrane failure determination in sterile filtration. The diffusion at a constant pressure and temperature of a given wetting liquid through a porous membrane is governed mainly by the extent of porosity on the membrane surface, the porosity in the membrane itself, and the thickness of the membrane. A swelling of the membrane with a decrease or increase in the membrane and pore dimensions therefore has a direct impact on the diffusion. In preliminary compatibility studies, the diffusion test proved to be very sensitive to structural changes in the membrane, but no correlation could be found between the diffusion test results, the swelling, and flow rate. The failure of the correlation may be based on various overlapping anomalous effects in all test procedures, which have already been discussed, as well as disturbing impacts of the test fluid. Further investigations of the relationship between the diffusion test and structural compatibilities are necessary.

Other preliminary studies showed a correlation between the extractables level of a membrane and the flow rate. The evaluation of the nonvolatile residue (NVR)

Table 6 Retention of Spores of *B. subtilis* by 0.2 μm Rated Cellulose Triacetate Membrane Filters[a]

	Bubble point		Percent retention
	Initial	After	
0.1% Peptone water (control)	55.3	56	100
10% Aq. vitamin C. preparation	45	45	100
Higher concentrate aq. vitamin C preparation	50.6	50	100
Hormonal preparation A in sesame oil containing 0.5% phenol	60	38	66
Hormonal preparation B in sesame oil containing 0.5% phenol	62	36	61.3

[a]Spore challenge: 8.5×10^4/100 mL, except for the hormonal preparations, for which it was 7.5×10^4/100 mL. Average of triplicate bubble points and triplicate runs for retention evaluation.
Source: Lukaszewicz and Meltzer (1980).

of a polyethersulfone (PESU) membrane showed a significantly higher extractable level, and the flow rate increased after exposure to various solvents. This can be explained by the fact that a membrane that starts to dissolve in a specific solvent or in which structural changes lead to a partial disruption of the polymeric matrix will cause higher amounts of particle shedding (membrane fractions) and extractables (decomposition products). A membrane that starts to deteriorate to such an extent will result in lower resistance to a flowing medium and yield higher flow rates. If the structural changes in the membrane do not result in destabilization of the polymer matrix, the extractable level should not be affected. However, if penetration of a membrane by a liquid leads to extreme swelling, the flow rate should decrease and the extractable level should rise due to the physical stress distortion of the membrane matrix. The experiments showed that with slightly decreasing or constant flow rates, no representative change in the NVR could be observed, whereas a strong decline in flow rate again showed higher extractable levels (Reif et al., 1995c). The preliminary data suggest that extractables analysis is a useful tool for the determination of filter compatibilities in a combination of several methods, but further studies regarding this extractables compatibility relation have to be performed.

Another important factor with respect to the structural suitability of filter media for the filtration of a liquid is the temperature at which the filtration is performed. Liquids that are compatible with the membrane materials at moderate temperatures may attack the polymer matrix at elevated temperature. Furthermore, with increasing temperatures the physical and chemical properties of the membrane polymers change, and the polymers eventually degrade. The extent of such changes depends on the type of polymer with its specific glass transition temperature and melting point (Mulder, 1991). Above these temperatures the properties of the membranes change even without any impact of a liquid. If the penetrating liquid causes structural deformation of the membrane matrix, the temperature stability of the polymer matrix may be even lower than the melting point or glass transition temperature of the dry polymer suggests. The factors influencing these relations are so numerous that it is impossible to predict the stability of a membrane by reference to the physical and chemical data. For each application, the thermal compatibility should be tested with respect to the specific application and solutions.

13 VALIDATION OF EXTRACTABLES AND FILTER COMPATIBILITIES

Summarizing the compatibility issue, it can be stated that the significance of the variations in the integrity data of filters to organism retention in processing contexts can be assessed meaningfully only by actual organism challenges. All other data and test methods regarding the compatibility of a filter are important and contribute to the evaluation of a filter for the specific process but cannot substitute for the bacterial challenge (BC) test. If the media to be validated do not allow the application of a BC test, it is advisable to apply all test methods available to ensure the compatibility of the filter with the challenging liquid.

Regarding the extractables of filters, in addition to the standard USP or BP procedures, all potential contaminants should be analyzed and identified. For this purpose, the extraction should be based on worst-case conditions, and the analytical methods should rely on the optimal, scientifically sound techniques. Due to the impossibility of predicting all fluid–filter interactions for the various solutions and mixtures in the pharmaceutical industry, the validation of a filter with a process fluid should always be performed with the specific fluid itself and under the exact conditions of the filter process operation.

REFERENCES

ASTM. (1984). Quantity of Water-Extractable Matter in Membrane Filters, ASTM Standard D-3861, American Society for Testing and Materials, Philadelphia.

Bordner, R., J. Winter, and P. Scarpino. (1978). Microbiological Methods for Monitoring the Environment, Document EPA-600/8-78-017, U.S. Environmental Protection Agency, Cincinnati.

Bower, J. P., and O. W. Kilham, (1978). Evaluation of organics contained in membrane filters and their effect on coliform bacteria, *Abstract of the Annual Meeting of the American Society for Microbiology*, Am. Soc. Microbiol., Washington, DC.

Brock, T. D. (1983). *Membrane Filtration*, Springer-Verlag, Berlin, Germany.

Cahn, R. D. (1967). Detergents in membrane filters, *Science*, *155*:195–196.

Chiou, L., and D. L. Smith. (1970). Adsorption of organic compounds by commercial filter papers and its implication on quantitative-qualitative chemical analysis, *J. Pharm. Sci.*, *59*(6):843–847.

Cooney, D. L. (1980). Interference of contaminants from membrane filters in ultraviolet spectrophotometry, *Anal. Chem.*, *52*:1068–1071.

Elias, H. G. (1993). *Makromoleküle*, Band 2, Hüthig a. Wepf, Basel, Switzerland.

Gandrud, B. W., J. C. Marshall, and T. H. Meltzer. (1969). Polymeric parameters of cellulosic support media affecting serum protein electrophoresis, *J. Appl. Polym. Sci.*, *13*:211–233.

Geldreich, E. E. (1975). *Handbook for Evaluating Water Bacteriology Laboratories*, Publication EPA-670/9-75-006, U.S. Environmental Protection Agency, Cincinnati.

Geldreich, E. E. (1977). Performance variability of membrane filter procedures, in *Proceedings of the Symposium on the Recovery of Indicator Organisms Employing Membrane Filters* (R. H. Bordner, C. F. Frith, and J. A. Winter, eds.), Publication EPA-600/9-77-024, U.S. Environmental Protection Agency, Cincinnati.

Lukaszewicz, R. C., and T. H. Meltzer. (1980). On the structural compatibilities of membrane filters, *J. Parenter. Drug Assoc.*, *34*(6):463–472.

Marvin, K. T., R. R. Proctor, and R. A. Neal. (1972). Some effects of filtration on the determination of nutrients in fresh and salt water, *Limnol. Oceanogr.*, *17*(5):777–783.

Mulder, M. (1991). *Basic Principles of Membrane Technology*, Kluwer, Dordrecht, Netherlands.

Olson, W. P. (1979). Validation and qualification of filtration systems for bacterial removal, *Pharm. Technol.* *3*:85–92.

Olson, W. P., R. O. Briggs, C. M. Garanchon, M. J. Quellet, E. A. Graf, and D. G. Luckhurst. (1980). Aqueous filter extractables: detection and elution from process filters, *J. Parenter. Drug Assoc.*, *34*(4):254–267.

Osada, Y., and T. Nakagawa. *Membrane Science and Technology*, Marcel Dekker, New York.

Pall Inc. (1994). *Guide to Extractables in Effluents from Pall P-Rated Ultipore N_{66} Filter Cartridges*, Publication TR-700a, Pall Industries, Glen Cove, NY.

Reif, O. W., P. Sölkner, and J. Rupp. (1995a). Analysis and evaluation of filter cartridge extractables for validation in the pharmaceutical downstream processing, *PDA J. Pharm. Sci. Technol.* submitted.

Reif, O. W., P. Sölkner, and J. Rupp. (1995b). A standard approach for the analysis of extractables, Poster presented at the PDA Fourth International Congress, Vienna, Austria.

Reif, O. W., J. Rupp, and P. Sölkner. (1995c). Correlation of chemical compatibilities and extractables of sterile filter membranes, in preparation.

Remberg G., H. Luttmann, G. von Unruh, and G. Spiteller. (1971). Über die Inhaltsstoffe von Filterpapieren-II, *Tetrahedron, 27*:5853–5859.

Robinson, J. W. (1995). *Undergraduate Instrumental Analysis*, Marcel Dekker, New York.

Rosenbluth, S. A., and G. W. Cribbs. (1969). Inhibitory effects of detergents in membrane filters, *J. Pharm. Sci., 58*(4):440–442.

Saad, H. Y., and W. I. Higouchi. (1965). Water solubility of cholesterol, *J. Pharm. Sci., 54*: 1205–1206.

Sartorius AG. (1995). *Validation Guide Srtobran P*, Publ. No. SPK 5712-d95061, Sartorius AG, Göttingen Germany.

Stone, T. E., V. Goel, and J. Leszczak. (1994a). Methodology for analysis of filter extractables: a model stream approach, *Pharm. Technol., 18*(10):116–130.

Stone, T. E., V. Goel, S. Gambale, R. Hegde, and C. Neville. (1994b). Overview of extractables testing of filtration devices used in the pharmaceutical industry, Poster presented at the Spring PDA Meeting, Chicago, IL.

Stone, T. E., V. Goel, and J. Leszczak. (1995). Methodology for analysis of filter extractables: a model stream approach, *Pharm. Technol. Eur., 7*(3):27–34.

Unger, K. K. (1989). *Handbuch der HPLC*, GIT Verlag, Darmstadt, Germany.

USP. (1995). *United States Pharmacopeia*, 23rd revision, U.S. Pharmacopeial Convention, Inc., Rockville, MD.

Winston Ho, W. S., and K. K. Sirkar. (1992). *Membrane Handbook*, Chapman & Hall, New York.

9

Bacterial Biofilms in Pharmaceutical Water Systems

MARC W. MITTELMAN

Centre for Infection & Biomaterials Research, The Toronto Hospital, Toronto, Ontario, Canada

1 INTRODUCTION

Bacterial contamination of purified waters continues to present a challenge to pharmaceutical, medical device, and cosmetics manufacturers. The presence of bacteria and their associated endotoxins (bacterial pyrogens) in pharmaceutical waters poses the single greatest threat to product quality. Regulatory recalls directly related to bacterial bioburden are often associated with contamination of purified water and water for injection; a review of the impact has been published by Mittelman (1995).

While the abiological particle loading of a given system usually remains relatively constant, small changes in environmental conditions can drastically influence the number and type of microorganisms present. Regardless of the prevailing conditions, however, the majority of bacteria in pharmaceutical water systems are associated with surfaces as biofilms. Biofilms may be described as surface accretions of bacteria, extracellular polymeric substances (slime), and entrained organic and inorganic detrital material. Desorption of bacteria and bacterial aggregates from biofilms gives rise to the majority of bulk-phase, or planktonic, bacteria in fluid-handling systems.

Although microporous membrane filters are designed to reduce or eliminate planktonic bacterial numbers, it is important to recognize that filtration efficacy and effective filter life are inextricably linked to bacterial biofilms associated with various surfaces. The high surface area/volume ratios associated with the many components of a purified water system create considerable niches for biofilms and, by extension, generate water system bioburden. It is this bioburden generated at surfaces that is most often responsible for transmembrane pressure increases resulting from fouling of microporous membrane feedwater surfaces.

2 THE MICROBIAL ECOLOGY OF PURIFIED WATERS

Virtually all bacteria isolated from purified water systems are gram-negative, nonfermentative bacilli. The gram-negative cell wall consists of multiple layers of phospholipids surrounded by a lipopolysaccharide (LPS) structure. This multilaminate structure may afford the cell protection from the extremely hypotonic environment that is intrinsic to purified water systems. These bacteria are heterotrophic, requiring the presence of reduced organic compounds as energy sources. Therefore, these compounds serve as limiting growth factors in purified water systems. The term ''oligotroph'' has been assigned to organisms that are capable of growth in media containing <1 mg/L organic carbon (Ishida and Kadota, 1981). In general, a positive correlation exists between assimilable organic carbon levels and planktonic bacterial numbers in purified waters.

Population densities in distilled water have been reported to exceed 10^6 colony-forming units per milliliter (CFU/mL) (Carson et al., 1973). McFeters et al. (1993) found 10^2–10^3 CFU/mL in a model laboratory water system, with many of the same system components (deionization beds, UV, and microporous membrane filters) that are seen in pharmaceutical grade purified water systems. Like a number of other workers (Martyak et al., 1993; Mittelman et al., 1987; Patterson et al., 1991), this group found that significantly greater numbers of bacteria (ranging up to 10^5 CFU/cm^2) were associated with various surfaces within the water production and distribution systems.

2.1 Starvation and Survival in Purified Waters

When one or more essential growth factors are limited, as is often the case in benthic environments and purified water systems, bacteria use a number of strategies designed to ensure their survival. In the short term, ''starved'' bacteria tend to use endogenous energy reserves for replication; therefore, one strategy for survival involves replication to increase the probability of species survival once additional energy sources become available (Novitsky and Morita, 1978). In marine systems limited in assimilable nutrients, some bacteria reduce their cell volume, forming ''ultramicrobacteria.'' Tabor et al. (1981) demonstrated that these organisms, many of which were <0.3 μm in diameter, were capable of passing through 0.45 μm pore microporous membrane filters. Their findings tend to corroborate the work of Christian and Meltzer (1986) and others regarding bacterial penetration of ''sterilizing grade'' microporous membrane filters.

2.2 Objectionable Organisms

The U.S. Pharmacopeia not only stipulates the maximum action limits for purified water and other pharmaceutical waters but also specifies that it not contain objectionable organisms. Included in this group are coliform bacteria, which by compendial requirement cannot exceed limits promulgated by the U.S. EPA. Currently, a limit of <1 CFU/100 mL total coliforms is in place. In addition, it is important to consider that changes in the microbial ecology of both the feedwater and the manufacturing environment may occur at any time. The significance of organisms in nonsterile drug forms requires an evaluation with respect to the product's intended use, the nature of the preparations, and potential hazard to the user.

Increasingly, however, noncoliform, heterotrophic bacteria previously considered "normal inhabitants" of purified waters are considered objectionable. Indeed, the prevailing view among manufacturers and the FDA is that objectionable organisms (other than the stipulated prohibition against coliform bacteria) are product application-defined. For example, purified water used in the manufacture of nonsterile ophthalmic preparations should be free of *Pseudomonas* spp, in particular, *P. cepacia* and *P. aeruginosa*. The definition of "objectionable organisms" in pharmaceutical waters is likely to broaden in the future: As new products and product applications are introduced, it follows that a number of existing and emerging environmental bacteria will be proscribed.

With an increasing recognition of the role bacterial biofilms play in the generation of water systems bioburden, it is likely that limits will eventually be placed on both "normal inhabitants" and "objectionable organisms" associated with surfaces. Current limitations associated with sampling and enumeration techniques for this significant subpopulation of water systems bioburden prevent the establishment of concern and action limits. Biofilms have been implicated as a reservoir for pathogenic bacteria in drinking water distribution conduits (Rogers et al., 1994; Wireman et al., 1993), hospital water systems (Alary and Joly, 1992), hemodialysis water systems (Phillips et al., 1994), and dental treatment units (Schulze-Robbecke et al., 1995; Shearer, 1996). However, as McFeters et al. (1993) noted, no comprehensive studies on the microbial ecology of pharmaceutical grade water systems—biofilm communities, in particular—have been carried out.

3 GENESIS OF BACTERIAL BIOFILMS

Perhaps the most significant adaptive mechanism used by nutrient-limited purified water bacteria involves adhesion to surfaces. Indeed, the majority of bacteria in a nutrient-limited environment, such as an ultrapure water system, are attached to surfaces (Fig. 1). Surfaces afford these organisms three major advantages over the bulk phase:

1. Trace organics, which can serve as nutrient sources, concentrate on clean surfaces shortly after their immersion.
2. Surface-associated bacteria tend to produce extracellular polymeric substances (EPS), which can further concentrate trace growth factors.
3. Bacteria in biofilms are afforded some protection from antagonistic agents such as biocides, heat treatments, and other inhibitory factors.

Several workers have shown that nutrient-limiting environments promote the attachment of bacteria to surfaces (Marshall, 1988; Mittelman et al., 1987).

The relatively high surface area/volume ratio associated with industrial water systems provides ample space for bacterial attachment. Any one of the many systems used in the purification of feedwaters is therefore a potential reservoir for contamination. In terms of biological contaminant generation, however, granular activated carbon columns (Collentro, 1986; Johnston and Burt, 1976), reverse osmosis (RO) and ultrafiltration membranes (Laurence and Lapierre, 1995; Ridgway et al., 1985), ion-exchange (DI) systems (Flemming, 1987), RO/DI water storage tanks (Collentro, 1996), and microporous membrane filters (Collentro, 1996) are the most significant

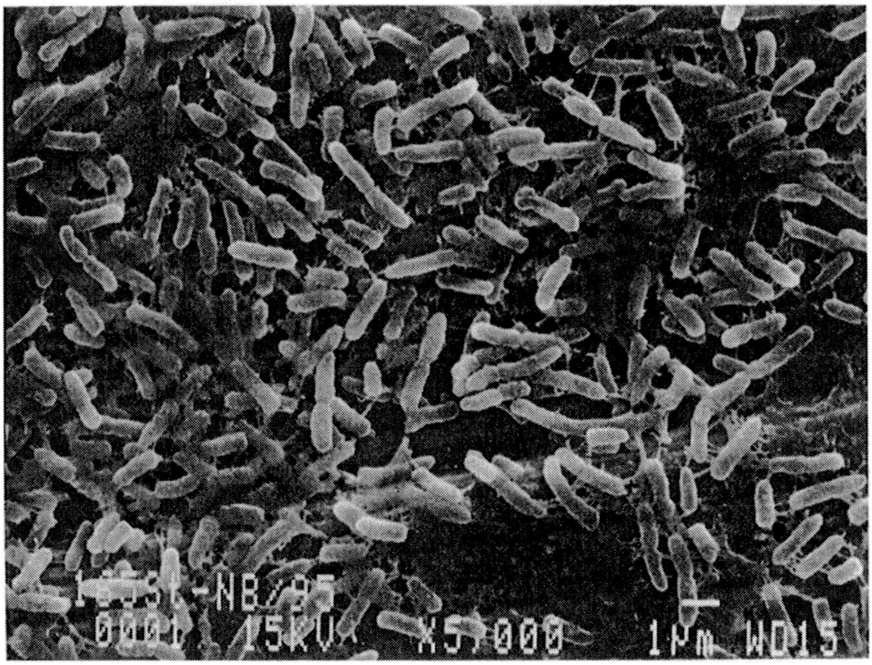

Figure 1 Scanning electron micrograph of a *P. aeruginosa* biofilm on 316 stainless steel.

areas of concern. Many of the same concerns surrounding biological contaminants in pharmaceutical waters have been reported in other industrial fluid-handling systems (Mittelman, 1991; Mittelman and Geesey, 1987).

3.1 Biofilm Development

Development of bacterial biofilms in aqueous environments proceeds in a three-step process: (1) accretion of trace organics on the surface, (2) primary (''reversible'') adhesion, and (3) surface colonization (growth of adherent bacteria). Bacteria form microcolonies on surfaces that may or may not be continuous in their distribution, as illustrated in Fig. 2. Although biofilms are known to be the source of bulk phase or planktonic bacteria in a water system, there is no discrete relationship known between the relative population sizes. This is due to the stochastic nature of adhesion, colonization, and desorption—all of which are affected by a number of interrelated physiocochemical factors (Table 1).

The elaboration of EPS by reversibly bound bacteria stabilizes the initial adhesion event. Extracellular polymeric substances often carry a strong net negative charge, which may be important in the stabilization of succeeding adherent organisms. Significantly, it is the presence of EPS that affords bacteria in pharmaceutical water systems protection from chemical treatments and, possibly, flowing steam/hot water treatment. EPS can constitute a significant fraction of the total surface biomass (bioburden) as is shown in Fig. 3.

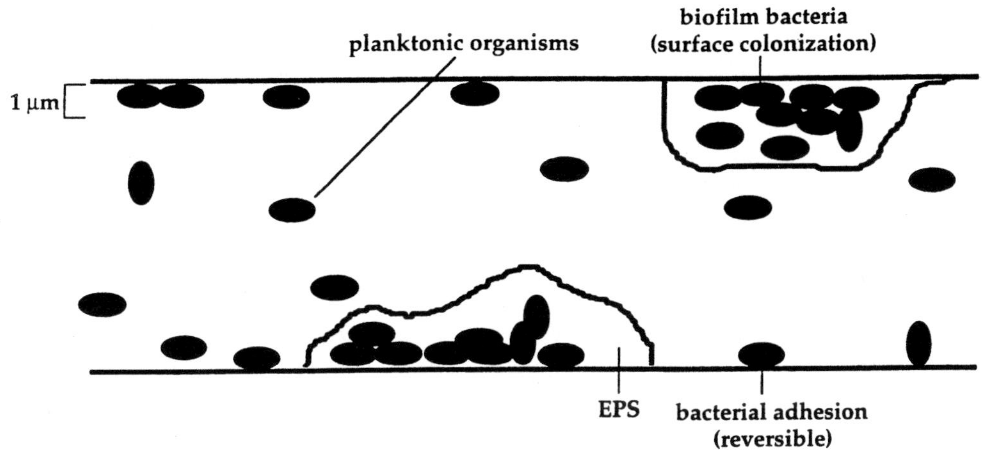

Figure 2 Genesis of bulk-phase and biofilm bacteria in a pipeline.

Table 1 Bacterial Adsorption to Surfaces in Purified Waters

Adhesion event	Mechanisms	Effect on adhesion	Key variables
Reversible phase	Balance between double-layer repulsion and van der Waals attractive forces.	Cells are maintained a finite distance from the surface; cells are loosely held and easily removed by mild hydraulic forces	pH; ionic strength; organic carbon concentration; fluid hydraulics
Irreversible phase	Adhesion is mediated by bacterial cell surface structures such as extracellular polymeric substances; hydrophobic interactions exist.	Cells are firmly adhered to surfaces; removal is effected by mechanical abrasion or alterations in the nature of adhesion factors	Electrostatic interactions; surface free energetics; temperature; hydrophobic interactions
Desorption	A stochastic event that may be dependent on cell–cell communication and surface density; bulk-phase physicochemical factors may be important.	Fluid hydraulic forces exceed adhesive forces; bacteria and/or their biomass constituents detach from the surface; desorbed bacteria can colonize downstream surfaces	Fluid hydraulics; temperature; ionic strength; surface tension; cell–cell signaling (quorum sensing)

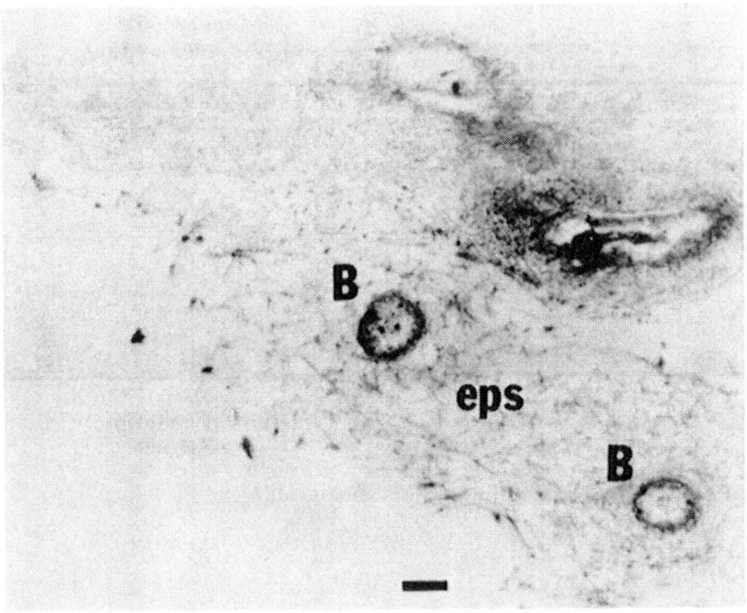

Figure 3 Transmission electron micrograph of a bacterial biofilm section adjacent to a 316 stainless steel surface. B = bacterial cell; eps = extracellular polymers. Bar = 1 μm.

3.2 Influence of Surface Characteristics

The influence of surface roughness and surface energetics on the development of bacterial biofilms has been examined by a number of investigators. Vanhaecke and Van den Haesevelde (1991) and Vanhaecke et al. (1990) reported that surface roughness can have an influence on the adhesion kinetics of some bacteria. They suggest that hydrophobic strains of *P. aeruginosa* show greater adhesion to electropolished stainless steel than strains possessing more hydrophilic cell surfaces. Indeed, the kinetics of adhesion for the former strain types were similar on 120 both polished and electropolished stainless steels. Other investigators reported significantly different "adhesion kinetics" for the same organisms (Pedersen, 1990; Quirynen et al., 1993; Verheyen et al., 1993).

There are no standardized methods for measuring bacterial adhesion under conditions designed to simulate those of the processing environment. Evaluations of surface effects on adhesion are very dependent on the methodologies employed. Evaluations are further complicated by the observation that adhesion kinetics are significantly influenced by a number of interrelated environmental and surface factors, some of which are listed in Table 2.

It is apparent that surface characteristics are important during the initial stages of adhesion (Dahlback et al., 1981; Marshall et al., 1971). It is unlikely, however, that surface structure or free energy considerations play important roles following the initial adhesion event. Following the initial adhesion event, succeeding bacteria may not contact the underlying surface. Similar findings have been reported for fluid hydraulic effects. Characklis (1990) showed that fluid hydraulics can affect the initial

Table 2 Environmental Effects on Bacterial Adhesion Parameters

Bulk-phase environmental parameters	Effect(s) on bacterial adhesion in aqueous environments	Conditions minimizing adhesion[a]	References
pH	Cell surface charge; adhesion to surfaces; binding capacity of cell surface; extracellular polymer stability	<6.	Characklis (1990); Herald and Zottola (1987); Richards et al. (1993)
Temperature	Metabolic activity; heat-shock protein synthesis	>40°C to minimize viscosity	Aranha and Meeker (1995); Hoadley (1981)
Ionic strength/ osmolarity	Cell surface charge; adhesion to surfaces	Greater ionic strength increases bacterial cell surface negative charge densities	Baldwin et al. (1988, 1995a, 1995b); Fletcher (1988); Geertsema-Doornbusch et al. (1993)
Assimilable carbon	Metabolic activity; organism size; cell surface hydrophobicity	Decreasing carbon and starvation result in shrinking cell size and increases in cell surface hydrophobicity	Dahlback et al. (1981); Morita (1982, 1985); Novitsky and Morita (1978); Nystrom et al. (1992)

[a]Surface- and organism-dependent.

rate of colonization; however, following this initial "lag" phase, biofilm development appears to proceed somewhat independently of fluid flow.

4 BIOFILM DETECTION

Since biofilm-associated bacteria are not detected by current test methodologies, serious underestimates of contaminating populations result. In addition, this inability to detect the major source of bulk-phase biological contaminants can result in an overestimate of treatment efficacies. Biofilm bacteria can be quantitatively recovered and enumerated from surfaces by using classical cultural techniques (Martyak et al., 1993; Patterson et al., 1991). Pipe surfaces may be swabbed with sterile cotton applicators, then plated onto the appropriate medium (R2A, etc.). However, the difficulty in reproducibly sampling surfaces has precluded more widespread testing of pharmaceutical systems. Currently, there are no commercially available biofilm samplers available for the pharmaceutical industry. Sacrificial pipe sections, including a modified Robbins device, have been used for recovery of biofilm bacteria in purified water systems (Martyak et al., 1993; Mittelman et al., 1987). However, these types of sampling systems and the associated analytical techniques are somewhat cumbersome and time-consuming.

In any process, it is important to monitor possible contamination so corrective action can be initiated as rapidly as possible. The ideal monitors should be nondestructive so they will not inhibit or damage the biofilm. If the test systems can be placed in supply lines or in the system ahead of purification/disinfection systems, then treatments can be modified to maintain microbiological control. A number of emerging on-line detection systems have previously been reviewed (Mittelman, 1994; Mittelman et al., 1993); three technologies with potential applications for the pharmaceutical industry are described herein.

4.1 Fourier Transform Infrared Spectrometry

Fourier transform infrared (FTIR) spectrometry operated in the attenuated total reflectance mode allows the detection of bacterial biofilms as they form on a crystal of zinc selenide or germanium (Nichols et al., 1985). The amide stretching of the proteins and ether stretch of the carbohydrates are clearly detectable when bacteria attach to surfaces. Often the nutrients attracted to the surface from the bulk phase are also clearly indicated by their infrared fingerprint. If the water system contained IR "windows," biofilm formation could be monitored and an indication of the chemical nature of the contamination would be apparent. Periodically, some mechanism for cleaning the "window" would have to be provided. A detection limit of $\approx 5 \times 10^5$ *Caulobacter crescentus* cells per square centimeter was obtained using a germanium substratum monitored in a ATR flow cell (Nivens et al., 1993a). This nondestructive technique holds promise as an on-line monitoring tool for bacterial colonization in purified water systems. The ability to monitor biomass "signature compounds" may be of particular utility in assessing chemical treatment efficacies against purified water system foulants.

4.2 Fluorimetry

The use of fluorimetry for on-line monitoring of biofilm development has been described for monitoring of antifouling (Mittelman et al., 1993) and uncoated stainless steel surfaces (Khoury et al., 1992). Reduced NAD compounds along with the aromatic amino acids (e.g., tyrosine and tryptophane) can be monitored as indicators of cell energy charge and biomass, respectively. As with FTIR spectrometry and quartz crystal microgravimetry (described below), this technique holds promise for application to monitoring purified water system fouling. Detection limits remain relatively poor, however, in the range of $\approx 10^5$ cells/cm^2.

4.3 Quartz Crystal Microbalance

The presence of material of a significantly different intrinsic viscosity than that of the water can be detected as a change in frequency of a vibrating quartz crystal in quartz crystal microbalance (QCM) technology. The surface can also be used as an electrode to produce both the microbalance and electrochemical signals (Deakin and Buttry, 1989). This technique was applied to monitoring biofilm formation in a simulated purified water system for the space station project. Detection limits of $\approx 10^5$ cells/cm^2 were obtained using an AT-cut quartz crystal (Nivens et al., 1993b).

5 TREATMENT

Inactivation and removal of bulk-phase bacteria following the most commonly employed physical and chemical treatments is usually complete. Within days or weeks of treatment, however, bulk-phase bacterial levels are often as high or higher than pretreatment levels. Bacteria existing in sessile biofilms are protected from the effects of antimicrobial agents and, to some extent, physical treatments (e.g., steam, hot water). A number of studies have shown that repopulation of purified and other industrial water systems is mediated by the presence of adherent bacterial populations (Mittelman and Geesey, 1987). The key to effective treatments, therefore, is inactivation and removal of this population of contaminating biological particulates.

5.1 Physical Treatments

Empirical experience has demonstrated the efficacy of frequent flowing steam or hot water treatments of pharmaceutical water systems (Agalloco, 1990). As with any type of antimicrobial treatment, the two key parameters are contact time and concentration (or temperature). Although there have been no reports of heat-resistant populations of bacteria in pharmaceutical water systems, problems with heat inactivation have been described for *Legionella* spp in distribution systems for potable water (Stout et al., 1986) and *Listeria monocytogenes* in dairy products (Lee and Frank, 1990).

While both flowing steam and hot water (80°C) appear to be effective at inactivating biofilm bacteria in pharmaceutical waters, neither treatment will effectively remove the biomass from surfaces, including extracellular polymeric substances (EPS) and constituent endotoxins. Depyrogenation of surfaces cannot be reliably accomplished using hot water or steam-in-place (SIP) treatments. Bacterial lipopolysaccharides are notoriously difficult to remove from surfaces (Ludwig and Avis, 1990; Novitsky, 1984). A significant number of problems with pyrogens have been reported in hemodialysis facilities with improperly treated purified water systems (Laurence and Lapierre, 1995; Murphy et al., 1987). Bacterial biofilms within various components of these systems are likely the major source of endotoxins (Vincent et al., 1989).

5.2 Chemical Treatment

The so-called bacterial regrowth phenomenon following chlorine treatments of purified and potable water systems is likely a function of biofilm formation rather than resistance in the classical sense of antibiotic resistance (LeChevallier et al., 1990; Wolfe et al., 1988). A combination of the polyanionic nature of many EPS moieties coupled with the inherent biocide demand associated with extracellular slime matrices may act as an inhibitor of various treatment agents. To date, the most effective chemical agents used in the control of bacterial biofilms in pharmaceutical grade water systems have been the oxidizing compounds such as chlorine, hydrogen peroxide, and, more recently, peracetic acid. Table 3 lists some of the more commonly applied chemical treatments along with typical dosage regimes.

The development of process- and product-compatible biofouling treatments has long evaded manufacturers of critical products that require purified water as a raw material. Of all the physical and biocidal treatments applied to pharmaceutical grade purified water systems, ozone appears to hold the greatest promise as an effective

Table 3 Chemical Treatment Regimes

Treatment agent	Dosage regime	Treatment time
Quaternary ammonium compounds	300–1000 mg/L	2–3 h
Chlorine	50–100 mg/L	2–3 h
Peracetic acid/peroxide	0.02–0.05% (v/v)	2 h
Iodine	50–100 mg/L	1–2 h
Hydrogen peroxide	10% (v/v)	2–3 h

Source: Mittelman (1995).

product-compatible biocide. With the development of fluoropolymer-based microporous membranes for pharmaceutical applications, ozone can be applied throughout a USP purified or water-for-injection (WFI) system. The technology is currently available for inactivation of residual ozone levels in situ via UV irradiation (Meltzer, 1993). Most of the problems with ozone application to purified water systems have been in the realm of component compatibility. Since ozone is an extremely reactive oxidant, its use is confined to systems constructed of such inert materials as Teflon and other fluoropolymers.

Hydrogen peroxide, a commonly employed purified water system treatment chemical, can also be readily degraded by ultraviolet light. However, it has relatively little activity against attached bacteria in biofilms. There is also evidence that suggests that hydrogen peroxide requires catalytic concentrations of Fe^{2+}, Ni^{2+}, or Cu^{2+} for optimal biocidal efficacy (Block, 1991).

Surfactants such as the quaternary ammonium compounds have excellent biocidal activity in addition to their intrinsic detergency. Synergistic combinations of chlorinated or brominated compounds with surfactants may provide additional activity against bacterial biofilm populations. Their ability to interact with surfaces does, however, create problems related to removal of these compounds following application. Larger volumes of rinse water are required for the surfactant compounds than, for example, for hydrogen peroxide.

Peracetic acid, 0.02% (v/v), has been found to be an effective treatment agent for both deionization resins and associated water system components (Alasri et al., 1993; Flemming, 1984). This compound is sometimes used in synergistic combinations with hydrogen peroxide and/or UV irradiation. Along with its true biocidal properties (i.e., sporocidal activity), peracetic acid is an effective depyrogenating agent and is used extensively in the hemodialysis industry, both for water system disinfection and for ultrafilter sterilization/depyrogenation.

As with any type of chemical treatment, the compatibility of water system components (including microporous membrane filters) should be verified with the appropriate manufacturers. Handling and disposal of water treatment and other chemical agents requires a familiarity with local health, safety, and environmental regulations.

REFERENCES

Agalloco, J. P. (1990). Steam sterilization-in-place technology, *J. Parent. Sci. Technol.*, *44*: 253–256.

Alary, M., and J. R. Joly. (1992). Factors contributing to the contamination of hospital water distribution systems by *Legionellae*, *J. Infect. Dis.*, *165*:565–569.

Alasri, A., M. Valverde, C. Roques, G. Michel, C. Cabassud, and P. Aptel. (1993). Sporocidal properties of peracetic acid and hydrogen peroxide, alone and in combination, in comparison with chlorine and formaldehyde for ultrafiltration membrane disinfection, *Can. J. Microbiol.*, *39*:52–60.

Aranha, H., and J. Meeker. (1995). Microbial retention characteristics of 0.2-microns-rated nylon membrane filters during filtration of high viscosity fluids at high differential pressure and varied temperatures, *J. Pharm. Sci. Technol.*, *49*:67–70.

Baldwin, W. W., J. T. M. Sheu, P. W. Bankston, and C. L. Woldringh. (1988). Changes in buoyant density and cell size of *Escherichia coli* in response to osmotic shocks, *J. Bacteriol.*, *170*:170–177.

Baldwin, W. W., R. Myer, T. Kung, E. Anderson, and A. L. Koch. (1995a). Growth and buoyant density of *Escherichia coli* at very low osmolarities, *J. Bacteriol.*, *177*:235–237.

Baldwin, W. W., R. Myer, N. Powell, E. Anderson, and A. L. Koch. (1995b). Buoyant density of *Escherichia coli* is determined solely by the osmolarity of the culture medium, *Arch. Microbiol.*, *164*:155–157.

Block, S. S. (1991). Peroxygen compounds, in *Disinfection, Sterilization, and Preservation* (S. S. Block, ed.), Lea & Febiger, Malvern, PA, pp. 167–181.

Carson, L. A., M. S. Favero, W. W. Bond, and N. J. Peterson. (1973). Morphological, biochemical, and growth characteristics of *Pseudomonas cepacia* from distilled water, *Appl. Microbiol.*, *25*:476–483.

Characklis, W. G. (1990). Microbial biofouling control, in *Biofilms* (W. G. Characklis and K. C. Marshall, eds.), Wiley, New York, pp. 585–633.

Christian, D. A., and T. H. Meltzer. (1986). The penetration of membranes by organism grow-through and its related problems, *Ultrapure Water*, *3*:39–44.

Collentro, W. V. (1986). Pretreatment. Part II: Activated carbon filtration, *Ultrapure Water*, *3*:39–44.

Collentro, W. V. (1996). USP purified water systems—case histories, Part I, *Pharm. Technol.*, September, pp. 148–168.

Dahlback, B., M. Hermannsson, S. Kjelleberg, and B. Norkrans. (1981). The hydrophobicity of bacteria—an important factor in the initial adhesion at the air-water interface, *Arch. Microbiol.*, *128*:267–270.

Deakin, M. R., and D. A. Buttry. (1989). Electrochemical applications of the quartz crystal microbalance, *Anal. Chem.*, *61*:1147–1154.

Flemming, H. C. (1984). Peracetic acid as disinfectant—a review, *Zbl. Bakt. Hyg.*, *179*:97–116.

Flemming, H. C. (1987). Microbial growth on ion exchangers, *Water Res.*, *21*:745–756.

Fletcher, M. (1988). Attachment of *Pseudomonas fluorescens* to glass and influence of electrolytes on bacterium–substratum separation distance, *J. Bacteriol.*, *170*:2027–2030.

Geertsema-Doornbusch, G. I., H. C. V. D. Mei, and H. J. Busscher. (1993). Microbial cell surface hydrophobicity. The involvement of electrostatic interactions in microbial adhesion to hydrocarbons, *J. Microbiol. Methods*, *18*:61–63.

Herald, P. J., and E. A. Zottola. (1987). Attachment of *Listeria monocytogenes* and *Yersinia enterocolitica* to stainless steel at various temperatures and pH values, *J. Food Protect.*, *50*:894 (abst.).

Hoadley, A. W. (1981). Effects of injury on the recovery of bacteria on membrane filters, in *Membrane Filtration: Application, Techniques, and Problems* (B. J. Dutka, ed.) Marcel Dekker, New York, pp. 413–450.

Ishida, Y., and H. Kadota. (1981). Growth patterns and substrate requirements of naturally occurring obligate oligotrophs, *Microb. Ecol.*, *7*:123–130.

Johnston, P. R., and S. C. Burt. (1976). Bacterial growth in charcoal filters, *Filtr. Separ.*, *13*: 240–244.

Khoury, A. E., R. Nicholov, S. Soltes, A. W. Bruce, G. Reid, and F. DiCosmo. (1992). A preliminary assessment of *Pseudomonas aeruginosa* biofilm development using fluorescence spectroscopy, *Int. Biodeterior. Biodegrad.*, *30*:187–199.

Laurence, R. A., and S. T. Lapierre. (1995). Quality of hemodialysis water: A 7-year multicenter study, *Am. J. Kidney Dis.*, *25*:738–750.

LeChevallier, M. W., B. H. Olson, and G. A. McFeters. (1990). *Assessing and Controlling Bacterial Regrowth in Distribution Systems*, American Water Works Assoc., Denver, CO.

Lee, S. H., and J. F. Frank. (1990). Resistance of *Listeria monocytogenes* biofilms to hypochlorite and heat, XXIII Int. Dairy Congr., Montreal, pp. 153.

Ludwig, J. D., and K. E. Avis. (1990). Dry heat inactivation of endotoxin on the surface of glass, *J. Parenter. Sci. Technol.*, *44*:4–12.

Marshall, K. C. (1988). Adhesion and growth of bacteria at surfaces in oligotrophic environments, *Can. J. Microbiol.*, *34*:503–506.

Marshall, K. C., R. Stout, and R. Mitchell. (1971). Mechanisms of the initial events in the sorption of marine bacteria to surfaces, *J. Gen. Microbiol.*, *68*:337–348.

Martyak, J. E., J. C. Carmody, and G. R. Husted. (1993). Characterizing biofilm growth in deionized ultrapure water piping systems, *Microcontamination*, *11*:39–44.

McFeters, G. A., S. C. Broadaway, B. H. Pyle, and Y. Egozy. (1993). Distribution of bacteria within operating laboratory water purification systems, *Appl. Environ. Microbiol.*, *59*: 1410–1415.

Meltzer, T. H. (1993). *High-Purity Water Preparation for the Semiconductor, Pharmaceutical, and Power Industries*, Tall Oaks Publishing, Littleton, CO.

Mittelman, M. W. (1991). Bacterial growth and biofouling control in purified water systems, in *Biofouling and Biocorrosion in Industrial Water Systems* (H. C. Flemming and G. G. Geesey, eds.), Springer-Verlag, Berlin, pp. 133–154.

Mittelman, M. W. (1994). Emerging techniques for the evaluation of bacterial biofilm formation and metabolic activity in marine and freshwater environments, in *Recent Developments in the Control of Biodeterioration* (D. Morse, ed.), Oxford Univ. Press, London, pp. 49–56.

Mittelman, M. W. (1995). Biofilm development in purified water systems, in *Microbial Biofilms* (H. L. Lappin-Scott and J. W. Costerton, eds.), Cambridge Univ. Press, London, pp. 133–147.

Mittelman, M. W., and G. G. Geesey. (1987). *Biological Fouling of Industrial Water Systems: A Problem Solving Approach*, Water Micro Associates, San Diego.

Mittelman, M. W., R. Islander, and R. M. Platt. (1987). Biofilm formation in a closed-loop purified water system, *Med. Device Diagn. Ind.*, *10*:50–55,75.

Mittelman, M. W., J. Packard, A. A. Arrage, S. L. Bean, P. Angell, and D. C. White. (1993). Test systems for evaluating antifouling coating efficacy using on-line detection of bioluminescence and fluorescence in a laminar-flow environment, *J. Microbiol. Methods*, *18*:51–60.

Morita, R. Y. (1982). Starvation-survival of heterotrophs in the marine environment, *Adv. Microb. Ecol.*, *6*:171–198.

Morita, R. Y. (1985). Starvation and miniaturization of heterotrophs, with special emphasis on maintenance of the starved viable state, in *Bacteria in the Natural Environments: The Effect of Nutrient Conditions* (M. Fletcher and G. Floodgate, eds.), Soc. Gen. Microbiol., London, pp. 111–130.

Murphy, J. J., L. A. Bland, B. J. Davis, R. W. Maxey, A. Light, M. S. Favero, and S. L. Solomon. (1987). Pyrogenic reactions associated with high-flux hemodialysis, *Proc. ICAAC* '87.

Nichols, P. D., J. M. Henson, J. B. Guckert, D. E. Nivens, and D. C. White. (1985). Fourier transform-infrared spectroscopic methods for microbial ecology: Analysis of bacteria, bacteria–polymer mixtures, and biofilms, *J. Microbiol. Methods*, *4*:79–94.

Nivens, D. E., J. Q. Chambers, T. R. Anderson, A. Tunlid, J. Smit, and D. C. White. (1993a). Monitoring microbial adhesion and biofilm formation by attenuated total reflection/Fourier transform infrared spectroscopy, *J. Microbiol. Methods*, *17*:199–213.

Nivens, D. E., J. Q. Chambers, T. R. Anderson, and D. C. White. (1993b). Long-term, on-line monitoring of microbial biofilms using a quartz crystal microbalance, *Anal. Chem.*, *65*:65–69.

Novitsky, J. A., and R. Y. Morita. (1978). Possible strategy for the survival of marine bacteria under starvation conditions, *Marine Biol.*, *48*:289–295.

Novitsky, T. J. (1984). Monitoring and validation of high purity water systems with the Limulus amebocyte lysate test for pyrogens, *Pharm. Eng.*, *4*:21–33.

Nystrom, T., R. M. Olsson, and S. Kjelleberg. (1992). Survival, stress resistance, and alterations in protein expression in the marine *Vibrio* sp. strain s14 during starvation for different individual nutrients, *Appl. Environ. Microbiol.*, *58*:55–65.

Patterson, M. K., G. R. Husted, A. Rutkowski, and D. C. Mayett. (1991). Bacteria: Isolation, identification, and microscopic properties of biofilms in high-purity water distribution systems, *Ultrapure Water*, *8*:18–24.

Pedersen, K. (1990). Biofilm development on stainless steel and PVC surfaces in drinking water, *Water Res.*, *24*:239–243.

Phillips, G., S. Hudson, and W. K. Stewart. (1994). Persistence of microflora in biofilm within fluid pathways of contemporary haemodialysis monitors (Gambro AK-10), *J. Hosp. Infect.*, *27*:117–125.

Quirynen, M., H. C. V. D. Mei, C. M Bollen, A. Schotte, M. Marechal, G. I. Doornbusch, I. Naert, H. J. Busscher, and D. V. Steenberghe. (1993). An in vivo study of the influence of the surface roughness of implants on the microbiology of supra- and subgingival plaque, *J. Dent. Res.*, *72*:1304–1309.

Richards, G. K., R. F. Gagnon, G. Obst, and G. B. Kostiner. (1993). The effect of peritoneal dialysis solutions on rifampin action against *Staphylococcus epidermidis* in the fluid and biofilm phases of growth, *Periton. Dial. Int.*, *9*:183–186.

Ridgway, H. F., M. G. Rigby, and D. G. Argo. (1985). Bacterial adhesion and fouling of reverse osmosis membranes, *J. Am. Water Works Assoc.*, *77*:97–106.

Rogers, J., A. B. Dowsett, P. J. Dennis, J. V. Lee, and C. W. Keevil. (1994). Influence of plumbing materials on biofilm formation and growth of *Legionella pneumophila* in potable water systems, *Appl. Environ. Microbiol.*, *60*:1842–1851.

Schulze-Robbecke, R., C. Feldmann, R. Fischeder, B. Janning, M. Exner, and G. Wahl. (1995). Dental units: An environmental study of sources of potentially pathogenic mycobacteria, *Tubercle Lung Dis.*, *76*:318–323.

Shearer, B. G. (1996). Biofilm and the dental office, *J. Am. Dent. Assoc.*, *127*:181–189.

Stout, J. E., M. Best, and V. L. Yu. (1986). Susceptibility of members of the family *Legionellaceae* to thermal stress: Implications for heat eradication methods in water distribution systems, *Appl. Environ. Microbiol.*, *52*:396–399.

Tabor, P. S., K. Ohwada, and R. R. Colwell. (1981). Filterable marine bacteria found in the deep sea: Distribution, taxonomy, and response to starvation, *Microb. Ecol.*, *7*:67–83.

Vanhaecke, E., and K. Van den Haesevelde. (1991). Bacterial contamination of stainless steel equipment, In *Sterile Pharmaceutical Manufacturing* (M. J. Groves, W. P. Olson, and M. H. Anisfeld, eds.), Interpharm Press, Buffalo Grove, IL, pp. 141–162.

Vanhaecke, E., J. P. Remon, F. Raes, J. Moors, D. DeRudder, and A. V. Peteghen. (1990). Kinetics of *Pseudomonas aeruginosa* adhesion to 304 and 316-L stainless steel: Role of cell surface hydrophobicity, *Appl. Environ. Microbiol.*, *56*:788–795.

Verheyen, C. C., W. J. Dhert, J. M. Blieck-Hogervorst, T. J. V. D. Reijden, P. L. Petit, and K. de Groot. (1993). Adherence to a metal, polymer and composite by *Staphylococcus aureus* and *Staphylococcus epidermidis*, *Biomaterials*, *14*:383–391.

Vincent, F. D., A. R. Tibi, and J. C. Darbord. (1989). A bacterial biofilm in a hemodialysis system. Assessment of disinfection and crossing of endotoxin, *Asaio Trans.*, *35*:310–313.

Wireman, J. W., A. Schmidt, C. R. Scavo, and D. T. Hutchins. (1993). Biofilm formation by *Legionella pneumophila* in a model domestic hot water system, in *Legionella*: *Current Status and Emerging Perspectives* (J. Barbace, ed.), Am. Soc. Microbiol., Washington, DC., pp. 231–234.

Wolfe, R. L., N. R. Ward, and B. H. Olsen. (1988). Inorganic chloramines as drinking water disinfectants: A review, *J. Am. Water Works Assoc.*, *76*:74–88.

10

Filtrative Particle Removal from Liquids

MAIK W. JORNITZ
Sartorius AG, Göttingen, Germany

THEODORE H. MELTZER
Capitola Consulting Company, Bethesda, Maryland

1 PARTICLE TRAPPING MECHANISMS

The sieve retention mode of particle capture is the one most evident in common filtration experience. It occurs whenever a particle is too large to pass through a filter pore. It is a geometric or spatial restraint. This type of particle arrest is considered absolute in that it is independent of the filtration conditions. It is not influenced by the applied differential pressure (unless, possibly, that level is so high as to deform either the particle or the filter pore, which can occur with mycoplasmas, for example). Sieve retention is also free of the influences of the particle challenge level. Regardless of the number of particles confronting the filter, if each is too large to pass the filter pores then none will be able to do so, and all the particles, regardless of number, will be retained. Additionally, the particle retention will be independent of the suspending liquid vehicle as defined by its ionic strength, pH, surface tension, temperature, viscosity, presence or absence of surfactant, etc. if it does not affect the filter's compatibility. (Figure 1 is an illustration of sieve retention known to many who have attended courses in membrane filtration.)

It is possible for a particle to be small enough to enter a filter pore and also to be too small to be restrained spatially within the pore. Nevertheless, the particle may be filtratively removed, imprisoned within the filter's tortuous passageway by adsorptive contact with the pore wall. The particle-arresting adsorptive force may arise from any of several origins. It is usually, but not always, in the nature of an electromagnetic charge. The term "adsorptive sequestration" has been used to refer to the particle capture effect that results from any such cause. Adsorptive sequestration, then, refers to any means of particle restraint other than sieve retention. That

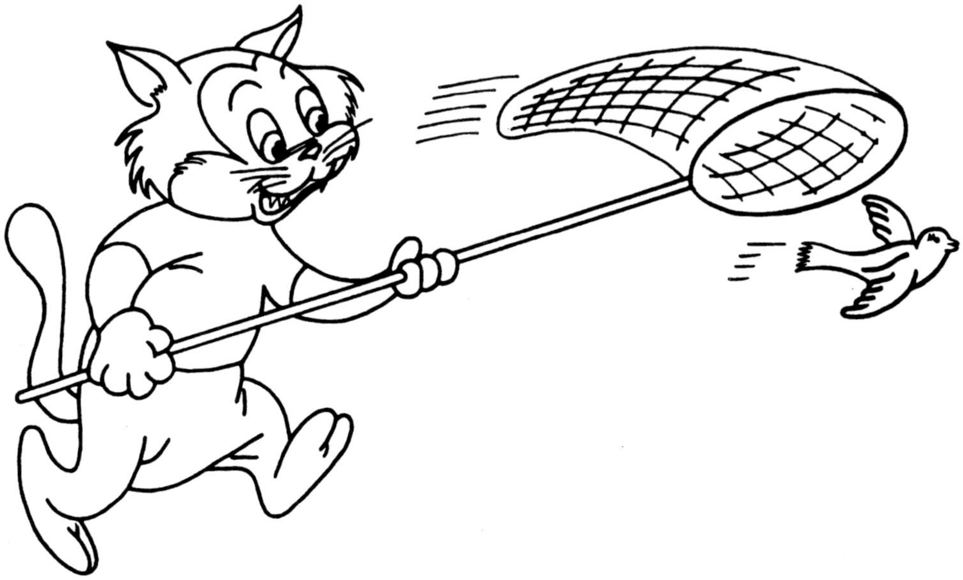

Figure 1 Solid–gas separation by sieve retention.

such adsorptive mechanisms are operative in membrane filtration has long been recognized (Zsigmondy, 1909; Elford, 1933; Ferry, 1935; Petras, 1967; Wallhäusser, 1995; Wallhäusser and Schmidt, 1967; Meltzer, 1987; Ostreicher, 1985; Sarry and Sucker, 1992; Meltzer et al., 1997).

2 ADSORPTIVE SEQUESTRATION

2.1 General Literature Background

As far back as 1909, it was pointed out that a filter surface has a certain adsorbing capacity whose affinity must first be satisfied before the dispersed phase may pass unhindered through the filter (Zsigmondy, 1909). Specific adsorptions of many entities have since been noted by numerous investigators. Elford (1933) reported that dyes could adsorptively be removed from true solutions by collodion membranes (cellulose nitrate). Lin (1973) elaborated on this finding. The strong adsorption tendencies of the cellulose nitrate polymer had also been noted by Elford (1931) in the case of viruses. Many investigators have since elaborated on virus adsorption (Smith and Doncaster, 1935; Farrah et al., 1976; Mix, 1974; Marzouk, 1976). The adsorption of oxyhemoglobin by cellulose nitrate membranes was early noted (Brinkman and Szent Gyorgi, 1923), and Hawker and Hawker (1975) investigated the adsorptive retention of radiotagged plasma proteins by various membranes. The use of membrane filters to adsorptively collect and isolate nucleic acids, enzymes, single-stranded DNA, robosomes, and proteinaceous materials in scintillation counting operations is well established. The adsorption of bovine serum albumin, antigens, antibodies, antibody complex (Skelley et al., 1973; Tanny and Meltzer, 1978) and specific binding and receptor protein (Millipore AB 304) to cellulose nitrate has been shown to occur. Berg et al. (1965) investigated the adsorption of both inorganic and organic compounds on polymerics such as cellulosic filter papers, nylon, polyethylene, and cellulose diacetate dialysis membranes. That water-soluble organics could be removed adsorptively from aqueous solutions by filters was observed by Chiou and Smith (1970). These investigators were thus led into a rather thorough study of such adsorption by filters. Chiori et al. (1965) found that cetrimide could be adsorbed onto microporous membranes in such concentrations as to inhibit the growth of *B. subtilis* on their surfaces. The adsorptive sequestration of preservatives from ophthalmic solutions undergoing filtrative sterilization was reported by Van Ooteghem and Herbots (1969).

Udani (1978) studied the adsorptive sequestration of such preservatives as benzalkonium chloride, chlorocresol, and chlorhexidine acetate from their solutions by membrane filters. The adsorptive removal of flu vaccine impurities and antibodies onto membrane filters was reported by Tanny and Meltzer (1978). Inorganic particulate matter can be removed filtratively through the adsorption mechanism (Johnston, 1975). Elford (1933) describes the retention of carbon black particles, and Kaczmarek et al. (1978) and Zierdt (1978) reported the adsorption of polystyrene latex particles by polycarbonate filters. Wrasidlo and Mysels (1984) enlarged on this occurrence with other filters, as had previously Wallhäusser (1975), Pall et al. (1980), and Wrasidlo et al. (1983). In chemotaxis studies, Wilkinson (1974) and Horowitz and Garrett (1971) established that the behavior of various living cells relative to filter barriers seems to be describable in terms of adsorption.

It is thus well documented that a myriad of molecules and materials can be adsorbed onto filters, to become filtratively removed thereby.

2.2 Various Aspects of Adsorptive Sequestration

Electrokinetic Effects and Positive Charge Filters

A counterpart to the electrostatic attractions that are known to be operative in gas media, depending on the humidity of the gas, are the electrokinetic attractions common to liquid media. Electrokinetic charges can be generated on filter surfaces by the liquid in contact with those surfaces. The charged sites serve to attract and filtratively remove particles of opposite electrokinetic charge from liquid streams.

When a solid particle is suspended in a liquid, the zeta potential charge characterizing its surface is a function of the dielectric constant values of both materials. Consider an aqueous suspension of silica. Water has a dielectric constant of 70; silica's is 2. Therefore, silica particles in aqueous systems have negative zeta charges. Asbestos, on the other hand, has a dielectric constant in excess of that of water. Consequently, asbestos in water assumes a positive zeta potential and maintains it over a large pH range.

Another way of looking at the matter is to consider the isoelectric point, the point of zero charge, of the filter material (Fiore and Babineau, 1979). Thus, asbestos has an isoelectric point at pH 8.3. It is therefore positively charged at pH below that value, including aqueous solutions of neutral pH.

Since most solid particles bear negative zeta potentials in water, their arrest by this particle capture mechanism requires filters with positive zeta charges. Asbestos is a superior filter material simply because, among other reasons, it naturally possesses this very property. Regrettably, certain forms of asbestos are carcinogenic. The use of asbestos materials is therefore effectively prohibited in pharmaceutical contexts.

Other materials are also known to have naturally positive zeta potentials or can be induced to have them. Membrane manufacturers offer filters with induced positive zeta charges for removing the lipopolysaccharides that are the seat of pyrogenic activity. This is done through use of the positive zeta charges that derive from quaternerization of amine groups present or grafted onto nylon and other filter surfaces, by coating filter surfaces with polyamines or other organic polyelectrolytes, or by coating particles or fibers with a cationic colloid (Ostreicher, 1977a, 177b, 1985).

These positively charged filters find numerous applications, particularly in water filtration and sometimes in pyrogen removal. Like all filters, these zeta-positive filters have their limitations. They bear a finite number of positive sites. Their particle-trapping properties are therefore stoichiometrically related to their charge density. Tolliver and Schroeder (1983) found that charge-modified membranes when challenged by a large number of particles progressively decreased in efficiency during the filtration from 90% to less than 20%. This is interpreted as being due to the lower probability of a particle encountering one of the decreasing number of remaining adsorption sites as the filtration progresses.

The user must make certain—for example, by a titration determination—not to overload the charge capacity of the filter; otherwise particle passage (''breakthrough'') or even desorption may occur. Such overload may not be signaled by an upturn in the resistance to flow, unlike the experience common to the usual filtrations, where loading the filter with particles has consequences in terms of flow rate diminution and the increase in applied pressures necessary to overcome it.

Parks (1967) showed that the zero or isoelectric point charge of a composite surface is the weighted average of the individual zero-point charges of the constituents (Fiore and Babineau, 1979). Therefore, the adsorption of charge-neutralizing entities onto the filter serves to diminish its remaining charge value. Raistrick (1982) states, therefore, that such charge-modified filters may have only limited usefulness for the filtration of complex fluids. Raistrick shows that such filters exhibit high removal efficiencies with latex particles (Sec. 8) suspended in aqueous acetate buffer but only low efficiencies with such particles suspended in potable liquids.

Raistrick's observations confirm AMF-Cuno findings that the adsorption of negatively-charged particles may shift the surface charge of positively charged filters. This may inhibit further negatively charged particle retention, leading to particle breakthrough or desorption, which would be disastrous in terms of endotoxin removal. A high peak of endotoxins in the filtered solution would be the result. Similarly, it has been indicated (Rossitto, 1983) that a charge-modified filter medium that is effective in removing a given species of particle from one solution medium may not be effective in removing the same particles from a second or different liquid composition. This is a consequence of charged particles of different species competing for the same adsorptive surface. Raistrick's finding relative to latex particle retention from potable liquids, mentioned above, is a case in point.

Charge-modified prefilters are characterized by a maximum pressure value above which they may not function properly due to the possibilities of desorption (unloading) and filter medium migration. The filter efficiency may actually decrease as the applied pressure increases. Therefore, when used with heavily loaded liquids, charge-modified filters should be preceded by prefilters. Otherwise, their maximum allowable pressure levels may become exceeded due to high loadings of particulates, whether trapped electrokinetically or by sieve retention, necessitating replacement. Excessive pressure surges must therefore also be guarded against. Also, moderation of flow rates may be required to optimize the removal of colloids, lipids, and endotoxins. The adequacy of fluid–filter contact time is an issue.

Particle size may influence the capture mechanism whereby charge-modified filters perform. Hou et al. (1980) neutralized the electrokinetic effectivity of such filters by operating at high pH. It was found that particles larger than approximately 1 μm were retained, but smaller particles retained at pH levels where positive charges were operative escaped capture at the high pH. It is concluded that the larger particles were captured by sieve retention when electrokinetic influences were absent, but that particles too small to be thus retained required charge interactions for their arrest.

Knight et al. (1982), by means of scanning electron micrography, established that 0.109 μm latex particles are captured within the pore passageways of positively charged filters of ratings too large to arrest them by sieve retention. Moreover, particles retained within these pores by mechanisms other than electrokinetic charge can be rinsed away; the charged filters alone retain their captured particles. This work demonstrates at once the effectiveness and strength of electrokinetic charged-induced particle captures.

It should be noted, however, that noncharged filters may also adsorptively remove particles from aqueous solutions and, at least in some cases, by mechanisms strong enough to resist aqueous rinsing (Zierdt et al., 1977). Additionally, a gradation in the electrokinetic strengths of the charged filters is possible, particularly as these become modified by adsorbed entities. What is to be expected, then, is a spectrum of electrokinetic charge effects in connection with charge-modified filters.

Removal of Pyrogens and Organisms by Charge-Modified Filters

Charge-modified filters are widely used, particularly in antibiotic manufacture, to remove pyrogenic endotoxin. This is an application whose success is widely attested to. Yet the operation requires care because charge-modified filters have finite capacities, can have their charge sites preempted by competitive adsorptions, and can even have their charge polarities reversed by such adsorptions. It is essential that both the solution and the filter be characterized in a validation exercise to ensure that the conditions favorable to a proper application of these useful filters do indeed obtain.

Carazzone et al. (1985) showed that charge-modified nylon membranes remove pyrogenic substances from solutions with an efficiency that depends on the composition of the liquid. The endotoxins used were extracted from *E. coli* 05:B5. The removed pyrogens are firmly adsorbed. They are not released during continuation of the filtration process. However, the charged nylon filters exhibit a finite adsorption capacity, the pyrogen removal efficiency decreasing with the successive aliquots being filtered. In the case of deionized water containing pyrogen concentrations comparable to 12 ng/mL of *E. coli* endotoxin, the adsorptive removal can be complete (depending on the filter). With 5% glucose solutions, pyrogen removal is not interfered with. However, 0.9% sodium chloride solution containing the same pyrogen concentrations is not depyrogenated to any extent by these charge-modified nylon membranes. Similarly, the presence of 2% peptone solution at a pH of either 3.8 or 8.3 inhibits the removal of endotoxin from solutions by the charged nylon filters.

Using 1 L aliquots of *Serratia marcescens* suspensions containing 1×10^7 CFU/mL filtered through 47 mm disk filters (15.9 cm^2 effective filtration area) at 6–10 psi (0.4–0.7 bar), Carazzone et al. (1985) found that organism retention is decidedly higher for positively charge-modified nylon filters than it is for conventional mixed esters of cellulose membranes of equal pore size ratings. Moreover, as in the case of endotoxin removal, the presence of electrolyte or peptone drastically reduces the efficiency of organism removal by the charge-modified membranes. The protein is seen as competing with the *Serratia marcescens* for the adsorptive sites and as successfully preempting them.

Carazzone et al. (1985) conclude, "Positively charged filter media are very interesting, but need careful preliminary studies in order to define their suitability and operational procedures."

Nowadays most of the pharmaceutical industry does not rely on charged filter membranes to remove endotoxins but tries to eliminate the causes of endotoxin buildup right at the beginning of the production process. Usually endotoxin levels can be kept low by keeping the bioburden level low at the early stages of the process, for example in the water purification. Sometimes ultrafiltration is used in water systems or low molecular weight solutions to separate endotoxin by sieve retention, if the necessity is seen (Flindt, 1983; Karbachsch et al., 1984; Woog, 1987).

It can be said that using a charged-modified filter at the end of the process to remove endotoxins is an excuse for the improper process conditions at the beginning.

Hydrogen Bonding

As stated earlier, electromagnetic attractive forces can arise from dipole–dipole interactions, which is to say from the unequal sharing of the electron pairs constituting chemical bonds. That these electromagnetic forces can serve to adsorb or fix one molecular entity to another is shown in the special case of the hydrogen bond in water. Given its low molecular weight of 18, water ought to be a gas at room temperature. However, due to strong dipole–dipole interactions, water molecules are joined by electrostatic interactions into a liquid polymer or gel. Each water molecule in the liquid is hydrogen-bonded to four neighboring water molecules, the intermolecular links being bent and stretched to produce irregular and varied networks. Within these arrangements, each water molecule offers two hydrogen atoms for bonding and accepts two in return, each oxygen atom providing a pair of unshared electrons (Tanford, 1980) (Fig. 2).

The hydrogen bond, although weak in its energy of attraction, figures importantly in many fields of chemistry. Its operation has strong influences in the associ-

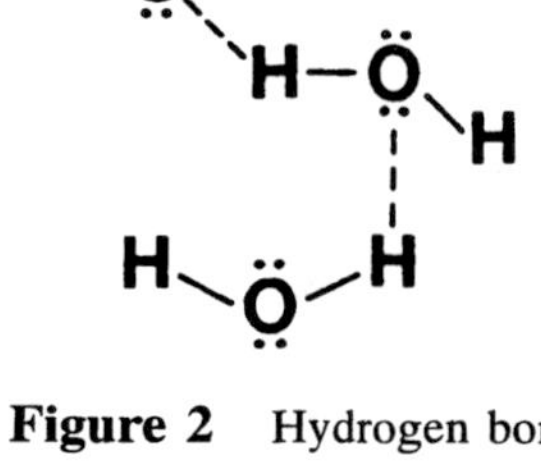

Figure 2 Hydrogen bonding.

ative bonding common to proteins and figures also in the action of wetting agents. It may well be that hydrogen bond formation is the force responsible for the adsorption to particular filter surfaces of, for instance, proteinaceous materials or other molecular species as characterized by active hydrogen atoms, as in amine groups, phenols, carboxylic acids, the hydroxyl groups of alcohols, etc. (Meltzer, 1984).

Secondary Valence Forces

The valence bond responsible for the chemical union of two atoms consists of two electrons shared by these atoms. If the two bonding electrons were shared equally, the two united atoms would be electrically neutral; there would be no residual charges. This equitable arrangement is seldom realized. Usually, one atom or the other in the chemical couple possesses a disproportionate share of the two bonding electrons. This unequal sharing can be the result of any of several causes, usually induced by the influence of neighboring atoms. The electronic dislocation may be permanent or fleeting. In every case, however, one atom has in its vicinity a greater density of the bonding electrons than the other. The two atoms are inextricably joined to one another, albeit the electrons creating the chemical union are unequally shared. The electron being the seat of electronegativity, the atom that possesses more than its share comes to bear a partial negative charge. Its deprived partner carries a partial positive charge (Fig. 3). The partial electric charges associated with the unequal sharing of the chemical bonding electrons are called secondary valence forces, van der Waals forces, etc. They serve to attract and bind entities of opposite charge. Being weak, they operate over only small distances. Although weak, these secondary or residual chemical bonds are important in their influences. Filters bearing such charges are capable of bonding molecules and particles of opposite charge that they encounter during filtration.

Hydrophobic Interactions

The secondary valence forces postulated above as forming the basis for the various adsorptive mechanisms are, like the chemical bonds themselves, electromagnetic. Thus, their attractive forces are responses to the allurements of opposite charges. There are, however, circumstances where noncharge considerations provide particle-arresting possibilities. These constitute a body of hydrophobic adsorptions independent of charge. The operational forces may involve solubility considerations, a molecular similarity in chemical bonding as expressed by a sameness or close matching

$$A:B$$

$$A^{\delta+}:B^{\delta-} \qquad A^{\delta-}\!: B^{\delta+}$$

cation $A^{+} + :B^{-}$ anion

$A\cdot + B\cdot$ free radicals

Figure 3 Bonding electron distribution.

in cohesive energy densities. It is likely that micellar groupings are involved under the influence of area-minimizing forces.

Hydrophobic Adsorption of Pyrogens

Robinson et al. (1982) showed that bacterial lipopolysaccharides (LPS; endotoxins) are adsorptively retained by hydrophobic membrane filters, presumably through the hydrophobic interaction between the uncharged filter surface and the lipid A core of the endotoxin.

Charge considerations are absent where hydrophobic filters such as PTFE (Teflon), polyvinylidene fluoride, and the polyolefins (e.g., polyethylene and polypropylene) are involved. These polymerics contain no ionizable substituent groups and are nonpolar. It is this nonpolarity that confers on them the property of hydrophobicity and renders them wettable by nonpolar liquids. Peters et al. (1973) showed that these hydrophobic interactions involve specific nonpolar binding sites within the proteins.

All known endotoxins have a hydrophobic lipid A core as well as a hydrophilic polysaccharide appendage. It is the lipid A core that is responsible for the pyrogenic activity of the endotoxin and for its hydrophobic character (Galanos et al., 1972). Its nonpolarity reflects the 16–20-carbon chain that comprises it. It is this nonpolar chain that furnishes the site for the hydrophobic interaction between the lipopolysaccharide and the like-bonded segments of the nonpolar polypropylene molecules.

In the case of the interaction between the fatty acids and serum proteins, the opportunity for hydrophobic interactions is increased by muting the polarity of the protein. This is done by adjusting the pH to the isoelectric point of the particular protein, because at that point the electrostatic forces inherent in the amphoteric protein molecules are neutralized. A similar opportunity exists to enhance the hydrophobic interaction of the polypropylene membrane–lipopolysaccharide combination.

The enclosed nonpolar lipid A core can come into contact with the nonpolar polypropylene pore walls and so become hydrophobically adsorbed upon rupture of the charged hydrophilic pellicle (Fig. 4). Underlying the hydrophobic effect is the entropically driven tendency of hydrophobic structures to interact with one another in order to reduce their contact with water. The probability of this occurrence is enhanced by a decrease in the pore size of the filter.

Table 1 illustrates that the adsorptive removal of the endotoxin is indeed inversely proportional to the pore size of the membrane. As the table also shows, disaggregation of the endotoxin micelles and vesicles by the action of ethylenediaminetetraacetic acid still results in the removal of the endotoxin by the nonpolar membrane but not by weakly polar cellulose triacetate membranes. These latter filters retained the aggregated pyrogens, but only because of size, through sieve retention, which would be the more appropriate and safer option than the use of charge-modified filters.

Example: Adsorptive Purification of Flu Vaccine

The literature cites a case in which the purification of a modified swine-type flu vaccine, strain A, by filtration through 0.45 μm rated membranes involved impurity removal by adsorption. Furthermore, the purified antibody was shown to adsorb preferentially to mixed esters of cellulose membranes, filters whose cellulose nitrate content predisposes them to hydrogen bonding with protein (Tanny and Meltzer, 1978).

That adsorptive sequestration of impurities was involved was deduced from flow decay data secured using 47 mm disk filters. The total volume of vaccine that

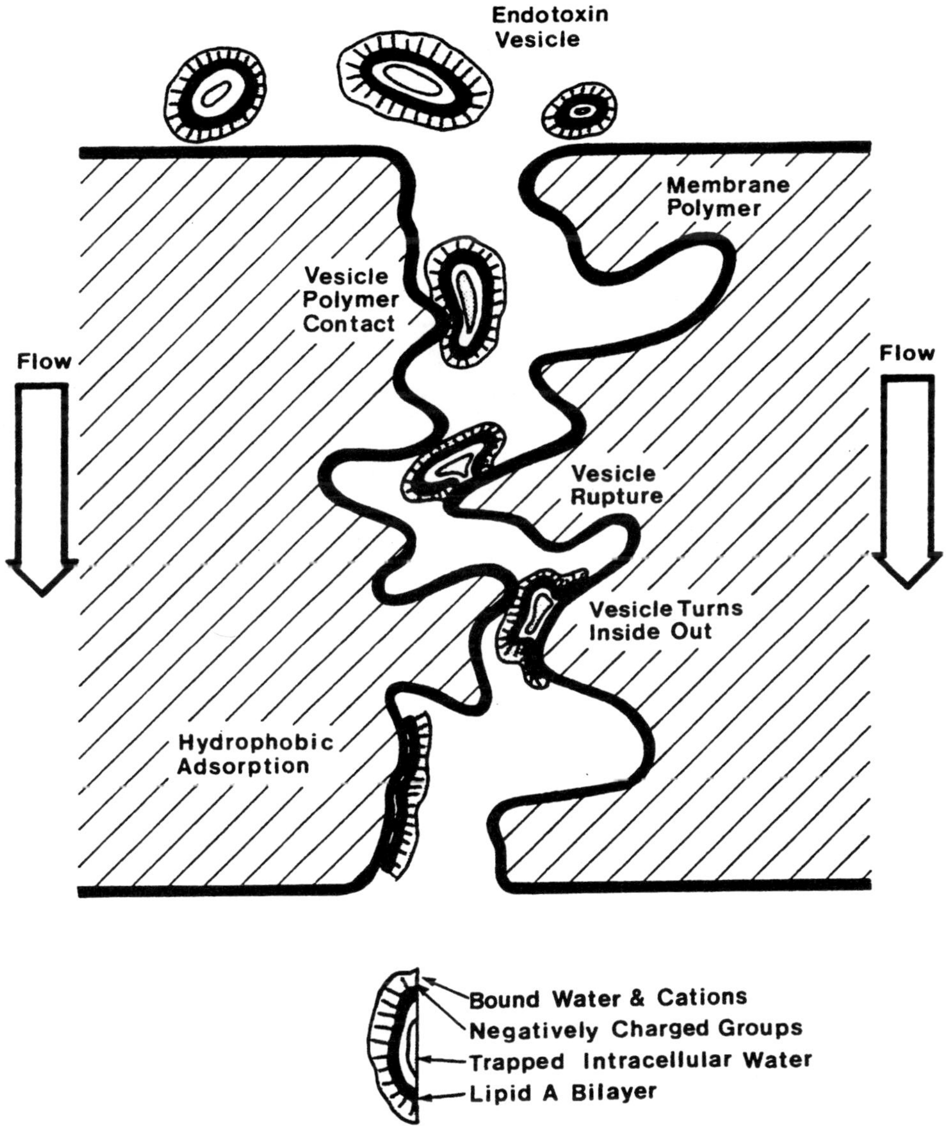

Figure 4 Hydrophobic adsorption mechanism. (From Membrana, Inc., Product Bulletin RD-102.)

was filtered as a function of total elapsed time was noted, readings being taken incrementally until flow all but ceased. Each datum point recorded the total flow volume in milliliters achieved to that total time point in seconds. Titer was determined on the final total volume of filtered vaccine using the chick cell agglutination method. The titer of the vaccine just prior to prefiltration was taken as being 100%.

Table 2 compares the flows achieved with each of four final filters. The vinyl chloride/acrylonitrile copolymer filters gave the greatest flow volumes sustained over the longest time intervals. The cellulose triacetate membranes performed almost as

Table 1 Influence of Pore Size and Endotoxin Aggregation State on Endotoxin Adsorption to Filters

Polymer type	Pore size (μm)	Endotoxin aggregation state[a]	Endotoxin LRV
Polypropylene	Prefilter	DI	0.1
	0.2	DI	1–3
	0.1	DI	3–4
Cellulose acetate	0.2	DI	0.1
	0.025	DI	3.0
Polypropylene	0.2	EDTA	1.0
	0.1	EDTA	1.0
Cellulose acetate	0.2	EDTA	0.1
	0.025	EDTA	0.1

[a] Deionized water (DI) solutions of endotoxin are mixtures of vesicular and micellar structures. 0.005 M EDTA solutions have only micellar structures.
Source: Robinson et al. (1982).

well. The membranes composed of the mixed esters of cellulose showed the poorest performance.

Even more significant than its limiting effect on volume throughput was the negative influence of the mixed esters of cellulose polymer on the titer of the filtered vaccine, a consideration of significant economic import. Table 3 compares the titers obtained using the mixed esters of cellulose membranes of four manufacturers. No appreciable dissimilarities are evident, the performance being inherent in the membrane's polymeric type.

Table 2 Flux Decline Data for Final Filters[a]

Manufacturer I			Manufacturer II		
0.45 μm Mixed cellulose esters			Mixed cellulose esters		
36/90	38/90	33/90	28/90	25/90	30/90
38/120	41/120	34/120	31/120	27/120	34/120
	(Titers 64, 65%)			(Titers 64, 65%)	
0.45 μm Cellulose triacetate			0.45 μm Vinyl chloride acrylonitrile copolymer		
40/90	46/90	40/90	64/90	48/90	52/90
42/120	50/120	41/120	70/120	53/120	57/120
45/180	55/180	43/150	78/180	57/180	63/180
	58/210		80/210		
	(Titers 91, 91%)			(Titers 89, 87%)	

[a] Volume in milliliters per second.
Source: Tanny and Meltzer (1978).

Table 3 Loss of Titer Using Mixed Cellulose Esters Membranes

Manufacturer	Titer (%)
I	64, 65
II	64, 65
III	67
IV	62

Source: Tanny and Meltzer (1978).

Table 4 summarizes the effects of each of the three subject types of membranes on the vaccine titer. Cellulose triacetate filters seem rather comparable to the vinyl chloride/acrylonitrile copolymer membranes. The mixed esters of cellulose are not suitable by comparison.

The flow decline data were subjected to mathematical analyses involving their fit to equations representing various idealized filtration models. An elucidation of the process involved in flu vaccine purification was sought in which the emergence of a straight line would indicate a "fit" to the model, whereas a deviation from linearity would indicate the inappropriateness of the model being tested.

Broadly speaking, idealized patterns of two different circumstances were considered. The first deals with the adsorptive process, a circumstance in which the particles are small enough to enter the filter pores. Particle retention by the sieve mechanism due to steric restraints inherent in the relative size of particles and pores is not involved here. Rather, a combination of van der Waals, hydrogen bonding, and electric field forces retain the colloidal entities or even sequester molecules from true solutions by adsorbing them onto the surfaces of pores larger than themselves in diameter.

Each time such a "particle" is thus captured or adsorbed within a pore, the pore diameter is decreased, and the pore will ultimately completely close up where pore bridging occurs. Intrapore sieve retention may also be involved. This leads to flux decline in accordance with the relation

Table 4 Loss of Titer on Prefiltered Vaccine Having a Titer of 95, 91, 96%

Polymer	Titer (%)	Percent loss in titer
Mixed cellulose esters	64, 65	30
Vinyl chloride/acrylonitrile copolymer	87, 89	7
Cellulose triacetate	90, 91	5

Source: Tanny and Meltzer (1978).

$$\frac{t}{V} \text{ versus } t$$

where t = time in minutes and V = volume in milliliters filtered over time t.

The second situation deals with the retention of discrete particles by sieving, i.e., by the spatial screening out of particles by filters having pores of smaller diameters at the filter surface. This model represents the case where a filter cake or layer of particles builds up on the filter surface to bring about flow decay. If conditions necessary to cake formation do not exist initially—namely, when the discrete particles are larger than the pores—they may nevertheless come about in response to intrapore pore clogging and bridging, as adsorbed material diminishes the pore diameters.

The flux decline relationship for sieving with cake formation is

$$\frac{t}{V} \text{ versus } V$$

where t = time in minutes and V = volume in milliliters filtered over time t.

The flow decay data for the flu vaccine filtration were plotted in accordance with t/V versus t, the adsorptive capture model, and with t/V versus V, the sieve retention model. A straight-line fit resulted from the adsorption model but not from the sieve retention model. This was taken to indicate that adsorptive sequestration, or at any rate intrapore blockage, not filter cake buildup, was the mode of filter operation in this instance (Figs. 5–7).

2.3 Adsorptive Sequestration of Organisms

There are several references in the literature pertaining to the retention of organisms by contact with solid (filter) surfaces. Pertsovskaya and Zvyagintsev (1971) report that different groups of different bacteria are adsorbed by films of such polymers as polyamide, polyacrylate, polyethylene, and cellulose triacetate. That various bacteria adsorb onto various surfaces was also disclosed by Gerson and Zajic (1978). Hjertin et al. (1974) found that cells of Baker's yeast are adsorbed on columns of nonionogenic hydrophobic agarose under conditions of elevated salt concentrations. Column adsorption of *S. typhimurium* takes place from 1 M ammonium sulfate solution, but a reduction of the salt content results in the elution of the organism. Zierdt et al. (1977) and Zierdt (1978) demonstrated that bacterial adsorption can take place on the surfaces of membrane filters whose pores are many times larger than the organisms.

Evidence of Organism Adsorptions

Zierdt et al. (1977) found that a higher percentage of bacterial retention occurs at low organism concentrations, about 500–1000 CFU/mL. At higher levels of 10^8–10^9 CFU/mL, increasing percentages of *E. coli* pass through the membranes, although a larger total number are retained. These phenomena accord with adsorption. Retention was investigated as a function of the filter pore size ratings. As expected, the larger the pore size ratings of the filters, the greater the amount of bacterial passage. At low bacterial numbers, 6.2×10^2 CFU for *E. coli* and 7.3×10^2 CFU for *S. aureus*, apparently no *E. coli* pass a 3.0 μm filter, nor *S. aureus* a 5.0 μm filter. They do begin to pass 5.0 and 8.0 μm filters, respectively. All of the above reflect

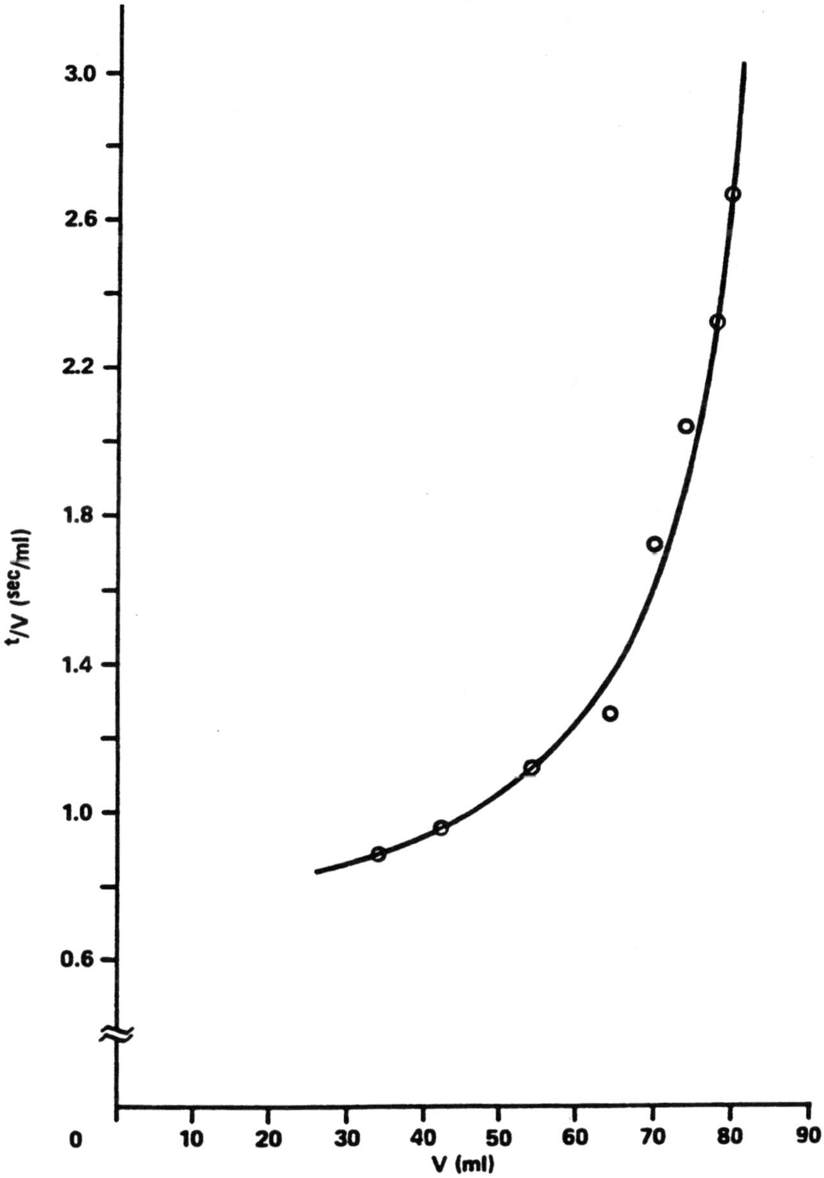

Figure 5 Fitting of flux decline data to filter cake model using vinyl acrylate copolymer membrane. [From Tanny and Meltzer (1978).]

the influence that organism concentration exerts on filter capture efficiency during adsorptive sequestrations.

That Zierdt and his associates are dealing with the adsorptive capture of bacteria is pictorially demonstrated in Fig. 8, where the 0.8 μm size *S. aureus* is shown, in a scanning electron micrograph of 5000× magnification, adsorbed on the surfaces of a polycarbonate membrane (Nucleopore) of 12.0 μm rated pore size. The bacterial

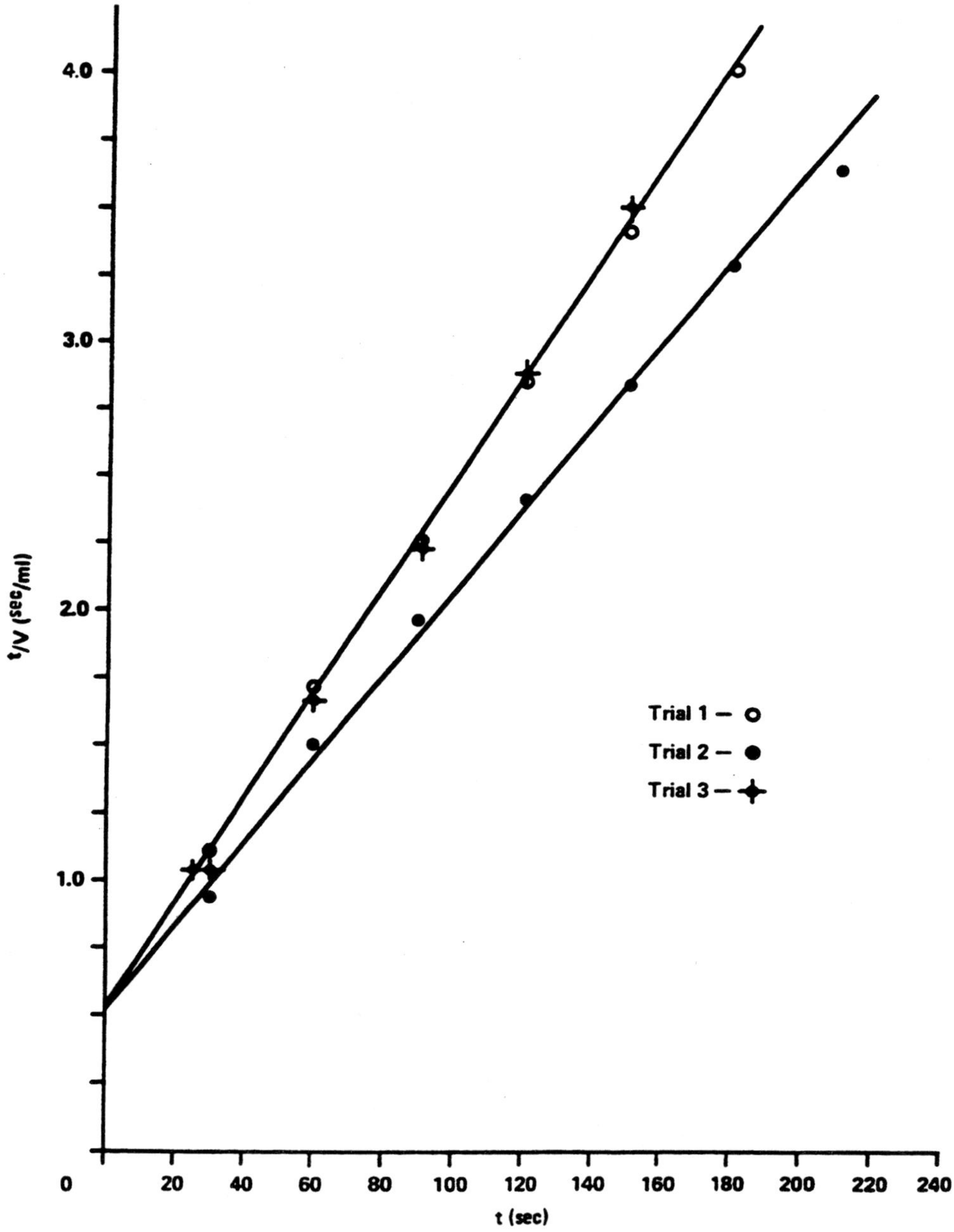

Figure 6 Fitting of flux decline data to intrapore deposition model using cellulose triacetate membrane. [From Tanny and Meltzer (1978).]

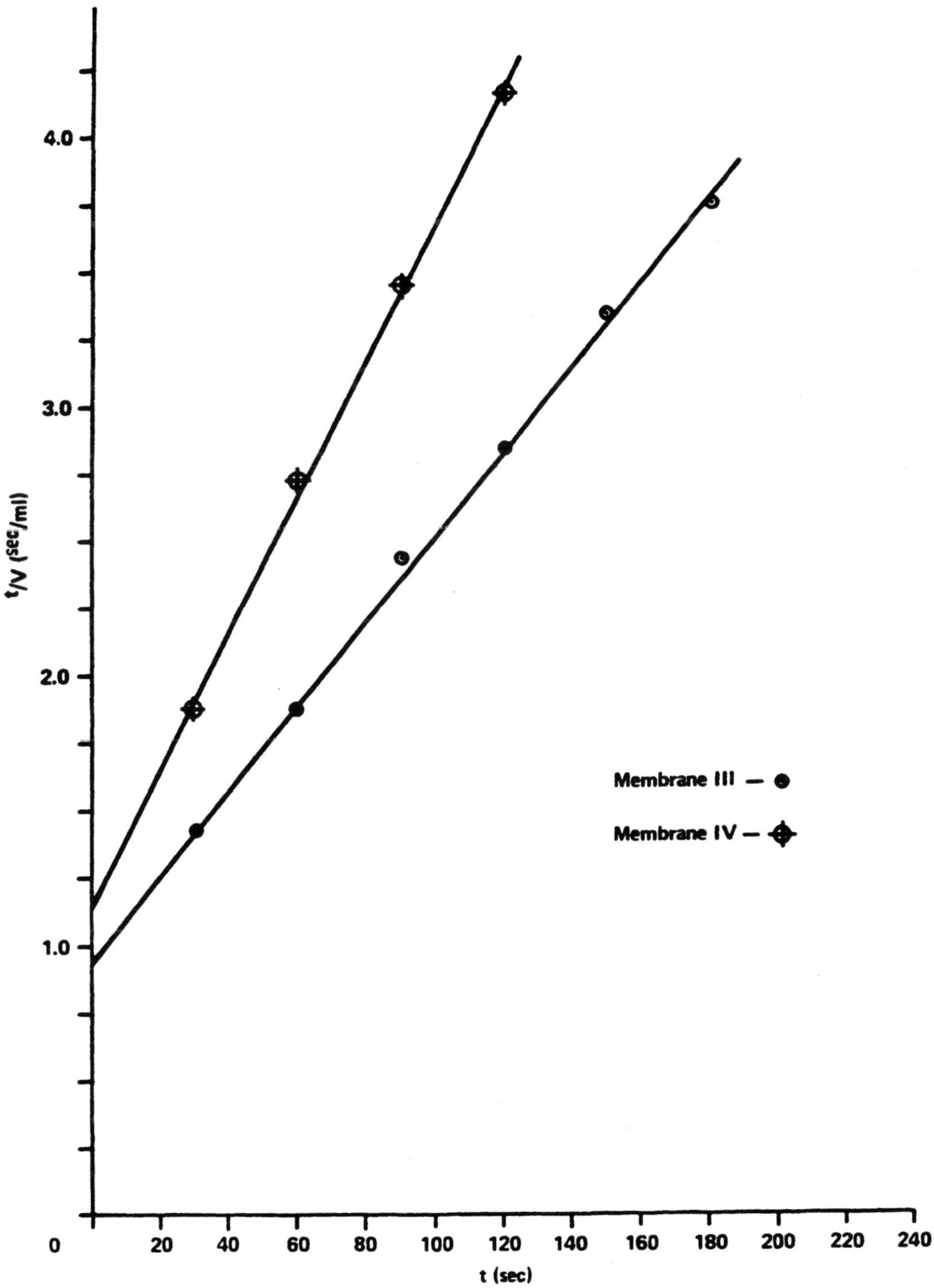

Figure 7 Fitting of flux decline data to intrapore deposition model using mixed esters of cellulose membrane. [From Tanny and Meltzer (1978).]

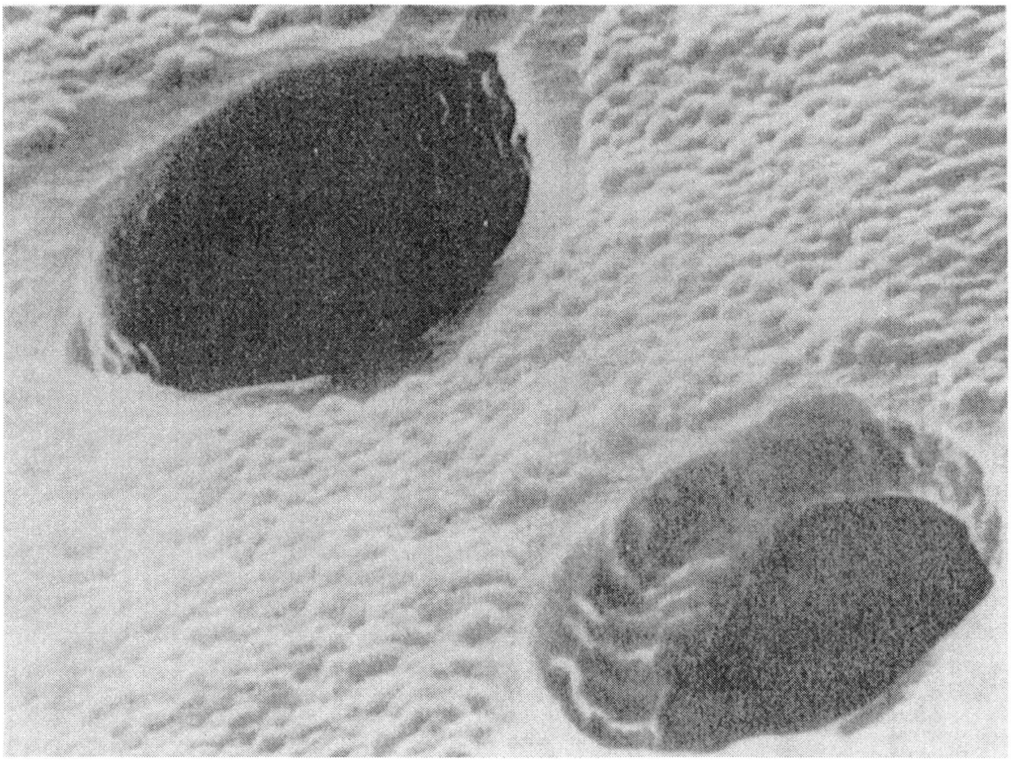

Figure 8 Adsorption of *S. aureus* on track-etch polycarbonate membrane. (Courtesy of Charles Zierdt, NIH Laboratories.)

plaque, apparently one cell thick, can be seen extending from the filter surface into the pores and over their inner vertical surfaces—a striking picture of bacterial adsorption on a membrane surface.

The scanning electron micrographs of Fig. 9 show the retention of *Pseudomonas diminuta* on a glass fiber filter. It is evident that many of the organisms are retained by contact capture rather than by sieve arrest; the filter pores, the spaces among the fibers, obviously are often too large to serve as retaining orifices. The pictorial evidence of adsorptive effects seems indisputable. This effect is often used to reduce bioburden levels by a first step prefiltration with glass fiber depth filters.

Dependence of Retention on the Organism Challenge Level

More than half a century ago, Elford sought to characterize membrane pore sizes by defining the operating circumstances under which a filter did or did not pass various entities. Although profoundly aware of adsorptive forces in filtration processes, Elford explained bacterial retentions on the basis of the sieve capture mechanism. Perhaps because they seemed mere confirmations of the common views, certain of his observations have gone relatively unnoticed. In his work with *B. prodigiosus*, now called *Serratia marcescens*, Elford defined the end point of a filter as being that pore size below which no organisms passed. He observed (Elford, 1933):

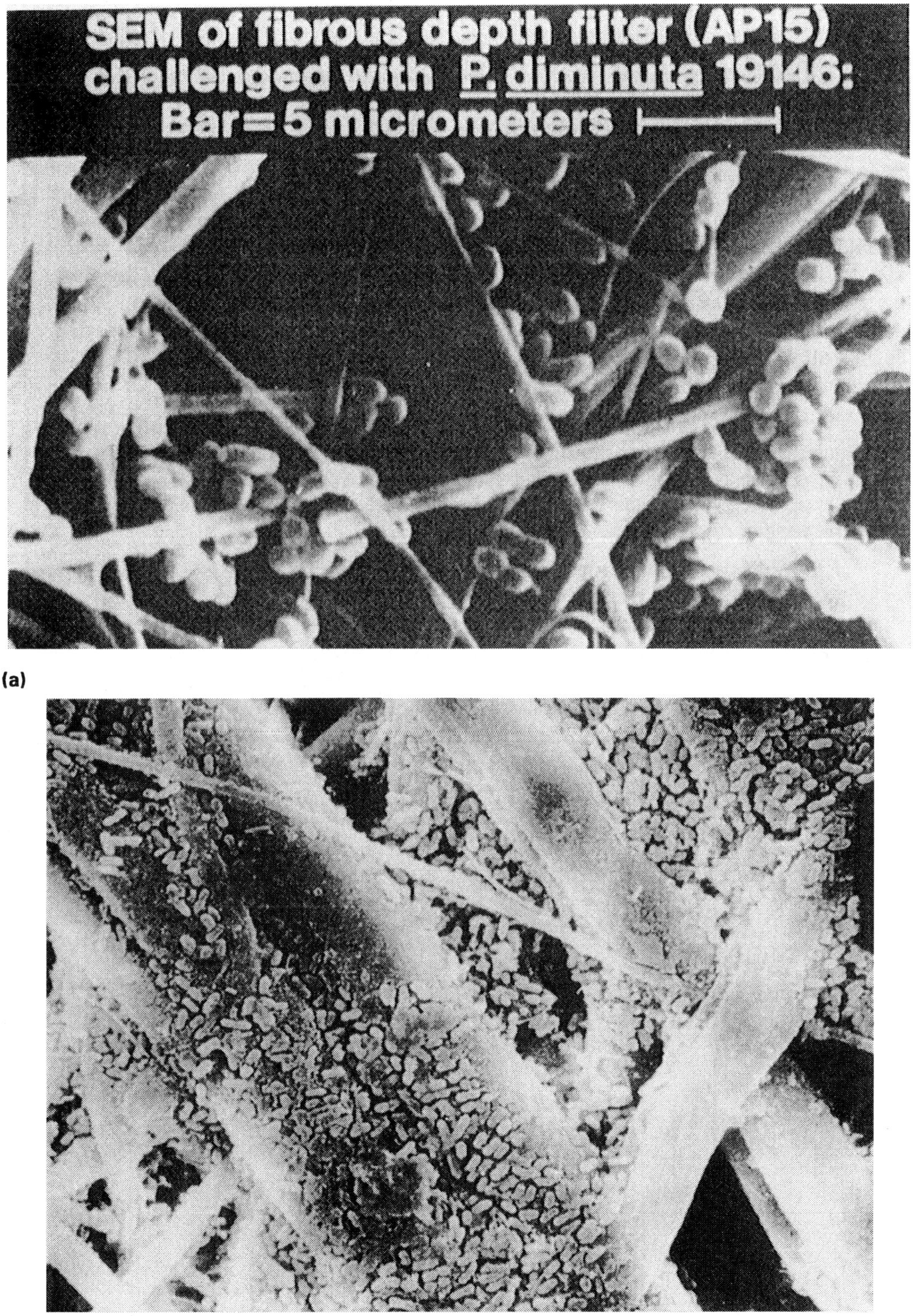

Figure 9 Adsorption of *P. diminuta* on glass fiber filter. (a, courtesy of Timothy J. Leahy, Millipore Corp., b, courtesy of Sartorius AG, Göttingen, Germany.)

> It is clearly indicated that above a certain porosity [larger] an active [i.e., nonsterile] filtrate is obtained even with a very weak suspension, but that between this porosity and the true end-point an active filtrate is only assured when the initial concentration of the dispersed phase exceeds a certain minimum value.

That Wallhäusser's later findings (1976) confirm Elford's observations is made plain by the latter's statement: "The initial concentration of the bacterial suspension is found, further, to be an important factor in determining the end-point." See Fig. 10.

Elford's work in the 1930s may also, at least in principle, have anticipated findings by Meltzer and his associates (Tanny et al., 1979) that the extent of organism passage, for a membrane of a given porosity (0.45 μm), is dependent on the applied differential pressure i.e., flow patterns and contact time. Elford, referring to his work with suspensions of *B. prodigiosus* in horse serum, stated,

> All membranes of calculated average pore-size less than 0.75 μm . . . have been found to retain the organism completely. . . . There is a range of permeability of 0.75–1.0 μm approximately where degree of filterability varies with the conditions obtaining, being determined by such factors as filtration pressure, concentration of organisms and nature of medium.

Elford's observations now find adequate explanation in the hypothesis concerning the adsorptive sequestration of bacteria by membrane filters. Adsorptive retentions are a probabilistic affair whose outcome reflects the particle (organism) challenge level and process conditions. The larger the number of particles, the higher the differential pressure, and the shorter the contact time, the more likely it is that some will escape capture. Additionally, influences of temperature, pH, ionic strength, and viscosity play an important role in the efficiency of capture by adsorption. Only at porosity sizes below that necessary for sieve retention is the efficiency of filtration

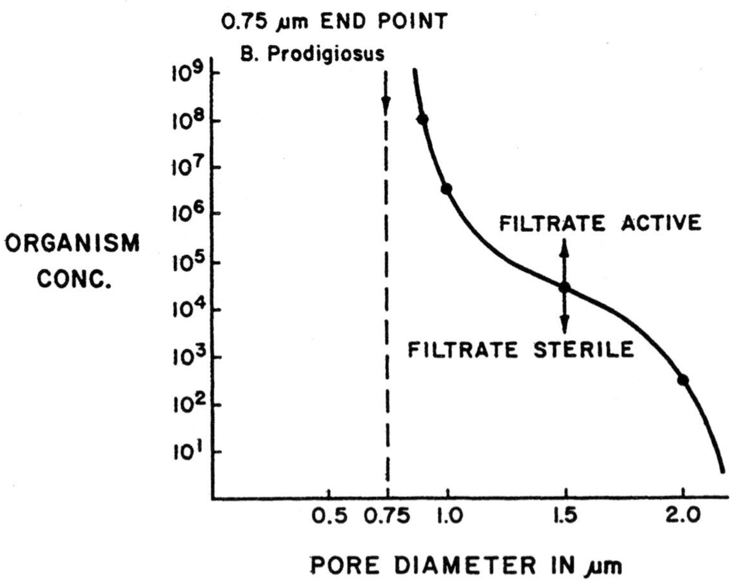

Figure 10 Pore diameter versus *Bacillus prodigiosus* concentration. Sterile or active effluent are a result of these parameters. [From Elford (1933).]

independent of the organism challenge level and the applied differential pressure. It is above that "end point," above that critical pore size, that adsorptive sequestration becomes an operational capture mechanism, reinforcing the effects of sieve retention but subject to the influence of the number of particles present. It is for this reason that filter efficiency is usually greatest where the challenge level is lowest. For this reason, too, final filters ideally fill the role of polishing filters, cleaning already rather clean liquids.

Dependence of Retention on the Applied Differential Pressure

Meltzer and his associates demonstrated that the completeness of *P. diminuta* retention by 0.45 μm rated cellulose triacetate membranes depended on the applied differential pressure level. (See Table 5.) This is because adsorptive captures are involved. Sieve retentions, whether on the surface or within the pore, reflecting only particle–pore size relationships, would be independent of the applied differential pressure. Tanny et al. (1979) showed by a mathematical fitting of flow decay data to equations representing the idealized models of filter cake buildup (surface retention or sieving) and of progressive pore clogging that adsorptive sequestration, or at least intrapore deposition, was the operational mode of organism trapping involved (at least for *P. diminuta* ATCC 19146 by 0.45 μm rated cellulose triacetate membranes).

In accordance with this view, the organisms are small enough to enter the pores of the 0.45 μm rated membranes and not be sieve-retained within the pore pathway. At that point they meet one of two fates (Fig. 11). An organism either traverses the entire pore passageway to emerge with the convective stream, or during its travel it encounters the pore wall and becomes arrested by adsorptive attraction. The probability of organism–pore wall encounter is, in the first instance, an expression of the residence time of the microbe within the filter: The longer the interval, the more probable the pore wall contact. The stream velocity within the pore essentially determines the residence time of the microbe within the pore passageway, and the

Table 5 Capture Efficiencies of 0.45 μm Cellulose Triacetate Membranes at Various Pressures[a]

Operating pressure (psi)	Organisms/100 mL 500 mL	1000 mL	1500 mL	2000 mL	Number of organisms/mL in filtrate	Capture efficiency E
5	0	0	0	0		
5	4	12	7200	7200	0	0.99995_0
5	0	0	0	0		
15	0	13	19	39		
15	3	2	0	7200	10–20	0.9999_0
15	6	15	12	11		
30	93	91	61	66		
30	38	34	39	52	50–100	0.999_5
30	7200	7200	7200	7200		

[a] Challenge concentration 1×10^5 organisms/mL or 2×10^7/cm^2 filter area.
Source: Tanny et al. (1979).

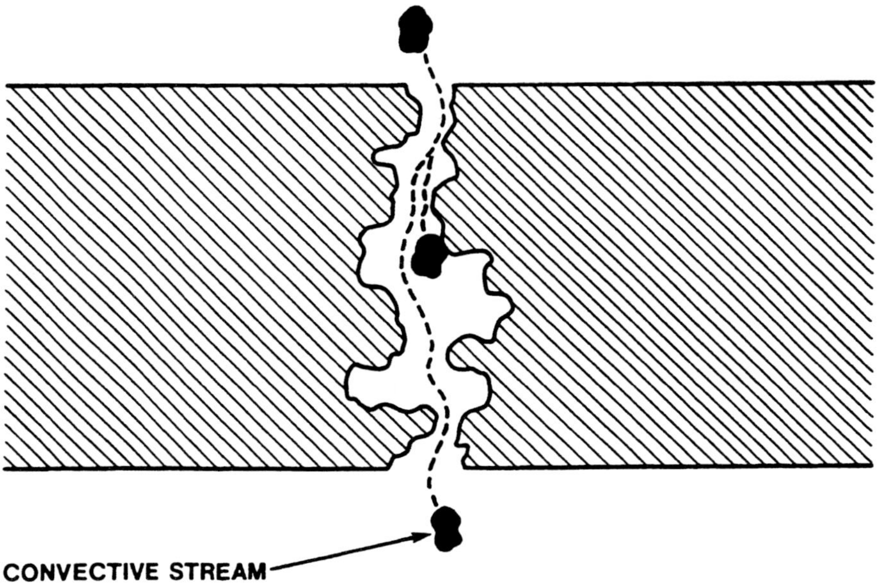

Figure 11 Alternative paths for particles entering pores.

applied differential pressure (in conjunction with the filter area) defines that parameter. Therefore, the lower the applied differential pressure (or the larger the effective filtration area), the greater the particle capture efficiencies of filters where adsorptive arrests are involved.

Pall and Kirnbauer (1978) showed that bacterial retention is directly proportional to filter thickness—up to a point. Their findings are in accord with the influence that greater effective pore lengths could be expected to have on bacterial retention through adsorptive sequestration. The longer the pore, the greater the residence time of the organism within it, and the greater its probability of encounter with the pore wall and consequent probability of capture. The same findings were reported by Osumi et al. (1996). Using SEM photomicrographs, evidence was given that *Pseudomonas* (now reclassified as *Brevundimonas*) *diminuta* is retained not only at the surface, but also within the first 30 μm of the membrane. For this reason filter membranes usually have a specified thickness, typically ≈150 μm.

Adsorptive sequestration also explains the influence of organism challenge levels on organism retention. Thus, it is a matter of probability whether the organism becomes captured by contact within the pore or emerges from the filter unscathed. Therefore, the larger the number of organisms that essay passage of the filter, the more will emerge untrapped.

Leahy and Sullivan (1978) provide a concise relationship among pore size ratings, applied differential pressures, and organism challenge levels for mixed esters of cellulose membranes. As shown in Table 6, mixed esters of cellulose membranes of 0.22 (0.2) μm rating exhibit log reduction values (LRVs) of 10 against *P. diminuta* ATCC 19146 challenges whether at applied differential pressures of 0.5 psi or 50 psi (0.33 or 3.3 bar). The same type of filter in its 0.45 μm rated manifestation shows an LRV of 8 at 0.5 psid, an LRV of 7 at 5 psid, and an LRV of 6 at 50 psid. The

Table 6 Effect of Pressure on the Passage of *P. diminuta* Through Membranes of Various Pore Sizes

Filter type	Pore size (μm)	β ratio 0.5 psid	β ratio 5 psid	β ratio 50 psid
GS	0.22	$>10^{10}$	$>10^{11}$	$>10^{10}$
HA	0.45	10^{8}	10^{7}	10^{6}
DA	0.65	10^{4}	10^{4}	10^{3}
AA	0.80	10^{2}	10^{1}	10^{0}

Source: Leahy and Sullivan (1978).

more open filter clearly shows the influence of the applied differential pressure level on the adsorptive sequestration of the organisms. The capture mode for the 0.22 (0.2) μm rated membrane in sieve retention, attested to by its freedom from the pressure differential influence. The 0.65 μm rated membrane and its 0.8 μm rated counterpart progressively show the increasing influence of the pressure differential as coupled with larger diameter pores, as would be expected of adsorptive arrests.

Alcholtz and Leahy (1985) again demonstrated the complete retention of *P. diminuta* ATCC 19146 by 0.22 (0.2) μm rated membranes, even at 55 psid (3.7 bar), which is a requirement of every HIMA retentive sterilizing grade filter. The HIMA (1982) document states that a sterilizing 0.2 μm filter has to retain 10^7 *P.* (now *Brevundimonas*) *diminuta* per square centimeter at a differential pressure of a minimum of 29 psid (2 bar) for a 47 mm disk filter. Furthermore, validation work on sterilizing grade filters in the industry has to be done by challenging the filter with the actual product under worst-case process conditions. This is done to ensure that the retentive mechanisms, whether sieve retention or adsorptive sequestration, are sufficient to produce a sterile effluent. If this is not the case, due to the product and process parameters, or for example, the adsorptive properties of the membrane filter being no longer effective, a filter with a pore size sufficiently smaller must be used to ensure sieve retention and therefore a sterile filtrate.

3 THE MODELING OF FILTER BLOCKING

It may be instructive to repeat the basis for the mathematical treatment leading to a distinction between the two organism capture mechanisms. The assumption is made that bacterial retention is the controlling event, the one leading to the eventual clogging of the filter. Flow decay or flux decline studies are performed in constant pressure filtrations. These studies are carried out by periodically plotting the volume or throughput as a function of time.

Flux decline during filtration will be a consequence of any retention mechanism but will follow different time–volume relationships depending on the mechanism governing the filter's clogging. The mode and rate of flow decay will differ depending on whether the flow decay is caused by sieve retention on the filter surfaces with resulting filter cake formation or by adsorptive arrest or other type of retention within the filter pores with consequent pore narrowing and blocking. It is possible to differentiate between these two sites of particle detention.

3.1 Sieve Retention

The most commonly used model (Ruth et al., 1933) for bacterial filtration by sieve retention is that of a porous matrix whose "holes" or pores are smaller than the organism (Fig. 12). In such a situation, the bacteria are retained on the surface of the membrane and create a filter cake that grows in thickness as the filtration progresses. Since this cake will add a hydrodynamic resistance to the flow at constant pressure, the instantaneous rate of filtration at time t, $J_v(t)$, and the total volume of filtrate up to time t, $V(t)$, will change in a disproportionate manner as a function of time. Assuming an incompressible cake (an assumption that is rather suited to more rigid particulates than bacteria), and with a constant pressure differential across the filter, the relation

$$\frac{t}{V(t)} = \frac{k}{2}\,[V(t) + 2V_f]$$

will be obeyed, where V_f is the volume of filtrate required to produce a change in total resistance equal to that of the filter. K is a "filtration constant" that depends on pressure ΔP, viscosity η, filter area A, cake resistance R_c, and particle concentration C in the following way:

$$K = \frac{2A^2\Delta P}{\eta C R_c}$$

From these simple relations, it follows that a plot of $t/V(t)$ versus $V(t)$ should yield a straight line with a slope of K and an intercept of KV_f. Such a plot constitutes

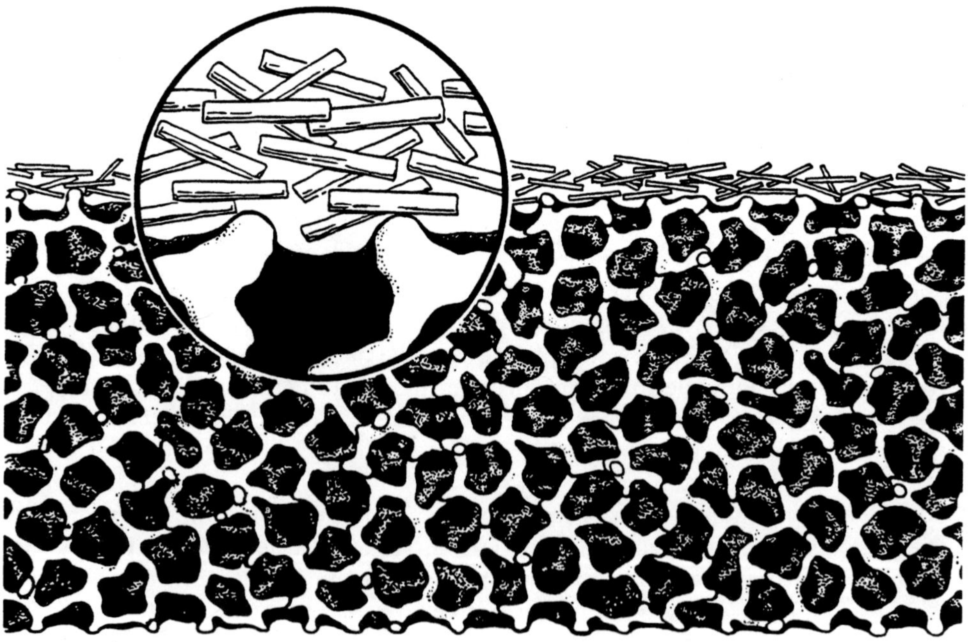

Figure 12 Filter cake formation.

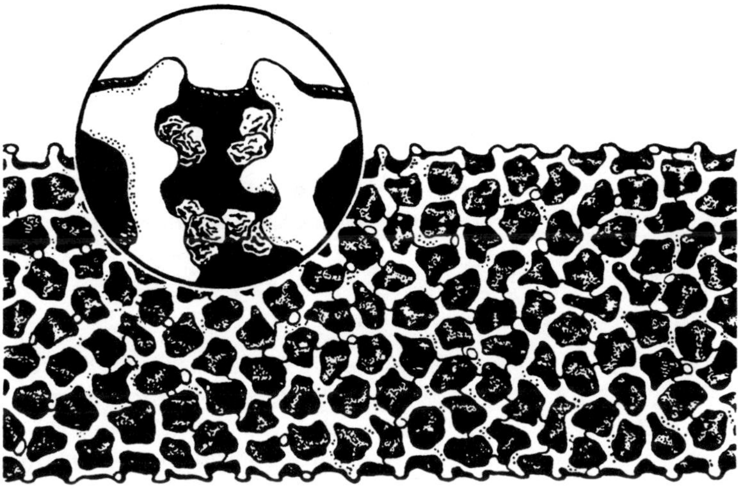

Figure 13 Clogging and bridging.

a first verification of the sieve retention or, more properly, the surface retention model.

3.2 Adsorptive Sequestration[1]

As depicted in Fig. 13, adsorptive capture, whether of a particle or of a soluble or near-soluble entity from solution, involves the entry of that particle, viable or otherwise, into the pore channel. (Intrapore sieve retention is also possible.) In these situations the body being adsorptively retained is smaller than the filter's pore. (Even though the pore entrance is larger than the organism, sieve statistics dictate that a substantial fraction of the bacteria will be excluded, approximately 99.9% for pores 10% larger in diameter than the particle.) The convective flow existing within the pores will tend to carry the particles that do enter through the membrane. However, the London–van der Waals interactions, the electrical double layer, and the hydrophobic attraction forces between the bacteria and the pore walls act against the convective flow and promote interception of the particles. In terms of the model, all these forces are combined and treated as a first-order reaction between the particle and the wall.

Each particle "reacting" within the pore cavity, i.e., being adsorbed, reduces the total pore volume. The equation expressing the adsorptive model of flux decrease is

$$\frac{t}{V(t)} = \frac{kt}{2} + \frac{1}{J_v(0)}$$

[1]This section is based on Hermans and Bredee (1936).

or

$$\frac{1}{J_\nu(t)} - \frac{1}{J_\nu(0)} = kt$$

where k is a filtration constant related to the internal pore area and the particle concentration. A plot of $t/V(t)$ versus t should yield a straight line with a slope of $k/2$, and such behavior constitutes a test of the model wherein the particles are retained within the pores.

3.3 Conclusions Concerning Blocking Mechanisms

The data reported by Wallhäusser (1979), when plotted in accordance with the equations representing the two retention models, were seen to accord with that of adsorptive capture. This is indicated by the linearity of that line (Figs. 14 and 15).

Additionally, flow decay experiments were made using *B. diminuta* suspension concentrations similar to those employed by Wallhäusser. These yielded data showing

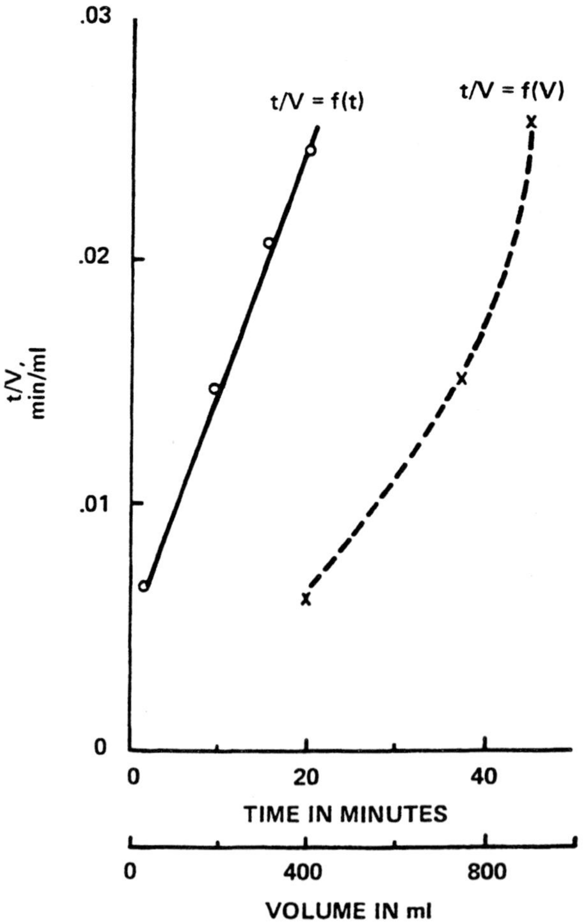

Figure 14 Plot of Wallhäusser data showing adsorptive effects. [From Tanny et al. (1979).]

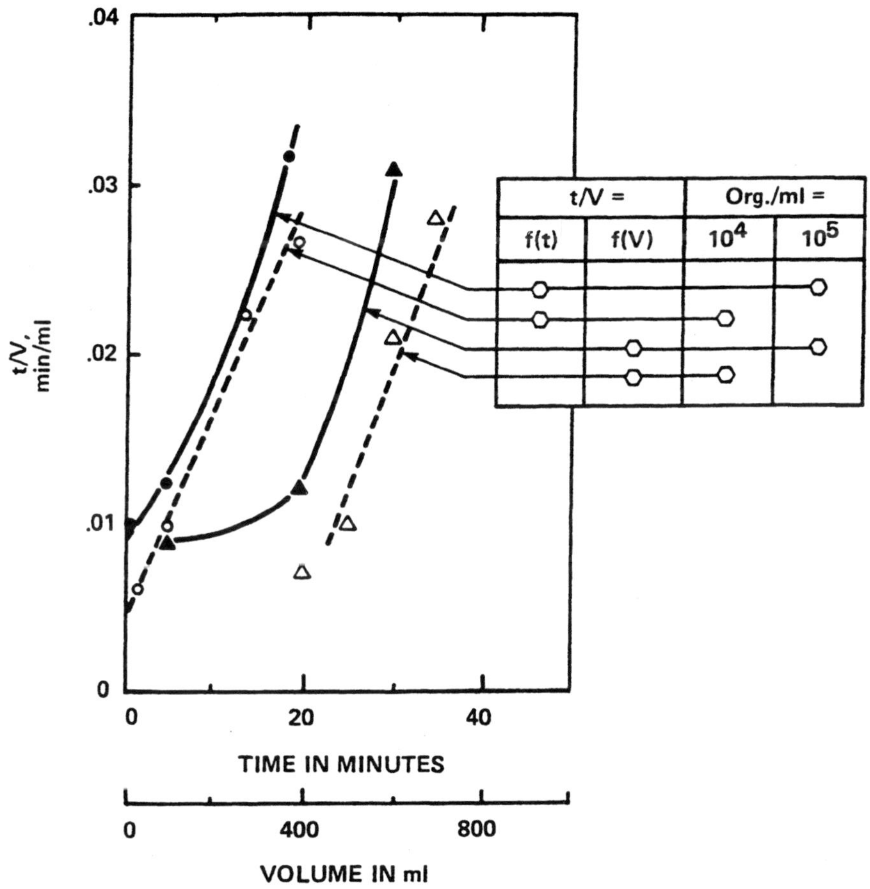

Figure 15 Plot of Wallhäusser data showing adsorptive effects. [From Tanny et al. (1979).]

that organism retention by 0.45 μm rated cellulose triacetate membranes also depended on the adsorptive sequestration mechanism.

The flux decline exhibited in Fig. 15 for the 0.45 μm cellulose triacetate membrane shows an almost straight line decrease, a consequence of its rather open porosity. By contrast, the flow decay of the corresponding 0.2 μm rated filter shows a more precipitous decrease, as the more finely sized pores become clogged more immediately.

The plotting of the data of Fig. 16 in accordance with the adsorption mechanism equation $(t/V)/t$ yields a straight line for the bacterial feed concentration of 10^4 mL^{-1} retained by the 0.45 μm rated filter. This straight line indicates that the site of the bacterial arrest is within the pore path. It is assumed, therefore, to be the result of adsorptive sequestration, although sieve retention can occur within the pore path as well in accordance with Williams' sinuous path scenario.

The line in Fig. 17 derived from the 0.45 μm rated membrane using a bacterial feed challenge of 10^5 mL^{-1} shows an initial straight line followed by the onset of a curve. This shape shows adsorptive retention, actually intrapore retention, leading to

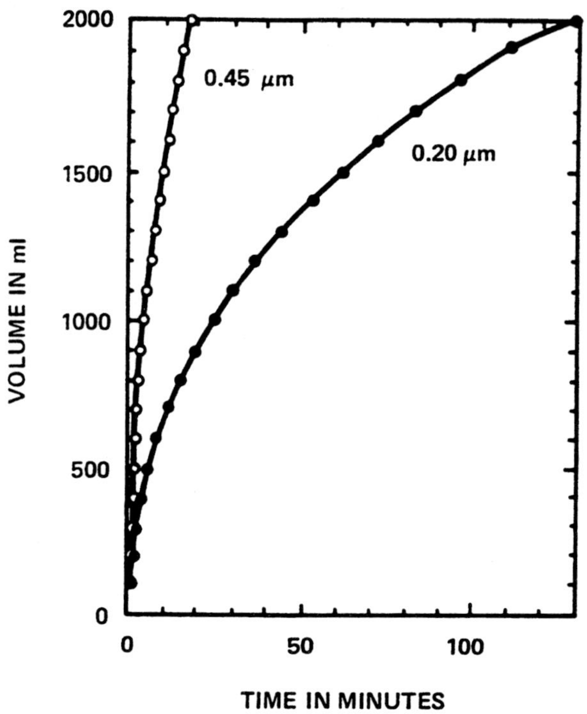

Figure 16 Flow decline data compiled for 0.2 μm rated and 0.45 μm rated membranes. [From Tanny et al. (1979).]

pore clogging (more rapidly realized as a result of the higher bacterial concentration), followed by sieve retention of the bacteria subsequently filtered out by the now clogged, and hence smaller diameter, pores.

By contrast, neither the thickness of the membrane, the concentration of particles, the fluid velocity, nor the applied pressure will affect the selectivity of a surface (filter cake) sieve-retaining filter toward bacteria. Only the pore size is important, and if all pores are equal in size to, or smaller than, the organism, the filter will be absolutely retentive. However, all commercial membrane filters have pore sizes distributed about some mean. Thus, it is conceivable that there exists at least one set of pores sufficiently large to allow the passage of a single organism. Hence the rationalization that if the number of organisms filtered per square centimeter of membrane approaches or exceeds the number of pores per square centimeter, the membrane is unlikely to prove absolutely retentive. Fortunately, taking the number of pores on a surface of a membrane filter into account or even the number of filter planes over the whole thickness, the bioburden needs to exceed 200 times the HIMA challenge level of 10^7 CFU/cm^2 (Mouwen and Meltzer, 1993). Osumi et al. (1996) showed that for a particular filter a challenge level of 5×10^8 *B. diminuta* per square centimeter is not sufficient to cover the membrane surface with a monolayer of microorganisms, i.e., every pore with an organism. To do so, a 5.000 L batch of product would have to be contaminated with 100 organisms/mL solution. Such a

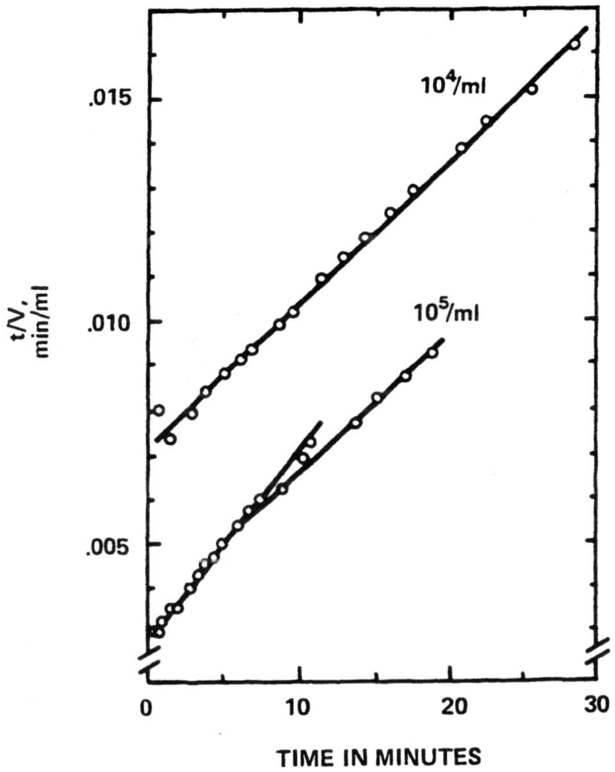

Figure 17 Retention of 10^4 and 10^5 organism/mL challenges by 0.45 μm rated membranes showing adsorptive sequestration. [From Tanny et al. (1979).]

bioburden would be unacceptable in any pharmaceutical process, with respect to endotoxin levels and product safety.

For sieve capture, the critical parameter for testing the absolute retentivity of the membrane is

$$\text{Total challenge} = \frac{\text{no. of organisms filtered}}{\text{area of filter}} = \frac{CV_{\text{total}}}{A}$$

where C represents the bacterial density per milliliter of solution, V is the volume of solution, CV is the total bacterial challenge, and A is the extent of filter area.

There are three reasons why the applied differential pressure influences a filter's efficiency and/or longevity or service life. Higher pressure levels detract from the filter performance when adsorptive arrests are involved. As stated, the higher differential pressures abbreviate the residence times of particles in the pore passageways, rendering less likely their encounter with pore walls and consequent adsorptive sequestration. Second, the polarized layer of particles built up during the filtration upstream of the filter becomes compacted under higher differential pressures. It thus offers greater resistance to fluid permeation. Third, the particulate matter deposited from the polarized layer as a filter cake may become impacted and even deformed under pressure to block the filter pore, thus shortening the filter's service life.

4 RELIABILITY OF ADSORPTIVE SEQUESTRATION

4.1 Definition of Absoluteness

Filters can be absolute in their retention of particles only when the smallest particle is larger than the largest pore of the filter. Under this circumstance, the filter efficiency of 100% is independent of the conditions under which the filtration is performed; the particles are all retained by sieve-type captures. However, only when *all* the particles of interest are so removed is there an identity between "absoluteness" and sieve retention. Otherwise, regardless of how small the fraction of particles captured through other mechanisms, the filtration conditions govern the filtration efficiency.

Where the pore size–particle size distribution relationships permit passage of a particle through a filter, particle arrest depends on the occurrence of adsorptive contacts between particle and pore wall. This situation is very much under the influence of the product and process conditions, and therein lies its lack of "absoluteness."

The term "absolute" in this context refers to the independence of particle capture from the operational conditions of the filtrative exercise. Particle capture may well be complete, whatever trapping mechanisms are involved. Thus, Tanny et al. (1979) showed that even 0.45 μm rated membranes could retain 2×10^7 *P. diminuta* ATCC 19146 per square centimeter of filter under stipulated conditions. The occurrence of complete particle removal does not necessarily depend exclusively on sieve retention. The purpose of the filter validation procedure is to ascertain the completeness of the removal of the particles of concern, such as organisms in a filtrative sterilization.

Absolute Filters and Filtration

It is common to hear of filters being defined as either absolute or nominal (Nicholaus, 1975; Bentley and Lloyd, 1992). Actually, this characterization does not describe an inherent quality of filters. Whether a given filter is absolute depends on the particle size distribution that confronts its pore size distribution. For instance, let us consider the wire mesh fence surrounding a tennis court. One of its functions is to keep tennis balls within the court. For this purpose it is an absolute filter. The ordinary wire mesh fence used for this purpose will reliably retain all standard size tennis balls. This type of fence is also an absolute filter for soccer balls, and indeed for any particle larger than its pores or holes. But the same fence may or may not retain golf balls or marbles that may be driven at it. The retention in these cases is therefore not absolute. The same fence, the filter in this case, is both absolute and not, depending on the size of the particle it encounters. Thus, a filter that is not absolute in one context may be absolute in another.

The term "absolute," as used relative to filters, implies a perfection in particle removal (of stipulated sizes) independent of the operational parameters of the filtration. Such a circumstance, as stated, exists only in the removal of given size particles solely by sieve retention in a situation wherein the smallest particle is larger than the largest pore. Today filter manufacturers classify their filters as sterilizing grade filters when they meet or exceed the requirements of HIMA (1982). Submicrometer particle filters are typically classified as mycoplasma-retentive filters; very few are called virus-retentive. Few filter vendors use the term "absolute" any longer; most specify the filters according to their retention capabilities. Prefilters are usually classified by retentive capabilities in percent for a certain particle size. The pore size label for membrane filters is often enough for administrative purposes. In the pharmaceutical industry, 0.2 or 0.22 μm rated membrane filters are usually sterilizing grade filters, which withstand the challenge level described in the HIMA guidelines.

4.2 Specific Aspects of Adsorptive Sequestration

As stated earlier, filter efficiencies involving adsorptive sequestration are influenced by such operational considerations as the particle challenge level and the applied differential pressure. Other factors must also be considered.

Desorption

Adsorption implies the possibility of desorption. Such may well be the case for depth filters, where the particulate unloadings occasioned by higher differential pressures may be ascribed to desorptions caused by higher liquid stream velocities. (These unloadings can also be attributed to fiber dislocations and channeling caused by the same forces.)

In any case, the published literature discloses no such incidents in the case of membrane filters. Here the higher differential pressures are not seen to cause the particle unloadings that would signal desorption. Nevertheless, there have been reports of desorption due to changes in pH and temperature as well as saturation of the adsorptive sites. It seems fair to say, however, that desorption from membrane filters, were it to occur, ought not in any case to be a surprise or uncontrolled happening. The possibility, like the event itself, would have become revealed in the filter validation exercise.

Finite Number of Adsorption Sites

In the classic adsorptions, such as the adsorption of gas or liquid molecules to the "active" sites of catalysts, there are specific loci where adsorption can occur. Moreover, there is a finite number of such sites. Once these are filled, no more adsorption can occur. Indeed, this is the case for the charge-modified filters, as discussed in Sec. 2.2, where a stoichiometric relationship exists between the positive zeta charge density and the quantity of material that can be removed by adsorption. The same phenomenon also holds true, at least frequently, in cases where protein is adsorbed onto surfaces. Thus, the prior coating with serum albumin of microporous membranes that are used in electrophoretic work serves to preempt the adsorptive sites to the exclusion of other protein adsorptions. In a reported instance, rinsing a polypropylene prefilter and cellulosic final filter with human serum albumin increased the recovery of Factor VIII blood clotting protein. The same was found when filter systems were rinsed with sodium chloride solution or buffers before the filter system was used for serum filtration. However, as Tanny and Meltzer (1978) found, there was no such exclusionary bar to the continued adsorption of protein when microporous membranes were used to purify crude flu vaccines. Here the adsorptive removal of protein continued, unrestricted by considerations of specific numbers of adsorption sites.

Whatever the circumstances in the case of charge-modified filters, where the adsorptive sequestration of *P. diminuta* by conventional microporous membrane filters is concerned, no limitations to organism removal are known to derive from considerations of a finite number of adsorption sites.

Leahy and Sullivan (1978) confronted the 0.45 μm rated membrane with 10^{10} *P. diminuta* organisms. At 0.5 psi (0.03 bar), only about 100 at most failed to be retained. At 50 psi (2.3 bar), some 10,000 escaped arrest. The difference in the numbers retained at 0.5 and 50 psi may be considered to be the number captured due to adsorption. Therefore, even for the 0.45 μm rated filter, retention of *P. diminuta* is essentially due to sieving. Adsorptive sequestration serves as a reinforcing mechanism, making more certain the removal of organisms by the filter.

Influences of the Liquid Vehicle

It is to be expected that the composition and conditions that define the liquid vehicle in which the particles are suspended might influence their adsorption. Its ionic strength and/or pH could modify the charge attractions. The presence of surfactant could coat the filter surfaces so as to alter their charge characteristics or imbue them with different cohesive energy density values. Surfactant could also coat the individual particles so as to change their surface chemistry, either to ensure the presence of discrete, unagglomerated organisms or to increase their size enough to prevent the mutual attraction between them and the filter surface by spatial buffering.

The interrelated influences of vehicle viscosity and temperature on adsorptive particle capture have been discussed. The hydrodynamic drag of a high viscosity liquid on a particle within a pore might keep it from diffusing to the pore wall where it might become contact-captured. Similarly, perhaps, such a drag might serve to desorb already sequestered particles. On the other hand, the slower rates of flow of viscous vehicles would permit longer residence times for particles within pore paths, increasing the likelihood of their adsorptive removal. Temperature is inversely related to viscosity. It might be expected, therefore, to have exactly opposite effects, except that at higher temperatures particle diffusion may become enhanced, such as by increased Brownian motion. This could lead to enhanced opportunities for particle–pore wall encounters and to greater possibilities for particle sequestration.

Meltzer et al. (1997) describe a comprehensive list of product and process parameters that can affect the separation mode of a filter system. Once more the reliability of sieve retention is underscored when the smallest particle or organism is larger than the biggest pore. Furthermore, influences on adsorptive sequestration by product-specific properties have been suggested. For this reason, product-specific bacterial challenge tests have to be performed.

Certainly another reason to view product- and process-specific parameters is their influence not only on a filter's separation capabilities but also on microorganism viability and size. Given this premise, one can comprehend why FDA inspectors require that the validation of the filter be performed for each drug vehicle being filtratively sterilized.

The Role of Validation

It is evident that many factors may influence the efficiency of particle removal by adsorptive sequestration. By contrast, where it occurs, the total removal of particles by sieve retention is uncomplicated in its straightforwardness. But the uncertainties that may beset adsorptive sequestration before its management is defined in no way reflect on its dependability once they are managed. The purpose of the filter validation is just that—to define whether and under what conditions the filter will yield dependable filtrative particulate removals regardless of the mechanisms involved.

Just as it is untrue that dependence on adsorptive particle arrest is unreliable, so too is it untrue that sieve retention can be relied on without question. Dependence on sieve retention also has its problems. How does one know whether all the particles of interest are indeed larger than the largest pores of the filter? As reported by Thomas et al. (1992) and Meltzer (1996), certain L forms of *Pseudomonas* are able to penetrate 0.2 μm membrane filters. Indeed, it begs the question to assume that *P. diminuta* is an apt model for any given pharmaceutical filtration. For this reason, product and production plant flora should be known to the drug manufacturer. Additionally, at a PDA meeting in June 1995, the FDA reported instances of *Pseudomonas* organisms penetrating 0.2 μm membrane filters due to their size being altered by the liquid product's properties.

Sieve retention is indeed simple in its mode of operation. Proving that it alone is the applicable particle removal mechanism would, however, be quite complicated. In the absence of such proof, it is inappropriate to assume its exclusive existence. For this reason, bacterial challenge tests should be performed with the product under worst-case process conditions.

Filter validation disposes of the complexities presented by considerations of the particle removal mechanisms. If the filter is validated to perform its designed function satisfactorily under stipulated, experimentally defined conditions, then the mechanisms of particle removal are of no consequence, and the filtration operation can be pursued unthreatened by theoretical vagaries. The adequacy of the validation, then, becomes the key to successful filter usage. Filter validations should also probe the constancy of the filter quality.

5 SUMMARY OF TRAPPING FORCES AND THEIR LOCI

The older literature refers to surface retention as if it were the consequence of particle arrest only by the sieve capture mechanism wherein the particle is larger than the pore. The evidence presented by Zierdt et al. (1977) (see Fig. 7) shows that adsorptive capture of, e.g., organisms can also result in surface retentions.

Even less correct are the implications that sieve retention, when it occurs, equates only with surface retention. The pore passageways are not uniform throughout their (tortuous) extents (Williams and Meltzer, 1983; Osumi et al., 1996). If anything, their restrictive bottlenecks probably occur more frequently within the depths of the filter than at its surface, if only as a matter of probability. This is particularly so if a filter is considered as a layered construction of individual filter planes each with its own pore size distribution (Piekaar and Clarenburg, 1967).

Surface retention, then, can result from the exercise of any particle capture mechanism and may involve particles larger or smaller than the pore sizes of the filter. But to enter a pore passageway the particle must be smaller than the pore entry. A particle that has entered a pore may encounter a restrictive pore area within the filter and may then be geometrically restrained by sieve retention. Sieve retention can be seen as being a "passive" restraint. Otherwise the particle may become arrested within the pore passageway by some mechanism involving an "active" attraction between particle and filter. All these, known and unknown in their nature, are described as adsorptive forces.

It follows, therefore, that the site of a particle's arrest reveals nothing necessarily definitive about its size relative to the size of the pores it encounters or about the mechanism involved in its capture. One can say, however, that if a noncompressible filter cake is built up according to the Ruth equation (Sec. 3.1), surface retention is involved; whereas if pore clogging results, in accordance with the Hermans–Bredee equation (Sec. 3.2), retention of the particles is taking place within the filter. In this connection it may be interesting to note that a given amount of particulate matter would more profoundly affect the filter flow decay if it were deposited *within* the filter pore passageways (pore clogging) rather than on the surface (filter cake buildup). The picture could change, however, if the surface deposit were capable of blocking the pores, for instance, by being deformed under the applied differential pressure.

The largest part of a membrane's surface constitutes its internal pore walls rather than its external areas, particularly because of the filter's high degree of porosity. To the extent, therefore, that surface retention due to adsorption can be ignored for membrane filters, surface retention does equate with sieve retention, and adsorptive captures can result only from the capture of particles small enough to enter pores. Intrapore sieve retention can also occur. Such possibilities reflect the matter of particle size and pore size distributions.

To recapitulate, "sieve retention" refers to a mechanical or spatial restraint resulting from a particle being larger than the restrictive pore area. "Adsorptive sequestration" refers to situations involving attractive forces between particle and filter surface. As stated, this can involve any number of particle-arresting mechanisms such as electrostatics, hydrogen bonding, electrokinetic effects, other charge-related phenomena, and noncharged hydrophobic attractions. These may differ in the intensity of their capture and in their resistance to desorbing forces such as the mechanics of fluid stream velocities. There is evidence that filters that bear induced charges arrest particles more tenaciously than do other adsorptive forces. No doubt, however, a gradation exists even within the phenomenon of electrokinetic charge attractions.

6 THE STERILIZING FILTER

6.1 Developmental Background

The microporous membrane originally designed for filtrative sterilization was the 0.45 μm rated filter. In some cases, protein solutions contaminated with organisms now identified as *Brevundimonas diminuta* were not sterilized by passage through such filters. To remedy this situation, the 0.22 (0.2) μm rated membrane was devised. Almost from its inception the 0.2 μm rated filter achieved undeniable success in the filtrative sterilization processing of pharmaceutical preparations. These filters acquired the reputation of being sterilizing grade filters; i.e., their retention was seen as being independent of the operating conditions, which today must be proven by product bacterial challenge tests.

It was known that depth filters, as well as the 0.45 μm rated membranes, were not absolute. They retained particles through the mechanism of adsorption whose efficiency or certainty of particle capture could vary with the conditions of the filtration. Depth filters were made with thicker constructions, in fact, in order to furnish ample sites on which adsorption could occur.

"Absoluteness," in contrast, meant freedom from operational constraints, an independence from challenge levels and from differential pressure considerations. Surface sieve retention offered the explanation as to why membrane filters seemed absolute. Microporous membranes, unlike depth filters, were thin. Obviously, the reasoning went, their upstream surfaces alone must be the sites for particle collection; there seemed not enough thickness for important amounts of adsorption to take place. Therefore, surface retention through sieving must be the mode of membrane action. The reason for the surface arrests by membranes was the narrowness of their pore size distribution, erroneously (Marshall and Meltzer, 1976) said to be only ± 0.02 μm about their mean pore size. Indeed, the spread between pore size rating and largest pore was so negligible that the distinction became blurred; the retention pore (the largest) and the mean pore size (the rated pore size) came to be considered identical. The doctrine of 0.2 μm absoluteness seemed established, but the terminology has since been corrected to refer to these filters as being of sterilizing grade.

Howard and Duberstein (1980) reported that naturally occurring *Pseudomonads* and other microbes in certain Long Island well waters were not completely retained by 0.2 μm rated membranes. They advocated that, at least in certain situations, the use of 0.1 μm rated membranes would better ensure sterilizations by filtration. The same was reported by Thomas et al. (1992). Mittelman et al. (1997) pointed out that such organisms can be typically found in high purity water systems.

6.2 Definition of Sterilizing Filter

A group representing membrane manufacturing organizations and various pharmaceutical houses who were users of membrane filters convened under the aegis of the Health Industries Manufacturing Association (HIMA) to define the term "sterilizing filter" and suitable methods for validating such filters. Practical approaches were sought. It was decided that membranes would be considered sterilizing filters if they could withstand challenges of 1×10^7 *P. diminuta* per square centimeter of membrane surface, delivered in the case of flat disks at applied differential pressures of 30 psi (2 bars) and in the case of cartridges at rates of flow of 3.86 L/min per 0.1 m^2 effective filtration area (to render practical the volume of culture medium required) (HIMA, 1982). A cartridge containing 7 ft^2 (6503 cm^2) effective filtration area would require a flow of 5.94 L/min.

The organisms were to be grown in saline lactose broth under conditions shown by Leahy and Sullivan (1978) to yield single microbes rather than rosette clumps. The challenge level was set to represent a worst-case situation. It was fixed at a magnitude higher than that which would be likely to exist in pharmaceutical preparations. Indeed, if such microbe counts were really present, then the pyrogenic endotoxin concentrations present in the solutions would be prohibitive. Furthermore, if such organism concentrations were encountered, they would first have to be reduced by prefiltration before the preparation was presented for final filtration. Most 5 ft^2 cartridges clog at total challenges of 10^{12}–10^{13}, equal to 10^8–10^9 per square centimeter of filter area.

Suggestions were made that the total organism concentration should supply at least one microbe per filter pore. The idea was impractical. Such a concentration of organisms would have caused organism crowding and overlap with concomitant diminution to the severity of their individual challenge. In fact, filter blockage would ensue before the required 1×10^9 or so organisms per square centimeter of filter surface could be reached. Also, the notion was ill-conceived. Johnston and Meltzer (1979) had pointed out the naivete of that suggestion. The challenge exercise would not really accomplish the uniform microbe disposition its champions expected. Rather, the distribution of organisms would reflect only the laws of probability. Interestingly enough, the laws of probability via the Poisson distribution [see, for example, Juran (1974)] show that in an attempt to lay down an average of two microbes, say, per square micrometer of area, one will end up with 15% of the squares still vacant, while another 15% will contain three or more organisms.

Moreover, squares 1 μm^2 in area seem excessively small from another point of view. As previously stated, a membrane filter can be considered to consist of a layered construction of individual filter planes, each with its own pore size distribution (Piekaar and Clarenburg, 1967). The overlapping of these planes yields a series of pore paths whose individual or intrapore pore size distribution, above a certain critical filter thickness (Pall and Kirnbauer, 1978) begins to approach the overall or interpore pore size distribution of the filter. If the thickness of a single such hypothetical plane is the dimension of its largest pore, and if the "largest pore" of a 0.2 μm rated membrane, in the pre-Williams terminology, is approximately 0.4 μm, double the mean flow pore value, then a 150 μm thick membrane will contain a series of some 300–400 such planes. However rough the arithmetic, it bespeaks a presentation of a series of successive pores to the permeating liquid, except where gross membrane damage might exist within the depths of the membrane. (The number of 0.2 μm rated pores would be even larger, depending on the pore size distribution.) It does not seem relevant, therefore, to be concerned with challenging surface squares having dimensions as small as 1 μm^2.

The hydrodynamics of filtration itself supplies a correction to the notion that the infrequent organism finds difficulty in locating the occasional large pore. On the contrary, the bulk of the flow bearing the organisms is self-directing toward the larger pores because that flow preferentially occurs through those larger pores, flow through a pore varying as the fourth power of the pore radius. Thus, the liquid flow, seeking the path of least resistance, finds the larger pores and carries the suspended organisms with it to preferentially challenge these larger pores.

At the 1×10^7 organisms/cm^2 surface challenge level, and excluding the Poisson distribution effect cited, the frequency of pore challenge per microbe is roughly 260 pores per organism, some two magnitudes of pores more than the number of organisms. Assuming the total porosity to consist only of 0.3 μm pores:

$$
\begin{aligned}
1\ \text{cm} &= 1 \times 10^4\ \mu\text{m} \\
\text{Surface of } 1\ \text{cm}^2 &= 1 \times 10^8\ \mu\text{m}^2 \\
\text{At } 80\%\ \text{porosity} &= 0.8 \times 10^8\ \mu\text{m}^2 \text{ of pores} \\
\text{Area} &= \pi r^2 \\
\text{Pore density for 0.2 pore} &= 3.14 \times (0.1\ \mu\text{m})^2 \\
&= 0.031\ \mu\text{m}^2 \text{ per } 0.2\ \mu\text{m pore} \\
&= \frac{0.8 \times 10^8\ \mu\text{m}^2}{0.031\ \mu\text{m}^2}
\end{aligned}
$$

$$\text{Pore density} = 2.6 \times 10^9 \text{ pores } (0.2\ \mu\text{m})/\text{cm}^2$$
$$\text{HIMA challenge} = 1 \times 10^7 \text{ organisms/cm}^2 \text{ filter surface,}$$
$$\text{Challenge} = \frac{1 \times 10^7 \text{ org/cm}^2}{2.6 \times 10^9 \text{ pores } (0.2\ \mu\text{m})/\text{cm}^2}$$
$$= \text{one organism per 260 } (0.2\ \mu\text{m}) \text{ pores}$$

The applied differential pressure level specification of 30 psi (2 bar), just like the organism challenge level, provides a safety margin. Filtrative sterilizations are seldom conducted at applied differential pressures in excess of 25 psi (1.7 bar). By the same token, however, those wishing to conduct operations consonant with the proposed HIMA sterilizing filter definition are obliged to constrain their applied pressure differentials to within the confines of the 30 psi (2 bar) maximum, unless the use of higher pressure has been validated. Additionally, some safety margin should be provided. The proposed HIMA recommendation imprimatur does not necessarily extend to "sterilizing filters" at applied pressure differentials above 30 psi, although the work of Leahy and Sullivan (1978) (Table 6) and the Tanny et al. findings of Table 7 indicate that 0.2 μm rated filters do have a sterilizing efficacy even at higher pressure differentials.

The proposed HIMA convention for defining a sterilizing filter has seemingly been endorsed by every filter manufacturer. This HIMA recommendation states that sterile effluent will issue from a sterilizing filter challenged with 1×10^7 organisms/

Table 7 Retention Performance of Cellulose Triacetate 0.20 μm Rated Membranes Challenged with *B. diminuta* Suspension of 10^5 organisms/cm[a]

Operating pressure (psi)	Organisms (per 100 mL) passing after			
	500 mL	1000 mL	1500 mL	2000 mL
5	0	0	0	0
5	0	0	0	0
5	0	0	0	0
5	0	0	0	0
5	0	0	0	0
15	0	0	0	0
15	0	0	0	0
15	0	0	0	0
30	0	0	0	0
30	0	0	0	0
30	185[b]	200[b]	16[b]	8[b]
45	0	0	0	0
45	0	0	0	0
45	0	0	0	0
45	0	0	0	0

[a][2000 mL over 9.6 cm^2 of available surface (47 mm disk); total organism challenge level 2×10^7 organisms/cm^2.]
[b]Colonies identified as contaminants, no *B. diminuta*.
Source: Tanny et al. (1979).

cm^2 filter surface at pressures up to 30 psi (2 bar). A sterilizing filter has come to be defined a bit more broadly, however, as one that effects a log reduction value (LRV) of 7 in the titer of a suspension of any unspecified magnitude of properly cultivated *B. diminuta* passed through it at applied differential pressures as high as 30 psi (2.1 kg/cm^2 or 2 bar). A sterilizing grade filter, in practical and newly defined terms, is a filter that retains 10^7 *B. diminuta* organisms suspended in the pharmaceutical product and challenged under worst-case process conditions, i.e., at specific pressure differential conditions, temperatures, contact times, etc.

Various terms have been used to represent the microbial removal efficiency of membrane filters. The term in common use now is the log reduction value, (LRV) adapted by HIMA to standardize the terminology.

The LRV is the logarithm to the base 10 of the ratio of the organisms in the influent stream to those that emerge in the filtrate. Thus, if a filter has an LRV of 7, it is capable of diminishing the organism test numbers by seven orders of magnitude. Expressed as a percent reduction in the number of microorganisms, the number would be 99.99999. To determine the specific LRV of a filter, such a test challenge level would have to be used as to cause some passage of organisms through the filter, in order to obtain a number for the denominator of the LRV expression. Sterilizing membrane filters, however, do not ordinarily permit the passage of test organisms. Therefore, the LRV of such filters is described solely in terms of the numerator—the influent or challenge level—namely, as being greater than $\log_{10}$ of that total challenge.

Not the least accomplishment of the HIMA effort was the joining together of the various filter manufacturers and important users in the attainment of this goal.

In summary, as stated, HIMA defines a sterilizing filter as one that does not permit the passage of any organisms when challenged with 1×10^7 organisms/cm^2 surface area. A simple extension of this definition has it that a sterilizing filter has an LRV of 7. Thus, if confronted by 1×10^8 organisms, it may permit the passage of 1×10^1 microbes. Nevertheless, this is not the case, as shown by Osumi et al. (1996). Furthermore, filter vendors usually challenge at $>10^8/cm^2$.

6.3 Microbes Smaller than *B. diminuta* ATCC 19146

The 0.2 μm rated membranes defined as sterilizing against *Pseudomonas diminuta* need not be absolute in their retention of smaller organisms. Thus, natural water-borne pseudomonads e.g., *P. cepacia* and *P. aeruginosa*, could conceivably penetrate such filters even at lower delta pressures and even at lower organism challenge levels. The same holds specifically true for the mycoplasmas periodically encountered in sera. To be absolute against such organisms, membranes with smaller pore size ratings would be required.

The designation of *B. diminuta* ATCC 19146 as the qualifying organism to be used by filter membrane manufacturers in their definition of "sterilizing filters" hopefully already bespeaks a worst-case situation for filter users. Pseudomonads are water-borne organisms. Their presence in water supplies, particularly in pharmaceutical manufacturing contexts, may signal that the Water for Injection is being manufactured improperly.

Whether a "sterilizing filter" is indeed suitable for the total organism removal required in a particular manufacturing process must be ascertained in the validation exercise by the filter user. That is the purpose of the validation. If a particular process does involve organisms smaller than *B. diminuta* ATCC 19146 and these are normal to that manufacturing practice, then filters of smaller pore size ratings may indeed be indicated. Their use may, however, be accompanied by reduced rates of flow. Such requirements have not been reported in the parenteral manufacturing experience (Robinson, 1984). For these operations the sterilizing 0.2 μm rated membrane filters seem to suffice. However, 0.1 μm rated microporous membranes are commercially available and find applications in mycoplasma removals and high purity water systems, and blow–fill–seal filling processes.

7 RETENTION OF LATEX SPHERES

7.1 Influence of pH and/or Surfactant on Latex Sphere Retention

In Pall et al. (1980) studies performed at pH 2.0, 3.7, and 9.8, it was established that the filter efficiency was influenced by pH. The relationship being essentially inverse, the lower pH values yielded greater retention values. From this it must be concluded that the larger hydronium ion concentrations served to increase the electrokinetic charge effects whereby adsorptive sequestration exerted a trapping influence on the latex particles. This effect was also reported by Wrasidlo et al. (1983) in their comparison study of several filter types using the latex spheres technique (Table 8).

As might have been expected, where adsorptive sequestration effects are operative, the surfactant influences the filter efficiency. Retentions were much lower when 0.1% Triton X-100 was introduced. Moreover, when Triton X-100 was omitted, the retention results, although better, were erratic. Therefore, Pall et al. (1980) used 0.1% Triton X-100 concentrations, the critical micelle concentration for that surfactant, in all of their comparative studies. Other surfactants gave results that showed slightly greater microsphere retention. Wrasidlo et al. (1983) encountered a similar influence on the part of surfactants on latex particle retention (Tables 9 and 10). As previously stated, the presence of surfactant was believed to assist microsphere passage of the filter by modifying surface adsorption propensities or, by coating the particle, increasing particle size to such an extent that adsorptive forces became too weak to operate. This is the steric stabilization effect previously discussed (Sec. 2.2), where the free energy barrier to its approach to the filter surface is raised, thus interfering with its adsorption. It is possible, however, that at least to some extent

Table 8 Percent Retention of 0.198 μm Latex for Various 0.2 μm Rated Membranes as a Function of pH

Filter type	Bubble point	pH 4	pH 6	pH 8	pH 9
Asymmetric polysulfone	51	100	100	100	100
Polycarbonate (track-etched)	63	100	100	100	100
Poly(vinylidene difluoride)	55	86.8	74.8	79.5	67.3
Cellulose esters	58	36.3	89.4	23.0	31.3
Nylon 66	45	99.9	82.1	23.7	28.4

Source: Wrasidlo et al. (1983).

Table 9 Retention of 0.198 μm Latex for Various 0.2 μm Rated Membranes as a Function of Surface Tension

Surface tension (dyn/cm)	75	50	34
Percent Triton X-100	0	0.001	0.05
Filter type		Percent retention	
Asymmetric polysulfone	100	100	100
Polycarbonate (track-etched)	100	100	100
Charge-modified nylon	100	100	100
Cellulose esters	89.4	17.1	25.1
Poly(vinylidene difluoride)	74.8	20.9	19.2
Nylon 66	82.1	38.5	1.0

Source: Wrasidlo et al. (1983).

surfactant served to disperse particles that might otherwise have been agglomerated. It might have been expected that where the suspending solutions had higher viscosities, their drag on the suspended particles might render adsorptive capture more difficult (Table 11). This effect was not clearly evident.

Both the Pall et al. and Wrasidlo et al. studies clearly demonstrated the influence on latex particle retention by those very factors that govern adsorptive effects. The conclusion seems inescapable that, at least where cross-linked polystyrene latex particles are concerned, adsorptive sequestration may play a part in their retention.

Wrasidlo and Mysels (1984) demonstrated that adsorptive effects are involved in the retention of 0.198 μm latex particles by most commercially available 0.2 μm rated membranes, the presence or absence of surfactant influencing the retention efficiency (Table 12). Retention is lowered in the presence of surfactant. The lack of such governance in the case of 0.1 μm rated membranes is taken to indicate particle trapping by sieve-type captures. Latex spheres 0.085 μm in size show the

Table 10 Retention of Various Size Latex Particles for 0.2 μm Rated Membranes[a]

	Latex particle size (μm)			
	0.091	0.198	0.305	0.460
Membrane type	Percent retention			
Asymmetric polysulfone	54.3	100	100	100
Charge-modified nylon	10.5	100	100	100
Polycarbonate (track-etched)	6.3	100	100	100
Poly(vinylidene difluoride)	23.4	19.2	84.5	100
Cellulose esters	17.7	25.1	48.6	100
Nylon 66	1.0	1.0	1.0	100

[a]All solutions were 0.04% latex in 0.05% Triton X-100.
Source: Wrasidlo et al. (1983).

Table 11 Retention of 0.198 μm Latex for Various 0.2 μm Rated Membranes as a Function of Solution Viscosity

Filter type	1	1.5	5	10
Viscosity (relative to water)				
Percent glycerin	0	10	50	60
Membrane type	Percent retention			
Asymmetric polysulfone	100	100	100	100
Polycarbonate	100	100	100	100
Charge-modified nylon	100	100	100	100
Poly(vinylidene difluoride)	74.8	95.9	99.5	100
Nylon 66	82.1	66.3	96.9	99.9
Cellulose esters	89.4	65.6	63.2	83.4

Source: Wrasidlo et al. (1983).

surfactant influence, an indication of adsorptive sequestration, in the case of both 0.1 and 0.2 μm rated filters.

Wrasidlo and Mysels (1984) defined the retention powers of various commercially available 0.2 μm rated membranes in terms of the size of latex particles retained to an extent of 99.0% in the presence and absence of surfactant. Table 13 shows surprising differences among similarly rated filters.

Table 12 Percent Latex Retention of Membranes

	0.198 μm particles		0.085 μm particles	
Membrane[a]	Triton X-100	Deionized H_2O	Triton X-100	Deionized H_2O
0.2 μm rated				
A Polysulfone	99	100	25	98
B Polysulfone	45	100	31	98
C Cellulosic	49	94	25	31
D Cellulosic	55	55	29	44
E Nylon	57	59	25	38
F Nylon (charged)	99[b]	96[b]	35	42
G Polycarbonate (track-etched)	96	100	10	20
H Polyvinylidene difluoride	40	78	25	29
0.1 μm rated				
I Polysulfone	100	100	99.7	100
J Nylon	89	99.4	38	40
K Polycarbonate (track-etched)	99.9	100	47	99.4

[a]A and I are highly asymmetric membranes; the others are conventional symmetric or slightly asymmetric membranes.
[b]Only initial retention; continued filtration gives substantial particle passage.
Source: Wrasidlo et al. (1983).

Table 13 Effect of 0.1% Triton X-100 Surfactant on Size of Latex Particles Retained 99.9% by Different Types of Membranes

	Latex radius (μm)		
Membrane	In distilled water	In 0.1% Triton X-100	Percent difference
Symmetrical cellulosic	0.165	0.298	81
Symmetrical PVF	0.178	0.235	32
Symmetrical nylon	0.218	0.315	45
Asymmetrical polysulfone	0.170	0.193	13.5

Source: Wrasidlo et al. (1983).

7.2 Utility of Latex Sphere Retentions

Schroeder (1984) used his investigation of latex particle retention, as did Wrasidlo and Mysels, to differentiate between sieving and adsorption by membranes in the capture of (latex) particles.

Other uses can also be made of latex sphere retention studies. Thus, Wrasidlo et al. (1983) use the technique to arrive at a flow–pore size distribution characterization of filters. The ability of a membrane to retain latex particles is plotted as a function of the various particle sizes. For example:

Retention data, latex particle diameter	Percent retention
0.050	0
0.091	40
0.198	97.8
0.305	99.98
0.412	100[a]
0.497	100[a]

[a] Test sensitivity ≥99.99.

The data obtained can be interpreted to reflect the flow–pore size distribution of the tested filter. By plotting these data, a pore distribution profile based on particle retention can be constructed (Fig. 18).

7.3 Comparisons with Organism Retentions

Regrettably, as will be seen, the implications of these studies do not translate directly to the retention of organisms. One thing these studies do demonstrate is the incorrectness of an earlier belief that membrane filters do not permit the passage of rigid particles larger by 0.2 μm or greater in size than their pore size ratings.

Tanny et al. (1979) ascribed the retention of *B. diminuta* by 0.45 μm rated membranes as being due to adsorptive sequestration. Experiments reported by Reti et al. (1979), do not seem to bear out the implications of such a conclusion. Reti and his associates found that mixed esters of cellulose membranes having bubble

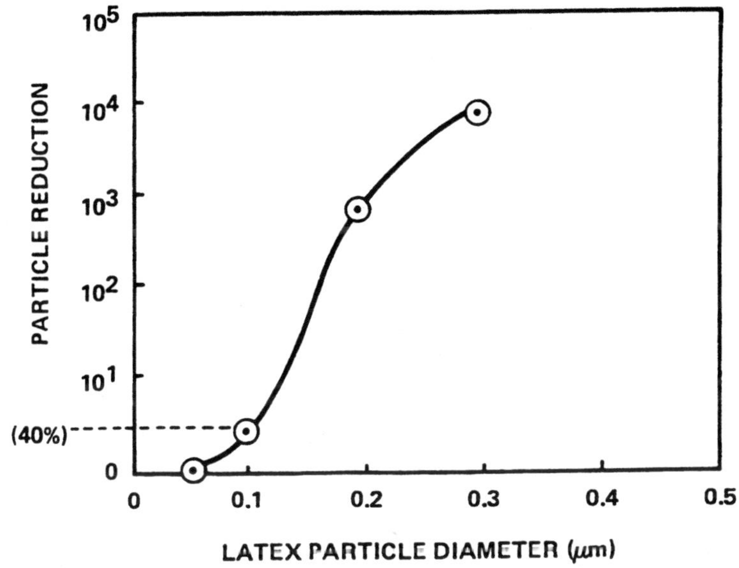

Figure 18 Flow pore size distribution of filters from latex retention studies of fibrous depth filter challenged with *P. diminuta*. [From Wrasidlo et al. (1983).]

point values of ≈2.3 bar, some 34 psi (traditionally taken to indicate the 0.45 μm rated filter for this polymer), were essentially uninfluenced in their retention of *P. diminuta* by high ionic concentrations or by the presence of surfactant (Table 14). Each of these two agencies would have been involved in adsorptions based on charge attractions (see Sec. 2.2). This finding is sometimes cited as evidence that membrane filters do not adsorptively sequester *P. diminuta*. However, in the same study, Reti et al. found that the extent of organism retention by the 0.45 μm rated membranes varied with the applied differential pressure, as would be expected for adsorptive arrest but not for sieve retention. The 0.45 μm rated filters exhibited log reduction values of between 1×10^5 and 1×10^6 at 50 psi (3.4 bar) and between 1×10^7 and 1×10^8 at 0.5 psi (0.034 bar). The challenge level of the *P. diminuta* varied between 4.7×10^{10} and 5.6×10^{10}. This cannot readily be explained on the basis of sieve retention.

It is possible that hydrophobic adsorptive effects cited in Sec. 2.2 are operative instead where *P. diminuta* capture is involved. These would not necessarily be influenced by ionic strengths or by surface-active agents. It could be hypothesized that mixed esters of cellulose membranes adsorb *P. diminuta* so strongly that ionic charge or surfactant has little effect. However, even if such a completely speculative view were true, that *P. diminuta* may be retained by adsorption to membrane filters but so strongly as to resist the liberating influences of pH, ionic strength, etc., such retentions independent of operating conditions would have to be judged to be absolute.

Robertson and DeVisser (1980) and Levy and Leahy (1985) confirmed that 0.2 μm rated mixed esters of cellulose membrane retained *P. diminuta* equally well regardless of the absence or presence of surfactant and independent of ionic strength.

Table 14 Passage Data for Various Fluid Chemistries[a]

Additive	Concn.	Bubble point (bar)	Initial challenge	Passage	$\beta = \frac{\text{challenge}}{\text{passage}}$	log β	Organisms	Membrane	Percent
None	—	2.3	2.0×10^{10}	5.2×10^{5}	2.0×10^{4}	4.58	−5.7	−11.5	−5.8
$MgCl_2$	0.01 M	2.2	2.0×10^{10}	4.8×10^{5}	2.0×10^{4}	4.62	+2.2	−6.2	−8.4
$MgCl_2$	0.10 M	2.3	2.0×10^{10}	3.6×10^{5}	2.0×10^{4}	4.75	+6.2	+1.8	−4.4
None	—	2.2	8.3×10^{10}	7.0×10^{5}	8.3×10^{5}	5.08			
$MgCl_2$	0.01 M	2.1	8.3×10^{10}	4.6×10^{5}	8.3×10^{5}	5.26			
$MgCl_2$	0.10 M	2.3	8.3×10^{10}	1.2×10^{6}	8.3×10^{4}	4.84			
None	—	2.3	1.9×10^{10}	1.7×10^{5}	1.9×10^{5}	5.04			
Pluronic F-68	0.0055%	2.3	1.9×10^{10}	9.0×10^{5}	1.9×10^{5}	5.32	−4.1	−6.9	−2.8
Pluronic F-68	0.10%	2.2	1.9×10^{10}	2.8×10^{5}	1.9×10^{4}	4.83	−1.4	−5.2	−3.8
None	—	2.3	6.0×10^{10}	1.2×10^{5}	6.0×10^{5}	5.70			
Pluronic F-68	0.0055%	2.3	6.0×10^{10}	4.6×10^{5}	6.0×10^{5}	5.11			
Pluronic F-68	0.10%	2.2	6.0×10^{10}	1.4×10^{5}	6.0×10^{5}	5.63			

[a]Transmembrane pressure = 3.4 bar, equivalent to 0.45 μm rating.
Source: Reti et al. (1979).

But that finding reveals little about adsorptive influences. These results can be imputed also to sieve retention of the organisms by the test filters because of the 0.2 μm pore size rating.

Pall et al. (1980) state that nylon and cellulose ester membranes that are 0.2 (0.22) μm rated on the basis of microbial retention would be rated 0.4–0.6 μm on the basis of latex particle capture and that a particular 0.1 μm rated nylon 66 membrane would, by latex particle retention sizing, be classified as a 0.286 μm rated filter. These authors agree that the ability of 0.2 (0.22) μm rated membranes to retain *P. diminuta* ATCC 19146 under "as severe challenge conditions as can be devised" is well established and confirmed, but suggest the contribution of adsorptive arrests to the retention picture.

These authors and others (Nakao, 1994; Bentley and Lloyd, 1992) tried to measure and specify pore sizes for membrane filters, specifically 0.2-μm filters. It is known that such filters have a pore size distribution that is typically of a Gaussian shape. It is important that this pore size distribution be narrow, ensuring that pores even bigger than 0.2 μm coincide with an underlying smaller pore. Besides, the labeling of the filters seems more an administrative convenience for filter manufacturers, which is more than understandable. The fact is, filter vendors must prove that their 0.2-μm-labeled filters withstand the HIMA challenge conditions. Moreover, they must meet the conditions found in the pharmaceutical process by challenging the filter with a minimum of 10^7 CFU/cm^2 of *B. diminuta* suspended in the product itself. Proper validation work and documentation eliminates the need for discussion of pore size labels.

7.4 Repetitive Filter Effects

Increasingly, final filters are being employed in a repetitive mode. It is a prudent practice. If all the particles were larger than all the pores, then the second filter would have no useful role to play. The potential efficacy of the repetitive filter means that there is a conceivable case of adsorptive particle sequestration in which capture by the downstream filter is due to an effectively longer pore path occasioned by the second layer of filter. It is for this reason that it is postulated that each filter layer can be characterized by a log reduction value and that such log reduction values become additive for filter assemblies with repetitive layers of filters (Sec. 6.2). Often two 0.2 μm sterilizing grade filters are used at critical filling lines, as a safety factor. Whether this is the right approach depends on individual opinion. Certainly the LRV of a sterilizing grade filter should be high enough to retain a sterile filtrate. The use of a second filter finds its logic in preventing a probable unsterility and therefore discard of the filled batch when the initial 0.2 μm filter fails the integrity test after filtration. This situation may obtain when the initial integrity test is done before steam sterilization of the filter, which usually is the most stringent situation for a membrane filter.

Two filters in series could mean, for certain applications, that product or product component yields can be greatly reduced owing to the higher nonspecific adsorption resulting from twice the effective filter area. Such an occurrence depends on the process conditions, pretreatment of the filter, and membrane filter material.

There is no doubt that prefilter cartridges of coarser pore size rating or retention rating will prevent premature blockage of the final filter, in some cases even reduce the bioburden. Such prefilter systems usually exhibit higher flow rate and throughput patterns and therefore can mean substantial costs savings for the filter user.

REFERENCES

Alcholtz, P., and T. J. Leahy. (1985). The effects of high pressure on the bacterial retention of membrane filters challenged with *Pseudomonas diminuta*, PDA, Philadelphia, November 1985, Poster Session.

Bentley, J. M., and P. J. Lloyd. (1992). Interpreting the rating of cartridge filters, *Filtr. Separ.*, *July/Aug*:333–335.

Berg, H. F., W. L. Guess, and J. Autian. (1965). Interaction of a group of low molecular weight organic acids with insoluble polyamides I. Sorption and diffusion of formic, acetic, propionic, and butyric acids into nylon 66, *J. Pharm. Sci.*, *54*(1):79–84.

Brinkman, R., and A. Szent Gyorgi. (1923). Studium Ober Die Physicalisch-Chemische Grundlagen Der Vitalen Permeabilität, *Biochem. Z.*, *139*:261–279.

Carazzone, M., D. Arecco, M. Fava, and P. Sancin. (1985). A new type of positively charged filter: Preliminary test results, *J. Parenter. Sci. Technol.*, *39*(2):69–74.

Chiori, C. O., R. Hambleton, and G. J. Rigby. (1965). Inhibition of spores of *B. subtilis* by cetrimide retained on washed membrane filters, *J. Appl. Bacteriol.*, *28*:322–330.

Chiou, L., and D. L. Smith. (1970). Adsorption of organic compounds by commercial filter papers and its implication on quantitative-qualitative chemical analysis, *J. Pharm. Sci.*, *59*(6):843–847.

Elford, W. J. (1931). A new series of graded collodion membranes suitable for general bacteriological use, especially in filterable virus studies, *J. Pathol. Bacteriol.*, *34*:502–521.

Elford, W. J. (1933). The principles of ultrafiltration as applied in biological studies, *Proc. Roy. Soc. (Lond.)*, *112B*:384–406.

Farrah, S. R., C. P. Gerba, C. Wallis, and J. L. Melnick. (1976). Concentration of viruses from large volumes of tap water using pleated membrane filters, *Appl. Environ. Microbiol.*, *31*:221–226.

Fiore, J. V., and R. A. Babineau. (1979). Filtration, an old process with a new look, *Food Technol.*, *33*:67–72.

Flindt, E. (1983). Pyrogenentfernung mittels ultrafiltration, Concept Symp. 8, June, Frankfurt, Germany.

Galanos, C. E., E. T. Rietschel, O. Ludertiz, O. Westphol, Y. B. Kim, and D. W. Watson. (1972). Biological activity of lipid A complexed with bovine serum albumin, *Eur. J. Biochem.*, *31*:230–233.

Gerson, D. F., and J. E. Zajic. (1978). The biophysics of cellular adhesion, in *Immobilized Microbiological Cells* (K. Ven Katsubramanian, ed.), American Chemical Society, Washington, DC, pp. 29–53.

Hawker, R. J., and L. M. Hawker. (1975). Protein losses during sterilizing by filtration, *Lab Pract.*, *24*:805–807, 814.

Hermans, P. H., and H. L. Bredee. (1936). Principles of the mathematical treatment of constant-pressure filtration, *J. Soc. Chem. Ind., Trans. Commun.*, *55*:1–4.

HIMA. (1982). *Microbiol Evaluation of Filters for Sterilizing Liquids*, Document No. 3, Vol. 4, Health Industry Manufacturers Association, Washington, D.C.

Hjertin, S., J. Rosengren, and S. Pahlman. (1974). Hydrophobic interaction chromatography: The synthesis and the use of some alkyl and aryl derivatives of agarose, *J. Chromatogr.*, *101*:281–288.

Horowitz, D. A., and M. A. Garrett. (1971). Use of leukocyte chemotaxis *in vitro* to assay mediators generated by immune reactions. I. Quantitation of mononuclear and polymorphonuclear leukocyte chemotaxis with polycarbonate (Nuclepore) filters, *J. Immunol.*, *106*:649–655.

Hou, K. C., C. P. Gerba, S. M. Gayel, and K. S. Zerda. (1980). Capture of latex beads, bacteria, endotoxin and viruses by charge modified filters, *Appl. Environ. Microbiol.*, *40*:892–896.

Howard, G., Jr., and R. Duberstein. (1980). A case of penetration of 0.2 μm-rated membrane filters by bacteria, *J. Parenter. Drug Assoc.*, *34*(2):95–102.

Johnston, P. R. (1975). Submicron filtration, *Chem. Eng. Process.*, *71*:70–73.

Johnston, P. R., and T. H. Meltzer. (1979). Comments on organism-challenge levels in sterilizing-filter efficiency testing, *Pharm. Tech.*, *3*(11):66–70, 110.

Juran, J. M. (ed.) (1974). *Quality Control Handbook*, 3rd ed., McGraw-Hill, New York, pp. 22–29; App. 2, p. 2.

Kaczmarek, A. J., E. Fochtman, and J. Klein. (1978). Private communication, IIT Research Institute, Chicago.

Karbachsch, M., G. Steinhoff, and H. Monzavi. (1984). Abtrennung von Pyrogenen aus Lösungen niedermolekularer Substanzen durch Ultrafiltration, *Pharm. Ind.*, *46*(4):399–402.

Knight, R. A., J. V. Fiore, and J. V. Rossitto. (1982). Microporous membranes as depth filters, *World Filtration Congress III*, Downingtown, PA, Vol. 2, pp. 472–483.

Leahy, T. J., and M. J. Sullivan. (1978). Validation of bacterial retention capabilities of membrane filters, *Pharm. Tech.*, *2*:65–75.

Levy, R. V., and T. J. Leahy. (1985). The effects of pH, viscosity, and additives on the bacterial retention of membrane filters challenged with *Pseudomonas diminuta*, PDA, Philadelphia, November 1985, Poster Session.

Lin, Y. (1973). Detection of wild yeasts in the brewery: A new criterion, *Brewers Dig.*, *48*(5)(-GL-):60–69.

Marshall, J. C., and T. H. Meltzer. (1976). Certain porosity aspects of membrane filters: their pore-distributions and anisotropy. *Bull. Parenteral Drug Assoc.*, *30*(5):214–225.

Marzouk, Y. (1976). Retrieval of poliovirus from water by different membranes, Private communication, Ministry of Health, Israel.

Meltzer, T. H. (1984). Polymeric surfaces and protein adsorption, Society of Manufacturing Engineers, Ann Arbor, MI, May.

Meltzer, T. H. (1996). *Pharmaceutical Water Systems*. Tall Oaks Publishing, Littleton, Colorado, pp. 235–236.

Meltzer, T. H., M. W. Jornitz, and M. H. Mittelman. (1997). Surrogate solution attributes and use conditions, PDA Conference, Osaka.

Mittelman, M. W., M. W. Jornitz, and T. H. Meltzer. (1997). Bacterial cell size and surface charge characteristics relevant to filter validation studies, *PDA J. Pharm. Sci. Tech.* (submitted).

Mix, T. W. (1974). The physical chemistry of membrane–virus interaction, in *Symposium on the Detection of Viruses in Waste and Other Waters, Developments in Industrial Microbiology*, Vol. 15 (G. Berg, Convener), Chap. 14.

Mouwen, H. C., and T. H. Meltzer. (1992). Sterilizing filters: Pore-size distributions and the $1 \times 10^7/cm^2$ challenge, *Pharm. Tech.*, *16*(7):28–32.

Nakao, Sin-ichi. (1994). Determination of pore size and pore size distribution 3. Filtration membranes, *J. Membrane Sci.*, *96*.

Nicholaus, N. (1975). What, when, and why of cartridge filters, *Filtration and Separation*, *12*(2):155–163.

Ostreicher, E. A. (1977a). Particulate filter medium and process, U.S. Patent 4,007,113.

Ostreicher, E. A. (1977b). Fibrous filter medium and process, U.S. Patent 4,007,114.

Ostreicher, E. A. (1985). Electrokinetics in liquid filtration—past, present and future, Hershey Conference, Hershey, PA.

Osumi, M., N. Yamada, and M. Toya. (1996). Bacterial retention mechanisms of membrane filters, *PDA J.*, *50*(1):30–34.

Pall, D. B., and E. A. Kirnbauer. (1978). Bacterial removal prediction in membrane filters, 52nd Colloid and Surface Symposium, Univ. Tennessee, Knoxville, June.

Pall, D. B., E. A. Kirnbauer, and B. T. Allen. (1980). Particulate retention by bacteria retention membrane filters, *Colloids Surf.*, *1*:235–256.

Parks, G. A. (1967). *Equilibria Concepts in Natural Water Systems*, Adv. Chem. Ser. 67, American Chemical Society, Washington, DC.

Pertsovskaya, A. F., and D. G. Zvyagintsev. (1971). Adsorption of bacteria on glass, modified glass surfaces, and polymer films, *Biol. Nauki*, *14*(3):100–105.

Peters, T., Jr., H. Taniuchi, and C. B. Anfinsen, Jr. (1973). Affinity chromatography of serum albumin with fatty acids immobilized on agarose, *J. Biol. Chem.*, *248*(7):2447–2451.

Petras, E. (1967). Comparative investigations of the efficiency of membrane filters, *Kolloid Z.*, *218*(2):136–139.

Piekaar, H. W., and L. A. Clarenburg. (1967). Aerosol filters: Pore size distribution in fibrous filters, *Chem. Eng. Sci.*, *22*:1399–1409.

Raistrick, J. H. (1980). "The Adsorptive Filtration of Liquids," *Recent Devel. Filter Media Their Appl. Proc. Internatl. Symp.*

Raistrick, J. H. (1982). The relevance of zeta potential to the filtration of small particles from potable liquids, *World Filtration Congress III, Vol. 1*, Downingtown, PA, pp. 310–316.

Reti, A. R., T. J. Leahy, and P. M. Meier. (1979). The retention mechanism of sterilizing and other submicron high efficiency filter structures, Second World Filtration Congress, London, pp. 427–435.

Robertson, J. H., and A. DeVisser. (1980). Microbiological qualification and validation of sterilizing membrane filters, *Interphex Abstracts*, Interphex, New York.

Robinson, J. R. (1984). The great filter-rating debate, *J. Parenter. Sci. Technol.*, *38*(2):47.

Robinson, J. R., M. D. O'Dell, J. Takacs, T. Barnes, and C. Genovesi. (1982). Removal of endotoxins by adsorption to hydrophobic microporous membrane filters, *PDA*, November 1982, Philadelphia.

Rossitto, J. (1983). Letter to *Liquid Filtration Newletter*, No. 50, October 10, 1983, The McIlvaine Company, Northbrook, IL.

Ruth, B. F., G. H. Montillon, and R. E. Montanna. (1933). Studies in filtration: Part I. Critical analysis of filtration theory, *Ind. Eng. Chem.*, 25:76–82.

Sarry, C., and H. Sucker. (1992). Adsorption of proteins on microporous membrane filters. Parts I and II, *Pharm. Tech. Int.* Oct./Nov.

Schroeder, H. G. (1984). Selection criteria for sterilizing grade filters, Society of Manufacturing Engineers, Philadelphia, May.

Skelley, D. S., L. P. Brown, and P. K. Besch. (1973). Radioimmunoassay, *Clin. Chem.*, *19*(2): 146–186.

Smith, K. M., and J. P. Doncaster. (1935). "The preparation of gradacol membranes and their application in the study of plant viruses, *Parasitology*, *27*:523–542.

Tanford, C. (1980). *The Hydrophobic Effect: Formation of Micelles and Biological Membranes*, 2nd ed., Wiley, New York.

Tanny, G. B., and T. H. Meltzer. (1978). The dominance of adsorptive effects in the filtrative sterilization of a flu vaccine, *J. Parenter. Drug Assoc.*, *32*(6):258–267.

Tanny, G. B., D. K. Strong, W. G. Presswood, and T. H. Meltzer. (1979). The adsorptive retention of *Pseudomonas diminuta* by membrane filters, *J. Parenter. Drug Assoc.*, *33*(1):40–51.

Thomas, A. J., H. H. Dürrheim, M. Alport, and P. Evers. (1992). Detection of L-forms of *Pseudomonas aeruginosa* during microbiological validation of filters, *Pharm. Tech. Int.*, March:34–44.

Tolliver, D. L., and H. G. Schroeder. (1983). Particle control in semiconductor process streams, *Microcontamination, 1*(1):34–43, 78.

Udani, G. G. (1978). Adsorption of preservatives by membrane filters during filtration sterilisation, Thesis for B.Sc. Honours (Pharmacy), School of Pharmacy, Brighton Polytechnic, Brighton, UK.

Van Ooteghem, M., and H. Herbots. (1969). The addsorption of preservatives on membrane filters, *Pharm. Acta Helv., 44*(6):602–610.

Wallhaüsser, K. H. (1975). Sterilizing by filtration in the pharmaceutical industry, *Pharm. Indu., 37*(1):10–17.

Wallhäusser, K. H. (1995). *Praxis der Sterilisation, Desinfection-Kouservierung*, Georg Thieme Verlag, Stuttgart.

Wallhäusser, K. H., and H. Schmidt. (1967). *Sterilisation, Desinfection Kouservierung, Chemotherapie*, Georg Thieme Verlag, Stuttgart.

Wilkinson, P. C. (1974). *Chemotaxis and Inflamation*, Churchill Livingstone, Edinburgh.

Williams, R. E., and T. H. Meltzer. (1983). Membrane structure, the bubble point, and particle retention: A new theory, *Pharm. Tech., 7*(5):36–42.

Woog, H. (1987). Abtrennung von Pyrogenen durch neuentwickelte Filter auf Basis der Ultrafiltration, Concept Symp., Dec. 7 to 8, 1987, Frankfurt, Germany.

Wrasidlo, W., and K. J. Mysels. (1984). The structure and some properties of graded, highly asymmetric porous membranes, *J. Parenter. Sci. Technol., 38*(1):24–31.

Wrasidlo, W., F. Hofmann, J. A. Simonetti, and H. G. Schroeder. (1983). Effect of vehicle properties on the retention characteristics of various membrane filters, PDA Spring Meeting, San Juan, PR.

Zierdt, C. H. (1978). Unexpected adherence of bacteria, blood cells and other particles to large porosity membrane filters, *Abstracts*, American Society of Microbiologists, 78th Annual Convention, Las Vegas, May, Article Q-93, p. 10.

Zierdt, C. H., R. L. Kagan, and J. D. MacLawry. (1977). Development of a lysis-filtration blood culture technique, *J. Clin. Microbiol., 5*(1):46–50.

Zsigmondy, R. (1909). *Colloids and the Ultramicroscope*, Chapman & Hall, London, p. 153.

11

Integrity Testing

MAIK W. JORNITZ
Sartorius AG, Göttingen, Germany
A. MARK TROTTER
Sartorius Corporation, Edgewood, New York
THEODORE H. MELTZER
Capitola Consulting Company, Bethesda, Maryland

1 INTRODUCTION—PROPOSED INTEGRITY TESTING OF FILTERS

In its proposed good manufacturing practices (GMPs) for large volume parenterals (LVPs), the Food and Drug Administration (FDA) established the requirements for the integrity testing of filters (*Federal Register*, June 1, 1976), as outlined below. Although never officially implemented—indeed, they were officially withdrawn in 1994—these proposed GMPs for LVPs have come to serve as the basis for FDA inspections. They have also been extended to small volume parenteral manufacture. In effect, then, whether formalized or not, there is the guideline requirement to integrity test 0.45 μm rated and 0.2 μm rated membranes used as "solution filters" or final filters both before and after the filtration operation.

212.721 Filters

(a) The integrity of all air filters shall be verified upon installation and maintained throughout use. A written testing program adequate to monitor integrity of filters shall be established and followed. Results shall be recorded and maintained as specified in 212.83.

(b) Solution filters shall be sterilized and installed aseptically. The integrity of solution filters shall be verified by an appropriate test, both prior to any large-volume parenteral solution filtering operation and at the conclusion of such operation before the filters are discarded. If the filter assembly fails the test at the conclusion of the filtering operation, all materials filtered through it during that filtering operation shall be rejected. Rejected materials may be refiltered using filters whose integrity has been verified provided that the additional time required for refiltration does not result in a total process time that exceeds the limitations specified in 212.111. Results of each test shall be recorded and maintained as required in 212.188(a).

2 BUBBLE POINT AND ORGANISM RETENTION

2.1 Sterilizing Membrane Rating

Of all the structural features characterizing a filter, none would seem more pertinent to particle retention, whether of viable or nonviable, than the pore size. In the early days of microporous filtration, 0.45 μm rated membranes were considered sterilizing filters, until Bowman et al. (1967) discovered an organism contaminating a protein solution that had consistently passed through 0.45 μm rated membranes. The 0.2 (0.22) μm rated filter was devised to retain that organism, later identified as *Pseudomonas diminuta*, ATCC 19146, as isolated and cultivated by Bowman.[1] The bubble point measurement was used to assure investigators that membranes about to be used in filtrative sterilizations were, indeed, 0.2 μm rated.

More recently, 0.1 μm rated membranes have been advocated as the filter media for at least some filtrative sterilizations of pharmaceutical preparations, for example, in high purity water systems and at some blow–fill–seal filling lines. The situation is complicated by nonstandardization of the pore-rating system (Robinson, 1984; Mouwen and Meltzer, 1993).

2.2 The Bubble Point Test

Hydrophilic microporous membranes will fill their pores with water by imbibing that liquid in accordance with the laws of capillary rise. The retained water can be forced from the filter pores by the impress of air. Liquid will be expelled first from the set of largest pores, in keeping with the inverse relationship of the applied air pressure P and the diameter of the pore, d, described in the bubble point equation

$$P = \frac{4\gamma \cos \theta}{d}$$

where γ is the surface tension of water and θ is the angle of wetting.

The voiding of liquid from the largest pores creates a pore passageway through which bulk airflow takes place, to be detected in the form of bubbles escaping downstream through a layer of water. The distinct pressure at which airflow through the filter commences, the bubble point, serves to characterize the size of the largest pores. Substitution of that air pressure value in the bubble point equation does not, however, yield an accurate numerical measure of the pore dimension. The values that are obtained do not, therefore, permit reliable predictions of particle retentions to be made (Lukaszewicz et al., 1978).

[1]As used in bacterial challenge work, this organism is indeed different from *Pseudomonas diminuta* as listed in Bergey's *Diagnostic Bacteriology* and is properly identified by the American Type Culture Collection Number 19146. More recently, based on DNA-rRNA hybridization studies, this organism has been shown to belong more properly to the genus *Brevundimonas* (Segers et al., 1994). It is here referred to by the genus name *Pseudomonas*.

The Capillary Rise Phenomenon

Water will rise in a capillary tube to an extent governed by the diameter of the tube. The narrower the diameter of the capillary, the larger the rise. Water will not, however, rise in a polyethylene tube or capillary, nor will mercury, for example, rise in a glass capillary. The reason for the rise of water in glass is that there is an attractive hydrogen bonding force between the water molecules and the silicate anions of glass that causes the spreading of the one over the other. The presence of such molecular allurements is signaled by the concavity of the liquid meniscus within the capillary. In the absence of an attraction to the solid surface, the liquid molecules would bond only to one another. Within the capillary this is manifested by a convex meniscus. Such attractive forces are absent for water–polyethylene or mercury–glass because of the dissimilarities (in the cohesive energy densities) of these molecules. The liquid rises only until it is balanced by the opposing force of gravity.

The rise is governed by the propensity of the liquid to wet the solid capillary surface, expressed by cos θ, where θ is the angle of wetting, or the contact angle, a measurement that reflects the avidity of liquid–solid attraction. This can be considered an adhesive force that bonds the water layer to the glass layer. Where the wetting is perfect, the angle of wetting is zero. When the attraction is less than perfect (mirroring differences in the cohesive energy densities between the liquid and solid molecules), the liquid tends to form droplets. Within a tube, a nonwetting liquid exhibits a convex meniscus, the upper curve of the free-falling drop. Where perfect wetting exists and the wetting angle or contact angle θ is zero, cos θ has a value of 1.

The water molecules that spread upward along the capillary walls are hydrogen-bonded to other water molecules and eventually, through a chain of hydrogen bonding, to water molecules removed from the attracting influences of the silicate walls. The mass of water is therefore lifted by these cohesive forces operating within the water bulk, as expressed by the surface tension γ of that liquid. Therefore, γ is a term of the equation describing the capillary rise.

The lifting of the liquid occurs at the capillary perimeter, the site of the liquid/solid interface. For a circular capillary the perimeter is expressed as $2\pi r$, where r is the radius of the capillary. The liquid rising is therefore described by

$$2\pi r\gamma \cos \theta$$

Opposing the rise is the mass of the liquid that has risen in the capillary. For a circular capillary, this is defined by the dimensions of the risen column, $\pi r^2 h$, the internal area of the capillary multiplied by its height.

At its equilibrium point, the capillary rise is thus described by the equation

$$2\pi r\gamma \cos \theta = \pi r^2 h$$

Rearranged, this becomes

$$h = \frac{2\pi r\gamma \cos \theta}{2\pi r^2} \quad \text{or} \quad h = \frac{2\gamma \cos \theta}{r}$$

If the capillary diameter is used instead of its radius, the equation becomes

$$h = \frac{4\gamma \cos \theta}{d}$$

The liquid height h becomes transformed into pressure units because of the force of gravity acting on the mass of the risen liquid:

$$P = \frac{4\gamma \cos \theta}{d}$$

For any given liquid, such as water, the numerator reduces to a constant (Table 1), and the equation becomes

$$P = \frac{K}{d}$$

For the purposes of the bubble point measurement it is assumed that the pores of microporous filters act as capillaries when they are wetted with water. To expel the water from the pores of such a membrane would require an added force to destabilize the capillary rise equilibrium. Air pressure applied to the surface of a wetted membrane contained in a suitable holder would be such a force. Enough pressure would have to be exerted to overcome the bonding forces anchoring the water molecules to the pore surfaces. The bubble point equation is therefore written as

$$P = \frac{4\gamma \cos \theta}{d}$$

where P is the pressure required to expel the liquid (test liquids other than water may be used) from the filter pore.

Consider pores of different diameters. In a wider capillary, less of the contained water is in contact with the pore walls. There is less of the water-bonding "wall effect." Because there are fewer bonds, the water rises to a lesser height. Also, less pressure is required to expel the water, as there are fewer bonding sites to overcome. In other words, if there were a series of capillaries of differing diameters, as there are pores of different sizes in membranes (because of the pore size distribution), then the impress of air would cause the liquid to be blown out first from the largest

Table 1 Characteristics of Liquids Commonly Used in Bubble Point Measurements

Wetting liquid	Surface tension (dyn/cm)	Conversion factor[c]
Water	72	30.0
Kerosene	30	12.5
Isopropanol	21.3	8.9
Freon TF	19.0	7.9
Silicone fluid[a]	18.7	7.8
Fluorocarbon fluid[b]	16	6.7
0.5% Triton X-100	30	12.5
0.1% Triton X-100	30	12.5

[a]Dow Corning 200 fluid, 2.0 cS.
[b]3M Company, Fluorochemical FC-43.
[c]Conversion factor divided by pressure in psi equals maximum pore in micrometers.

(in terms of diameter) capillaries. This is expressed mathematically in the bubble point equation by the inverse relationship of P and d:

$$d = \frac{4\gamma \cos \theta}{P}$$

Pore Shape Factor

The reason for the difference between the calculated and measured dimensions (or pressure levels necessary to cause liquid expulsion from the pores) derives, as stated, from the assumption inherent in the equation that the pores are circular in cross section.

Shown in Fig. 1 is a scanning electron micrograph (SEM) of a "typical" inverse-phase microporous membrane. The convoluted shapes of the pores make it impossible to directly measure their perimeters or the areas they enclose.

A capillary rise equation that more generally treats the shape of the pore includes a shape factor l for the length of the pore perimeter and A for the area it encloses instead of $2\pi r$ and πr^2, terms correctly applicable to circles alone.

$$P = \frac{l\gamma \cos \theta}{A}$$

In the one instance where calculations based on the shape factor can be performed —namely, for woven metallic cloth of the Dutch twill design—wherein the pores are skewed equilateral triangles, calculated and measured values agree (SAE, 1968).

When water is used, the wetting angle must first be determined (Sec. 7.1). Water gives a contact angle of 60–90° with polycarbonate. When poly(vinyl pyr-

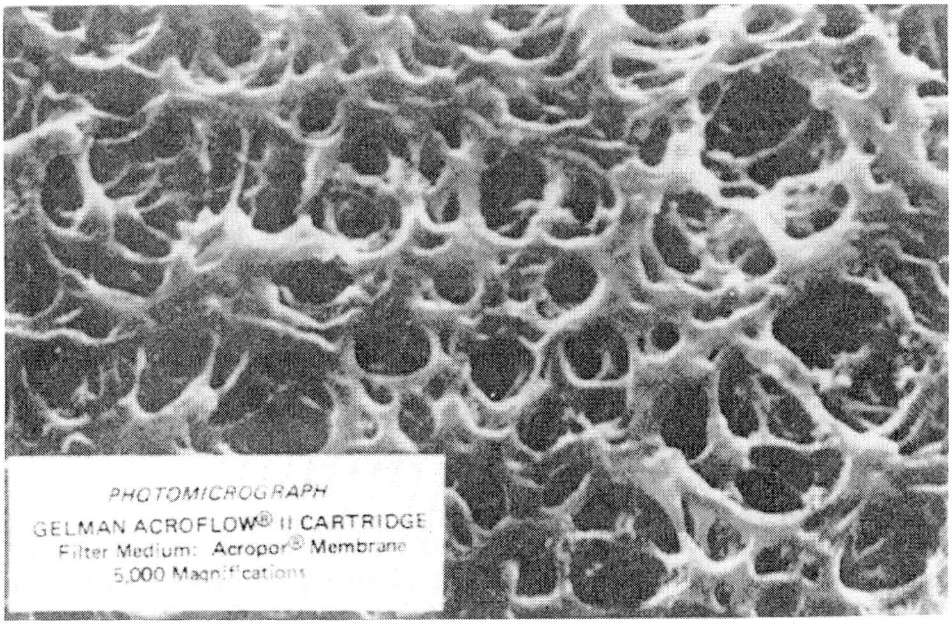

Figure 1 Inverse-phase membrane SEM, 5000X. (Courtesy of Gelman Science Inc.)

rolidone) is used as a wetting agent, the angle of wetting becomes 50–70°. If the median value of 60° is used, $\cos \theta = 0.50$. The use of this value in conjunction with the surface tension of the wetting solution is stated to approximate closely the calculated theoretical bubble point value of about 100 psi ($208 \times 0.50 = 104$ psi).

The pore shapes, then, importantly influence the pore diameter values. Pores having the irregular outlines that characterize membrane voids are smaller in their extent of open volume than are openings of a similarly-sized circular periphery. This is so because the area of a circle is the largest expanse that can be enclosed by its size perimeter. If the same size perimeter assumes any shape other than circular, the area it encloses must be smaller. It is therefore safe to say that particles much smaller than the numerical pore ratings will be sieve-retained by the membrane filters (Ferry, 1935; Petras, 1967). In any case, the bubble point procedure or mean flow–pore method based on the capillary rise experience yields only relative values. Indeed, as the Aerospace Recommended Practice (SAE, 1968) on the bubble point procedure states: "No bubble point test measures actual pore size, but only allows correlation of the measured capillary pressure with some dimensional characteristics of the pore structures."

The numerical pore size values assigned by membrane manufacturers are commonly based on a combination of the HIMA bacterial challenge test correlation and bubble point testing. 0.2 μm rated membrane filters are often referred to as sterilizing grade filter membranes.

2.3 Correlation of Bubble Point and Retention

At best, the bubble point determination can provide only an indirect measure of retention of organisms. It is considered more suitably pertinent to directly measure membrane organism retention efficiencies. Unfortunately, the assessment of filter efficiency by means of organism retention measurements, although commendably unambiguous, leads to destruction of the filter; the filter cannot be used after it has been tested. What is required, then, is a nondestructive test of a filter that correlates with its organism retention capabilities. Once a dependable relationship has been established, the former can usefully serve as a surrogate test for the latter, more pertinent test of applicational interest. Once employed to determine (rather questionably) the pore size rating of a given filter, the bubble point measurement is now used to verify the equivalency of pore size of the filter used in the filtration to that employed by the membrane vendor in the challenge test with *P. diminuta* (ATCC 19146) and its ability to retain a minimum 1×10^7 concentration per square centimeter of filter area.

While the emphasis in bubble point measurement centers on its correlation with organism retention in the case of sterilizing filters, the method is applicable to all filters. The bubble point values reflect the "largest pore size" in accordance with the above capillary rise equation.[2]

Using retention data and corresponding bubble point values reported in the literature, Johnston and Meltzer (1979) plotted correlations between these two measurements. Reti et al. (1979), Elford (1933), and Pall and Kirnbauer (1978) had

---

[2]See Pall (1975) for calculations relating to total number of pores and to numbers of pores of different sizes.

recorded such data. From these were plotted the microbe reduction ratio versus the bubble point of membranes that differed only in bubble point or average pore diameter. Elford reported pore diameters, and the reciprocals of his values were arbitrarily employed to convert them to bubble points. Since the other investigators who reported bubble points did not describe the details of how they performed this measurement (which is hardly standard in its execution), these bubble point values were simply plotted on a logarithmic scale with the understanding that each must be multiplied by some constant appropriate to each bubble point investigation before the results of one experimenter can be compared to those of another. The different plots, therefore, did not yield a single line, but such a line resulted from a multiple superposition of all the individual plots.

Figure 2 shows the plots. All three groups of data suggest straight lines of the same slope. The slope (m) of that line appears in the mathematical expression.

$$R = me^{aB}$$

where

R = the microbe reduction ratio
B = the bubble point of the membrane
a = the constant that reflects the method of measuring the bubble point and the kind of microbes involved
m = slope of the line

Figure 2 is in fact a plot of

$$\ln (\ln R) = \ln a + m \ln B$$

To understand the significance of the constant a, one must recall that the bubble point is a function of the surface tension of the liquid wetting the pores of the membrane. This was different (and unspecified) in each of the investigations. Additionally, this constant is a function of that rate of airflow through a unit area of membrane that constitutes what is called the first perceptible flow of air. This quantity might also differ according to the individual experimenter's sensitivity of perception. Further, one must understand that while Elford employed the microbe *Bacillus prodigiosus*, now known as *Serratia marcescens*, the other investigators used *P. diminuta*.

All three lines of Fig. 2 can be combined into the single line of Fig. 3 where on the x axis can be added a scale showing the relationship between membrane permeability to water as a (relative) function of bubble point. (Such information appears in the product literature and validation guides of various membrane manufacturers.) Figure 3 shows that a 10% change in bubble point (and subsequent changes in permeability and pore size) results in a tenfold change in the microbe reduction ratio. Figure 3 suggests the obvious conclusion: When one attempts both to measure such large reduction ratios and to reproduce the results ±10%, one should expect to see tenfold variations in the microbe reduction ratio. In other words, if 10^7 is a true value, one may find numbers anywhere between 10^6 and 10^8 because of the uncertainties of the bubble point measurement, as ordinarily conducted.

222

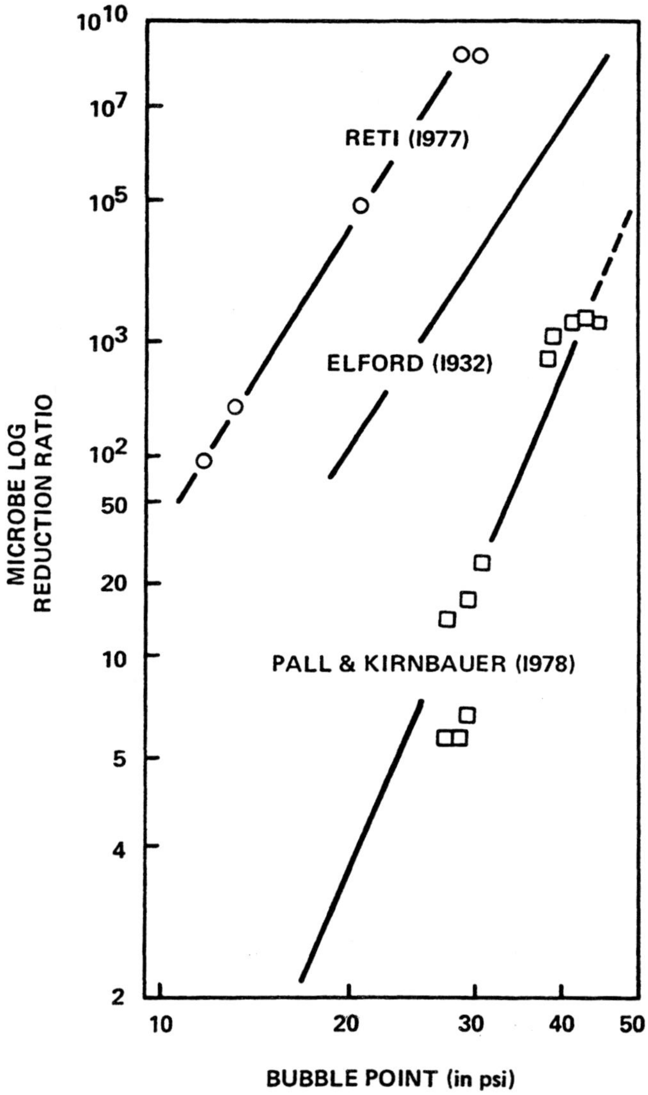

Figure 2 Correlation of bubble points and organism retention (from data reported in the literature). [From Johnston and Meltzer (1979).]

In separate test runs involving four different 0.2 μm rated membrane filters from four different manufacturers, Wallhäusser (1979) fed a 21 L/min stream of water containing *P. diminuta* at a concentration of 10^9 L^{-1}. During the course of each run, he sampled 1 L portions of the filtrate to obtain their microbe counts. His results, illustrated in Fig. 4, reveal the kind of reproducibility that Fig. 3 suggests; that is, his data indicate a microbe reduction ratio between 10^7 and 10^9, with an average

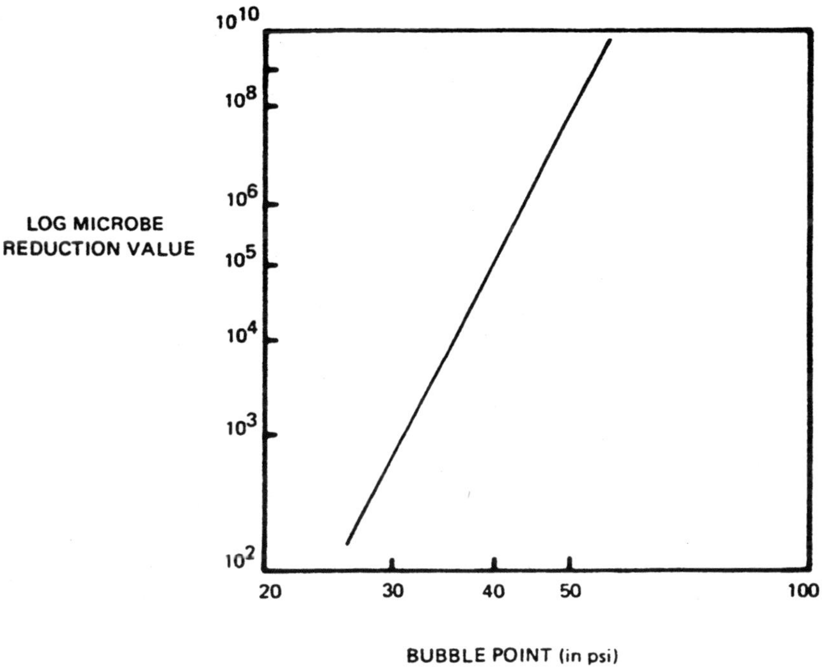

Figure 3 General curve relating microbe retention to bubble point, where ln ln R = ln a + 2 ln P, $R = e^{aP^2}$, $R = 10^{aP^2}$, and a = experimental constant reflecting how the bubble point is measured, volumetric flow rate, differential pressure, filter area, duration of the filtration, the types and numbers of the microorganisms being filtered, etc. [From: Johnston and Meltzer (1979).]

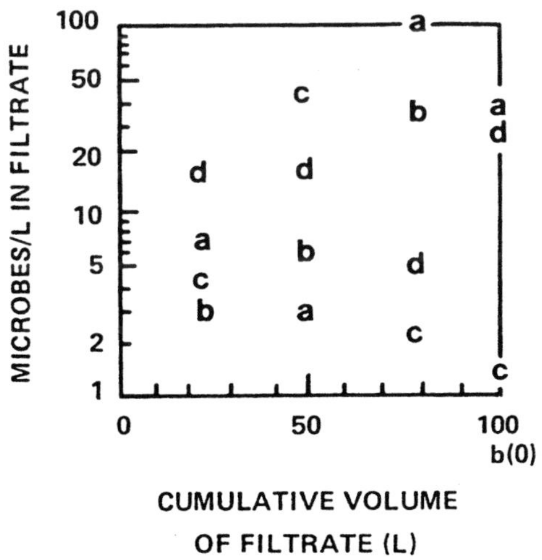

Figure 4 Plot of experimental bubble point–organism retention data showing random scatter. [From Johnston and Meltzer (1979).]

near 10^8. Obviously, from the foregoing, these data do not demonstrate that any one of the filters Wallhäusser tested is better than another, nor do they reveal for any of these filters a change in filtration efficiency with time. In other words, Fig. 4 constitutes a plot of random numbers.

Because of the randomness introduced into the correlation of large numbers (i.e., the organism retention values) with a measurement (bubble point) that may vary by ±10%, one must exercise caution in judging the filters. Thus, if 1×10^7 constitutes a passing retention value, then 9.9×10^6 does not constitute failure. (Conversely, if 9.9×10^6 constitutes failure, 1×10^7 does not signify acceptability.) Both values are within the experimental error of the experimentally established correlation. To ensure a minimum of 1×10^7 retention value, an LRV of 7, an experimentally established LRV of 8 would be required, unless, of course, one wishes to assume, or can ensure, that the bubble point measurement has less than a 10% variation.

In manual bubble point testing, the end point takes the form of a steady stream of bubbles rising through a liquid (or by measurement of the volume of liquid displaced by the bubbles). But a bubble is some finite volume of air, formed by the coalescence of microquantities of the airflow, and the size necessary for its detection may reflect the subjective sensitivity of the observer. Some observers will see bubbles before others do, or, to put it another way, some will detect smaller bubbles, lesser volumes of air, than others. For this reason filter manufacturers developed sophisti-

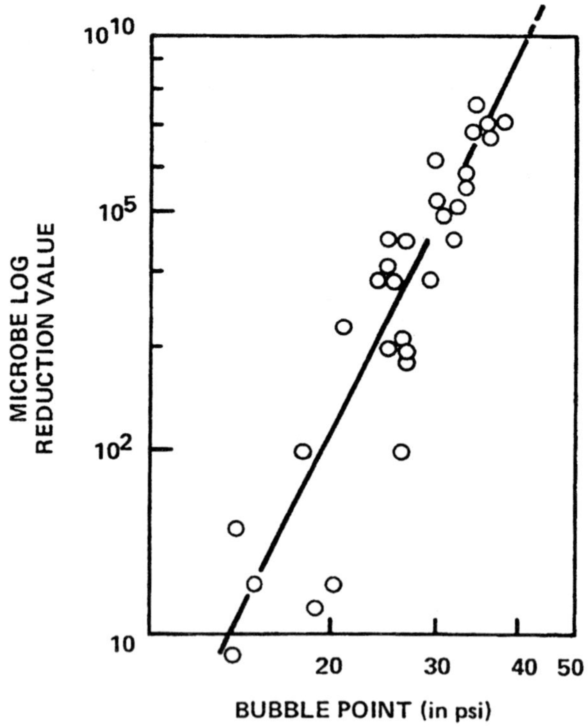

Figure 5 Correlation of bubble points and organism retention. [From Leahy and Sullivan (1979).]

cated, automated integrity test machines that measure the bubble point automatically and compare it with an installed minimum allowable bubble point. Automatic test machines have the benefit of reducing human failure and providing proper documentation of the test results.

The experimentally established correlation of bubble point values with organism retention values as set forth by Johnston and Meltzer (1979) is confirmed by data from Leahy and Sullivan (1978) (Fig. 5) and from Reti et al. (1979) (Fig. 6). The slope of the line is invariant; it has a steep slope of 2, confirming the large alterations in filter LRV with small changes in bubble points.

The bubble point value as an indication of filter organism retention derives its authority from this relationship rather than from any fancied indication of any particular pore size, whether 0.2 μm or whatever. The bubble point measurement is useful as a convenient nondestructive indicator of a filter's efficiency vis-à-vis particle retention. The size implications of the bubble point speak primarily to sieve retention. However, it is also relevant to adsorptive particle arrests, as pore diameters influence them as well. In filtrative sterilizations, the standard particle of interest is the *P. diminuta* organism, ATCC 19146.

Given how little is known about microporous membrane structure, it cannot be assumed that all sterilizing grades of membranes, whether from one or from another of the several manufacturers, have the same organism retention characteristics unless the organism retention is known to be solely the result of sieve-type capture. It is

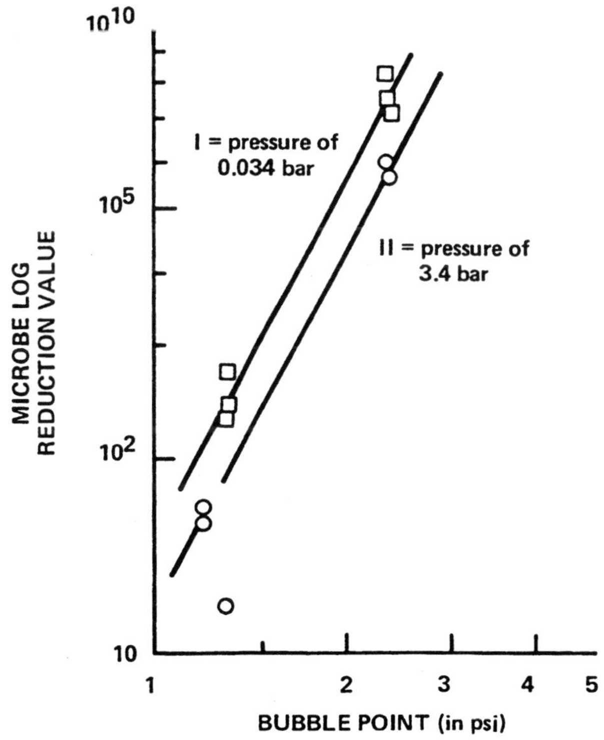

Figure 6 Correlation of bubble points and organism retention. [From Reti et al. (1979).]

therefore important in the filter validation program that each membrane type be evaluated for the adequacy of its organism retention. The filter user may rely on the elucidative work performed by the filter manufacturer, which is primarily based on water bubble point values. Such reliance should not, however, be in the nature of an act of faith. The user should request in advance of testing the detailed evaluation protocol and validation data for placement in his FDA file. The filter user is, in any case, responsible for the pertinent validation studies.

3 CAUSES OF BUBBLE POINT DEVIATIONS

3.1 Operator Subjectivity

The subjectivity that may be involved in the manual performance of a bubble point measurement has already been remarked on. Rigid adherence to an established test protocol can serve to minimize errors from this source. Bubble point readings are most valuable in yielding relative comparisons before and after testing. It is doubly important, therefore, that operator subjectivity be minimized. The use of automated integrity test machines is recommended.

3.2 Product as the Wetting Liquid

It has been observed that contact between certain membranes and various pharmaceutical preparations can produce depressed bubble points compared with the values for water. Thus, it was early noted that 0.45 μm rated cellulose ester membranes, whether of mixed or triacetate composition, after contact with dilute sodium bicarbonate or sodium heparinate solutions show bubble point values of some 18–20 psi (1.26–1.40 bar), down from the water bubble point of 32 psi (2.24 bar). In comparison, the kerosene bubble point of 14 psi (0.98 bar) is not affected by bicarbonate or heparin solution contact. The depressed bubble point can be restored, more or less, but mostly less, by copious washing of the filter with water. Some subtle wetting effects involving product ingredients may be at work here whose surface physics is not comprehended. In addition, the surface tension differences between the product and water are contributory to the anomaly.

Often, efforts are made to flush the filter with water before running the final integrity test, so that before-and-after bubble point tests using water are obtained for comparison. However, even copious water flushing may not restore the water bubble point. In such cases, before-and-after comparisons may usefully be performed using product-wet filters. The displacements in bubble values being ascribed to unknown wetting effects, but largely to the influences of the surface tension values of the product, are assumed not to reflect on the organism removal capabilities of the membrane.

However reasonable this assumption, it falls short of the proof required by validation. Therefore, prudence requires that validation of the filter be conducted using appropriate organism challenge levels in conjunction with the very solution being manufactured.

Parker (1986) determined the acceptable minimum bubble point for a given type of filter using product in accordance with the formula

$$P_{\mathrm{p}} = \frac{P_{\mathrm{o}}}{P_{\mathrm{w}}} P_{\mathrm{m}}$$

where P_p is the minimum acceptable product bubble point, P_o is the observed bubble point using product, P_w is the average of the water bubble points observed for samples of the filters, and P_m is the filter manufacturer's stated minimum allowable bubble point. Enough filters or filter devices are secured from each lot of the subject filter type to yield an acceptable average value. Testing is performed for each product being filtered using 47 mm disk filters or small-scale pleated filter devices.

More recently, Desaulnier and Fey (1990) confirmed Parker's findings. Both Parker and Desaulnier and Fey describe the exact protocols by means of which the product bubble point may be determined. The latter authors also describe an apparatus suitable for the purpose.

Usually the evaluation of the so-called product integrity test values requires three filter membranes or devices of three different lots, i.e., nine tests in total. Nowadays one of these filter lots must be close to the minimum allowable water bubble point value given by the filter manufacturer to ensure retentive capability at the established limit values.

3.3 Procedure for Prewetting Filters

In prewetting membrane filters preparatory to performing an integrity test, the filter manufacturer's protocol should be followed exactly. There is no uniform standard procedure. Usually, soaking the filter (placing cartridges into a container of water) will not suffice. A dynamic water flow is required. One manufacturer stipulates that the 10 in. filter cartridge should be soaked in the housing for 5 min under enough water pressure to expel all the air and fill the housing, as evidenced by water exiting from the vent valve. Water should then be flowed through the housing for 2–3 min at 15–30 psi (1–2 bar) with the downstream valve so regulated as to permit a flow of 2–3 gpm (8–12 L/min). Recalcitrant cases may benefit from the use of hot water (100–200°F; 38–84°C). The use of an alcohol such as 70% isopropanol, followed by a water flush (promptly, to prevent drying out of the alcohol) is a very effective means of achieving wetting.

Virtually each membrane cartridge is alleged to have been integrity-tested by the manufacturer prior to release. For this reason alone, low bubble point values obtained by the user can be suspected to have arisen from incomplete wetting rather than from integrity test failures. Initial integrity test failures should be rechecked to make certain they are not caused by incomplete filter wetting. Effects of imperfect wetting are described by Meltzer (1987). In imperfect wetting, a pore channel may be so partially filled with the liquid as to give any "bubble point" value between zero and the true bubble point magnitude.

3.4 Effects of Relative Polymer Hydrophobicity

It would seem reasonable that the greater the reluctance of the polymeric filter to become wetted by water, the greater the possibility of imperfect wetting. Not surprisingly, therefore, it is found that there is a greater variability in the bubble point of unmodified microporous fluorocarbons, even when a wetting agent is used, than there is for more wettable polymerics.

3.5 Effect of Filter Area

The size of a filter does not affect its intrinsic bubble point, reflecting the size of the largest pores inherent in the filter. However, it does influence the amount of air passing through the filter at the intrinsic bubble point, simply as an expression of the number of largest pores present. Filter area, then, could conceivably affect the perceived bubble point, the instance when enough air has passed the filter to coalesce into a visible bubble. Perhaps for this reason most catalogs list cartridges as having lower bubble point values than disk filters composed of the same polymers.

Figure 7 (Johnston et al., 1981) shows that at an airflow of 16 mL/min (the logarithmic average of the 5 and 50 mL/min observations), the same membrane in its 47 mm disk size appears to have a bubble point of 44 psi, while in the form of a pleated cartridge (4545 cm^2 of filter), it appears to have a bubble point of 33 psi.

The intrinsic bubble point (the knee or theoretical infection point on each curve) is invariant, regardless of the filter size. *This true bubble point correlates with a filter's organism retentivity characteristics.* But the apparent bubble point as perceived by the observer will differ. This occurs because, given acceptable membrane

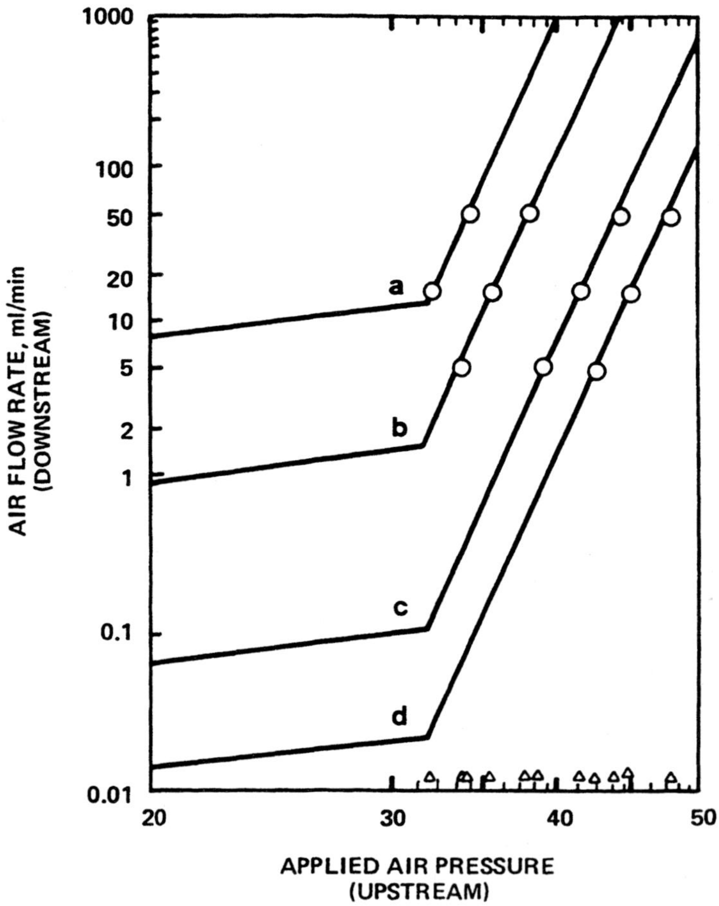

Figure 7 Apparent shift in bubble point as a function of filter dimension. For different areas of a 130 μm thick, 0.2 μm rated, membrane: a = 4545 cm^2 in a pleated cartridge, b = 589 cm^2 in a 293 mm diameter disk, c = 44 cm^2 in a 90 mm disk, d = 9.6 cm^2 in a 47 mm disk.

homogeneity, although the proportion of the largest pores remains constant regardless of the membrane area, their number and the volume of air they pass per unit time at the intrinsic bubble point increase in direct proportion to the filter area.

A larger filter simply permits the passage of more air, due to a higher diffusive airflow through the water layer. Simply put, the rate of air passage is proportional to filter area.

Filter area significantly affects the diffusion test. Schroeder and DeLuca (1980) demonstrated consistent tenfold increases in airflow for successive tenfold increases in filter area—a very predictable dependency. However, the practical contribution of filter area to bubble point test values may be rendered uncertain. If bubble points were determined for all filters as they are for the 47 mm disk, as open bubbles arising from it, then the influence of filter size would definitely be a factor [complicated, however, by the diffusional effect that is significant for larger area filters (Reti, 1977)]. However, 293 mm disks and cartridges, both singly and in their multiple forms, are bubble point tested in their housings (also with some subjectivity), from which quantities of liquid must first be expelled before air bubbling becomes evident. If the airflow at 40 psi is 10 mL/min, then it will require 10 min to see the bubbles if the volume downstream, in the cartridge core and/or holder, is 100 mL. By then, the operator may well have increased the test pressure in the belief that the bubble point had not yet been reached. While great refinement may be used in such contexts, the mechanics of the manual bubble point operation do dispose toward override of the intrinsic bubble point. In such cases, the operator may not allow quite enough time at a given air pressure level for the flow of bubbles (already in progress, but invisible within the filter holder) to manifest itself, whether as bubbles or as displaced liquid flow, before raising the air pressure further. When the delayed bubbles do appear, they are mistakenly ascribed to the higher pressure then registering on the gauge. It may be that the filter area effect, tending to give bubble points perceived as lower for the larger filter areas, is partly offset by the bubble point override possible for the same filters. A degree of balance may cancel out both spurious effects.

Should the filter area effect be shown to have practical significance, it can be neutralized by normalization of the airflow data. This can be done by describing airflow rates as a function of pressure and filter area. The airflow rate units would then be milliliters per minute per square centimeter.

3.6 Effect of Membrane Multilayering

Pall and Kirnbauer (1978) observed that for membranes of equal pore size ratings, increases in thickness increase the bubble point values (what the authors designate as the K_L pressure readings). Wrasidlo and Mysels (1984) noticed the same effect with intimately superimposed membrane multilayers, but not where the layers are separated, in which case each membrane acts independently. It should be noted that the surface smoothness of the anisotropic polysulfone membranes used by Wrasidlo and Mysels lends itself to a very close superpositioning with minimum space in between.

Johnston (1985) comments that the pore size distributions of filters resemble a log-normal distribution with a characteristic geometric standard deviation. Like Piekaar and Clarenburg (1967), Johnston views a filter as consisting of superimposed theoretical planes of homogeneous filter medium, each with its pore size distribution. The theoretical plane has some "unit" thickness, and the statistical meaning of the size of an individual pore is the two-dimensional view of the ratio of pore perimeter to cross-sectional area. The filter medium as a whole consists of a stack of these planes. A large pore in one plane is not necessarily adjacent to a large pore in the next plane. What constitutes the largest pore (as measured by the bubble point) is tied to what cumulative sum of the log-normal distribution one wishes to consider. Therefore, the bubble point will increase, up to a point, the greater the number of theoretical unit plates that are superimposed on one another.

Whatever the pore nature of membranes, they are seen to provide passageways through which fluid flow occurs. The term "pore" is thus used to refer to those individual passageways that in their totality comprise the filter. Each passageway, however, is a composite of many different regions having widths of varying dimensions. The more restrictive of these regions have the greater effects on fluid flow and are also referred to as "pores," in an unfortunate example of the current ambiguity in filter terminology. It is, of course, this latter intrapore size distribution that finds reflection in the interpore size distribution that, overall, describes a given filter.

When two layers of filter are made intimately congruent, the likelihood is increased that passageways having different degrees of restriction will be joined to one another to create longer (or thicker) passageways of narrower intrapore size distributions. Thus, the overall interpore size distribution is narrowed, and the resulting thicker filter is more retentive. The above describes why such multilayered arrangements should have higher sieve retention efficiencies. The loci of such added sieve retentions are internal, however, not surface. By the same token, their more extensive pore wall areas serve also to increase retentions involving adsorptive sequestration.

3.7 Effect of Rapid Pressure Rise

In the manual performance of the bubble point measurement, the end point under observation is the appearance of an unbroken stream of bubbles rising through liquid—a flow of gas in liquid. In a suitable protocol, the wetted filter is subjected incrementally to increasing levels of air pressure. Ultimately, a pressure is reached that suffices to eject the water from the set of largest pores present. The flow of bulk air that exits from the vacated pores manifests itself in the form of bubbles rising through a depth of water overlying (or a pool of water downstream of) the wetted membrane. Hence the term "bubble point."

After each increase of the inlet air pressure, that level is maintained for some finite period of time while the advent of bubbles is awaited. When none is noted, the differential pressure is further raised, followed by a period of waiting, until the bubble point is reached. The duration of the waiting period is a product of experience. It may also be tempered into brevity by subjective impatience. In such cases, the actual bubble point pressure may be overridden. Bubbles caused by an earlier, lower pressure setting may become evident only after a higher pressure is being recorded and be erroneously ascribed to that higher pressure. To shorten the time required for determination of the bubble point, it is common to raise the pressure rather rapidly, to obtain some impression of where the bubble point pressure level lies. The procedure is then repeated, with a rapid pressure rise to just below the bubble point, followed by more careful and smaller pressure adjustments coupled with longer waiting periods to secure accurate readings.

Since the assurance of a minimum bubble point is often being sought, one that will ensure an adequacy of organism retention, an alternative procedure is to almost immediately register the inlet pressure to the minimum acceptable bubble point and await the outcome of this go/no-go test. Membrane manufacturers almost always furnish filters that exceed the stipulated minimum bubble point, thus making this procedure possible.

As performed in the laboratory characterization mode, the bubbles escaping the horizontally positioned membrane to its up side (downstream) are immediately visible in the supervening water layer. In processing contexts, however, enough air must emerge from the filter to push the water out of the filter housing on the downstream side before bubbles become evident. This can create enormous overrides in the bubble point pressure reading unless adequate time is allowed, on the basis of experience, at each newly registered pressure level near the expected bubble point. To minimize such happenings, cartridge housings should be mounted in such a position that liberated air will rise to the outlet tube where its appearance will be detected sooner. At the very least, sightglass sections ought to be installed in line as close to the exit from the housing as possible to enable early spotting of the stream of bubbles. While such arrangements minimize the errors of override, they do not eliminate them.

More sophisticated observers look not for bubbles, the movement of air in liquid, but rather for liquid flow caused by air displacement, liquid movement in air. When pressure is first applied to the housing, water flows through the membrane from its upstream side, to emerge as a liquid flow. That flow ceases as all the upstream water is expelled. As pressure is increased, an uneven liquid flow will resume due to the compression of the cartridge pleats and to the spatial adjustments of the various layers comprising the cartridge. This will abate, and perhaps even cease entirely, if an ample waiting period is observed. Some liquid trickle may persist, the product of liquid displacement from the reservoir in the housing downstream of the filter as occasioned by diffusional airflow. Whatever this rate of persistent liquid flow, it is eclipsed by the subsequent faster liquid displacement caused by bulk air passage at the bubble point. It is this more vigorous liquid flow, not difficult to recognize with some experience, that is taken to be the bubble point indicator.

3.8 Effect of Temperature

Hofmann (1984) discussed the effect of temperature on the bubble point and diffusive airflow values. A 10°C temperature increase was found to translate to a 2% decrease in the bubble point value owing to lower surface tension of the test liquid. The effect of temperature on nitrogen gas diffusion was found to be more complex, depending on two factors, the solubility of the gas in the liquid and the diffusion coefficient of the gas. The solubility of gas in liquid decreases with increases in temperature. The reverse is true for the diffusion coefficient, a quantity that reflects the viscosity of the liquid, which decreases with temperature. Below 60°C, nitrogen gas diffusion increases with decreasing liquid viscosity at a faster rate than does the solubility of the nitrogen in the solution. The result is an overall increase in diffusion as temper-

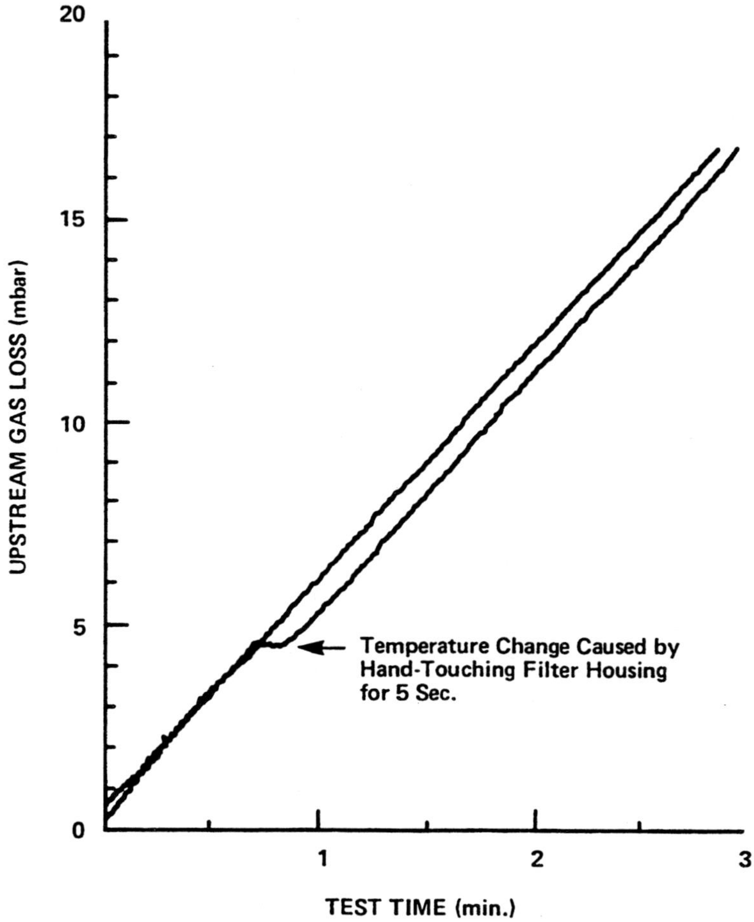

Figure 8 Temperature effect on diffusion point sensitivity. [From Hofmann (1984).]

ature increases, until the 60°C level is attained. Above 160°C, gas diffusion decreases with increases in temperature because the solubility of nitrogen gas in the liquid decreases more rapidly than does the liquid viscosity and the value of the diffusion coefficient it occasions. The upshot is that the integrity tests should be run within the temperature range (20–25°C) recommended by the filter manufacturers. Temperature deviations are possible, provided they are maintained for the duration of the test, but need to be correlated to the allowable limit values, at 20°C, given by the filter manufacturers.

An upstream pressure change caused by temperature can be calculated:

$$\Delta P = \frac{(P_{test} + P_{atm})(T_t - T_0)}{T_0}$$

where

ΔP = upstream pressure change (mbar)
P_{test} = diffusion test pressure (mbar)
P_{atm} = atmospheric pressure (mbar)
T_0 = absolute temperature (K) at time 0
T_t = absolute temperature (K) after time t

A temperature change in the system from 20 to 21°C (68 to 70°F) at a test pressure of 40 psi (2.7 bar) results in a pressure change of 12.7 mbar, a significant quantity.

Figure 8 (Hofmann, 1984) illustrates the temperature effect on pressure change that was caused simply by hand-touching a 10 in. (25.4 cm) sanitary test housing for about 5 s.

3.9 Polymer Contribution to Bubble Point Values

It is generally comprehended that microporous membranes composed of a given polymeric material will exhibit different bubble point values according to the liquid used. As described by Meltzer (1987), not only the changes in surface tension of different wetting media but also the interactions of the media with the different polymers of membranes have an influence on the bubble point measurement. The cosine of the wetting angle, cos θ, changes with the change in the membrane polymer and/or the wetting medium, owing to differences in the solid–liquid interactions, i.e., the work of adhesion. Therefore, since the bubble point test values reflect the invisible combination of both solid and wetting liquid, one can neither arbitrarily set a standard bubble point test liquid to characterize all membranes nor regard the resulting bubble point test value as an independent parameter for the purpose of characterizing the filter performance of all membranes.

4 BUBBLE POINT MEASUREMENT

4.1 Bubble Point Measurement Protocol

It is evident that there are numerous ways in which the manual bubble point measurement is conducted. As remarked earlier, however, the numbers obtained have significance only in that they have been shown, *specifically for that type of filter*, to correlate with the completeness of organism retention (Pall and Kirnbauer, 1978). The bubble point protocol employed by filter users must therefore imitate exactly the procedure practiced in establishing the correlation. Where the data establishing the relationship of organism retention and bubble point values derive from filter manufacturer efforts, the manufacturer's procedure for bubble point determinations should be followed.

It is possible to recommend a manual bubble point measurement protocol (see Table 2):

1. Observe the filter manufacturer's directions.
2. Flush the filter to wet it thoroughly, in accordance with the manufacturer's recommendations. Flushing adequacy should also address the removal of extractables, as stated by the USP 23 (1995).

3. Raise pressure quickly to just below the expected bubble point, and follow with an interval of waiting to permit equilibration of the liquid flow at that pressure.
4. Thereafter raise the pressure progressively to the end point in 1 psi increments, and wait for equilibration of the liquid flow after each pressure boost (approximately 30 s).
5. The end point to be observed is an equilibrated liquid flow that is more vigorous than its predecessors at the lower pressure settings followed by a steady stream of bubbles.

Table 2 Procedure for Performing Manual Bubble Point Measurements

1.0 *Purpose*

To establish filter integrity and define pore size.

2.0 *Materials*

- 2.1 Regulated clean, dry compressed gas
- 2.2 Diluent: Water for injection, absolute alcohol, or as appropriate for application and product to be filtered
- 2.3 Calibrated pressure gauge, 0–60 psig
- 2.4 Tubing
- 2.5 "Y" connector
- 2.6 Collection vessel
- 2.7 Hose clamps
- 2.8 Tubing clamp or valve
- 2.9 Filter assembly

3.0 *Method*

- 3.1 Assemble the test apparatus per the accompanying diagram.
- 3.2 Close the gas supply line and product transfer line.
- 3.3 Initiate diluent flow through the filter to the bubble point line at a rate of approximately 2 mL/cm^2 area at low pressure [2 L/(min. ft^2), 0.5 gpm/ft^2, 2.5 gpm/5 ft^2 cartridge).
- 3.4 Open the vent of the housing to allow displacement of all discharged air. Close the vent when fluid flows through the vent.
- 3.5 Flush the filter with at least 10 mL/cm^2 area (10 L/ft^2, 2.5 gal/ft^2, 12.5 gal/5 ft^2 cartridge to ensure complete wetting.
- 3.6 Turn off the diluent flow and open the gas supply source.
- 3.7 Pressurize the filter assembly to 5 psi. Fluid will flow initially as the gas displaces the diluent in the housing. When fluid flow stops, hold the pressure for 1/2 min and observe the bubble point line for continuous bubbling. This will verify the integrity of the seals.
- 3.8 If bubbles are not observed, increase the pressure at a rate of 10 psi/min up to 50% of the bubble point value. Hold the pressure for 1/2 min again, observing for continuous bubbling in the collection vessel.
- 3.9 Increase the pressure to 80% of the bubble point at a rate of 10 psi/min. Hold for 1/2 min and observe for continuous bubbling.
- 3.10 Increase the pressure up to the bubble point value at 10 psi/min. Hold for 1/2 min and observe for continuous bubbling. If continuous bubbling is not observed, increase the pressure until the actual bubble point is seen.

4.2 Manufacturer's Bubble Point

Discussions of the bubble point necessarily focus on its definition and its measurement. The bubble point probing of significance to the user of a commercial filter, however, is not necessarily the intrinsic bubble point elucidation of a particular filter but rather the "bubble point" value determined by the filter manufacturer to correlate with reliable total organism retention. In any case, filter manufacturers do not necessarily list as the minimum acceptable bubble point the intrinsic bubble point values of filters but rather levels that provide a margin of safety.

The price to be paid for this margin of safety as contributed by "tighter" filters is some reduction in the rate of flow. Manufacturers of filters that exhibit enhanced rates of flow, as of thinner or anisotropic membranes, are obviously at an advantage in this regard, although they generally exhibit lower bubble point values. Membranes of such structures can be tightened to give a margin of safety to their degree of retention while remaining competitive in flow characteristics.

The manufacturer's stipulated bubble point value is uncomplicatedly free of intimations that it relates to any particular pore size measurement, whether 0.2 μm or whatever. It emphasizes the correlation of the bubble point value with the desired certainty of organism retention, as exemplified by the removal of *P. diminuta* from liquid suspensions. It implies that higher bubble point values may be required to certify the filtrative retention of smaller organisms.

Advanced by the filter manufacturer as a value that correlates with a particular level of organism removal, the bubble point value bespeaks dependable validation work rather than the elucidation of an elusive break in an air passage curve.

Freed from the need to precisely define the onset of viscous airflow through a wetted filter, membrane manufacturers could, by offering filters that exceed their recommended bubble point values by as little as 1 psi, enable filter users to integrity test them by the speedy technique of rapidly bringing the air pressure to that minimum to see whether or not air passes in an uncomplicated go/no-go type of test.

Underlying the manufacturer's recommended minimum bubble point value is its correlation with organism retention, as in conformity with the HIMA standard, for instance. It bears repeating that a membrane filter should not be used until it has been ascertained that such a correlation does indeed exist. A critical examination of the correlative data should be made prior to the user accepting or undertaking validation of the filter.

4.3 Rating of Membranes by Bubble Point

Membrane comparisons on the basis of bubble point magnitudes have value to membrane manufacturers who use this measurement as an index of manufacturing control. It bears repeating, however, that the practice of rating membrane filters by the similarity of their bubble points is a technical absurdity when extended to prognostications of similarities in terms of flow characteristics or particle retentions. These latter performance characteristics reflect the pore shapes and sizes and their distributions. These find indistinct revelations in the bubble point.

4.4 Effects of Pore Size Distribution

When the differential air pressure applied to a wetted filter is sufficient to vacate its set of largest pores, the bubble point is reached. That point marks the convergence of the diffusive airflow, soon to be discussed, with the bulk or viscous airflow. Each of these flows is characterized by rates that are straight line with respect to the differential pressure, albeit of much different slopes. It might be expected, therefore, that their point of intersection would be sharp. Such, however, is seldom the case.

After the set of largest pores has been vacated of liquid, the succeeding sets of next smaller pores sequentially follow, resulting in progressively larger rates of airflow. However, the air pressure increments required for these successive pore openings are small. Therefore, the line describing the airflow rates through the consecutively vacating pores as a function of increasing differential pressure is curved. The arc of the curve reflects the pore size distribution of the filter. Pall and Kirnbauer (1978) report obtaining for a nylon 66 membrane a plot of airflow rate versus differential pressure wherein the straight lines representing the diffusive airflow and the bulk airflow meet so sharply as to almost form a point, a consequence of the narrow pore size distribution of that filter. Usually, however, the pore size distribution produces a curve of wider latitude. The line curves upward from the bubble point and becomes linear only after all the pores are blown dry. As will be seen, the diffusion curve that joins at the bubble point is also curved. Therefore, the bubble *point* usually lies on a curve, a reach wherein the accuracy of measurement is of necessity clouded by the rapid change in the slope of the line. These curves can be accurately measured by automated test machines using the multipoint diffusion test, as described by Waibel et al. (1996).

5 DIFFUSIVE AIRFLOW

The bubble point is also obscure because, lying at the confluence of the diffusive airflow and the viscous airflow, the true magnitude of the latter is inevitably masked by contributions from the former. Hofmann (1984) points out that while both diffusive and bulk airflow lines are linear with respect to the applied differential pressure for most experimental experiences, bulk or viscous airflow is actually a nonlinear function. It is proportional to the product of differential pressure and the ratio of absolute upstream pressure to absolute downstream pressure. The diffusive airflow is linearly reflective of the applied differential pressure in that the latter causes the pressure-dependent gas solubility whose concentration gradient across the membrane is the cause of the diffusive airflow.

The air pressure applied to the wet membrane in the search for the bubble point serves to dissolve air in the liquid layer in accordance with Henry's law, which states that the amount of gas dissolved in a liquid is a function of the partial pressure of that gas above it. The dissolved air is in a true state of solution, individual molecules of the gas(es) being dispersed among the molecules of liquid. Different regions of this solution interface regimens of dissimilar differential pressure, however. On one side, the solution of air in liquid is confronted by the high in-line pressure. On the other side of the membrane it faces the weaker downside pressure. This defines the total transmembrane pressure. However, a decrease in the applied differential pressure is progressively sustained by the successive layers of the solution of air in liquid throughout the entire thickness of the membrane. Therefore, as dictated by Henry's law, the air becomes less and less soluble in the liquid regions as these come to be positioned nearer the downstream surface of the membrane. Increasingly released from solution by the progressive decrease in differential pressure throughout the membrane's depth, the molecules constituting the air emerge in their gaseous state to form bubbles, microquantities of bulk air. The rate of such air diffusion, following Fick's law, is a direct function of the applied differential pressure, as shown by the left part of the curve in Fig. 9. The rate of diffusive airflow is quite low compared to the rate of bulk airflow through pores emptied of water, as on the right side of the curve of Figs. 9 and 10. However, at the higher differential pressure levels, and for larger areas of filter, it can be enough to obfuscate the true beginnings of the

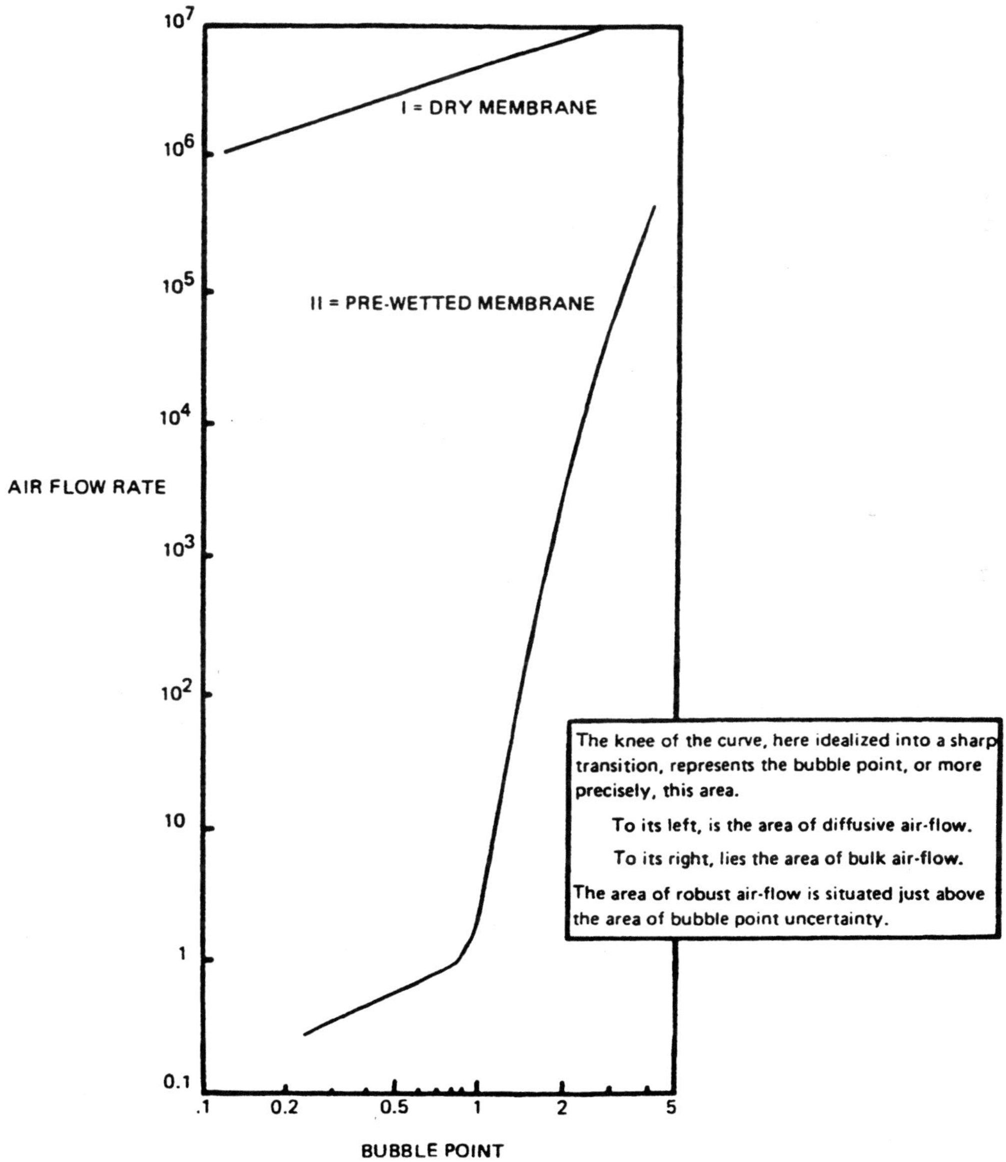

Figure 9 Airflow versus applied differential pressure. [From Johnston and Meltzer (1980).]

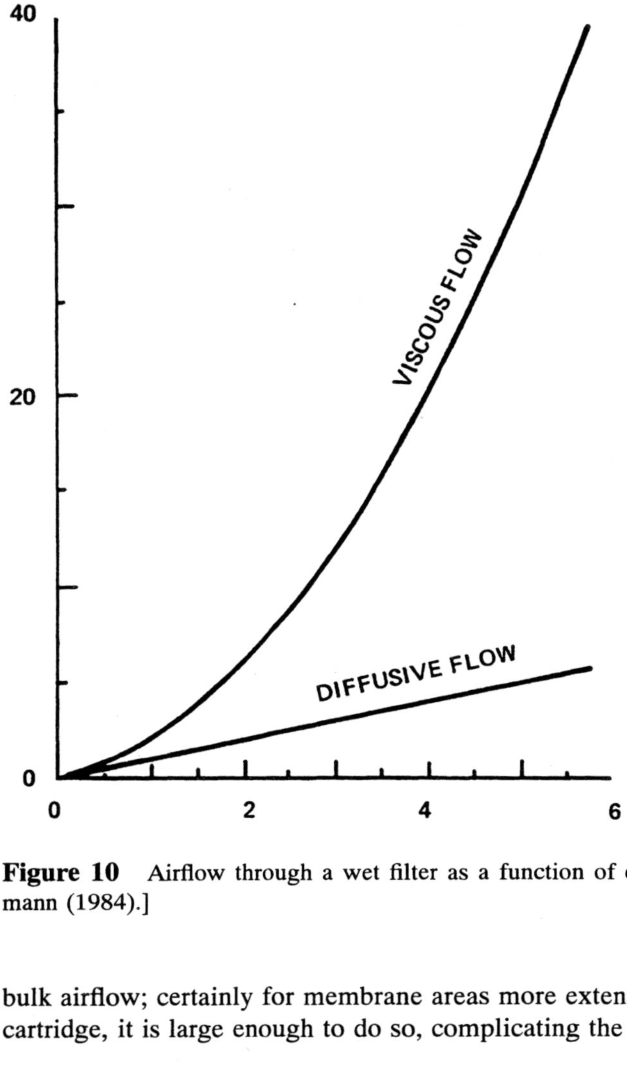

Figure 10 Airflow through a wet filter as a function of differential pressure. [From Hofmann (1984).]

bulk airflow; certainly for membrane areas more extensive than that of a 10 in. filter cartridge, it is large enough to do so, complicating the detection of the bubble point.

5.1 Effects of Diffusive Airflow

As stated, for large area filters, the diffusive airflow may serve to mask the bubble point, the beginning of viscous airflow. Hofmann (1984) quantifies the effect. When larger filter areas are involved, the increasing contribution of gas diffusion diminishes the contribution of the viscous flow to the total airflow. Thus, determination of the bubble point of a 47 mm disk is not complicated by diffusive airflow. The bubble point will involve gas flows of about 20–50 μL/min. If the diameter of the downstream tubing is 2 mm, the linear gas test flow within the tubing will be 6–16 mm/min. To achieve the same 20–50 μL/min sensitivity with a 296 mm disk or with a 10 in. (24.9 cm) cartridge (both of 0.2 μm rating) would require that the observer detect this small viscous airflow in addition to diffusive airflows of 1.5 and 12 mL/min, respectively.

Be that as it may, in actual plant operations it is found possible to integrity test by bubble point multicartridge assemblies [seven rounds, each 20 in. (50 cm) high, having a bubble point of 45 psi (3 bar)] without noticeable interference from air diffusion. The air pressure is increased to the bubble point value in 5 psi (0.33 bar) increments over a period of 1 min, allowing too little time for diffusional influences. Again a multipoint diffusion test with an automatic tester, which checks the diffusive flow across the liquid layer in the membrane matrix at different test pressures, can detect a clear bubble point, due to the automated and defined steps of measurement. The resulting graphic, printed by the test machine, will show the higher diffusive flow values due to the increased filtration area, but also the clear beginning of bulk flow.

5.2 Diffusive Airflow as an Indicator of Integrity

The wetted membrane provides, in effect, a liquid layer across which the diffusive airflow occurs in accordance with Fick's law of diffusion. In an experimental elucidation of the factors involved in the process, Reti (1977) simplified the integrated form of Fick's law to read

$$N = \frac{DH(p^1 - p^2)}{L} \times \rho$$

where N is the permeation rate (moles of gas per unit time), D is the diffusivity of the gas in the liquid, H is the solubility coefficient of the gas, L is the thickness of liquid in the membrane (equal to the membrane thickness if the membrane pores are completely filled with liquid), P is the transmembrane pressure, and ρ is the void volume of the membrane, its membrane porosity (its effective permeation area divided by the tortuosity factor of its pores, in the conventional view; the liquid pathway through the contiguous polyhedra and their interconnecting apertures, in the Williams view).

It should be noted that the sizes of the pores do not enter into the equation; in their aggregate they comprise L, the thickness of the liquid layer, the membrane being some 80% porous. The appearance of a flaw, in effect a joining of smaller pores already extant, would not increase the thickness of this liquid layer. Nevertheless, at the bubble point pressure, the larger opening would become revealed. Such a large pore could manifest its presence in another way. It could result in a larger diffusive airflow because at elevated pressures (but still below that sufficient to cause bulk airflow, i.e., below the true bubble point), the liquid layer within that large pore might thin to provide a lesser impediment to diffusion. The shape of the void might be important. Consider it to be, at least roughly, funnel-shaped, with its larger diameter upstream. The pressure would cause liquid to flow out of the funnel, narrowing the liquid layer, until a smaller diameter corresponding to the applied differential pressure was reached. At that point, further flow would cease until the bubble point of that narrower diameter was exceeded. Actually, the liquid height in that larger pore or flaw would subside progressively as the applied air pressure mounted. Were the funnel shape to be reversed, the pore would retain its full complement of liquid until the pressure exceeded the bubble point level of its smaller upstream diameter (Fig. 11).

Such partial emptying of larger pores would detract from the linearity of the diffusive airflow rate expected of the unflawed membrane with its uniform liquid thickness, for diffusive airflow through the thinner water layers would be greater.

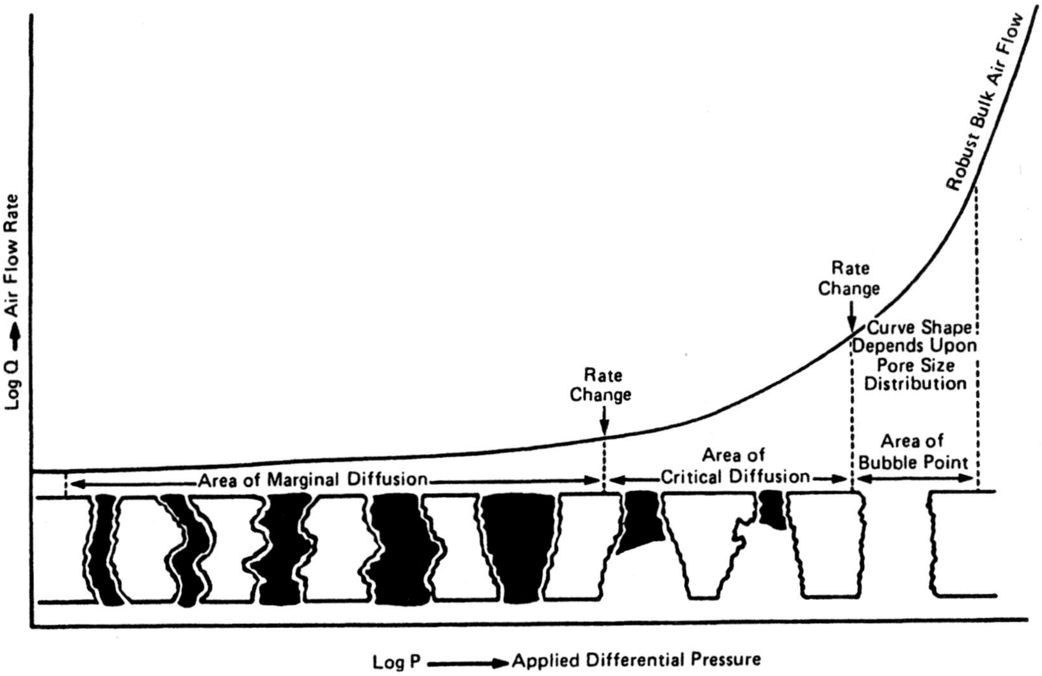

Figure 11 Rate of airflow through a wetted filter.

Thinning of the liquid layers commences only near the bubble point. Reti (1977) estimates that at 80% of the bubble point value, the diffusive airflow is still linear. But the diffusive airflow line begins to curve before the bubble point is reached. Therefore, if membrane filters are measured for diffusive airflows at pressure levels some 20% below their bubble points, they should yield that volume of the air per unit time that would reflect Fickian diffusion across a uniform water layer thickness at that transmembrane pressure. The line would be straight. Higher volumes of diffused air would signal a departure from linearity as caused by liquid thinning in pores larger than the filter is supposed to have.

Diffusive airflow tests intended to distinguish between membranes of different pore size ratings should be conducted at pressures between the corresponding bubble points. Membrane manufacturers recommend different test pressures because of the different bubble point values of the different polymers used.

A filter element that shows less diffusion will not necessarily retain better. It may mean only that this filter element contains less membrane area or that the membrane has a reduced total porosity or that it is thicker than stated.

As in bubble–point measurement, the numbers obtained from diffusive airflow tests have significance only because they can be correlated with organism retention. The measurements are usually stipulated to be performed at some minimum pressure that was used in securing the correlation, usually at 80% of the bubble point value.

The diffusive airflow integrity test does not measure air diffusion solely through the set of largest pores present or through a single flaw. Rather, it measures the flow diffused through all the available pores.

5.3 Effects of Membrane Anisotropy

The "funnel-shaped" pores that are the cause of enhanced flow properties also exaggerate the effects that applied pressures below the bubble point have on the diffusive airflow rate as a result of thinning the liquid layers resident within these pores. By definition, the bubble point lies at the nexus of the diffusive airflow and bulk airflow curves. Membrane anisotropy with its attendant water-layer thinning bestows a more generous arc to the diffusive airflow curve, causing it to meet the bulk airflow curve, still at the same invariant bubble point but at an airflow level that alters the perceived bubble point value (Fig. 12). In other words, for anisotropic membranes, the higher rates of diffusion sufficiently alter the perceived bubble point as to mask the intrinsic bubble point with a falsely lower value.

For those accustomed to conventional membranes, the bubble point and diffusive airflow testing of anisotropic filters bring uncommon test values that for conventional membranes would be indicative of integrity failures. Nevertheless, the integrity test numbers for these types of filters do correlate with organism retention experience. Those who refrain from the use of anisotropic filters on the basis of feelings of insecurity induced by the unaccustomed low bubble point or high diffusive airflow values forego unnecessarily the processing advantages of these filters.

Anisotropic membranes have heightened possibilities for departures from the linearity of their air diffusion curves because their "funnel"-shaped pores predispose toward thinning of their occluded liquid layer. The knee regions of the curves de-

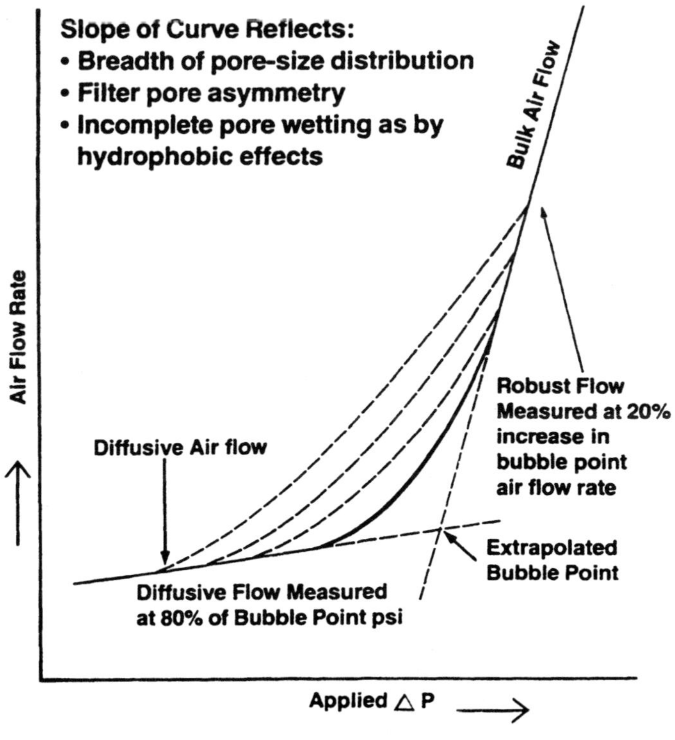

Figure 12 Air passage through wetted membranes; influence of anisotropy.

scribing air passage by such filters are therefore notably extended. Here the multipoint diffusion test can be a valuable help in integrity testing such membranes reliably. At least one manufacturer of anisotropic filters constructs cartridges to contain repetitive membrane in a back-to-back posture so that the downstream filter is positioned with its smallest pores upstream. In this arrangement, the cartridge exhibits the diffusive air permeation characteristics normal to nonanisotropic membranes. However, some of the flow advantage offered by the anisotropic structure is lost thereby.

The first microporous membranes were usually in the form of flat disks of diameters up to 293 mm. Their integrity could usually be determined unambiguously by way of bubble point determinations, measurements whose magnitude had been correlated to organism retentions in terms of log reduction values (LRVs). When, however, the effective filtration area of the microporous membrane came to exceed that of the 293 mm disk, as in the case of pleated cartridges, it was found that the flow of air diffusing across the filter obfuscated the clarity of the bubble point (Reti et al., 1979). Correlations were developed between the diffusive airflows and organism retention values, permitting the former to serve as surrogates for the latter and allowing the diffusive airflow measurement to be used as an integrity test.

5.4 Interfering Diffusive Airflows

Whether the diffusive airflow given by a filter interferes with the accurate determinations of the filter's bubble point depends on the effective filtration area of the filter and the length of time necessary to arrive at the bubble point. During the progressive pressure increases on the way to the bubble point, diffusive airflow will be taking place. If in the interval over which the bubble point is reached enough air becomes diffused to substantially match the free airflow at the bubble point, the latter determination becomes uncertain. This effect becomes more noticeable when liquids of lower surface tension, such as solvent–water mixtures, are involved. Generally, the diffusive airflows from 10 in. cartridges begin to interfere significantly with the bubble point as it is commonly run. However, even multiple 10 in. cartridges can be and are successfully bubble point tested provided the pressure is rapidly brought to just below the minimum allowable bubble point (as previously correlated to the HIMA bacterial retention test) and then carefully, but not leisurely, raised to the actual bubble point. There are limits even to this helpful technique. At some point the area of the filter is sufficiently large to provide diffusive airflows that will interfere with the bubble point regardless of how expeditiously the test is performed. The relevant area will differ for different filters and has therefore not been defined.

Consider a 10 in. cartridge with a diffusive airflow of 15 mL/min. At its bubble point it will have a certain free airflow far in excess of 15 mL/min, perhaps about 540 mL/min. Three such cartridges joined into one 30 in. assembly would have a diffusive airflow of 45 mL/min but the same free airflow at the bubble point, namely, about 540 mL/min if only a single section were involved. An assembly of three 30 in. cartridges would have a diffusive airflow of about 136 mL/min and free airflow at the bubble point of 540 mL/min or so. (If the bubble point is simultaneously reached at more than a single cartridge, the airflow would be proportionately greater.) The difference between 135 and 540 mL/min is large enough not to confuse the two different airflows provided the time to reach the bubble point is minimized. If, however, it takes 4–5 min to reach the bubble point, then the diffusive airflow will not be distinguishable from the bubble point because the total diffusive airflow and the free airflow (at the bubble point) will be equal. The latter will be confused by the former. An assembly of twelve 30 in. cartridges will have a diffusive airflow of 540 mL/min. No matter how fast the bubble point is determined, it will be interfered with by the diffusive airflow emanating from the filter arrangement.

There is, therefore, occasion to use either the bubble point or the diffusive airflow or both in characterizing the integrity of filters, depending on the circumstances.

5.5 Preference for Bubble Point or Diffusive Airflow

There can be a legitimate preference for the bubble point integrity test over the diffusive airflow method in situations where either can be performed. The bubble point test does relate to the size of the largest pores present in the filter. The implications for the retention of particles, viable or otherwise, are direct. The diffusive airflow measurement reflects a filter's total porosity, however, not just the largest pores. Its implication for organism retention is solely by way of empirically defined correlations. There are those who hold, however, that bubble point readings usually overstate their actual pressure levels by being performed too rapidly, causing them to appear better than they are. Then, too, there is the possibility of inexactness caused by diffusive airflow interference, depending on how the bubble point is actually performed.

In the bubble point determination, air comes to flow through the largest pores of the filter. It is possible that, as has been alleged, in some instances and with certain filters this may result in a drying out of the pore passageways, making it difficult to rewet the pore surfaces. This may cause failures in succeeding bubble point measurements. In other instances it is possible that the membrane can be damaged due to the pressure required to perform a bubble point measurement over a single emptied pore. Diffusive airflow determinations may be preferred for any such reasons.

5.6 Single-Point Testing

The precise bubble point (Fig. 2) lies somewhere on the curved portion of the line joining the diffusive airflow to the frank or viscous airflow. At a certain moment, before the bubble point, the rate of diffusive airflow increases due to thinning of the water layer in asymmetrically shaped pores (Reti, 1978). Beyond the bubble point, the rate of air passage continues to rise as the progressively increasing pressure causes succeedingly smaller pores to become emptied of water. The inherent bubble point need not be defined with the greatest exactitude because the perceived bubble point is correlated with the necessary organism retention experience (Johnston and Meltzer, 1979).

In determining the diffusive airflow, however, care is taken not to perform measurements in the region of the curved line. Measurements falling on curved lines are less reliably reproduced. They are therefore avoided if possible. Single-point diffusive airflow determinations are usually performed at about 80% of the bubble point pressure level.

Test at 80% of the Bubble Point Value

The convenience of single-point diffusive airflow integrity testing has its advantages. It has its utility in proper settings. However, as previously stated, testing at 80% of the bubble point, as at any level lower than the bubble point, leaves the region above the test point, between it and the bubble point, untested, so the integrity of that region is not ensured.

In those cases where the diffusive airflow line extends straight and unbroken to the bubble point, there is a correlation between the bubble point and the diffusive airflows measured at any pressure, however low. This correlation extends also to the implications of organism retention as defined by the bubble point. What is not made certain at lower test pressures, however, is that the undefined portion of the diffusive airflow line extends unbroken beyond the test pressure to the bubble point. It is for this very reason that forward flow (diffusive airflow) testing, initially performed at lower pressures, underwent procedural modifications calling for testing at 80% of the bubble point.

This means, however, that the certainty of integrity testing by diffusive airflows cannot be ensured beyond the point generally tested, i.e., at 80% of the bubble point. This is analogous to testing a filter's bubble point to only 80% of its expected value and concluding that the filter is integral.

Filter integrity measured to 80% of the bubble point level is usually assumed to extend to the unassayed remaining 20%. Actually, the most that can be claimed for a filter that passes a responsibly tight diffusive airflow specification is that its bubble point is, to some undetermined extent, above the pressure selected for the diffusive airflow test. Precisely to eliminate this area of uncertainty, multipoint diffusive airflow testing through the bubble point is advocated. Nevertheless, testing is and has long been performed at this single level. Generally, the results do correlate with the HIMA challenge value. The history is a positive one.

There are those who argue, in favor of single-point testing, that a ''filter that has passed a bacterial challenge test will pass a 'diffusive airflow' test, and that a filter that has failed a bacterial challenge test will fail a 'diffusive airflow' integrity test'' (Haughney, 1992). The truth of that statement reflects favorably, however, on the process control of filter manufacturing, not on the revelations imparted by the integrity testing. The argument is reversed in its logic. It is the constancy of the integrity test values that attests to the uniformity of filter manufacture. That sameness of manufacture may not be assumed. It is the very purpose of integrity testing to affirm that constancy in the case of the particular filter being examined. Those who *assume* that single-point testing to the 80% level of the bubble point leads to safe conclusion may, however, be justified by experience dependent on reliable manufacturing practices.

Limitations of Single-Point Diffusive Airflow Testing

In an effort to provide a safety margin, filter manufacturers may provide cartridges that have diffusive airflows of less than the maximum acceptable rate, say 15 mL/min at the given test pressure. Consider an assembly of nine 10 in. cartridges. Assume that eight of these elements have acceptable diffusive airflows of 10 mL/min but the ninth one, lacking integrity, has a diffusional airflow rate of 55 mL/min. The total diffusive airflow rate for the nine-element assembly would be 135 mL/min, undistinguishable from the 135 mL/min expected for the integral nine 10 in. cartridge arrangement. A single-point diffusive airflow determination would not reveal the presence of the flawed cartridge. However, multipoint diffusive testing, as shown in Fig. 3, could make evident a single filter's flaw even within a multielement arrangement (Waibel et al., 1996). The rate of flow differs with pressure and also as the fourth power of the pore radius. Therefore, at higher pressure levels the flows through the flaw would increase markedly. If, consequently, the diffusive airflows are plotted from multipoint pressure data, the rate of climb of the resulting curve may reveal what a single point cannot.

In diffusive airflow integrity testing, a filter is judged integral if its diffusive flow rate does not exceed the manufacturer's specified maximum values. If, however, the diffusive airflow measurement is at a higher level, it is judged to be a failed membrane; the higher rate of air passage is assumed to be due to a departure from linearity caused by the effect of larger pores, presumably at or near the bubble point. A lower diffusive airflow rate is taken as indicating an acceptable filter, one not characterized by oversized pores or flaws.

To be sure, for gross filter damage, the damaged area would typically not be limited to a small area or small number of pores but to a significant portion of the filter. This damaged area would exhibit higher diffusive flow compared with the initial observations.

The diffusive airflow rate is a function of the filter's total porosity. This may certainly undergo change as the filter becomes at least partially clogged and blocked by particle accretion. In effect, therefore, one is dealing with different filters in the pre- and postfiltration contexts in terms of total porosities. The diffusive airflow rates as a function of applied pressure require experimental definition for each of these filters within each of these contexts. A single measurement point is incapable of such definition. Multipoint measurements should be made before and after filtration, particularly for filters with long service lives such as those used in sterile venting or water system applications.

Once the proper diffusion curve limit is defined by multipoint testing, as in a validation exercise, the reliability of the single-point diffusive airflow becomes established. It is then safe to depend on single-point diffusive airflow measurements in the production context.

When a drug product is used to wet the filter, the bubble point will change, usually decreasing, due to the difference in the surface tension of that product compared to that of water. Consequently, 80% of the bubble point level when water is the wetting fluid may represent a different level when product is used as the wetting liquid. The product-specific bubble point value has undergone a shift from the water bubble point because of the surface tension effect and possible changes in the angle of wetting (Parker, 1986; Tröger and Kolmann, 1988; Desaulniers and Fey, 1990). A simple numerical displacement may not, however, be assumed in deriving the single-point diffusive airflow. The diffusive airflow displacement not only reflects the shift in bubble point occasioned by the liquid's surface tension but may also be raised or lowered by the solubility of air (or nitrogen, where this is used) in the product compared to that in water. Product-specific values are involved. It may be that in any given case the factors other than surface tension that influence the diffusive airflow displacement are minor. Indeed, that is *assumed* by one filter manufacturer, who therefore assigns the diffusive airflow level for the drug product the same value it has for water. Given the more complex influences on the diffusive airflow, as compared to the bubble point, such assumptions, albeit convenient, may not be prudent where judgments regarding filter integrity are at stake. These influences are generally due to the complex nature of the drug product where the solubility of the test gas into and out of the drug product, coupled with the diffusivity of the test gas in the drug product, will have an effect on the diffusive flow characteristics during the integrity test.

Definition can be achieved by determining the actual slope of the diffusive airflow portion of the air permeation curve, using the drug product and multipoint diffusion testing. This would unambiguously establish the correct level of the diffusive airflow (Fig. 11).

To determine the appropriate single-point diffusive flow integrity test limit to be used as a routine test for membrane filters wetted with drug product in the production setting would require conducting the appropriate validation testing. The validation of this integrity test limit would follow a pattern similar to the determination of the minimum required bubble point. The basic principle is to test filters of three different lots wetted with water. By performing the multipoint diffusion profile and determining the water-wetted bubble point for this filter, one obtains a baseline value for the integrity test results for the given filter membrane. Subsequently removing the water from the filters and wetting them with the drug product in question will allow one to determine the corresponding multipoint diffusion profile and product-specific bubble point for the given test filters wetted with drug.

The product-specific minimum required bubble point, as previously discussed, relates importantly to the differences in surface tension between water and the product in question. This product minimum can easily be calculated from a ratio. Using 80% of this test pressure to perform a single-point diffusion test is of limited use. Although this will be the value that is used for the test pressure in the case of the single-point diffusion test, the actual maximum allowable diffusion test limit is still unknown. Because of the differences in the solubility of the test gas in water and in the drug product coupled to the diffusivity of the test gas in the liquid, the actual maximum allowable limit for diffusion at the 80% of bubble point test pressure needs to be evaluated. In contrast to the bubble point, where the single factor of surface tension and the subsequent ratio to water can be used to validate the product-specific test limit, the characterization of the maximum allowable diffusion test at the 80% test pressure must be validated. Simply using 80% as the test pressure and the maximum allowable diffusion limit for membranes wetted with water does not take into account the differences with respect to diffusive gas flow of the product. By examining the multipoint diffusion profile, one can determine if the product, at the product-specific test pressure, has higher or lower diffusion than the same test filter wetted with water and tested at the pressure required for water diffusive airflow testing.

It is only through such a validation exercise that one can determine the minimum product bubble point limit and the true value for a single-point diffusive airflow test at a pressure of 80% of that "new" bubble point test limit.

5.7 Advantages of Diffusive Airflow Testing

Microporous membranes may have pore sizes that are so small, generally less than 0.1 μm rating, that the applied pressures necessary to determine their bubble point may be too great for the filter construction or membrane to withstand. Where such applied pressures may damage the filter's retentive properties, diffusive airflow measurements are indicated. Similarly, capsule filters and others contained in polymeric shells or housings may not be designed to endure high pressures. Integrity testing these filter devices at the lower pressures involved in diffusive airflow determinations is an acceptable alternative.

As stated, the bubble point reflects only the largest pores; the diffusive airflows mirror the filter's total porosity. It is the latter that figures in the flow of fluids through a filter. Therefore, phenomena reflecting the clean water flow of filters ought better to be revealed by diffusive airflow measurements than by bubble point data. Once again, however, useful intimations of comparative clean water flows would be derived from a comparison of complete diffusive airflow curves, as plotted from multipoint data; single-point comparisons will not serve.

Implications regarding better water flows for filters having higher diffusive airflows should be made with caution. The greater viscosity of liquids (water) compared to air would minimize the effects. More especially, the unelucidated pore size distributions could be very influential, flow being a function of the pore radius to the fourth power. Nevertheless, both diffusion and flows are consequences of total porosity, not just of largest size pores.

Multipoint diffusive airflow testing repeated over a period of time can reveal the progressive involvement of the smaller pores of a filter with wetting and with subsequent water flow. All the pores of a filter do not necessarily wet out all at once; the smaller ones may do so with greater reluctance. Therefore, as a function of time a newly installed filter may exhibit a decreasing diffusive airflow, occasioned by a progressive intrusion of wetting water into previously empty (unblocked) pores. Where this occurs, it becomes revealed by a comparison of the diffusive airflow curves taken over time. The phenomenon has implications for filter wettability and filter flow, but only in contexts where pore blockage by accretions is not taking place. The ongoing periodic determinations of diffusive airflows (involving pores smaller than those detected by bubble point testing) can be used to gauge the completeness of a clean membrane's wetting, the efficacy of wetting adjuncts where used, and changes in the degree of hydrophilicity of the membrane itself.

Periodic multipoint diffusive flow determinations may also be useful where filters are in long-term use, particularly when damage may result in a progressive, subtle manner. A multipoint integrity test could indicate a trend of increasing diffusion over time that might be overlooked with single-point diffusion testing and even through bubble point testing. Take as an example the case of a hydrophobic vent filter cartridge on a water-for-injection tank. If the system is in-line steam-sterilized daily, potentially stressing the filter membranes with each cycle, the filter may eventually lose its integrity and fail both a single-point diffusive airflow test and a bubble point test. The bubble point value in this example may also never quite decrease to the point at which the filter actually loses its integrity. The same may be true for the case of single-point diffusion testing. However, a trend may be elucidated if a reduction in membrane integrity is demonstrated as a function of time and not as a single stressful incident. Better estimates of the service life of these vent filters may be made available through such validation of the filters over their operating service life.

Gross incompatibilities between membranes and fluids may be easy to discern. Subtle effects can be judged by the influence of the medium being filtered on the bubble point of the filter (Lukaszewicz and Meltzer, 1980). Any indication that contact between the filter and fluid tends to enlarge the pores is clear evidence of incompatibility. Diffusive airflow measurements may here offer an even more sensitive indicator of incompatibility than bubble point measurements. The bubble point values reflect the largest pores. Changes in the smaller pores do not become registered. However, the diffusive airflow readings mirror the influences of all the pores (total porosity). Therefore, diffusive airflow measurements indicate potential fluid–filter incompatibilities with greater sensitivity than bubble point determinations alone.

More certain implications for retention based on definition of the largest pores present in a filter may be seen where bubble point testing is possible. Where diffusive airflows interfere with bubble point determinations, the diffusive airflow measurements themselves, correlated to organism retentions, serve as integrity tests.

Diffusive airflow measurements have their advantages in addition to serving as indicators of filter integrity. They can more precisely reveal filter incompatibilities. They can be used to gauge the completeness of a filter's wettability, and they are more revealing of a filter's clean water flow properties.

In almost all its applications, however, diffusive airflow integrity testing requires that the diffusive airflow curve be defined by way of multipoint measurements using the liquid product in question. This is especially true in filter validation contexts where product-specific testing is required.

Once the full diffusional airflow curve has been elucidated, single-point diffusional flow testing is warranted, as in production integrity testing settings. Single-point diffusive flow testing can be used as a standard integrity test method in the pharmaceutical production environment.

5.8 Sensitivity of Diffusive Airflow Tests

Schroeder (1984) proposes to calculate "pessimistic" LRVs from theoretical considerations that apply to wet flow porosimetry. Consider, for example, a sterilizing cartridge that is characterized by an airflow of 10^8 mL/min at 40 psig (2.70 bar). If this filter is to be "validated" at this pressure by the diffusive airflow test (to see whether or not it is integral in accordance with the linearity of its diffusive airflow, as discussed above), then the resulting LRV value will depend on the accuracy with which the diffusive airflow test is performed. Any diffusive airflow values experimentally found that are above the predicted diffusion level can be considered the "error" in the determination. The corresponding "pessimistic" LRV can be calculated:

$$\text{Pessimistic LRV} = \frac{\text{total potential airflow}}{\text{``error'' airflow}}$$

$$= \frac{10 \text{ mL/min}}{\text{airflow above mL/min predicted}}$$

Airflow rate error (mL/s)	"Pessimistic" LRV
None	
0.1	9
1.0	8
10	7
100	6

Every tenfold error in the reading of the diffusive airflow translates to an increase in the uncertainty of the LRV of the filter by one full order of magnitude, a powerful argument for accurate test results.

Encouragingly, an "error" in the diffusion test will not automatically mean that organisms will pass through the filter. It has been remarked that membrane filters perform better than predicted, possibly as a consequence of their Williams structure. However, passage of organisms could well be the result of lack of sensitivity in the test procedure, even to a 10-fold extent.

Johnston and Meltzer (1980) found that for the relationship between bubble point values and organism retention, each 10% decrease in bubble point reading accuracy translates to a "pessimistic" LRV value one order of magnitude less than that inherent in the filter.

6 PRESSURE HOLD TEST

In the performance of the diffusive airflow integrity test, a wetted filter sealed into its housing is subjected to a continuously maintained level of air pressure on its upstream side, and the volume of air that diffuses during a stated time interval is collected and measured. If the housing is improperly sealed, air will leak out. Small leaks may even go undetected, even though they provide opportunities for contaminants to enter into the system. If the pressure level is sufficiently well maintained, which is not too difficult in the case of small leaks, the volume of air collected downstream may not be affected.

The pressure hold test is a variant of the diffusive airflow test. All is arranged as in the diffusion test except that when the stipulated applied pressure is reached, the pressure source is valved off. The decay of pressure within the holder is then observed as a function of time. The decrease in pressure can come from two sources, the first being diffusive loss across the wetted filter. Since the upside pressure in the holder is not maintained, it decreases progressively all the while diffusion takes place. The rate of diffusion is therefore progressively decreasing. As a result, the volume of air collected is less than in the diffusive airflow test. The second source of pressure decay is that caused by faulty filter/housing assembly. Indeed, one virtue of the pressure hold test is that it tests the integrity of the plumbing. That is why it is often used as the initial integrity test. However, the pressure hold measurement can serve as an integrity test only when it correlates the organism retention capabilities of the filter with a precise measure of air pressure diminution.

The pressure hold test measures the loss of air from within the holder that houses the filter(s). The perfect gas law governs the air loss measurement.

$$PV = nRT$$

where n is the moles of gas, R is the universal gas constant, T is temperature, V is gas volume, and P is the gas pressure.

The decrease in gas pressure is influenced strongly by the volume of the filter holder. It depends on the particular holder–filter combination and the exact details of the filter and housing being used. Even the placement of the valve and any tubing volume must be considered, because this can affect the total volume within which the pressure decay takes place. Changing either the filter or the housing necessitates a redetermination of the diffusive airflow loss under the pressure hold conditions, for this may change the total volume surrounding the filter in its housing.

In the semiconductor industry, where integrity tests are used to signal conformation to the filter's specifications (rather than to reflect precise organism retention levels as required by FDA regulations in pharmaceutical processing), the pressure hold test can serve very well, provided that the measurement of the pressure decay is sensitive enough and that a use history is developed for the given holder/filter employed.

As stated, to be an integrity test reflective of a filter's organism retention capabilities, the test measurement, as of pressure decay, must be demonstrably correlated to that property.

Hango et al. (1989) describe the use of the pressure hold method as an integrity test under conditions of having the exact volume of the holder/filter and the relevant diffusive airflow defined by the filter supplier (Fig. 13). Under these circumstances, the pressure decay measured under pressure hold conditions (in the absence of

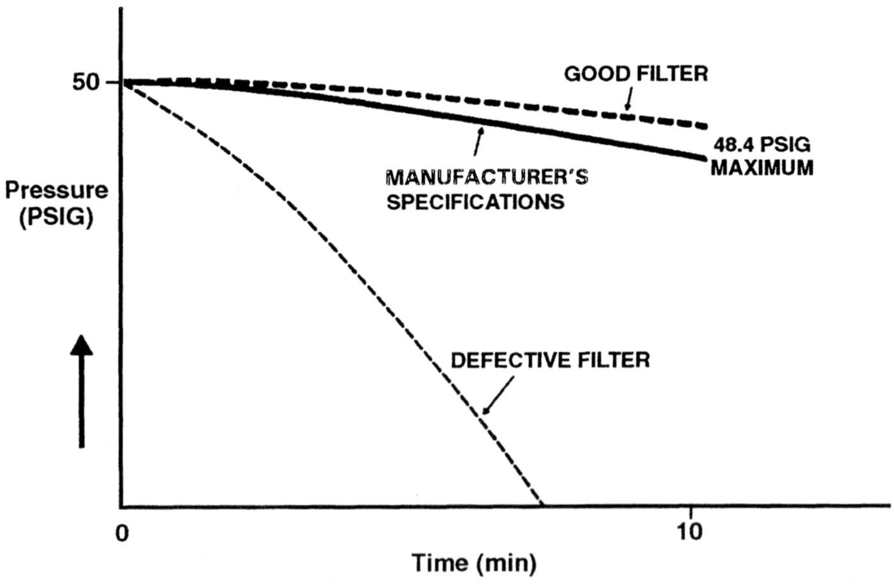

Figure 13 Filter integrity testing; pressure hold. From Hango et al. (1989); courtesy of the Semiconductor Pure Water Conference.

plumbing leaks) can be correlated to ordinary diffusive airflow data that are in turn correlated with specific organism retention values.

The translation of the pressure-hold (decay) curve into the straight line of the diffusive airflow plot that relates to organism retention can be accomplished mathematically. It is, however, automatically performed by the automated test machines designed for integrity testing. Moreover, these devices have the sensitivity essential for detecting the small pressure losses that may be involved.

Determinations of the pressure decays by means of the gauges normally employed in the manual pressure hold tests are woefully inadequate. According to Hofmann (1984), pressure gauges commonly require pressure losses of at least 40 mbar/min in order to record the event. Such a loss in a 10 in. cartridge would be forthcoming from a flaw 50 μm in size (or an aggregate of flaws to that size) at a pressure level of 40 psig. Conventional pressure gauges lack the requisite sensitivity for application to the pressure hold test. Nevertheless, at least one filter manufacturer believes it is adequate to use gauges of 1.5 in. diameter where small volumes are involved. If there are no sealing leaks, the pressure in the housing will decline about 1 psig over a 10 min period. After 20 min, it is to be hoped that such a drop can be noticed even on 1.5 in. gauges. In the event of system leaks, the pressure drops more precipitously. Such small pressure drop readings may be of value in determining whether filter seating or housing O-ring leaks exist. Such readings are too insensitive to reveal much about the filter. Larger diameter gauges would be more useful, but these and their periodic calibration are expensive.

In measuring the pressure losses from the filter housing, it is not necessary to measure the large air volumes (or their water displacements) that are so burdensome to the use of the diffusive airflow test on multicartridge housings. Most of the automated integrity test devices use mass pressure transducers to measure the flow of air into the housings to replace the air lost or else they measure the in-line gas flow. These measurements can be made with great accuracy. Pressure transducers have a sensitivity of ± 1 millibar. That is why the automated instruments have requisite detection sensitivity. Such a sensitivity is required because the pressure hold test, even more than the diffusive airflow method, is strongly influenced by temperature. In the former case, temperature is a factor in the perfect gas law. In the latter, the solubility and diffusivity of the gas (as well as the volume it occupies) are influenced by temperature.

To accommodate the requirement for constant temperature conditions in the pressure hold test, the appropriate automated testers include equipment to determine whether the temperature is within the acceptable range. If it is not, the machine displays a warning.

One advantage of the pressure-hold test is that it is capable of revealing imperfections in the assembly and sealing of the housing and filters and disclosing flaws in the filters. This is particularly useful in initial integrity testing for the early disclosure of filter seating failures or housing sealing leaks, avoiding a profitless undertaking of the filtration in the first place.

A second advantage is that the pressure decay reading central to the pressure hold test can be made on the upstream side of the filter, on the housing itself, without compelling invasion of the downstream side of the system. Aseptic invasions and connections are common; they are successfully made every day. They do, however, portend risk to the system and are best avoided where possible.

The use of automated test devices helps avoid downstream invasions during the performance of the more conventional integrity tests.

7 WATER INTRUSION INTEGRITY TEST

For integrity testing, the hydrophobic vent filter can be wet out with alcohol and an alcohol bubble point test performed. Isopropyl alcohol in 60% aqueous solution or 25% aqueous *tert*-butanol are both satisfactory. The alcohol is then removed by drying prior to the filter being autoclaved. Polysulfone filters may stress-crack under alcohol drying. For such polymers, removal of the alcohol by water flushing is indicated. The sterilized vent filter is then installed aseptically.

It is also possible to define the largest pores of a hydrophobic membrane by the pressure needed to force water into such pores. Obviously, as is known from mercury porosimetry work, for instance, higher pressures are required to force a nonwetting liquid into pores of narrower diameter. Therefore, a measurement of water intrusion into a hydrophobic membrane will reflect the entrance, or incipient entrance, of water into the largest pores of the filter. The upstream side of the hydrophobic filter cartridge housing is flooded with water. Nitrogen gas pressure is then applied by way of an automatic integrity tester to a level of 2.5 bar (36 psig). A period of pressure stabilization takes place over some minutes, during which the cartridge pleats adjust their positions under imposed pressures. After the pressure drop thus occasioned stabilizes, any further pressure drop in the upstream pressurized gas volume, as measured by the automatic tester, signifies a beginning of water intrusion into the largest (hydrophobic) pores, water being incompressible. The automated integrity tester is sensitive enough to detect the pressure drop (Fig. 14). A correlation has been demonstrated between the observed pressure drop and the organism retention characteristic of the hydrophobic membrane (Tarry et al., 1993; Dosmar et al., 1993; and Tingley et al., 1995) (Figs. 14–16). This empirically es-

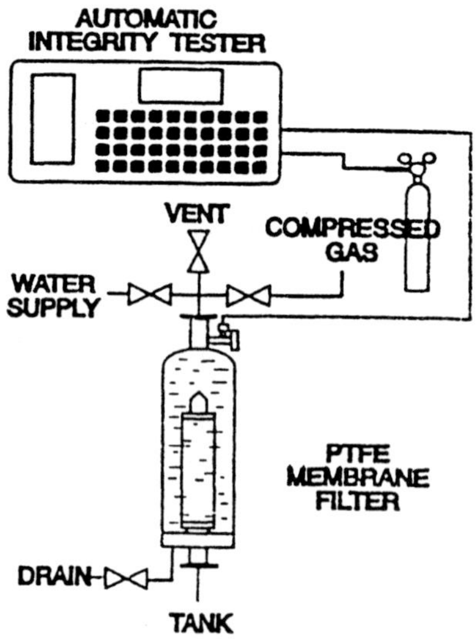

Figure 14 Water intrusion test setup. From Tarry et al. (1993); courtesy of *Ultrapure Water*.

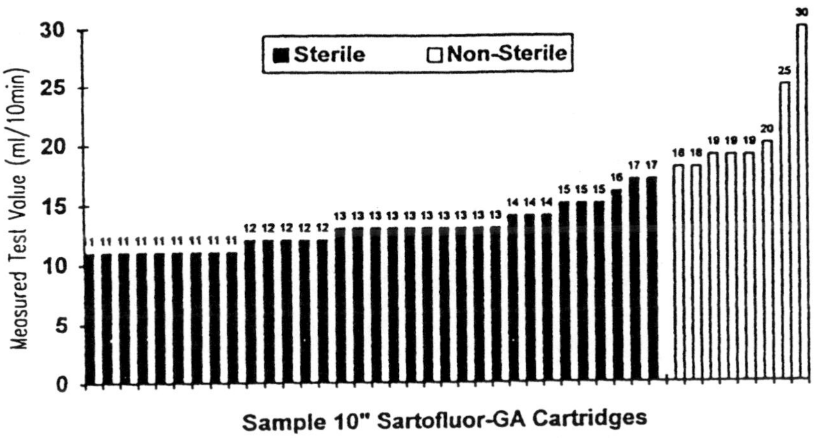

Figure 15 Bacterial challenge correlation in the water intrusion test. From Tarrey et al. (1993); courtesy of *Ultrapure Water*.

tablished correlation serves as the validating authority for the water intrusion test. By way of this procedure, hydrophobic vent filters can be integrity tested in situ without the use of alcoholic solutions and without risk to downstream filter asepsis.

Tingley et al. (1995) confirmed the suitability of the water flow methodology to the in-line testing of hydrophobic filters. These investigators confirmed correlation between their water intrusion point pressures and log reduction values for organism retentions, as shown in Table 3. The test, like other integrity tests, is sensitive to temperature and to the water purity in terms of surface tension. It is, however, less

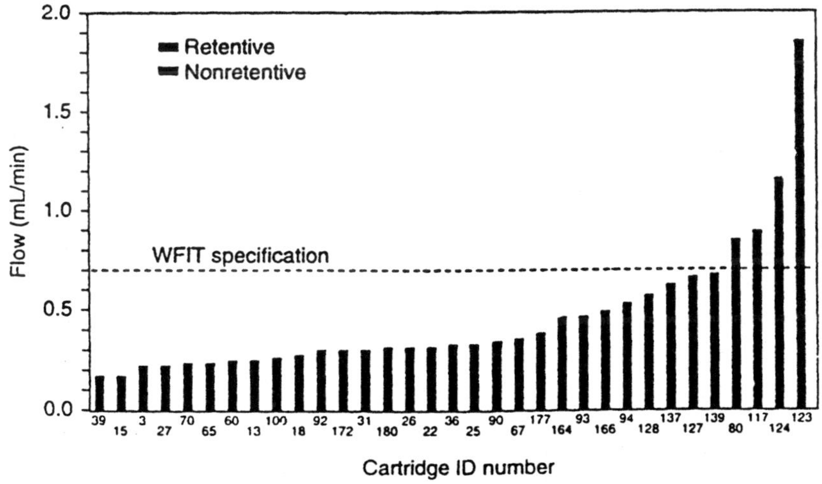

Figure 16 Water flow values correlation to bacterial retention (Aervent cartridges at 38 psi test pressure); test value-LRV correlation achieved with a flow specification of 0.7 mL/min water (Aervent cartridges at 38 psi test pressure). From Tingley et al. (1995); courtesy of *Pharmaceutical Technology*.

Table 3 Retention LRV as a Function of Water Intrusion Pressure[a]

Water intrusion point pressure (psi)	Retention LRV
21.5	9.42
22.5	9.45
23.5	10.0
25.0	10.5
25.5	9.01
27.0	9.81
27.0	10.8
32.5	10.9
32.5	11.3[b]
36.0	11.3[b]
26.0	11.4[b]
37.0	11.3[b]

[a]10 in. Aervent filter cartridges challenged with *P. diminuta* per HIMA methodology.
[b]Sterile effluent.
Source: Tingley et al. (1995).

sensitive to temperature variations than the bubble point and forward-flow (diffusive airflow) measurements because of the large thermal mass represented by the water in the housing. Tingley et al. (1995) demonstrated that the water intrusion or water flow test was as robust as the alcohol-based bubble point measurement test.

The basis for this integrity test has already been discussed. Correlations have been established between the organism retentions exhibited by a filter and the rates of pressure drop from a given pressure level as caused by water intruding into a hydrophobic filter (Fig. 17). The larger the rates of pressure drop, the greater the extent of water intrusion into the pores, as measured by pressure drop over a given time interval. The lower the pressure drop, the narrower the pore and the more retentive the filter. The principle underlying this integrity test is the same as that which is the basis for mercury in a nonwettable (to mercury) glass capillary, except that pressures too low to cause polymeric pore distortions are involved. Nonintegral filters will actually have water in them; integral filters will not. The automatic test machine is sensitive enough to detect the small pressure decrease rate that accompanies incipient water entry into integral filters.

Since the water intrusion test involves wetting phenomena, it will reflect, in common with the other integrity tests, the influences of surface tension (therefore, water purity), temperature, and pore wettability. The importance of these factors in the operations of the bubble point, diffusive airflow (forward-flow), and pressure hold integrity tests has been detailed by Scheer et al. (1993).

The influence of the pore wettability bears mention. The wettability of a polymeric surface by water depends on its critical surface tension (CST). Water has a surface tension of 72 dyn/cm at ambient temperatures. To be wetted by water requires a polymer to have a high CST, one that approaches the surface tension of water.

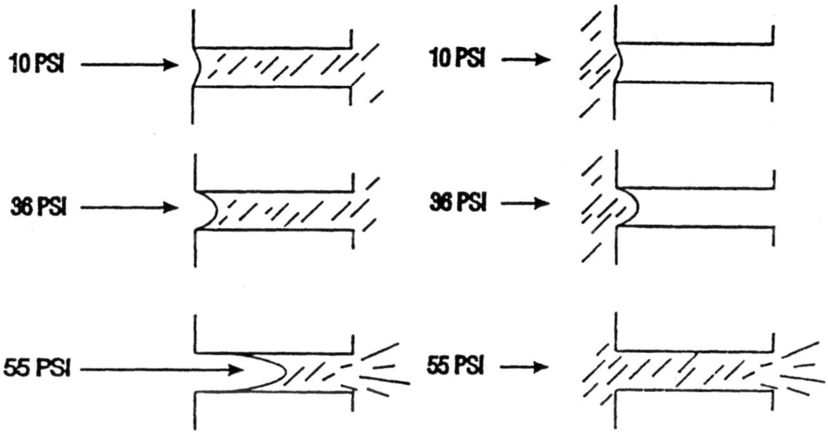

Figure 17 Water bubble-point test (left), and water pressure integrity test (right), 0.2 μm pore. From Tarry et al. (1993); courtesy of *Ultrapure Water*.

Polytetrafluoroethylene (PTFE) has an extremely low CST. It will have extreme reluctance to be wet by water; aqueous alcoholic solutions have lower CSTs than water and therefore wet PTFE filters more readily. Vent filters made of PVDF and of other hydrophobic polymers have higher CST values than PTFE. They will more readily be wetted by water. Therefore, filters composed of less hydrophobic substances can be expected to exhibit water pressure integrity test values different than those given by PTFE filters. Even more, polymers having CSTs of 19–21 can be expected to vary greatly in their wettability. Some authorities believe that CST values of 45 dyn/cm are required for wetting. In any case, because of their lower CST values, PTFE filters may show more steadfastness of water intrusion test (WIT) values than vent filters of not so low CST.

7.1 Air Filter Hydrophobicity

As stated earlier, condensation of water within the pores of vent and air filters would block the flow of air. To minimize this interference and its untoward consequences, hydrophobic membranes are used. Water is more easily expelled from such filters. However, a film of moisture, not necessarily enough to block the pores, may still be present. Air filters undergo repeated use because they are ordinarily little consumed in a single processing operation. Before reuse they are steamed to resterilize them. They are then integrity tested to determine their continuing suitability to retain organisms. Steam sterilization can leave a film of water on local portions of the hydrophobic filter surface, rendering them hydrophilic. This can lead to organism penetration of the air filter as a function of time. It would be wise to ensure the proper drying of the steamed air filter. This achievement can be tested by use of the same water intrusion test that is used to establish the integrity of hydrophobic filters.

The water intrusion test depends on and reflects the hydrophobicity of the filter. Only the experimentally demonstrated correlation of its values with the entrance of water into the hydrophobic pore structure suits it to act as an integrity test. But the basic measurement of filter hydrophobicity is itself an inherent requirement in its pertinence to air filter reuse. Consider an integral air filter that contains hydrophilic accretions or deposits on its surface. Their presence may encourage microbial growth and, ultimately, organism penetration. Solely ensuring air filter integrity, however essential, is not enough. The filter's full hydrophobicity must also be assessed to ensure freedom from compromising hydrophilic impurities.

As previously stated, in the usual air filtration or vent filter applications, the filter is so little exhausted by the depositions it collects that its reuse is compelled for economic reasons. Hence the need to verify its integrity before and after each individual use—ideally without removing it from its installation and usually after steam sterilizing it. The filter may remain integral, but if it collects, as it well may, deposits of hydrophilic matter, then as localized and limited as these may be, they can serve as loci for organism growth and penetration, defeating the very purpose intended by the use of a hydrophobic filter. If the intention of the integrity test in air filtration applications is solely to assess filter integrity, then the water intrusion test may, on occasion, be misleading and may be responsible for the discard of integral filters. If, however, the purpose of examining the filter is to gauge its suitability as a longer term air filter, as in fermenter operations for example, then the water intrusion test is sovereign for the purpose because it simultaneously measures the integrity and the hydrophobicity of the filter, both of which are required.

When the water intrusion test indicates an integral filter, the filter may be used (or reused) with confidence, even in long-term air applications. Failure to pass the water intrusion test signals a need for further filter assessment. A bubble point test subsequently performed and passed successfully may indicate that the filter is not sufficiently free of deposits to permit its safe reuse in spite of its integrity. Then, if considered desirable, a suitable filter-refurbishing effort may be undertaken (Meltzer et al., 1994).

8 INITIAL INTEGRITY TEST

8.1 Before or After Sterilizing

Whether the initial integrity test is to be performed before or after sterilization of the filter, such as by autoclaving, depends on the purposes of the test. If the purpose is to check on whether a 0.2 μm rated or a 0.45 μm rated filter is being used, then presterilization testing is acceptable. If, however, comparison with the postfiltration integrity test value is being sought, then the initial integrity test should follow the sterilization.

It is known from experience that most cartridges that undergo loss of integrity do so after sterilization, not during filtration. This means that the decision to accept a filter on the basis of an initial integrity test should be made after the filter has been sterilized.

It seems prudent to subject filters to initial integrity testing. Filtration time and the costly cleaning of equipment would be spared should it turn out finally that the cartridge has lost integrity prior to the filtration. Furthermore, initial integrity testing conforms to the proposed good manufacturing practices (GMPs) for large volume parenterals (LVPs) (*Federal Register*, 1976). However, initial integrity testing is not without its disadvantages. As usually performed, it may serve to compromise the sterility of the system, and where product is used as the wetting liquid it is wasteful of product. There is, therefore, some reluctance to performing initial integrity tests, although in the main they are highly advisable. The FDA inspectors intend that they are performed.

8.2 The Need for Initial Testing

Regardless of the success of the initial integrity testing of a filter, which is performed before filtration commences, failure of the final integrity test, which is carried out after the filtration is completed, necessitates nonacceptance of the product. At the very least, refiltration is required. This is so because final integrity test failure implies damage to the filter during the filtrative process, the initial test having ensured that the filter was integral at the start.[3] It would seem prudent, therefore, as has been stated, to subject filters to initial integrity testing.

In LVP manufacture it is a common practice to perform an initial integrity test on the filter and to also carry out integrity tests periodically during the entire course of the filtration (although this practice is increasingly omitted where repetitive or serial final filters are used). A final integrity test is also performed. The (successful) periodic integrity testing attests to the integrity of the filter to that point in time and justifies the manufacturers risking an additional quantity of product to the action of the filter whose fallibility is assumed until proven otherwise by its passing the final integrity test. In this view, then, manufacturers perform the initial integrity test solely to eliminate their own risk in utilizing a filter that may be flawed to begin with.

In small volume parenteral (SVP) production, both initial and final integrity tests should be performed as an extension of the proposed LVP practice. However, it is not uncommon in SVP production to store the filtered product in a sterile holding tank prior to the tank being filled. If the filter fails its final integrity test, or for any other reason, the batch can expeditiously be refiltered at this point. Given that the penalties attendant upon the risks devolve upon the SVP manufacturer, it could be argued that it ought to be his option to use initial integrity testing or not. It is not altogether unheard of in small volume parenteral manufacture, therefore, for the initial integrity testing of the filter to be omitted.

Although undertaking risk in choosing to forego initial integrity testing, the SVP manufacturer does not exercise a gamble in the sense involved in a game of chance. Membrane filters are presumably released by their manufacturers only in accordance with meaningful quality control procedures designed to ensure, among other properties, the integrity of these filters. However, no filter manufacturer, it is true, can certify that every single filter he purveys will meet his minimum standards upon use, if only because the shipping, storing, handling, sterilization, and installation are beyond the manufacturer's control. Also, mistakes can and do occur.

It would seem that sterility testing ought to be relied upon. The problem is that in sterility testing, conclusions regarding the suitability of a batch may be drawn from tests performed on only 20 or so individual samples withdrawn from that batch as filled over a 24 h period. The correlation of sterility with the integrity test is based more substantially on the sterility testing of the entire filtrate volume that has passed

[3]Because of the imperfections inherent in integrity testing, some companies subject "failed" filters to straightforward organism challenges as a more direct method of verifying failures. This procedure, however, requires specialized microbiological facilities and is expensive and arduous to perform.

through the filter. Hence the reluctance to release a filter on the basis of final sterility testing and the desire to depend on the authority of the integrity test.

The focus, then, is on the adequacy of the filter validation work. This work should reflect possible filter variability, both interbatch and intrabatch, and should involve the bioburdens, organisms, and fluids germane to the particular drug manufacturing process. More especially, filter validation work should establish the reliable area of integrity test–organism retention correlation by clearly defining the organism challenge retention–bubble point correlation over an extended experience, not merely as a go/no-go value.

The situation is not one marked with great certainties. Therefore, however speculative the FDA thesis, prudence as well as legal requirements dictate the performance of initial integrity tests. They should not be neglected.

9 PRESENT STATUS OF INTEGRITY TESTING

Integrity tests are by far the most reliable and least ambiguous when performed using an automated test device. These instruments have the additional considerable advantage of not requiring the invasion of the system downstream of the filter.

The integrity testing of a given filter should be carried out in conformity with its manufacturer's protocol.

The bubble point test is the only integrity test with theoretical underpinnings to the largest pore size. It loses reliability as the effective filtration area increases.

Single-point diffusive airflow testing relies on empirically established correlations to organism retentions. Multipoint testing through the bubble point correlates directly with retention.

As commonly performed without benefit of automated instruments, both the bubble point and diffusive airflow measurements necessitate invasion of the system downstream of the filter, risking asepsis.

The pressure hold test does not violate downstream system integrity. It can be a useful indicator of system leaks, whether of seals or filters or both. Its readings must be correlated with retention levels. Its performance needs the sensitivity of automated testing devices.

The water intrusion test is suitable for the determination of hydrophobic membrane integrity.

Integrity testing can be used to investigate filter compatibility.

Initial integrity tests should be performed. As a matter of practicality, the pressure hold test can serve the need of initial integrity testing when performed by automated devices.

In common with all test methods, the various integrity test procedures have their limitations. Where their positive implications are not overstated, they provide useful and dependable indications of a filter's suitability. That is their purpose. They should be used nonritualistically, however, with an understanding of their limits. So performed, they provide dependable conclusions.

10 AUTOMATED FILTER INTEGRITY TESTING

Pharmaceutical and healthcare-related industries are accelerating the incorporation of microprocessors and microelectronic circuitry and equipment into their manufacturing processes. In the aseptic processing of pharmaceuticals, verification of the integrity of sterilizing grade filters by automated integrity test instruments (see Fig. 18) is a highly developed technology used to provide accurate and reproducible filter integrity test results.

The computerized systems used to control pharmaceutical manufacturing process, although not fundamentally different from those used in automated integrity test instruments, are required to undergo detailed software and hardware validation. Not so the test instrument. The reasoning behind this difference is the indirect, auxiliary role fulfilled by an integrity test instrument relative to actual manufacturing control and monitoring performed by computer-aided manufacturing systems. Because of the critical nature of the testing provided by these automated integrity test instruments, most regulatory and industry validation groups require these units to meet minimum qualification requirements. These standards and specifications, as detailed below, are usually provided by the integrity test manufacturer in its support documentation and service.

Filters perform a critically important role in pharmaceutical production. The removal and retention of particulates and microorganisms must be ensured to provide safe and effective high quality products. The integrity testing of filters must also be part of the qualification and validation process. Validation is defined as

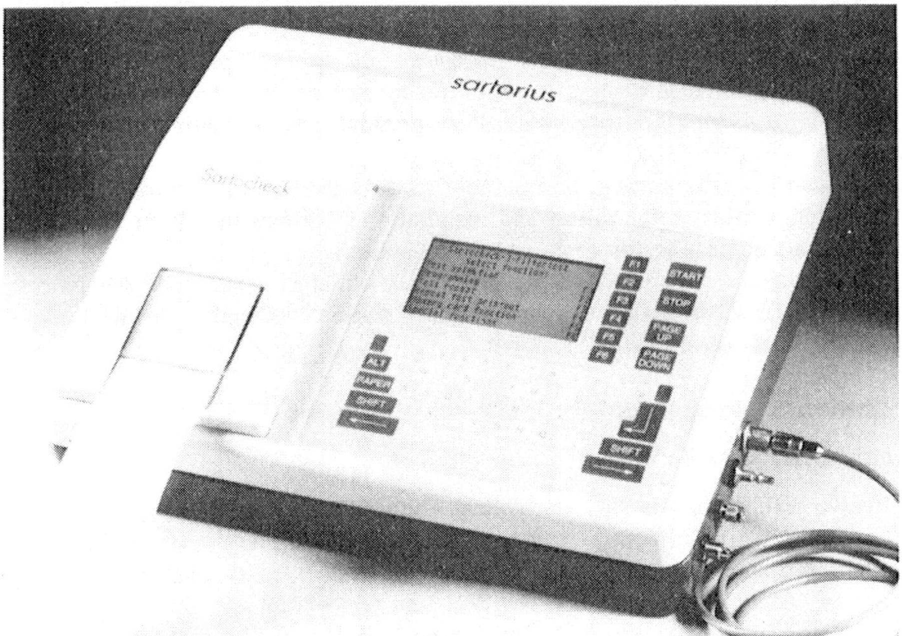

Figure 18 Automatic filter integrity test instrument.

> Establishing documented evidence which provides a high degree of assurance that a specific process will consistently produce a product meeting its predetermined specifications and quality attributes.

Relating this statement to the validation of a filter integrity test instrument, this would mean documenting that when one instrument performs the test it follows a specified operating procedure, uses the correct test parameters, and provides accurate results. Computer-related system validation (RSV) is defined as

> The procedure to establish documented evidence that provides a high degree of assurance that a specific computer-related system will consistently operate in accordance with predetermined specifications.

These validation procedures and protocols are well documented by filter integrity test instrument manufacturers. The following sections describe these processes in detail and outline the testing and documentation needed to fulfill the instrument qualification in the current regulatory and industrial environment.

Integrity test instruments are electropneumatic devices that use mass flow meters or pressure transducers as their primary measurement transducers. Most of these instruments use pressure decay test methods. The current preference for the use of pressure transducers is based on their having greater measuring resolution, wider measurement range coupled with reliable field experience, and less temperature sensitivity than mass flow meters. Mass flow meters, although more sensitive to environmental influences—e.g., temperature fluctuations and clean, dry air supply—perform in real time, demonstrating measurement accuracy equally as high as that of pressure transducers and also perform the standard accepted integrity tests, e.g., diffusive airflow and bubble point measurements.

Test methods and testing protocols vary with the type of electropneumatic measurement device used, pressure decay or mass flow transducers, and the device manufacturer's specific testing sequence, measurement, and test parameters. The integrity test instrument, regardless of manufacturing source, is connected to the upstream side of the filter/housing system to prevent any potential downstream contamination.

Automated integrity testing, like manual tests, determines the construction integrity and proper micrometer rating and installation of filters in a filter system as well as the leak-tightness of the piping and connections.

All instruments perform integrity tests that are widely accepted and recognized by regulatory and industrial agencies and advisory bodies—diffusive airflow, bubble point, and water intrusion tests.

10.1 Automated Filter Integrity Test Methodologies

Automated Diffusive Airflow Pressure Hold Test

The Diffusive airflow or pressure decay test quantitatively measures the diffusive airflow through the wetted pores when a predetermined air pressure is applied to a wetted filter. Pressure decay on the upstream side is measured after isolating the incoming gas supply. The pressure decay is a function of the gas flow through the filter. If the airflow through the filter membrane is below the maximum allowable value, then the filter unit passes the test. If there are a number of pores larger than a specified size, then the airflow and resultant pressure decay will exceed the maximum allowable value. A liquid filter test assembly is shown in Fig. 19 and the diffusion test sequence in Fig. 20.

The diffusive airflow pressure decay test is performed by an automated filter integrity test instrument as a modified version of the upstream diffusive airflow test. Pressure decay is measured on the upstream side of a liquid-wetted, sterilizing grade filter inserted into a housing. The upstream side is connected to the instrument, all other valves on the upstream volume are closed. The downstream connections of the system need not be disturbed with this method, and thus the test can be performed before or after the sterile filtration process without compromising the sterility of the downstream system. An advantage of this test is that it confirms the integrity of the entire test assembly.

The filter housing and upstream connections are pressurized to a predetermined setting, then isolated from the pressure source. Once the pressure setting is reached, the air pressure in the system is allowed to stabilize for 5–10 min. During the diffusive airflow test, the inlet volume of the upstream filter system is determined after half of the stabilization phase has elapsed. This upstream volume determination is used to accurately calculate the diffusive airflow as a direct function of pressure decay in a closed system.

The pressure phase is maintained for a period of time and is followed by a quantitative measurement of pressure decay, which is a function of total gas flow through the filter. The accuracy and reproducibility of this test requires eliminating leaks and maintaining constant temperature within and around the filter test system, housing, and device. The accuracy of measurements of the actual pressure decay and the critical upstream volume calculations may otherwise be compromised by radical temperature fluctuations (see environmental discussion that follows).

The interpretation of the measured value is based on a mathematical relationship involving differential pressure, atmospheric pressure, diffusive flow, test time, and upstream volume of the filter housing and testing system. The test results are interpreted by the device by comparison with preprogrammed pass/fail values for that particular filter and housing system. The device determines the calculated values, and if they are less than the maximum diffusion rate the filter is declared integral and passes the test; however, if the value exceeds the maximum allowable value, the device reports the filter failure.

The integrity test instrument manufacturer must supply a validation guide and instruction manuals that detail the gas law formulas, calculations, and correlations to empirical studies.

Automated Bubble Point Test

In the visual bubble point test, a filter disk is wetted and air pressure is applied and slowly increased until water is expelled from the largest pores and bubbles appear from a submerged tube in a downstream collection vessel. Vigorous bubbling or bulk airflow, as opposed to diffusive airflow or occasional bubbles, is indicative of reaching the bubble point.

The automated modified bubble point integrity test is performed in four phases in the same sequence as the diffusive test—pressurization, stabilization, measurement, and final venting.

The integrity test instrument performs the bubble point test by pressurizing the upstream side of a wet filter with the test gas. Using the diffusion versus pressure

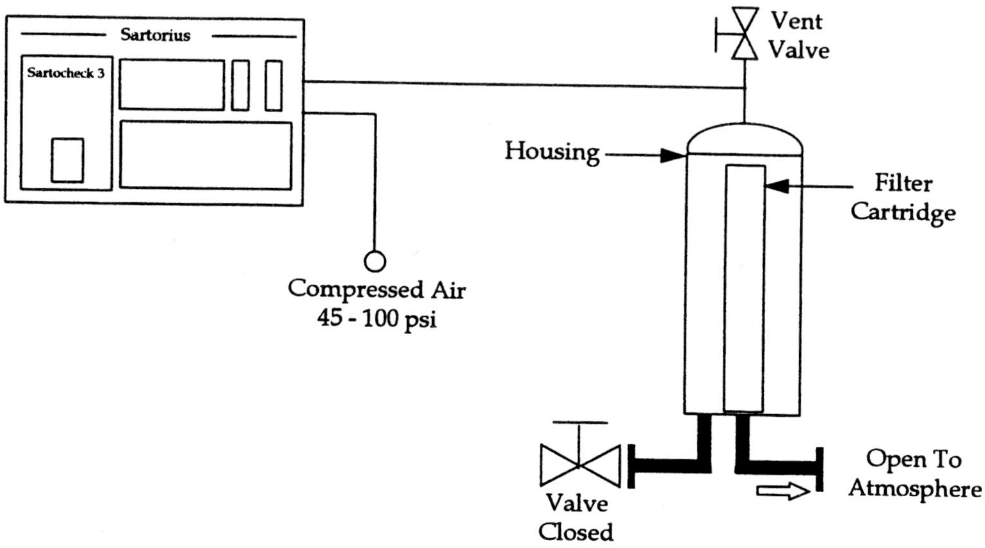

Figure 19 Liquid filter test assembly.

relationship, the unit calculates the maximum allowable pressure loss at that pressure and measures the pressure decay for a predetermined time. If this pressure decay window, usually 50 mbar or less, is not exceeded, then the integrity test instrument increases the test pressure, calculates a new maximum decay value, and measures the pressure decay again. This cycle is repeated until the measured pressure decay exceeds the maximum allowable value. When the maximum pressure decay for a given pressure has been exceeded, there will be bulk airflow through the filter mem-

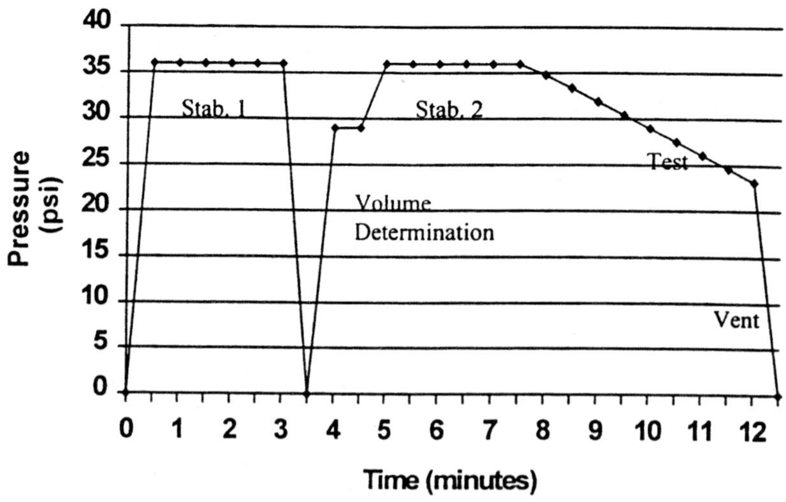

Figure 20 Diffusion test sequence.

brane, and, by inference, the bubble point value for that particular membrane has been reached.

In an airtight system, after the stabilization phase is successfully completed, the instrument automatically begins the measurement test phase. As described above, the upstream volume is slowly pressurized in incremental steps, usually less than 1.0 psi (0.07 bar). Between each step and the next, the system is monitored for several seconds for any pressure decay. This sequence of pressurization and monitoring is repeated for each successive step. The process continues until the pressure transducer detects a sudden and rapid pressure loss, qualified as exceeding the pressure decay window. This value is used as the first indication that the system has detected bulk airflow through the filter medium and is referred to as the bubble point.

If rapid pressure loss is detected when an attempt is made to further increase pressure, the instrument confirms the inability to maintain pressure and prints the pressure value at which the first rapid pressure decay was detected. The entire system is vented to the atmosphere, while the printer completes the test report.

Should the bubble point pressure value fail to meet or exceed the minimum preprogrammed value, the integrity tester, upon comparing these values, will fail the filter. If the bubble point pressure value is higher than this limit, then the filter passes and is considered integral. The bubble point test sequence is shown in Fig. 21 and diffusion and the bubble point test sequence in Fig. 22.

Automated Water Intrusion Test

The water intrusion test (WIT) is a water-based integrity test for hydrophobic membrane filter cartridges. Due to its ease of use, a variety of air/gas filter systems, vacuum breaks, fermentor air, etc. may be tested in situ.

The primary advantage of the WIT test is the elimination of alcohol in the testing of hydrophobic filters and the substitution of pharmaceutical grade water in its place. The elimination of alcohol increases the number of applications that use hydrophobic filters that now can be tested in situ. Additional advantages include significant reduction in the emissions of volatile organic carbons (VOCs), the elimination of potential fire and health hazards, and the prevention of accidental alcohol contamination of the downstream system.

The automated test sequence is similar to that of a conventional diffusion test. The test differs significantly in the use of water as a test medium. Rather than actually wetting out the filter membrane, water is used to fill the upstream side of a filter housing that contains a dry hydrophobic filter membrane. The filter membrane, being hydrophobic by nature, will resist being wetted out by this flood of water. There will remain a small upstream air volume as a cap in the filter housing. This critical air volume will be automatically calculated by the integrity test device during the stabilization time.

To sufficiently compact the filter element's pleat pack, the integrity test unit automatically pressurizes the upstream side to an initially higher preprogrammed pressure. This will act to force the "air-filled" PTFE membranes to compress to their maximum. This process drastically reduces or eliminates the apparent pressure decay and thus prevents apparent water flow from interfering with actual flow calculations.

During the measurement phase, the pressure drop is measured on the upstream side when the water intrudes into the hydrophobic membrane's microporous struc-

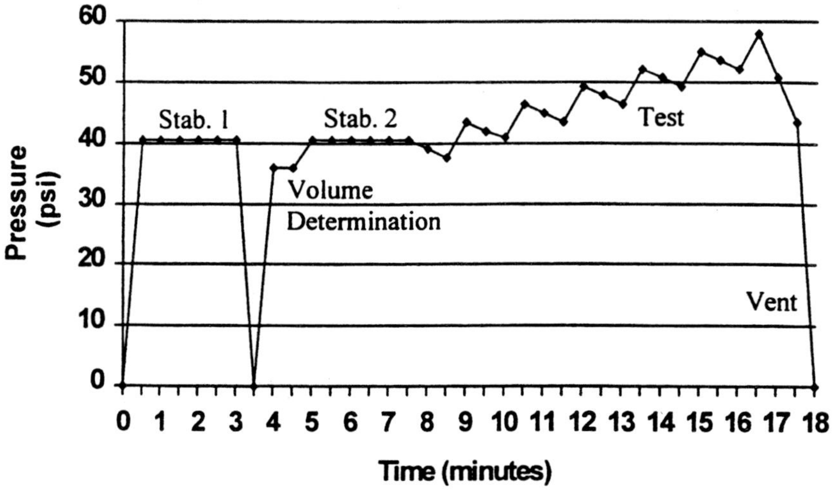

Figure 21 Bubble point test sequence.

ture, initially through the larger pores. Analogous to the diffusion determination, the resulting pressure drop and the upstream volume are used to calculate the water intrusion rate.

"Water intrusion" is defined as that pressure value where water begins to enter into and permeate the microporous structure of a hydrophobic membrane. The permeation of water during the intrusion stage shows a linear response to increasing pressure. The "water penetration" value, as opposed to the water intrusion value, is where water permeation departs from linearity, the hydrophobic membrane becomes wetted, and water begins to flow freely.

During a test with a defective filter, the integrity test instrument will measure the actual water flow through the defect(s) and the perceived flow due to compres-

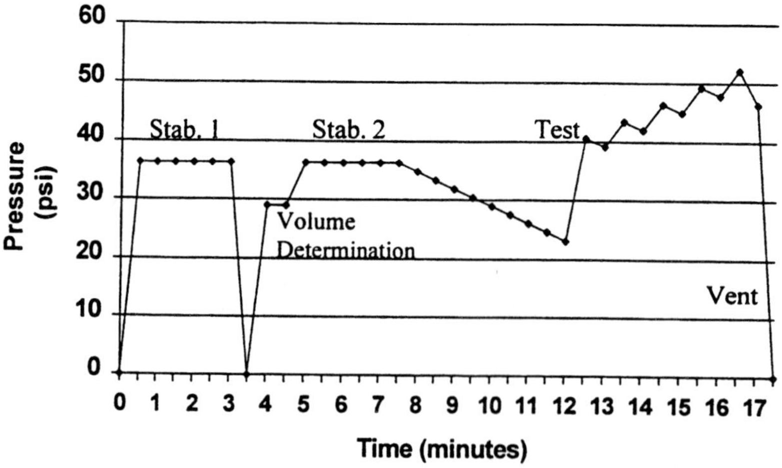

Figure 22 Diffusion and bubble point test sequence.

sion. The key to conducting a successful automated water-based test is to choose a measurement device that has sufficient resolution to measure the small flow rates associated with this type of test. While mass flow meter systems provide high accuracy and reproducibility, as do pressure transducer–based systems, the sensitivity to temperature fluctuations requires additional insulation and stability precautions. Figure 23 depicts a typical device.

Intrusional flow is a function of time. Therefore the test device must be programmed to the individual system under test. Parameters such as the test and stability times, test pressures, pass/fail limits, and initial pressure drop (pressure drop is translated into flow) are determined on the basis of several factors, including (1) wetting of the outer polypropylene drainage layer of the cartridge and (2) compression and settling of the filter pleats.

The total test time is usually 20 min. The first step is the stabilization phase, which is followed by an upstream volume determination step that calculates the volume of the air cap. This initial time period is referred to as the stabilization phase and depending on system parameters can be reset when reprogramming the integrity test instrument. After the volume determination procedure, the integrity test instrument increases the pressure of the system to the test pressure and measures the pressure decay resultant from water intrusion or permeation for the duration of the test. Usually after 20 min the test is completed, the pressure decay is determined, and the device then calculates the water intrusion values. (See Fig. 24.)

Automated Multipoint Diffusion Test

The multipoint diffusion test (Fig. 25) is a routine integrity test that is used to characterize filter membranes by their diffusive flow at varying test pressure levels. The test evaluates a single-point diffusion value and incorporates a complete

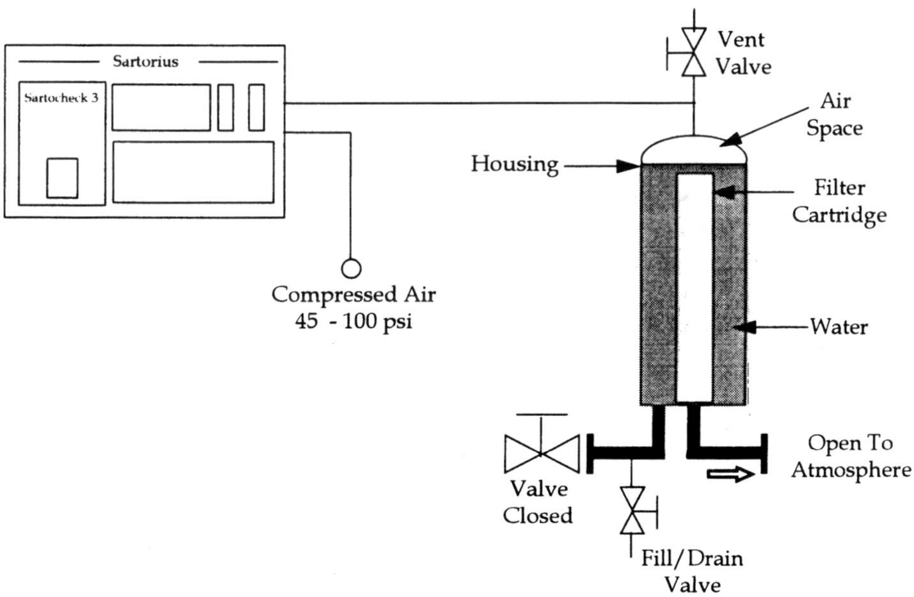

Figure 23 Water intrusion test assembly.

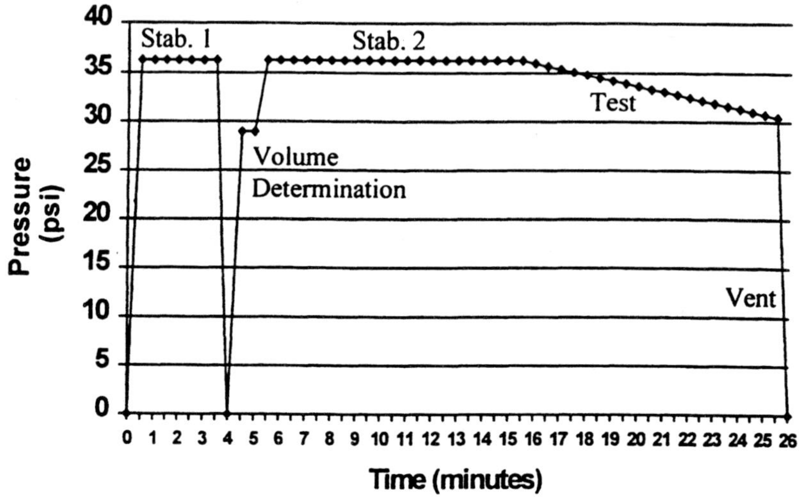

Figure 24 Water intrusion/flow test sequence.

pressure–diffusion profile over a preprogrammed pressure range. The pressure range and the number of pressure steps or the intervals between the pressure steps are selectively programmed into the integrity test instrument.

The automated test determines test parameters for fluids (liquids) with different surface tensions than that of water. The test allows for the determination of actual product-specific maximum allowable diffusion limits for product-wetted filters. Should processing conditions require the filter to be integrity tested at elevated temperatures, a multipoint diffusive air flow test can assist in determining the proper integrity test limits for production process control.

10.2 Factors Affecting Automated/Manual Integrity Tests

The most important requirement for obtaining correct test results is to consider specific environmental and test factors that affect final test results. These factors include temperature, leaktight conditions of the system, surface tension of the wetting fluid, the type of test gas, and the system upstream volume. Knowledge of what corrective action should be taken and how to take it can mean the difference between passing and failing an integral filter and thus preventing unnecessary and time-wasting retesting of otherwise integral filters.

Temperature

Since all integrity test methods are ultimately based on measuring the pressure on the upstream side of a filter system, they are also subject to the Boyle–Mariotte general law concerning gases. This law demonstrates that any changes in temperature during the individual measurements with a constant gas volume cause the pressure to change accordingly, which in turn results in incorrect data.

Another term that one may encounter that applies mostly to atmospheric conditions is the adiabatic effect, which describes the interrelationship between temperature and pressure in air/gas systems. In other words, temperature fluctuations can

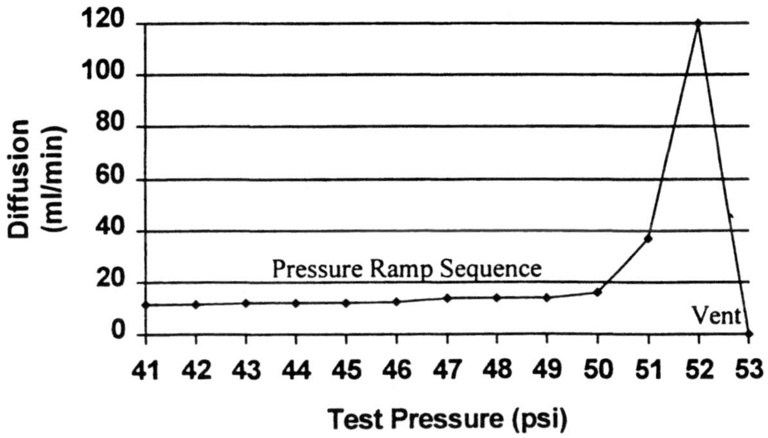

Figure 25 Multipoint diffusion test sequence.

affect the final test results. Therefore, one is cautioned that substantial temperature drift during a measuring phase must always be avoided. The following conditions must be attained during an integrity test:

Temperature of test gas = temperature of wetting fluid
= temperature of test area

Leak-Free Condition of the Filter System

One should consider it practical to routinely check the filter system regularly for leaks and poor piping connections. This process can be accomplished by using the automatic integrity tester to measure the pressure drop without a filter element installed in the housing and with the downstream system outlet closed. Any resultant pressure drop in the system will be due to leaking seals and/or piping connections. This preprocessing step will prevent needless false failure analysis and retesting due to system leaks and connection defects.

Surface Tension of the Wetting Fluid

The test pressure value depends on the surface tension of the wetting fluid. Since the parameters and limits specified by filter manufacturers are based on a standard wetting fluid (e.g., water for hydrophilic filter elements), new limits must be established when different wetting fluids are used.

Type of Gas

If a gas other than air is used, the test parameters must be reset accordingly or obtained from the filter manufacturer. The most commonly substituted gas is nitrogen, which exhibits different diffusive flow characteristics than air. The automated test units may be reprogrammed to account and adjust for the various gas test media used. This can be readily accomplished through the programming function.

Upstream Volume Determination of the Filter System

Integrity test instruments can deliver correct results only if the test parameters are in the proper relation to the upstream volume of a filter system. This volume must be kept constant during the testing phase. Any changes could and most likely will affect the final test results, thereby leading to questionable test results. The automated test device usually determines the upstream volume before each test, thus eliminating the potential of small innocuous changes or large volume changes affecting these critical final test results.

Measurements for Multielement Systems

It can be difficult to interpret the results of integrity tests (excluding the bubble point test) performed for multielement systems because the values measured are always the sum of the individual values per filter element. The high values of slightly defective filter elements may be masked by the lower values of the other elements. A reliable test evaluation can be obtained in these cases only by individually testing the elements before they are installed in a system. The total value obtained for the multielement system must approximately equal the sum of the individual values. One advantage of the automated system is its objectivity, and reproducible testing sequences can reduce or eliminate retesting by providing a consistent testing protocol with high sensitivity so marginal false failure reports are also reduced.

Stabilization Phase Time

The stabilization phase reduces the influence of adiabatic effects and permits temperature equalization within and around the filter system. Constant test and environmental conditions must be attained prior to beginning the testing phase. During this time, fluctuations in pressure caused by compaction of the filter element(s) and/or temperature drift are automatically compensated for by the automated device. Here are a few examples of optimal settings for the stabilization time:

Disk filters	3 min
Minicartridges and disposable cartridges	4 min
Standard cartridges	5 min
Special systems	5–10 min

Test Phase Time

During the test time, the pressure drop caused by diffusion within the filter system is determined and is used to calculate the diffusion rate. Based on the integrity tester's programmed accuracy for measuring the pressure drop, the test time must be selected so that a sufficiently high pressure drop is attained. The shorter the test time selected, the higher the measuring error will be.

Here are a few examples for selecting optimal test time settings:

Disk filters	3–5 min
Minicartridges and disposable cartridges	3–5 min
Standard cartridges	5 min
Special systems	5–10 min

10.3 Hardware Components and Component Interfacing

The hardware of an automated integrity test device basically consists of a central processor unit (CPU) board and a printer circuit board for the pneumatic components. Located on the CPU board are a microprocessor chip, memory chips, a real-time clock, a battery, and interface and driver chips. The CPU board is connected to various components: to the memory card slot via a flat cable, to the keypad, to the display via a controller board, to the serial interface, to the printer via a controller board, and to the board for the pneumatic components through an expansion bus.

The pneumatic components of the automated integrity test device vary in the number of valves and pressure transducers and in the type of flow meter based on the structural hierarchy and design function. Such design considerations may include 2/2-way and 3/2-way solenoid valves for controlling the flow of compressed air through the internal and external pneumatic system. A proportional valve and/or automatic pressure regulator for controlling the airflow is needed to obtain the preprogrammed test pressure. A pressure sensor measures the system pressure. This test pressure is the parameter that the integrity test device is usually programmed to use to perform the integrity test sequence. An internal stainless steel pressure vessel serves as the reference volume, usually 1000–2000 mL, for measuring the upstream volume of the system.

A temperature sensor prevents the automated integrity test device from performing integrity test measurements beyond the defined temperature range. The temperature measured by the sensor is transmitted to the board for the pneumatic components and is checked before each integrity test is run.

The pneumatic components circuit board functions as the input/output (I/O) server for pneumatic control of the device. This board receives analog signals from the temperature sensor and the pressure sensor, converts these signals into digital information, and transmits this information to the CPU board. In addition, the valves are activated through driver transistors according to the signals received from the CPU board.

A proportional valve, which requires a pulse-width-modulated square-wave voltage, permits accurate and precise absolute pressure levels to be obtained by feedback loops and microprocessor control. This voltage is supplied to the proportional valve through a digital-to-analog converter and a pulse-width modulation chip.

The integrity test device should have a bidirectional RS-232 interface, which enables it to communicate with third-party computational devices such as an external computer or PLC. The communication process is controlled by a chip located on the CPU board.

The integrity test device display is usually a liquid crystal display (LCD) unit, which may have upwards of 640 × 200 pixels. Smaller and larger LCD readouts offer varying levels of information that can be displayed at one time. Most commonly, the test parameters, product and production area information, and final test results are readily displayed. The LCD is connected through a controller board to the CPU.

The test device may have an alphanumeric keypad that can be a standard off-the-shelf QWERTY keyboard, but more splashproof security is afforded by sealed-membrane type keypads. These keypads and keyboards enable the operator to use single function keys for specific programming commands. This greatly reduces the number of keystrokes required and minimizes the potential for error. The keypad is connected to the CPU board.

Automated integrity test devices may have a memory card and card connector and card slot. This design configuration permits the end user to easily store test programs directly onto the memory card and greatly increase the efficiency and ease of access without the need to connect to third party computer and external storage devices. The memory card connector is directly connected to the CPU board.

For printing test parameters, test data, and final integrity test results, an automated integrity test device must be equipped with a printing unit. An internal dot matrix printer is usually the preferred design, with splashproof safeguards to protect its components. The printer is activated by the CPU board via the printer control board.

The device is powered by a switching power supply with a wide range of voltage inputs to supply the various voltage requirements of the internal and external components. The power supply must be shielded from external radio-frequency (rf) emissions and other sources of electromagnetic force (emf). In addition to this shielding against radio interference, the fuse holders, power socket, and power switch are shielded by a brass plate to reduce interference generated by the power cable. The external power and data transmission ports should be splashproofed. The device housing may be constructed from a variety of materials including extruded aluminum, sheet metal, and polystyrene. The housing should be shielded by the metallized interior surfaces.

10.4 Integrity Tester Do's and Don'ts

Do:

Use filter supplied with integrity tester on compressed gas source.
Connect tester to the *top* of the test housing to prevent contamination of the instrument.
Use a water trap between the tester and the housing for additional safety from contamination.
Follow cleaning instructions if the integrity tester becomes contaminated.
Confirm that the integrity tester is calibrated before testing.
Perform integrity tests only at a constant temperature.
Use manufacturer's recommended test parameters.
Follow manufacturer's instructions for system preparation.
Completely drain the test housing before each test.
Save test programs on the memory device immediately after writing.

Verify that the test pressure is in proper proportion to the system volume.
Verify with supervisor that system parameters are optimized for application.

Don't:

Open any connections while the test is in progress.
Attempt to connect the integrity tester to a pressurized housing.
Use a wetting fluid that is not at room temperature.
Use compressed gas that is not at room temperature.
Use any unnecessary connections or fittings that increase system volume.
Place small objects near the vent port.
Reduce stabilization time to speed up the test without considering the recommendations in the manual.
Permit excessive or rapid temperature changes during the integrity test procedure.
Use city or tap water to perform integrity tests.

What Can You Expect from a Modern Integrity Tester?

Table 4 is a checklist of features and performance benefits that should be evaluated to determine which devices best meet your integrity test operational requirements.

10.5 Instrument Validation

During the development and manufacture of the integrity test instrument, each component and major subassembly must undergo functional qualification as part of the complete assembled operating device. Also the software development and functionality must undergo the same scrutiny to check the implementation and performance of the standard and special operating procedures carried out by the instrument. Finally, one must analyze and document through empirically derived values that the test parameters used and test results obtained are qualified and validated.

Validation Process

Three fundamental operations are needed to confirm and qualify the proper operation of the integrity test instrumental systems, both hardware and software. This qualification is achieved through the well-established methodology accepted by the industry and by regulatory agencies. The names may change in various global markets; however, the terms of installation qualification (IQ), operational qualification (OQ), and performance qualification (PQ) are most commonly used to describe the validation of equipment, instrumentation, and software used in the pharmaceutical and associated industries.

Installation qualification requires the inspection, verification, and documentation that the facility support utilities, air/gas, water, etc., meet or exceed minimum specifications, that the environment is suitable and meets or exceeds requirements and specifications, and that the integrity test unit's hardware and software systems, once installed and connected, will perform to specifications.

Operational qualification requires checking, verification, and documentation that the test device will provide correlatable results. A series of qualification

Table 4 Checklist for Product Performance

Feature	Benefit
User-friendly with easy-to-use operating/command functions	Clear, candid, and easy-to-follow readout of programming functions, i.e., input of test parameters. No special programming or operating codes; menu-driven with self-explanatory functions.
	Error and trouble-shooting functional details with comprehensive instructional manual.
	Large LCD readout with QWERTY type keypad; function keys for easy programming and operation.
Microprocessor control	Objective and reproducible testing process, eliminates operator subjectivity and consistency.
	Easy data management for test result storage and quick recall of previous test results.
	Fast calibration and functional verification.
	Data transmission to third party devices.
	Housing and I/O ports splashproofed.
Designed for process conditions	Printer and keypad dust-, dirt-, and water-resistant.
High level of reliability	Unit qualified tested to stringent factory test requirements, substantiated by QA certificates and factory calibration reports.
Highly accurate and reproducible results	Provides security and high confidence of critical testing functions and test results.
Validation and qualification guide	Comprehensive guide for step-by-step IQ, OQ, and PQ testing protocols to meet regulatory and industry requirements and standards.
	Technical support and on-site assistance in verification and performance of these protocols.
Instruction manuals and technical support documents	Detailed manual describes in flowcharts and logic diagrams the functional operations and programming for ease of use and fast-track training.

tests are performed in the process environment. These tests establish operational certification by empirically checking and testing against the manufacturer's recommended test sequences all the critical operational and functional features and performance specifications of the device. The test reports act to certify that the device meets or exceeds the manufacturer's specification and that the operation is qualified in the process environment.

Performance qualification requires the end user to establish a testing and qualification process that documents the continued testing and maintenance of the device in the user's production environment. These records include batch records, routine calibration, and performance checks, either by the manufacturer or by certified metrology personnel. Maintenance and continued testing and verification are the responsibility of the end user, who may seek assistance from the device manufacturer or its own metrology department.

These three fundamental qualification processes are repeated during each phase of the validation process. In the qualification phase a baseline level of performance information is obtained from the component manufacturers' data and test results, structural testing of the software, and the associated vendor documentation.

Documenting a Validation Program for an Automated Integrity Test Instrument

Integrity test instrument manufacturers provide documentation for the instrument qualification and validation, as various design features and functions may be considered proprietary information. The documentation should include a comprehensive validation guide that details the above installation and operational qualification processes and an instruction manual that provides exact information that permits end users to validate the operation of the instrument with their products and conditions of use as described in the previous section.

Finally, integrity test instrument operators must establish documentation systems to serve as part of this validation and qualification process. For example, they should maintain a historical log of integrity test parameters and test results traceable to batch records, training records, calibration records and establish annual review procedures.

10.6 Installation Qualification Protocols

The following installation qualification protocols must be completed satisfactorily.

Document inspection
Physical inspection
Facilities requirements check
Software version and calibration date check

Document Inspection

Purpose: To ensure that all validation package documentation has been supplied.

A. Standard documents supplied with the integrity tester

1. Installation and operating instructions
2. Brief instructions

3. Test certificate
4. Calibration certificate

B. Documents supplied with the integrity tester validation package

1. Confidentiality
2. Installation and operating instructions
3. Software development and structure
4. Verification document
5. Certificates
   a. Certificate of compliance
   b. Sample test certificate (blank)
   c. Sample calibration certificate (blank)
   d. Supplier component documentation
   e. Test and release directions
6. Mechanical components
7. Electronic components

Physical Inspection

Purpose: To ensure that the integrity tester unit supplied is integral and undamaged.

1. There are no scratches, cracks, or other signs of damage to the instrument casing:
2. All external pneumatic and electrical ports are tight and undamaged.

Facility Requirements Check

Purpose: To ensure that the appropriate support facilities are available to operate the integrity tester.

1. Power supply = 85–240 V (47–440 Hz)
2. Minimum inlet (operating) pressure = 3000 mbar
3. Environmental considerations
   a. Temperature ranges
   b. Humidity control
   c. Air supply quality
   d. Air circulation
   e. Water supply quality

Software Version and Calibration Date Check

Purpose: To record the current integrity tester software version number and the most recent calibration date.

Method and Results: Refer to the integrity tester installation and operating instructions.

Operation Qualification Protocols

The following operation qualification protocols must be completed satisfactorily.

Valve function test
Printer function test
System security functions

Valve Function Test

Purpose: To ensure that the internal valves operate correctly.

Method: Refer to integrity tester installation and operating instructions.

Acceptance criterion: The valve function is correct if the valve can be heard to be opening and closing.

Printer Function Test

Purpose: To ensure that the printer operates correctly.

Method: Refer to integrity tester installation and operating instructions.

Acceptance criterion: The printer function is correct if all characters printed out in black and red.

Test Selection Accuracy

Purpose: To ensure that the test selected with the test selection function and that the correct test parameters are used.

Method: Refer to integrity tester installation and operating instructions.

Acceptance criterion: The integrity tester should perform the test selected with the programmed parameters.

Program Selection Accuracy

Purpose: To confirm program selection and print out the preprogrammed test parameters and limits.

Acceptance criterion: The program data and printout match.

Performance and Reproducibility

Purpose: To ensure that the unit will perform all test types and perform them reproducibly.

Acceptance criteria

1. The measuring accuracy of the diffusion test should be ±5%.
2. The measuring accuracy of the bubble point test should be ±50 mbar.
3. The measuring accuracy of the pressure drop should be ±5%.
4. The measuring accuracy of the water intrusion test should be ±5%.
5. The measuring accuracy of the water flow test should be ±5%.

Comparison with Manual Testing and Calculation Accuracy

Purpose: To ensure that the unit will produce the same results (within the limits of reproducibility) as tests done manually and that the calculations from pressure drop measurements are accurate.

Acceptance criteria

1. The automatic and manual pressure drops should agree within ±5%.
2. The automatic and manual bubble points should agree within ±50 mbar.
3. The calculation of pressure drop to diffusion/water intrusion/water flow should agree to within ±5%.

Filter Failure Detection

Purpose: To ensure that the unit will detect a filter failure.

Acceptance criterion: The test results and evaluation should indicate a filter integrity test failure.

Timer Clock Function

Purpose: To ensure that the integrity tester timer clock is accurate.

Acceptance criterion: The integrity tester time clock and stopwatch results should agree within ±3 s.

Volume Measurement Accuracy

Purpose: To ensure that the integrity tester measures the test system upstream volume accurately.

Acceptance criterion: The measuring accuracy of the volume determination function should be ±4%.

Test Pressure Accuracy

Purpose: To ensure that the integrity tester measures the test pressure accurately.

Acceptance criterion: The measuring accuracy of the test pressure should be ±10 mbar.

Test Record Accuracy

Purpose: To ensure that the test record printout corresponds accurately to the screen display.

Acceptance criterion: The test record printout and screen display data should be identical.

Repeat Test Accuracy

Purpose: To ensure that the integrity tester will accurately repeat a test after F3 is selected from the Main Menu when no data have been changed.
Acceptance criterion: The program parameters used for the repeated test should be identical to those in the original test.

Repeat Test Printout Accuracy

Purpose: To ensure that the integrity tester will accurately repeat a test printout after F4 is selected from the Main Menu when no data have been changed.

Acceptance criterion: The printout of the repeated test should be identical to that of the original test.

Changes in Measurement Units—Pressure and Diffusion

Purpose: To ensure that the integrity tester will accurately convert the diffusion and pressure units on repeated test printouts.

Acceptance criterion: The units of diffusion and pressure should be accurately changed from mL/min and mbar to mL/t and psi, respectively, on the repeated test printout.

System Security Functions

Purpose: To ensure that the integrity tester will allow or prevent access to password-protected functions.

Acceptance criterion: A correct password should allow access to all functions except the Service Menu (which is protected by a separate password known only to Sartorius Separations Technology Service personnel). An incorrect password should prevent access to all functions.

REFERENCES

Barton, A. F. M. (ed.). (1984). *Handbook of Solubility Parameters and Other Cohesion Parameters*, CRC Press, Boca Raton, FL.

Baszkin, A., D. J. Lyman, and T. H. Meltzer. (1978). Theoretical considerations of bubble point measurement: Solid/liquid wetting interaction, *Pharm.-Tech. Int.*, *2*(1):22–31.

Bowman, F. W., M. P. Calhoun, and M. White. (1967). Microbiological methods for quality control of membrane filters, *J. Pharm. Sci.*, *56*:453–459.

Code of Federal Regulations. (1976). Human drugs—"CGMPs for LVPs and SVPs," *Fed. Reg.*, *41*(106), 21CFR, Part 212, 22202–22219, June 1.

Desaulniers, C., and T. Fey. (1990). The product bubble point and its use in filter integrity testing, *Pharm. Tech.*, *42*(10):42–52.

Dosmar, M., P. Wolber, K. Bracht, H. Troeger, and P. Waibel. (1992). The water intrusion integrity test for hydrophobic membrane filters, *J. Parenteral Sci. Tech.*, *46*(4):102–106.

Dupre, A. (1869). *Theorie Mechanique de la Chaleur*, Gauthier-Villars, Paris.

Elford, W. J. (1933). The principles of ultrafiltration as applied in biological studies, *Proc. Roy. Soc. (Lond.)*, *112B*:384–406.

Guastalle, J. (1952). Contribution a l'etude du mouillage, *J. Chim. Phys.*, *49*:250–261.

Hango, R. A., W. A. Syverson, M. A. Miller, and M. J. Fleming, Jr. (1989). DI water point of use filter program for 1-MB DRAM semiconductor manufacture, Transcripts of Eighth Annual Semiconductor Pure Water Conference, Santa Clara, CA, January 18–20, pp. 73–94.

Hansen, C. M., and A. Beerbower. (1971). Solubility parameters, in *Encyclopedia of Chemical Technology*, Suppl. Vol. (Kirk and Othmer, eds.), Wiley-Interscience, New York.

Haughney, H. (1992). Letters to the editor, *J. Parenteral Sci. Tech.*, *46*(1):19–24.

Hildebrand, J. H., and R. L. Scott. (1950). *Solubility of Non-Electrolytes*, Rheinhold, New York.

Hofmann, F. (1984). Integrity testing of microfiltration membranes, *J. Parenter. Sci. Technol.*, *38*(4):148–158.

Johnston, P. R. (1986). Another view of the integrity test (bubble point) applied to fluid filter media, in *Fluid Filtration*, Vol. 2, ASTM-STP 975, (P. R. Johnston and H. G. Schroeder, eds.), ASTM, Philadelphia, PA.

Johnston, P. R., and T. H. Meltzer. (1979). Comments on organism-challenge levels in sterilizing-filter efficiency testing, *Pharm. Tech.*, *3*(11):66–70, 110.

Johnston, P. R., and T. H. Meltzer. (1980). Suggested integrity testing of membrane filters at a robust flow of air. *Pharm. Tech.*, *4*(11):49–59.

Johnston, P. R., R. C. Lukaszewicz, and T. H. Meltzer. (1981). Certain imprecisions in the bubble point measurement, *J. Parenter. Sci. Technol.*, *35*(1):36–39.

Kesting, R. E., A. S. Murray, K. Jackson, and J. M. Newman. (1981). Highly anisotropic microfiltration membranes, *Pharm. Tech.*, *5*(5):52–60.

Leahy, T. J., and M. J. Sullivan. (1978). Validation of bacterial retention capabilities of membrane filters, *Pharm. Tech.*, *2*:65–75.

Libby, D. V., J. J. Cronin, and L. L. Cunningham. (1981). The effect of anisotropy on mixed ester microfiltration membranes, *J. Parenter. Sci. Technol.*, *35*(6):276–280.

Lukaszewicz, R. C., and T. H. Meltzer. (1980). On the structural compatibility of membrane filters, *J. Parenteral Drug Assoc.*, *34*(6):463–472.

Lukaszewicz, R. C., G. B. Tanny, and T. H. Meltzer. (1978). Membrane filter characterizations and their implications for particle retentions, *Pharm. Tech.*, *2*(11):77–83.

Marshall, J. C., and T. H. Meltzer. (1976). Certain porosity aspects of membrane filters: Their pore-distributions and anisotropy, *Bull. Parenter. Drug Assoc.*, *30*(5):214–225.

Mehta, D. V., D. I. Hauk, and T. H. Meltzer. (1979). The influence of wetting agents on the bubble points of membrane filters, Proc. Second World Filtration Congress, London, pp. 387–396.

Meltzer, T. H. (1987). *Filtrated in the Pharmaceutical Industry*, Marcel Dekker, New York, pp. 255–259.

Meltzer, T. H. (1992). The insufficiency of single point difference air flow integrity testing, *J. Parenter. Sci. Technol.*, *46*(1):19–21.

Meltzer, T. H., M. W. Jornitz, and P. J. Waibel. (1994). The hydrophobic air filter and the water intrusion test, *Pharm. Tech.*, *18*(9):76–87.

Meltzer, T. H., and T. R. Meyers. (1971). The bubble point in membrane characterization, *Bull. Parenter. Drug Assoc.*, *25*:165–173.

Odlaug, T. E., D. A. Ocwieja, K. S. Purohit, R. M. Riley, and W. E. Young. (1984). Sterility assurance for terminally sterilized products without end-product sterility testing, *J. Parenter. Sci. Technol.*, *38*(4):141–147.

Olson, W. P., L. A. Gatlin, and C. R. Kern. (1983). Diffusion and bubble point testing of microporous cartridge filters: Electromechanical means, *J. Parenter. Sci. Technol.*, *37*(4):117–124.

Olson, W. P., E. O. Martinez, and C. R. Kern. (1981). Diffusion and bubble point testing of microporous cartridge filters: Preliminary results at production facilities, *J. Parenter. Sci. Technol.*, *35*(6):215–222.

Pall, D. B. (1975). Quality control of absolute bacteria removal filters, *Bull. Parenter. Drug Assoc.*, *29*(4):192–204.

Pall, D. B., and E. A. Kirnbauer. (1978). Bacterial removal prediction in membrane filters, 52nd Colloid and Surface Symposium, University of Tennessee, Knoxville, June 12.

Pall, D. E., E. A. Kirnbauer, and B. T. Allen. (1980). Particulate retention by bacteria retention membrane filters, *Colloids Surf.*, *1*:235–256.

Parker, J. H. (1986). Establishment and use of minimum product bubble points in filter integrity testing, *Pharm. Manuf.*, *3*:13–15.

Piekaar, H. W., and L. A. Clarenburg. (1967). Aerosol filters—Pore size distribution in fibrous filters, *Chem. Eng. Sci.*, *22*:1399–1408.

Price, J. M., and W. A. Pauli. (1976). Utilization of new integrity test for membrane filter cartridges, *Bull. Parenter. Drug. Assoc.*, *30*(1).

Reti, A. R. (1977). An assessment of test criteria in evaluating the performance and integrity of sterilizing filters, *Bull. Parenter. Drug Assoc.*, *31*(4):187–194.

Reti, A. R., T. J. Leahy, and P. M. Meier. (1979). The retention mechanism of sterilizing and other submicron high efficiency filter structures, *Proc. Second World Filtration Congress*, London, pp. 427–435.

Robinson, J. R. (1984). The great filter rating debate, *J. Parenter. Sci. Technol.*, *38*(5):47.

Schroeder, H. G. (1984). Selection criteria for sterilizing grade filters, Society of Manufacturing Engineers, Philadelphia, May 23–24.

Schroeder, H. G. (1985). Microbial retentive filtration, Society of Manufacturing Engineers, Philadelphia, March.

Schroeder, H. G., and P. P. DeLuca. (1980). Theoretical aspects of sterile filtration and integrity testing, *Pharm. Tech.*, *4*(11):80–85.

Tarry, S. W., J. Henricksen, M. Prashad, and H. Troeger. (1993). Integrity testing of ePTFE membrane filter vents, *Ultrapure Water 10*(8):23–30.

Tingley, S., S. Emory, S. Walker, and S. Yamada. (1995). Water-flow integrity testing: a viable and validatable alternative to alcohol testing, *Pharm. Tech.*, *19*(10):138–146.

Troeger, H., and T. Kolmann. (1988). Methods for determining integrity test parameters for various wetting liquids. Sartorius AG, Publication No. FP 4501e, Dec., Goettingen, Germany.

Tuttle, J., and S. Chrai. (1985). An automated method for integrity testing of membrane filters, *PDA*, Philadelphia, PA, November, Poster Session.

USP (1985). Potassium permanganate—volumetric solutions, USP 21, United States Pharmacopeial Convention, Inc., Rockville, MD, p. 1432.

Waibel, P. J., M. W. Jornitz, and T. H. Meltzer. (1996). Diffusive airflow integrity testing, *PDA J. Pharm. Sci. Tech.*, *50*(5):311–316.

Wallhäusser, K. H. (1979). Is the removal of microorganisms by filtration really a sterilizing method?, *J. Parenter. Drug Assoc.*, *33*(3):156–171.

Wallhäusser, K. H. (1985). Sterility assurance based on validation and in-process control for microbial removal, filtration, and aseptic filling, *Pharm. Ind.*, *47*(3):314–319.

Williams, R. E. (1984). Bubble point testing and its importance to the end user, Filtration Society, Monterey, CA, March.

Williams, R. E., and T. H. Meltzer. (1983). Membrane structure, the bubble point and particle retention, *Pharm. Tech.*, 7(5):36–42.

Walber, W. P., D. Beech, and M. McAllister. (1988). Validation of computerized membrane integrity test systems, *J. Parenter. Sci. Technol.*, 106–110.

Wrasidlo, W., F. Hofmann, J. A. Simonetti, and H. G. Schroeder. (1983). Effect of vehicle properties on the retention characteristics of various membrane filters, PDA Spring Meeting, San Juan, P.R.

Wrasidlo, W., and K. J. Mysels. (1984). The structure and some properties of graded, highly asymmetric porous membranes, *J. Parenter. Sci. Tech.*, 38(1):24–31.

Young, I. (1855). *Miscellaneous Works*, Vol. 1 (G. Peacock, ed.), Murray, London, p. 418.

Zisman, W. A. (1964). Relation of equilibrium contact angle to liquid and solid constitution, *Adv. Chem. Ser.*, 43:1.

12

Sizing Microporous Membrane Filter Systems

HARWOOD GREEN
Becton Dickinson and Company, Franklin Lakes, New Jersey

LARRY A. SCHEER
Pall Corporation, Ann Arbor, Michigan

1 INTRODUCTION

Filtration is the practice that frees fluids, whether liquid or gaseous, from their contaminating viable or nonviable particulate matter via flow driven by differential pressure. In the process, the solid particles are removed and collected by the filter, which in consequence becomes progressively blocked by the particles. The progressive decrease in effective filtration area results in progressively diminishing flow rates for constant applied differential pressure filtration and in increasing applied differential pressures for the operations where flow rates are kept constant. In either case, the ultimate blockage of the filter determines throughout, i.e., the total liquid volume that becomes filtered.

The flow of fluid through a filter is dependent on many factors. The cross-sectional dimensions of the filter passageways are of influence because for micrometer and submicrometer orifices, flow varies as the fourth power of the radius. Porosity (number of pores per unit area or void volume per unit area) defines the proportion of the filter supporting flow. Flow through such pores varies inversely with the viscosity of the fluid, which in turn varies inversely with temperature. For most liquids, flow through the filter pores also varies directly with the applied differential pressure. The longer the pore passageways and the more complex their convolutions, the greater their impediment to fluid flow due to frictional forces. The thinner the filter and the more numerous the pore paths, the greater its rate of flow.

Therefore, the total porosity of the filter, the thickness, and the extent of filter surface directly affect the flow properties of a filter. Time is also a factor in any practical consideration of filtration, and the term ''flux'' may be used to define the volume flow through a unit area of a given filter per unit of time. The purpose of filtration is of prime importance, as well as filter testing requirements, chemical characteristics of the fluid, and equipment consideration.

The discussion that follows presents a simple mathematical treatment of membrane filter system sizing based on assessing flow decay, the reduction of the rate of flow of a filter that is caused by the buildup of retained particulate matter. This treatment provides a uniform method of system sizing that can be used by anyone familiar with the basics of filtration and will result in an orderly approach to the problem, yielding consistent and accurate solutions. Topics are included that review the background concepts. The discussion and examples are for cartridge filters, as larger cartridge systems are the most difficult to size. However, the methods are entirely applicable to smaller disk or capsule systems.

Filtration is an expensive process, and proper design and sizing of a system is necessary for a cost-effective solution.

2 INFORMATION REQUIREMENTS

The first step in the process of designing and sizing a membrane filtration system is to obtain information on the attributes of the application, fluid, and system.

Application Attributes

Purpose of the filtration, such as sterilization, clarification, bacterial reduction, particulate removal.

Final filter pore size, if not inherent in the application, such as ''sterilizing'' filtration, which requires a 0.2 μm rated membrane.

Sterilization, sanitization, cleaning methods, frequency, conditions.

Integrity testing methods.

Fluid Attributes

Chemical composition providing information on the properties of the fluid and compatibility issues with the materials to be used.

Fluid viscosity, which directly affects flow rates.

Surface tension, which affects the results of integrity testing.

Fluid temperature, which affects viscosity and material properties.

Pretreatment of the fluid, such as prefiltration, deionization, and reverse osmosis.

Prior experience with the solution, such as filters used, flow rate, throughput.

System Conditions

Flow rate required, whether average, constant, or peak.

Pressure available, including inlet pressure, initial differential pressure, and maximum differential pressure.

Throughput and change frequency whether a function of batch size, operating life, or differential pressure increase.

Equipment requirements, including provisions for peak demand, future batch size or flow rate changes, and physical limitations.

3 DIFFERENTIAL PRESSURE

The addition of a filter into a fluid stream creates resistance to flow. To overcome the resistance to flow, a higher pressure must be applied upstream of the filter than exists downstream of the filter. The difference in pressure levels between the upstream and downstream sides of the filter is the applied differential pressure. It is the driving force of filtration.

The applied differential pressure bears a straight-line relationship to the rate of fluid flow through the filter. Applied differential pressure, not inlet or line pressure, controls the flow rate through the filter. The filter is affected only by the difference between the upstream and downstream sides.

Pressure definitions are given in Table 1.

3.1 Closed Systems

In a closed filtration system (see Fig. 1) such as pumping to a filling machine, gauges are used before and after the filter to measure upstream and downstream pressures. The applied differential pressure is the difference between the two gauge pressures.

3.2 Open Systems

An open or freely vented system (see Fig. 2) is a special case of a closed system where the downstream pressure is equal to ambient pressure. When gauge pressure is used, downstream pressure equals zero, and differential pressure is equal to inlet pressure. However, if valves or piping follow the filter in an open system, there may be a downstream pressure loss, so the open system must be treated as a closed system. For this reason a downstream pressure gauge is always recommended.

Table 1 Pressure Definitions

Inlet pressure The pressure entering the inlet side of the filter. Also called upstream pressure or line pressure.

Outlet pressure The pressure existing the outlet side of the filter. Also called downstream pressure.

Ambient pressure Pressure at ambient conditions. Also called atmospheric or standard pressure.

Gauge Pressure The pressure measured by a pressure gauge. Pressure above ambient pressure. Symbolized psig.

Absolute pressure The pressure above an absolute vacuum. One atmosphere (14.7 psi) greater than gauge pressure. Symbolized psia.

Differential pressure The difference between inlet pressure and outlet pressure. Also called delta $P(\Delta P)$, psid, pressure drop or applied differential pressure.

Maximum differential pressure The maximum differential pressure available for filtration as defined by pump limitations and system restrictions. This is typically greater than the differential pressure actually used for filtration. Also called available differential pressure.

Initial differential pressure The differential pressure at the start of filtration before particles are deposited on the filter. Also called clean differential pressure.

Final differential pressure The differential pressure at the conclusion of filtration. Also called dirty differential pressure.

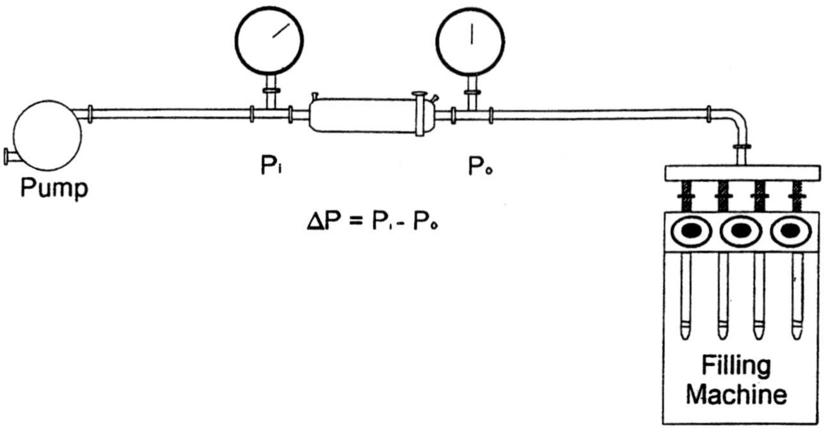

Figure 1 Closed system.

3.3 Parallel Filtration

A selected filtration system will be constructed of standard available filter units where cartridges or disks are assembled to provide the required effective filtration area. Where many cartridges are required, they may be contained within a multicartridge housing. The need for many disk filters may require the use of a multiple disk housing. Alternatively, several single-cartridge or -disk housings may be joined to provide the required filtration area.

In all of these filter configurations, the flow pattern will involve the concurrent passage of fluid through several filter units. This is known as parallel filtration. Regardless of the number of parallel or replicating flow paths, the applied pressure differential is constant. However, the total flow rate and differential pressure are equally distributed across each filter. For a given flow, the total differential pressure will be reduced proportionately by the number of parallel filters.

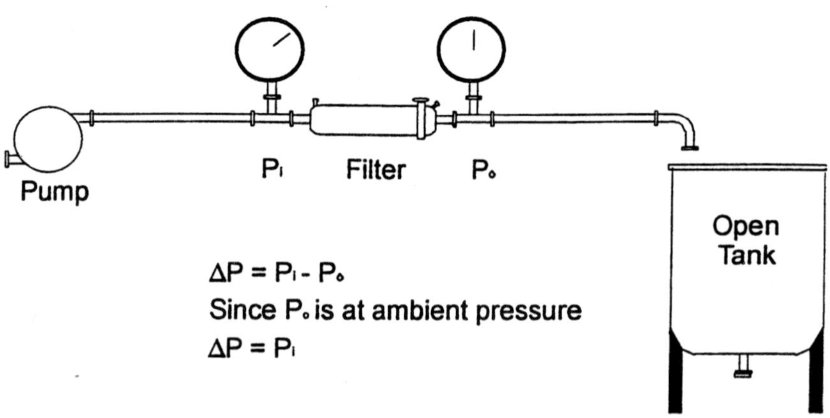

Figure 2 Open system.

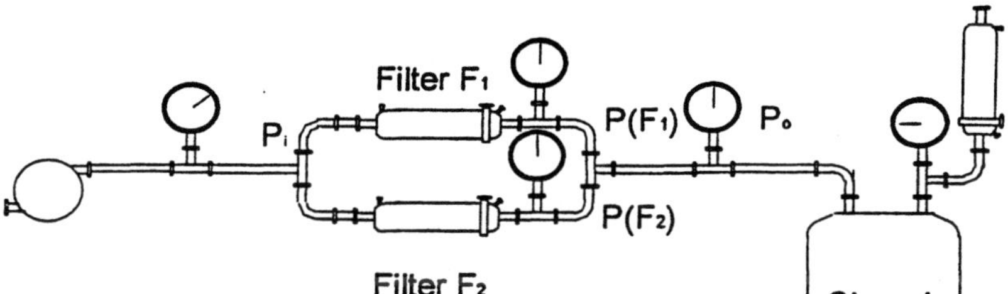

$$\Delta P(F_1) = \Delta P(F_2)$$
$$\Delta P(F_1) = P_i - P(F_1)$$
$$\Delta P(F_2) = P_i - P(F_2)$$
$$\Delta P(\text{total}) = [\Delta P(F_1) + \Delta P(F_2)] / [2 \text{ Filters}]$$
$$= P_i - P_o$$

Figure 3 Parallel filtration.

In Fig. 3 two parallel filters are shown. However, the principle and arithmetic may be extended to three or more filters.

Parallel flow is used to increase the effective filtration area of a system and thus system flow and throughput. A system scale-up from a disk to a cartridge is a basic form of parallel flow through increasing area.

3.4 Series Filtration

The significance of parallel flow is that the total applied differential pressure is not a value dependent on the number of filters operating in parallel. That is not the case in a series arrangement, where the fluid flows first through one filter then through the next (see Fig. 4). Here the total differential pressure is the sum of the differential

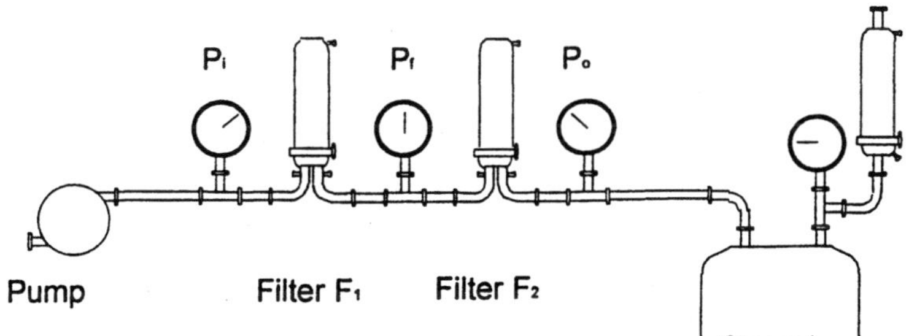

$$\Delta P(F_1) = P_i - P_f$$
$$\Delta P(F_2) = P_f - P_o$$
$$\Delta P(\text{total}) = P_i - P_o$$
$$= \Delta P(F_1) - \Delta P(F_2)$$
$$= (P_i - P_f) + (P_f - P_o)$$

Figure 4 Series filtration.

pressures across the individual filters. Prefilters and final filters in combination are the most common examples of series filtration. Redundant filtration, where two filters of the same pore size rating are used to increasing system reliability, is another example. Pleated devices containing multiple layers are a simple case of series filtration.

Because of the additivity of the individual differential pressures in series filtration, more filters should not be added without good reason. Additional filters may require an increase in pump size and energy and greater fluid loss in the system. Also, the increment of applied differential pressure may, given the finite rating of any pumping system, limit the degree of completeness to which the filters might otherwise have been utilized.

3.5 Pressure Levels

In filtration operations, the rate of fluid flow is directly proportional to the applied differential pressure. Accordingly, higher levels of differential pressure will generally result in more rapid rates of filtration. However, the shape of the flow decay curve may also depend on the differential pressure, because elevations in the level of that driving force may increasingly promote the rate of filter blockage and hence decrease throughput (see Fig. 5).

The lowest possible differential pressure level is generally preferred for process filtration. Throughput volume and filter longevity will usually be greater, which improves filtration economics. The lower rates of flow will be compensated for by greater duration of flow. This is particularly true for fluids with semirigid particles such as polymers, dextrose, serum, or gels and for fluids with a high degree of particle loading.

The longevity of membrane filters is promoted by the use of lower applied differential pressure levels. At low levels, the particulate matter being removed forms a diffuse layer adjacent to the filter face. The fluid being filtered finds little resistance in permeating this diffuse layer. At higher differential pressure levels, the velocity

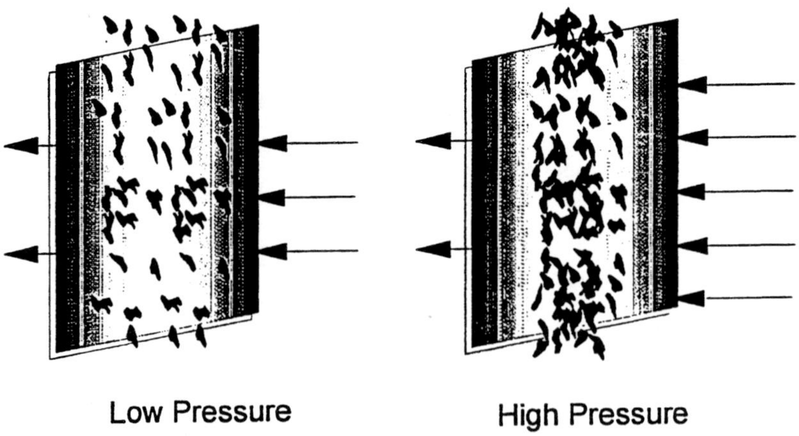

Figure 5 Effect of differential pressure on throughput.

of the particles may be such that the layer becomes impacted, offering an increased resistance to fluid flow.

If the removed particular matter impacts the filter surface and passes into the filter matrix, it will plug the filter's pores and block fluid flow. This is particularly possible where gelatinous or other deformable depositions are involved that can extrude into the pores. Flow may be prematurely diminished and throughput reduced as a consequence. Such an occurrence may more than offset the advantages of increased initial flow rates that derive from the use of higher differential pressures.

For membrane filters, particle retention is largely a result of sieve type capture: i.e., particles larger than the pore size are retained on the surface of the membrane filter. This retention characteristic is virtually unaffected by differential pressure. However, when the particles are small enough to enter the filter's pores, and when their retention then depends on their making contact with the pore walls, the probability of their capture is inversely proportional to the applied differential pressure. The probability of an encounter between the particle and the pore wall depends on the residence time of the particle in the pore. This primarily depends on the fluid velocity in the pore, which is a direct function of the differential pressure. Therefore, except where the particle size distribution completely exceeds the largest of the filter pores in dimension, the efficiency of particle capture will vary inversely with the applied differential pressure. Cognizance of this effect is important to ensure the efficiency of depth filters regardless of particle size.

Since they do not have a defined pore structure, depth filters, particularly those composed of unbonded fibers, can change structure under high pressures and flow velocities. In addition, high particle burdens can cause depth filters to unload over time, reducing their useful life.

As a practical measure, higher rates of flow and greater throughput volumes should be sought in process filtration contexts through the use of larger effective filtration areas rather than by the employment of elevated applied differential pressures.

4 FILTER BLOCKING

The purpose of filtration is to remove particulate matter from a liquid or gas. As particles are removed, they become deposited on or within the filter medium, thereby occluding the pores. As filtration proceeds, the filter becomes increasingly loaded with particles and the pores become increasingly blocked. Thus the effective filtration area (EFA) is progressively reduced and flow diminishes.

Flow rate is directly related both to differential pressure and to effective filtration area. For a constant flow rate, differential pressure and effective filtration area are inversely related. For constant differential pressure, flow and effective filtration area are directly related. It follows that in actual filtration, changing one of these parameters alters at least one of the others. (See Table 2.) These relationships are proportionate. Changing one parameter by some percentage or multiple will necessitate a change in a second parameter by the same percentage or multiple. This follows from the knowledge that flow rate per unit of differential pressure per unit of effective filtration area is a constant value.

If the flow rate remains constant and the differential pressure doubles, then the effective filtration area must be half its initial value because of filter blocking by the

Table 2

Effective filtration area	Flow	Differential pressure
Decrease	Constant	Increase
Increase	Constant	Decrease
Increase	Increase	Constant
Decrease	Decrease	Constant
Constant	Increase	Increase
Constant	Decrease	Decrease

removed contaminants. Alternatively, if the differential pressure remains constant and the effective filtration area doubles, the flow rate will double. If the flow rate is reduced by half, then either differential pressure or area must be reduced by half. (See Table 3.) Using these proportions, an increase in the differential pressure of a filtration system not only indicates that the filter is becoming blocked but also shows how much of the filter is unblocked and still available. (See Table 4.)

The figures in Table 4 demonstrate that each time the differential pressure doubles the available filtration area is halved. Expressed mathematically,

Table 3

Effective filtration area		Flow (gpm)	Differential pressure (psi)
Initial area	5 ft^2	10	10
Double area	10 ft^2	10	5
		20	10
Half area	2.5 ft^2	10	20
		5	10
Quarter area	1.25 ft^2	10	40
		5	20

Table 4

Multiple of differential pressure	Percent blocked
1 × (initial clean condition)	0%
2 ×	50%
3 ×	67%
4 ×	75%
5 ×	80%
8 ×	88%

$$\% \text{ EFA available} = \frac{100\%}{\text{multiple of clean differential pressure}}$$

$$\% \text{ EFA blocked} = 100\% - \% \text{ EFA available}$$

$$\% \text{ EFA blocked} = 100\% - \frac{100\%}{\text{multiple of clean differential pressure}}$$

When plotted, the second equation provides a curve that is increasing at a steadily decreasing rate. The curve illustrates the law of diminishing returns, with the maximum efficacy of use at 80% filter blockage. It is for this reason that filters are usually replaced at this point, either where, at constant pressure, the flow has diminished to 20% of its initial rate or where, at constant flow rate, the required differential pressure has increased fivefold.

In the fivefold increase of the original applied differential pressure to the point of diminishing returns on the flow decay curve lies the economical optimization of filter use previously discussed. To permit its achievement, the original differential pressure must be as low as possible. (See Fig. 6.)

Whether necessitated by the use of a long series of prefilters and final filters or by the desire for a high initial flow rate, elevated initial differential pressures are sometimes used. In such cases, the possibilities of manyfold pressure increases may be forfeited. Restrictions on the extent of pressure increase may also be imposed by limitations in the capacity of the system's pump. In that event, the filter system will not be usable to the 80% level of its capacity.

Different characteristics may be desired in a filter system depending on its operational purposes. In a continuous filtration mode, or where the batches are very large, the extreme durability of the filter system is usually sought to minimize the frequency of interim filter changes. These changes are always disruptive and time-consuming. Their avoidance is always desired.

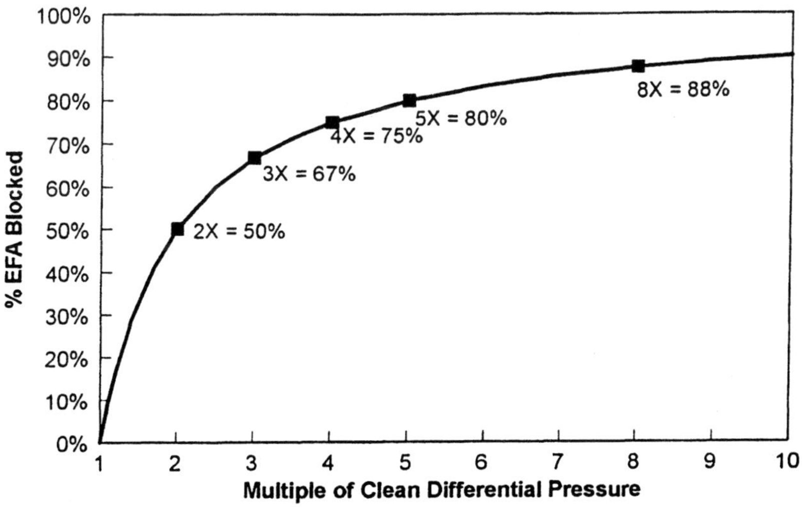

Figure 6 Filter blocking versus increasing differential pressure.

It has already been discussed that savings in filtration time are best achieved by increasing the system's effective filter area. Parallel filter arrangements may be advantageously be used to this end.

When batch filtration is used, it is helpful if the filter's exhaustion is coincident with the completion of the batch. When the batch size is so small as not to deplete the filter capacity, and when, to prevent batch cross-contamination, reuse of the filter is not allowed, the operation offers the possibilities of using higher initial differential pressures to attain peak flow rates or reducing processing times. In such cases, compromise of filter longevity becomes less important.

5 FLOW DECAY

How rapidly a filter will block during the filtration of a given fluid can be determined only by experimentation. Before beginning the design of a system involving large volumes of fluids, some prior indication of the fluid filterability is desirable as a means of avoiding mismatching process expectations and performance. It should be kept in mind that both undersizing and oversizing a filtration system can have costly ramifications.

Although general experience can be a good guide, flow decay measurements will provide a more accurate method to yield optimal system design. The purpose of a flow decay is to provide information on the particle distribution of the fluid to be filtered and on the interaction between the fluid and the filtration medium. This then provides an estimate of expected filter life. Filtration experiments are performed on small fluid volumes and small filter areas to provide an estimate of flow rate and throughput characteristics. From the effective filtration area of the small filter and the flow rate, throughput, or pressure changes it yielded, an arithmetical proportion will reveal the effective filtration area necessary to the complete processing of larger volumes or flows of that particular fluid.

A flow decay is the most cost-effective method for selecting filter types, pore sizes, and filter areas, particularly for a new system. Flow decays can be performed quickly and easily in a matter of hours using small disk filters, whereas the alternative often will require experimentation with large filter systems for days or weeks. A flow decay provides fairly accurate data leading to the choice of proper prefilter and final filter combinations as well as the proper ratio of filter areas.

Flow decay evaluations are commonly conducted on liquid solutions but are rarely conducted for gas or vent filtration applications because of the relative cleanliness and consistency of gases. However, a flow decay can be performed for gas or vent filtration, particularly if the air to be filtered is from an environment that is known to be dirty.

5.1 Final Filters

The first filter to be considered is always the final filter. The final filter is usually specified, at least indirectly, by the application, fluid, and system conditions, so the starting point for a flow decay is clear. The filter will be selected on the basis of pore size rating, porosity, composition, and other factors to provide the treated fluid with the ultimate degree of purification required.

The pore size rating selected for the final filter will be in accordance with the purposes of the filtration. Thus, visible particle removal may employ a 5 μm rated membrane, bacterial reduction will use a 0.45 μm rated filter, and sterilization modeled by *Pseudomonas diminuta* (*Brevundimonas diminuta*) will require a 0.2 μm rated filter.

In the rare case where the choice of final filter is not clear, preliminary filter and fluid qualification testing should be performed to determine the most viable candidates for in-depth evaluation.

Membrane filters are usually used as final filters because their narrow pore size distributions suit them for the ensured retention of particulate matter. When correctly selected for an application, the largest pores of a membrane pore size distribution will be smaller than the smallest particles of the particle size distribution they are required to retain. Particles are retained on the surface because they are too large to enter the membrane pores. (This is a gross simplification of the complexities of filtration dynamics.)

The smaller the membrane's pores, the lower the flow per unit area that will be supported at a given differential pressure. Thus, it is important to closely match a filter's pore size rating to the particle distribution of the fluid. A filter's pores will most readily be plugged by particles that are close to the pore size. The membrane filter may become prematurely blocked, thus reducing flow rate and curtailing throughout. Especially where fluids involving high particulate contents are involved, prefilters must be employed to remove the bulk of particles.

5.2 Prefilters

When flow decay studies on the final filter show too large a drop in flow rate resulting from a rapid blockage of the membrane surface by particulate loading, prefiltration is indicated. Combining the final filter with a prefilter will prolong the period of acceptable flow rates. (See Fig. 7.) A second prefilter, protective of the first, can give an additional period of useful life to the filtration system.

After obtaining initial data on the unprotected final filter, a prefilter of the next logical pore size should be added and the test repeated on that prefilter. Generally,

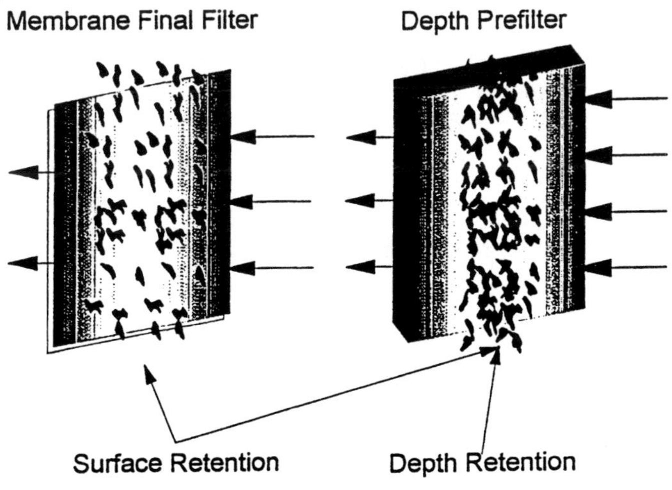

Figure 7 Prefilter and final filter combination.

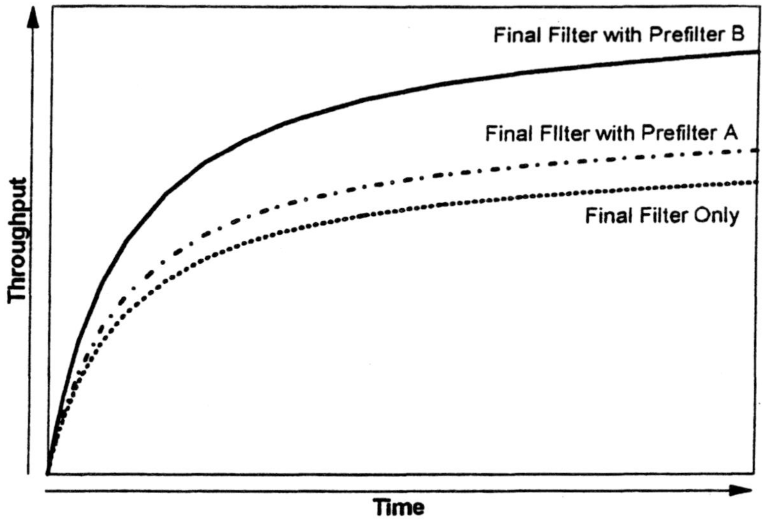

Figure 8 Extending filter life with prefiltration.

the prefilter first tried should be of a pore rating somewhat greater than that of the final filter in order to remove particles that may just fit, and therefore completely block, the final filter's pores. Progressively, prefilters of increasingly larger pore ratings are tried.

Prefilters are often of the depth construction, although membranes are also used. The larger pores of the prefilter remove the larger particles, thus protecting the final filter and extending its life. Depth prefilters have the added feature of broader pore size distributions that invite penetration by particles smaller than the pores. Small particles may be retained within the pores of the prefilter, utilizing its vast inner surfaces.

Retention within the matrix of a filter accounts for the prefilter's ability to accommodate a large loading of particles. Unfortunately, another outcome of prefilter pore penetration is incomplete, and frequently inconsistent, particle retention. These particles emerge to confront the final filter. The load on the final filter is, however, reduced by the prefilter, and the useful life of the final filter is increased. A balance of retentivity and permeability for the prefilter is needed so that it removes the bulk of the particles and significantly prolongs the life of the final filter.

If the chosen prefilter has throughput similar to the tested final filter, then its pore size rating is too small. (See Fig. 8.) A large pore size rated prefilter is indicated. If very little flow decay is seen with the prefilter, or if the flow decay of the final filter is not improved by the prefilter, then the prefilter has a pore size rating that is too large.

5.3 Test Parameters

There are many methods that may be used to conduct a flow decay test. The recommendations that follow may take longer to conduct and may use more equipment than other methods that could be suggested. However, these recommendations will provide a maximum of useful information and greater assurance of accuracy than simpler methods. The filtration system that results will thereby be of a more optimal design than might otherwise be obtained.

1. Use a separate holder to simulate each filter. Flow decays are sometimes conducted by placing as many different prefilter and final filter disks in a singler holder as will fit while still providing adequate sealing. This method is faster and simpler than using multiple holders but will not yield as much useful data. The flow decay will provide information on the proper pore size, material selection, and throughput. However, in using a single-disk holder, the flow decay will, by experimental design, yield equivalent areas for the prefilters and final filter. Instead, a separate holder should be used for each simulated filter to obtain data on the individual assembly. The effluent from each assembly is collected in a clean vessel and filtered through the next assembly in the series. This approach will generate the maximum data from the flow decay.
2. Using a single holder to simulate multiple-layer filters. When a serial or double-layer design cartridge filter is being considered, this construction must be reflected in the flow decay test. In this case, the multiple layers should be placed in the same disk holder because this will automatically yield the equivalent areas inherent in the serial cartridge design.
3. Conduct the test under normal operating conditions. The flow decay should be performed at the differential pressure fluid temperature to be used in the final system. The fluid age and temperature should be the same as those normally used in the process. This allows the interaction between the filter and fluid to simulate operating conditions. Changing these parameters, e.g., accelerating the flow decay by raising the pressure, may adversely affect the accuracy of the data owing to factors such as particle impaction.

   Flow decays are conducted almost exclusively at constant pressure with variable flow. However, many applications require constant flow with variable pressure. Where practical, variable pressure should also be used for the flow decay.
4. Repeat the test to accommodate variability. Two factors that can seriously affect the accuracy of the tests are changes in particle distribution/burden of the fluid and fluid/system dynamics. If equipment, operating range, or materials change or are known to be variable, then trials should be repeated to accommodate the variability. Because fluid batches and system conditions can vary even in the most controlled environment, repeating the flow decay with different batches of fluid is always a good practice that can eliminate later problems.
5. Use the largest reasonable effective filtration area. Flow decays are most commonly performed on 47 mm disks. However, smaller disks may be used on clean solutions such as deionized water to shorten the time interval to filter blockage. Using a smaller disk, decreasing filtration area, and reducing testing times will sacrifice accuracy. The largest filtration area that is reasonable with respect to accuracy, time, and expense should be con-

sidered. In some cases, a flow decay conducted on capsules or small cartridge filters may be appropriate.

5.4 Test Evaluation

The flow decay can be monitored by various methods, and the results can be graphed.

1. Flow rate versus time in a constant differential pressure system. The test is complete when the flow is one-third to one-fifth the initial rate. The system is then sized for average flow rate, minimum flow rate, or throughput.
2. Differential pressure versus time in a constant flow rate system. The test is complete when the differential pressure reaches 3 to 5 times its initial value. The system is then sized for flow rate or throughput.
3. Throughput versus time in constant pressure systems. The test is complete when a predetermined fluid volume has passed through the filter or a predetermined time has passed. This is the least common method of monitoring the test but may be useful in sizing a system for batch processing using elapsed time or throughput.

The flow or pressure data sets can be converted into throughput by evaluating the area under the curve, or throughput can be estimated by multiplying the average flow by the test duration. Throughput data can be converted into flow data by calculating volume changes over time. These relationships can be described through mathematical integration and differentiation.

$$\text{Throughput} = \int \text{flow rate } d(\text{time})$$

$$\text{Throughput} = \text{differential pressure } d(\text{time})$$

$$\text{Flow rate} = \frac{d(\text{throughput})}{d(\text{time})}$$

When the system is sized, its effective filtration area will usually reflect the most stringent demands such as the peak flow rates. Accommodating these conditions requires a larger filter area than would an average or more modest constant rate of flow. There are, however, alternatives such as the use of an intermediate storage vessel that may permit system sizing on the basis of average rates of flow. The filter requirements would then be reduced.

Where the particle content is not excessive, the system may be designed to use only a final filter. However, prefilters may still serve to decrease the final filter area and to protect the final filter from unusual events. Prefiltration delays blockage of the final filter, thus influencing the filter's rates of flow and throughput. Prefilters are less expensive than final membrane filters and may be economically justifiable.

5.5 Flow Decay Example

Application

Purpose of the filtration: Removal of submicrometer particles in water
Final filter pore size: 0.2 μm rated

Sanitization: Weekly with 85°C water
Integrity testing methods: None required
Pretreatment: Tap water treated with chlorine and passed through activated carbon and deionizing beds to 1 MΩ resistivity
Prior experience with the solution: Filtration through 1 μm string-wound cartridge that does not block

Fluid

Chemical composition: Water with low bacteria counts and a high level of submicrometer particles
Viscosity: 1 cP
Surface tension: Not required
Fluid temperature: Ambient

System Conditions

Flow rate: 10 gpm
Pressure: 30 psig inlet filtering to ambient
Throughput/change frequency: As needed

Equipment Requirements

There are no system requirements.

Test 1

The first step in the design process is to conduct the flow decay determination. Two 0.2 μm cartridges were chosen for evaluation, one containing a 0.45 μm prefilter layer, and the second containing a 0.8 μm prefilter. The 0.2 μm layer was the same material in both cartridges.

The 0.2 μm rated filter was placed into a 47 mm holder, and the test was conducted at the specified operating conditions. Flow rate readings were taken at 5 min intervals.

Time	Flow Rate	Throughput
Start	210 mL/min	0 mL
5 min	200 mL/min	1025 mL
10 min	100 mL/min	1775 mL
15 min	90 mL/min	2250 mL
20 min	70 mL/min	2650 mL
25 min	50 mL/min	2950 mL
30 min	40 mL/min	3175 mL

Flow decay of 80% was reached, and the test was terminated.

Test 2

The 0.45 μm rated membrane was added to a new 0.2 μm rated membrane in the same holder to simulate the dual-layer 0.45 μm over 0.2 μm cartridge. Note that the 0.45 μm filter must be the upstream layer.

Time	Flow rate	Throughput
Start	140 mL/min	0 mL
5 min	130 mL/min	675 mL
10 min	110 mL/min	1275 mL
15 min	100 mL/min	1800 mL
20 min	80 mL/min	2250 mL
25 min	70 mL/min	2625 mL
30 min	60 mL/min	2950 mL
35 min	50 mL/min	3225 mL
40 min	30 mL/min	3425 mL

Flow decay of 80% was reached and the test terminated. This test showed a decrease in initial flow rate due to the increased pressure drop incurred by adding the 0.45 μm rated filter. The data indicate that most of the particles that blocked the 0.2 μm rated filter also blocked the 0.45 μm rated membrane, and throughput was increased by under 10%.

Test 3

For a third test, the 0.8 μm rated membrane was tried with a new 0.2 μm filter in the same holder. This simulated the 0.8 μm over 0.2 μm cartridge configuration. Table 5 gives the results.

Flow decay of 80% was reached, and the test was terminated. The 0.8 μm over 0.2 μm filter combination provided a 55% increase in throughput with only a 15% flow rate reduction over the 0.2 μm membrane alone. The 0.8 μm rated layer appears to provide a good separation of the particle distribution so that neither membrane layer is overburdened with particulate matter.

Thus, the final filter will be a cartridge comprising a 0.2 μm rated final membrane with an integral 0.8 μm rated membrane as a prefilter. However, the system may not yet be optimized.

Table 5

Time	Flow rate	Throughput
Start	170 mL/min	0 mL
5 min	150 mL/min	800 mL
10 min	140 mL/min	1525 mL
15 min	130 mL/min	2200 mL
20 min	110 mL/min	2800 mL
25 min	100 mL/min	3325 mL
30 min	90 mL/min	3800 mL
35 min	70 mL/min	4200 mL
40 min	50 mL/min	4500 mL
45 min	40 mL/min	4725 mL
50 min	35 mL/min	4913 mL

Table 6

Time	Flow rate	Throughput
Start	800 mL/min	0 L
5 min	800 mL/min	4 L
10 min	700 mL/min	8 L
15 min	600 mL/min	11 L
20 min	600 mL/min	14 L
25 min	500 mL/min	17 L
30 min	400 mL/min	19 L
35 min	300 mL/min	21 L
40 min	250 mL/min	22 L
45 min	200 mL/min	23 L
50 min	160 mL/min	24 L

Test 4

A prefilter with a pore size rating of 1 μm will be tried. Two possibilities are available: a 1 μm rated membrane cartridge and a 1 μm rated glass fiber depth medium. The membrane filter has the inherent advantages of surety of retention and nonfibrous construction. The nominally rated depth filter has the characteristic of high dirt-holding capacity. Since the application does not proscribe the use of fibrous medium, the glass fiber is chosen for trial.

A 47 mm disk of the glass fiber media is placed in a holder. A second holder is prepared with the 0.8 μm over 0.2 μm membrane configuration to simulate the final filter cartridge. A flow decay study is conducted on the glass fiber filter alone. The results are listed in Table 6.

Flow decay of 80% is reached, and the test is terminated.

The collected 1 μm filtered solution is now filtered through the 0.8/0.2 μm membrane combination. The results are given in Table 7. Flow decay of 80% is reached, and the test is terminated.

The glass fiber prefilter has increased the throughput of the 0.8 μm over 0.2 μm combination by 25%. Together the glass fiber prefilter and the 0.8 μm membrane filter have doubled the throughput of the 0.2 μm rated membrane.

The fact that the 1 μm string-wound cartridge did not clog in the application indicates that continuing testing to larger pore size filters is unnecessary. However, as evidenced by the 1 μm glass fiber having a definite clogging factor, pore size ratings by industrial depth-type medium manufacturers may not be the same as the ratings by membrane manufacturers. In this case, a trial of a 3 μm membrane demonstrated no appreciable flow decay after 2 h and was considered ineffective in further prolonging the life of the 0.2 μm rated filter.

Using the final flow decay data and equations, the theoretical flow rate and throughput for each cartridge can now be calculated.

Table 7

Time	Flow rate	Throughput
Start	180 mL/min	0 mL
5 min	170 mL/min	875 mL
10 min	160 mL/min	1700 mL
15 min	150 mL/min	2475 mL
20 min	140 mL/min	3200 mL
25 min	130 mL/min	3875 mL
30 min	120 mL/min	4500 mL
35 min	110 mL/min	5075 mL
40 min	100 mL/min	5600 mL
45 min	80 mL/min	6050 mL
50 min	60 mL/min	6400 mL
55 min	30 mL/min	6625 mL

5.6 Sizing the Final Filter

The final filter is a 0.8 μm over 0.2 μm membrane cartridge, 10 in., 6.5 ft^2.

Step 1. Determine throughput per cartridge.

$$\frac{\text{Throughput per disk}}{\text{cm}^2\ \text{EFA per disk}} \times \frac{6.45\ \text{cm}^2}{\text{in.}^2} \times \frac{144\ \text{in.}^2}{\text{ft}^2} \times \frac{\text{ft}^2\ \text{EFA}}{\text{cartridge}} = \text{throughput per cartridge}$$

$$\frac{6625\ \text{mL throughput}}{9.6\ \text{cm}^2\ \text{EFA per 47 mm disk}} \times \frac{6.45\ \text{cm}^2}{\text{in.}^2} \times \frac{144\ \text{in.}^2}{\text{ft}^2} \times \frac{6.5\ \text{ft}^2\ \text{EFA}}{\text{cartridge}} \times \frac{\text{liter}}{10^3\ \text{mL}} \times \frac{\text{gal}}{3.791} = 1100\ \text{gal throughput per 10 in. cartridge}$$

Step 2. Determine clean flow rate per cartridge at differential pressure.

$$\frac{\text{Clean flow per disk}}{\text{cm}^2\ \text{EFA per disk}} \times \frac{6.45\ \text{cm}^2}{\text{in.}^2} \times \frac{144\ \text{in.}^2}{\text{ft}^2} \times \frac{\text{ft}^2\ \text{EFA}}{\text{cartridge}} = \text{clean flow per cartridge}$$

$$\frac{180\ \text{mL/min flow}}{9.6\ \text{cm}^2\ \text{EFA per 47 mm disk}} \times \frac{6.45\ \text{cm}^2}{\text{in.}^2} \times \frac{144\ \text{in.}^2}{\text{ft}^2} \times \frac{6.5\ \text{ft}^2\ \text{EFA}}{\text{cartridge}} \times \frac{\text{liter}}{10^3\ \text{mL}} \times \frac{\text{gal}}{3.791} = 29\ \text{gpm clean flow rate per 10 in. cartridge}$$

Step 3. Determine clean flow rate per unit differential pressure.

$$\frac{\text{Clean flow per cartridge}}{\text{Flow decay pressure}} = \text{clean flow per unit differential pressure}$$

$$\frac{\text{29 gpm clean flow}}{\text{30 psid}} = \text{1.0 gpm/psid per 10 in. cartridge}$$

Step 4. Determine average flow rate per cartridge.

$$\frac{\text{Throughput per cartridge}}{\text{Flow decay time}} = \text{average flow rate per cartridge}$$

$$\frac{\text{1100 gal}}{\text{55 min}} = \text{20 gpm average flow rate per cartridge}$$

5.7 Sizing the Prefilter

The prefilter is a 1 μm nominal glass fiber cartridge, 10 in., 4.5 ft^2.

Step 1. Determine throughput per cartridge.

$$\frac{\text{Throughput per disk}}{\text{cm}^2\text{ EFA per disk}} \times \frac{6.45\text{ cm}^2}{\text{in.}^2} \times \frac{144\text{ in.}^2}{\text{ft}^2} \times \frac{\text{ft}^2\text{ EFA}}{\text{cartridge}} = \text{throughput per cartridge}$$

$$\frac{24\text{ L}}{9.6\text{ cm}^2} \times \frac{6.45\text{ cm}^2}{\text{in.}^2} \times \frac{144\text{ in.}^2}{\text{ft}^2} \times \frac{4.5\text{ ft}^2}{\text{cartridge}} \times \frac{\text{gal}}{3.791} = \text{2800 gal throughput per 10 in. cartridge}$$

Step 2. Determine clean flow rate per cartridge at differential pressure.

$$\frac{\text{Clean flow per disk}}{\text{cm}^2\text{ EFA per disk}} \times \frac{6.45\text{ cm}^2}{\text{in.}^2} \times \frac{144\text{ in.}^2}{\text{ft}^2} \times \frac{\text{ft}^2\text{ EFA}}{\text{cartridge}} = \text{clean flow per cartridge}$$

$$\frac{800\text{ mL/min}}{9.6\text{ cm}^2} \times \frac{6.45\text{ cm}^2}{\text{in.}^2} \times \frac{144\text{ in.}^2}{\text{ft}^2} \times \frac{4.5\text{ ft}^2}{\text{cartridge}} \times \frac{\text{liter}}{10^2\text{ mL}} \times \frac{\text{gal}}{3.791} = \text{92 gpm clean flow rate per 10 in. cartridge}$$

Step 3. Determine clean flow rate per unit differential pressure.

$$\frac{\text{Clean flow per cartridge}}{\text{Flow decay pressure}} = \text{clean flow per unit differential pressure}$$

$$\frac{\text{92 gpm}}{\text{30 psid}} = \text{3.1 gpm/psid per 10 in. cartridge}$$

Step 4. Determine average flow rate per cartridge.

$$\frac{\text{Throughput per cartridge}}{\text{Flow decay time}} = \text{average flow rate per cartridge}$$

$$\frac{\text{2800 gal}}{\text{50 min}} = \text{56 gpm average flow rate per cartridge}$$

6 SIZING LIQUID SYSTEMS

This section introduces system sizing equations through examples of various systems. The techniques provide a uniform method for the design of filtration systems.

There is always an area of uncertainty regarding the accuracy of extrapolating the results of small trials to larger operations. Flow decay measurements are no exception. It is common practice to oversize filtration systems by factors of 1.5–2. The intention is to avoid underdesign, which leads to premature filter changes and insufficient housing capacity. Although the practice is justified, oversizing a system should not serve as a substitute for drawing conclusions from careful flow decay determinations and analysis of other available data. Decisions on oversizing should in every case be a result of consultation with the end user and risk–benefit analysis.

It is very possible that the degree of overdesign may become stimulated by the filter housing. If a water purification system were to require five 10 in. cartridges in parallel to deliver the necessary flow, then a seven-cartridge housing may be indicated (assuming that five- or six-cartridge housings were not readily available). Automatically, the five-cartridge system would become oversized by two cartridges or 1.4 times. Here the degree of overdesign would be permitted to rest, particularly if the next larger available housing was for 14 cartridges.

The practice of reasonable oversizing may be prudent to provide a safety factor against the vagaries of solution variability and to avoid the interruption of critical operations.

In the examples that follow, oversizing is indicated by equipment requirements after sizing is completed rather than by being built in to the calculations. This is the recommended approach.

Given the eventuality that systems will be designed without data being available from a flow decay exercise, the examples in Secs. 6.1 and 6.2 use known values from catalogs, and only a final filter is sized for simplicity. In the example in Sec. 6.3, the catalog flow decay data are used for both prefilter and final filter.

6.1 Liquid System

This example is for a deionized water system flowing into a vented tank at 20 psig line pressure. The filter chosen has a flow rate of 1 gpm/psid as indicated in the manufacturer's literature.

Step 1. Determine the maximum available differential pressure.

Inlet pressure = outlet pressure = available differential pressure

30 psig inlet − 10 psig outlet = 20 psig available differential pressure

Step 2. Determine initial clean differential pressure.

$$\frac{\text{Maximum available differential pressure}}{\text{Multiple of clean differential pressure}} = \text{initial clean differential pressure}$$

Starting the filtration at the maximum available differential pressure leaves no room for additional pressure increases. As soon as the flow decreases to 80% of its initial value, the filter must be discarded.

If the initial clean differential pressure is not specified by the user, and the maximum available differential pressure is known, the clean differential pressure should be chosen as one-third to one-fifth of the maximum available differential pressure. Then the denominator on the left-hand side of the equation in 3–5. Only for a constant pressure and variable flow application such as batch processing should clean differential pressure be selected to equal the maximum available differential.

A constant pressure, variable flow rate condition is assumed in this example, so clean differential pressure is equal to the maximum available differential pressure of 20 psig. If the application were for constant flow and variable pressure, one-third to one-fifth the maximum available differential pressure would have been chosen.

Step 3. Determine flow rate per unit effective filtration area at the clean differential pressure.

Flow per unit EFA at unit differential pressure × clean differential pressure = flow per unit EFA

1 gpm/psid × 20 psid = 20 gpm per cartridge at 20 psid

This calculation is carried out using the slope of the flow rate curve from the manufacturer's catalog data. Flow rate at a specific clean differential pressure can also be determined from the manufacturer's flow rate graphs.

Step 4. Correct the flow rate for fluid viscosity.

$$\frac{\text{Flow rate per unit EFA at clean differential pressure}}{\text{Viscosity}} = \text{viscosity-corrected flow rate}$$

$$\frac{\text{20 gpm at 20 psid}}{\text{1 cP}} = \text{20 gpm per cartridge at 20 psid}$$

Since the fluid is aqueous, the viscosity is equal to 1 cP, and a viscosity correction is not needed.

Step 5. Determine the number of filtration units.

$$\frac{\text{System flow rate requirement}}{\text{Viscosity-corrected flow rate per unit EFA at clean differential pressure}} = \text{number of filtration units}$$

$$\frac{\text{10 gpm}}{\text{20 gpm/10 in. cartridge at 20 psid}} = \text{0.5 10 in. cartridges}$$

The system chosen will consist of one 10 in. cartridge.

Step 6. Recalculate the actual clean differential pressure.

$$\frac{\text{System flow rate requirement}}{\text{Viscosity-corrected flow rate per unit EFA at unit differential pressure} \times \text{number of units}} = \text{actual clean differential pressure}$$

$$\frac{\text{10 gpm}}{\text{1.0 gpm/psid} \times 1} = \text{10 psid clean differential pressure}$$

Step 7. Determine the percentage of filter blocked at the change point.

$$\frac{\text{Maximum available differential pressure}}{\text{Actual clean differential pressure}} = \text{multiple of clean differential pressure}$$

$$\frac{20 \text{ psid}}{10 \text{ psid}} = 2$$

$$100\% - \frac{100\%}{\text{multiple of clean differential pressure}} = \%\ \text{EFA blocked}$$

$$100\% - \frac{100\%}{2} = 50\%\ \text{EFA blocked}$$

Step 8. Review the system for possible competing factors of flow rates, throughput, and economics.

An initial premise of this example was that it involves a constant pressure and variable flow application. Under this condition, steps 6 and 7 are not needed in that the pressure will be 20 psig and the initial flow rate will be 20 gpm. The filter will be used until it stops flowing.

One alternative recommendation might be to begin at 10 psi and increase the pressure as the filter blocks and flow rate declines. Under these conditions, 50% of the filter will be blocked at the change point as shown above. A second alternative would be to recommend a 20 in. cartridge. The clean differential pressure would then be 5 psi. This allows for a multiple of 4 in pressure increase, resulting in 75% filter blockage at the change point.

6.2 High Flow Rate System

Using filters with a large pore size and high flow rate or designing systems with high differential pressures can yield very high theoretical flow tests. Based on extrapolating graphs in catalogs, it may appear that a high flow rate system (e.g., 100 gpm) could be designed with one or two 10 in. cartridges. This design, however, would not take into account the resistance to flow of the filter housings and piping or the effects of turbulence.

Filter manufacturers publish graphs of flow rates that are fairly linear within a reasonable operating range. Within this range, most of the differential pressure is being used to drive the fluid through the filter and only a small portion is used to overcome the flow resistance of the housing. However, when the recommended flow range is exceeded, differential pressure will increase in a curvilinear fashion at a level higher than predicted by straight-line extrapolation. Although the filter may still behave in a linear manner, because of the small orifices involved the housing inlet, cartridge core, and outlet become increasingly restrictive to fluid flow.

Filter efficiency and throughput may be decreased due to the high velocity impaction of particles on the filter media. Also, the increased frictional losses and turbulence can generate heat. This can denature certain biological solutions and components.

Considering these restrictions, certain filter flow rate limitations can be recommended. These recommendations are based on generally accepted fluid velocity through pipes and orifices.

The flow per cartridge/housing interface should be maintained at 5–15 gpm, and the maximum flow rate per cartridge/housing interface should be 25 gpm. These values are based on fluid velocities that will be sufficient to completely wet the filter while maintaining a fluid velocity of under 10/s (through a 1 in. diameter orifice). Thus a single-cartridge housing should have a flow rate not exceeding 25 gpm whether the cartridge length is 10, 20, or 30 in. If a flow rate of 25 gpm can be achieved with a 10 in. cartridge, increased lengths should be used to increase throughput rather than flow rate. Equivalent maximums for three-round and seven-round housings should be 75 gpm and 175 gpm, respectively.

The next example is to design a system for filtration of an aqueous solution into a high flow filling machine. The pump upstream of the filter is producing 30 psig. There is a pressure requirement of 10 psig downstream into the filling machine. A constant flow rate of 50 gpm is needed. The filter is a 5 μm membrane construction with 4.5 ft^2 of effective filtration area. The manufacturer's catalog data indicate that the cartridge has a flow rate of 5 gpm/psid.

Step 1. Determine the maximum available differential pressure.

Inlet pressure − outlet pressure = available differential pressure

30 psig inlet − 10 psig outlet = 20 psig available differential pressure

Step 2. Determine the initial clean differential pressure.

$$\frac{\text{Maximum available differential pressure}}{\text{Multiple of clean differential pressure}} = \text{initial clean differential pressure}$$

$$\frac{\text{20 psig maximum differential pressure}}{4} = \text{5 psig initial clean differential pressure}$$

To allow for filter blockage, clean differential pressure of one-fourth the maximum available, or 5 psig, will be chosen.

Step 3. Determine the flow rate per unit effective filtration area at the clean differential pressure.

Flow per unit EFA at unit differential pressure × clean differential pressure = flow per unit EFA

10 gpm/psid × 5 psid = 50 gpm per cartridge at 5 psid

Step 4. Correct the flow rate for fluid viscosity.

$$\frac{\text{Flow rate per unit EFA at clean differential pressure}}{\text{Viscosity}} = \text{viscosity-corrected flow rate}$$

$$\frac{\text{50 gpm at 5 psid}}{\text{1 cP}} = \text{50 gpm per cartridge at 5 psid}$$

Since the fluid as aqueous, the viscosity is equal to 1 cP, and a viscosity correction is not needed.

Step 5. Determine the number of filtration units required.

$$\frac{\text{System flow rate requirement}}{\text{Viscosity-corrected flow rate per unit EFA at clean differential pressure}} = \text{number of filtration units}$$

$$\frac{50 \text{ gpm}}{50 \text{ gpm/10 in. cartridge at 5 psid}} = 1.0 \text{ 10 in. cartridge}$$

Theoretically, the system will work with one 10 in. cartridge. However, at this flow rate, the velocity through the filter is too great and will adversely affect filter performance and life. Since the cartridge has 4.5 ft^2 filtration area, the flow rate should be a maximum of 22.5 gpm, preferably 4.5–13.5 gpm. Therefore, we must have at least three 10 in. cartridges and preferably four 10 in. cartridges. Following this line of thought, one 30 in. or 40 in. cartridge should be sufficient. However, there is a second limitation on flow rate through the cartridge/housing interface and housing outlet. The flow rate per interface should be 25 gpm maximum, preferably 5–15 gpm. A 30 or 40 in. cartridge will not suffice, and a three-round housing or four single housings in parallel must be used.

While four assemblies are preferred, there is not a four-round housing available. Consultation with the user indicates that four single housings in parallel is not viable for the installation. Thus, limitations in equipment, space, and connections dictate that a three-round housing with three cartridges in parallel will be selected. The flow rate per cartridge will now be 17 gpm.

Step 6. Recalculate the actual clean differential pressure.

$$\frac{\text{System flow rate requirement}}{\text{Viscosity-corrected flow rate per unit EFA at unit differential pressure} \times \text{number of units}} = \text{actual clean differential pressure}$$

$$\frac{50 \text{ gpm}}{10 \text{ gpm/10 in. cartridge per psid} \times 3 \text{ cartridges}} = 1.7 \text{ psid clean differential pressure}$$

Step 7. Determine the percentage of filter blocked at the change point.

$$\frac{\text{Maximum available differential pressure}}{\text{Actual clean differential pressure}} = \text{multiple of clean differential pressure}$$

$$\frac{20 \text{ psid}}{1.7 \text{ psid}} = 12$$

$$100\% - \frac{100\%}{\text{multiple of clean differential pressure}} = \%\text{ EFA blocked}$$

$$100\% - \frac{100\%}{12} = 92\% \text{ EFA blocked}$$

Step 8. Review the system for competing factors of flow rate, throughput, and economics.

The clean differential pressure is much lower than strictly needed. However, equipment and engineering considerations have dictated the final configuration. Although the cost is high in terms of filter usage, this system virtually ensures that the filters will perform well without blocking throughout its service life.

6.3 Prefilter and Final Filter Combination

Ideally, system sizing should always be completed using test data from a flow decay study. This becomes increasingly important in large systems where one or more prefilters must also be sized. Unfortunately, performing flow decay studies is not always possible, and reliance on other sources of information such as prior experience with the fluid and its probable cleanliness assumes a greater role.

In the case of a complete absence of data, other approaches can be used:

1. Size the prefilter and final filter systems for the same clean differential pressure. This approach makes the assumption that there is a uniform particle distribution that will result in concurrent prefilter and final filter blocking. Since prefilters generally have a lower differential pressure per unit flow rate than final filters, this assumption will result in the use of fewer prefilters than final filters.
2. Size for the same number of prefilters and final filters. This approach simplifies inventory and hardware requirements. Generally this will result in a lower differential pressure for the prefilter than for the final filter.
3. Size two prefilters for every final filter. This approach follows from the fact that the function of a prefilter is to protect a final filter and will therefore accumulate greater particle loading. Prefilters are also considerably less expensive than final filters and thus can be discarded with less economic loss.
4. The ratio of prefilters to final filters may be determined respecting a desire for system versatility, which may dictate that the same housing be used for each. System design should include provisions for peak load versus average demand. Future plans for batch size or flow rate scale-up should also be considered.

There is merit to each one of these approaches, although the sizing solutions are less than optimal. It should be remembered that ideally prefilters and final filters should block concurrently to maximize area utilization and minimize change frequencies.

This example uses the flow decay data obtained in Section 5.5.

System Requirements

Flow rate requirement = 10 gpm

Maximum available differential pressure = 30 psid

Final Filter, 10 in.

Throughput = 1100 gal

Clean flow rate = 29 gpm at 30 psid = 1.0 gpm/psid

Prefilter, 10 in.

Throughput = 2800 gal

Clean flow rate = 92 gpm at 30 psid = 3.1 gpm/psid

Step 1. Determine ratio of prefilters to final filters.

$$\frac{\text{Final filter throughput per unit EFA}}{\text{Prefilter throughput per unit EFA}} = \text{number of final filters per prefilter}$$

$$\frac{\text{1100 gal/10 in. final filter}}{\text{2800 gal/10 in. prefilter}} = \text{0.4 prefilter per final filter}$$

This calculation assumes data from a flow decay assay. If the arbitrary ratio is chosen, that ratio should be substituted.

The unit effective filtration area was chosen as one 10 in. cartridge in each case. However, square feet or other units may also be used.

Step 2. Determine the maximum available differential pressure. In this case it was specified as 30 psi.

Step 3. Determine the initial differential pressure.

$$\frac{\text{Maximum available differential pressure}}{\text{Multiple of clean differential pressure}} = \text{initial clean differential pressure}$$

$$\frac{\text{30 psig}}{4} = \text{5 psig initial clean differential pressure}$$

Step 4. Determine the differential pressure of the corrected unit effective filtration area of the combined assembly to meet system requirements.

$$\frac{\text{System flow requirement}}{\text{Final filter flow per EFA unit differential pressure}} + \frac{\text{system flow requirement}}{\text{prefilter flow per EFA unit differential pressure}}$$

$$= \text{clean differential pressure at flow rate of unit combined assembly}$$

$$\frac{\text{10 gpm}}{\text{1.0 gpm/psid}} + \frac{\text{10 gpm}}{\text{3.1 gpm/psid}} = \text{10.0 psid final filter} + \text{8.1 psid prefilter}$$

$$= \text{18.1 psid unit combined assembly}$$

Step 5. Correct the clean differential pressure for viscosity.

$$\frac{\text{Flow rate per unit EFA at clean differential pressure}}{\text{Viscosity}}$$

$$= \text{viscosity-corrected flow rate}$$

A viscosity correction is not needed because the flow decay automatically accounted for viscosity.

Step 6. Determine the number of filtration unit assemblies required.

$$\frac{\text{Combined unit assembly differential pressure}}{\text{System differential pressure}} = \text{number of combined unit assemblies}$$

$$\frac{\text{18.1 psid unit assembly combined}}{\text{7.5 psid system clean differential pressure}} = \text{2.4 combined assemblies}$$

Number of unit assemblies × number of filters per assembly

= number of filters

2.4 Assemblies × 1.0 10 in. final filter per assembly = 2.4 10 in. final filters

2.4 Assemblies × 0.4 10 in. prefilter per assembly = 1.0 10 in. prefilters

Since the cartridges must be complete units, a 30 in. final filter would be selected. A 20 in. prefilter would also be recommended to compensate for the added final filter area so that the prefilter will not block prior to the final filter. The unused area in the prefilter is acceptable given the low cost of the prefilter compared to the final filter.

Step 7. Recalculate the actual clean differential pressure of system.

$$\frac{\text{System flow requirement}}{\text{Filter flow per unit differential pressure} \times \text{number of filters}} = \text{filter clean differential pressure}$$

$$\frac{\text{10 gpm system flow requirement}}{\text{1.0 gpm final filter flow per psid} \times \text{3 final filters}} = \text{3.3 psid clean differential pressure}$$

$$\frac{\text{10 gpm system flow requirement}}{\text{3.1 gpm prefilter flow per psid} \times \text{2 prefilters}} = \text{1.6 psid clean differential pressure}$$

Final filter clean differential pressure + prefilter clean differential pressure

= system clean differential pressure

3.3 psid final filter + 1.6 psid prefilter

= 4.9 psid system clean differential pressure

Step 8. Determine percentage of filter blocked at change point.

$$\frac{\text{Maximum available differential pressure}}{\text{Actual clean differential pressure}} = \text{multiple of clean differential pressure}$$

$$\frac{\text{30 psid}}{\text{4.9 psid}} = 6.1$$

$$100\% - \frac{100\%}{\text{multiple of clean differential pressure}} = \%\ \text{EFA blocked}$$

$$100\% - \frac{100\%}{6.1} = 84\%\ \text{EFA blocked}$$

Step 9. Review the system for possible competing factors of flow rate, throughput, and economics.

The designed system results in a greatly oversized prefilter to compensate for a mildly oversized final filter. Given the limitations of 10, 20, and 30 in. units, a 30 in. final filter must be used. As was indicated, the 20 in. prefilter ensures that premature blocking will not occur. Economically, this is reasonable. However, other alternatives are available to the user. A 10 in. prefilter could be selected along with the 30 in. final filter, increasing the clean differential pressure to 6.5 psi. This theoretically will allow 78% filter utilization before the differential pressure reaches 30 psi and necessitates changing the filter. The disadvantage to this approach is that the prefilter may block prematurely, thus preventing full utilization of the final filter.

Another alternative design would be to use 20 in. units for both the prefilter and final filter. This has the advantage of simplifying hardware and providing versatility. For this case, the clean differential pressure will be 6.6 psi, allowing 78% filter blocking. However, the final filter may block prematurely, preventing full utilization of the prefilter.

7 SIZING COMPRESSED GAS SYSTEMS

Sizing compressed gas systems differs from the sizing of liquid systems in one important way. Unlike a liquid, gases are highly compressible (see Fig. 9).

Since flow is volume per unit time, gas at a given flow rate measured at ambient pressure will occupy less volume when compressed. Standard cubic feet per minute

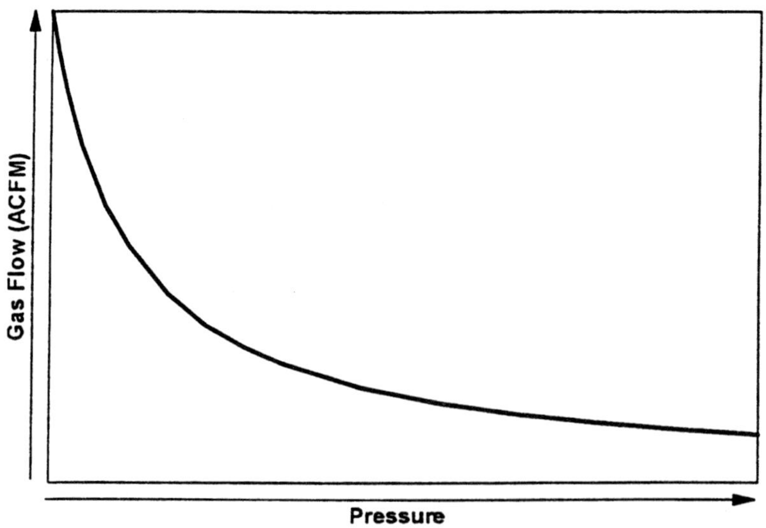

Figure 9 Gas compression under pressure.

(or standard liters per minute) is the measure of flow rate or volume at ambient pressure (1 atm). The compressed flow in actual cubic feet per minute (or actual liters per minute) should be used for filter sizing. This can result in significantly smaller compressed gas filtration systems than might otherwise be specified.

Compressed gas may be sized using the following equation. This equation is derived from the real gas law, and the derivation follows the examples.

$$\frac{\text{Volume at 1 atm} \times \text{1 atm}}{\text{Inlet pressure} + \text{1 atm} - \text{differential pressure}} = \text{volume at actual pressure}$$

Compressed gas systems rarely require prefiltration due to low particular levels and the high relative areas used to keep the pressure drop low. However, particularly in compressed air systems, care should be taken to ensure that the gas is dry and oil-free through pretreatment with a dryer and oil coalescer.

Compressed gas systems usually include 0.2 μm pore size rated filters due to the availability of high flow cartridges. However, it should be recognized that in gas filtration, particles one-third to one-tenth of as large as the liquid pore size rating will be retained. Gas retention is improved due to Brownian motion and an increase in the static forces as gas molecules flow through the filter. Static forces are largely neutralized in liquids.

Compressed gas filters are also usually hydrophobic. Should there be any moisture in the system, hydrophobicity prevents the filters from getting wet, thus avoiding bacterial growth and flow reduction. Compressed gas filters are usually resterilized and reused, in contrast with liquid filters, which are typically single-use. Historically, hydrophobic filters have been able to withstand more sterilization cycles than their hydrophilic counterparts, thereby decreasing cost per use.

7.1 Compressed Air

In this example, a compressed air system is required to deliver 500 scfm (standard cubic feet per minute) sterile air into a fermenter. Line pressure at the fermenter is 50 psig. Temperature is 80°F (300 K). The differential pressure is specified to be 1 psi clean and 5 psi the maximum allowable. The cartridge used will contain a PTFE membrane and flow at 20 cfm/psid.

Step 1. Determine the maximum available differential pressure.

The maximum differential pressure is specified as 5 psi.

Step 2. Determine the initial clean differential pressure.

The clean differential pressure is specified as 1 psi.

Step 3. Convert the flow rate from standard temperature and pressure units to actual units.

$$\frac{\text{System standard flow requirement} \times \text{1 atm}}{\text{Inlet pressure} + \text{1 atm} - \text{differential pressure}} \times \frac{\text{ambient absolute temperature}}{\text{actual absolute temperature}} = \text{system actual flow}$$

$$\frac{\text{500 scfm} \times \text{14.7 psia}}{\text{50 psig} + \text{14.7 psia} - \text{1 psid}} \times \frac{\text{293 K}}{\text{300 K}} = \text{113 actual cfm (acfm)}$$

Step 4. Determine flow rate per unit effective filtration area at the clean differential pressure.

Flow rate per unit EFA at unit differential pressure × clean differential pressure = flow rate per unit EFA

20 cfm per 10 in. cartridge per psid at 1 psid × 1 psi = 20 cfm per 10 in. cartridge

Step 5. Determine the number of filtration units required.

$$\frac{\text{Actual system flow requirement}}{\text{Flow rate per unit EFA at clean differential pressure}} = \text{number of filtration units}$$

$$\frac{\text{113 acfm}}{\text{20 cfm per cartridge at 1 psid}} = \text{5.6 10 in. cartridges}$$

Reviewing available equipment, a seven-place multicartridge housing is found to be the proper housing. Therefore, seven 10 in. cartridges will be used.

Step 6. Recalculate the actual clean differential pressure of the final system.

$$\frac{\text{System flow requirement}}{\text{Flow rate per unit EFA per unit differential pressure} \times \text{number of units}} = \text{actual clean differential pressure}$$

$$\frac{\text{113 acfm}}{\text{20 cfm per cartridge at 1 psid} \times \text{7 cartridges}} = \text{0.8 psid clean differential pressure}$$

Step 7. Determine the percentage of the filter blocked at the change point.

$$\frac{\text{Maximum available differential pressure}}{\text{Actual clean differential pressure}} = \text{multiple of clean differential pressure}$$

$$\frac{\text{5 psid}}{\text{0.8 psid}} = 6.3$$

$$100\% - \frac{100\%}{\text{multiple of clean differential pressure}} = \%\ \text{EFA blocked}$$

$$100\% - \frac{100\%}{6.3} = 84\%\ \text{EFA blocked}$$

Step 8. Review the system for possible competing factors of flow rate, throughput, and economics.

Compressed gas filters are the one case in pharmaceutical applications where the filter will be repeatedly sterilized and placed in the system. When the system is well maintained to produce dry, oil-free air, the burden of viable and nonviable particles removed by the filter will be small. Also, unlike liquid systems, there is no appreciable risk of pyrogens. Thus, compressed air filters are rarely replaced because of filter blockage. Typically, they are replaced as a part of a routine maintenance schedule or for integrity failure as a consequence of too many sterilization cycles. As a result of these factors, point-of-use filters in a high quality compressed air system usually do not require significant oversizing.

7.2 Derivation of Formula

The ideal gas law, $PV = nRT$, where nR is a constant, shows that at constant temperature and for a defined mass of gas, volume is inversely proportional to pressure, i.e.,

$$V = nRT/P$$

If pressure increases, then volume decreases. (In fact, as absolute pressure doubles, the volume is halved, which happens to be the inverse of the filter blocking curve.) The ideal gas law is used to account for compressibility as follows:

$$\text{Pressure} \times \text{volume} = \text{constant}$$

$$\text{Volume at 1 atm} \times \text{1 atm} = \text{constant}$$

$$\text{Volume at actual pressure} \times \text{actual pressure} = \text{constant}$$

$$\text{Volume at 1 atm} \times \text{1 atm} = \text{volume at actual pressure} \times \text{actual pressure}$$

$$\frac{\text{Volume at 1 atm} \times \text{1 atm}}{\text{actual pressure}} = \text{volume at actual pressure}$$

$$\text{Actual pressure} = \text{Inlet pressure} + \text{1 atm} - \text{differential pressure}$$

$$\frac{\text{Volume at 1 atm} \times \text{1 atm}}{\text{Inlet pressure} + \text{1 atm} - \text{differential pressure}} = \text{volume at actual pressure}$$

Although not usually necessary, flow requirements can further be adjusted for temperature above or below ambient temperature (20°C or 68°F or 293 K). Again using the ideal gas law, where volume and flow are inversely related to pressure, they are directly related to temperature (for a constant pressure and mass of air), i.e.,

$$V = \frac{mR}{P} \times T$$

If absolute temperature doubles, then volume will double. The adjustment can be made using the ratio of ambient absolute temperature to actual absolute temperature in kelvins. Because the base number is so large, a large temperature change is required to make a noticeable volume change.

8 SIZING CHAMBER VENTS

Chamber vent sizing may be applied to saturated steam sterilizer (autoclave) vents, ethylene oxide (EtO) sterilizer vents, and vents on a vessel such a carboy to be sterilized inside a varying pressure environment. The environment surrounding the vent filter is wet, so hydrophobic filters are always used. Care must be taken to locate the filter and housing in such a way that condensate can drain freely on either side of the filter. Generally, the cartridge core drains back into the chamber and an inlet side drain on the housing is left open and pointed down. The amount of condensate collected can be minimized by heat tracing the housing or be distancing the filter from the tank with a condensing coil or simple run of pipe. In designing vent filter systems, prefiltration is rarely needed and filter blockage by particles is rarely an issue. However, care must be taken so that design and sizing are such that condensate blockage is prevented or accounted for.

Sizing the filter system is somewhat difficult due to the fact that the differential pressure driving flow starts as some degree of vacuum that subsequently approaches ambient pressure at a decreasing rate as the chamber void is replaced with air. The decreasing differential pressure at a decreasing rate follows an exponential function.

Chamber vents may be sized using the equation below. This equation is derived from the ideal gas law, and the derivation follows the examples.

$$\text{Chamber volume} \times \frac{\ln[(\text{Starting differential pressure})/(\text{ending differential pressure})]}{\text{Filter flow per unit pressure} \times \text{ambient pressure} \times \text{time}} = \text{number of filtration units}$$

It would be expected that the differential pressure will be zero when venting is completed, i.e., chamber pressure equals outside pressure equals ambient pressure of 1 atm.

Since ending differential pressure is a divisor in the equation, zero differential pressure results in the need for an infinite number of filters (or an infinite time) for any application of this type. To size a usable filtration system, a value for the ending differential pressure greater than zero must be arbitrarily assumed. This must be a differential pressure (vacuum) that will allow the chamber door to be readily opened.

It is suggested that 0.1 psid be used for the ending differential pressure. The smaller the value of the ending differential pressure, the greater the number of filters required. If initial evacuation approaches an absolute vacuum, then setting the ending differential pressure equal to 1 psid results in half as many filters and setting the ending differential pressure equal to 0.01 psid results in 1.5 times as many filters.

8.1 Autoclave Vent

A 1000 ft^3 autoclave is completely evacuated to remove steam after completion of the sterilization cycle. The chamber doors must be able to be opened 10 min after cycle completion. A cartridge filter containing a PTFE membrane with a flow rate of 20 cfm/psid per 10 in. length will be used.

$$\text{Chamber volume} \times \frac{\ln[(\text{starting differential pressure})/(\text{ending differential pressure})]}{\text{filter flow per unit pressure} \times \text{ambient pressure} \times \text{time}} = \text{number of filtration units}$$

$$1000\ \text{ft}^3 \times \frac{\ln[(14.7\ \text{psid})/(0.1\ \text{psid})]}{20\ \text{cfm/psid per cartridge} \times 14.7\ \text{psid} \times 10\ \text{min}} = 1.7\ \text{cartridges}$$

One 20 in. cartridge filter is recommended.

8.2 EtO Sterilizer Vent

A 150 ft^2 EtO sterilizer is evacuated to 10 in. Hg to remove the EtO gas. The sterilizer is 10 ft high. The chamber is expected to be at ambient pressure within 5 min. A cartridge filter containing a PTFE membrane with a flow rate of 20 cfm/psid per 10 in. length will be used. Before determining the requirements, the chamber volume is calculated and the pressure converted into common units of measure.

$150\ \text{ft}^2\ \text{area} \times 10\ \text{ft height} = 1500\ \text{ft}^3\ \text{volume}$

(10 in. Hg)/(2.0 in. Hg/psid) = 5 psid

$$\text{Chamber volume} \times \frac{\ln[(\text{starting differential pressure})/(\text{ending differential pressure})]}{\text{filter flow per unit pressure} \times \text{ambient pressure} \times \text{time}} = \text{number of filtration units}$$

$$1500\ \text{ft}^3 \times \frac{\ln(5\ \text{psid}/0.1\ \text{psid})}{20\ \text{cfm/psid per cartridge} \times 14.7\ \text{psid} \times 10\ \text{min}} = 2.0\ \text{cartridges}$$

One 20 in. cartridge filter is recommended.

8.3 Carboy Vent

A 40 L carboy can be sterilized in an autoclave. The chamber will be evacuated to 20 in. Hg, then saturated steam will increase the chamber pressure to 15.0 psig within 5 min. A vent is required to prevent explosion or implosion of the carboy during the sterilization cycle. A 47 mm PTFE disk filter with a flow rate of 200 mL/(min·cm^2·psid) is selected. A 47 mm disk has an effective filtration area of 9.6 cm^2, yielding 1920 mL/min per disk.

20 in. Hg × 0.49 in. Hg/psid = 9.8 psid

The total change in differential pressure must be calculated as the sum of the vacuum and gauge pressure.

9.8 psig/atm + 15 psid = 24.8 psia

The differential pressure may also be calculated in terms of absolute pressure.

14.7 psig/atm + 15 psig = 29.7 psia

(30 in. Hg − 20 in. Hg) × 0.49 psig per in. Hg = 4.9 psia

29.7 psia − 4.9 psia = 24.8 psid

The filter must be sized for the total differential pressure.

Chamber volume

$$\times \frac{\ln[(\text{starting differential pressure})/(\text{ending differential pressure})]}{\text{filter flow per unit pressure} \times \text{ambient pressure} \times \text{time}}$$

$$= \text{number of filtration units}$$

$$40 \text{ L} \times \frac{\ln(24.8 \text{ psid}/0.1 \text{ psid})}{1.92 \text{ L/min per psid per disk} \times 14.7 \text{ psid} \times 5 \text{ min}} = 1.6 \text{ disks}$$

Two 47 mm disks are recommended.

8.4 Derivation of Formula

The ideal gas law, $PV = nRT$, demonstrates that volume is directly proportional to the number of moles of gas and inversely proportional to pressure. The sizing equation is derived from the ideal gas law using the following definitions.

F = flow rate of filter at unit pressure
n = number of moles of gas
P_a = absolute pressure outside chamber (1 atm)
P_t = absolute pressure inside chamber at time t
Q = number of filters
t = time
V = volume

Flow is equal to the change in gas volume per change in unit time:

$$\frac{\Delta V}{\Delta t} = QF\Delta P$$

where $\Delta P = P_a - P_t$ so that

$$\frac{d(V)}{d(t)} = QF(P_a - P_t)$$

The gas quantity flowing into the filter may be defined as

$$P_a\Delta V = \Delta nRT \qquad \text{or} \qquad \Delta n = \frac{P_a\Delta V}{RT}$$

$$\frac{d(n)}{d(t)} = \frac{P_a}{RT}\frac{d(V)}{d(t)}$$

Substituting flow for volume per unit time,

$$\frac{d(n)}{d(t)} = \frac{P_a}{RT}[QF(P_a - P_t)]$$

The pressure within the chamber may be defined as

$$\Delta P_t V = \Delta nRT \qquad \text{or} \qquad \Delta P_t = \frac{\Delta nRT}{V}$$

$$\frac{d(P_t)}{d(t)} = \frac{d(n)}{d(t)}\frac{RT}{V}$$

Substituting flow for the change in gas quantity,

$$\frac{d(P_t)}{d(t)} = \left\{\frac{P_a}{RT}[QF(P_a - P_t)]\right\}\frac{RT}{V} = \frac{QFP_a}{V}(P_a - P_t)$$

The equation is rearranged to yield

$$d(P_t) = \frac{QFP_a}{V}(P_a - P_t)\, d(t)$$

or

$$\frac{d(P_t)}{P_a - P_t} = \frac{QFP_a}{V}\, d(t)$$

Integrating both sides gives

$$\int_{P_t=0}^{P_t=t} \frac{d(P_t)}{P_a - P_t} = \frac{QFP_a}{V}\int_{t=0}^{t=t} d(t)$$

Evaluating the integral,

$$-\ln(P_a - P_t)\Bigg|_{P_t=0}^{P_t=t} = \frac{QFP_a}{V}\, t\,\Bigg|_{t=0}^{t=t}$$

$$-\ln(P_a - P_{t=t}) - -\ln(P_a - P_{t=0}) = \frac{QFP_a}{V}\, t - \frac{QFP_a}{V} \times 0$$

The equation is rearranged:

$$\ln(P_a - P_{t=0}) - \ln(P_a - P_{t=t}) = \frac{QFP_a}{V}\, t$$

$$\ln\left(\frac{P_a - P_{t=0}}{P_a - P_{t=t}}\right) = \frac{QFP_a}{V}\, t$$

Since $P_a - P_{t=0} = \Delta P_{t=0}$ and $P_a - P_{t=t} = \Delta P_{t=t}$, substitution yields

$$\ln\left(\frac{\Delta P_{t=0}}{\Delta P_{t=t}}\right) = \frac{QFP_a}{V}\, t$$

which rearranges to the final equation:

$$Q = V\,\frac{\ln(\Delta P_{t=0}/\Delta P_{t=t})}{FPt}$$

9 SIZING TANK VENTS

Tanks are vented with membrane filters so that the solution inside the tank is free from external contamination. Many of the difficulties encountered with chamber vents are also experienced with tank vents. The environment surrounding the vent filter is wet, so hydrophobic filters are always used.

Care must be taken to locate the filter and housing so that condensate can drain freely on either side of the filter. Condensate can block the filter quickly and completely, rendering the vent useless and allowing the tank to collapse. Condensate is always of particular concern during a steam-in-place operation and is equally problematic when the solution is heated such as is common in water-for-injection holding tanks. Generally, the cartridge core drains back into the chamber and an inlet side drain on the housing is left open and pointed down. The amount of collected condensate can be minimized by heat tracing the housing or by distancing the filter from the tank with a condensing coil or simple run of pipe.

When a tank is to be steam sterilized, the air volume needed to return the tank to ambient pressure after poststerilization steam collapse will typically define the maximum air flow requirement. A constant used to calculate this requirement is derived following the examples. The use of this constant assumes that the tank is not insulated or jacketed and that the outside environment is constant within the range 60–80°F. Tank insulation may slow the steam collapse, thus making the constant more conservative. A tank jacket may either slow or speed steam collapse.

If a tank is located outside, wind may speed steam collapse, requiring the use of more sophisticated formulas. Variable heat from the sun and daily temperature changes may also be factors.

Tank vents are typically designed as static devices. For a static vent, a filtration system is placed on the tank and air flow is governed by vacuum and pressure gradients within the tank. Dynamic vents are increasingly common, particularly in tanks with minimal vacuum ratings, because they require fewer filters. Dynamic vents are designed to always have the tank operate under a slight positive pressure, thus eliminating the possibility of tank collapse and providing an additional barrier to external contamination of the fluid. For a dynamic vent, a compressed gas line is connected to a second filtration system. A dynamic vent connected to a nitrogen source can be used to provide an inert atmosphere over the solution in the tank.

To size a tank vent, the following information is needed:

Maximum solution flow into tank
Maximum solution flow out of tank
Maximum positive pressure rating
Maximum negative (vacuum) pressure rating
Tank height and diameter
Maximum sterilization temperature
Minimum operating temperature

9.1 Static Vent

For an example of a static vent, a 7500 gal water-for-injection holding tank has a diameter of 10 ft and a height of 15 ft. Fill rate is 10 gpm, and peak use rate is 25 gpm. The tank will be sterilized at 125°C and allowed to cool to ambient temperature (20°C). The tank is operated at 30°C (86°F) and has a vacuum rating of 5 in. Hg (2.5 psi) and a pressure rating of 100 psig. The cartridge to be used has an air flow of 18 cfm/psid and contains a PTFE membrane.

Step 1. Convert maximum fluid inflow and outflow to air flow.

10 gpm fluid inflow × 0.1337 ft^3/gal = 1.3 scfm inflow

25 gpm fluid inflow × 0.1337 ft^3/gal = 3.3 scfm inflow

Step 2. Determine tank surface area.

$$\pi \times \left[\frac{(\text{diameter})^2}{2} + (\text{diameter} \times \text{height})\right] = \text{tank surface area}$$

$$\pi \times \left[\frac{(10\ \text{ft})^2}{2} + (10\ \text{ft} \times 15\ \text{ft})\right] = 628\ \text{ft}^2\ \text{tank surface area}$$

Step 3. Determine temperature change between maximum sterilization and minimum operating conditions.

Maximum temperature − minimum temperature = temperature change

125°C − 20°C = 105°C temperature change

Note that the temperature change in degrees Celsius is the same as the temperature change in kelvins and 5/9 the temperature change in Fahrenheit. The change in Fahrenheit is therefore 189°F.

Step 4. Determine air flow rate from steam condensation after sterilization.

Surface area × temperature change × constant = air flow

$628\ \text{ft}^2 \times 189°\text{F} \times 10^{-3}\ \text{ft/(°F}\cdot\text{min)} = 119$ scfm air flow

Note that the constant is defined within the section on derivation of the formula.

Step 5. Determine the smaller *of the tank's pressure rating and vacuum rating and divide by 2.*

The vacuum rating usually defines the allowable differential pressure. A tank can be rated for at most a full vacuum of 1 atm (14.7 psi), which is the case for ASME-coded vessels. This is an area where conservation must prevail. While it is highly unlikely that tank pressure will build to a point where the tank will explode, it is not at all unlikely that a poor design could cause a non-ASME-coded tank to collapse due to excess vacuum. To guard against this possibility, the minimum of the vacuum or pressure rating is usually divided into 2 for safety, so that the vent is automatically 100% oversized for expected initial conditions. This is the one case where oversizing is built in to the calculations.

In this case, 100 psid allowable pressure is considerably in excess of the 5 in. Hg (2.5 psid) vacuum rating. The differential pressure to be used is one-half the 2.5 psid vacuum rating, or 1.2 psid.

Step 6. Select the largest *air flow requirement from among fluid inflow, fluid outflow, and steam collapse.*

As is the case in this example, the air flow due to steam collapse (119 cfm) usually exceeds the air flow from fluid inflow (1.3 cfm) and fluid outflow (3.3 cfm). Thus, the filter will be sized for 119 cfm.

Step 7. Calculate the number of filters required.

$$\frac{\text{System air flow requirement}}{\text{Filter flow per unit differential pressure} \times \text{differential pressure}} = \text{number of filters}$$

$$\frac{\text{119 scfm required}}{\text{18 scfm per cartridge per psid} \times \text{1.2 psid}} = \text{5.5 10 in. cartridges}$$

A three-round 20 in. high housing and a seven-round 10 in. high housing are two alternatives for this application. The seven-round often offers the advantages of lower differential pressure and less risk of filter blockage by condensation due to the wider distribution of cartridges. However, the three-round housing will be considerably easier to install and is chosen for the application.

Step 8. Recalculate the actual clean differential pressure.

$$\frac{\text{System flow rate requirement}}{\text{Flow per unit EFA at unit differential pressure} \times \text{number of units}} = \text{clean differential pressure}$$

$$\frac{\text{119 scfm}}{\text{18 scfm per cartridge per psid} \times \text{6 cartridges}} = \text{1.1 psid clean differential pressure}$$

Step 9. Review the systems for possible competing factors of flow rate, throughput, and economics.

The selected system is within half the allowable vacuum and can be expected to function acceptably with an adequate safety margin.

9.2 Dynamic Vent

As with the static vent, this example is for a 7500 gal water-for-injection holding tank that has a diameter of 10 ft and a height of 15 ft. Fill rate is 10 gpm, and peak use rate is 25 gpm. The tank will be sterilized at 125°C and allowed to cool to ambient temperature (20°C). The tank is operated at 30°C (86°F) and has a vacuum rating of 5 in. Hg (2.5 psi) and a pressure rating of 100 psig. The cartridge to be used has an air flow of 18 cfm/psid and contains a PTFE membrane.

An available compressed air source of 50 psig has been added. Note that the compressed air pressure chosen must be less than the tank's pressure rating. The compressed air is at ambient temperature. These calculations are essentially a combination of the equations for compressed air with the equations for a static vent.

Step 1. Determine the differential pressure to be allowed for the dynamic vent.

The dynamic vent will be sized for 1 psid. This represents the goal of ensuring high compressed air flow into the tank to alleviate the potential for vacuum within the tank.

Step 2. Convert the maximum flow rate from standard temperature and pressure units to actual units.

$$\frac{\text{System standard flow requirement} \times \text{1 atm}}{\text{Inlet pressure} + \text{1 atm} - \text{clean differential pressure}} \times \frac{\text{ambient absolute temperature}}{\text{actual absolute temperature}} = \text{system actual flow}$$

$$\frac{119 \text{ scfm} \times 14.7 \text{ psia}}{50 \text{ psig} + 14.7 \text{ psia} - 1 \text{ psid}} \times \frac{273 \text{ K} + 20°\text{C}}{273 \text{ K} + 20°\text{C}} = 27 \text{ acfm flow}$$

The system flow of 119 scfm is determined in the static vent example, steps 1–4.

There is no correction for temperature because the compressed air temperature is ambient (20°C) flowing into the tank. Since the tank temperature is above ambient, the gas will expand within the tank and be able to displace more than the calculated volume; however, this factor will be additional oversizing incorporated into the result for safety.

Step 3. Determine the number of filtration units required for the dynamic vent.

$$\frac{\text{Actual system flow rate requirement}}{\text{Flow rate per unit EFA} \times \text{clean differential pressure}} = \text{number of filtration units}$$

$$\frac{27 \text{ acfm system flow}}{18 \text{ cfm per cartridge per psid} \times 1 \text{ psid}} = 1.5\ 10 \text{ in. cartridges}$$

Two 10 in. cartridges will be used for the dynamic vent.

Step 4. Recalculate actual clean differential pressure.

$$\frac{\text{Actual system flow rate requirement}}{\text{Flow rate per unit EFA at unit differential pressure} \times \text{number of filtration units}} = \text{actual clean differential pressure}$$

$$\frac{27 \text{ acfm}}{18 \text{ cfm per cartridge per psid} \times 2 \text{ cartridges}} = 0.8 \text{ psid clean differential pressure}$$

Using the dynamic vent, the pressure inside the tank will be ambient during the poststerilization steam collapse. However, during operation tank pressure will be subject to 50 psig compressed air. Flowing into the tank is 119 scfm compressed air plus the equivalent of 1.3 scfm in liquid flow. This condition is acceptable but not desirable.

A static vent will be added to reduce the tank pressure.

Step 5. Determine the differential pressure to be allowed for the static vent and the tank.

The static vent will be sized for 5 psi, since a small positive pressure within the tank is a benefit in preventing external contamination.

Step 6. Determine maximum flow for the static vent during operation.

Compressed air flow + liquid inflow air equivalent = maximum air flow

119 scfm + 1.3 scfm = 120 scfm

Step 7. Convert the maximum flow rate from standard temperature and pressure units to actual units.

$$\frac{\text{System standard flow requirement} \times 1 \text{ atm}}{\text{Inlet pressure} + 1 \text{ atm} - \text{differential pressure}} \times \frac{\text{ambient absolute temperature}}{\text{actual absolute temperature}} = \text{system actual flow}$$

$$\frac{120 \text{ scfm} \times 14.7 \text{ psia}}{5 \text{ psig} + 14.7 \text{ psia} - 5 \text{ psid}} \times \frac{273 \text{ K} + 30°\text{C}}{273 \text{ K} + 20°\text{C}} = 124 \text{ acfm}$$

Inlet pressure is equal to differential pressure in this case. Temperature is corrected for tank operating conditions of 30°C versus 20°C ambient.

Step 8. Determine the number of filters required for the static vent.

$$\frac{\text{System air flow requirement}}{\text{Filter flow per unit differential pressure} \times \text{differential pressure}} = \text{number of filters}$$

$$\frac{124 \text{ scfm}}{18 \text{ scfm per cartridge per psid} \times 5.0 \text{ psid}} = 1.4 \text{ 10 in. cartridges}$$

Two 10 in. cartridges will be used for the static vent.

Step 9. Recalculate actual clean differential pressure.

$$\frac{\text{System flow rate requirement}}{\text{Flow per unit EFA at unit differential pressure} \times \text{number of units}} = \text{clean differential pressure}$$

$$\frac{124 \text{ scfm}}{18 \text{ scfm per cartridge per psid} \times 2 \text{ cartridges}} = 3.4 \text{ psid clean differential pressure}$$

Step 10. Review the system for possible competing factors of flow rate, throughput, and economics.

The static vent requires six cartridges versus the four required by the dynamic venting system, two each for the dynamic and static portions. This savings in filters must be compared to the additional cost of a second vent port on the tank and the cost of supplying compressed air.

9.3 Derivation of Formula

The highest air flow rate into a tank is usually during the phase change after steam sterilization when the steam changes to water. A constant to calculate this flow is derived below based on the heat losses due to convection and radiation. The use of this constant assumes that the tank is not insulated or jacketed and that the outside environment is constant within the range 60–80°F. The constant is calculated at 212°F because this is the temperature where steam changes from the gas phase to the liquid phase. Above 212°F, the tank will be under pressure, so venting air flow is not needed.

The following terms are used:

a, *b*, and *m* are empirically derived values.
Other terms used are defined in Sec. 10.

Heat loss due to convection is defined by the Nusselt equation,

$$N_{\mathrm{Nu}} = a(N_{\mathrm{Gr}}N_{\mathrm{Pr}})^m = \frac{h_c L}{k}$$

where the Grashof and Prandtl numbers are

$$N_{\mathrm{Gr}} = \frac{L^2\rho^2 g\beta\Delta T}{\mu^2} \qquad \text{and} \qquad N_{\mathrm{Pr}} = \frac{c\mu}{k}$$

Substituting into the Nusselt equation gives

$$N_{\mathrm{Nu}} = a\left[\frac{L^3\rho^2 g\beta\Delta T}{\mu^2}\left(\frac{c\mu}{k}\right)\right]^m = a\left[\frac{(\rho^2 g\beta c\mu)(L^3\Delta T)}{\mu^2 k}\right]^m = \frac{h_c L}{k}$$

Expanding terms,

$$N_{\mathrm{Nu}} = \frac{h_c L}{k} = a\left(\frac{\rho^2 g\beta\mu}{\mu^2 k}\right)^m\left(\frac{L^3\Delta T}{\mu^2 k}\right)^m$$

$$= a\left(\frac{\rho^2 g\beta c\mu}{\mu^2 k}\right)^m\left(\frac{L^3}{\mu^2 k}\right)^m\left(\frac{\Delta T}{\mu^2 k}\right)^m$$

$$= a\,\frac{(\rho^2 g\beta c\mu)^m}{\mu^{2m}k^m}\left(\frac{L^{3m}}{\mu^{2m}k^m}\right)\left(\frac{(\Delta T)^m}{\mu^{2m}k^m}\right)$$

which rearranges to

$$h_c = ka\,\frac{(\rho^2 g\beta c\mu)^m L^{3m-1}(\Delta T)^m}{\mu^{2m}k^m}$$

A simplified form of the equation may be used by substitution:

$$h_c = b(\Delta T)^m L^{3m-1}$$

The empirically derived values *m*, *a*, and *b* are determined as functions of the product of the Grashof and Prandtl numbers. When these values are used to calculate h_c, the term $b(\Delta T)^m$ varies from 0.9 to 1.0, and the term L^{3m-1} varies from 0.5 to 1.0 for tank heights up to 20 ft. Thus the value for h_c varies from 0.5 to 1.0.

Heat loss due to radiation is defined for a surface where ε is emissivity of the steel surface, *T* is temperature in degrees Rankine, and σ is the Stefan–Boltzmann constant (0.17×10^{-8}):

$$q = h_r\Delta TA$$

$$h_r = \frac{\sigma T^4}{\Delta T}$$

$$q = \sigma\Delta T^4 A$$

Substitute for the temperature between surfaces and emissivity of the surface:

$$T^4 = \varepsilon(T^4_{max} - T^4_{min})$$

$$h_r = \frac{T^4_{max} - T^4_{min}}{T_{max} - T_{min}} \sigma\varepsilon$$

Assuming stainless steel surfaces, $\varepsilon = 0.55–0.66$, so the value of h_r varies from 0.8 to 1.0.

The heat loss due to convection and radiation ($h_c + h_r$) will then be 1.3–2.0.

At 212°F, steam has a heat of vaporization of 970 Btu/lb and a volume of 28 ft^3.

$$\frac{28 \text{ ft}^3/\text{lb}}{970 \text{ Btu/lb}} = 0.028 \text{ ft}^3/\text{Btu}$$

The total heat loss from the tank, where flow is in cubic feet, is

$$q \frac{\text{Btu}}{\text{h}} = (h_c + h_r) \frac{\text{Btu}}{\text{h} \cdot \text{ft}^2 \cdot {}^\circ\text{F}} \times A \text{ ft}^2 \times \Delta T{}^\circ\text{F}$$

$$\frac{\text{ft}^3}{\text{h}} = q \frac{\text{Btu}}{\text{h}} \times 0.028 \frac{\text{ft}^3}{\text{Btu}} = 0.028(h_c + h_r) \frac{\text{ft}^3}{\text{h} \cdot {}^\circ\text{F}} \times A \text{ ft}^2 \times \Delta T{}^\circ\text{F}$$

$$\frac{\text{ft}^3}{\text{min}} = \frac{\text{ft}^3}{\text{h}} \times \frac{\text{h}}{60 \text{ min}}$$

$$\frac{0.028}{60} (h_c + h_r) \frac{\text{ft}^3}{\text{h} \cdot {}^\circ\text{F}} \times A \text{ ft}^2 \times \Delta T{}^\circ\text{F} = 4.7 \times 10^{-4}(h_c + h_r) \frac{\text{ft}^3}{\text{h} \cdot {}^\circ\text{F}} \times A \text{ ft}^2 \times \Delta T{}^\circ\text{F}$$

$$\text{Constant} = 4.7 \times 10^{-4}(h_c + h_r) \times A \text{ ft}^2 \times \Delta T{}^\circ\text{F}$$

$$\frac{\text{ft}^3}{\text{min}} = \text{constant} \frac{\text{ft}^3}{\text{min} \cdot {}^\circ\text{F}} \times A \text{ ft}^2 \times \Delta T{}^\circ\text{F}$$

When $h_c + h_r$ is within the range 1.3–2.0, the constant ranges from 6.1×10^{-4} to 9.3×10^{-4}. Since conservatism must prevail in sizing tank vents, the value for the constant is chosen to be 10×10^{-4}, or 10^{-3}.

10 ABBREVIATIONS

A	Surface area
acfm	Actual cubic feet per minute
atm	Atmosphere
β	Coefficient of thermal expansion
Btu	British thermal units
c	Specific heat of air
°C	Degree Celsius
cfm	Cubic feet per minute
cP	Centipoise
ΔP	Differential pressure
ε	Emissivity of radiative surface

EFA	Effective filtration area
EtO	Ethylene oxide
g	Acceleration of gravity
gpm	Gallons per minute
H_2O	Water
h	Hour
h_c	Heat transfer by convection
h_r	Heat transfer by radiation
k	Thermal conductivity of air
L	Liter
L	Length or height
min	Minute
μm	Micrometer
μ	Viscosity of air
n	Number of moles of gas
N_{Gr}	Grashof number
N_{Nu}	Nusselt number
N_{Pr}	Prandtl number
P	Pressure
psi	Pounds per square inch
psia	Pounds per square inch, absolute
psid	Pounds per square inch, differential
psig	Pounds per square inch, gauge
q	Total heat loss
°R	Degrees Rankine (Fahrenheit absolute)
R	Universal gas constant
scfm	Standard cubic feet per minute
t	Time
T	Temperature
V	Volume
ρ	Density of air
σ	Stefan–Boltzmann constant

11 CONVERSION FACTORS

11.1 Length

Multiply	by	To obtain
centimeters	38.3213	inches
centimeters	0.01	meters
centimeters	10	millimeters
feet	30.48	centimeters
feet	12	inches
feet	0.3048	meters
inches	2.540	centimeters
inches	0.0833	feet
meters	100	centimeters
meters	3.281	feet

Multiply	by	To obtain
meters	39.37	inches
meters	10^6	micrometers
meters	10^3	millimeters

11.2 Area

Multiply	by	To obtain
cm^2	1.076×10^{-3}	ft^2
cm^2	0.1550	$in.^2$
cm^2	10^{-4}	m^2
ft^2	929	cm^2
ft^2	144	$in.^2$
ft^2	0.09290	m^2
$in.^2$	6.45	cm^2
$in.^2$	6.944×10^{-3}	ft^2
$in.^2$	645.2	mm^2
m^2	10^4	cm^2
m^2	10.76	ft^2

11.3 Volume

Multiply	by	To obtain
ft^3	7.481	gal
gal	28.32	L
gal	0.1337	ft^3
gal	3.785	L
L	0.03531	ft^3
L	0.2642	gal

11.4 Pressure

Multiply	by	To obtain
atm	14.7	psi ($lb/in.^2$)
atm	1.033	kg/cm^2
atm	1.01	bars
atm	1.013×10^6	dyn/cm^2
atm	76	cm Hg
atm	29.92	in. Hg
psi	2.036	in. Hg
psi	0.703	kg/cm^2
kg/cm^2	14.22	psi
bars	14.5	psi
cm Hg	0.1934	psi
H_2O	0.03613	psi

11.5 Temperature

Kelvin = °C + 273
Kelvin = [(°F − 32)/1.8] + 273

°Celsius	=	kelvin − 273
°C	=	(°F − 32)/1.8
°Fahrenheit	=	(°C × 1.8) + 32
°F	=	[(kelvin − 273) × 1.8] + 32

12 REAGENT PROPERTIES

Values at Ambient Temperature

Reagent	Surface tension (dyn/cm)	Viscosity (cP)
Acetic acid	28	1.2
Acetone	24	0.3
Aniline	43	4.4
Benzene	29	0.7
Benzyl alcohol	39	5.8
Butyl alcohol	25	2.9
Carbon tetrachloride	27	0.9
Chloroform	27	0.6
Ethyl alcohol	23	1.2
Ethyl ether	17	0.2
Formamide	58	3.3
Freon TF	17	0.7
Glycerol	63	1,500
Isopropyl alcohol	22	2.5
Isopropyl ether	10	0.3
Methyl alcohol	23	0.6
Nitric acid	80	1.3
Propyl alcohol	24	2.3
Sulfuric acid	55	25
Toluene	32	0.6
Water (distilled)	72	1
Xylene	28	0.7

REFERENCES

Cole, J. C., and R. H. Shumsky. (1977). Filter sizing for economics: Liquid systems, *Pharm. Technol.*, *1*(11):39–41.

Johnston, P. R., and D. L. Beals. (1980). Constant pressure liquid filtration: Mathematical models for fast plugging of the filter medium, *J. Testing Eval.*, *8*(2):57–62.

Lukaszewicz, R. C., P. R. Johnston, and T. H. Meltzer. (1981). Prefilters/final filters: A matter of particulate/pore size distribution, *J. Parenter. Sci. Technol.*, *35*:40–47.

Meltzer, T. H., and R. C. Lukaszewicz. (1979). *Quality Control in the Pharmaceutical Industry*, Vol. 3, Academic, New York, 1979.

Meltzer, T. H. (1987). *Filtration in the Pharmaceutical Industry*, Marcel Dekker, New York.

Perry, R. H., and D. W. Green (eds.). (1984). *Perry's Chemical Engineer's Handbook*, 6th ed., McGraw-Hill, New York.

Trasen, B. (1981). Designing microfiltration systems, *Pharm. Technol.*, *15*(11):62–69.

Weast, R. C. (ed.). (1986). *CRC Handbook of Chemistry and Physics*, 67th ed., CRC Press, Boca Raton, FL.

13

Filter Housing Materials and Surface Finish

JOHN GULLIFORD
Pall Corporation, Pleasanton, California

1 INTRODUCTION

The 3-A Sanitary Standards (1984) developed by the International Association of Milk, Food and Environmental Sanitarians cover the proper design, materials, and construction of milk distribution systems. 3-A Standard 10-03 is for filters using disposable filter media. This standard calls for the product contact surface materials to be AISI 300 Series stainless steel or other metal that under conditions of intended use is at least as corrosion-resistant as stainless steel of the foregoing type and is nontoxic. This standard also calls for all product contact surfaces to have a finish at least as smooth as a No. 4 ground finish on stainless steel sheets. Filter housings for use in critical pharmaceutical applications are required to be of sanitary design and must comply with this 3-A standard. The correct selection of material and surface finish plays a vital role in minimizing corrosion of filter housings. This will help ensure a long, contamination-free service life.

2 MATERIALS OF CONSTRUCTION

There are two primary criteria for selection of filter housing materials. The first is corrosion resistance, and the second is cost. There is no one perfect material that is immune to all types of corrosion. All materials corrode to some degree. The material must be matched to its environment. In almost all cases, materials with high corrosion resistance will cost more than the less corrosion resistant materials.

2.1 Corrosion Resistance

Corrosion is the return of any metal to its most stable thermodynamic state. It is the reaction of a metal with its environment to form a stable oxide, sulfide, amine, amide, sulfate, carbonate, nitrate, or any other compound related to the environment. Corrosion alters the metal's physical dimensions and reduces its strength and ductility. This can lead to fatigue or stress corrosion failure.

Since no material is immune to all types of corrosion, it is essential to match the proper material with the environment. Materials are attacked by five basic types of corrosion: uniform corrosion, galvanic corrosion including pitting and crevice corrosion, intergranular corrosion, stress corrosion cracking, and microbiologically influenced corrosion.

Uniform Corrosion

Metals form a protective oxide or other compound on their exposed surfaces. It is this layer that gives the metal its corrosion resistance. On some metals, this layer is only several molecules thick and does not increase in thickness until some event, such as an increase in temperature, upsets the equilibrium. This is called a passive layer, and it occurs in such metals as stainless steel, titanium, chromium-nickel alloys, aluminum, and zirconium. Other metals form their protective layer by allowing it to grow to a finite thickness, at which time the outer layer sloughs off and allows oxygen or other corrodent to reach the base metal. A new layer is formed, and the sloughing off process is repeated. This is called an active layer, and given enough time the metal will be consumed by its environment. This active layer formation is typical of copper and its alloys, cast iron, carbon steel, and zinc.

Uniform corrosion is the uniform breakdown of the passive layer or the accelerated formation or removal of the active layer over the entire surface of the metal. It is expressed as a regular rate of metal loss over the entire surface. If a corrosion allowance is made in a design, it is for this type of corrosion loss only. Uniform corrosion can be minimized by choosing the proper materials that are resistant to the environment.

Galvanic Corrosion

A factor known as the *solution pressure* is obtained by immersing a metal into a 1 molal (1 *m*) solution of one of its salts and measuring the electrical potential that must be applied to prevent any action. A listing known as the galvanic series of metals and alloys is made by listing metals in order of their solution pressures (see Table 1).

When two dissimilar metals in contact are suspended in an electrolyte, the one that is above the other in the galvanic series will become anodic, suffer corrosion, and protect the other metal, which becomes cathodic. The cathodic metal shows no corrosion loss even though it could if it were not in contact with the other metal. This can be seen in the use of sacrificial zinc in protecting ship hulls and in galvanizing.

Pitting is a form of galvanic corrosion in which the passive layer breaks down in isolated spots. Note that stainless steel occupies two positions in the electromotive force series. Pitting corrosion of stainless steel is galvanic corrosion where both the anode and cathode exist on the same surface. Rapid attack can occur because the cathode area is large and can create high current densities at each pit, especially in acidic chloride solutions. Stainless steels that are high in chromium and molybdenum have excellent resistance to pitting.

Table 1 Galvanic Series of Metals and Alloys

Least noble or corroded (Anodic)
↑ Magnesium
Beryllium
Aluminum
Manganese
Zinc
Chromium
Mild steel
Cast iron
Stainless steels (active), Alloy 20Cb-3 (active), Hastelloy C (active)
Cadmium
Nickel [includes nickel (active), Inconel (active), Hastelloy B (active)]
Tin
Lead
0 Hydrogen
Copper [includes brasses, copper, monel, nickel (passive), Inconel (passive), stainless steel (passive), alloy 20Cb-3 (passive)]
Mercury
Silver
Stainless steel Type 430 (passive)
Stainless steel Type 304 (passive)
Stainless steel Type 316 (passive)
Palladium
Platinum
↓ Gold
Most noble or protected (Cathodic)

A form of pitting corrosion found in pharmaceutical water-for-injection (WFI) systems is known as *rouge*. Rouge takes many forms such as a yellowish-green powder over a dense brown deposit on a black layer, a reddish-brown deposit over a black layer, or a dry upper crust over a gelatinous hydrated bottom layer. This type of corrosion can be very destructive to austenitic stainless steel. It can be generated by a number of contaminants such as martensitic or carbon steel in the system; excessive heat tint produced during welding, grinding, or electropolishing; or improper passivation. Rouge cannot be simply wiped off and must be removed chemically either through electropolishing or by repassivation in nitric acid or chelant solution. If possible, the cause of the rouge should be found and eliminated.

Crevice corrosion is another form of galvanic corrosion. It is caused by local differences in the oxygen concentration within a crevice. The crevice can be under deposits on the surface such as paint, or under gaskets, lap joints, or bolt heads. Crevice corrosion can progress very rapidly and is more severe with acidic halide solutions. The stainless steels that are high in molybdenum are often used to minimize the problem.

Intergranular Corrosion

When austenitic stainless steels that contain carbon are heated or cooled through the range of 850–1650°F (427–899°C), chromium along the grain boundaries will combine with carbon to form chromium carbides. This process is called sensitization or carbide precipitation. The carbide formation requires more chromium than is available immediately around the carbon atoms and takes chromium from the surrounding area. This creates an area that is too low in chromium to form the protective passive layer. Rapid grain boundary attack can then occur through galvanic corrosion. Sensitization can occur from improper heat treating wherein the entire piece is affected or from welding, which affects a narrow band along the weld known as the heat-affected zone or HAZ.

Intergranular corrosion in austenitic stainless steels can be prevented by the following methods:

1. Use metal in the annealed state with no welding.
2. When the metal has been sensitized by welding, redissolve the carbides by annealing after fabrication. This involves heating to 2000°F and rapid quenching to prevent the carbides from re-forming.
3. Use low carbon (0.030% maximum) stainless steel for welded fabrication. This is denoted by the L grades 304L, 316L, and 317L. Their low carbon content prevents carbide precipitation during the short heat exposure of welding. They still may become sensitized during prolonged exposure to temperatures above 1000°F.
4. Use a stainless steel alloy that contains titanium (Type 321), or columbium (niobium) (Type 347). The protection is formed by the greater affinity of titanium and columbium for carbon compared to chromium.

Stress Corrosion Cracking

Three conditions are needed for stress corrosion cracking to occur: a sensitive metal, a tensile stress, and a suitable environment. Many alloys are known to experience stress corrosion cracking: brass in ammonia, aluminum in seawater, stainless steel in chloride solutions, titanium in methanol, and even gold in acetic acid. The solutions do not need to be concentrated; often just a few parts per million are all that is necessary. High levels of nickel increase the resistance of stainless steels to stress corrosion cracking. Also, as the molybdenum content increases, the resistance to stress corrosion cracking also increases.

Microbiologically Influenced Corrosion

Bacterial action can cause corrosion by producing compounds such as carbon dioxide, hydrogen sulfide, ammonia, and acids that attack metals. Bacteria can also produce products that act as catalysts for corrosion. Bacteria have been known to concentrate manganese from the environment, which when combined with chlorine produces hydrochloric acid that can rapidly attack stainless steel.

2.2 Cost

Corrosion-resistant materials cost more than those that corrode (see Table 2). The difference in cost can usually be justified on the basis of savings in downtime, lost product, and replacement cost.

Table 2 Material Cost Comparison[a]

Alloy	Ratio	Alloy	Ratio
Carbon steel	0.24	310S	3.03
Brass	0.94	904L	3.31
304	1.00	Titanium Gr2	3.85
90-10 Cu-Ni	1.10	825	4.09
409	1.14	20Cb3	4.38
316L	1.14	G3	4.59
439	1.22	800	4.67
321	1.35	7-Mo PLUS	4.91
18-2	1.43	800 Seamless	5.32
317L	1.43	17-7PH	5.73
347	1.51	625	5.90
70-30 Cu-Ni	1.80	200	6.14
317LM	1.80	C-276	6.14
430	1.88	X	6.55
2205	2.21	Invar 36	6.55
SEA CURE	2.41	600	6.63
309S	2.62	B-2	8.19
AL-6XN	2.86		

[a]Cast ratio based on Type 304 stainless steel = 1.00. This is a relative comparison only and should not be construed as a price schedule.
Source: Data furnished courtesy of Trent Tube, East Troy, WI.

2.3 AISI 300 Series Stainless Steel

The AISI 300 Series stainless steels are known as austenitic stainless steels, and they contain chromium and nickel. The 31 stainless steels in this group have different properties and compositions. They have excellent corrosion resistance and good workability. They are nonmagnetic and cannot be hardened by heat treatment.

Type 304 stainless steel is the most common commercially used member of this series. It is also known as 18-8 stainless. At ambient temperatures and pressures it is resistant to a great variety of corrosive agents. It is very susceptible to chloride stress corrosion cracking, especially in the unannealed, cold-worked, or as-welded condition. When welded, Type 304, which contains 0.08% carbon, may develop a heat-affected zone that is sensitized. If this area is exposed to active electrolytes, intergranular corrosion may occur. The use of Type 304L, which contains less than 0.03% carbon, will minimize this problem. Type 304 or 304L should not be used in salt water or other high chloride solutions as pitting or crevice or stress corrosion cracking may occur. Type 304 or 304L can be protected from galvanic corrosion by joining with aluminum, Types 410 and 430 stainless steels, lead, carbon steel, and Babbit bearing metal. If any mineral packing containing sulfur, Monel, titanium, platinum, or silver is used with Type 304 or 304L stainless steel, accelerated galvanic corrosion will occur.

Type 316 stainless steel is most commonly used in pharmaceutical applications. It offers the best combination of high corrosion resistance with a minimal cost increase. It has better corrosion resistance than Type 304 due to its slightly higher nickel content and the addition of molybdenum. It is slightly more resistant to chloride stress corrosion cracking, but it is still susceptible at temperatures above 150°F. When welded, Type 316, which contains 0.08% carbon, may develop a heat-affected zone that is sensitized. If this area is exposed to active electrolytes, intergranular corrosion may occur. The use of type 316L, which contains less than 0.03% carbon, will minimize this problem. Types 316 and 316L have a higher critical crevice corrosion temperature (CCT) in chloride solutions than Types 304 and 304L. The critical crevice corrosion temperature is the temperature below which crevice corrosion will not occur but above which it will occur. Crevice corrosion always occurs at temperatures less than those required for pitting. The CCT is directly related to the crevice and pitting resistance equivalent (PRE).

The pitting resistance equivalent is calculated by the formula PRE = % Cr + (3.3)(% Mo) + (16)(% N). The PREs for several materials are listed in Table 3. This equation and Table 3 show the relationship of molybdenum content to pitting resistance. The higher the molybdenum content of a metal, the higher the PRE, the higher the CCT, and the less susceptible the metal is to pitting and crevice corrosion. This increased corrosion resistance for Type 316 stainless steel increases the material cost only about 14% over that of Type 304 (see Table 2).

Type 317 stainless steel has more chromium and molybdenum than Type 316. This gives Type 317 a higher CCT than Type 316 and even greater resistance to pitting in chloride solutions. Type 317L is available to minimize intergranular corrosion after welding. This increase in corrosion resistance increases the material cost by 43% over that of Type 304 (see Table 2). Type 317L is sometimes used as a welding filler metal when welding Type 316L. The Type 317L filler metal provides a higher molybdenum content to the weld joint and increases the corrosion resistance in this sensitive area.

2.4 Other Corrosion-Resistant Metals

For applications that require higher corrosion resistance than is afforded by Type 316 stainless steel, there are a number of other choices. For environments that require high pitting or crevice corrosion resistance, there are SEA-CURE, AL-6XN, and

Table 3 Pitting Resistance Equivalent

PRE	Material	Percent Mo
18.0	304	0
19.6	304N	0
22.6	316	2.0–3.0
24.2	316N	2.0–3.0
25.6	20Cb-3	2.0–3.0
27.9	317	3.0–4.0
31.8	317LMN	4.0–5.0
42.7	AL-6XN	6.0–7.0
46.4	625	8.0–10
73.9	C-276	15.0–17.0

20Mo-6. For applications requiring high chloride stress corrosion cracking resistance, there are 20Mo-6, 7-Mo PLUS, SEA-CURE, 2205, and AL-6XN. For use in strong reducing agents, there are B-2 and titanium. These alternative materials raise the cost by 221–819% over that of Type 304 (see Table 2).

3 SURFACE FINISH

Surface finish is expressed by using several different terminologies and obtained by using various mechanical and chemical methods. To select the proper surface finish for a pharmaceutical filter housing, it is necessary to understand what these different terminologies and methods are and the differences between them.

3.1 Mechanical Surface Finishing

There are three primary means of classifying surface finish. The first is called the Standard Mechanical Sheet Finish and is given with a number and letter that indicates a process sequence used in the manufacture of stainless steel sheet. The second type of classification is by grit or mesh size. For example, 180 grit indicates the smallest size abrasive used in the surface finishing procedure. The third is by surface finish measurement using a device such as a profilometer.

Sheet Finish

The sheet finish number refers to the manufacturing processes that the mill used to manufacture the sheet (see Table 4). It is a designation of that process only and is not a quantitative measurement of the surface. Sheet finishes No. 2B, No. 4, and No. 7 are commonly found in pharmaceutical filter housing manufacture.

Mill Finish No. 2B

The most commonly used material for filter housing shells has a No. 2B mill finish. This material has a bright finish that to the naked eye appears very smooth, but when viewed under a scanning electron microscope (SEM) it is seen to be very rough surface (see Fig. 1). The grains can be seen to be clearly separated by deep valleys. This is caused by the pickling process that uses chemicals that attack the surface. The grain boundaries are very reactive and are attacked to a higher degree than other areas, leaving these valleys between the grains. The flattened grain tops are caused by the light roll after pickling. It is these flat grain tops that give the bright finish. This rough cold-worked surface is known as the Bielby layer. The surface may also contain contaminants such as carbon steel particles pressed into it during the final cold-rolling operation. This surface finish is unsuitable for critical pharmaceutical filtration and must receive further finishing before use. Also, if this surface is scratched, the original finish cannot be restored.

Mill Finish No. 4

This finish is often referred to as a sanitary finish. It is the finish specified in the 3-A standard. It is produced by grinding a No. 2B with a progressively finer series of abrasives, finishing with a 150–180 grit. This finish is visibly grained, and when viewed with a scanning electron microscope (see Fig. 2) reveals a surface with no visible grain boundaries. The surface is now covered with many small ridges and valleys. These ridges and valleys are several micrometers in height and width. These

Table 4 Standard Mechanical Steel Finishes

Unpolished finishes	
No. 1	A rough, dull surface produced by hot rolling to the specified thickness, followed by annealing and descaling.
No. 2D	A dull finish produced by cold rolling to specified thickness, followed by annealing and descaling. May also be accompanied by a final, light roll pass on dull rolls.
No. 2B	A bright finish commonly produced in the same way as No. 2D, except that the annealed and descaled sheet receives a final, light roll pass through polished rolls. This is the general-purpose cold-rolled finish and is more readily polished than the No. 1 or No. 2D finishes.
No. 2BA	A bright mirrorlike finish produced by cold rolling then annealing in a controlled atmosphere furnace. This is followed by a single light skin pass through a cold mill over highly polished rolls.
Polished finishes	
No. 3	An intermediate polished finish obtained by finishing with a 100 grit abrasive. Generally used where a semifinished polished surface is required. A No. 3 finish usually receives additional polishing during fabrication.
No. 4	A polished finish obtained by finishing with 120–150 grit abrasive following initial grinding with coarser abrasives. This is a general-purpose bright finish with a visible "grain" that prevents mirror reflection.
Buffed finishes	
No. 6	A soft satin finish having lower reflectivity than No. 4 finish. It is produced with a greaseless compound, No. 200 grit, top dressed with white rouge or chromium green compound on a No. 4 finish.
No. 7	A highly reflective finish produced by buffing finely ground surfaces, but not to the extent that existing grit lines are removed.
No. 8	The most reflective surface; obtained by polishing with successively finer abrasives and buffing extensively until all grit lines from preliminary grinding operations are removed.

Source: Stainless steel industry data.

are not the visible grain lines. There are no flat reflective surfaces. The rough, jagged edges of the ridges can break off and become a source of particles in the system. This finish is a procedural specification only and does not have any measurable quality requirements. Therefore it can vary greatly from vendor to vendor and even from lot to lot.

Mill Finish No. 7

This mirror-bright surface appears to the naked eye to be almost perfect. There are no visible scratches, pits, or flaws. It is produced from No. 4 finish sheet that has been further finished by using cloth buffing wheels and buffing compounds. The buffing compounds may or may not be greaseless. The greaseless compounds contain water, glue, and abrasives such as silicone carbide. The other buffing compounds contain a binder and an abrasive. The binder can consist of one or more materials taken from animal or vegetable fats as well as petroleum and similarly derived products. Animal fats are such materials as fatty acids, tallows, and glycerides. Waxes can be from vegetable-, insect-, or petroleum-based products. Petroleum-based or

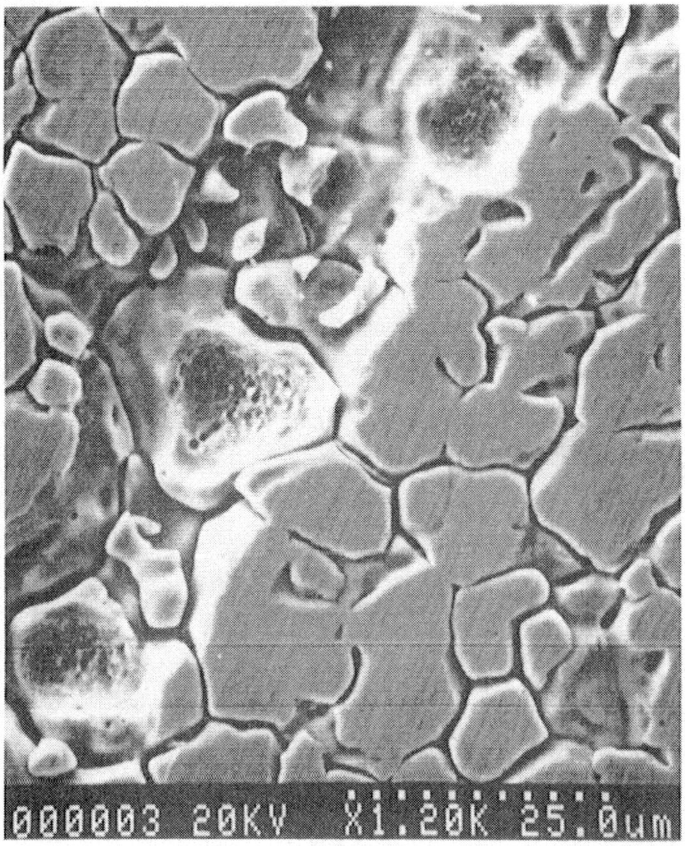

Figure 1 Scanning electron micrograph of No. 2B mill finish (×1800).

vegetable-based oils can also be used. The animal and vegetable materials are more saponified and will produce a water-soluble soap when combined with alkali. Petroleum, mineral oils, and waxes are unsaponified and therefore might create subsequent cleaning problems.

The buffing wheel is run perpendicular to the grain in the No. 4 finish. When the No. 7 finish is viewed with a scanning electron microscope (see Fig. 3) it can be seen that the buffing process has smeared the ridges in the grain over the valleys and produced a very flat surface. This accounts for the high degree of reflectance. But due to the variation in the grain in the No. 4 finish, every so often there is a valley that was too wide or too deep to smear over. This produces grooves in and tunnels under the surface. These tunnels may trap buffing compound and other contaminants that cannot be cleaned. These may in time leach out and contaminate the system. Due to these tunnels, a No. 7 finish should never be used on a product contact surface.

Grit Finish

When a surface finish is referred to as some number grit finish such as "180 grit," the number refers to the smallest abrasive grain size used in producing that finish.

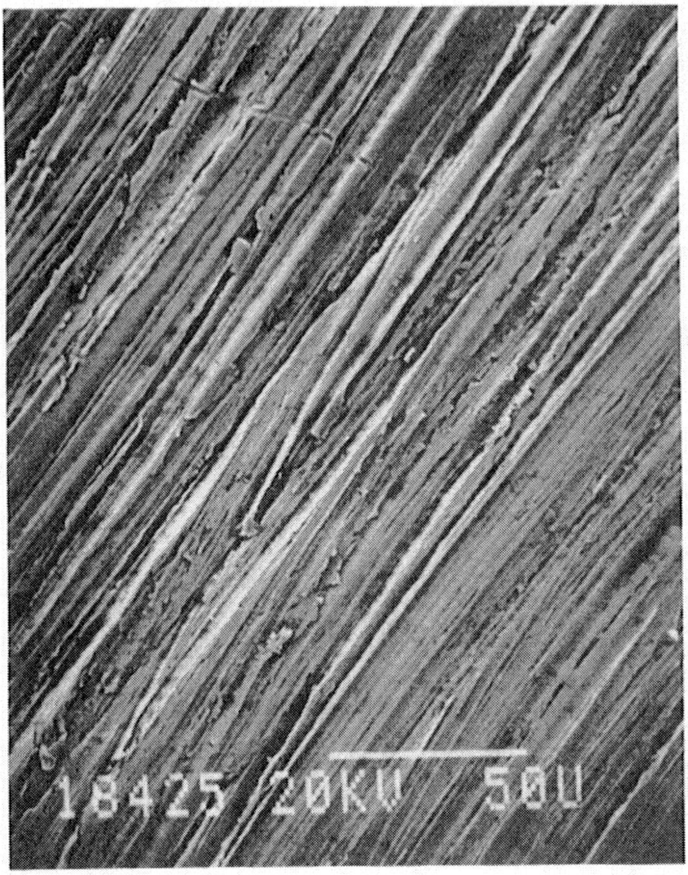

Figure 2 Scanning electron micrograph of No. 4 ground finish (×680; the line near the bottom = 50 μm).

Grinding and sanding abrasives start out as large chunks. These are then crushed, and the resulting grains are then separated into standard particle sizes using screens made from silk threads of an exact size and number per square inch. The grit number (mesh number) represents the approximate number of openings per linear inch in the final screen. The Coated Abrasive Manufacturers Institute has a grading specification called CAMI grades to which the coated abrasive manufacturers adhere. A comparison of grit particle size to CAMI grade is listed in Table 5.

Like the standard mechanical sheet finish, the grit finish number is a procedural specification and does not have any measurable quality specifications. The finish can vary with choice of abrasive materials, whether hand or machine ground, and duration of each grinding step. To finish stainless steel to a 180–400 grit finish, it is necessary to proceed in steps, starting with a coarse abrasive such as 80 grit to remove the original mill finish, then repeating with 120 grit and 180 grit and so forth until the final grit necessary to produce the desired finish. If the housing manufacturer takes shortcuts and skips these preparatory steps, the final surface could still contain the impurities of the original mill surface.

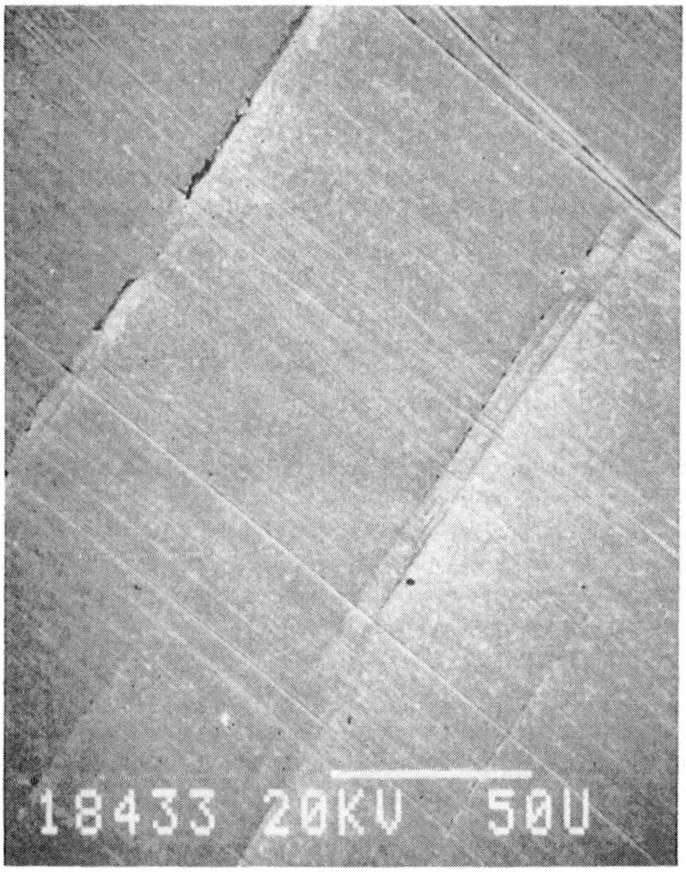

Figure 3 Scanning electron micrograph of No. 7 buffed finish (×680).

Surface Finish Measurement

Advances in electronics during the past few years have produced instruments that can directly measure the surface finish. The most common device consists of a precision drive with a probe and stylus mounted on one end. The stylus has a diamond-ground tip with a rounded conical shape. The drive draws the probe across the surface, perpendicular to the grain, and the stylus tip follows the surface contour. Electronic signals from the tip are amplified, filtered, and delivered as roughness output. There are also new devices that employ laser and optical sensors.

The most common unit of surface roughness measurement is average roughness, R_a, which is the average value of the departures from its centerline of the sampling length expressed in microinches. The centerline is such that the sum of the areas within the profile above the line is equal to the sum of those below the line. A difficulty in using this measurement is that many different surface profiles can have the same R_a value. Another common unit is R_{rms} or R_q, which is based on the statistical deviation of root mean square and expressed in micrometers (μm) or microinches (μin.). This unit weights the surface's predominant features. An approxi-

Table 5 Abrasive Grain Size

Particle size		
in.	μm	CAMI grade
0.00092	23.6	400
0.00140	36.0	320
0.00209	53.5	240
0.00304	78.0	180
0.00452	116.0	120
0.00749	192.0	80

mate comparison between various finishes produced using different grit sizes and the resulting R_{rms} and R_a values is given in Table 6.

When using a surface finish measurement device, several measurements must be taken at different locations. This is due to the fact that a measurement is being made on a very small site and a local anomaly can have a large effect on the measurement and not be representative of the entire surface.

Chemical Surface Finishing

The three most commonly used chemical surface treatments for stainless steels are pickling, passivation, and electropolishing. The three processes employ different chemistries and have markedly different effects on the metal surfaces.

Pickling

Pickling is the process of immersing a metal into a solution of acids to remove metal, metal oxides, heat-treat scale, and foreign metals from the surface. It generally leaves the surface chemically clean and ready for further processing. Stainless steel, nickel alloys, and titanium are usually pickled in a bath of nitric and hydrofluoric acids. Hydrochloric acid can be used but can cause intergranular attack, and residual chloride ions may cause stress corrosion during service. Pickling leaves a rough surface as seen on the SEM of No. 2B sheet (see Fig. 1).

Table 6 Surface Finish Comparison

Grit size	R_{rms} (μin.)	R_{rms} (μm)	R_a (μin.)
36	160	4.06	142
60	98	2.49	87
80	80	2.03	71
120	58	1.47	52
180	34	0.86	30
240	17	0.43	15
320	14	0.36	12

Passivation

Passivation of stainless steel is the formation of the protective layer of nickel and chromium oxides that prevents the formation of iron oxide (rust). Stainless steel self-passivates when exposed to air. This process can be inhibited by surface contaminants such as dirt or oil and by the presence of carbon steel particles. The process known as passivation is actually an acid cleaning process that removes these surface contaminants and allows the stainless steel to form an integral passive layer when reexposed to air. There are several different passivation procedures depending on the alloy. These are covered by federal specification QQ-P-35. Passivation does not change the surface appearance or profile.

Electropolishing

Electropolishing is a method of imparting brilliance to a surface by removing a thin surface layer. The work to be electropolished is the anode in a cell containing a suitable electrolyte. Electropolishing may be considered as the opposite of electroplating. It is also known as electrolytic polishing, anodic lustering, bright finishing, bright pickling, or superpassivation. The 300 Series stainless steels are most com-

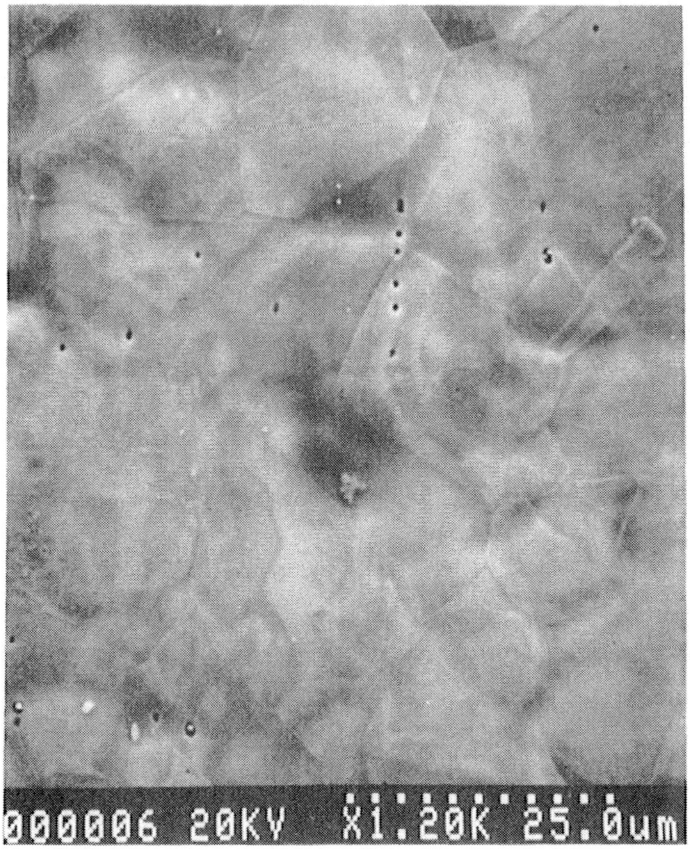

Figure 4 Scanning electron micrograph of No. 2B mill finish after electropolish (×1800).

monly electropolished, but many other metals can also be electropolished by using the proper electrolytes and procedures.

Electropolishing produces a surface that is extremely smooth. This minimizes the adherence of debris on the surface. This is especially important in pharmaceutical applications because contaminants can ruin an entire batch. The smooth surface also shortens cleaning time, as hydroblasting can be accomplished using less pressure and in less time.

Electropolishing removes the Bielby layer (cold-worked metal) that seems to attract corrosives, including bacteria. Compare the surfaces shown in Figs. 1 and 2, which show No. 2B and No. 4 finishes with Figs. 4 and 5, which show the same surfaces after electropolishing. Note that the electropolished No. 4 surface shown in Fig. 5 is almost totally devoid of physical features.

Removal of the Bielby layer also removes most imperfections that act as microstress risers. These stress risers can lead to poor fatigue strength, premature mechanical failure, or, in some cases, stress corrosion cracking.

Electropolishing removes the ferrite ions from the surface and 25–50 Å deep into the metal. This produces a layer that is richer in chromium and nickel than the

Figure 5 Scanning electron micrograph of No. 4 ground finish after electropolish (×680).

base metal. The extra chromium and nickel combine with oxygen to form a passive layer of chromium and nickel oxides that is thicker and denser than the layer found on nonelectropolished surfaces.

4 SUMMARY

In choosing the proper material and surface finish for a pharmaceutical filter housing, there are a number of factors to consider. To minimize corrosion and contamination of the solution being filtered, the materials of construction must be compatible with the solution being filtered and the environment in which they are being used. 316L stainless steel has the best combination of corrosion resistance and low cost and is the most commonly used pharmaceutical filter housing material. Due to the vagueness of the various methods of specifying a surface finish, no one current method alone will suffice even if the manufacturer should furnish surface finish measurement certificates. A surface should be specified by a combination of factors such as 180 grit progressively ground finish, using no buffing compounds, with $32R_a$ maximum followed by electropolishing.

REFERENCES

3-A sanitary standards, *J. Food Protect*, May, 1984.

American Iron and Steel Institute. (1983). *Finishes for Stainless Steel*, AISI, Washington, DC, June.

Coleman, D. C., and R. Evans. Corrosion investigation of 316L stainless steel pharmaceutical WFI systems, *Pharm Eng.*, *11*(4):9–13.

Dickman, A., and B. Millman. Polishing and buffing, *Metal Finish.*, *94*(1A):16–33.

Nickel Development Institute. (1991). *Design Guidelines for the Selection and Use of Stainless Steel*, Toronto, Ontario, Canada.

Trent Tube. (1996). *Stainless Steel & Alloy Tubular Products Handbook*, East Troy, WI, February.

Tverberg, J. C. (1994). Choosing the Proper Stainless Steel, Trent Tube, East Troy, WI.

Tverberg, J. C. (1994). Electropolished Tubing Pharmaceutical Quality, Trent Tube, East Troy, WI.

14

Filter Housings for Biotechnology and Pharmaceutical Applications

STANLEY W. TARRY
Sartorius Corporation, Edgewood, New York

1 INTRODUCTION

Filter housings designed for critical applications found in the pharmaceutical and biotechnology industries must adhere to numerous national and international standards. Applications such as clarification, sterile liquid filtration, sterile venting, and sterile supply of bulk gases require validated processes and validated equipment. Accepted regulations and standards set forth include cGMP/FDA (current Good Manufacturing Practices of the Food and Drug Administration), the 3-A Sanitary Standards, the USP (United States Pharmacopeia), and the ASME BPVC Section VIII, Division 1 (American Society of Mechanical Engineers Boiler and Pressure Vessel Code). Manufacturers of filter housings must ensure that designs are in compliance with current revisions of each standard. Filter housings are supplied by filter cartridge manufacturers as well as independent suppliers. Universal designs are available that allow for use of any vendor's filters.

2 APPLICATIONS OF FILTER HOUSINGS

Filter housings are generally used when the cost associated with cleaning validation does not outweigh that of using a completely disposable device such as a capsule filter (see Fig. 1). For example, in a laboratory, sterile air can be supplied by using a disposable, hermetically sealed stainless steel housing. Enclosed within the housing is a 0.2 μm Teflon membrane cartridge. While this may appear to be an expensive "throwaway" device, the simplicity and longevity of the device makes it a viable alternative to a multipiece cartridge housing with a replaceable cartridge. When considering sterile filtration of SVPs (small volume parenterals), quite often it is more

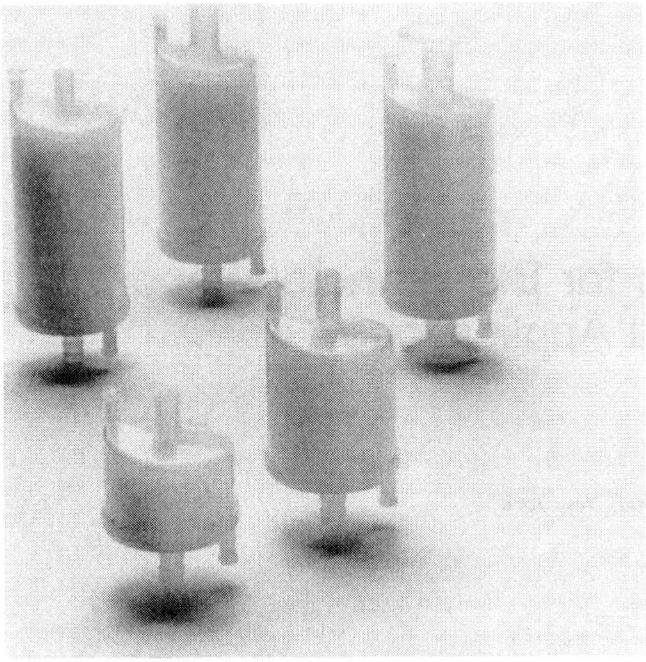

Figure 1 Disposable capsule for point of use.

cost-effective to use disposable capsule filters for the final stages of filtration because capsule filters eliminate the need for cleaning of a reusable filter housing.

3 TYPES OF FILTER HOUSINGS

3.1 Disk Filter Housings

The commonly accepted definition of a filter housing is that of the stainless steel type. However, in a laboratory setting where flat sheet (individual membrane) housings are used, the material of construction may be polycarbonate, Teflon, polypropylene, or stainless steel. When a longer life is needed, a commonly used material for flat sheet membrane filter housings is 316L stainless steel. The holders are commonly available to house membranes with diameters of 47, 90, 142, and 293 mm. Although the 293 mm device was commonly used in the past for production scale filtration, it has largely been replaced by the introduction of sterile disposable capsule filters. A typical disk filter holder design is shown in Fig. 2.

This design consists of a filter base with supporting legs, a drainage screen, a support screen, an upstream support plate, the top inlet plate, isolation O-rings, and vent/sample valves. The filter membrane is sandwiched between the upper and lower support plates with an O-ring acting to prevent any bypass of liquid around the edges of the disk. Care must be exercised when tightening the disk filter housing to prevent permanent deformation of the O-ring. The general procedure for use of disk filter housings is to wet the membrane with buffer, water, or product and gently place it on the lower support screen. The upstream compression O-ring is placed on top of

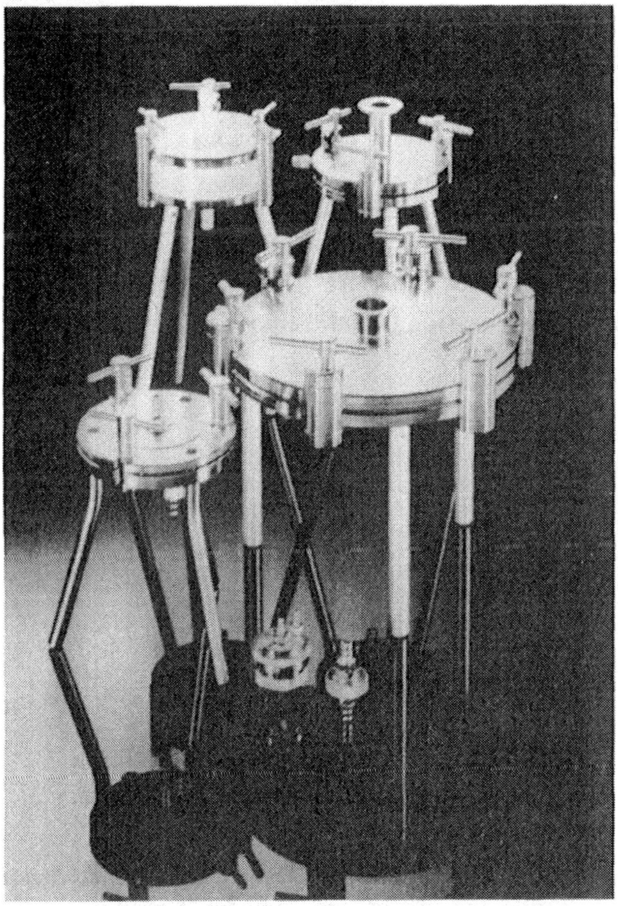

Figure 2 Typical disk filter holder designs.

the membrane, followed by the top plate. The top plate is secured by tightening the T-bolts in an alternating pattern. If an integrity-testable membrane is being used, the filter assembly may be integrity tested by the bubble point method once the assembly is properly closed. After testing, unfiltered liquid is introduced to the top plate. Excess air will become trapped and may denature proteins, so most devices come equipped with a manual sanitary vent valve. In addition to the sanitary vent valve, some designs are also equipped with a drain/sample valve on the lower casing. This can be used to facilitate cleaning or for sampling the filtered product during the filtration operation.

3.2 Stacked Disk Filter Housings

Stacked disk filter housings are currently being offered to the pharmaceutical industry by various manufacturers. This type of filter cartridge contains various types of depth filtration media on a support structure. Multiple disks are stacked on a central filtrate column. Generally available in 10 in. stacks of five or six disks, the individual stacks

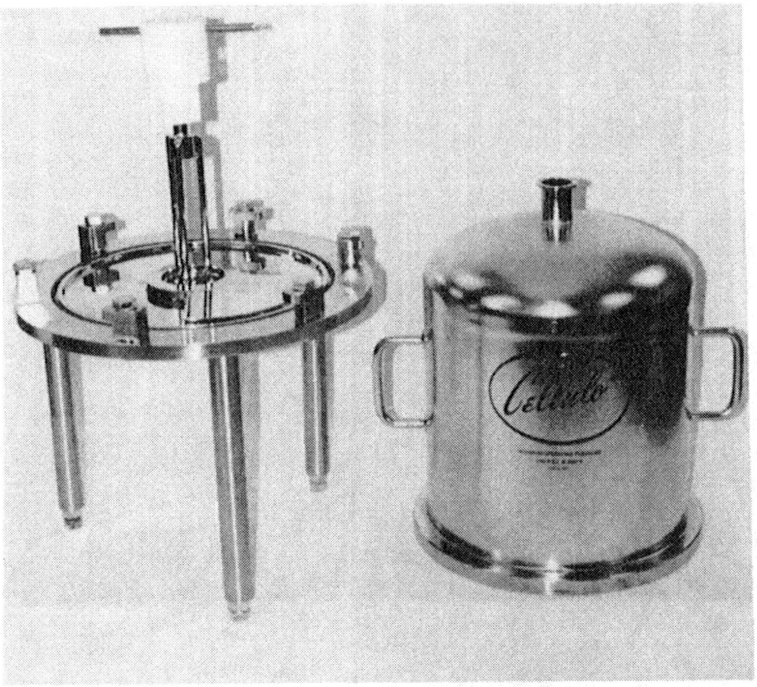

Figure 3 Typical housing and filter design.

may be combined to form elements up to 40 in. in height. The designs of the element lock differ for each company, requiring the use of one company's product solely with each filter housing. Adapters are available to allow for conversion to another supplier's filters, but this adds an additional component to the piece of equipment. Figure 3 illustrates a typical housing and filter stack design.

This type of housing is usually manufactured in a T-line configuration, where the inlet and outlet are both on the base of the housing. Custom configurations are available from most manufacturers to suit specific installation requirements.

3.3 Cartridge Filter Housings

The majority of filter housings used in the pharmaceutical industry are designed to accept cartridge filters. Cartridge filters come in standard lengths of 10, 20, 30, and 40 in. and are generally slightly less than 3 in. in diameter. Some suppliers offer a 5 in. version with a universal interlock, while others maintain a design specific to their filters alone. Filter housings are designed for a single cartridge or for multiple parallel cartridges. Multicartridge housings and single-cartridge housings are available in several configurations. The most common are described below.

T-Line

T-line housings, or T-style as they are often referred to, are designed for installation into fixed piping systems. A typical design is shown in Fig. 4. The housing base

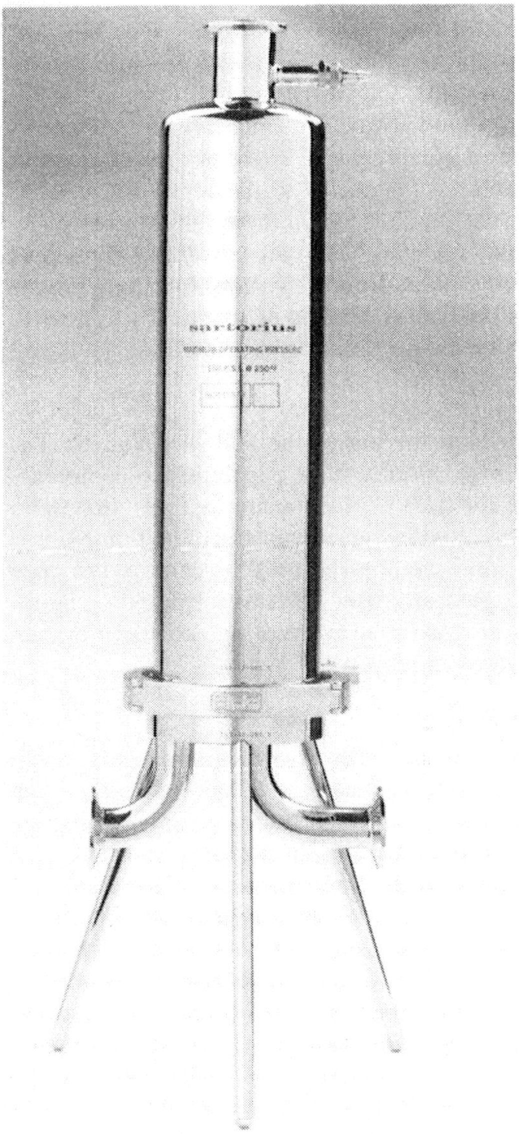

Figure 4 T-style filter housing commonly found in the biopharmaceutical industry.

plate has elbows for feed and filtrate, allowing for ease of cartridge change-out at the end of the filtration process. Since the bell will usually have only a pressure gauge and a vent valve, it can be removed without breaking any piping connections. This design is well suited for skid mounting, as the span of piping occupied by the filter housing is generally small (5–12 in. based on housing size). The housing bell (or bowl as it is sometimes referred to) can be changed to a larger or smaller size should production requirements change. This change would not affect the fixed base installation. The bell of the housing will typically have a vent valve and, if a sterilizing grade filter is used, an integrity test port. This port might serve the dual function of holding a pressure gauge during the process. Since the pressure is typically monitored on the upstream, nonsterile side, the top of the bell is ideal for this purpose. Automated integrity test devices should always be connected to a high point on the housing because the final function of an automatic device is to vent the filter housing of pressurized air. If the test device is connected to the lower inlet elbow, residual liquid may be brought into the device and contaminate the internal pneumatics. T-style housings will normally have a sanitary vent valve to allow for removal of air and a low point drain valve. The low point drain will allow for emptying the housing completely prior to opening the assembly. This is of practical merit when the cartridge becomes plugged and must be changed during the batch.

In-Line

The inlet connection on in-line housings is at the top of the bell (see Fig. 5). The flow is parallel and through to the cartridge. In-line filter housings are commonly used for tank venting applications where the base of the housing is fixed directly to a connection on the top of the tank. When used in systems that are hard piped, it is more difficult to access the cartridge because the housing must be removed to open the assembly. Since tank vent filters are generally used for several months, the inconvenience is minimized. In-line filters are also used for venting and water system applications where the elements are changed infrequently.

Steam Jackets and Electrical Heat Tracing

In certain applications, water vapor can condense when it comes into contact with the inside wall of the housing bell. Small amounts of water may be removed through the low point drain in the housing base, either to a steam trap or simply to a waste line. Water must not accumulate inside the filter housing in the case of a tank vent as it will ultimately blind off the surface area of the filter cartridge. This could lead to a vacuum condition inside the vessel. A second circumstance that can blind off a vent filter occurs during the sterilization cycle of a bioreactor. When steam traps are used and the lines have all come up to temperature, the steam flow is reduced to replace only the heat lost due to radiation and natural convection losses from process piping. When the tubing is insulated, the losses can be minimized. The loss from the housing bell may be significant and can result in excessive condensation of the water vapor within the matrix of the vent filter. This will blind off the downstream piping until the pressure within the vessel exceeds the bubble point of the membrane or until the condensate is revaporized. With steam and a 0.2 μm filter, this will occur at about 15 psig (1 bar). This pressure differential on the filter at 121°C may damage the membrane of the filter cartridge.

Each of the above circumstances can be avoided through the use of steam jacketing (Fig. 6) or by heat tracing the housing bell. The choice of the utility is based on facility constraints. Steam may not be available in the location of the filter housing, and it may be less expensive to provide electricity for the heat trace. Heat tracing should include either self-regulating heat tape or a process controller with a thermocouple. When steam jackets are used, the pressure rating of the jacket should be equal to that of the unregulated plant steam unless the system includes a pressure relief valve rated below the jacket design pressure. In the case of a steam jacket, the jacket pressure should be maintained as low as possible to minimize thermal deg-

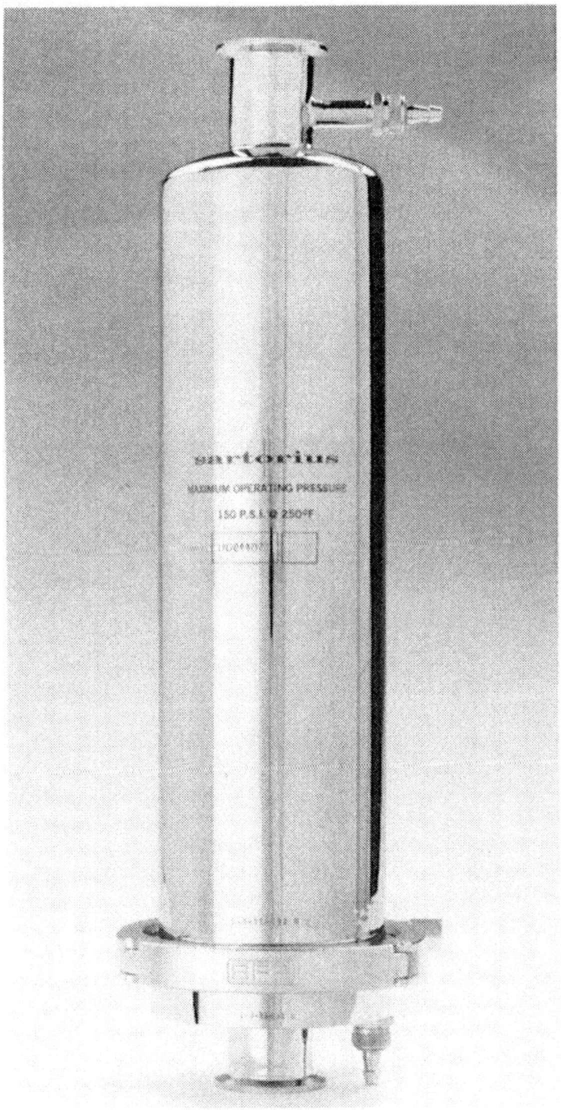

Figure 5 A commonly used in-line filter housing.

radation of the cartridge. The same holds true for heat-traced housings. In both cases, the heat supplied to the housing should be cut off when the housing is not in use. Filter cartridges will oxidize through long-term exposure to dry heat. This will significantly reduce the life of the filter.

Multiround Housing

Filter housings are available that hold multiple cartridges in parallel. Some common sizes are 3-, 5-, 6-, 7-, 12-, and 21-round for cartridges ranging in length from 10 to 40 in. Where a sanitary design is required, the base consists of two pieces, a

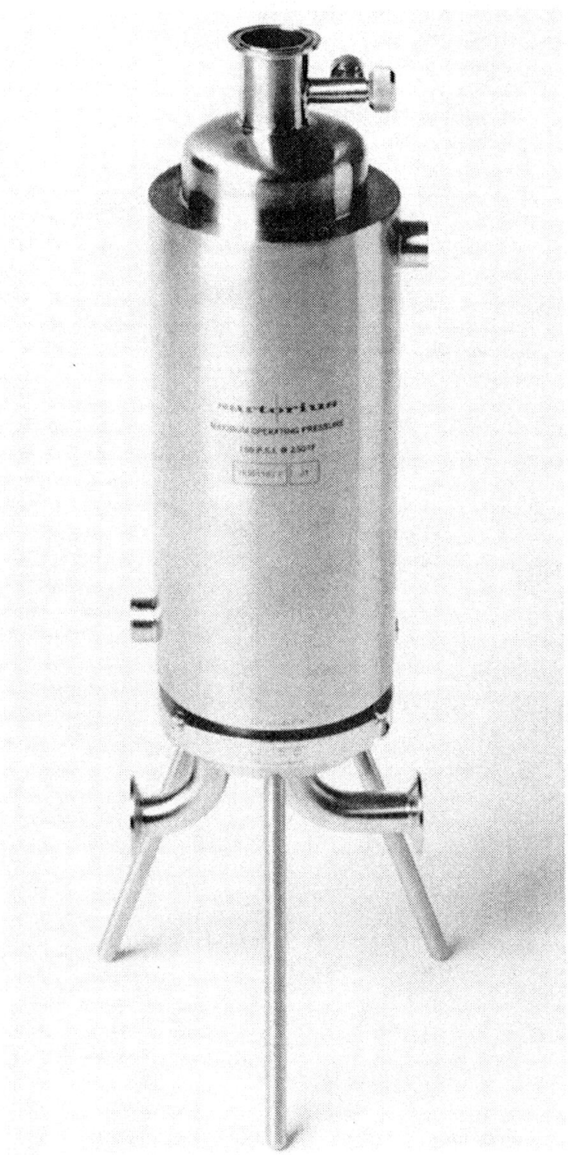

Figure 6 Steam-jacketed housing.

receiver plate and the base plate. The cartridges are inserted into the receiver plate, which is sandwiched between the housing bell and the base plate. O-rings isolate the filtrate fluid from the feed fluid. In the three-round version, one design shown in Fig. 7 provides a three-round housing sanitary construction in a single-piece base. The recommended closure where cleaning in place is required is one with sanitary gaskets as opposed to O-rings. This type of seal when properly tightened provides a flush mating of the surfaces. If O-rings are used, it is important for the groove to

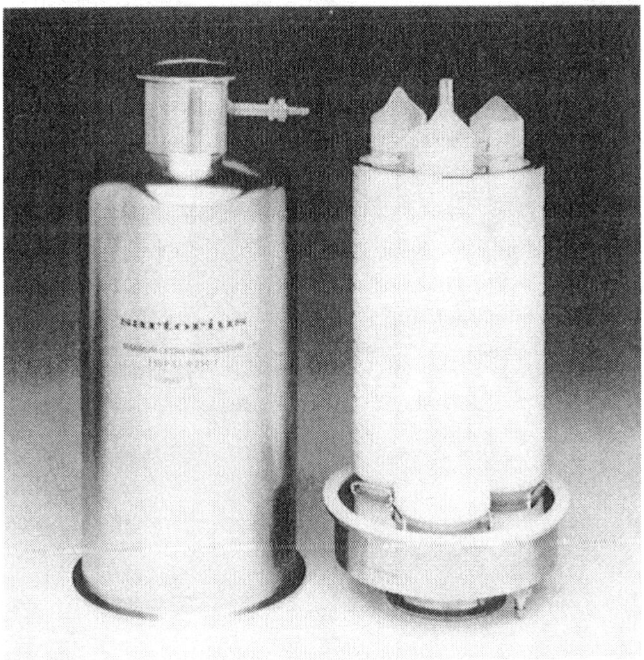

Figure 7 Three-element multiround housing design.

have a relied cutaway on one side to allow cleaning solution to access the seal. Where feed fluid is to be isolated from filtrate, such as with a T-style five-round design, some manufacturers use a double outer O-ring on a post to seal against the bore in the receiver plate. This type of seal provides added assurance that bypass will not occur. Some earlier designs relied on a single O-ring squeezed between the receiver plate and the base to isolate feed from filtrate. This can lead to bypass as the O-ring wears with age. Housing O-rings, as well as cartridges in long-term use, need to be visually inspected on a regular basis.

Swing bolts or cam locks are the most common means of securing the bell to the base, as either one can be designed to meet the requirements of the ASME code. On non-Code vessels, V-band clamps or two-piece clamps can be used for liquid applications. The recommended closure for vessels greater than 6 in. in diameter is one of multiple swing bolts or cam locks.

Retainer rods or tie rods secure a retainer plate to the top of the cartridges and prevent unseating of, for example, Code 8 cartridges (nonlocking, plug-in style) and also prevent the cartridges from twisting under the force of the initial flow of product into the housing. The retainer rods in sanitary design housings either must be welded to the base or use an O-ring type of arrangement to isolate any threads. Designs have been used with the threaded hole in the receiver plate and an O-ring seated just above the threads on the retaining rod. This method is adequate, but ultimately product may get into contact with the threads. The recommended design is one in which threads are eliminated. The mechanism that secures the retainer plate to the rods should also be thread-free for sanitary design housings.

Custom Designs

Filter housing manufacturers offer designs to suit specific installation constraints. These modifications include

Special vent and drain connections
Bells with removable caps for cartridge change-out and CIP considerations
Changes to inlet and outlet connection type and size
Exotic materials of construction and/or vessel lining
Special surface finishes
Specific testing, documentation, and handling

An example of a custom housing is shown in Fig. 8. This particular filter housing has autoweld fittings that reduce the risk of contamination and a removable

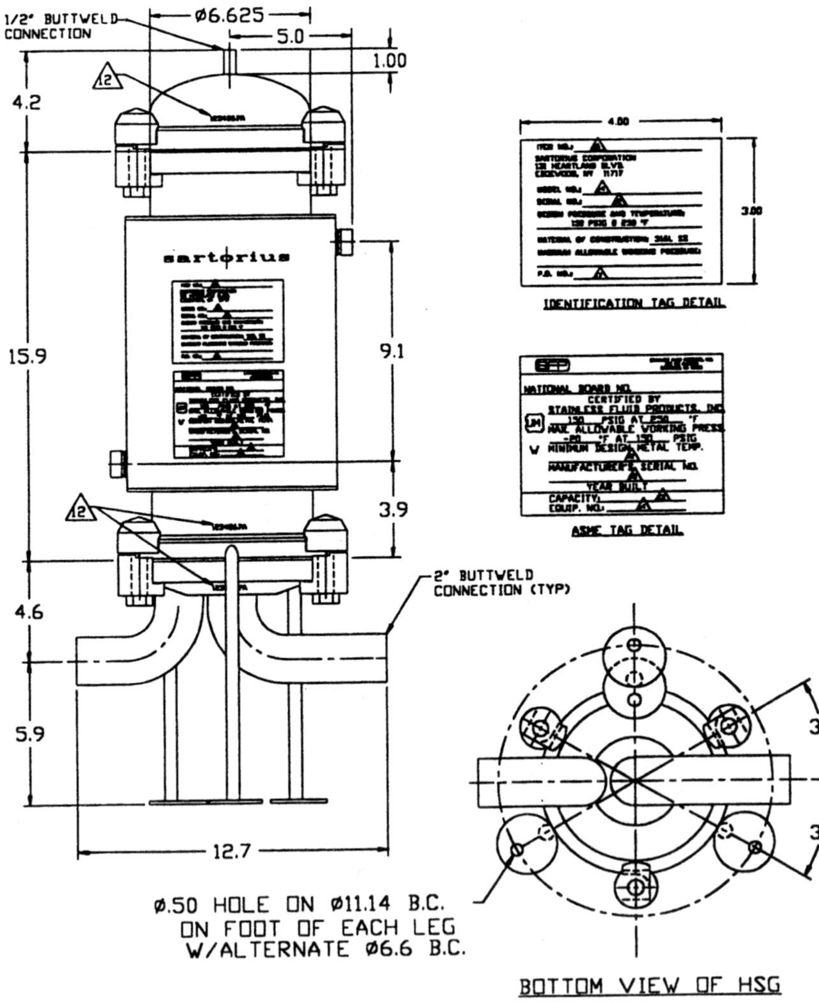

Figure 8 Custom-designed housing.

cap for access to the cartridges. The steam jacket prevents the vapor from condensing when it comes in contact with the inside wall of the housing.

4 DESIGN CRITERIA

The design criteria of any filter housing need to meet specific requirements for the application they are used in. It does not make sense to use a pharmaceutical grade housing in an intermediate crude chemicals filtration step, because criteria other than mirror polishing—for example, housing closure—need to be fulfilled.

The specific design criteria have to be specified by the user of the housing and need to be well documented to meet design qualification (DQ) purposes. The documentation and thorough description of the criteria are important to the housing manufacturer to meet all requirements and DQ. For pharmaceutical grade housings, the main criteria are

Low surface roughness
Good cleanability
Low dead volume
Secure sealing mechanisms
Low shear forces due to optimized flow patterns
Good drainability
Easy maintenance

5 INDUSTRY CODES AND STANDARDS

Current good manufacturing practices (cGMPs), the 3-A Sanitary Standards, the ASME (American Society of Mechanical Engineers) codes, and USP 23 provide the general requirements for filter housings used in the manufacture of biopharmaceuticals in the United States. Although some of these standards are accepted by other countries, local codes and standards may be the primary concern. Following is a summary of some of the main points of each standard as they relate to filter housings.

5.1 cGMPs

Filter housings must be validated.
Filter housings should be easy to clean.
Materials of construction to be nonreactive.
Materials of construction must not affect product.
Housings must be designed to prevent product contamination.

As part of the validation procedure, all documents must be provided by the manufacturer to enable the validation team to verify if the housing received meets the specification. Documents that may accompany a new filter housing can include QC certificates, material certificates from the steel mill, as-built drawings, design calculations, equipment tags, heat numbers, installation and operating instructions, and spare parts lists. Vessel labels should be legible and include serial numbers for full traceability.

5.2 3-A Sanitary Standards

Filter housings must be constructed of 300 series stainless steel or other acceptable material.
All surfaces must be capable of CIP or be easily dismantled for cleaning.
Welds are to be ground smooth and flush and be free of pit cracks, crevices, and inclusions.
Product contact surfaces must be self-draining.
Product surfaces must be at least No. 4 polish.
No threads shall be in contact with product.
Non-product surfaces must have a smooth cleanable finish.
All materials must be inert, nonporous, nonabsorbent, nontoxic, nonrusting, nonreactive, nonadditive, and insoluble.

Since materials of construction are addressed in a separate chapter, we accept the current standard as Type 316L stainless steel. This material has proven to be relatively easy to machine and meets the requirements cited above.

5.3 ASME BPVC Section VIII, Division 1

Vessels containing nonlethal gas at a pressure greater than 15 psi and having an inside diameter > 6 in. require stamping. This simply means that vessels that have dimensions or service conditions below those cited in the code are excluded from the scope of the code. These vessels can still be designed, built, and stamped in accordance to the code. The ASME code includes requirements for materials of construction, vessel inspection, vessel design, stamping of the vessel, fabrication, and pressure relief devices. In most states, the Uniform Building Code or OSHA (Occupational Safety Health Act) requires companies to adhere to ASME requirements for pressure vessels or to follow "good engineering practice." In most cases, the ASME code is the accepted standard because it is not left open to interpretation. The insurance carrier for the pharmaceutical company may require the use of vessels that are in compliance with the ASME code. This further protects the carrier against injury claims.

Where vessels for nonhazardous liquid filtration are required, vessels stamped in accordance with the ASME code are required when the pressure exceeds 300 psi or the temperature exceeds 210°F, regardless of vessel size. Since many pharmaceutical liquid filters require integrity testing before and after use, even liquid filter housings will be pressurized with gas beyond the 15 psig limit. Additionally, many housings are steamed in place at 15–30 psig and as a result still fall under the requirements for ASME code design.

Typically, single-round housings are not designed to code because the preferred closure is a 4 in. triclamp ferrule that does not meet the design requirements of the code with respect to the thickness of the ferrule in comparison to the extension out of the bell. Most end users prefer a quick-release closure that is not accepted by the ASME. Closures must have a backup in case of a single-component failure. One type of clamp that is marketed to address this constraint falls short of meeting code requirements because the diameter of the bolts is 3/8 in. The minimum bolt diameter on closures must be 1/2 in. These high pressure clamps are recommended for high pressure service such as plant air even when single-round housings are used.

"U" vs. "UM" Stamp

To manufacture vessels and stamp them in accordance with the ASME code, the facility must first be approved by the insurance underwriter. This approval process includes a detailed review of the quality system, quality control, engineering design, manufacturing procedures, and documentation for the given facility. The approval can be given to manufacture with a "U" stamp or a "UM" stamp and also to repair code-stamped vessels. The "U" stamp is applied to vessels over 5 ft^3 in volume and with a design pressure of 250 psig or 1.5 ft^3 in volume and 600 psig design pressure. The "U" stamp is applied by an independent AI (ASME inspector) after review of design calculations, materials, witness of welding, and witness of hydrostatic test. The "UM" symbol may be stamped on vessels that fall below the limits set for the "U" symbol. In this case, the manufacturer must maintain all documentation for regularly scheduled audits by the AI. The stamp is applied by a designated inspector within the manufacturing organization after review of all procedures and documents.

An ASME coded vessel is shown in Fig. 9.

5.4 Baseler Norm

The Baseler norm is not an official standard but is used broadly in Europe to specify housing design parameters. It was created by the Baseler Industries, Hoffmann La Roche, Sandoz, and Ciba Geigy. The Baseler norm specifies the following parameters:

1. Housings must be made from 316L stainless steel.
2. The weldings must be flush and polished.
3. The ferrite content of the welding must be < 1%.
4. The inside surface must have an average surface roughness of $R_a \leq 0.5$ μm.
5. The outside surface should have an $R_a \leq 1.6$ μm.
6. The housing specifications must conform with common European pressure vessel regulations and 3.1B certification.

6 DESIGN PRESSURE AND TEMPERATURE

Filter housings must be operated within the design ratings on each vessel. The rating applied to the vessel should cover the range of operation during processing, cleaning, and sterilization. Since the temperature for steaming in place has increased to 300°F in many cases, it is recommended that the vessel be rated at 300°F (149°C) for many applications.

Most vessels have carried a pressure rating at 250°F (121°C). The pressure rating is not generally affected significantly by the temperature, so moving the rating from 250°F to 300°F does not increase the pressure substantially in most conditions. Jacketed vessels must provide ratings for the filter housing as well as the steam jacket. If the vessel is rated to full vacuum (FV), that should be so stated on the vessel housing.

7 HOUSING SEALING MECHANISMS

Housing closure mechanisms vary widely. Among the most common are the three-segment sanitary clamp, ferrule, and gasket assembly; swing bolts; cam lock closures;

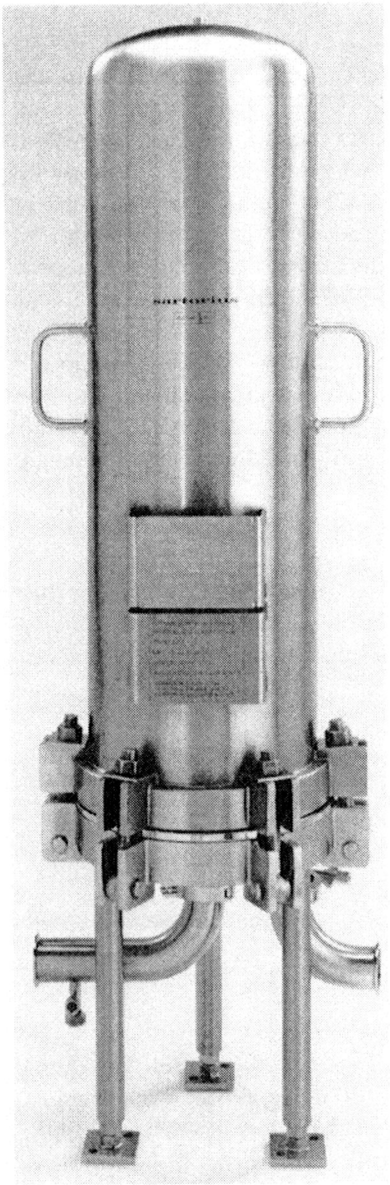

Figure 9 ASME-coded housing.

and V-band clamps. Sanitary clamps are most commonly used on single-element housings because they allow easy opening of the housing. The use of sanitary ferrules to form the seal between the bell and the base on single-round housings is recommended over the use of a flared bell seating against an O-ring. Sanitary ferrules will in most cases hold their shape better under the rigorous handling conditions of the production environment. Slight deformation of the sealing surface, especially due to heat set found with EPDM O-rings, can lead to false integrity test failures during processing. When this happens just a few times, the money saved on the less expensive flared closure may be lost. For the same reason, the heavier machined base is recommended over those of lighter, thinner design. Multiround housings usually use one of the other closure mechanisms. In all cases, specific torque settings should be used to ensure safe operation of the housing. All O-rings and gaskets should be inspected on a regular basis.

8 ELASTOMERS

Elastomers are found in several places within the filter housing, and it is critical that the materials be properly suited for the application. Chemical compatibility charts are available for most fluids. The proper elastomer material must also be selected for the cartridge seal O-rings. Within the housing, the bell-to-base I/O connections, vent/drain valves, retaining rods, and receiver plates are all locations where elastomers are used. The common types of elastomers are

Silicone: Standard elastomer in the biopharmaceutical industry
EPDM: Compatible with a wider range of chemicals
Viton: Greater chemical and thermal resistance
PTFE encapsulated Viton/EPDM: Provides excellent resistance to corrosion while maintaining some elasticity

Solid PTFE gaskets frequently leak due to cold flow properties and long-term deformation. Slight damage to the housing components from normal usage can result in leaks. It is recommended that PTFE gaskets be used only when others are not suitable.

9 SURFACE FINISHES

The surface finish of product contact surfaces for sanitary design housings is typically less than 25 μ-in. (0.6 μm) R_a. In certain applications where the product is particularly difficult to remove, 15 μ-in. (0.4 μm) R_a may be selected for improved ease of cleaning. One of the most important aspects of surface finish is the uniformity of finish. It is of little use to have a base plate with a mirror polish when the inside of the housing bell has deep swirl lines on the cap. The internal surface finish should be measured with a profilometer and not specified as a grit finish. Grit finish measurements will vary when using a profilometer depending on the age of the abrasive. Measurement of the actual finish is of the greatest importance because it is directly related to one's ability to clean the surface.

10 VENT AND DRAIN VALVES

Vent and drain valves should be designed to have minimal dead legs between the sealing surface and the bulk fluid within the housing. These dead legs are difficult to clean and can become a site for contamination. A typical sanitary vent valve is shown in Fig. 10. The threads are isolated from the product by the O-ring on the valve stem. A center channel provides the pathway for fluid to exit the housing once the Teflon tip is backed off the valve seat.

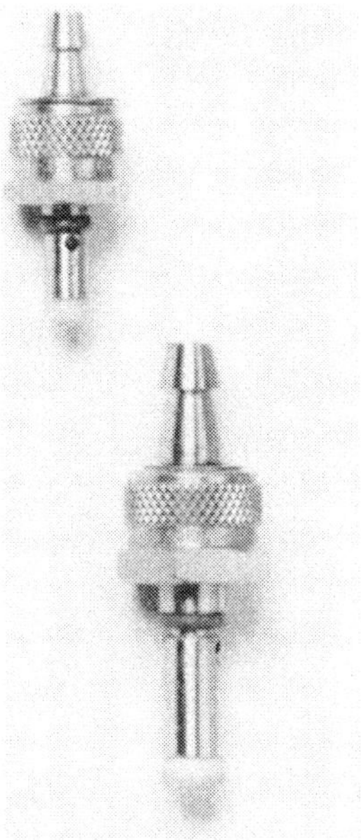

Figure 10 Design example for vent and drain valves.

11 CARTRIDGE SEALING MECHANISMS

The means by which cartridges seal to the filter housing can be divided into three main types.

Double 226 Type O-Rings with Locking Tabs (Code 7, Double Bayonet). This is the accepted standard for cartridge filters. Each filter manufacturer serving the biopharmaceutical marketplace offers cartridges with this type of interlock. Cartridges range from 5 to 40 in. in length. The twist lock is facilitated by two small wings positioned slightly above the O-rings. The base plate of the housing may have a machined groove down into which the tabs slide and are twisted, or the housing may have surface features as those shown in Fig. 11 into which the cartridge locks into place. The benefit of the recessed groove is in the smaller dead volume of the housing. The disadvantage of this design is that it is difficult to clean and verify the cleanliness of the recessed machined groove. The design shown in Fig. 11 offers easy access to the lock-down region for cleaning purposes.

Double 222 Type O-Rings Without Tabs (Code 8, Plug-In Style). Slightly smaller than the Type 226 O-rings and without the locking tab, the Type 222 cartridge is still widely used in existing installations. In most cases, housings are switched over to the Code 7 design unless inventory constraints limit the number of different filter elements to be stocked by the pharmaceutical company. Usually either Code 8 housings are equipped with a spring mechanism to prevent dislodging of the filter from backpressure or the length of the bell is such that it holds the cartridge firmly in place upon closure. The latter may limit use to one vendor's cartridges because cartridge manufacturers'

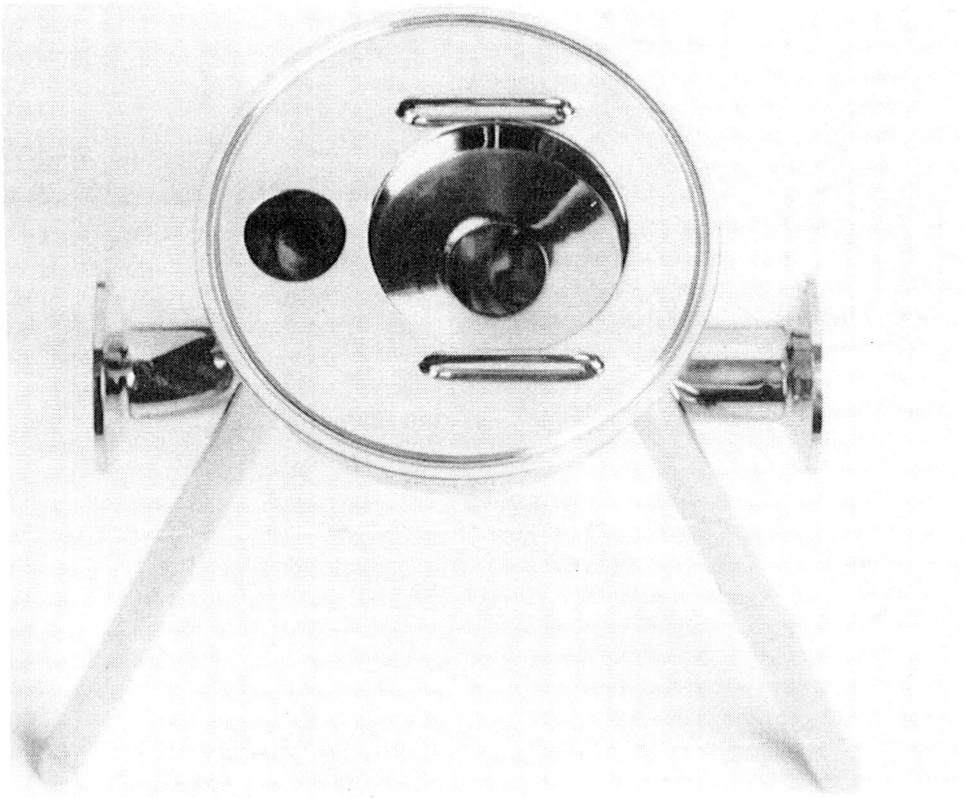

Figure 11 Double-bayonet, double O-ring cartridge adapter.

filters may vary slightly in overall length. Since a locking tab does not exist, the base plates are similar among manufacturers.

Knife-Edged Seals. The housing is usually equipped with a cup that accepts a Type 222 (Code 8) cartridge, or the edge of the cup can act as the knife to form the seal against the filter medium or against a gasket. This type of seal is commonly used for initial clarification steps on city water or for other nonsanitary applications. The filter can be a nonpleated element where the knife cuts into the side of the medium, or if it is a pleated filter, a flat gasket is used against the cartridges.

15

Detection and Measurement of Particles in Pharmaceutical Liquids

ALVIN LIEBERMAN
Particle Measuring Systems, Inc., Fremont, California

1 INTRODUCTION

This chapter deals with the problems and the means of measuring particulate material in pharmaceutical liquids. Both process and product liquids must be as clean as possible. Particulate material is a contaminant that must be minimized in the liquids. For purposes of this discussion, the question of particle viability is not pertinent. The particles present are considered to be inert debris that must be eliminated because of chemical, physical, or mechanical interference with product quality. At the same time, it is realized that even inert particles may have some effect on patient morbidity, making it even more important to keep pharmaceutical liquids as clean as possible.

An important step in cleaning liquids is to define the material to be removed from the liquid in terms of particle size, concentration, and chemical and/or physical properties. With this information, the optimum "purification" process needed for the particular liquid of concern can be defined more easily. This definition process does not necessarily consider sterility requirements and is seldom concerned with chemical composition of the particles to be removed. It is not necessary to specify all parameters of the particle–liquid system for every cleanliness definition.

Selection of the particle system parameters to be measured depends on the product quality standard that is applied. In some cases, in-house company standards are all-controlling, especially when those specifications are more severe than any imposed by an external regulatory agency such as the Food and Drug Administration (FDA). In other situations, externally produced standards are used as the basis for liquid cleanliness requirements. In the United States, two specifications are universally applied for essentially all pharmaceutical production. The first standard is the document defining the criteria for good manufacturing practices for parenteral products [1]. This standard specifies environmental conditions and documentation required to validate that the specified conditions are present. The second standard is the document on particulate matter in injections [2]. This standard specifies the maximum concentrations of inert particles of specified sizes in large volume injections and in small volume injections. It also defines procedures to measure the particle concentrations in the liquids.

Typically, the standard or specification that is used will define the maximum particle concentration per unit volume of liquid for specific particle size ranges. The standard may also state the method and protocol to be used for sample procurement, observation, or measurement as well as for data interpretation. As an example of a procedure for developing pharmaceutical product standards, consider current practices for United States Pharmacopeia (USP) standards and test methods. First, a committee-written draft is published in *Pharmacopeial Forum* for comment. After comments are received and reviewed, a revised draft is then published, with revisions based on committee evaluation of the comments. If no further pertinent comments are received, the revised draft is published and is normally used by the pharmaceutical industry as a test method. It is often referenced by the FDA as a required standard for a particular product.

The problems involved in accurate definition of particle size and concentration are difficult and sometimes subtle in terms of the methods for procurement of good data. The sizes of the particles of concern range from 2 μm to a millimeter or so in diameter. Since the sources of potential pharmaceutical contaminant particles are widely varied, the particles are of widely varying shapes and composition. This aggravates the problems of defining size for materials of widely varying shape and composition. Essentially all of the instruments used in particle measurement respond to system parameters other than only the "size" of the particle of concern. Therefore, successful instrument operation requires procedures of instrument setup and calibration as well as sample preparation and handling that must be well understood by the technicians making the measurements.

Considering the variety of potential sources of contaminant particles, the reasons for some of the measurement problems become apparent. The sources include atmospheric silica or vegetation fragments normally present in the air, metal particles from nearby industrial production, carbonaceous materials from fossil fuel power generation or from vehicle exhausts, abraded metal or polymer materials from a process control valve, fibers from a damaged filter element, and skin flakes from personnel. Particles may be deposited into process vessels from the surrounding atmosphere during filling or flushing operations. Particles may be produced by chemical reactions occurring in liquids during processing operations. Each type of particulate material can react with the particle measuring device in a different manner. Even so, most commercially available particle measuring devices produce data that appear to be totally unambiguous and that are affected only by the size of the particle being examined. The operators tend to have blind faith in the data that are produced and frequently do not realize the problems that must be solved and the caveats that must be accepted in interpreting data from these instruments.

This discussion is prepared to aid the reader in understanding both the capabilities and limitations of instrumental particle-measuring systems in use with pharmaceutical product liquids. The discussion covers some of the sample acquisition and handling problems common to all particle measurement methodology. These must be solved for any of the particle measurement instruments to operate to the best of their ability. Performance and operation requirements, limitations, and problem areas for present particle measuring devices are then discussed.

2 SAMPLE ACQUISITION

2.1 Sample Collection Considerations

For convenience, the discussion on sample handling is subdivided in terms of in situ or on-line sampling and batch sampling. The first step in the liquid cleanliness measurement process is selection of the specific standard that will be used to define requirements. In the United States, most pharmaceutical manufacturing facilities use the USP 23 < 788 > [2] for injectable materials or the GMPs for most other products or process liquids [1]. In some facilities, an in-house standard may be used that is more rigorous than a government-imposed standard. If products are being produced for shipment to foreign areas, then the product cleanliness standard used may be based on requirements of a foreign customer, which may be more or less severe than the U.S. standards.

Once the standard has been selected, questions of particle size and/or concentration ranges to be measured are answered. Next, knowledge of the overall process or product variation to be expected in a specific facility is useful in defining the range of capability needed for the sample handling and particle measuring systems to be used there. A system should be chosen that will produce the data required by the selected standard. The system should also provide data that will identify operations approaching or actually out of accepted limits.

Suitable facilities should be established for sample preparation, handling, storage, and measurement. These may include an area with sample container storage and cleaning and processing equipment if batch samples are to be observed; they may include product sample storage and/or observation systems; they may include modifications to an assembly or filling system to permit on-line observation or process materials or product samples and disposal of materials that have been measured and cannot be returned to the production line.

2.2 Batch Sampling

In situ sampling has some advantages over batch sampling in terms of fewer sample handling problems and container cleaning requirements. However, particle measurement in many pharmaceutical products is best handled by analysis of batch samples.

For example, particle measurement in either large volume or small volume injections must be carried out using the product containers in accordance with compendial requirements, as specified in USP 23 < 788 >. Care is required in carrying out batch sample acquisition, handling, storage, and measurement. Otherwise data can display excessive variability from one sample container to another in the same batch or even within a series of aliquot samples from the same container.

Product container size and configuration for sample measurement in many pharmaceutical liquid products is usually in the range from 1 mL to 1 L. Where product samples are being measured, standard product packages must be used. For many liquid products, containers are used that may be fitted with a single-use or reusable closure. If the closure inner surfaces are coated with low reactivity coatings, then contamination from the closures is minimized. When plastic or glass containers are used, they are often heat-sealed; the product is accessed by carefully penetrating the container. The sample must be taken using the same procedures as are used for normal product handling in use.

Some product system sample acquisition procedures to be considered follow:

Large volume injectable products are normally contained within glass or plastic containers. The container exterior, particularly the area around the closure (if present), is cleaned with a stream of clean water and dried. The contents are mixed or a clean stirring bar added before the closure is removed or the container penetrated for sample removal.

Small volume injectable products are normally contained within glass containers with closures or in sealed ampules. For a container with closure, the procedure is essentially the same as that used for the large volume injectable product. For the sealed ampules, the first step is to clean the outer surface of the ampule. Next, score the glass, rinse any chips from the outer surface, and remove the top portion of the ampule. The contents can be withdrawn with a cleaned syringe and needle. Some glass chips will most likely fall into the liquid. This can be minimized by using a pencil point torch to open a hole in the ampule through which the contents can be withdrawn.

The required number of containers from a batch of product can be selected in accordance with statistically accepted sample size requirements in use. Table 1 illustrates the recommended numbers of bottles to be sampled from various lot sizes. With these sample quantities, confidence limits of 95% or more for any measurement data are ensured.

It may also be necessary to collect batch samples from a process liquid line for later examination. This may be the situation when water-for-injection (WFI) cleanliness is to be verified or filter performance is to be determined by taking upstream and downstream batch samples simultaneously for later examination. The sample container filling process can be quite simple. If at all possible, samples from a flowing line should not be taken as soon as flow begins or a sample valve is opened. Such samples can be contaminated by debris entrained from line surfaces

Table 1 Container Samples for Various Lot Sizes

Number of bottles per lot	Number of bottles to be sampled
2–8	2
9–15	3
16–25	5
26–50	8
51–90	13
91–150	20
151–280	32
281–500	51
501–1200	80

Source: Ref. 3.

by an initial flow liquid surge or generated from the valve operation. Thus, a period of 10 s or so should elapse between the time of starting the sample line flow and collecting the sample in order to flush the sample valve and line. When a sufficient volume of liquid has entered the sample container, remove the container from the liquid stream before shutting off the flow.

After batch samples have been acquired, they may be stored for some time before any particle measurements are made. In this situation, precautions are necessary. Before a sample container is opened, the exterior surfaces should be cleaned carefully, especially in the closure area. Then the liquid should be well mixed by shaking, inverting repeatedly, or stirring. Samples are withdrawn from containers by either pouring the liquid into a smaller container or removing it by vacuum or by pressure through a sample line to the point of measurement. If a sample line removal method is used, the liquid should be stirred before and during removal. The sample should never be stirred during removal at a rate fast enough to result in formation of a vortex. If a vortex is formed, air is aspirated into the vortex and bubbles are drawn into the sample stream. Similarly, when pouring from one container to another, the technician should take care to minimize bubble generation and splashing caused by pouring too rapidly. However, the liquid should not be poured so slowly that a film of liquid adheres to the outer surface of the container and collects container surface debris before entering the smaller container.

A typical procedure can be summarized in stepwise manner for sample measurement from a single 1 L container:

1. Clean container exterior by flushing with a stream of clean water.
2. Mix container contents by inverting at least 10 times.
3. Carefully remove closure and insert cleaned magnetic stirring bar.
4. Place opened container into pressure container of sample feeding system or on vacuum feed system aspirator platform with cleaned sample feeder tube inserted to a level 2–4 cm above container bottom. The container should be centered on the magnetic stirrer.
5. Note that the particle measuring device or sample collector is placed between the sample feed tube and the sample volume measuring device.
6. Set particle size ranges to be observed by particle measuring device or verify placement of clean sample collecting element.
7. Set sample volume and feed rate controller of sample feeding system and start stirrer at a rate that will not generate a vortex.
8. Flush entire sample measurement system with 20–50 mL of liquid and discard the liquid. If the sample collecting element is a filter patch, remove the filter during this flush and replace following the flush.
9. Pass sample through particle measuring device or sample collector and retain data or particles.
10. Repeat step 9 as required, within limits of sample size and total volume in container.
11. Record particle concentrations in required size ranges for each replicate measurement, and process data as required.
12. If an automated sample acquisition system is used, repeat steps 1–3 for each container to be sampled before installing it. Set the automated system to carry out steps 8–11 for each container.

13. Flush entire system with clean diluent liquid and shut down. Depending on particle measuring device or sample collector used, either dry the flow elements with filtered dry air or seal with clean liquid remaining in system.
14. Dispose of the sample residues and flush materials in a safe and approved manner.

Establishment and implementation of a standard protocol will permit generating good data by techniques that minimize the effects of procedural variations. Similar protocols can be established for collection of data from small volume injections, from medical device flushing systems, from on-line systems, from filters or other component test loops, etc. Any variable or erratic data produced will result from actual sample variability rather than from procedural errors.

2.3 In Situ Sampling

There are several areas where in situ sampling is important in pharmaceutical applications. These include the operations where water for injection (WFI) and product container cleaning water is being processed and areas where product materials are prepared for processing. Another area, although not as widely used, for in situ sampling is filter system performance verification. Measurement of filter penetration or of filter medium degradation has been found more reliable if in situ samples rather than batch samples are taken for later observation [4]. The possibility of artifact production as a result of sample handling is reduced when in situ sampling is used. However, because of this same problem, in situ sampling is seldom used to characterize the cleanliness of bottled products; any artifacts introduced by the product container become part of the product, no matter how clean the material in the filling line may have been.

With these points in mind, one may then begin considering the requirements for in situ sampling. The first step is to decide the location for meaningful sample acquisition. This is done by examining the system handling the liquid of concern. This examination should allow the sample system designer to define the points where the cleanliness of the system may be degraded. These include supply lines for raw materials, flow control, and fluid cleaning components; special processing component elements (heat exchangers, stirrers, vent lines, filters, pumps, etc.); and any points where personnel access is required. Figure 1 shows an idealized flow system containing a liquid reservoir, a fill port, a pump and filter system, a reaction chamber, and fill line. Some obvious critical sample points are shown on the diagram. The cleanliness of the supply liquid refilling the system will affect filter life at several points; a sample point downstream of a filter is of concern in that it verifies acceptability of the liquid entering or leaving the reaction chamber; the fill line point is used to ensure that acceptable product is being filled. Similar logic can be used in systems with other components.

Next, a sampling schedule and sample size base should be defined. Depending on the process for which the system is designed, the fluid flow rate, and uniformity of use, a sampling frequency can be established. Sample collection intervals can range from continuous sampling to regular intervals of up to 1 week or longer. For intermittent operations, sampling is carried out only when the system is in operation.

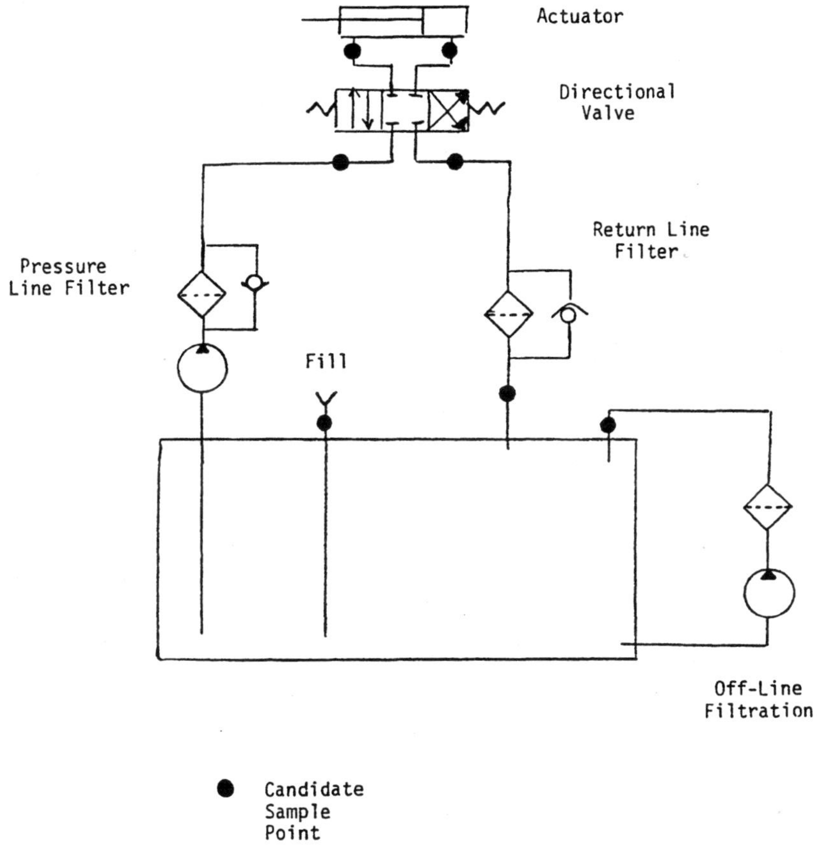

Figure 1 Idealized flow sample selection points.

The sample size depends on the requirements of the measurement system and the level of particulate contamination that is expected. For example, a measurement system based on collection of particles on a 47 mm membrane filter or on commercially available light extinction particle counters will not be capable of handling more than a few hundred milliliters per minute. For clean liquids with no more than 10 particles per liter, a minimum sample volume of approximately 10 L is required for generation of sufficient data to permit establishing an acceptable confidence limit when characterizing the liquid cleanliness. For very clean samples, the operator must expect that sample times may be quite long. The measurement instrument that is used and the sample point configuration must take into consideration the liquid flow rate at the point of sampling. This is particularly important when energy transfer analyzers (optical, electrical, etc.) are being used. For these devices, the effects of particle residence time and residence time variation in the instrument's sensitive volume on the response of electronic components must be considered.

The in situ analyzer measures particles within a portion of the main stream in a nonintrusive manner, typically using an energy transfer system that observes flow within a portion of a flowing stream. The particle measurement methodology is based on transmission of either optical or acoustic energy into and out of a flow system to determine the size and number of particles in the liquid flowing therein. An acoustic system with a convergent–divergent cone-shaped sensing volume had been developed and was evaluated in 1981 [5]. The particle position and the varying acoustic energy level in that volume prevented any differentiation between particles with sizes varying by a factor of less than 2. The authors who evaluated the system stated "the effective sensing volume for 19.8 μm spheres is 22 times that for 9.8 μm spheres." This observation indicates that it would indeed be difficult to define the concentration in which any sample is observed if there is a range of particle sizes in that sample.

At this time, available in situ particle measurement systems use light scattering to observe the central portion of the stream. Either a gas laser or a solid-state laser is used as the energy source. The sensitive zone or the illuminated volume of the main stream must be well defined, and the light energy level must be constant. The sensitive zone must be small enough that the probability of more than one particle being present in that volume at any time is acceptably low. The volume must be large enough that particles pass through that volume at rates sufficient to provide statistically valid data in a reasonable time. Counting rates in the range of 10–1000 particles/s are sought. At lower rates, sample measurement time becomes excessive; at higher rates, the probability of two or more particles being present within the illuminated volume at the same time becomes excessive.

For operation of a practical in situ optical particle counter, the problem of defining the sampled volume within the entire stream must be addressed. An early in situ optical counter used a telecentric laser beam that passed into the liquid stream through a window in the flow line. Light scattered from a particle was collected from a volume defined by the placement and optical design of the collecting lens located just behind an observation window in that line. In such a counter, exact definition of the sampled volume is limited only by edge effects. That is, when a large particle passes through the edge of the illuminated volume, it may produce the same signal as a small particle passing through the center of the volume if the portion of the large particle moving through the illuminated volume is as large as the entire small particle entirely within the illuminated volume. A technique was developed to reduce the uncertainty. The light scattered from any particle in the illuminated volume is first passed through a beam splitter, which produces two image planes for two detectors. The reflected image splitter face is masked with a vertical slit to block the transmission of the central image during particle transit. The second face is not masked. The images from the two faces are compared. The use of double-pulse-height analysis provides a means for defining whether or not the particle is in or at the edge of the sample volume [6].

Another, more recent technique [7], shown in Fig. 2, involves comparison of "S" and "P" polarized beams of light from a single polarized laser source to define the sampled volume. These laser beam components are shaped to produce beams of circular (S) and elliptical (P) cross section in the sensitive volume. The smaller circular beam is aligned so that when a particle traverses both beams it must have crossed the center of the elliptical beam, as shown in Fig. 3. This defines the sample volume in one dimension. The other dimension, based on system depth of field, truncates naturally because the circular S beam converges and diverges more rapidly than the elliptical P beam near the focal plane. When the scattered light signals from the two polarized beans are compared, those particles within the defined sampled

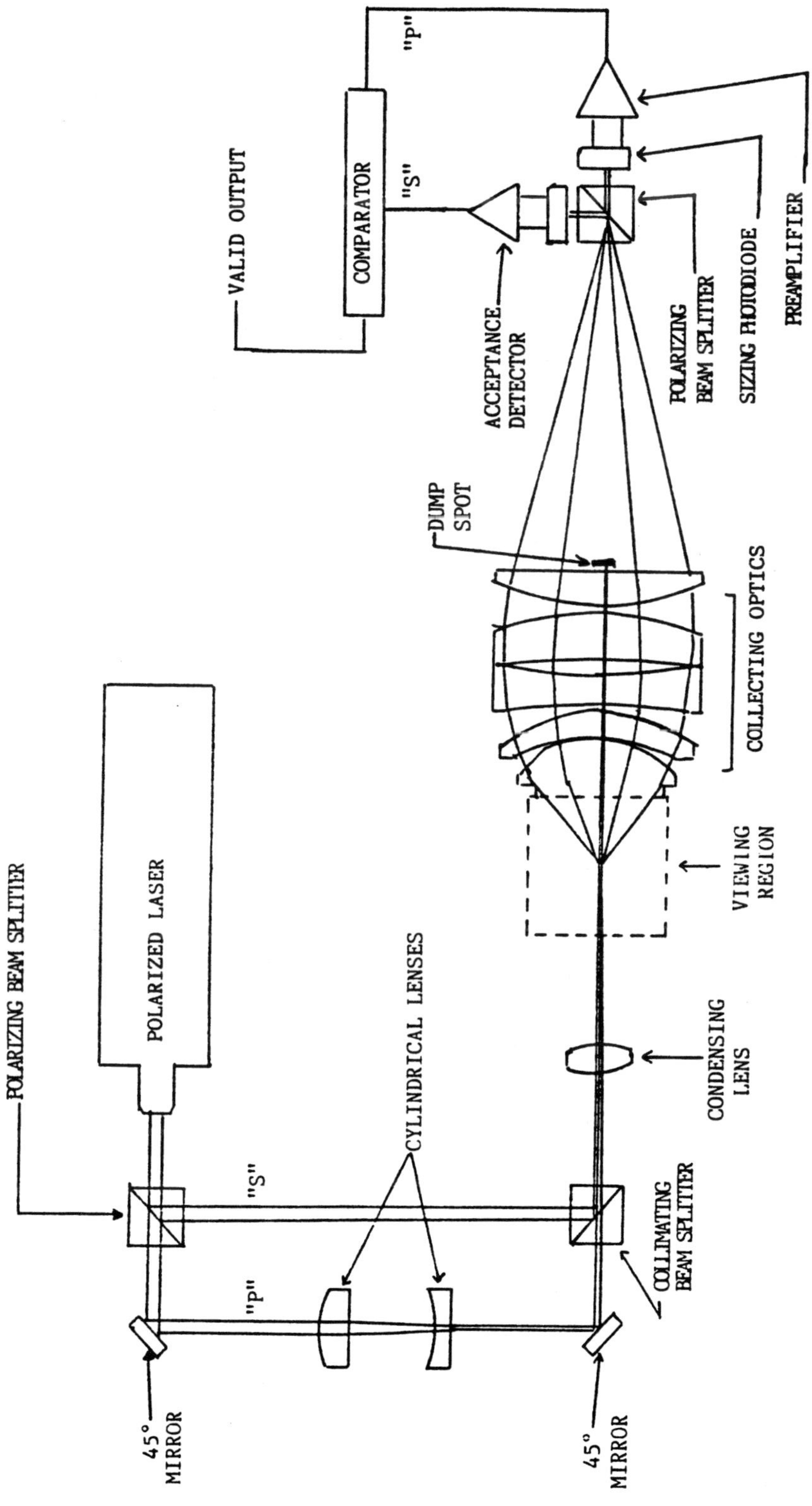

Figure 2 Polarized light system to define in situ sample volume.

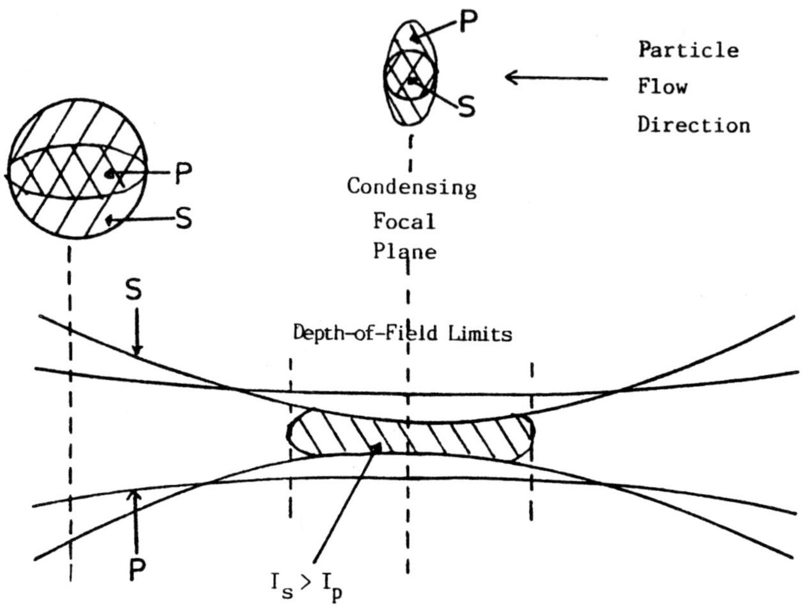

Figure 3 Beam paths for polarized light system.

volume are accepted and counted only if the S scattering signal exceeds the P scattering signal. Particle sizing is accomplished by analysis of the scattering signal.

Both methods provide information on the sample fraction of the total volume of liquid in the line being sampled. However, it is still necessary to know either the volumetric flow rate of the liquid in the line or the liquid velocity at the point of measurement. Otherwise it is not possible to define particle concentration in terms of particles per unit volume of liquid in the sampled line. Generally, it is assumed that the particles observed by the in situ counter are in equilibrium with the liquid streamlines. Normal practice is to determine stream flow by independent means of flow measurement. The illuminated volume is usually located in the center of the flow stream. The main line velocity profile is defined on the basis of the stream velocity, line dimensions, and fluid characteristics. For laminar flow, the velocity profile is parabolic, with the stream velocity at the center of the line being twice the average stream velocity. For turbulent flow, the velocity profile is nearly uniform across the entire stream. It is usually assumed that the velocity profile does not include any irregularities. For this reason, in situ sample points should be located 12 diameters or more downstream of valves, elbows, or any other flow elements that will produce line dimension changes.

2.4 Side Stream On-Line Sampling

Sometimes there is a choice between the use of an in situ analyzer and an on-line analyzer to measure liquid flowing in a side-stream line. The side-stream line samples a portion of the main stream flow for particle measurement. When particles are to be measured in a flowing fluid from which a sample is to be removed, the question of isokinetic sampling usually arises. This question arises because the need to remove a sample from the main body of fluid without changing either the main body of fluid or the particle content in the sample is paramount. Isokinetic sampling is required for that purpose. Isokinetic sampling means that the sample line inlet velocity (both speed and direction) is identical to the fluid velocity in the sampled line at the point of sampling. Both flow speed and flow direction must be considered. The side stream sample line inlet should face into the sampled liquid flow and should collect liquid isokinetically or at least isoaxially if the flow rate in the main liquid line may vary. If the entire side stream line flow is passed through a particle measurement device, a flow rate of 1–100 mL/min will probably be used. Sample probe lines ranging from 2 to 6 mm in diameter will handle adequate liquid flow velocity to minimize the deposition and settling of most particles within horizontal portions of the side stream flow line. Even so, the line should be as short and direct as possible to minimize any deposition. Figure 4 illustrates some side stream sample probe configurations. Since the probe dimensions (particularly the radius of curvature for any bends in the probe) are smaller than those of the line being sampled, particle deposition by centrifugal force onto the probe walls must be avoided by minimizing probe line curvature. That is why straight probe lines facing into the flow with minimum curvature to the point of measurement are favored over the common Pitot tube sample probe configuration, even though the Pitot tube types require smaller ports in the sampled flow line.

In situ measurement involves no sample removal; thus isokinetic sampling is not a concern. For side stream on-line measurements, isokinetic sampling is not a

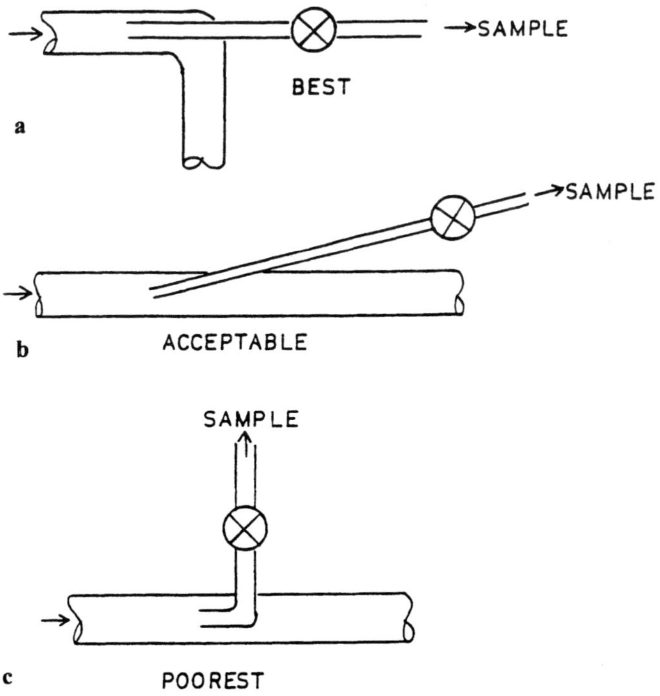

Figure 4 Side-stream sample probe configurations. (a) Best; (b) acceptable; (c) poorest.

concern during the measurement process, but the side stream removal from the main body stream must be carried out isokinetically to ensure that the measurement data will represent conditions in the main body of liquid as well as they do that of the side stream material. For most liquids, particle divergence from streamlines due to changes in process liquid stream flow rate or direction is important only for particles larger than approximately 5 μm. As liquid density or viscosity increases, the relaxation time (time for a particle to accommodate to velocity change in the liquid) for particles decreases and particles tend to remain within the liquid streamlines. For liquids with viscosity similar to that of water, particles larger than 10 μm or so can diverge from the liquid streamlines rapidly.

After the side stream sample has been acquired, it must be transported to the point of measurement. Sample transport problems are associated with particle loss due to settling or entrapment, with the introduction of artifacts due to ingestion of debris or release of extraneous materials from the process line, or with the generation or release of dissolved components in the liquid due to flow inhomogeneities. Particle losses due to settling in transport lines can be minimized by keeping the flow turbulent. Reynolds numbers of at least 5000 are satisfactory. Particle loss by entrapment is controlled by selecting components with minimum trapping configurations —smooth-wall tubing, fittings with uniform cross section, ball or diaphragm valves, etc. Avoid intermittently used dead lines; in addition to trapping particles, these may also become sources of microbiological contaminants. Whenever a valve is operated, abrasion products may be released from the valve components. If a valve located upstream of the particle measuring device is operated, then it is necessary to wait until the locally generated debris has been flushed from the line before recording any particle data. If the liquid in the line contains significant quantities of dissolved materials, then any line segments with abrupt dimensional changes can produce velocity and pressure changes in flow that can result in the formation of bubbles or the precipitation of dissolved materials. The bubbles will be reported as particles. Solids that precipitate out of solution may dissolve very slowly. Understanding these problems and establishing uniform sample acquisition and handling protocols will reduce the problem effects.

2.5 Sample Validity Considerations

Whether batch or in situ samples are used, it is necessary to ensure their validity. The definition of "sample" is "a portion or piece taken or shown as representative of a whole." This means that the samples must be representative of the total quantity of liquid being sampled, that the sample is not distorted by collection and handling processes, that the sample provides sufficient data that an acceptable confidence limit can be stated, and that the measurement device is capable of handling the sample correctly.

Following the procedures in accepted particle measurement standards documents will usually ensure that samples are truly representative of the liquid being analyzed. In general, the larger the sample, the better it will represent the population from which it came. At the same time, the operator must keep in mind that liquids with high concentrations of particles can be characterized with small volume samples, as the number of particles required to provide valid data are present in a small sample. In addition, excessively large samples may require so long a sampling time that normal process operations may cause variations in the liquid being sampled during very long sample periods.

Most particulate material is resistant to physical or chemical changes caused by liquid handling. However, the disposition of particles in a liquid can be significantly affected by the handling process. Particulate material is not an integral part of a liquid and is usually not in equilibrium with the liquid. It may settle out of the main body of liquid, or it can deposit on container surfaces; it can agglomerate or disperse within the liquid; it may dissolve in or react with the liquid. An obvious precaution in storing liquid samples can be emphasized here. Containers may be left over a long weekend in an area that is overheated or may be exposed to freezing temperatures. This may cause emulsion breakage or suspension agglomeration. Containers may be left insecurely closed. This may result in evaporation of volatile liquids, with resulting increase in particle concentration. It may also result in ingression of atmospheric particles or of water vapor into a large container that "breathes" with temperature changes. Secure, stable sample container storage should be provided when the samples cannot be analyzed as soon as they are received.

The requirement that a sample provide sufficient data for adequate characterization of the population from which it came arises from the fact that the particle distribution in any liquid will vary from point to point and from instant to instant. For this reason, most measurement standards include requirements for some sample replication and for sufficient data in the samples that an acceptable confidence limit can be stated for the particle content of the material being sampled. In most instances, the number of replicate measurements is less than five or so. Where particle concentrations are low, larger samples may be required simply to ensure an adequate confidence level for the data. Statistical considerations are applicable.

Most pharmaceutical production facilities have a competent statistical staff to define data requirements in detail. However, some obvious points are presented here to emphasize the need for good data. For particles in liquid, a Gaussian spatial distribution can be expected. The standard deviation, defining the variance (ratio of standard deviation to the mean) of data for a series of samples, will be nearly equal to the square root of the mean values for the samples. As an example, for a series of samples from a large population with particle counts averaging 1000 per sample, the variance is $\pm 3\%$. For a mean count of 100, the variance is $\pm 10\%$. The confidence limit for data values that fall within ± 1 standard deviation (SD) is 85%. For a more preferable confidence limit of 95%, the range of data is the mean ± 1.66 SD. Figure 5 shows the range of uncertainty for data at count levels up to 1000.

It is also possible that the particle size distribution reported by any particle measurement device can be truncated by the device limitations. The smallest particle detectable by a device will be reported as the smallest particle present in the sample, even though there may be many more smaller particles present. This is not a serious problem in characterizing parenteral liquid cleanliness; essentially all of the modern particle measuring devices are capable of counting and sizing particles ≥ 2 μm and up to some 50–100 μm in diameter. Most acceptable parenteral liquids are much cleaner than the specified limit values. The effective dynamic range for accurate particle counting and sizing is adequate for most liquid contaminant particle measurement. For liquids with contamination levels close to the limit values, however, excessive quantities of "subcountable" particles may be reported as particles larger

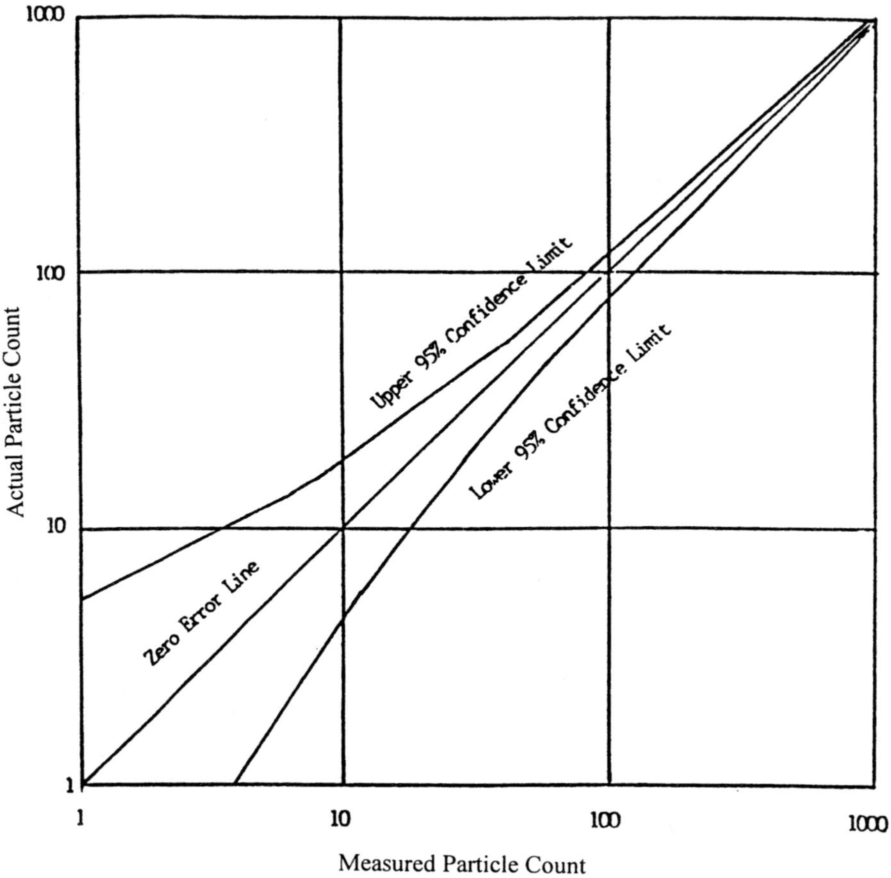

Figure 5 Variation of 95% confidence limit range with data quantity.

than their true size because of coincidence effects in the single-particle counting device.

The majority of particle measuring devices used to characterize pharmaceutical liquid cleanliness are single-particle sizing and counting instruments. They respond to the effect of a phenomenon occurring within a defined sampling volume that is assumed to result from the passage of a single particle. The capability of the particle measuring device to handle samples is affected by the probability that the observed effect may be caused by more than a single particle within that volume. Since particles in any liquid are distributed randomly and are in motion, the instantaneous particle concentration at any point can vary about the average value. If the average concentration becomes too high, then two phenomena occur that can cause undercounting errors. More than one particle can be present within the viewing volume, or the signal from individual particle passages can occur so rapidly that the electronic data processing circuits cannot distinguish individual pulses. The first error is described as *particle coincidence*, and the second error is described as *electronic saturation*. Fortunately, saturation problems are not of great concern, as modern pulse counting and sizing circuitry is capable of good operation at rates up to 100 kHz.

The coincidence problem, however, continues to limit applications of single-particle counting devices. If all of the particles being considered are insignificant in dimension compared to any dimension of the viewing volume, then the probability that one or more particles can be present in the viewing volume can be calculated from an equation derived from statistical probability theory. An accepted reduced version of this equation [8] states that the ratio of indicated to true particle concentration is equal to 1 minus one-half the product of the true concentration and the sensing volume. This product reflects the long-term average sensing volume population level. The reduced version is valid up to a concentration where the probability of one or more particles being present in the sensing volume population is 10%. When particle concentration increases beyond this point, then the reported concentration values begin to decrease significantly. Eventually the measuring device indicates nearly zero concentration when the true concentration is so high that one or more detectable particles are present in the sensing volume at all times. The signal level from the sensing volume never decreases to the point where the counting circuitry can reset to indicate another count. An example of this effect is shown in Fig. 6 [9], which describes data taken with an optical extinction single-particle counter on a series of sequentially diluted samples. As particle concentration in the sensing volume increases to the point where multiple particles are present in that volume, the counter indicates those particles as a single, larger particle. The total reported particle concentration is less than the true concentration of all particles, even though the reported number of large particles is greater than the true number of large particles.

When the particles being measured are large enough that their size approaches one of the dimensions of the sensitive volume of the single-particle counter, then the simple Poisson relationship to define coincidence loss is not longer applicable. A more complex relationship must be used that is based on the fact that the electronic system will not respond to a particle until the one moving out of the sensing volume is out of that volume far enough that the detector signal is less than that from the smallest particle to which the counter will respond [10].

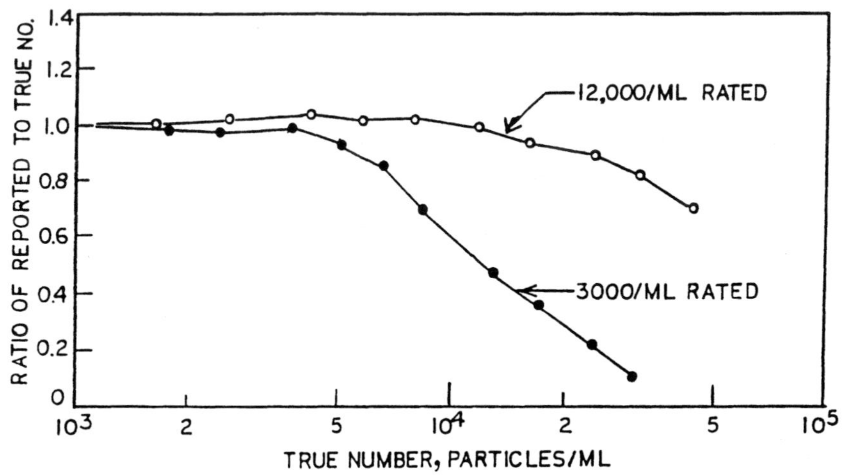

Figure 6 Coincidence loss effects on counting accuracy.

3 PARTICLE MEASUREMENT METHODS FOR PHARMACEUTICAL LIQUIDS

Particles in pharmaceutical liquids can be measured either while they are suspended in the liquid or after they have been removed to a suitable substrate surface for observation. This section describes some measurement methods now in use. It discusses the operating basis for each method, the capabilities and limitations of the methods, and how to use the methods best.

3.1 Manual Visual Observation of Sealed Containers

A brief discussion of techniques used for measurement of particles in transparent sealed containers is presented here. For more detailed discussion of some of the problems, procedures, and methods used for detection and measurement of particles in this manner, see refs. 11–13.

The first system used for definition of particles in pharmaceutical liquid containers was a manual method of visual observation of the containers by personnel trained to detect particles within the containers. The personnel are placed before a diffusely illuminated white screen; they scan containers against the screen background illumination to detect particles by naked-eye observation. It is generally accepted that particles larger than 50 μm in diameter may be detected by the naked eye. For vials or ampules, diffuse background illumination aided by a magnification of 2–3× may be used.

Testing has shown a 50% probability that inspectors with good visual acuity can detect 20 μm particles after adequate training [11]. For 100% probability of detection, the particle size is 55 μm. The effect of particle concentration on the effectiveness of the method is difficult to quantify, though there appears to be noticeable interaction between particle size and concentration in visual detection of particles. It is generally concluded that the larger the particles and the greater their concentration, the more likely will be their detection. The method is quite subjective.

The major advantages of the method are that it has been in use for a very long time, the capital costs are very low, and the requirement that "no visible particles be present" is stated in the 1980 release of one compendial standard for pharmaceutical liquids [2]. The major problems with the method are that it is not truly quantitative and a large number of variables can affect particle detectability, including the color of the particles and liquid, the level and type of illumination, container surface conditions, and personnel health, mood, and visual acuity.

3.2 Automated Observation of Sealed Containers

Once it was realized that manual container inspection could result in data that were not deterministic but strictly probabilistic and highly subjective, procedures for replacing the manual methods with more automated systems were initiated in the early 1980s [12]. Automated versions of the conventional manual inspection methodology were investigated. A robotic inspection method was developed that caused particles to move about within the sealed container. Observation of particles is carried out with a system that includes a servo-controlled bottle spinner to agitate the liquid, a constant intensity light source, and a forward-scattered light detector that responds

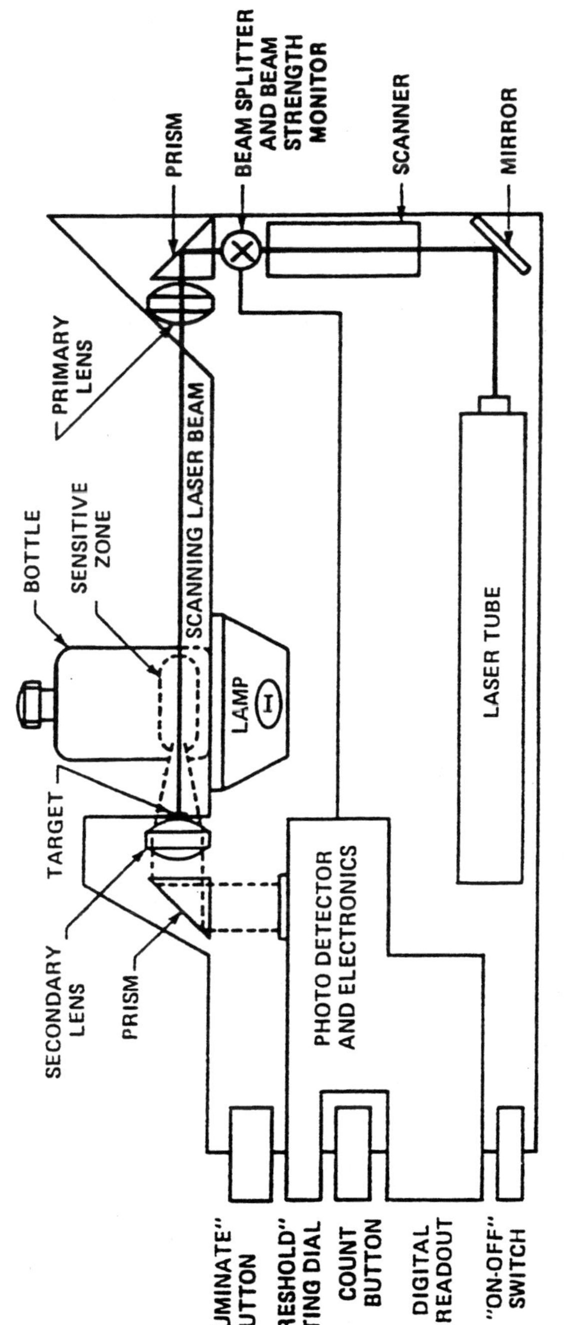

Operation of Prototron enclosed bottle particle counter.

Figure 7 Prototron counter (for in-container particles).

to moving particles. This system was reported to be capable of detecting 10 μm particles in sealed vials at a rate of some 10,000 vials per hour.

Another system has since been developed for counting and sizing particles within transparent closed containers [13]. The Prototron counter passes a laser beam through the walls of the container or through a transparent tube. The beam is moved in a circular pattern so that the beam path outlines a cylindrical pattern within the container. The direct beam is blocked by a circular dump spot, and the light scattered in a near-forward direction is collected on an annular lens surrounding the dump spot. The optical layout of this system is shown in Fig. 7. The sensitive volume for this system consists of a hollow cylinder approximately 2 cm long that is defined by the beam scanning pattern and the depth of focus of the collecting lens. Any particles present within the sensitive volume will scatter a pulse of light with flux proportional to the size of the particle. The pulse signals are processed to provide size and count data for the particles within the sensing volume. Particles on the container interior or exterior walls do not provide measurable signals because they are not in the sensitive volume defined by the optical system. However, variations in bottle wall thickness or glass seams affect the beam adversely and can cause errors in measurement.

The Prototron counter is described as being capable of detecting particles of ≈1–100 μm in size. Containers with inside diameters of 20–200 mm can be scanned. The sensitive volume is 1 mL. Since the scanning system illuminates only a small fraction of the sensitive volume at any time, particle concentrations of up to a few thousand per milliliter can be counted with low coincidence error. In the size range from 1 to 17 μm, sizing resolution to 1 μm is reported; resolution to 5 μm is reported over the rest of the instrument's dynamic range.

The advantages of the instrument are its capability for nonintrusive operation and its ease of operation. The instrument can be used with transparent containers or transparent tubing. The particles in the container should be reasonably well mixed before measurements are made. Almost any liquid can be used, but changes in liquid opacity or refractive index must be accounted for in the readout or by calibration for specific liquids. As long as the sample container is reasonably clean and of uniform wall thickness with no distinct seams in the light path, interferences do not seriously affect the particle data. The major disadvantages of the instrument are its susceptibility to wall interferences that can distort the light beam path and a potential problem in defining low concentrations of large particles. The effects of small particles recirculating through the sensitive volume while large particles settle out of the beam more rapidly must also be considered. As with any single particle counting instrument that does not image the particles, the response to gas bubbles cannot be distinguished from the response to particles; thus, care is required in agitating the containers before measurement.

3.3 Collection and Microscopic Observation

Membrane Filters

Particles can be removed from liquids and deposited on any one of a number of substrates by filtration. The filter systems used to characterize particles in pharmaceutical liquids are usually based on the use of a membrane filter to collect particles from liquid batch samples. Although a large variety of filter media are available, membranes are frequently chosen. Filter media consisting of porous membranes are available with a wide selection of pore size distributions. The pore shapes are tortuous in cross section through the membrane, thus resulting in very high retention efficiency, with most particles collected on or near the top surface of the membrane. Membrane materials can be chosen from a wide range of materials. Easily soluble organic materials or relatively insoluble materials such as metals or fluorinated hydrocarbons can be selected depending on the nature of the liquid to be characterized. Many membranes are produced by formation of a porous gel. A class of membranes known as ''track-etched'' filters are produced by placing thin sheets of a polymer such as polycarbonate in a neutron flux. The neutron penetration results in localized damage to the polymer. Subsequent chemical etching dissolves the polymer at the points of damage so that relatively uniform straight-through pores are produced with diameters from ≈0.2 μm to 10–20 μm.

Microscopic Observation

After particles have been collected on the chosen substrate, the numbers and sizes of particles can be determined by microscopic observation. If the U.S. compendial limits effective in 1994 for injections [2] are used, then particles with effective linear dimensions of either 10 or 25 μm and larger are observed and counted. Present limits in other areas (and probable future U.S. limits) require definition of particles as small as 2 μm.

The measurement method uses oblique incident illumination and low power (100×) magnification. In some facilities, a stereoscopic microscope is used with an operator observing the particles and recording data. In other facilities, an automated microscopic measurement procedure uses an image analyzer for particle sizing and data reduction. These types of microscopic observation are of great use when detailed characterization of the particles is desired. Information on particle morphology and composition can be obtained in addition to particle size data. A description of the techniques and equipment to carry out such measurements is not within the scope of this chapter; they are dealt with in detail in most standard optical texts and journals. Only general comments are given here.

The optical microscope is a convenient and very useful instrument for characterizing particulate material. It has frequently been used as a referee method for calibrating measurements from other particle measuring systems. The material it has been used to examine can be retained for future measurements and for both subjective and objective examinations. A light microscope can be used for magnifications of approximately 1000 times the numerical aperture of the objective lens. The smallest particles that can be sized accurately are ≈0.3 μm in diameter. Refractive index data can be determined with the light microscope by simple comparison methods. Particle size can be determined by use of an eyepiece reticle that has been calibrated against a stage micrometer traceable to the National Institute of Science and Technology (NIST). The reticle can be calibrated in terms of linear dimensions for operation in accordance with American Society for Testing and Materials (ASTM) Method E20 [14]. A fundamental method is described there for use and operation of the optical microscope to determine particle size of subsieve materials to the extent that particle shape and refractive index will permit.

Manual measurement of microscopic images can be carried out with acceptable accuracy for time periods up to an hour or so. Operator error begins to increase after that period because of fatigue unless a break is taken. When a skilled microscopist makes the measurements, reasonable counting and sizing accuracy can be expected. A basic ASTM procedure for measurement of particles ≥5 μm on membrane filters specifies that repeatability of ±25% is acceptable for repeated measurements by the same operator [15]. For these reasons and for greater speed, automated systems using sophisticated image analyzers are used to count and size particles on the membrane filter surfaces.

Image analysis involves conversion of the normal analog images produced by a microscopic optical system to digital images and the use of a computerized digital data processing system to define the images for the desired particle size and population functions. In operation, a microscope field is scanned by a video camera and the image is digitized for subsequent computer processing. Particles can be counted and sized at speeds up to several thousand per second, with measurements made of any desired size parameter. Data output can be alphanumeric or graphical, with statistical evaluation of the data, as desired. Evaluation of modern image analysis systems [16] indicates that automated particle count measurements using image analysis techniques are more accurate than manual measurements.

Particle Collection and Measurement Procedure

The sample of liquid to be characterized is normally stored in a suitable sample container. The sample may be one of a batch of large-volume or small-volume injection products, or it may be a container of liquid sampled from a process line. Online sampling for microscopic evaluation is seldom used, since the filtration rate through membranes of submicrometer pore size may vary due to partial filter blockage as particles are deposited on the filter surface. Flow control to define the sampled liquid volume can be difficult.

In operation, a membrane filter is first cleaned by flushing with clean water. It is then placed in a filter funnel attached to a suitable vacuum source such as a filter flask or a direct connection to a trap-equipped vacuum line. The sample container is agitated sufficiently to ensure that large particles that may have settled during storage will be dispersed throughout the container. An aliquot sample of 25–100 mL is placed in the filter funnel and the liquid is drawn through the membrane. The filter funnel walls are then washed with clean liquid, which is also drawn through the membrane. After the membrane is essentially dry, it is removed from the filter funnel, covered with a clean, dry cover slip, and taken to the microscope for particle measurement.

The particle size range that can be defined accurately and with good resolution is approximately 2–200 μm. Bright-field or dark-field overhead (episcopic) illumination can be used for measurement of particles in pharmaceutical products with good sizing accuracy and resolution. The concentration range that can be measured is very broad. The major limitation is a requirement that no more than 10% of the membrane surface be covered with particles so that particle overlap is low, minimizing visual coincidence. By adjusting the liquid volume that flows through the membrane, the well-defined particle concentration can vary from a few hundred per liter to several hundred thousand per milliliter. This is done by counting a few hundred or a few thousand particles per measurement, knowing the fraction of the membrane surface measured and the fraction of the total sample that passed through that membrane surface. Calculation of the particle concentration can then be carried out.

The potential for accuracy for the membrane filter–microscope method is limited only by the amount of skill and care applied to carrying out the procedure. The accuracy of particle sizing is nearly 100%, especially when image analyzing systems are used. However, the overall accuracy of the method can be degraded by procedural errors. The distribution of material on the filter surface must be random and nearly uniform or the possibility arises that the operator may not select truly representative fields for examination. This is particularly serious when the particle population on the filter surface is large enough that only a few fields need be examined to supply a statistically valid measurement. This problem can be minimized by making sure that preferred flow paths are not established during the filtration process and while the filter funnel walls are being flushed. Microscopic observation should be carried out with the membrane completely flat on the slide to avoid sizing errors. When specific fields are being examined, a consistent and unambiguous basis for accepting or rejecting particles on the boundary of a field must be established and maintained for all measurements. Other errors that can affect the accuracy of the method can arise from the many manual operations inherent in the procedure. These operations exist in sample handling before and during filtration as well as in handling the filter before and during observation. The possible errors during these actions are not easily quantified.

The particular advantages of the membrane–microscope measurement method result from the nondestructive measurement process. The particles can be observed repeatedly and are retained on the membrane for reference and/or other analysis at any time. If it becomes desirable at any time to determine particle composition, the retained samples can be analyzed by any of a variety of wet or dry analytical methods. The sample size can be adjusted to a level that will produce any desired quantity of particles on the membrane surface, as long as the operator can select sample collection durations and/or adjust dilution ratios as desired. The capital costs for the components are relatively low unless a very sophisticated image analysis system is used. Overall system reliability is good, because there are no complex mechanical, optical, or electronic components. Storage and operating space for materials and equipment is quite small, requiring only a few cubic feet of clean storage space and part of a clean bench for measurements unless a complex image analysis system is used.

The major problem with the method is that it is primarily a manual operation. Measurements of sample volumes, setting up and cleaning the systems, conclusions as to system tares and background data, microscope settings for particle types, selection of fields to measure, etc. are generally subjective rather than objective decisions.

3.4 Electrical Sensing Zone Analysis

Conductive liquids have been analyzed for particle content for many years using electrical sensing zone measurement techniques [17,18]. In operation, liquid is passed through a small orifice placed in a nonconducting barrier such as the wall of an orifice tube. Electrodes are located in the liquid at each side of the barrier, and an electric current is passed through the liquid. Figure 8 illustrates the operation of an

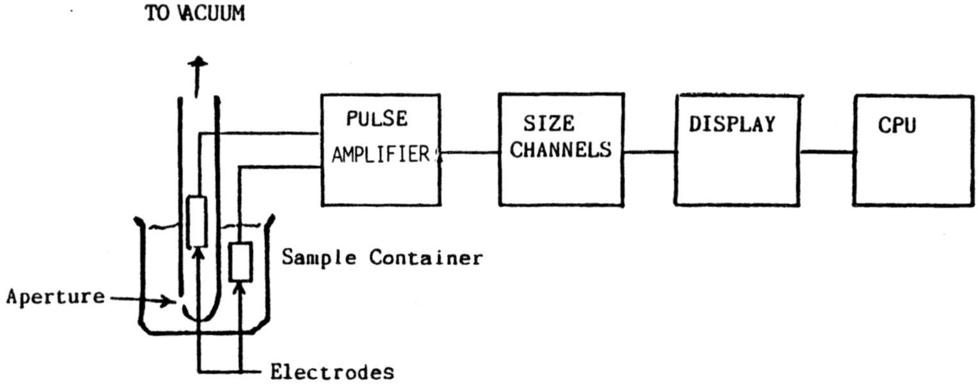

Figure 8 Operation of electrical sensing zone counter.

electrical resistance particle counter, including a flow control system and an indication of a data processing and control system. As each particle passes through the orifice, a momentary change in impedance occurs in the electrical path through the orifice. The current pulse caused by passage through the orifice of a particle of less conductivity than the liquid can be related to particle volume. By recording the pulse height distribution and comparing that distribution against previous calibrations of pulse height produced by particles of known size, a particle size distribution for material passing through the orifice can be derived. The size parameter is expressed as the diameter of a sphere of the same volume as the particle being measured. Multichannel models of the instrument are available with microprocessor control and data processing systems that provide particle size and concentration data in almost any format.

Underlying assumptions in interpreting particle size data from this device are that the system response is directly proportional to particle volume and that no other system parameter affects response. However, both particle resistivity and shape, as well as position within the orifice during passage, can affect response. Particle resistivity is a parameter whose effect is rarely observed, because the normal oxide films on conductive metals or the Helmholtz electrical double layer on most other materials results in sufficient difference in conductivity from that of the suspension liquid that most particles can be considered almost equally nonconductive. Particle shape can affect response, particularly if the surface has many convolutions or other shape factor extremes. For example, flakes are usually oversized, and porous particles may be reported as having volumes larger than the skeletal volume. Where particles are highly conductive or porous, special care in calibration is required to avoid erroneous undersizing for these materials [19].

Another factor that affects response is the location of the particle within the aperture during passage. This occurs because the apertures are normally cylindrical with a length-to-diameter ratio of ≈ 2, and the current density is usually higher around the orifice edges. Heavy or large particles that may not remain within the liquid streamlines moving through the orifice are often oversized. The degree of oversizing is not great but may be of importance for materials that have a narrow size distribution. This problem can be minimized by using a flow system with a hydrodynamically focused orifice that directs all particle flow through the center of the orifice, where current density is uniform [20]. The only difficulty with this procedure is the requirement for the addition of special, noncommercial flow control components to the device.

Apertures are available with diameters ranging upward from 20 μm. For the smallest aperture, 0.5 μm particles are defined with good resolution. The particle sizing range for any single aperture is usually considered to be 2–40% of the aperture diameter. In some circumstances, the linear sizing range can be extended upward to 80% of the aperture diameter [21]. The upper size for particles measurable by the method is generally limited only by the capability of keeping particles in suspension in the liquid moving to the orifice and by the dimensions of the orifice in use. The lower measurable size for any aperture is limited by background noise and possible electromagnetic or radio-frequency interference; the upper size is limited by possible plugging of the aperture. For a 30 μm orifice, a size range of 0.6–12 μm is recommended; at 5% coincidence, this orifice can handle a particle concentration to 1.5×10^6 particles per milliliter, and a sample volume per measurement of 0.05 mL is recommended. For a 600 μm orifice, a size range of 12–250 μm is recommended; at 5% coincidence, this orifice can handle a particle concentration of 250 particles per milliliter, and a sample volume size of 2 mL is recommended. The term "sample size" refers to the volume of liquid passed through the orifice for each measurement. This volume is an aliquot sample of the total liquid sample in the container into which the orifice tube is placed.

In operation, the instrument is placed in a clean environment free of electrical noise that may cause erroneous counts. Noise can be reduced by enclosing the instrument within a grounded Faraday cage; a wire mesh screen can be used for this purpose. The sample should be a liquid with conductivity adequate to result in an orifice resistance of 5000–100,000 Ω at the rated instrument current flow. If the liquid to be analyzed is not sufficiently conductive, then additives can be used to increase conductivity. A list of electrolyte solutions useful for work with electrical sensing zone analyzers is shown in one of the British standard methods for particle sizing [22]. A liquid sample in a suitable clean container is placed on the analyzer platform. Continuous stirring and avoidance of a flat-bottomed container is recommended strongly; otherwise the sample withdrawal rate may be so low that turbulence due to horizontal stirring effects and aspiration of the liquid alone may not be sufficient to keep the particles adequately dispersed. The orifice tube and stirrer are inserted into the container, and stirring is begun at a rate that will not produce a vortex. The orifice dimensions are selected for the particle size range of concern; this selection also defines the volume of the measured aliquot sample. The desired aliquot samples are drawn through the orifice, and data on particle size and number per aliquot sample are recorded. If flow rate disturbance or distorted pulse shape is noted, then data from that aliquot sample may have to be discarded, the flask may have to be moved for better mixing control, or the orifice may have to be cleaned if inspection with the built-in inspection microscope shows partial or total blockage of the orifice.

The electrical sensing zone analyzer has several advantages. The response is less affected by system parameters other than the reported one than any other automated system. Sizing resolution is excellent, as the response to particle volume (a third-power function of diameter) rather than to a first- or second-power function produces a broad signal response to small changes in size. Counting rates up to 5000 s^{-1} are easily achieved. An extensive library of software for processing particle count and size data is available. The method is used extensively for blood cell counting and sizing, and many data have been developed for measurements in pharmaceutical facilities. Operation of the device is not very difficult, and the instrument vendors provide training programs that permit laboratory personnel to work with a wide variety of materials.

One disadvantage of the electrical resistance method is that the liquid being characterized must be conductive. Otherwise a particle-free conductive solvent must be available that is miscible with the liquid to be tested and that will not modify the particles present in that liquid. ''Large'' particles can block flow through the aperture, and the long electrical path through the liquid can pick up any stray electrical noise from external sources. Measured aliquot sample volumes are very small, particularly for the detection of small particles. The low measured sample flow causes difficulty in keeping dense particles dispersed well enough that they will be reliably aspirated into the orifice. In very noisy areas, the instrument must be operated within a Faraday cage; otherwise, electromagnetic interference may produce erroneous data.

3.5 Acoustic Response Detection

Characterization of particle content in liquids usually calls for the removal of a sample from the main body of the liquid or modifies the particles in some way. Therefore, a nonintrusive, nondestructive analytical procedure has long been sought. Shortly after World War II, the successful application of acoustic detection techniques for submarine location led to studies of acoustic response for particle measurement in the liquids used in the aerospace industry. The Sperry Corporation developed an acoustic echo-sounding system for detection of particles in nearly opaque liquids [23]. Liquid samples could be placed in a container fitted with a piezoelectric crystal at its base, or the crystal could be located in the wall of a liquid flow line. The crystal functioned as both an emitter and receiver for the sonic energy. A pulse was emitted in a converging beam focused at the center of a defined sensitive volume. Immediately after pulse generation, the crystal function was changed so that it acted as a receiver. When the energy beam reached a particle in the liquid, some energy was reflected back to the crystal. Only those pulses that were returned to the crystal after a time required for transmission to and from that volume of liquid located in the central portion of the container would be accepted. This time gate allowed definition of a specific volume of liquid from which particle signals would be accepted. The reflected energy is proportional to the size of the particle that produced the echo and the energy flux present at the particle location.

Operation of the acoustic response counter is shown in Fig. 9. In use, careful calibration is required because of the nonuniform energy distribution in the conical beam. Some problems were also noted because of false signals from turbulence and bubbles in the liquid. The smallest particle that could be measured by this device was $\approx$25 μm in diameter. A system using a higher frequency (15 MHz) crystal emitting microsecond pulses was later used for measurement of in vivo blood flow [24]. This device was applied to measurement of contaminant particles in other liquids but could not detect individual particles smaller than 13.5 μm. In addition, sizing resolution was poor. A large angle of convergence is used to provide high

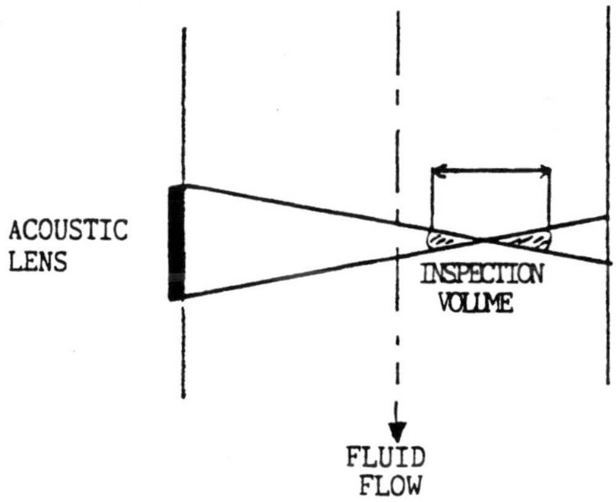

Figure 9 Acoustic response counter operation.

energy in the acoustic beam focal zone. This results in low level signals from large particles at the outer portion of the sensitive zone. These signals are confused with equal energy level signals from small particles within the zone. Thus it is practically impossible to define the size of individual particles producing signal information or the liquid volume from which the data were produced [5].

The major advantage of the method is that it is indeed nonintrusive and it can detect changes in particulate contamination levels. However, the disadvantages of poor size sensitivity and the difficulty of defining particle size or concentration in the widely divergent acoustic beam make it very difficult to define particle size or concentration consistently. Poor size resolution and the requirement that the speed of sound be known for the liquid in use in order to define particle size and sample volume for each liquid makes the device strictly a gross contamination indicator rather than a true particle measurement system. This instrument should not be used for accurate particle size definition where particles as small as 10 μm are of concern.

3.6 Optical Interaction Measurement Methods for Particle Arrays

Photometric Observation

At this time, the most widely used methods for detecting and counting particles in pharmaceutical liquids are based on optical interaction effects. Most particle measurement in the pharmaceutical industry is carried out to define the number of particles in various size ranges. However, there are some occasional requirements for defining overall levels of particulate material in liquids. In these situations, information on particle size distribution is not required. Photometric and turbidimetric devices are used to obtain information on total particle loading in many liquids. A primary application area for these instruments is in ensuring acceptable levels of particle content in potable water. The instruments are also useful in verifying uniformity of colloidal suspensions in the pharmaceutical industry.

These instruments define the quantity of light removed from a direct beam by a suspension of particles in liquid. Photometers can record the reduction in light level caused by the combination of scattering out of the direct beam and the absorption of light by the particles in the liquid. The removal of light by a particle is

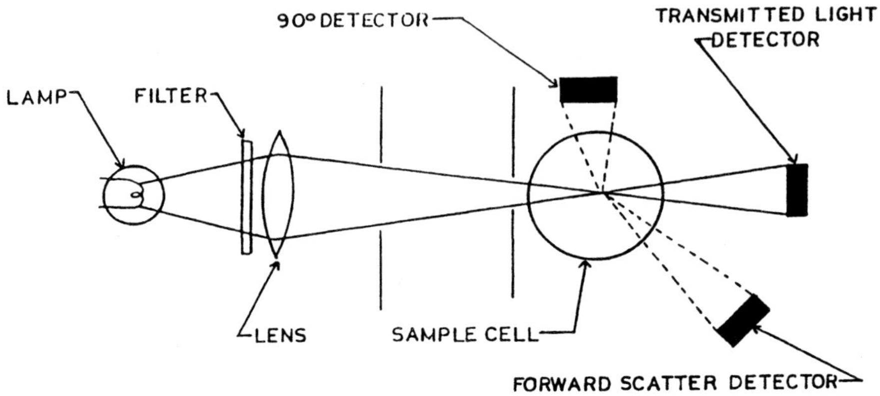

Figure 10 Optical system for ratio turbidimeter.

referred to as light extinction or absorption. When reductions in light levels are measured, the instrument is referred to as an absorption analyzer or a turbidimeter. The reduction in light flux is a function of the total projected area of the particles and the particle extinction coefficient. The particle extinction coefficient is defined as the ratio of total light flux scattered and absorbed by a particle to the light flux incident on that particle. In a polydisperse particle suspension, the relationship between particle area and concentration will vary with the particle size distribution function. The coefficient varies with particle size and refractive index. Absorption analyzers (turbidimeters) are usually used to define particle concentrations up to approximately 1000 ppm. Nephelometers are available that record only the light flux that is scattered out of the beam at a specific solid angle. Depending on the observed angle, the scattering analyzers can be used to define concentration levels up to 10–15% solids in liquid. Particle size information is not defined with either instrument type.

For measurement of turbidity in relatively clean liquid, the ratio of light scattering at a specific scattering angle to light extinction is used. Figure 10 shows the optical system for a commercial ratio turbidimeter. Instruments of this type can be used to observe turbidity in either flowing liquid streams or batch samples. They are sensitive to turbidity levels as low as 0.001 nephelometric turbidity units (NTU). One nephelometric turbidity unit is equivalent to approximately 1 ppm of particulate contamination in a liquid. For particles of density near 2.5, the number concentration of 10 μm particles is approximately 1000 mL^{-1}; for 1 μm particles, the concentration increases by three orders of magnitude. Multirange systems can be set to indicate levels as high as 2000 NTU. Waters with turbidity less than 1 NTU can be measured in this way [25].

Fraunhofer Diffraction Analyzers

Figure 11 illustrates the optical design of a Fraunhofer diffraction analyzer system. A stream of fluid containing the particles to be measured is passed through a sensing zone illuminated by a collimated laser beam. Particles in the size range from ≈ 0.7 to 700 μm in diameter scatter light in the forward direction at angles inversely proportional to size at intensities proportional to size. The scattered light pattern

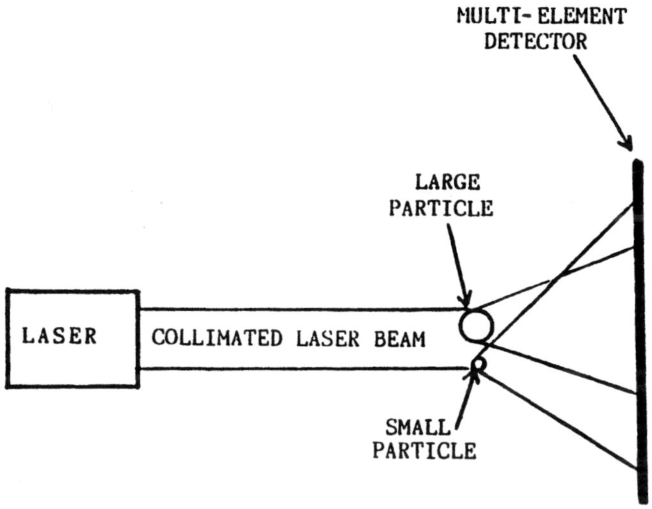

Figure 11 Fraunhofer diffraction analyzer optical system. The diffraction angle is small for large particles and large for small particles.

from each particle in the sensing zone can be thought of as producing a number of Airy patterns, each consisting of concentric bright and dark rings. The scattered light is collected by a Fourier optical system and focused on a radial photodiode array detector. In this way the pattern of scattered light intensity as a function of scattering angle can be defined. By assuming one of several possible particle size distribution functions, an algorithm can be used in a high speed data processing system to deconvolute the data and convert the light intensity and scattering angle data to particle size distribution and concentration data [26]. Experience has shown that only a few particle size distribution functions are adequate to characterize most of the particle size distributions appearing in nature. Concentrations up to a few percent by volume can be measured over the size range of the system. Difficulty can arise if detailed information is needed on particles in the tails of the distribution. The instrument readout may not record these particles at all.

Operating procedures are quite simple. Modern instruments incorporate automated and well-controlled sample handling, dilution, and mixing systems. Either liquid suspensions or dry powder can be handled in the flow and mixing system. The scattered light measurement system is programmed to operate with very little manipulation, and the data reduction program is almost completely automatic. Formats for several common size distribution functions are programmed into the system, which seeks a best fit to one of the formats. The advantages of the system are the capability of handling large samples in an extremely wide concentration range, the repeatability demonstrated in operation, and the wide particle size range that can be handled. The system is capable of particle measurement in either gas or liquid suspensions. The major disadvantage is the assumption that the particles being measured will fit one of the assumed size distribution functions. Even this is not a problem unless quite detailed information on specific particles is required; most real particle size distributions fit one of the installed standard two- or three-constant distribution functions such as a log-normal or a log-probability function.

3.7 Optical Interaction Measurement Methods for Single Particles

Interferometric Response from Single Particles

A recent development in optical particle counting has been described that uses interferometry to count and size particles in liquids [27]. The instrument developed does not measure the intensity of scattered light from a particle but rather the phase shift caused by that particle. In a manner similar to the operation of a Mach–Zehnder interferometer, an incoming laser beam is divided into two equally intense beams by a beam splitter. One beam passes through the sensitive volume of the particle flow path, and one beam undergoes a 90° phase change. A second beam splitter combines the two beams, which are 180° out of phase. The intensities of the out-of-phase beams are measured. When no particles are present, these intensities are equal. The presence of a particle causes a phase shift related to particle size. When the refractive index of the particle is greatly different from that of the substrate liquid, the phase shift is close to a function of the ratio of the indices; when the two indices are not greatly different, the phase shift is a function of the difference between the two. It is suggested that this effect will allow discrimination between gas bubbles and particles, because the bubbles have lower refractive index than the liquid. Since particle indices are normally larger than that of the liquid, particle signals should have polarity opposite to that of signals from bubbles. The instrument is too new to provide complete comments as to its advantages or problems. However, some studies point out advantages in its capability to distinguish between particles and bubbles and to detect particles with refractive index near that of the liquid [28].

One problem that has been noted is that the device requires very intense light, with laser beam focusing to a very small sensing volume, so that the observed volume will also be very small. Questions have also been raised regarding the instrument's effective dynamic range and resolution when particles with significant absorption are present. It appears that these particles result in excessively polytonic response from an interferometric system, making it essentially impossible to characterize the nature of contaminant particles larger than 1–2 μm in diameter. That problem resulted in withdrawal of this instrument from the market in 1995.

Light Interaction with Single Particles

Optical particle counters (OPCs) used for counting and sizing particles in a liquid use either light extinction or light scattering to characterize the particles. Light extinction methods are used for particles in the size range from ≈1 to 100 μm, while light scattering is used for particles in the size range 0.03–20 μm. Operation of either OPC type is neither as simple as might be indicated by the brief summary that is presented here nor as complicated as might be expected from consideration of the light interaction theory and the fluid dynamic and electronic considerations involved in the operating OPCs.

For light extinction optical systems, when a collimated beam of light is passed through a liquid, any particle present in the beam's path will remove some of the light by absorbing some and by scattering some out of the beam. The removal of light from the beam moving through the liquid is called extinction. The relationship between incident and transmitted light is

$$I/I_0 = \exp(-AEt)$$

where

I = transmitted light
I_0 = incident light
A = particle projected area
E = particle extinction coefficient
t = beam path length

For particles larger than approximately 5 μm in diameter, the extinction coefficient value is 2, resulting in an extinction signal level proportional to the particle's projected area. For smaller particles, the extinction coefficient varies sufficiently that direct calibration is required for such smaller particles.

Light scattering is complex. The particle reflects some light at the interface between the particle and the suspending medium, diffracts light at the particle boundary, and may absorb some of the light passing through the particle, as shown in Fig. 12. The amount of scattered light will vary with the illumination wavelength, particle

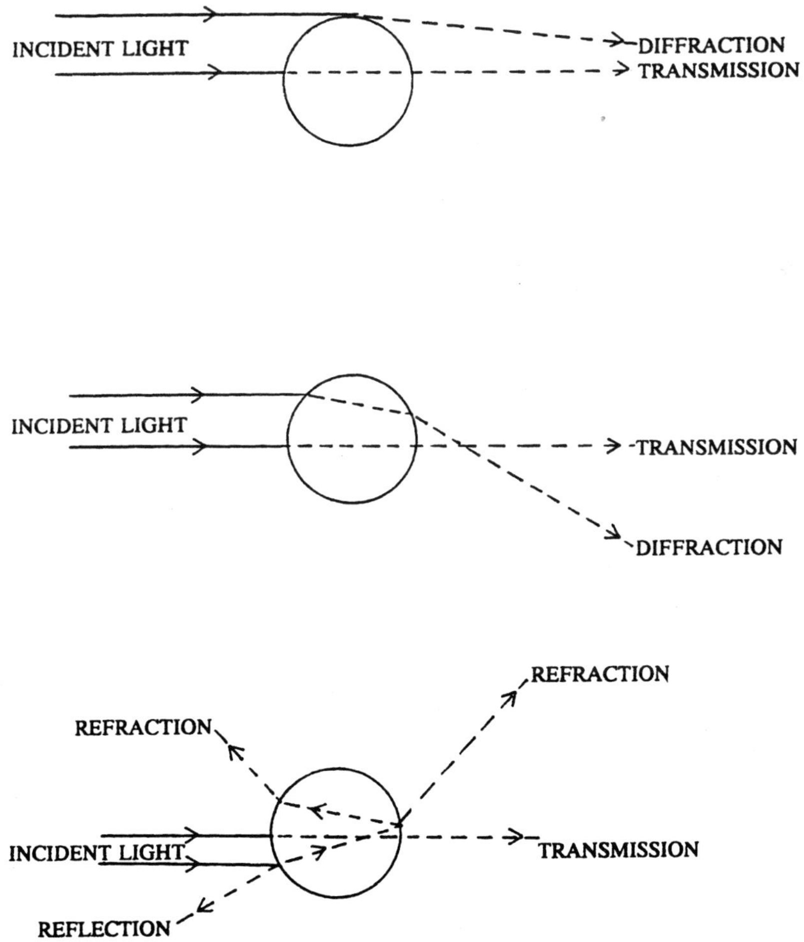

Figure 12 Beam paths in geometric light scattering.

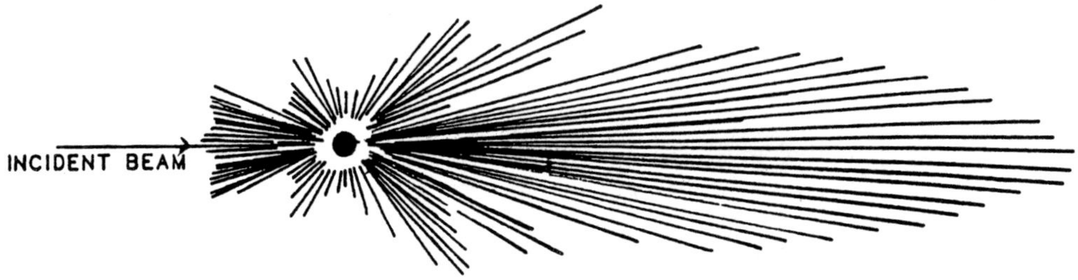

Figure 13 Scattered light pattern from large particle.

size, shape, and refractive index. The amount of light that is collected and measured will vary with the optical design of the instrument and the performance of the optical and electronic components. As a result of these phenomena, the intensity of light scattered from a particle appreciably larger than the wavelength of the illumination varies over a range of scattering angles, as shown in Fig. 13.

4 OPTICAL SINGLE-PARTICLE COUNTER PERFORMANCE PARAMETERS

4.1 Optical Assemblies

There are two general types of OPCs used with liquids. An in situ system measures the particles within a larger stream that may be flowing through the OPC optical system and is usually a scattered light system. A volumetric system observes the complete volume of the sample moving through the OPC. Light extinction OPCs are volumetric counters only, whereas light scattering OPCs can be designed as an in situ or volumetric system.

Figure 14 shows volumetric sensor optical systems in which the entire sample flow passage is illuminated. Two of the illuminated sample boundaries include the flow path boundaries as well. Rectangular flow passages with cross-sectional dimensions ranging from a few tens of millimeters to a few millimeters are used. The third dimension is defined by the illumination beam masked to a height of a few tens of micrometers and a width that extends across one of the flow path boundaries. Either light scattering or light extinction measurement can be used with this system. Liquid flow rates from a few millimeters per minute to liters per minute can be accommodated. At the lower flow rates, light scattering permits measurement of particles as small as 0.1 μm. For systems with larger flow rates, the operating mode is to measure particles larger than 1 μm up to millimeters in diameter by light extinction. The dynamic range for any of the optical systems is approximately 1.5 orders of magnitude from the smallest to the largest particle that is sized. Above the dynamic range upper limit, the larger particles will be detected but are sized only as being equal to or larger than the upper limit size.

Light scattering optical systems for in situ measurements are often used for counting and sizing submicrometer particles. The in situ optical system observes a portion of the liquid stream that is isolated from the illumination beam entrance and exit windows. This isolation is made possible by either focusing a collecting optical system at a point away from the scattered light exit window or orienting the col-

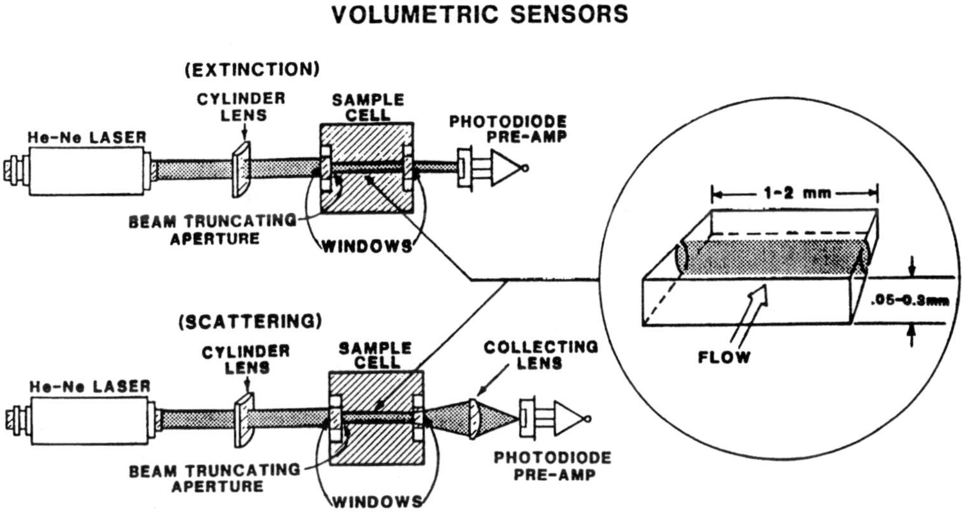

Figure 14 Volumetric sensor optical systems.

lecting optical system at 90° to the illumination beam axis. In this way, collection of light scattered by defects or debris on the windows is greatly reduced and instrument sensitivity is nearly that imposed by the background scattering from the liquid alone. The near-forward-scattered light collection system shown in Fig. 15 uses helium-neon laser illumination. It is capable of detecting 0.1 μm particles at observed sample liquid flow rates of a few milliliters per minute. The right-angle collection system [29] shown in Fig. 16 has a sensitivity of 0.05 μm at observed sample flow rates of a fraction of a milliliter per minute. The higher sensitivity is obtained by observing a smaller sensitive volume and using a solid-state laser source that is more

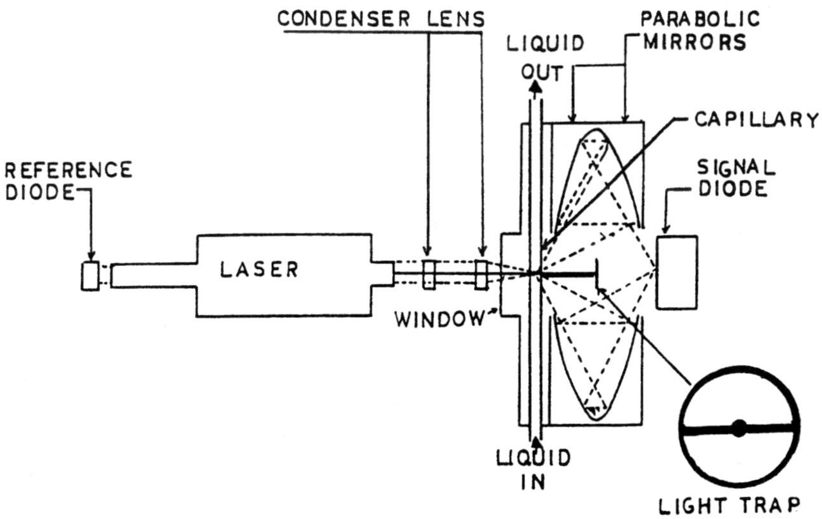

Figure 15 High sensitivity light scattering optical system.

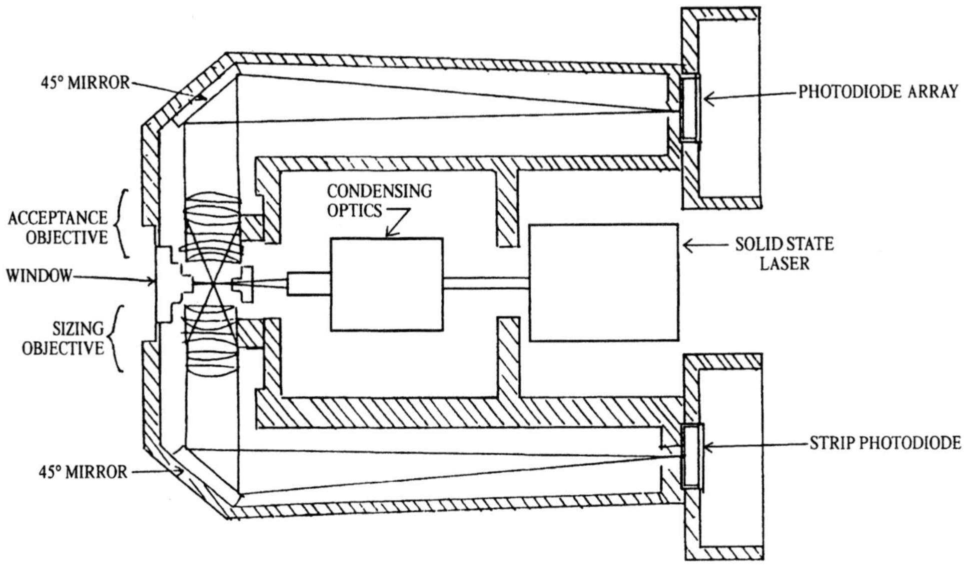

Figure 16 Ultrahigh sensitivity light scattering optical system.

powerful than the gas laser. The system of Fig. 15 observes a sample of several milliliters per minute within a stream flowing at several hundred liters per minute, using a conventional 5 mW He-Ne gas laser for illumination. The system of Fig. 16 observes a sample of 0.3 mL/min flowing within a stream flowing at 300 mL/min, using a 50 mW solid-state gas laser for illumination.

Aside from sensitivity and convenience in physical layout, the performance of the system will depend on the choice of right-angle or near-forward collection optical systems. Either a gas laser or a solid-state laser can be used with both systems. Conveniently sized He-Ne gas laser power levels are in the 5–10 mW range, whereas solid-state laser power levels are nearly an order of magnitude higher. The gas laser emits 633 nm radiation, and the diode laser emits 780 or 840 nm radiation. Wavelength changes over these levels will not change signal levels to a great degree; however, the scattered light signal versus particle size response function oscillates at any wavelength, particularly for particles larger than a few tenths of a micrometer; the location of the oscillations shifts somewhat with wavelength. The near-forward collection optical system is limited to a smaller solid collection angle than is the right-angle collection system. Particle size resolution is significantly better for instruments with larger solid collecting angles. Changes in slope of the response curve are of minor concern as long as the curve does not reverse.

To maximize the signal level, the beam may be focused to a smaller cross section to increase intensity. The uniphase TEM_{00} laser mode emits a beam with a Gaussian energy distribution; even a multimode laser beam, normally considered to have a relatively uniform intensity beam, has a zone where intensity decreases at its edges. For this reason, the amplitude of the scattered light signal from a particle will always depend on its location when it passes through the beam. An in situ measurement sensor does not control the location of particles that are present in the liquid. Thus a large particle may pass through the edge of the illumination beam where very low intensity exists. Only part of that large particle may be illuminated, and it will still produce a signal as large as that from a smaller particle passing through the center of the beam. When a particle monitor is used, it responds to signals with amplitudes equal to and greater than a preset threshold level; these signals may be produced by particles passing through any part of the illuminated volume. For this reason, the effective sample volume in which a particle will be detected can be considered to increase to some extent with particle size. (The location of a particle is usually defined as the position of its center.) Either special optical and electronic components are used to reduce the detection volume change with particle size or the counter detection volume is reduced by discarding data from the beam edges. When a segment of a particle much larger than the threshold limit size sensitivity for the particle monitor passes through the edge of the illumination beam for a monitor, the segment may be as large and scatter as much light as a threshold limit size particle. This can occur even though its center may not be outside the defined sample volume for the monitor simply because the particle is sufficiently larger than the specified threshold size in a size range where response varies with the sixth power of particle size.

A complete description of the operating principles and limitations of all OPCs is beyond the scope of this presentation, but OPC vendors provide detailed design information on their products and there is extensive information in the literature on particle physics. The following discussions on procedures for selecting, setting up, and operating the OPC should be considered as recommendations for selecting, using, and establishing satisfactory operation of the OPC that will be used to characterize the liquids of concern.

5 OPTICAL PARTICLE COUNTER OPERATION

5.1 Selection Considerations

In selecting an OPC for use in characterizing pharmaceutical liquids, the criteria that should be considered for selection are relatively straightforward. The OPC should be capable of meeting any regulatory agency requirements in terms of performance and reliability. The OPC should be capable of making the required measurements at minimum cost. Both capital expense for the OPC and operating costs for personnel and consumable items should be considered.

In terms of the regulatory agency requirements, consideration of the specifications for particle size sensitivity as stated for small volume and large volume injections means that the OPC must be sensitive enough to permit counting and accurately sizing particles as small as 2 μm in diameter and size the particles with good size resolution. It should be fitted with a sample feeding system that will feed batch samples to the OPC with accurate volume and flow rate control. If the same OPC is to be used to verify the performance of filters used to prepare water for injection, then submicrometer particle sizing capability may be required. The difference in cost between an OPC with 2 μm sensitivity and one with submicrometer sensitivity can be thousands of dollars, depending on the required size sensitivity.

Accurate particle sizing is required because essentially all measurement requirements state the maximum permitted particle population in a sample in terms of the number of particles as large as or larger than a specified particle size. If the OPC does not size the particles accurately, then the typical particle size distribution function seen in many contaminant suspensions will magnify the sizing error significantly. Figure 17 illustrates how a 5% sizing error can result in a 15% counting error when measuring a particle size distribution where the concentration varies inversely with the third power of the particle size. Figure 18 shows how an OPC with poor sizing resolution makes it almost impossible to determine particle size for particles whose dimensions differ by a large ratio. At this time, OPC producers supply OPCs with particle sizing resolution that will not increase the reported relative standard deviation for measurement of monosize particles by more than 5%.

Accurate sample volume determination for measurement of batch samples is ensured by use of syringe pump sample feeding systems that allow the use of a precision syringe to control aspiration of a sample through the OPC sensitive volume. These devices are ideal for most injectable liquids and for liquids with viscosities similar to that of water. For liquids with higher viscosity, the aspiration process can reduce the pressure in the OPC sensitive volume to the point where any dissolved gases can form bubbles when passing through that sensitive volume. In that situation, the OPC reports the bubbles as particles. It is necessary to pressurize the liquid before aspiration occurs or to use a feeding system that operates by pressure rather

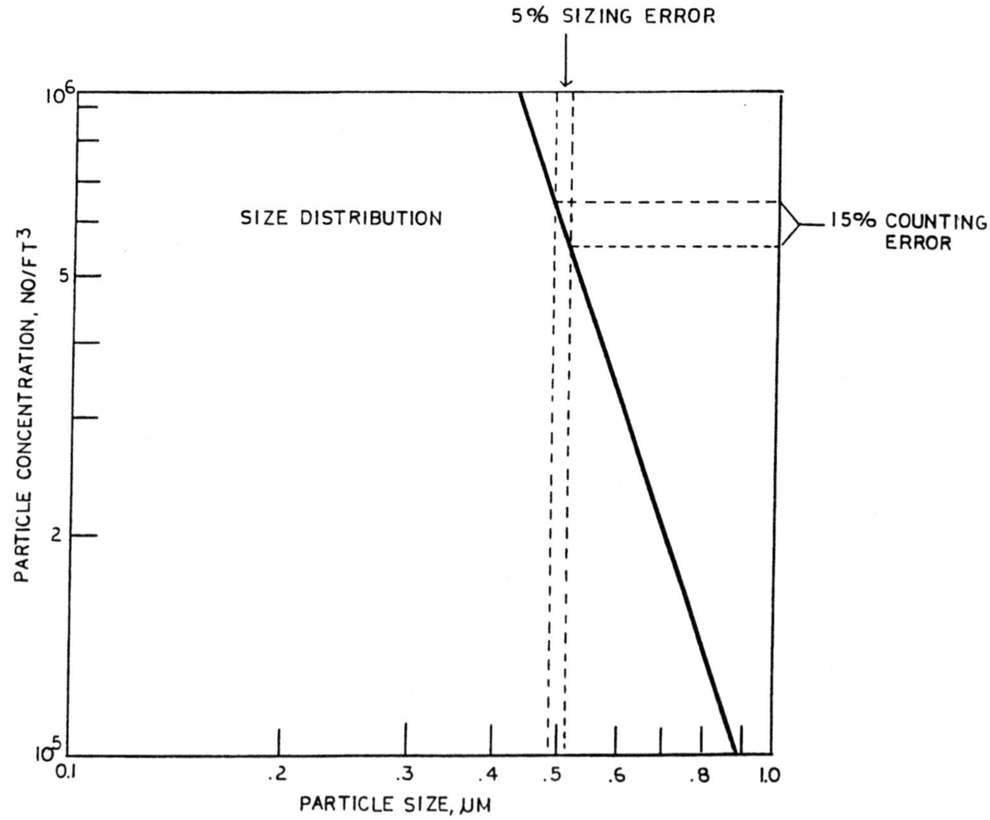

Figure 17 Counting error as a function of sizing error.

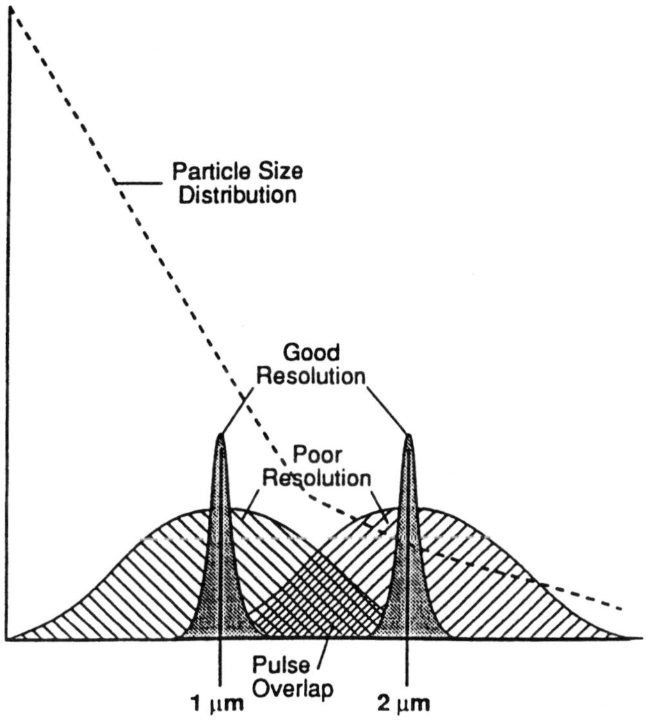

Figure 18 Effects of sizing resolution on particle size indication.

than vacuum and measures sample volume by means of a buret or mass measurement after passage through the OPC.

5.2 Calibration Bases and Methods

Calibration is carried out by determining the response of the OPC to spherical isotropic particles of known size and refractive index. The calibration procedure is described in detail in ASTM F658-87 [30]. That method describes the procedure for determining particle sizing accuracy, sizing resolution, and counting accuracy for OPCs whose response varies with the particle's projected area. This is typical for extinction counters that are specified as the compendial measurement device in USP 23, < 788 > [2]. The calibration particles normally used are monodisperse latex spheres of refractive index 1.6 with zero absorption for visible light. They are available in diameters ranging from less than 0.1 μm to several millimeters with relative standard deviations less than 1% for particles smaller than 5 μm and no more than 5% for larger particles. Sizes of particles of other refractive index and/or shape can be expressed in terms of an "equivalent optical diameter" when the instrument response to such a particle is compared to that of the calibration base material.

5.3 Sample Measurement and Data Collection

When making measurements in some pharmaceutical products, it may be necessary to dilute the sample to avoid coincidence errors in the particle measurement device.

If this is required, then a first step is to determine the tare or background level of particles in the diluent, sample container, and sample handling system. The procedure is to use a quantity of diluent equivalent to that which is used to transport the diluted sample. The particle concentration and size distribution measured during this tare determination should be recorded even it if is essentially zero. Next, the selected number of aliquot samples is taken and the particle size distribution and concentration in these aliquot samples are determined. The data are recorded for each sample.

The next step in the procedure is to determine the liquid sample quantity to be measured. This will require placing the sample container into the sample feeder with which the counter is fitted. When doing so, it may be necessary to agitate the sample to mix the particles thoroughly and then to deaerate the sample so as to remove the air bubbles that may have been generated during the mixing process. A brief exposure to low power ultrasonic energy, followed by a brief evacuation, may be adequate. The sample is then placed in or on the sample feeder with a clean stirring bar placed in the sample. Stirring should continue during the time the sample is fed through the OPC, but stirring should be controlled so that no vortex is allowed to form. If a vortex forms, then air may be drawn into the liquid and bubbles can be generated. The sample can then be fed through the counter for particle measurement.

Most commercially available sample feeders can be adjusted to feed liquid at a rate of 1–100 mL/min. The maximum concentration before coincidence in many single-particle counters becomes a problem is in the range of 3000–10,000 particles/mL. A desirable total particle count to permit reasonable description of most size distributions and concentrations with acceptably low variability between aliquot samples is approximately 10,000 particles per sample. Thus, if the concentration of particles in the sample will permit measurement within these parameters (e.g., 30–100 mL aliquot samples with 100–3000 particles/mL), then an aliquot sample volume can be determined easily. If the original sample is a suspension in which the particle concentration is appreciably lower than the range above, then the largest possible volume is selected. Once the volume has been selected, the measurements are made and the data are recorded for that sample. If at all possible, several aliquot samples are measured for each liquid sample. A typical practice is to measure three to five aliquot samples from each liquid container and determine the standard deviation for the number of particles counted in each size range measured. If only one measurement can be made because of the small quantity of liquid available, it is recommended that the data be considered as a mean value and that a standard deviation be defined as the square root of the mean. This assumes that the single measurement represents a mean value and that additional measurements would produce a Gaussian data distribution.

5.4 Data Handling and Reporting

Most OPCs have the capability of allowing selection of data presentation in either differential or cumulative mode. The devices accumulate data in the differential mode, and their built-in pulse height analyzer/counter assemblies are fast enough to permit a calculator program to convert the data to a cumulative format. Where a small number of particle size ranges are specified, a cumulative data format presentation may be most useful. Where a larger number of size ranges are available and the system sizing resolution justifies it, the differential format can permit examination of the particle size distribution in detail to permit observation of multimodal or otherwise atypical size distributions.

In addition to the simple initial data presentation format, the availability of sophisticated computer programs makes it possible to report the data with warning and alarm levels if excessive particle concentrations may be of concern during production operations and to carry out statistical processing to verify data conditions. In addition, sample identification and conditions, environmental conditions during measurement, counter condition and status, along with many other conditions can be reported, and data can be stored as required.

Most present-day optical particle counters for pharmaceutical liquids are fitted with a precision syringe pump liquid feeder to permit precise control of aliquot sample volumes and feed rates. A precision stepper motor draws a sample from the stirred sample container and moves it at a constant rate through the sensor portion of the counter. Volumetric accuracy of ± 0.1 mL is common for sampling volumes that range from 1 mL to 1 L. The counter units are often fitted with software that runs in a Windows environment. The operator can observe particle concentrations in as many as 15 size channels that range from 2 to 125 μm. Multiple threshold settings within this range can be chosen. The sensor can be calibrated at flow rates selected to permit system operation over a range of liquid viscosities. The calibration procedure is performed by passing a series of monodisperse latex sphere suspensions through the sensor, as specified in ASTM F658-87 [30], entering the labeled size and standard deviation for each suspension and setting the software program to the calibrate mode. The calibration procedure using such software is completed in less than 30 min. The response curve and sizing resolution of the counter system are stored in the system memory.

5.5 Sample Changeover, System Cleaning, and Shutdown

Most discussions of particle measurement with an OPC cover measurement of single samples. In practice, a series of samples are usually measured. Samples in production facilities are most often measured during a single shift. In some development facilities, an OPC will be used over a long period with a variety of liquid materials. Inter- and intrasample interferences can cause problems unless good laboratory practices are followed. Problems may be caused by chemical or physical reactions between different liquids. If two liquid samples are immiscible, then colloid droplets may form and will be reported as particles. When changing from one liquid to another, it is advisable to use a mutually miscible liquid to flush out the first sample material before adding a second material to the liquid handling components. If the two liquids can react to form a hazardous material, then the first liquid should be removed completely from the flow system before the second one is added. In addition to chemical reaction products, hazards can occur if heat of solution or reaction results in temperatures so high as to cause damage to seals or other system components.

When an OPC is shut down for a weekend or any extended period, it should be flushed with an inert solvent and a final clean water fill left in the system so that no liquid with appreciable vapor pressure is left in the liquid handling system. In this way there is no possibility of a film of nonvolatile residue being deposited on critical optical or mechanical elements that could cause problems. During any of these flushing operations, both in-plant occupational safety requirements and external environmental concerns must be satisfied. The nature and quantity of liquids to be disposed of must satisfy municipal and in-plant safety regulations.

REFERENCES

1. Code of Federal Regulations. Current Good Manufacturing Practice in Manufacturing, Processing, Packing and Holding of Large Volume Parenterals. 21 CFR, Part 212, *Fed. Reg.*, *41*(106):22202–22219 (1976).
2. United States Pharmacopeia, Vol. 23, < 788 > Particulate Matter in Injections. *Pharmacopeial Forum*, *19*(2):4939–4942 (1993).
3. Sampling Procedures and Tables for Inspection by Attributes, MIL-STD-105D, U.S. Navy Publishing and Printing Office, Philadelphia, PA, 1989.
4. S. H. Goldsmith and G. P. Grundelman, In situ method for evaluating filter cleanliness, *Pharm. Manuf*, *1*(9):37–43 (1984).
5. L. A. Gatlin and S. L. Nail, Initial evaluation of focused ultrasound for in situ measurement of small particles in flowing water streams. *J. Parenter. Sci. Technol.*, *35*(5): 227–230 (1981).
6. R. G. Knollenberg, In situ optical particle size measurements in liquid media, Proceedings of the Second Pure Water Conference, San Jose, CA, 1982.
7. R. G. Knollenberg, Monitoring systems for semiconductor fluids, in *Handbook of Contamination Control in Microelectronics* (D. L. Tolliver, ed.), Noyes, Park Ridge, NJ, 1988, pp. 257–300.
8. K. Willeke and B. Y. H. Liu, in *Aerosol Generation, Measurement, Sampling, and Analysis*, B. Y. H. Liu, editor, p. 44, Academic Press, New York, 1976.
9. A. Lieberman, Flow rate and concentration effects in automatic particle counters, Proceedings National Conference on Fluid Power, Chicago, IL, 1975.
10. J. Z. Knapp and L. R. Abramson, A new coincidence model for single particle counters, Part I: Theory and experimental verification, *J. Pharm. Sci. Tech.*, *48*(3):110–134 (1994).
11. N. Leelarasamee, S. A. Howard, and H. J. Baldwin, Visible particle limits in small volume parenterals, *J. Parenter. Drug Assoc.*, *34*(5):167–174 (1980).
12. J. Z. Knapp and H. K. Kushner, Particulate inspection of parenteral products: From biophysics to automation, *J. Parenter. Sci. Technol.*, *36*:121 (1982).
13. Y. Chung, Suspended particulates in ocean waters—Abundance and size distribution as determined by a laser particle counter, *Proc. Geol. So. China*, *25*:102–110 (1982).
14. ASTM E20-85, Practice for Particle Size Analysis of Particulate Substances in the Range 0.2 to 75 μm by Optical Microscopy, Am. Soc. Testing and Materials, W. Conshohocken, PA, 1985.
15. ASTM F-312-69, Methods for Microscopical Sizing and Counting Particles from Aerospace Fluids on Membrane Filters, Am. Soc. Testing and Materials, W. Conshohocken, PA, 1980.
16. T. A. Barber, M. D. Lannis, and J. G. Williams, Method evaluation: Automated microscopy as a compendial test for particulates in parenteral solutions, *J. Parenter. Sci. Technol.*, *43*:27 (1989).
17. W. H. Coulter, Means for counting particles suspended in a fluid, U.S. Patent 2,656,508 (1953).
18. S. Kinsman, Instrumentation for filtration tests, *Chem. Eng. Prog.*, *7*(3):48–50 (1974).
19. G. Van der Plaats and H. Herps, A study on the sizing process of an instrument based on the electrical sensing zone principle. Part 1: The influence of particle material, *Powder Technol.*, *36*(1):131–136 (1983).

20. R. Davies, R. Karuhn, J. Graf, and J. Stockham, Studies on the Coulter counter, Part 2: Investigations into the effect of flow direction and angle of entry of a particle on both possible volume and pulse shape, *Powder Technol.*, *12*(2):157–166 (1975).
21. J. G. Harfield, Response of the Coulter counter Model ZM to spheres, *Part. Charact.*, *1*(1):32–36 (1984).
22. British Standard Methods, Determination of Particle Size in Powders, No. 3406, Part 5. Recommendations for Electrical Sensing Zone Method, British Standards Institution, London, UK, 1963.
23. C. Alberson, Detection of particles in liquids by the use of ultrasonics, Proceedings of the First National Symposium on Nondestructive Testing of Aircraft and Missile Components, San Antonio, TX, February 1960.
24. L. R. Abts, Computerized discrimination of microemboli in extracorporeal circuits, *Am. J. Surg.*, *135*:535 (1978).
25. C. Hach, Measurement of color and insoluble matter in reagent chemicals, *Am. Lab.*, *15*(6):42–48 (1983).
26. C. A. Daniels and A. A. Etter, Latex particle size analysis by the Coulter nano-sizer: Response to synthetic mixture of sizes, outsize particles and comparison with other methods, *Powder Technol.*, *34*(1):113–119 (1983).
27. D. B. Blackford and D. C. Grant, Evaluating a novel liquid-borne particle counter based on interferometry, *Microcontamination*, *11*(2):27–32, 66 (1993).
28. J. S. Batchelder and M. A. Taubenblatt, Evaluating a novel liquid-borne particle counter based on interferometry. 3. Comparison detection of nearly index-matched particles, *Microcontamination*, *11*(4):35–39, 61 (1993).
29. R. G. Knollenberg and D. L. Veal, Optical particle monitors, counters, and spectrometers: Performance characterization, comparison, and use, *J. IES*, *35*(2):64–81 (1992).
30. ASTM F658-87, Defining Size Calibration, Resolution, and Counting Accuracy of a Liquidborne Particle Counter Using Near-Monodisperse Spherical Particulate Material, Am. Soc. Testing and Materials, West Conshohocken, PA, 1987.

16

Crossflow Ultrafiltration

MICHAEL DOSMAR
Sartorius Corporation, Edgewood, New York

DANIEL BROSE
Chemica Technologies, Inc., Bend, Oregon

1 INTRODUCTION

In 1991 it was reported by the Pharmaceutical Manufacturer's Association (PMA) that the number of biopharmaceutical products had grown by more than 63% over 4 years. These biopharmaceutical products include monoclonal antibodies, vaccines, interferons, interleukins, and growth factors, among others. Of these, monoclonal antibodies represent the largest production volume. It has been predicted that U.S. biotechnology sales will rise to $7.4 billion by 1997 (Anon., 1992), with human therapeutics dominating the market and accounting for two-thirds of total sales (Thayer, 1991).

Biotechnology products are cell-derived, and as a result separation technology plays an important role in the processing scheme. Crossflow filtration is often the primary process used for purification of biotechnology-derived products. Crossflow filtration is distinguished from conventional "dead-end" filtration in that the fluid to be filtered flows parallel to the filters surface rather than perpendicular to the filters surface (see Fig. 1). The crossflow generates shear that limits the thickness of the filter cake or gel layer. In conventional dead-end filtration the filter cake thickness increases with time, resulting in the eventual cessation of flow.

Crossflow filtration offers distinct advantages over other separation technologies. These include improved throughput relative to dead-end filtration, elimination of aerosols (as generated in centrifugation), elimination of filter aids (as used in conventional filtration), and the lack of a requirement for phase changes (as in freeze-drying) (McGregor, 1990). Because of these and other advantages, crossflow ultrafiltration is widely used in biopharmaceutical manufacturing.

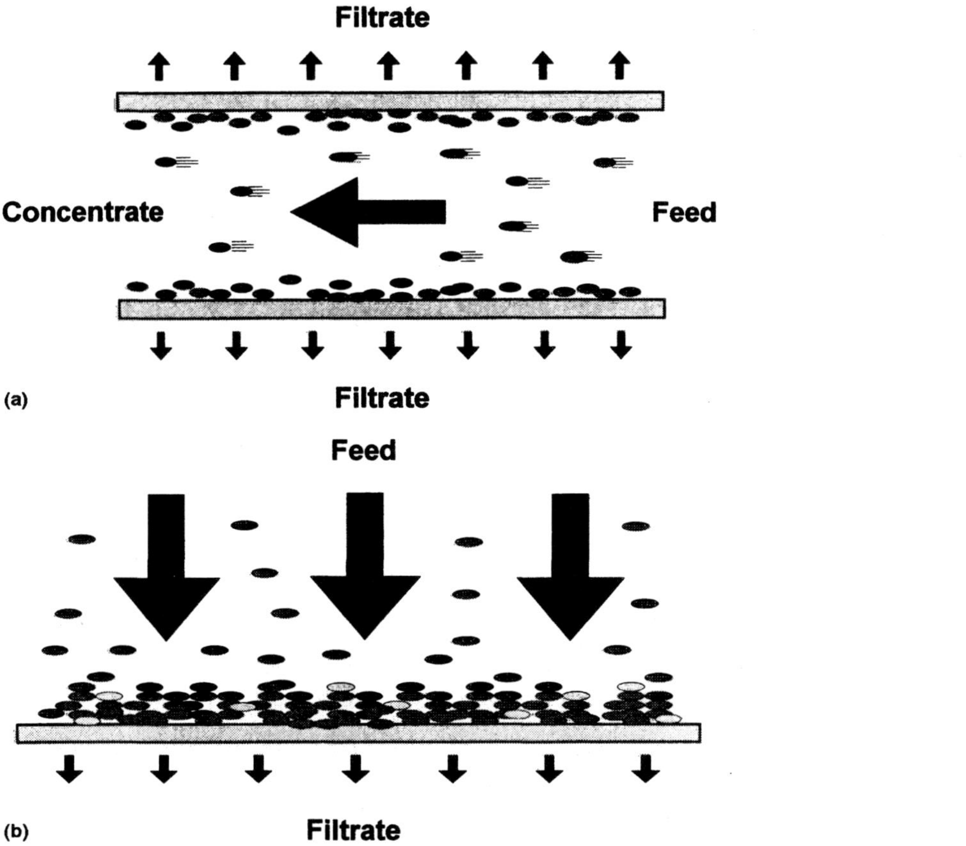

Figure 1 Comparison of (a) crossflow filtration and (b) dead-end filtration.

Crossflow filtration membranes had their origins in the 1950s when reverse osmosis membranes were developed for water desalination (Michaels, 1986). The Loeb–Sourirajan process of membrane formation by phase inversion created the first asymmetric membranes for reverse osmosis. The asymmetric membrane's rejection layer was one-thousandth the thickness of a symmetric membrane (Cheryan, 1986; Loeb, 1981). The development of asymmetric membranes by Loeb and Sourirajan (see preface to Cheryan, 1986) made it practical to use crossflow filtration for industrial applications. It is this development, coupled with the development of new ultrafiltration membranes, that gave birth to crossflow filtration in the biotechnology and biopharmaceutical industries (Michaels, 1986).

In the pharmaceutical industry, crossflow filtration is used for both microfiltration and ultrafiltration. Figure 2 shows the effective membrane pore sizes for membranes used in reverse osmosis (RO), nanofiltration (NF), ultrafiltration (UF), and microfiltration (MF). Ultrafilters are generally highly asymmetric (anisotropic); the membrane's rejecting layer is thin (0.1–5 μm) with very small pores, and the underlying support structure is thick (~100 μm) with much larger pores (see Fig. 3). The materials used in UF membranes vary widely, and some of the common membrane polymers (from most hydrophilic to most hydrophobic) are regenerated cel-

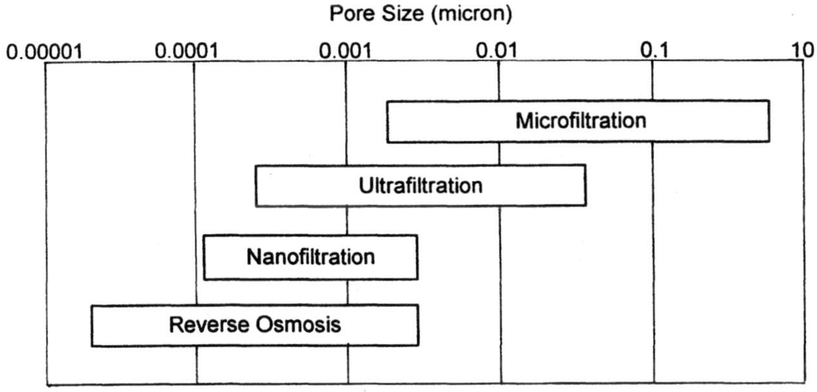

Figure 2 Typical pore sizes for membranes used in reverse osmosis, nanofiltration, ultrafiltration, and microfiltration.

lulose (RC), cellulose acetate (CA), modified poly(vinylidene difluoride) (PVDF), modified polysulfone (PS), polyethersulfone (PES), natural PS, nylon, polypropylene (PP), natural PVDF, and polytetrafluoroethylene (PTFE). Membranes made of these materials have been successfully used for isolation and purification of biopharmaceutical products by crossflow filtration.

2 CROSSFLOW ULTRAFILTRATION THEORY

In crossflow ultrafiltration the feed stream flows parallel to the surface of the membrane, that is, the feed flows across the flow or tangentially to the permeate or filtrate stream. A small fraction of the feed stream permeates the membrane; the remaining fraction is retained by the membrane and exits as the retentate or concentrate stream. When little solute is present in the feed stream, flow through the membrane is accurately modeled by the Hagen–Poiseuille equation, which describes liquid flow through cylindrical pores (Cheryan, 1986):

$$J = \frac{\varepsilon r^2 \Delta p}{8\eta \Delta x} \tag{1}$$

where

J = liquid flux
ε = membrane porosity
r = mean pore radius
Δp = transmembrane pressure
η = liquid viscosity
Δx = pore length

This equation states that liquid flux is proportional to the transmembrane pressure and inversely proportional to the liquid viscosity, which is controlled by the solute concentration and the temperature. Therefore, increasing the pressure or the temperature results in an increase in the flux. The Hagen–Poiseuille equation accurately predicts clean water flux through ultrafiltration membranes.

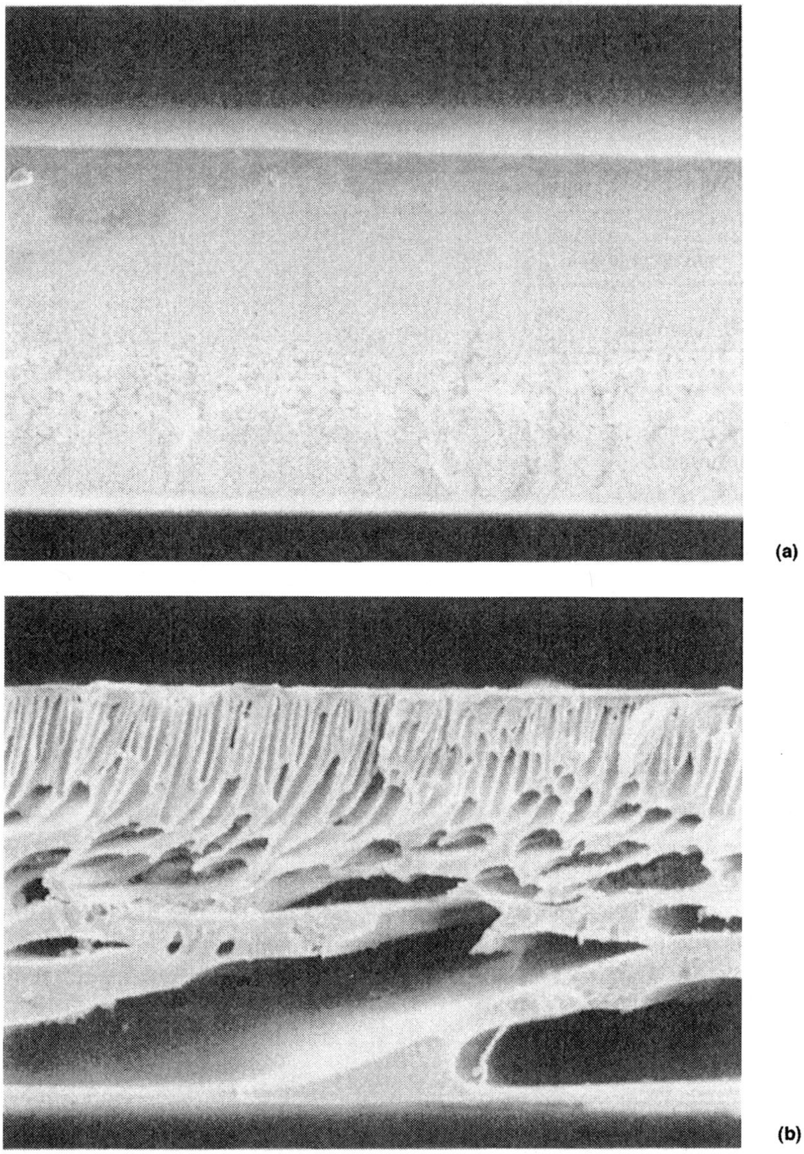

Figure 3 Scanning electron micrographs of asymmetric ultrafiltration membrane. (a) Foam structure; (b) finger structure.

When solute is present in the feed stream, liquid that permeates the membrane drags solute and debris toward the membrane surface by convective flow. Retained solute builds up on the membrane surface and forms a gel (or cake) layer; solute can back-diffuse through this layer via Brownian motion into the tangentially flowing aqueous stream. The flowing aqueous stream also acts to sweep the material brought to the membrane surface back into the bulk flow via inertial lift (Fig. 1a).

Once a gel layer forms, the gel often contributes the greatest resistance to liquid flow through the membrane. This increase in resistance causes a reduction in flux from that predicted by the Hagen–Poiseuille equation (Cheryan, 1986). The gel layer can also have a profound influence on the membrane's selectivity. The thickness of the gel layer is dependent on a number of factors, including (1) the rate at which permeating liquid brings solute to the membrane surface, (2) the rate at which solute back-diffuses into the feed stream, and (3) the hydrodynamic shear of the tangentially flowing stream. If the retained solute on the membrane surface can be dispersed back into the bulk fluid, then the membrane can be used much more economically. Successful exploitation of membranes in crossflow filtration is largely dependent on effective fluid management techniques (Porter, 1981). Belfort (1987) states, "By using hydrodynamic considerations, polarized solutes [can] be sheared from the membrane surface, thereby increasing the back diffusion and reducing the decline in performance."

The interrelationship of process variables in crossflow ultrafiltration can be understood by considering the physical model shown in Fig. 4. When the feed stream flows past the solid membrane surface, a stagnant boundary layer develops. The boundary layer is a result of the friction between the membrane surface and the liquid nearest the surface. This friction causes a reduction and stagnation of flow at the membrane surface. The gel layer forms in this stagnant boundary layer and grows until the rate of solute deposition by convective flow equals the rate of solute diffusion back into the feed stream. Once this steady state is established, a solute concentration gradient exists, with the highest solute concentration nearest the membrane surface and the lowest solute concentration in the bulk feed stream (see Fig. 4). This polarization of solute from the membrane surface to the feed stream is commonly referred to as concentration polarization. The polarization layer (gel layer)

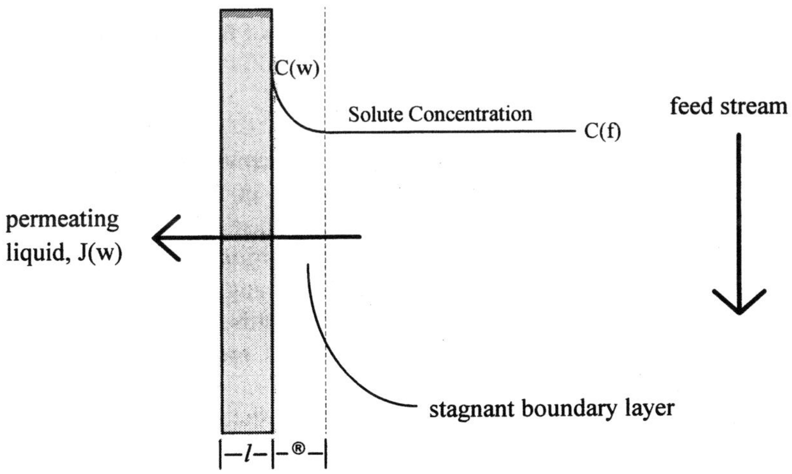

Figure 4 Physical model of concentration polarization and mass transport in a crossflow membrane application.

in biopharmaceutical separations is generally viscous and gelatinous, being composed of large molecular weight species.

Assuming that solute is completely rejected by the membrane and that the steady state has been achieved, the rate of solute convection into the boundary layer exactly equals the rate of diffusion out of the boundary layer (Nakao and Kimura, 1981; Cheryan, 1986):

$$J_w C = D \frac{dC}{dx} \qquad (2)$$

where

J_w = water flux through the membrane
C = solute concentration
D = solute diffusivity (diffusion coefficient)

This equation is integrated from the outside edge of the boundary layer ($x = 0$), where the concentration is equal to the feed concentration ($C = C_f$) to the membrane surface ($x = \delta$), where the concentration is equal to the wall concentration ($C = C_w$), resulting in the relationship

$$J_w = k \ln[C_w / C_f] \qquad (3)$$

where k is the mass transfer coefficient,

$$k = \frac{D}{\delta} \qquad (4)$$

δ is the thickness of the stagnant boundary layer adjacent to the membrane surface.

Equation (3) holds for a given transmembrane pressure drop (Δp). Each time Δp is increased, a new equilibrium is reached at the membrane surface, with an attendant increase in the steady-state value of C_w. As Δp is further increased, C_w reaches the point at which gelation or precipitation of solute occurs at the membrane surface. At this point, C_w equals the gelation concentration of the retained solute (C_g) and Eq. (3) becomes (Blatt et al., 1971)

$$J_w = k \ln[C_g / C_f] \qquad (5)$$

Further increases in Δp cannot increase the wall solute concentration beyond C_g, and so flux becomes independent of Δp. Though an increase in Δp at this point does temporarily increase flux through the membrane, this increase is short-lived because it causes the gel layer to thicken proportionally. Figure 5 demonstrates the flux versus pressure relationship for ultrafiltration of bovine serum using a 100,000 molecular weight cutoff (MWCO) polyethersulfone membrane.* As this figure shows, at pressures greater than 25 psi the flux becomes independent of pressure, indicating that a gel layer has formed on the membrane surface.

Equation (5) can be used to experimentally determine the gelation concentration C_g, which is constant for a given feed solution. J_w is plotted versus $\ln C_f$, and C_g is determined from the x intercept of the resulting line. Figure 6 shows experimental data plotted in this format, which the data were obtained from the ultrafiltration of

* MWCO is discussed in Sec. 4.1.

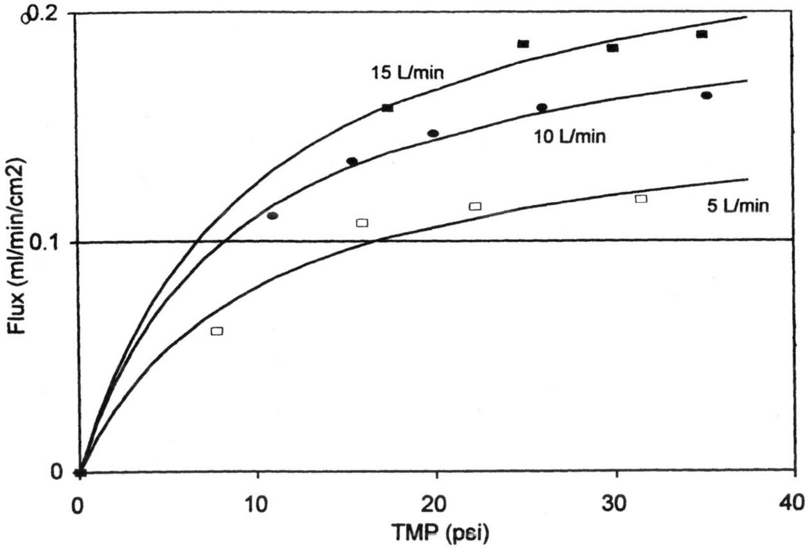

Figure 5 Flux versus transmembrane pressure (TMP) for ultrafiltration of bovine serum using 100,000 MWCO polyethersulfone membrane at three different crossflow velocities. (Courtesy of Sartorius Corp.)

bovine serum using a 100,000 MWCO polyethersulfone membrane. As these data demonstrate, C_g = 23% and is independent of solution flow rate.

The mass transfer coefficient k can also be determined from this plot, as the slope of the line is proportional to k. As demonstrated in Fig. 6, k is a strong function of crossflow velocity, increasing as crossflow velocity (flow rate) increases.

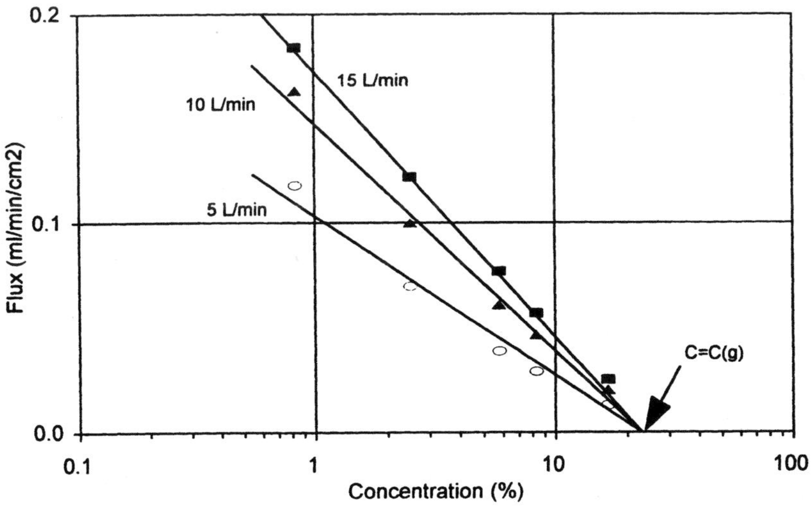

Figure 6 Flux versus $\ln(C_f)$ for ultrafiltration of bovine serum using 100,000 MWCO polyethersulfone membrane at three different crossflow rates. (Courtesy of Sartorius Corp.)

The dependence of the mass transfer coefficient on crossflow velocity has been accurately correlated (Blatt et al., 1971; Cheryan, 1986). For laminar flow the correlation is

$$k = 0.816 \left[\frac{\gamma}{L} D^2\right]^{0.33} \tag{6}$$

where γ is shear rate (γ = 8v/d for flow through tubes and γ = 6v/h for flow through rectangular channels, where v is solution velocity, d is tube diameter, and h is channel height), L is length of the membrane flow path, and D is solute diffusivity.

When flow is turbulent, the mass transfer coefficient is proportional to velocity raised to the 0.80 power instead of to the 0.33 power:

$$k = 0.023 \left(\frac{1}{d_h}\right)^{0.20} \left(\frac{\rho}{\mu}\right)^{0.47} D^{0.67} v^{0.80} \tag{7}$$

where d_h is the hydraulic diameter [=4 × (cross-sectional area)/(wetted perimeter)], ρ is liquid density, and μ is liquid viscosity. Because of the greater dependence on velocity when flow is turbulent, improved benefits in flux can be realized when flow is increased. The relationship between flux and velocity for both laminar and turbulent flow is shown in Fig. 7.

Mass transfer coefficients determined from the slopes in the semilog plots of flux versus solute concentration (Fig. 6) can be correlated to fluid velocity and used in the design of crossflow processes. Such correlations, although device-dependent, allow prediction of scale-up from one device to another. To illustrate, experimental evaluation of crossflow devices results in the following correlations for effective area of 60, 1000, or 7000 cm^2.

For 60 cm^2 cassettes,

$$J_w = 0.216 \left(\frac{1}{\mu/\rho}\right)^{0.47} D^{0.67} v^{0.40} \ln\left[\frac{C_g}{C_f}\right] \tag{8}$$

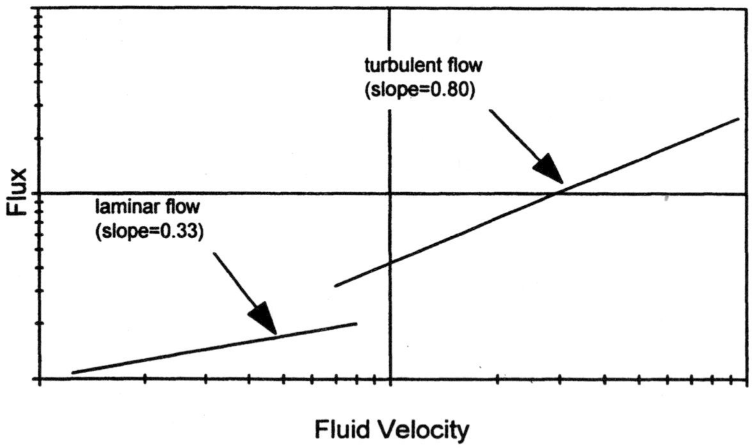

Figure 7 Flux as a function of fluid velocity for laminar and turbulent flow in crossflow ultrafiltration. (Courtesy of Sartorius Corp.)

For 1000 and 7000 cm^2 cassettes,

$$J_w = 0.373 \left(\frac{1}{\mu/\rho}\right)^{0.47} D^{0.67} v^{0.55} \ln\left[\frac{C_g}{C_f}\right] \tag{9}$$

Using the correlations in Eqs. (8) and (9), one can evaluate a feed solution at small scale using the 60 cm^2 device to determine D and C_g and then insert these values into Eq. (9) to predict performance with much larger crossflow devices. Similar scale-up conversion factors may be found in vendors' literature.

3 CROSSFLOW MODULE DESIGN

To achieve the goal of minimizing the polarizing gel layer and increasing the rate of mass transfer (and thus flux), a number of issues must be considered in designing a crossflow module.

3.1 Design Considerations

Turbulence-Promoting Insertions

Insertion of static mixers into the flow path enhances the transition of the flow from laminar to turbulent. Screens or meshes are used as static mixers between membranes in a variety of crossflow devices. Screens are used in spiral-wound cartridges and in some plate-and-frame designs. These mesh-like spacers can cause considerable turbulence and have been shown to improve flux (Cheryan and Chiang, 1984). There is some debate as the nature of the flow through these systems. Belfort (1987) considers the flow to be laminar through systems with screened channels, whereas Cheryan (1986) reports the flow as turbulent based on the pressure drop within the flow channel. This matter, though, can be resolved in a straightforward manner by experimentally determining the slope of a log-log plot of flux as a function of velocity as shown in Fig. 7.

There are potential downsides to the indiscriminate use of turbulence-promoting insertions for biopharmaceutical filtrations. Specifically, product may hang up on the mesh, creating a cleaning problem as well as causing potential occlusion of the flow channel (Cheryan, 1986). If particulates tend to either hang up on the mesh or occlude the flow channel, then pretreatment of the feed is required. Usually 50–200 μm prefiltration of the feed will alleviate this problem.

Flow Path Length

The way to control gel polarization is to maintain high velocity and shear at the membrane surface. The length of the flow path (L) has direct and indirect bearing on these hydraulic forces. First, as shown in Eq. (6), when flow is laminar the flux is proportional to the quantity $(1/L)^{0.33}$. Therefore, increasing the flow path length has the effect of decreasing flux. In turbulent flow, the length of the flow path does not have a direct bearing on flux. Second, the flow path length has an indirect bearing on flux for both laminar and turbulent flow because pressure drop through the crossflow device is proportional to the flow path length because of frictional forces at the fluid/membrane interface. Therefore, the longer the flow path, the greater the pressure drop and the lower flux. Third, because fluid is continually permeating the membrane, as the flow path length increases, the volumetric flow and velocity of the feed solution decreases; and according to Eqs. (6) and (7), decreasing velocity causes a reduction in flux. Therefore, both direct and indirect reasoning lead to the conclusion that increasing the length of the flow path lowers the flux.

Flow Channel Height

The flow channel height also has direct and indirect bearing on flux in crossflow ultrafiltration. As Eqs. (6) and (7) show, in laminar flow flux is proportional to the quantity $(1/d_h)^{0.33}$, and in turbulent flow flux is proportional to $(1/d_h)^{0.20}$. Therefore, as the channel height (or hydraulic diameter) increases, the flux will decrease. The indirect consequence of changing channel height is to cause a change in the crossflow velocity, assuming constant volumetric flow rate. That is, the cross-sectional area of the flow channel divided by the volumetric flow rate gives the fluid velocity in the flow channel. By increasing the flow path channel height, the cross-sectional area is increased, resulting in a decrease in the velocity and the flux.

Increasing the volumetric flow rate in order to increase velocity may result in the need for very large pumps. Running pumps at high speeds results in high shear in the pump and the generation of excess heat. The channel height should be as small as possible. However, care must be taken not to select a channel height that might trap recirculating particles or require a pump that might destroy existing particle aggregates in the attempt to achieve sufficient crossflow rates (Devereaux and Hoare, 1985).

3.2 Crossflow Module Types

As discussed previously, the ability to create shear and reduce concentration polarization is affected by the inherent design of the membrane module. There are numerous module designs to select from for crossflow filtration. The traditional ''process'' designs used in the pharmaceutical industry are cassette (plate-and-frame) modules, spiral-wound modules, hollow-fiber and tubular modules, and rotating surface modules.

Cassette Modules

Cassette modules consist of flat-sheet membranes mounted into a framework (Fig. 8). In the assembly of these systems each flow path is made up of two membranes that are facing each other (see Fig. 9). The upstream flow path must be sealed from the downstream permeate side of the membrane. Stacks of pairs of membranes are layered one on top of the other, and the permeate side of each membrane is supported by a rigid and porous spacer plate. In systems making use of preassembled modules, the membrane is generally glued onto the spacer plate. The spacer plate may be smooth or have surface features that give the membrane an uneven surface to promote turbulence. Flow paths are usually open; they may be parallel and or in series. In an alternative design not using rigid plates, the membrane's support is achieved by the dynamic interaction of the membranes above and below the permeate's flow path.

Feed flow paths can be open, but most do use screens. Feed enters at one end of the module through a series of inlet ports and exists the other end of the module through the outlet ports. Permeate flow exists through a series of permeate ports. Preassembled cassettes come in a variety of sizes from 0.06 to 25 ft^2. Systems using these designs may have surface areas as high as 1000 ft^2.

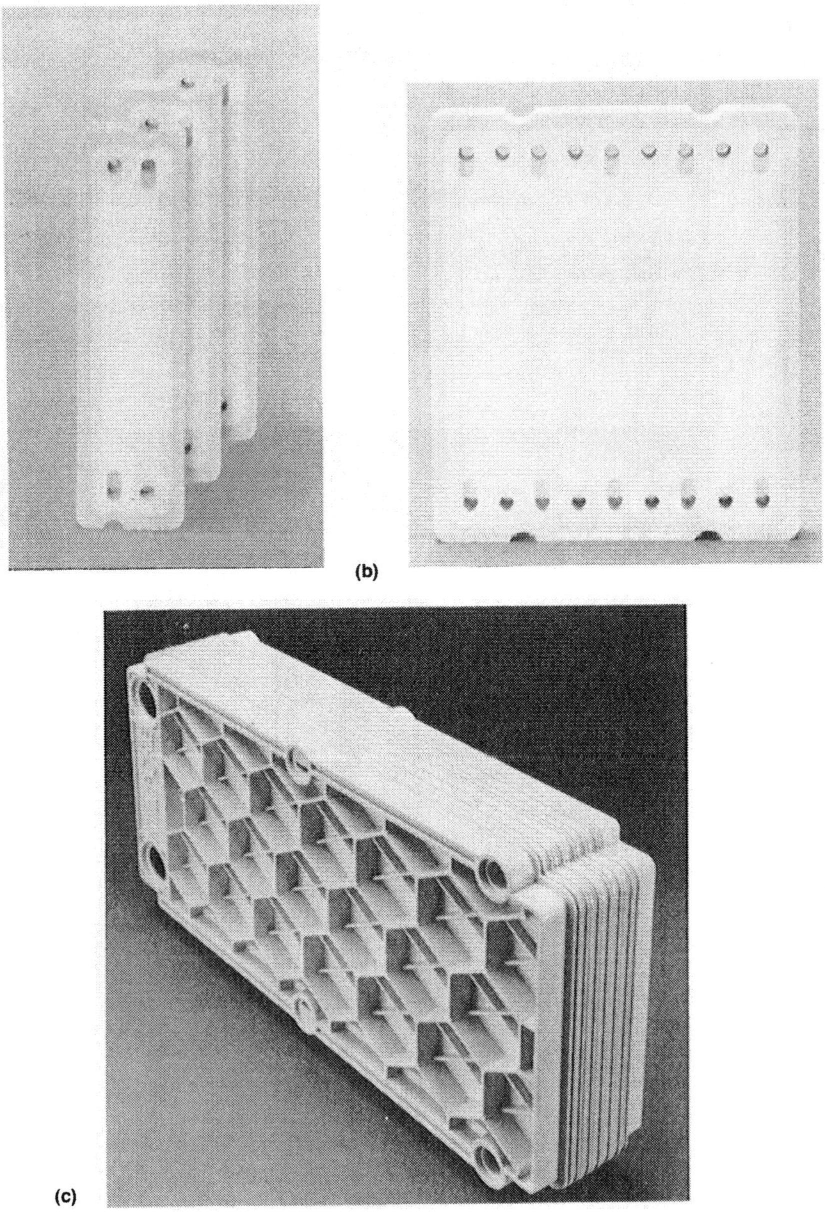

(a) (b) (c)

Figure 8 Crossflow filter cassettes. (a) Screened channel cassette of 1 ft^2 surface area. (b) Screened channel cassette of 7 ft^2 surface area. (c) Open-channel cassette. (a, b: Courtesy of Sartorius Corp. c: Courtesy of Millipore Corp.)

The filter holders for these designs are usually constructed of stainless steel, though acrylic versions are available for the laboratory market. The filters are sealed into the holder between two plates via a compression seal. Closure is achieved by tightening tie rods that are attached to the back plate and go through the front plate

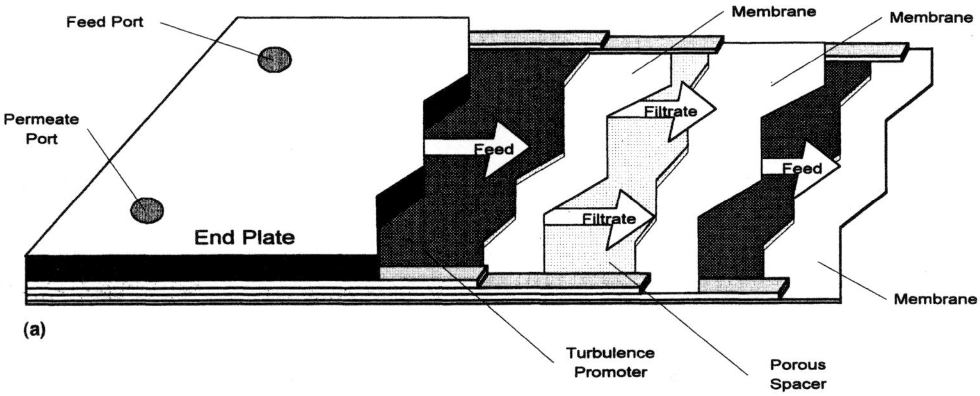

(a)

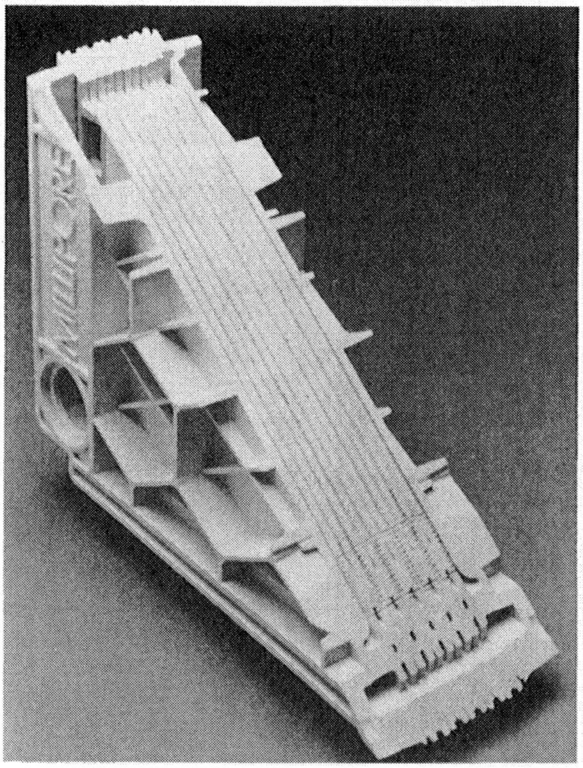

(b)

Figure 9 (a) Schematic description of flow paths in screened channel cassette. (b) Cross section of an open-channel cassette. (Courtesy of Millipore Corp.)

(Fig. 10). Larger systems achieve compression by using a hydraulic cylinder that exerts a force onto a movable front plate, thereby compressing the modules in the middle.

Plate-and-frame systems are generally easy to clean, have relatively high packing densities, support a wide variety of membrane materials, are amenable to incorporating turbulence-promoting spacers, and provide good crossflow performance. Drawbacks to this design are that fabrication of modules can be labor-intensive and thus expensive, and packing densities are not as great as those of hollow-fiber modules. However, the advantages to plate-and-frame systems outweigh the disadvantages, and this design is widely used in the biopharmaceutical industry.

Spiral-Wound Modules

Spiral-wound modules use pairs of flat sheet membranes bounded on the up- and downstream sides by screens similar to those in cassette systems. As shown in Fig. 11, the membrane sandwich is sealed at three edges so that the feed is isolated from the permeate. The fourth side (the unsealed side) of the membrane sandwich is attached to a perforated permeate collection tube. The membrane pairs are then rolled around the perforated collection tube, thereby creating the spiral.

Feed enters at one end of the spiral, flows tangentially along the axis of the cartridge, and is discharged at the other end. Permeate flows at a right angle to feed flow toward the center of the spiral and is collected in the core of the spiral. Spiral-wound modules are available in a variety of surface areas, from 1 to 50 ft^2. Surface area can be increased by increasing the number of membrane pairs, increasing the diameter of the spiral wrap, or increasing the length of the flow path. Spiral cartridges are placed in snug-fitting housings. The cartridge is sealed to the housing wall via an O-ring or brine seal. Feed flow on the outside of the cartridge is either blocked by an O-ring or restricted by a screen so as to provide the same resistance to flow as in the feed flow channels between the membranes. Laboratory devices are available that are encapsulated in polysulfone housings.

Spiral-wound modules can be ganged together to make filter systems of varying surface areas. Spiral systems feature relatively high membrane packing densities and are inexpensive. This design is extremely successful for particulate-free process streams but the modules are difficult to clean when particulates clog the flow paths or collect at the O-ring seals. Other drawbacks to this design are that spiral systems are difficult to sterilize and their long flow paths make high flow with low pressure drop impossible.

Hollow-Fiber and Tubular Modules

The fundamentals of hollow-fiber and tubular crossflow systems are essentially the same, the difference being that tubes are considerably larger in diameter than hollow fibers. Figure 12 is an electron micrograph of a hollow fiber. Fiber lumen diameters range in size from 0.5 to 3.0 mm. Tubular systems may also be configured with removable tubes that are inserted into individual tube holders. In ceramic tubular systems the membrane is cast as part of the ceramic tube array.

The "rejecting" layer of a hollow fiber or tube can be on the inside, as in Fig. 12, or outside of the fiber, with the wall of the fiber functioning to support and strengthen the rejecting layer. Liquid permeates the fiber wall, as with a flat-sheet membrane, and permeate is collected on the opposite side of the fiber. Hollow fibers and tubes are grouped and sealed into tubular shells to form modules as shown in Fig. 13. In the case where the rejecting layer is on the inside (lumen) of the fiber, the feed solution enters the lumen of the fiber at one end and flows down the length of the fiber, and retentate exists at the other end. Permeate is collected on the outside (shell side) of the fiber.

Hollow fibers are generally defined as having an inner diameter of less than 1 mm. These fibers have greater pressure drop than tubular modules; however, they

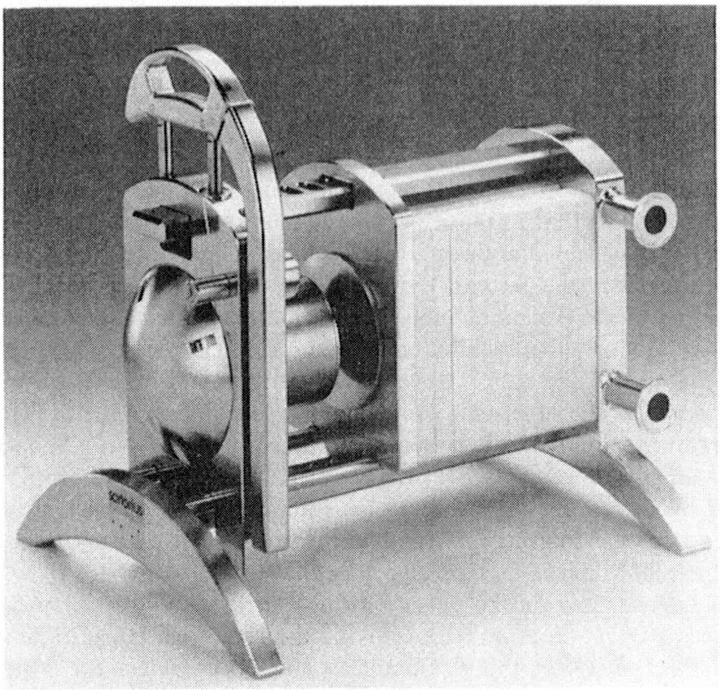

(a)

Figure 10 Cassette holders and systems. (a) Hydraulic cassette holder. (b) Hydraulic cassette holder on a filter skid. (c) Hydraulic system on a filter skid. (a, b: Courtesy of Sartorius Corp. c: Courtesy of Millipore Corp.)

also have much greater membrane surface area per volume. Hollow-fiber modules are also cheaper than tubular modules. Ceramic and tubular modules have low packing densities, but because of their large lumen they are able to handle very high particle loads. Because of the large lumen they require very high flow rates to maintain high velocity. Ceramic tubular systems have very high initial installation costs, but because they use inorganic membranes they have extremely long membrane life.

Spinning Disk Modules

Spinning disks are used in modules to create shear and turbulence by Taylor and Dean vortices, which are instabilities created when fluid flows around a curved or rotating surface. (See Chapter 27 in this volume.) A commercial membrane module based on this principle is shown in Fig. 14. As the disk spins, the fluid is destabilized and Taylor vortices are created. The rate of shear is a function of the velocity of the disk, which increases as fluid moves away from the center along a radial line. The driving force (transmembrane pressure—TMP) is created by the spinning disk, and that force also increases with increasing distance from the center. Whether these systems can be optimized so that the changes in pressure and shear offset each other has not been adequately investigated to date.

The theoretical advantage of spinning disk modules is that shear at the membrane surface becomes uncoupled from the feed volumetric flow rate. In practical application, though, spinning disk systems generate a great deal of heat as a result

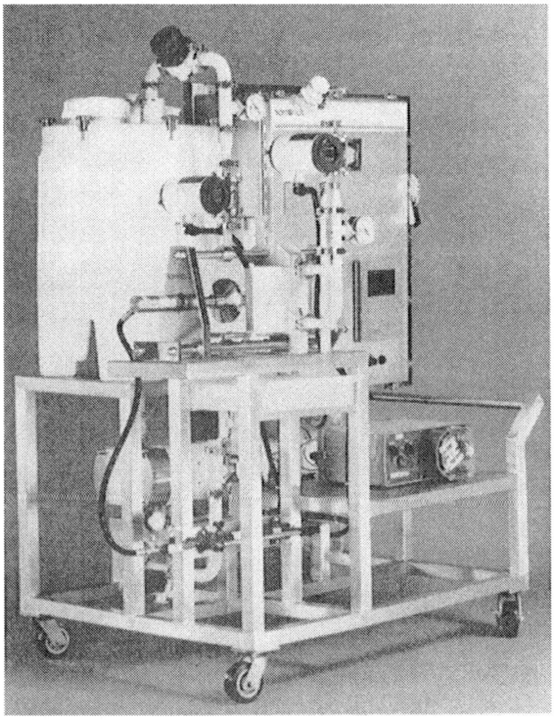

(b)

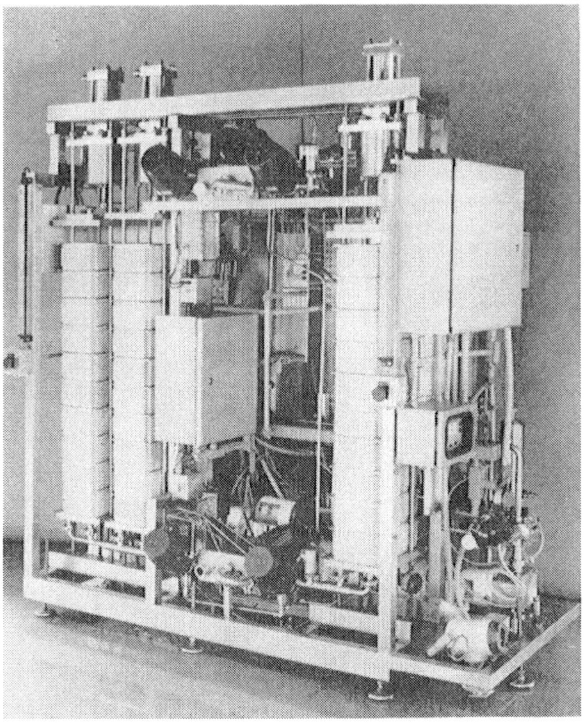

(c)

Figure 10 Continued

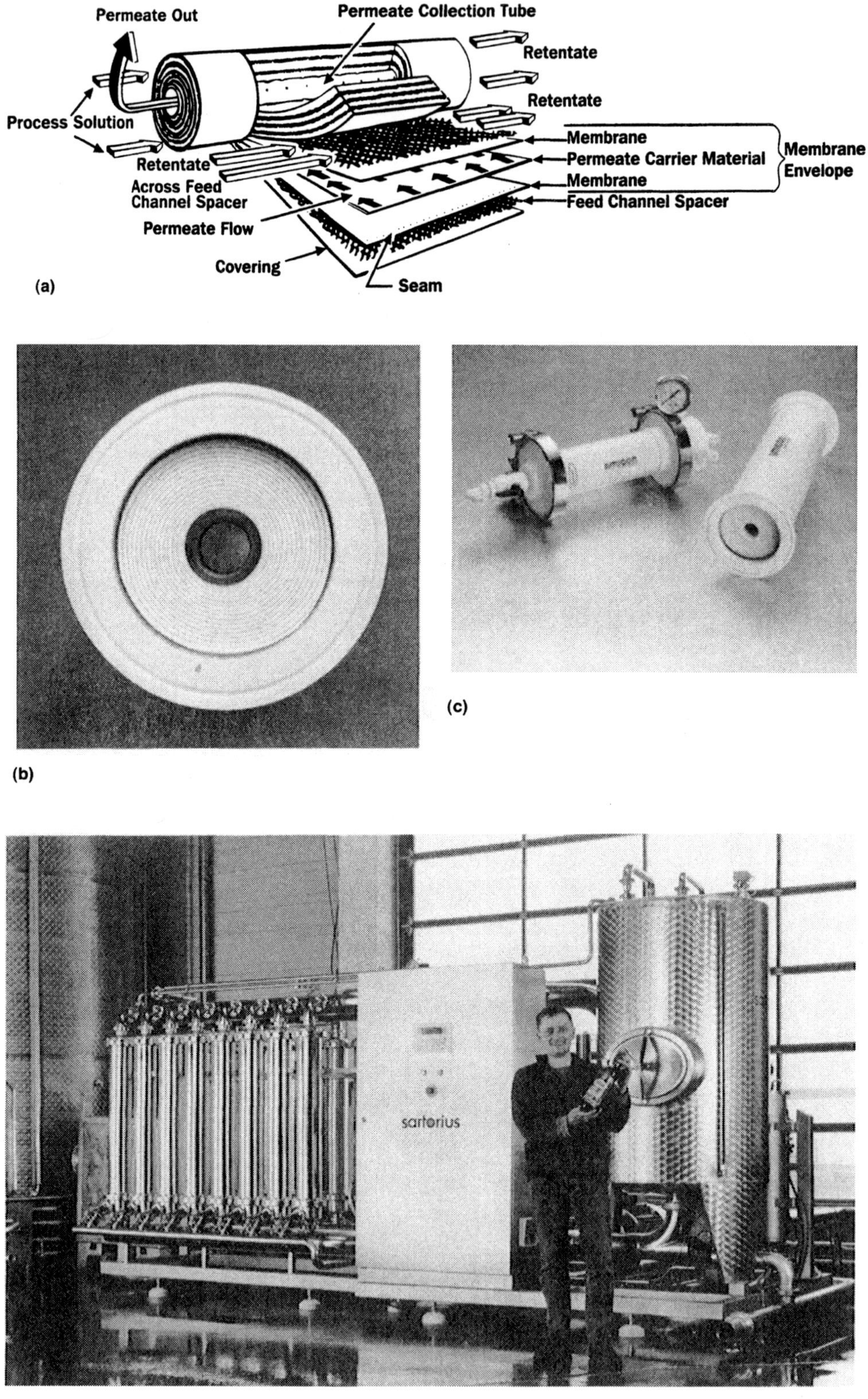

Figure 11 (a) Diagram of a spiral-wound crossflow module. (b) End view of spiral cartridge. (c) Spiral-wound cartridges. (d) Spiral-wound system. (a–c: Courtesy of Amicon Corp. d: Courtesy of Sartorius Corp.)

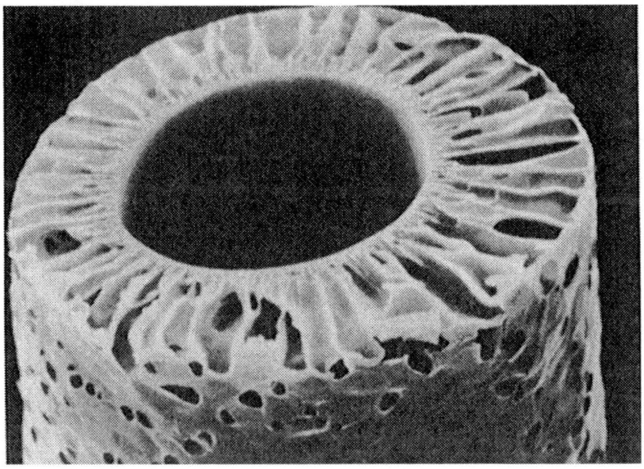

Figure 12 Electron micrograph of a hollow fiber.

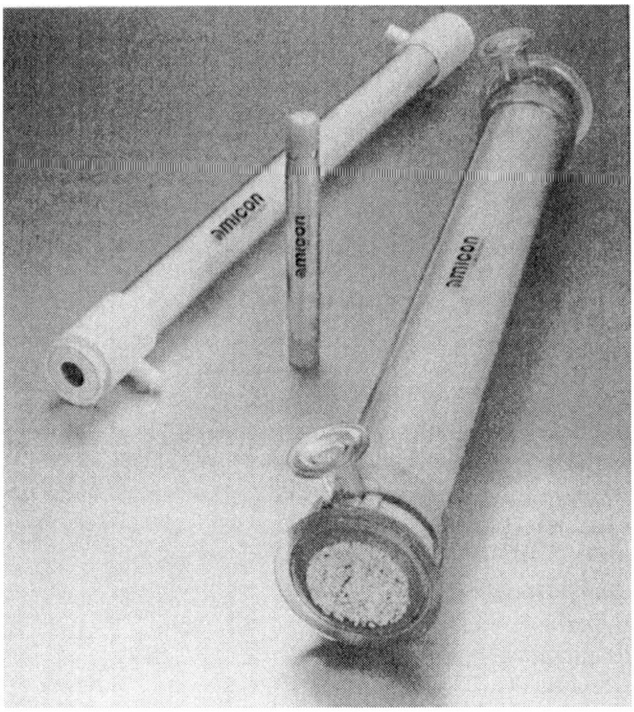

Figure 13 Hollow-fiber cartridge. (Courtesy of Amicon Corp.)

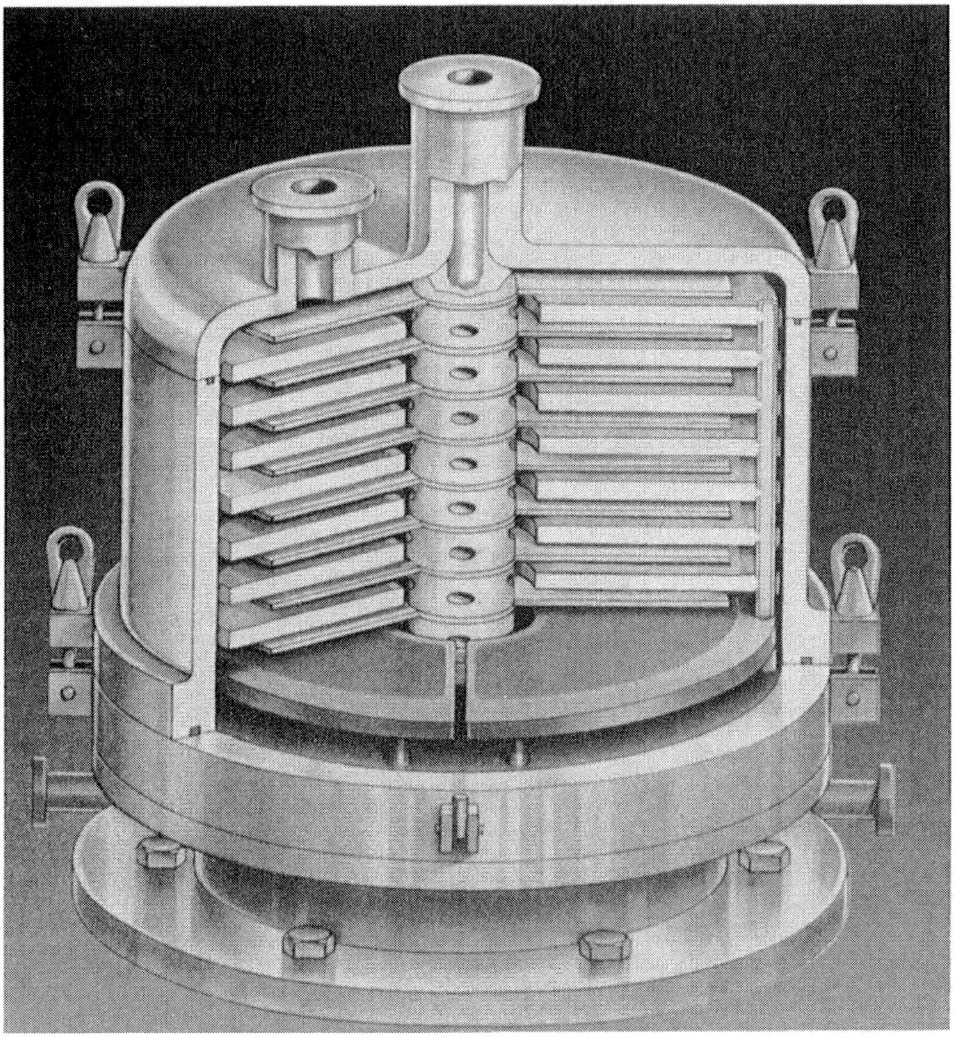

Figure 14 Spinning disk membrane module. (Courtesy of Pall Corporation.)

of the friction between the fluid and the membrane. To dissipate the heat, high fluid flows are required. This fluid flow may be as high as or higher than that required in conventional systems. In addition, at the very center of the disk there can sometimes be a net negative pressure, especially if there is any back pressure on the permeate. The negative pressure differential results in backflow of permeate into the retentate stream (starling flow). For systems using a rotating cylinder of fixed radius, pressure and shear do not change along the membrane's surface. The limitation of these systems is that they are mechanical devices that may be subject to containment failures (leakage) because of the extensive use of dynamic seals and bearings. Furthermore, system scale-up cannot be linear, because changes in the radius of either design results in changes in the internal forces.

4 CROSSFLOW MEMBRANES

As discussed in the Introduction, ultrafiltration membranes are highly asymmetric, with the rejecting layer consisting of a tight skin (5–10 μm thick) supported by a thick spongy structure of much larger pore size. Flow must generally be in the direction of the tight skin side toward the open side of the ultrafilter; flow in the reverse direction can result in the delamination or separation of the skin from the rest of the membrane.

4.1 Characterization of Ultrafiltration Membranes

Ultrafiltration membranes are rated with a nominal molecular weight cutoff (MWCO). However, there are no standardized guidelines for determining the MWCO of an ultrafilter. The rated MWCO and actual MWCO can differ by as much as 50–98% (McGregor, 1986; McGregor and Shah, 1980; Wolber and Dosmar, 1987). Current convention for the rating of ultrafilters uses specific protein markers. Depending on the membrane manufacturer, a retention of somewhere between 50% and 95% of the protein marker is the criterion for establishing a membrane's MWCO. Retention of protein is defined as

$$\text{Retention} = 1 \frac{C_p}{C_f} \tag{10}$$

where C_p is protein concentration in the permeate and C_f is protein concentration in the feed.

Typically, a marker protein is filtered through a membrane, and retention is determined using Eq. (10). The use of single proteins as markers has many disadvantages. Proteins of the same molecular weight vary in size, shape and structure, isoelectric point, and lypophilicity. Consequently, a membrane's retention of a single protein provides limited information with regard to its retention of other proteins.

For most applications, variation in the retention profile between vendors can be tolerated without any adverse impact on the process yield. However, if the process is sensitive to the membrane's retention profile, it may then be necessary to characterize the retention profile relative to the actual process. From a process and validation standpoint, actual retention coefficients would be best determined by end users filtering actual process streams.

It has been suggested in the literature that rather than using protein markers, polydispersed dextran solution should be used as the challenge solution (Tkacik and Michaels, 1991). Using this approach, a single challenge solution can be used to test membranes of 10,000–1,000,000 MWCO. The analysis of permeate and retentate samples via size-exclusion chromatography can be translated into a retention curve. However, when two or more solutes are being filtered, the retention of the smaller solute will be increased by the presence of the larger solute. Both Gergen et al. and Tam and Tremblay demonstrated that heterogeneous dextran mixtures and heterogeneous PEG mixtures, respectively, resulted in a membrane's retention shifting toward higher MWCO values (see Marshall et al., 1983).

The matter of retention rating, regardless of the method employed, should be viewed only as a guideline for the end user, because retention will be affected by the nature of the feed stream.

4.2 Membrane Types

Membrane polymers differ in their useful pH ranges, temperature ranges, pressure ranges, surface charges, protein adsorptivity, and degree of hydrophilicity. Some common ultrafiltration (UF) membrane materials and their characteristics are shown in Table 1. No one membrane polymer is suitable for all applications, and care must be taken to consider the nature of the membrane, the process fluids, and the operating conditions when selecting the membrane.

4.3 Protein Adsorption on UF Membranes

A consequence of protein adsorption is a decrease in membrane permeability accompanied by an increase in membrane fouling. Numerous studies in the literature support this observation (Marshall et al., 1993; Levy and Shehan, 1991). It has been shown that protein adsorption is greater on hydrophobic membranes than on hydrophilic membranes. The chemical nature of a membrane is further influenced by the nature of the deposited protein. For example, globular or spherical protein deposits influence flux decline less than does deposition of protein sheets. Freeze-fracture and deep-etching techniques have shown that bovine serum albumin (BSA) is deposited onto a hydrophilic regenerated cellulose membrane in the form of spheres. The size of the deposited spheres is consistent with the accepted size of the BSA molecule. However, BSA deposited onto a hydrophilic polysulfone membrane is filamentous. The conclusion is that the tertiary structure of the protein is disrupted through the interaction of the solute and the membrane (Marshall et al., 1993).

Similarly, Truskey et al. (1987) measured protein adsorption, circular dichroism, and biological activity of insulin, IgG, and alkaline phosphatase before and after passing through a variety of membranes. Shifts in circular dichroism and decreases in the activity of the enzymes are the result of conformational changes of the protein structure. This study clearly shows that membranes with the greatest degree of hydrophobicity had the greatest effect on protein adsorption and protein deformation (Truskey et al., 1993). The result of such protein–membrane interactions is that the protein's internal hydrophobic sites become exposed. These exposed hydrophobic surfaces then serve as sites for further protein binding, leading to an increase in the rate of membrane fouling. This phenomenon is greatest when protein concentration

Table 1 Membrane Polymers and Pertinent Operating Data

Membrane material	MWCO pore size range	pH	Maximum temp. (°C)
Cellulose acetate	1000 MWCO–5 μm	4–8	50–121
Regenerated cellulose	0.45 μm–1000	1–13	121
Cellulose nitrate	8.0 μm–10,000	4–8	121
Polyethersulfone	1000 MWCO–0.65 μm	1–13	121
Polypropylene	0.1–8 μm	1–13	121
Polysulfone	1000 MWCO–0.45 μm	1–13	121
PVDF	6000 MWCO–0.65 μm	1–10	121

is low, which is often the case for conditioned media arising from harvest broths in which cells are grown in the absence of serum.

Membrane surfaces may range from very smooth to rough. Increasing surface roughness results in increasing the relative surface area of the membrane and may also result in an increase in protein adsorption. On the other hand, increased roughness decreases gel layer formation because of increased turbulence at the membrane surface.

A membrane's porosity, pore size, and pore size distribution also influence performance. As the membrane's pore size is increased, the resistance to flow is decreased, but the tendency toward fouling increases because of the increase in flow through the larger pores. Devereaux and Hoare (1985) showed that the decline in flux through a 0.2 μm membrane was greater than that through a 50,000 MWCO membrane when the same feed stream was being filtered. These results have been attributed to the greater internal surface area of the microfilter relative to the ultrafilter. It has also been shown that though the initial retention values for various proteins on a microfilter may be low, over time their retention will increase. These observed values, however, may be minimized subject to the management and optimization of the operating conditions (Wolber et al., 1988).

4.4 Membrane Fouling

The long-term loss of performance (flux) in crossflow ultrafiltration is due to a process known as fouling. Fouling, unlike concentration polarization, is considered an irreversible process. The fouling process can be attributed to membrane compaction and to the deposition of macromolecules onto or in the membrane pore structure. Membrane compaction is the result of high transmembrane pressure (TMP), resulting in a decrease in the membrane's permeability. The deposition of feed stream components is the result of the adsorption of solutes such as protein to the membrane, causing the formation of a monolayer either on the membrane surface or in the pores. These fouling depositions are the result of membrane–solute interactions and, unlike concentration polarization, are not affected by concentration or velocity. These initial deposits are important and will determine the subsequent buildup of fouling layers or cakes (Romero and Davis, 1988; McGregor, 1990).

The decline in flux occurs in three phases, being due in part to both concentration polarization and membrane fouling. The rapid drop in flux that is observed over the first minute of operation is usually due to concentration polarization. The ensuing decline in flux over the next hour is the result of solute adsorption. First, a monolayer is formed; second, material is deposited onto the monolayer; and third, when steady state is achieved, more material is slowly deposited onto the membrane and the fouling layer becomes consolidated (Marshall et al., 1993). The deposition of material onto the membrane leads to changes in the behavior or retention characteristics of the membrane. Over time there may be an apparent shift to a lower MWCO, and the membrane selectivity will therefore decrease as the membrane's retention increases.

When the fouling process is the result of product adsorption onto the membrane surface followed by the deposition of material onto the adsorbed monolayer, a secondary membrane is formed. When this happens, the intrinsic properties of the membrane remain unchanged, though the behavior of the system is due to the secondary membrane. When fouling is within the pore structure, then the ensuing reduction in the membrane's pore size dominates the membrane's behavior. This reduction may be calculated by the Hagen–Poiseuille law. It is likely that these processes occur simultaneously (Marshall et al., 1993).

The nature of the feed stream's depositions (proteins) affects the membrane permeability. Spherical depositions, e.g., those laid down by γ-globulin, hinder membrane permeability less than the deposition of protein sheets, e.g., BSA. Since feed streams are usually complexes of many proteins, the result is the formation of protein cakes made up of lattice-like structures in which larger components form an infrastructure and the smaller components fill the interstitial spaces (Marshall et al., 1993). The nature of this cake is influenced by hydrodynamic conditions, and the cake compacts over time. Because of the consequences of fouling, it is useful to minimize the effect of fouling though the careful selection of membrane polymers and operating conditions.

4.5 Membrane Cleaning

Crossflow membranes are generally designed to be reused. Thus it is generally necessary to clean the membrane when fouling occurs or between filtration batches, so that there is no cross contamination between batches. Furthermore, the methods used to clean the membranes must not damage or alter the membrane, and the cleaning agent must be completely removed from the membrane before reuse.

The goal of the cleaning procedures is to remove product from the membrane and to return the membrane's flux as close to the original starting flux as possible. The selection of a cleaning protocol must take into account the nature of the product and the agent responsible for fouling the membrane. It is critical to examine the interaction of membrane foulant and cleaning agent, because it is possible to irreversibly fix fouling proteins to a membrane or to render a membrane unsuitable for the application for which it is intended by leaving a residual charge on its surface. It is also critical to the process to be able to test for the presence of any residual cleaning or sanitizing agents because of their deleterious effects on subsequent runs (Kirsch et al., 1993).

Cleaning may be considered from the perspective of time, temperature, and cleaning chemicals. As a rule, the longer a cleaning agent is allowed to work, the more effective it is. This is especially true when the cleaning agent contains proteases. The higher the temperature, the more reactive the cleaning agent. The limitation on raising the temperature must be balanced between the reactivity of the cleaning agent and the stability of the fouling proteins. Too high a temperature can lead to protein denaturation. When proteins become denatured and precipitate on or within the membrane matrix, cleaning becomes considerably more difficult. The proper selection of cleaning chemicals and their proper use will result in the desired effect (Table 2). Just as one must optimize the operating parameters for production, one must optimize the operating parameters for the cleaning process.

The cleaning procedure should begin immediately after the end of the filtration run. Allowing protein-containing solutions to remain in a drained membrane system can lead to protein denaturation and adsorption at the protein/membrane/air interfaces. It is generally advisable to rinse out as much of the product as possible at the end of the run prior to introducing the cleaning agents. One needs to be cognizant of the solutions used to rinse out the solution because of potential fouling by residual protein or antifoamants as a result of pH, temperature, or ionic strength. For protein-

Table 2 Biological Foulants and Recommended Membrane Cleaning Agents

Foulant	Cleaning agent
Antifoamant	1. Cold water + P3 Ultrasil 53 or Calgonite CMR or P3 Ultrasil 11 or P3 Ultrasil 91
	2. Sodium hydroxide
Biopolymers and proteins	1. Isotonic saline or urea or citrate tetraborate or sodium hydroxide
	2. P3 Ultrasil 11
	3. P3 Ultrasil 91
Blood	1. Citrate solution + isotonic saline
Cell debris and denatured proteins	1. Isotonic saline solution
	2. P3 Ultrasil 11 or Calgonite CMR
	3. Sodium hydroxide
	4. P3 Ultrasil 91
Lipids	1. P3 Ultrasil 53 or Calgonite CMR
	2. P3 Ultrasil 11
	3. P3 Ultrasil 91
Polysaccharides	1. Citrate tetraborate hypochlorite solution
	2. P3 Ultrasil 53 or Calgonite CMR
	3. Sodium hydroxide
	4. Hypochlorite

containing solutions it is generally recommended that the membranes be rinsed with an isotonic solution.

Membrane pretreatment can also have profound effects on product yield. Prewashing polysulfone 100,000 MWCO membranes with a buffered bleach solution followed by a 0.1 N NaOH rinse gives considerably higher yields in the purification of polio virus than the use of NaOH alone (M. Prashad, personal communication). Divizia et al. (1989) improved yields of polio virus by preblocking potential membrane-binding sites using a variety of buffers of varying concentrations.

5 EFFECT OF PROCESS OPERATING CONDITIONS

To this point we have considered the effect of membrane and membrane module design on the performance of a crossflow UF process. However, process operating conditions such as feed stream composition, flow rate, temperature, pressure, and pH or ionic conditions can play equally important roles in the performance of a crossflow process.

5.1 Feed Stream Composition

The nature of the feed stream can have profound effects on the retentivity of a crossflow system. The presence of large molecular weight components can increase the retention of smaller molecular weight components. Blatt et al. (1971) demonstrated that the retention of human serum albumin (67,000 daltons) on a 100,000 MWCO membrane was nearly zero. However, when γ-globulin (160,000 Da) was added to the feed stream, the albumin retention rose. Albumin retention showed a linearly increasing correlation to increasing concentrations of the γ-globulin (Blatt et al., 1971). Porter

(1981) similarly showed that the retention of ovalbumin, chymotrypsin, and cytochrome c are increased when a 1% solution of albumin is added to the feed mixture. Furthermore, it was shown that the retention of the smallest component was most dramatically affected—having a retention of less than 5% in the absence of the albumin and 70% in its presence. As discussed in Sec. 4.1, actual retention coefficients for a specific membrane and feed mixture should always be experimentally determined on a small scale before designing large-scale UF processes.

5.2 Flow Rate

High shear rates generated at the membrane surface tend to shear off deposited material and thus reduce the hydrodynamic resistance of the fouling layer (Cheryan, 1986). Increasing the rate of recirculation increases the flow velocity and shear rate. If the flow rate is sufficiently high, the flow will become turbulent, further increasing the shear rate. When high feed velocities are maintained, lateral lift at the membrane surface can exceed the oppositely directed membrane permeation velocity (Green and Belfort, 1980). It is important to properly select a pump for the delivery of the desired flow rates. Devereaux and Hoare (1985) showed that when pump speeds are high, feed stream aggregates can be broken up, leading to fouling of the membrane pores. This problem can be overcome by selecting a pump that will deliver the required flow at low revolutions per minute.

The pulsing of flow in the flow channel may result in the destabilizing of the gel layer, thereby minimizing its thickness. Most pumps used in crossflow operations pulse to some extent. The advantage of pulsed flow, if any, is likely offset by the reduction in membrane life that results from the added stress that the oscillations impose. Flow reversal has also met with mixed success. Though this technique has been used with great success in some beverage applications, its effect is short-lived in biotechnological applications (Woods et al., 1990). This is most likely due to the fouling action of protein streams.

5.3 Temperature

The effect of temperature on flux can be simply explained by the changes in solution viscosity. Temperature has a direct effect on viscosity. As temperature is increased, viscosity decreases; and as viscosity decreases, flux increases. As described previously, in turbulent flow the mass transfer coefficient (and thus the flux) is inversely proportional to the viscosity of the feed solution.

Biopolymer polarizing gels that are formed during crossflow filtration are gelatinous. The plasticity of these components is affected by the temperature of the solution. When the solution is kept cold and viscosity is high, they behave like rigid particles; when they are warmed, they are free to deform from the stresses of the filtration process. As discussed earlier, a polarizing gel forms as the filtration proceeds. Polarizing gel layers are compressible, and the pressure of filtration can cause the gel layer to collapse and completely clog the membrane. The temperature of the solution influences the compressibility of the gel layer. When the solution is kept cold (e.g., 4°C) the gel layer is less compressible than when it is warm. Because of the issue of cake compressibility, biopolymer filtration proceeds far better when the solution is kept cold. The increased throughputs when running cold far outweigh the reduction in flux as a result of the increased viscosity of the solution.

Temperature also influences the solubility of certain proteins. Cryoglobulins are a class of serum proteins that precipitate when the temperature of the solution is lowered to a critical limit. Freezing and thawing of protein solutions also results in the generation of protein precipitates. Adding heat to the solution can cause the disruption of hydrogen bonding, causing some portions of the protein to unfold, which in turn results in the formation of aggregates that may precipitate.

If the temperature is raised, protease activity may be activated or accelerated, which will result in protein degradation and precipitation of the proteolytic fragments. Finally, at higher temperatures the adsorption of protein to the membrane is enhanced, resulting in greater membrane fouling.

5.4 Pressure

The driving force for liquid flow through the membrane during crossflow filtration is the pressure driving force—the TMP—which is an average difference in pressure from the feed to the permeate. TMP is defined as

$$\text{TMP} = \frac{P_i + P_o}{2} - P_f \tag{11}$$

The flow of liquid into the feed channel is at some positive pressure (P_i). As the solution exits the flow channel (at pressure P_o) there is a loss of energy to the system. This loss of energy is due to the loss of product mass, because a portion of the liquid permeates the membrane. Energy is also lost due to fluid drag at the membrane surface, resulting in a pressure drop in the flow channel (ΔP_{fc}):

$$\Delta P_{fc} = P_i - P_o \tag{12}$$

The appropriate inlet pressure, outlet pressure, and TMP must be determined through experimentation. Generally it is not practical to fully develop flux versus pressure profiles, but it is necessary to determine some operating conditions that are reproducible. As a rule of thumb, the greater the TMP, the greater the tendency toward membrane fouling. It is important to note that as flux decreases because of the increased resistance to flow through the gel layer, any increase in pressure attempting to overcome the loss in driving force only serves to compress the gel layer. This then increases the gel layer's density, which increases its resistance to flow, further reducing flux.

Coupled to the issue of the effects of pressure on the density of the gel layer, one must also consider the effect of pressure on the membrane itself. When a membrane is subjected to a pressure differential it will tend to compress and become more dense. As this occurs, solvent flux will decrease. Measuring solvent flux after a filtration run may lead to the erroneous conclusion that the membrane is fouled because it has failed to return to its preuse solvent flux. Allowing the membrane to rest overnight may allow it to return to its preuse flux. McGregor (1986) reports observing membrane hysteresis with a variety of membranes.

5.5 pH and Ionic Conditions

Protein solubility increases or decreases as one moves away from or toward its isoelectric point, respectively. As one approaches the isoelectric point of a protein it will begin to precipitate from solution, fouling the membrane. Moving the pH too far one way or the other from the isoelectric point charges the protein, increasing protein–membrane or protein–protein interaction. Under these conditions, proteins may start to agglomerate or bind to the membrane, which will adversely affect the product and the process. Changes in the proteins' conformation and stability affect their adsorption to membrane surfaces. McDonogh et al. (1990) showed that protein fouling is maximized at the protein's isoelectric point and that the phenomenon is concentration-dependent. Changes in the protein's effective size also alter the porosity of the secondary membrane, thereby influencing flux.

Buffer exchanges and diafiltrations (see Sec. 6.3) are common in the processing of protein solutions. It is important to maintain an ionic equilibrium in the solution. The salt concentration, like pH, profoundly affects the protein solubility. When a buffer or salt is exchanged, one must be sure that all the components remain in solution during the exchange process. Failure to do this may result in fouling of the system. This is especially true when protein concentration is taking place, because if the salts concentrate with the proteins the proteins may start to salt out. Likewise, if the salt level falls too far, protein precipitation may also take place. Calcium and phosphate are directly implicated with the formation of insoluble calcium salts that serve as bridging agents for protein deposits (Marshall et al., 1993).

Removal of certain ionic species will also result in the formation of precipitates. This happens when the quaternary protein structure is lost as the result of the removal of cations such as magnesium, which serve to bridge the subunits. When serum proteins are dialyzed against distilled water, flocculation occurs as a result of the precipitation of a class of proteins called euglobulins, primarily IgM.

6 PROCESS APPLICATIONS

The traditional applications for crossflow filtration may be grouped into three basic types of operations: concentrations, fractionations, and diafiltrations. Crossflow systems are also used in specialized upstream applications for media and gas exchange in cell culture systems, as bioreactors, enzyme reactors, and as part of a cell recycling system in continuous fermentation operations. However, these specialized applications are not discussed here.

6.1 Concentration Processes

Concentration is the process of decreasing the solvent content of a solution to increase the concentration of solute. Typical examples of processes where this technique is used are the separation of cells from cell culture broth, the dewatering of proteins and peptides, and the harvesting of viruses. The degree of concentration is given as a concentration factor (CF):

$$\mathrm{CF} = \frac{V_0}{V_r} \tag{13}$$

where V_0 is the initial feed volume and V_r is the retentate volume.

Cell harvesting may be applied to bacterial and yeast fermentations, the culture of mammalian cells, and the separation of blood cells from plasma. The separation of cells from culture media can be successfully employed regardless of whether the fraction of interest is in the cell mass or in the broth. When using crossflow filtration for this application it is important to evaluate all aspects of the crossflow process because it rarely is acceptable to disrupt the cells during the process. If cells are disrupted during this step, the release of intracellular products such as organelles, nucleic acids, and proteins (especially proteolytic enzymes) may have a negative impact on the separation process. Cellular disruption is usually shear stress–induced and can be avoided by the proper selection of pump and line sizes. Cell harvesting can be accomplished by using either microfilters or ultrafilters, though it has been shown in the literature that microfilters are more likely to foul than ultrafilters (Devereaux and Hoare, 1995; Wolber et al., 1988).

Protein, peptide, and virus concentration with ultrafilters are fairly straightforward processes. Product yields, however, may be affected by the cleaning process, and each process must be evaluated as a unique application.

6.2 Fractionation Processes

Fractionation may be described as a separation process during which a fraction of the process fluids is separated from the bulk. Examples of membrane fractionation are depyrogenation, lysate clarification, and molecular weight separation of polydispersed polymers such as proteins and carbohydrates.

Depyrogenation of low molecular weight solutions such as buffers and pharmaceutical preparations is accomplished by retaining the contaminating LAL reactive material in the retentate and allowing the pyrogen-free product to pass through the membrane. Typically, 10,000–20,000 MWCO membranes are used for this application (Brown and Fuller, 1993); however, for products of molecular weights greater than 10,000 Da, membranes with MWCOs of 100,000–1,000,000 have been successfully employed (Wolber and Dosmar, 1987). [This is because pyrogens range in size from 10,000 to 1,000,000 Da (Pearson, 1985).] The actual size of the pyrogens has to do with their degree of dispersion in solution. If they are highly monodispersed, they will pass through the larger MWCO membranes. Endotoxin aggregation and filter retention increase with increasing ionic strength and decreasing pH (Brown and Fuller, 1993).

Clarification of cell lysates is the fractionation or separation of cellular debris from the products of interest. Lysates are prepared in biotech applications where cells are coaxed into producing a quantity of a particular protein that is retained intracellularly. To release the product from the cells, the cells must be disrupted. Usually the disruption process is carried out after the cell mass has been harvested and concentrated to a manageable volume. After disruption, the solid phase is separated from the liquid phase via filtration. Lysates can be very fouling, and the success of the operation is very much affected by the selection of the appropriate membrane, pore size, and operating parameters (Sartorius Corporation, unpublished data).

6.3 Diafiltration Processes

Diafiltration is a term combining the words dialysis and filtration. In most dialysis operations the goal is to exchange one or more components in a bulk solution for another. In biotechnology this is usually the exchange of one buffer for another prior to a column exchange step. Diafiltration is also used for the washing of cell harvests and products when, after concentration, a fraction of the product still remains in the concentrate. Regardless of the specifics of the application, the intent is to remove one or more components from a mixture.

Diafiltrations may be run as either continuous or discontinuous operations. Continuous diafiltration is a constant-flow wash where diafiltrate buffer feed is matched to the rate of permeate flow. In discontinuous diafiltration, the batch is concentrated and then diluted with buffer in a stepwise operation. Aliquots of buffer are added after each successive concentration until the desired dilution is reached. The amount of diafiltrate required to achieve the desired end point is greater for continuous than discontinuous diafiltration. The degree of dilution in a continuous diafiltration is given by the equation

$$C_s = C_{s,0} \exp[-(V_d/V_0)] \quad (14)$$

or

$$V_d = V_0 \ln(C_s/C_{s,0}) \quad (15)$$

where

C_s = concentration of microsolute remaining after diafiltration
$C_{s,0}$ = original microsolute concentration
V_d = total volume of diafiltrate
V_0 = volume of retained product

Solving Eq. (15) for a typical application where 99% removal of microsolute is desired results in a requirement for 4.6 volumes of diafiltrate. The component being washed out of the bulk becomes progressively diluted, so that each volumetric exchange reduces the concentration of that component. Table 3 gives the percentage of microsolute removal for each volume of diafiltrate added.

The practical application of diafiltration usually involves concentration of the bulk solution prior to the diafiltration step. Because the volume of diafiltrate required is directly proportional to the volume of the bulk, the greater the initial concentration factor the smaller the volume of diafiltration buffer required. The optimal concentration factor prior to starting the diafiltration, though, must consider the effect of solute concentration on the flux. As described previously, flux is a logarithmic function of solute concentration, where flux declines as the concentration of the solute increases. At low concentration, flux will be high, but so will the volume required for diafiltration. At high concentration factors, both the flux and diafiltration volumes will be low. The optimal value here can be solved by determining the shortest pro-

Table 3 Microsolute Removal During Diafiltration as a Function of Diafiltrate Volume

Diafiltrate volume, V_d/V_0	Removal of microsolute (%)
1.0	63.2
2.0	86.5
3.0	95.0
4.0	98.2
5.0	99.3

cessing time to accomplish the diafiltration. Ng et al. (1976) solve the mathematical derivations for the optimal concentration factor, which is given as

$$C_b = C_g/e \tag{16}$$

where C_b is the optimal concentration and C_g is the gel concentration. So, in a typical application where $C_g = 25\%$, $C_b = 9.2\%$, which is the concentration to which the batch should optimally be concentrated before adding diafiltrate and repeating the concentration process.

After a cell harvest or lysate clarification, a portion of the product may remain associated with the concentrate. Washing or diafiltering the concentrate is desirable at this point in order to recover the remaining product. Diafiltration is also used for washing the product. For example, after liposome encapsulation of a drug, free unencapsulated drug often remains in the mixture. Diafiltration of the liposome solution results in the removal of the unincorporated drug from the liposome preparation.

7 PROCESS DESIGN AND SCALE-UP

Aside from standard engineering practices, there are certain considerations specific to crossflow systems that should be taken into account in a system design. The interrelationship of system components such as tanks, valves, pumps, crossflow module, and instrumentation can have a significant impact on the process performance and yield. The development of a complete crossflow process is often begun on a relatively small scale, and the process is sequentially scaled up as the product proceeds from clinical trials to full production runs. In the earliest stages of a process, when the batch size is small, the process may use laboratory equipment such as peristaltic pumps, flexible tubing, and glass vessels. As the batch size increases, so must the capabilities of the crossflow system. At the same time, the equipment cost, membrane cost, and product value increase. In order to ensure cost-effective and successful scale-up from laboratory scale to full production runs, it is important to perform incremental design and scale-up as described in this section.

7.1 Laboratory-Scale Process Characterization

Before any considerations are given to designing a full-scale crossflow process, it is vital to characterize and optimize the process at the laboratory scale. In the laboratory, one can characterize the process with regard to crossflow velocities, TMP, membrane surface area to batch size ratio, MWCO required, gelation concentration C_g, protein diffusivity D, and mass transfer coefficient k. Simply using pressure profiles to scale up a crossflow process can lead to erroneous conclusions with respect to the scaled-up process (Wolber et al., 1988). A full understanding of the above process parameters will lead to successful scale-up and process design.

Using a laboratory-scale apparatus similar to that shown in Fig. 15, a crossflow process can be characterized in the laboratory. Initially, the optimum membrane type should be determined, where tests are conducted using the laboratory-scale apparatus to determine that there is sufficient retention of the desired solute from the feed solution. Subsequently, the apparatus in Fig. 15 should be used with a small laboratory-scale crossflow module to optimize flux as a function of the TMP and the crossflow rate (Wolber et al., 1988). Once the optimum TMP (i.e., that TMP above

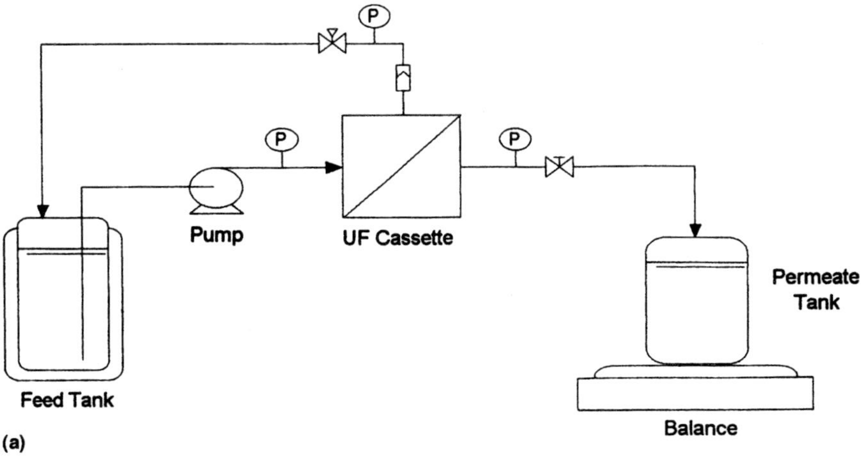

(a)

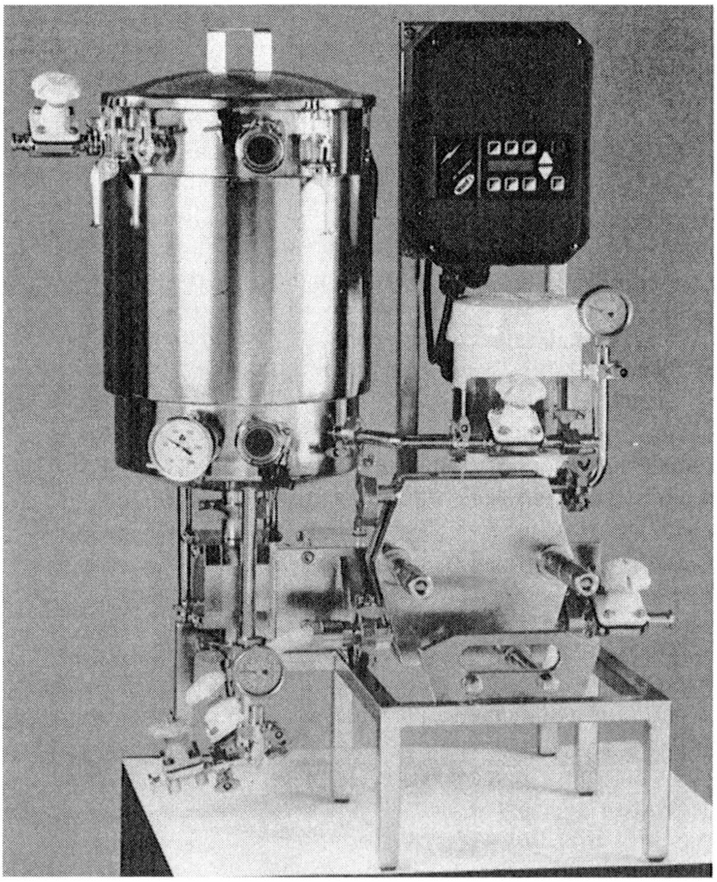

(b)

Figure 15 (a) Schematic of apparatus for testing and characterization of crossflow cassettes. (b) Test skid.

which no further improvement in flux is realized) is determined, the crossflow process should be characterized to determine flux as a function of retained solute (e.g., protein) concentration. Solute concentration experiments should be conducted at a number of different crossflow rates, as shown in Fig. 6 (Sec. 2). From these experiments, mass transfer coefficients (k) and gel concentrations (C_g) can be determined (Brose et al., 1996).

7.2 Crossflow Scale-Up Procedures

Once laboratory-scale characterization and optimization is performed, one can use scale-up correlations to predict the performance of larger scale devices and aid in the evolving design process. Scaling from a laboratory-scale crossflow device to a pilot- or production-scale device often requires changes in the fluid flow path geometry, i.e., length, height, and width of the flow channel. When these changes are made, solution velocities and shear will also change, and if not taken into account the scaled-up process will fail to perform as required. For this reason, it is critical to know the performance correlations of crossflow devices used at small scale and large scale and adjust crossflow velocity accordingly to achieve the desired performance.

As an example of proper scale-up of crossflow UF devices, consider the scale-up of open-channel disposable crossflow devices (60 cm^2) to pilot/process-scale cassettes (7000 cm^2). Equations (8) and (9), which describe the precise correlations for these devices, are repeated here:

For 60 cm^2 cassettes,

$$J_w = 0.216\left(\frac{1}{\mu/\rho}\right)^{0.47} D^{0.67}v^{0.40}\ \ln\left[\frac{C_g}{C_f}\right] \tag{8}$$

For 1000 and 7000 cm^2 cassettes,

$$J_w = 0.373\left(\frac{1}{\mu/\rho}\right)^{0.47} D^{0.67}v^{0.55}\ \ln\left[\frac{C_g}{C_f}\right] \tag{9}$$

These equations show the dependence of flux on solution viscosity, solution density, crossflow velocity, protein diffusivity, gel concentration, and solute concentration in the feed.

To scale up from the small-scale 60 cm^2 laboratory device to the much larger scale 7000 cm^2 cassette, the following specific procedure is recommended. Table 4 shows the relationship of recirculation rate, velocity, and surface area to the different device sizes.

Table 4 Characteristics of Ultrafiltration Devices Relative to Size

Device	Surface area (cm^2)	Velocity (cm/s)	Crossflow rate (L/min)
Small	60	16.9	0.5
Medium	1083	16.7	3.5
Large	7000	16.7	10

Step 1. Using the small-scale device, concentrate the process solution.

Operate at fixed feed flow rate (v = 15–30 cm/s). It is important to keep the flow rate constant throughout the run.

Optimize transmembrane pressure. While recirculating permeate to the feed tank, increase retentate pressure by slowly and stepwise closing the retentate valve. Monitor the permeate flow rate at each pressure step, and continue until permeate flow does not increase further; this pressure is the optimum TMP, where flux becomes independent of the TMP and dependent on the recirculation velocity, and should be used for further operation (Porter, 1981).

Perform concentration run. With temperature, feed flow rate, and retentate pressure at predetermined optimized values, measure permeate flow rate (mL/min) prior to any concentration of feed. Concentrate to approximately 2×; adjust temperature, feed flow, and retentate pressure to original values; and again measure permeate flow rate, noting the exact concentration of solute in the feed (i.e., the original solute concentration times the concentration factor). Concentrate again by approximately 2×, and repeat permeate flow measurement. Concentrate a fourth time, and repeat permeate flow measurement.

Step 2. Convert permeate flow rates to fluxes by dividing permeate flows by membrane area and plot permeate flux versus feed concentration as semilog plot (as in Figs. 5 and 6).

Determine C_g. After plotting data on a semilog plot, place the best straight line through the data and determine the x and y intercepts of the line. The x intercept equals C_g.

Determine k. Choose one point on the best-fit line (C_f, J_w), and insert this data point and C_g into the following equation to determine k in units of milliliters per minute per square centimeter (the same units as flux):

$$k = \frac{J_w}{\ln[C_g/C_f]} \quad \text{mL/(min} \cdot \text{cm}^2) \tag{17}$$

Convert k to units of centimeters per second as follows:

$$\left(k \frac{\text{mL}}{\text{min} \cdot \text{cm}^2}\right) \times \left(\frac{1\ \text{cm}^3}{1\ \text{mL}}\right) \times \left(\frac{1\ \text{min}}{60\ \text{s}}\right) = k\ \text{cm/s} \tag{18}$$

C_g and k will be used next to perform scale-up.

Step 3. Determine diffusion coefficient (D) for the process solution.

Determine the kinematic viscosity. Determine the appropriate value for kinematic viscosity (μ/ρ) in units of square centimeters per second for the process solution. If this value cannot be determined experimentally or found in a reference, use the kinematic viscosity of water at 70°F (μ/ρ = 0.010 cm^2/s).

Calculate D. Using the value for k determined in step 2, the value for μ/ρ, and the appropriate solution velocity, calculate D using Eq. (19) if k was found for a 60 cm^2 cassette or using Eq. (20) if k was found using a cassette.

For 60 cm^2 cassettes:

$$D = \left[\frac{4.63k(\mu/\rho)^{0.47}}{v^{0.40}}\right]^{1.5} \tag{19}$$

For 1000 cm^2 cassettes:

$$D = \left[\frac{2.68k(\mu/\rho)^{0.47}}{v^{0.55}}\right]^{1.5} \tag{20}$$

where k has units of cm/s, μ/ρ has units of cm^2/s, v has units of cm/s, and D has units of cm^2/s.

Step 4. Determine flux for the scaled-up device.

Calculate initial flux. Using Eq. (21) and the solution constants determined in previous steps (D, C, and μ/ρ), calculate initial flux [mL/(cm^2·s)] at the initial feed concentration (i.e., before concentration of feed) using the appropriate velocity:

$$J_i = 0.373\left(\frac{1}{\mu/\rho}\right)^{0.47} D^{0.67}v^{0.55}\ln\left[\frac{C_g}{C_i}\right] \tag{21}$$

where all variables have the same units as described previously.

Calculate final flux. Use Eq. (22) to calculate the final flux at the final feed concentration:

$$J_f = 0.373\left(\frac{1}{\mu/\rho}\right)^{0.47} D^{0.47}v^{0.55}\ln\left[\frac{C_g}{C_f}\right] \tag{22}$$

Calculate average flux. Use Eq. (23) to calculate the average flux throughout the concentration run:

$$J_{avg} = \frac{J_{initial} - J_{final}}{\ln(J_{initial}/J_{final})} \tag{23}$$

Calculate average process filtrate flow rate. Using the following equation, calculate the average flow that can be expected per cassette over the course of a concentration run:

$$\text{Average process flow} = J_{avg} \times (\text{surface area}) \tag{24}$$

To test the scale-up method described above, the procedure was used to predict the performance of 1000 and 7000 cm^2 cassettes using solution data obtained with concentration tests conducted with a 60 cm^2 device. Figure 16 shows the actual and predicted data for filtration of a globulin-containing cell culture medium. As this figure shows, the predicted results are very close to the actual results.

7.3 Crossflow System Engineering Design

The procedure described in Sec. 7.1 is used to determine the optimum TMP and solution flow rates for operation of a scaled-up crossflow process. Once this determination has been made, particular process components can be specified. In this section we give general guidelines for the design and specification of individual system components.

Pump Design

When sizing a pump for use in a crossflow system, one should consider all stages of the crossflow process. For example, the maximum flow for the recirculation (cross-

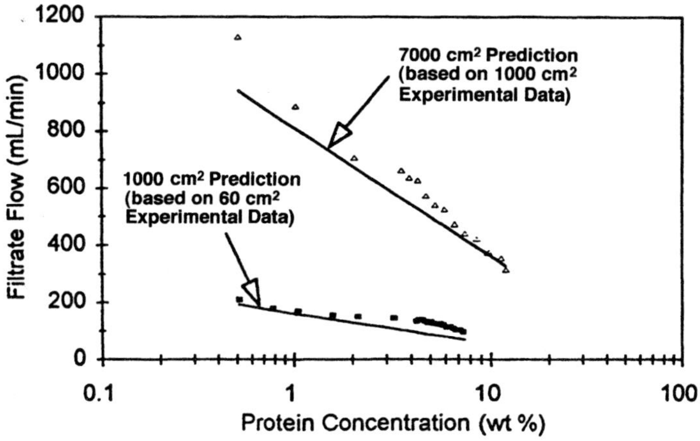

Figure 16 Actual and predicted filtrate flow as a function of total protein concentration for ultrafiltration of a globulin-containing cell culture media using a 1000 cm^2 cassette at a crossflow rate of 6 L/min and using a 7000 cm^2 cassette at a crossflow rate of 10 L/min.

flow) pump is generally required during the cleaning cycle. One should calculate the pump's output to ensure that all parts of the system piping are in full turbulent flow during the cleaning cycle. This flow requirement should be compared to that calculated in Sec. 7.1, and a comparison should be made to determine which is greater. In any event, the pump must be controllable so that flows lower than the pump maximum can be attained. It is also important to consider that pump slippage occurs with many types of pumps, and pump slippage will generally be highest during the cleaning process.

There are a variety of pumps available in the marketplace. These include rotary lobe, centrifugal, peristaltic, diaphragm, and neutating. In the pharmaceutical industry it is generally a requirement that the pump be capable of being cleaned in place (CIP). This requirement limits the field to the types of pumps just listed. Other CIP designs exist but are not generally used for crossflow applications.

Rotary lobe pumps are frequently used for pumping biological solutions. These pumps offer very good flow control, but they are expensive. Not accounting for pump slippage, at a given rotational speed the pump produces a constant flow rate regardless of the head pressure. Flow rate is controlled by controlling the rate of rotation of the rotary lobes. Depending on the rotor style and the rate of rotation, the pump produces flow with little to moderate pulsation. Rotary lobe pumps come in a variety of sizes and styles. Rotor designs include bi-lobe, tri-lobe, five-lobe, and scimitar-lobe configurations. The timed rotors turn in opposite directions inside a rotor housing, thereby creating an expanding cavity at the pump inlet and a collapsing cavity at the pump discharge. Because these pumps create a vacuum at the pump inlet, it is imperative that the pump inlet be flooded at all times so that cavitation does not occur (vaporization of the fluid). Rotary lobe pumps can deliver relatively high pressures, so pressure relief valves or pressure cut off switches are advisable.

Cavitation results in the foaming and denaturation of protein solutions and cell disruption if whole cells are being pumped. It most often occurs when there is a long restricted flow path on the pump inlet side. As a rule of thumb, the tank discharge port, valves, and hoses leading to the pump should be sized to the pump's inlet dimensions. If this is not possible, restrictions should be kept to a minimum. Current convention for the orientation of rotary lobe pumps is that they discharge vertically. This orientation makes it possible for the pump and associated hardware to drain freely.

Scimitar rotors are an improvement over standard lobe designs because they have a longer sealing path, which can improve the overall efficiency of the pump by reducing pump slip. On the other hand, shear at the metal/metal interface may be higher than in conventional rotor designs.

Centrifugal pumps operate by moving product along spinning veins. They are relatively inexpensive. These pumps operate at fixed pressures. They have no ability to pull a vacuum at the pump inlet, so if the pump is starved for product at the inlet, the rotor will spin freely without dispensing product. If a head pressure is applied to the discharge of the pump, flow will decrease and may stop. Centrifugal pumps are used less often than rotary lobe pumps on biological products. Centrifugal pumps are often used on water systems and in processing shear-insensitive products. Flow through these pumps is nonpulsing.

Diaphragm pumps have a great deal of pulsation, which can be reduced through the use of a pulse dampener. Their use on crossflow systems is limited.

Tank Design

Tank size and design will vary considerably. However, there are certain guidelines that make it easier to operate a crossflow system. It is usually best to use a conical tank bottom, because this results in the minimum operating volume and maximum concentration capability. Dished bottom tanks will also work well for many crossflow applications.

Sufficient intrusions should be included in a tank to allow it to be cleaned, vented, charged with product, fitted with a recirculation line and sight glasses, and accept instrumentation, and it should have at least one spare port for future needs. The discharge port should be matched to the recirculation pump inlet. This will ensure sufficient flow to the pump to avoid cavitation. One can always reduce the discharge nozzle, but it is generally not practical to increase the tank discharge dimension after the tank has been fabricated.

Tank jacketing is an excellent way to provide a heat exchange surface to remove heat that is added to the process by the recirculation pump. At the start of the process the volumes are greatest, so the added heat is not greatly noticed as a temperature rise. As the product concentrates, the volume decreases and the viscosity increases. The heat input from the pump becomes increasingly noticeable as a temperature increase of the solution. Jacketing the bottom of the tank ensures that the solution can be sufficiently cooled and that the temperature will not rise at the end of the process.

Pump, Tank, and System Interaction

Systems are often required to operate over a wide range of process volumes. It should be noted that the required pump and associated interconnecting tubing for a system makes it impossible to achieve the concentration factors required for batch sizes below a critical value. Typically, volume will be reduced by 90–99%. A starting volume of 1000 L will therefore have an ending volume of 10–100 L. To achieve the desired ending volume, the system's minimum operating volume should ideally be less than the desired ending volume.

Product value is greatest when the product has been concentrated in solution. Simply draining the system at this point will leave considerable material behind. A successful strategy for optimal recovery and for achieving the desired concentration factor is to overconcentrate the product (if possible) by an amount equal to the system's minimum operating volume, draining the system and then flushing it with a bolus of a suitable buffer. When possible, tubing runs should be as short as possible so as to minimize the system fill volume. The pump discharge should also be located such that the inlet is always flooded and so there are no points in the tubing that do not drain by gravity.

Line Sizing

Because the system volume increases as the line size increases, the line size should be kept as small as possible without restricting flow or generating turbulence during normal processing. Table 5 helps approximate system volume as a function of size and length of the process tubing.

Membrane Area Sizing

Required membrane area is generally determined by dividing the total permeate flow rate by the process flux [Eq. (25) is a revised version of Eq. (24)].

$$A_p = \frac{V_t/t}{J} \tag{25}$$

where

V_t = total permeate volume
t = processing time
V_t/t = average permeate flow rate
J = average flux
A_p = membrane surface area required

As the processing time t decreases, membrane surface area requirements increase. As surface area requirements increase, so do the recirculating flow rates, associated line sizes, and minimum operating volumes. At this point in the design process it is necessary to determine what the minimum system volume must be. It

Table 5 Tube Volume

Tubing size	Volume per foot
4 in.	2.27 L
3 in.	1.23 L
2 in.	545 mL
1½ in.	298 mL
1 in.	122 mL
¾ in.	63 mL
½ in.	23.5 mL

may be necessary to make some compromises with respect to the system size and processing time in order to meet all of the product requirements.

Control Options and Instrumentation

The crossflow process is dynamic. The product concentration, viscosity, flow rates, and pressure profiles are all subject to change during the operation of the process. It may therefore by advisable to provide protective control options on the system.

Pressure Control

As the solute concentration increases, so will the pressure at the membrane inlet. A safety pressure switch, alarm, or loop controller interlocked to the pump controller can safeguard the process and membranes by either shutting down or slowing the pump when a maximum allowable pressure is reached. Retentate and permeate back pressure and TMP can be controlled either manually or by using loop controllers.

Temperature Control

Temperature will increase as a result of the heat input from the pump. A temperature switch or loop controller can be installed to either alert the operator or provide coolant to the heat exchanger.

Flow Rate Control

Process flow rates may change as a result of changes in system back pressures and product concentration. Flow meters can be used to monitor or control the process. Permeate flow meters can be configured to provide batch volume control signaling a desired end point.

UV, pH, and Conductivity

The use of UV, pH, or conductivity monitors can be used to indicate or signal process end points.

Control of System Operation

A typical crossflow system may have seven or more process steps, including

1. Rinse storage solution out of system.
2. Equilibrate system with buffer.
3. Operate the crossflow process.
4. Recover concentrated product.
5. Rinse system with buffer.
6. Clean and sanitize the system.
7. Fill the system with storage solution.

These various steps may be carried out manually or they can be automated through the use of loop controllers or PLCs. Automation of the process will reduce the risk of operator error and subsequent product loss.

Hardware geometry also contributes to the performance of a crossflow system. Considering the effect of crossflow velocity on performance, failure to provide uniform flow through each flow channel will result in less than optimal performance. Liquid flow will always favor the path of least resistance, so care must be taken to ensure that flow resistance is uniform throughout the filter's flow path.

8 VALIDATION ISSUES

The validation of crossflow systems is in principle no different than the validation of any other pharmaceutical process—that is, ''establishing documented evidence which provides a high degree of assurance that a specific process will consistently produce a product meeting its predetermined specifications and quality attributes'' (FDA, 1987). There are numerous documents detailing the specifics of crossflow validation. The PDA Technical Report No. 15 (PDA, 1992) deals specifically with this topic by providing an industrial perspective on the validation of crossflow filtration. Specific validation issues that may be considered to be critical to crossflow filtration need to be addressed. These fall into two groups: process-specific and application-specific validation issues.

8.1 Process-Specific Validation Issues

The compatibility of a membrane system that is reused depends on the effects of reuse on the membranes with regard to any changes in extractables after prolonged exposure to all of the fluids that the process will encounter. These include the storage, rinse, cleaning, sanitizing, and process solutions. Membrane integrity must be monitored both by direct testing of the membrane's integrity and by continued achievement of the desired product yield and product quality. Furthermore, the membrane's retention coefficient should also be monitored over the life of the membrane.

Retention coefficients as discussed in Sec. 4.1 are highly subjective. It may be best to specifically determine the membrane's retention coefficient with the products of interest by using these products in the presence of normal process fluids. This then provides a practical reference by which to evaluate performance.

Membrane cleaning and sanitization from a validation standpoint must be determined to be effective. It must also be demonstrated that the cleaning agents can be removed prior to reuse. The ability to demonstrate this is important, especially considering the potentially deleterious effects of residuals on product yield and product purity (Kirsch et al., 1993). Validation of cleaning cycles can be performed through the analysis of permeate and retentate effluents after each stage of the operation. Analysis should include specific assays for compounds that have been introduced into the system. Alternative approaches are to flush the system with water for injection (WFI) and determine whether the effluents continue to meet the WFI specifications. Total organic carbon (TOC) analysis of effluent rinses offers yet another approach to this problem. Direct physical inspection of membrane systems provides further confirmation that cleaning procedures are adequate. After the membranes have been cleaned it is suggested that a WFI or buffer flux be determined. Clean water flux or buffer flux determinations can serve as a benchmark for subsequent cleanings. Generally the flux from an unused membrane will not be achieved after the first production run followed by the first cleaning. It is not uncommon for the flux to drop by 20%, though this reduced value should be retrievable after subsequent use and cleaning cycles.

8.2 Application-Specific Validation Issues

During a concentration process, low level contaminants may suddenly become problematic. Two specific contaminants are of particular interest. First, protein solutions may have low levels of contaminating proteases. Though the rate of proteolysis may be undetectable in the unconcentrated bulk form, after concentration the rate may be increased by the square of the concentration factor (PDA, 1992). The effect of proteases on product yield can be devastating to the process. Second, endotoxins may be concentrated from below detectable limits to levels high enough to cause product lot rejection. Apparent endotoxin content can be also influenced by the nature of the ionic content of the process fluids, which means that they may appear only after a buffer-exchange step.

9 CONCLUSION

Crossflow filtration has application in a wide variety of processes. Numerous articles can be found within the literature that specifically address these process applications. Crossflow filtration has also found use as an adjunct with other methods such as the removal or clearance of viral contaminants (Bechtel et al., 1988). Crossflow systems are also employed as membrane bioreactors and in continuous cell culture operations.

Future developments in the area of crossflow filtration will primarily be in the areas of improved geometries for fluid flow management, new membrane developments, and development of novel applications for membranes. The field of membrane science is fertile, and researchers continue to propose new and improved ways for applying crossflow filtration.

REFERENCES

Anon. (1992). Biotech is coming into its own, *Chem. Week*, *150*:29.

Bechtel, M. K., A. Bagadsarian, W. P. Olson, and T. N. Estep. (1988). Virus removal or inactivation in hemoglobin solutions by ultrafiltration or detergent/solvent treatment, *Biomaterials*, *16*(1–3):126–128.

Belfort, G. (1987). *Adv. Biochem. Eng.*

Blatt, W. F., A. Dravid, A. S. Michaels, and L. Nelsen. (1971). Solute polarization and cake formation in membrane ultrafilters: Causes, consequences, and control techniques, in *Membrane Processes in Industry and Biomedicine* (M. Beir, ed.), Plenum, New York, p. 57.

Brose, D. J., M. Dosmar, S. Cates, and F. Hutchinson. (1996). Studies on the scale-up of crossflow filtration devices. *J. Pharm. Sci. Technol.*, *50*(4):252–260.

Brown, S., and A. C. Fuller. (1993). Depyrogenation of pharmaceutical solutions using submicron and ultrafilters, *J. Parent. Sci. Technol.*, *47*(6):285–288.

Cheryan, M. (1986). *Ultrafiltration Handbook*, Technomic Publishing Company, Lancaster, PA.

Cheryan, M., and B. H. Chiang. (1984). In *Engineering and Food*, Vol. 1 (B. McKenna, ed.), Applied Science, London, UK.

Devereaux, N., and M. Hoare. (1985). *Biotechnol. Bioeng.*, *28*:422–431.

Divizia, M., A. L. Santi, and A. Panà. (1989). Ultrafiltration: An efficient second step for hepatitis A virus and poliovirus concentration, *J. Virol. Methods*, *23*:55–62.

FDA. (1987). Guidelines on the General Principles of Process Validation, Prepared by the Center for Drugs and Biologics and the Center for Devices and Radiological Health, Food and Drug Administration.

Green, G., and G. Belfort. (1980). Fouling of ultrafilter membranes: lateral migration and particle trajectory model, *Desalination*, *35*:129.

Kirsch, L. E., R. Riggin, D. A. Gearhart, D. F. Lefber, and D. I. Lytle. (1993). In-process protein degradation by exposure to trace amounts of sanitizing agents, *J. Parent. Sci. Technol.*, *47*:155–160.

Levy, P., and J. Shehan. (1991). Performance characteristics of polysulfone and cellulose membranes for the ultrafiltration of biological process streams, *Biopharm.*, *April*:24–33.

Loeb, S. (1981). The Loeb–Soirirajan membrane: How it came about, in *Synthetic Membranes*, Vol. 1 (A. Turbak, ed.), ACS Symp. Ser. 153, Am. Chem. Soc., Washington, DC, p. 6.

McDonogh, R. M., H. Bauser, and N. Stroh. (1990). Concentration polarisation and adsorption effects in cross-flow ultrafiltration of proteins, *Desalination*, *79*(2/3):217–231.

McGregor, W. C. (1986). Selection and use of ultrafiltration membranes, in *Membrane Separations in Biotechnology* (W. C. McGregor, ed.), Marcel Dekker, New York.

McGregor, W. C. (1990). Advances in primary separations with membranes, in *Biologicals from Recombinant Microoganisms and Animal Cells: Production and Recovery* (M. D. White, S. Reuveny, and A. Shafferman, eds.), Proceedings of the 34th Oholo Conf., Eilat, Israel.

McGregor, W. C., and P. Shah. (1980). Factors in the selection and use of ultrafilter membranes, Proceedings of Interphex.

Marshall, A. D., P. A. Munro, and G. Trägårdh. (1993). Effect of protein fouling in microfiltration and ultrafiltration on permeate flux, protein retention and selectivity: A literature review, *Desalination*, *91*:65–108.

Michaels, A. S. (1986). Foreword to M. Cheryan, *Ultrafiltration Handbook*, Technomic Publishing Company, Lancaster, PA.

Nakao, S. I., and S. Kimura. (1981). Effect of gel layer on rejection and fractionation of different-molecular-weight solutes by ultrafiltration, in *Synthetic Membranes*, Vol. 2 (A. Turbak, ed.), ACS Symp. Ser. 153, Am. Chem. Soc., Washington, DC, pp. 119–132.

PDA. (1992). Industrial Perspective on Validation of Tangential Flow Filtration in Biopharmaceutical Applications, Tech. Rep. 15, *J. Parent. Sci. Technol.*, *46* Suppl.

Pearson, F. C. (1985). Endotoxin: Its Structure and Function with Respect to Depyrogenation, Parenteral Drug Assoc. Tech. Rep. 7, pp. 1–14.

Porter, M. C. (1981). The effect of fluid management on membrane filtration, in *Synthetic Membranes*, Vol. 1 (A. Turbak, ed.), ACS Symp. Ser. 153, Am. Chem. Soc., Washington, DC, p. 407.

Romero, C. A., and R. H. Davis. (1988). Global model of crossflow microfiltration based on hydrodynamic particle diffusion, *J. Membrane Sci.*, *39*:157–185.

Thayer, A. M. (1991). Biopharmaceuticals overcoming market hurdles, *Chem. Eng. News*, *69*: 27–28.

Tkacik, G., and S. Michaels. (1991). A rejection profile for ultrafilter membranes and devices, *Bio/Technology*, *9*:941.

Truskey, G. A., R. Gabler, A Dileo, and T. Manter. (1987). The effect of membrane filtration upon protein conformation, *J. Parent. Sci. Technol.*, *41*(6):180–193.

Wolber, P., and M. Dosmar. (1987). Depyrogenation of pharmaceutical solutions by ultrafiltration: Aspects of validation, *Pharm. Technol.*, *11*(9):38–46.

Wolber, P., M. Dosmar, and J. Banks. (1988). Cell harvesting scale-up: Parallel-leaf crossflow microfiltration methods, *Biopharm.*, *1*(6):38–45.

Woods, W. J., J. Horne-Shaw, and G. E. Frost. (1990). Industrial-scale crossflow membrane technology in downstream processing of bacterial antigens, in *Fermentation Technologies: Industrial Applications* (P.-L. Yu, ed.), Elsevier Applied Science, Elsevier Science Publishers Ltd., Barting, Essex, England, pp. 427–432.

17

Protein Adsorption in Microporous Membrane Filtration

SRIKANTH SUNDARAM
Pall Corporation, Port Washington, New York

1 INTRODUCTION

Membrane filtration processes are being increasingly integrated into existing reaction, isolation, and recovery schemes for the production of valuable biological molecules, primarily owing to the limitations of competing technologies [1,2]. For example, membranes are used for air and aqueous feed stream sterilization; for recovery, purification, and sterilization of bioproducts or treatment of wastes; for extractive fermentation processes; as a support to immobilize biocatalysts; and in affinity crossflow filtration design. Membranes are particularly suited for bioprocesses involving the cultivation of microorganisms of cells, in which the product of interest is secreted extracellularly. Such extracellular product based processes require cell separation, product recovery, and concentration and use microfiltration and ultrafiltration extensively. Typically, microfiltration of protein solutions (i.e., biological fluids) is used in the biotechnology industry for clarification (primary cell/debris removal) and sterilization of such solutions [1,2], and more recently for removal of viral contaminants [3–6]. Unlike ultrafiltration, which is most commonly used in the biotechnology industry for concentration and/or diafiltration of the product and where the protein molecules are normally retained at the membrane surface, transport of the protein through the membrane is required in microfiltration. Most microporous membranes that are used for clarification and sterilization purposes have tightly controlled pore size distributions and a high degree of porosity resulting in high internal surface area. Hence, interactions of proteins with microporous membranes is a significant phenomenon that can have a substantial influence on the recovery of filtered proteins.

Adsorption of proteins can occur whenever any solid surface comes in contact with a protein solution. The phenomenon of protein adsorption is thus not unique to membrane filtration but affects the performance of many materials and processes, in areas ranging from medicine to biochemical engineering [7]. In medicine, a major area in which protein interactions with solid surfaces is of importance is that of biocompatible materials and implantable medical devices. In this case, adsorption of proteins from surrounding fluids strongly affects the cellular interactions with foreign surfaces, thereby determining biocompatibility. In *in vitro* cell culture and biotechnology applications, adhesion of the cells to the substrate is usually mediated by an adsorbed layer of protein. Diagnostic applications, such as solid-phase immunoassays, depend on the adsorptive immobilization of an antibody or other specific proteins. Traditionally, the separation and purification of proteins is accomplished by solid–liquid chromatography, which largely depends on the adsorptive interaction of proteins with a solid chromatographic support. In pharmaceutical applications, interaction of the active peptide or protein agent with container surfaces can lead to its depletion from solution [8]. In view of the enormous scope of protein adsorption, several reviews are now available [9–12], underscoring the importance of understanding and controlling the interaction of proteins with solid surfaces in a number of fields.

In recent years, there has been increasing interest in the characterization of the protein-binding properties of microfiltration membranes. This has been driven largely by the desire of manufacturers of high value protein preparations to obtain the highest possible yields of these substances. In addition, international regulatory guidelines for the pharmaceutical and biotechnology industry require that the composition of the product be unaffected by any of the manufacturing processes employed (including sterile filtration). In such applications, concerns have been expressed about the possible adsorptive loss of these valuable proteins during filtration.

2 PRINCIPLES OF PROTEIN ADSORPTION—PHENOMENOLOGICAL ASPECTS

An understanding of the basic principles governing protein adsorption is essential to the proper design and operation of microfiltration applications involving dilute protein solutions. Thus, a general discussion of the principles and phenomenological aspects of protein adsorption to solid surfaces serves as an appropriate starting point. The information needed to understand and control the phenomenon includes (1) the amounts of protein adsorbed as a function of the bulk solution concentration (the classical adsorption isotherm); (2) the amount adsorbed as a function of time (the adsorption kinetics); (3) the desorption/exchange properties when the protein solution is removed and replaced with either a buffer or other protein solution; and (4) the organization of the adsorbed protein layer and the effect of adsorption on the conformation of the protein. The aforementioned topics are discussed in this chapter in terms of single-protein systems where they are much better understood. The adsorption characteristics of complex protein mixtures such as serum and plasma (competitive adsorption) are discussed separately.

2.1 Adsorption Isotherms

The steady-state amount of protein adsorbed on a unit area of a solid surface is often reported as a function of the protein concentration in solution—the so-called adsorption isotherm. Figure 1a shows a typical adsorption isotherm where the amount of protein adsorbed initially increases with increasing bulk (solution) protein concentration before reaching a well-defined plateau at dilute or semidilute protein concentration in solution. At this concentration, all the available sites on the solid surface are bound, resulting in no further increase in protein binding. Usually this plateau value corresponds closely to a well-packed monolayer of protein. In some cases, the plateau value can be considerably lower due to either the formation of an incomplete monolayer or the spreading of the adsorbed protein at the solid surface. Occasionally, as observed with some proteins at various surfaces, the occurrence of kinks or steps in the adsorption isotherm is seen (Fig. 1b), suggesting different modes of binding at high and low concentration (i.e., sites of varying affinities or different orientations of the adsorbed molecules at different concentrations). At low protein concentrations, binding occurs primarily through sites on the solid surface that have a high affinity

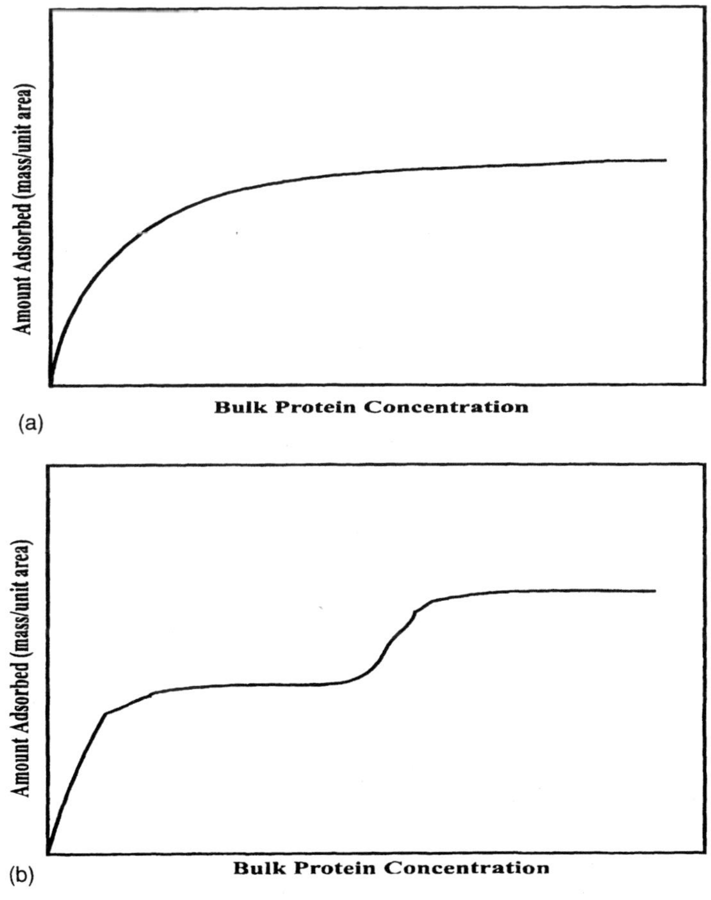

Figure 1 (a) Typical adsorption isotherm. The amount of protein adsorbed (in mass per unit area) is plotted as a function of the bulk (solution) protein concentration (expressed as either percent or mass per unit volume). (b) Adsorption isotherm showing the presence of steps, indicating rearrangements at higher protein concentrations.

for the protein; as the protein concentration increases, binding begins to occur through sites of lower affinity, resulting in an increase in the amount of protein bound.

The adsorption isotherm and the extent of protein adsorption depend on a number of factors, including the nature of the protein, the solution and/or process conditions, and the membrane surface chemistry. Table 1 lists the protein, solution (or process), and membrane surface variables that are important in the study of protein adsorption.

The similarity of the experimentally determined protein adsorption isotherms to the classical Langmuir adsorption isotherm has frequently led to the application of the latter in analyzing protein adsorption data, especially if the solution is sufficiently dilute. In the case of protein adsorption, the Langmuir isotherm is usually written as

$$m_{\text{ads}} = \frac{m_{\text{max}} c}{K_{\text{ads}} + c} \tag{1}$$

where m_{ads} is the amount of protein adsorbed per unit area, m_{max} is the amount of protein adsorbed at saturation, K_{ads} is the adsorption equilibrium constant, and c is the bulk protein concentration.

Although in most cases the experimental data are described reasonably well by the Langmuir isotherm, it must be noted that the similarity is entirely fortuitous, as virtually none of the assumptions involved in the Langmuir theory are satisfied in the case of protein adsorption [13]. The Langmuir treatment of gas (or solute) adsorption assumes that adsorption occurs reversibly on identical sites on a surface, without any lateral interaction between the adsorbing molecules. In addition, the adsorbing molecule also has only one site, and each site on the surface can adsorb only one molecule. On the other hand, protein adsorption is generally not reversible (see below), and both the protein molecule and the surface are usually heterogeneous, in that they have two or more classes of binding sites. In addition, the rates of

Table 1 Factors Important in the Study of Protein Adsorption

Protein	Solution/process	Solid surface
Isoelectric point	pH	Surface composition (chemistry)
Net change	Ionic strength	Surface potential
Charge distribution	Buffer composition	Surface topography and heterogeneity
Nature and placement of hydrophobic groups	Protein concentration	Passivation/pretreatment
Rigidity/shape—conformational variability and dynamics	Nature and concentration of other proteins	
Degree of hydration	Temperature	
Degree of aggregation	Pressure	
Binding of low molecular weight ligands (or other proteins)	Hydrodynamics (flow)	
Labeling (if any)	Shear	
	Interfacial surfaces (air)	

adsorption and desorption are determined by complex and multiple (nonidentical) interactions between the surface and the protein as well as lateral interactions between the adsorbed molecules. Despite this, several investigators have fit experimentally derived data to a Langmuir curve; however, the physical meaning of values for the Gibbs energy of adsorption derived from such an analysis is questionable.

2.2 Structure of the Adsorbed Protein Layer

The structure of the adsorbed protein layer can be discussed either at the level of organization of the protein layer as a whole or in terms of the structure of the adsorbed protein molecules individually. As stated earlier, globular protein molecules form a more or less fully packed monolayer at saturation wherein the thickness of the monolayer approximates the dimensions of the native molecule [13]. For example, using a light-scattering technique, Morrissey and Han [14] concluded that the thickness of a layer of γ-globulin on polystyrene latex was 21.6 nm; given the dimensions of the γ-globulin molecule, this is consistent with a monolayer of end-on oriented molecules. Under conditions of strong electrostatic interaction and at hydrophobic surfaces, however, protein molecules tend to collapse and flatten upon adsorption to form a very dense layer [15].

The application of techniques normally used for protein structure determination in solution such as nuclear magnetic resonance (NMR) spectroscopy, circular dichroism (CD), and infrared (IR) spectroscopy, is fairly limited in the case of adsorbed proteins. Thus, much of the evidence for conformational changes in the protein molecule upon adsorption is indirect. These include the reduction of biological activity upon adsorption, the reduction in the thickness of the adsorbed protein layer to a value smaller than the shortest dimension of the molecule in solution, and the entropic nature of adsorption as reflected by the influence of temperature on adsorption isotherms [16–18].

In recent years, progress has been made in applying total internal reflection fluorescence (TIRF) spectroscopy; CD spectroscopy, Fourier transform infrared (FTIR) spectroscopy, and electron spin resonance (ESR) spectroscopy to adsorbed proteins [19–26]. Thus, direct CD spectral measurements of coagulation factor XII adsorbed on quartz showed evidence of conformational changes, whereas fibrinogen did not [19]. The experimental difficulties associated with direct CD measurements of proteins in the adsorbed state has led to the examination of the adsorbed proteins after their removal from the substrate. CD spectra of proteins eluted after different contact times (of up to 10 days) with the surface showed a direct relationship between contact time and the degree of conformational change. Similar measurements with polypeptide surfaces of varying charge density revealed that the helical content of albumin was greatly reduced, while that of fibrinogen only slightly reduced upon elution [20]. In contrast to the direct CD measurements mentioned above, the helical content of fibrinogen eluted from glass was found to be reduced by about 50% [21]. This discrepancy indicates that in cases where structural changes have been observed in the eluted molecules, it is not clear whether they are induced by adsorption or desorption; it is also possible that elution (desorption) is accompanied by a partial restructuring toward the native form. In an example of the application of TIRF spectroscopy, the adsorption of fibronectin on a hydrophobic surface resulted in a shift in the fluorescence maximum from 321 nm to 326 nm, suggesting conformational changes [22]. The effect of hydrophilicity of the surface on conformational rearrangements is unclear; for example, fibronectin showed no change in the fluorescence maximum upon adsorption to hydrophilic silica, while the fluorescence maximum of albumin shifts from 342 nm to 333 nm upon adsorption to a hydrophilic quartz [23]. It appears that adsorption on hydrophobic surfaces is likely to be accompanied by conformational changes, whereas on hydrophilic surfaces, conformational changes are less likely. In addition, the characteristics of the protein are also known to be important in determining both the likelihood and extent of conformational changes that can occur upon adsorption; for example, a 1992 study suggests that the extent of conformational changes upon adsorption increases with increased structural flexibility of a protein as indicated by its adiabatic compressibility [27].

2.3 Kinetics of Protein Adsorption

The typical time profile for the adsorption of proteins is usually shown by plotting the amount adsorbed as a function of time as shown in Fig. 2a. There is initially a period of rapid adsorption, followed by a slower approach to a limiting value; the time profile thus mirrors the adsorption isotherm. In some cases, an "overshoot" has been observed in the time profile; in these cases, after a steady increase over some period, the amount adsorbed decreases significantly to reach a constant limiting value (Fig. 2b).

Any adsorption process may be divided into the following steps: (1) transport to the surface, (2) binding or attachment to the surface, (3) structural rearrangements in the adsorbed state, (4) detachment of the adsorbed molecule from the surface (desorption/exchange), and (5) transport away from the surface. Any one of these steps can, in principle, be the rate-limiting step and thus control the overall rate of the adsorption process.

Transport to (and away from) the surface is essentially controlled by diffusion; even in flow systems there is a stagnant layer (boundary layer) at the solid surface. The thickness of the boundary layer depends to some extent on the temperature and on the interface itself but primarily on the flow system; it can range from 0.1 cm in unstirred systems to 0.001 cm in vigorously stirred systems (and thinner in the case of flow through submicrometer-rated microporous membranes). Proteins have very low diffusion constants (typically on the order of 10^{-7} cm^2/s), and thus diffusional transport to the interface is most likely to be the rate-limiting step at low bulk concentrations and at low surface coverage. At high protein concentrations or at high surface coverage (as saturation progresses), the protein–surface interactions may become rate-limiting. In some systems, the surface reaction can be rate-limiting throughout the process, irrespective of surface coverage and/or concentration; in these cases, there is usually an energy barrier to adsorption, such as electrostatic repulsion between a charged surface and a like-charged protein.

Both surface-induced conformational changes and desorption of the adsorbed protein are time-dependent. Soderquist and Walton [28] proposed a widely accepted model in which the adsorption process is characterized by three stages:

1. Short times (on the order of a few minutes) where adsorption is rapid and is reversible with little chance for conformational changes; thus, a pseudo-equilibrium is present. The protein is adsorbed in a random arrangement at low (less than 50% of theoretical monolayer) surface coverage; at greater

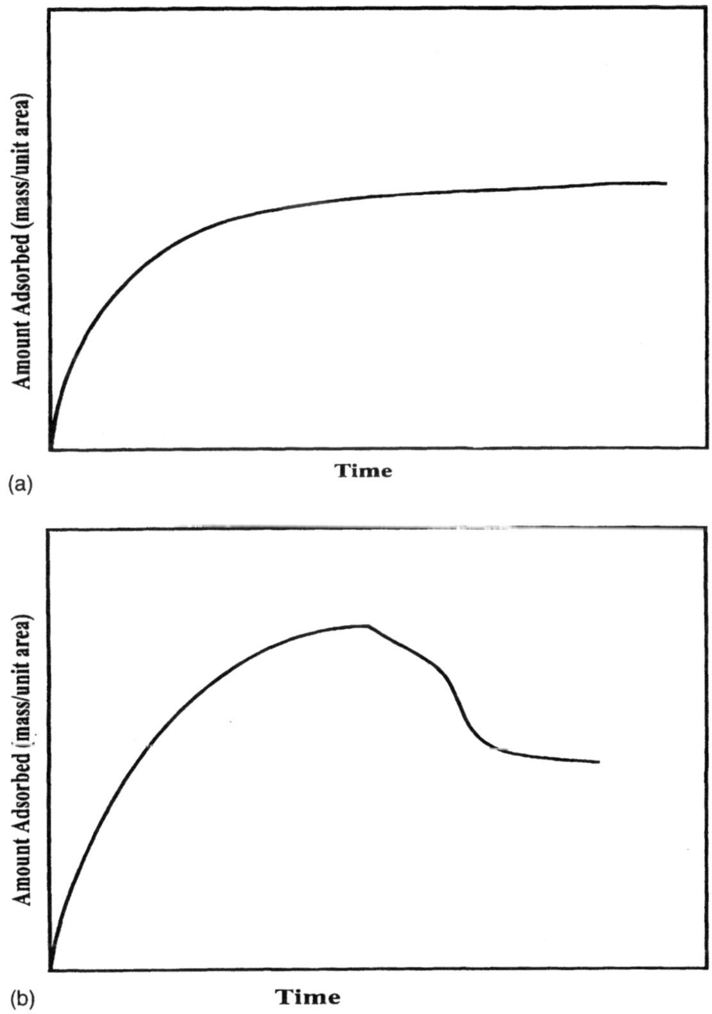

Figure 2 Kinetics of protein adsorption. (a) Typical time profile. (b) Overshoot phenomenon seen with some systems.

surface coverages, surface transitions and ordering may develop, resulting in more efficient packing and increased adsorption (seen as a kink in the adsorption isotherm).

2. Given sufficient time, adsorbed proteins undergo slow conformational changes leading to increased surface interaction. During this process, proteins less optimally adsorbed can desorb, leading to the overshoot seen in some adsorption time profiles. The process is no longer completely reversible, with desorption decreasing.
3. At long times, the conformational change of the adsorbed protein molecule is complete. Adsorption is now essentially irreversible, and the amount adsorbed reaches a saturation/limiting value.

2.4 Reversibility of Protein Adsorption

When considering reversibility of protein adsorption, it is convenient to distinguish between (1) reversibility upon dilution of the solution and/or upon changing external conditions such as pH, ionic strength, and temperature and (2) exchange of protein molecules between the adsorbed state and dissolved state and/or displacement of adsorbed protein by other proteins and/or small molecules [29].

It has been observed that desorption of proteins upon dilution frequently does not occur on a reasonable time scale; dilution of the system with solvent (or replacement of the protein solution with solvent) does not result in any significant desorption from the surface. Similarly, although the extent of protein adsorbed can almost always be increased by changing solution conditions (such as pH, ionic strength, and temperature) appropriately, desorption of proteins by reversing such a change once adsorption has occurred is frequently not realized or only partly realized. Usually, protein desorption upon dilution or upon changing solution conditions is more likely to occur with hydrophilic surfaces than with hydrophobic ones, presumably because proteins are less tightly bound at hydrophilic surfaces [13,29].

Although the protein may be irreversibly adsorbed with respect to dilution, the exchange of proteins between the adsorbed and dissolved states as well as the displacement of adsorbed protein by other proteins and/or small molecules has been observed [29]. This seemingly anomalous behavior is typical of multisite binding and can be explained in terms of a high activation energy barrier for desorption. Upon adsorption, the protein molecule attaches to the surface via several segments (or binding sites), and consequently the molar free energy of adsorption is quite high. In the adsorbed state, the protein molecule may rearrange its structure to optimize its interaction with the surface, thereby further contributing to the adsorption free energy. In order to desorb, the protein molecule has to overcome the combined free energy of adsorption and rearrangement; consequently, the activation energy barrier for desorption is large. Furthermore, for desorption to occur, the protein molecule must detach from the surface at all of its bound segments at the same time, which is statistically improbable.

On the other hand, displacement of an adsorbed protein molecule by another one of the same kind (exchange) or by another component (competitive adsorption) can be accomplished by a sequential detachment of segments of the adsorbed molecule in favor of the attachment of segments of the newly arriving molecule. The activation energy for exchange is determined by the adsorption energy of a single segment and is therefore significantly lower than that for desorption.

After desorption, the protein molecule may regain its native conformation either completely or partly or may persist in the (different) conformation attained upon adsorption. In the latter case, the surface can be regarded as a catalyst facilitating a structural transition. Persistence of the desorbed protein molecule in the conformation attained upon adsorption does not necessarily mean that the desorbed molecule has a lower free energy than the native molecule, but rather that the activation energy for the transition back to the native conformation may be too high for it to occur [13,29].

2.5 Adsorption from Protein Mixtures

The adsorption behavior of protein mixtures such as blood and plasma has been studied extensively [30–32]. When a surface is exposed to plasma or complex protein mixtures, different proteins from the mixture adsorb on the surface. The exact composition of the adsorbed layer depends on the concentration of the various proteins, the nature of the proteins and the surface, the adsorption time, and, in the case of plasma, the degree of dilution of the sample. The change in the composition of the adsorbed layer as a function of time reflects the relative rates of adsorption of the different proteins and the exchange processes between different proteins at the solid surface. In the case of plasma, it has been shown that extensive exposure of various surfaces to undiluted plasma results in a relatively limited adsorption of some proteins from even less concentrated pure solutions [32]. Vroman et al. [32] showed that the exchange hierarchy for plasma proteins adsorbing on glass and metal oxides is

$$\text{Albumin} \rightarrow \gamma\text{-globulin} \rightarrow \text{fibrinogen} \rightarrow \text{fibronectin}$$
$$\rightarrow \text{Factor XII} \rightarrow \text{high molecular weight kininogen (HMWK)}$$

The exchange processes noted above are consistent with classical binding theory, which dictates that the protein that initially adsorbs is the one that is present at the highest concentration; however, this can be replaced by a scarce component that has a higher affinity for the surface. In such a model, dilution generally should not cause a qualitatively different behavior (except at highly dilute bulk solutions where adsorption of scarce components could lead to its depletion from the bulk phase), but only make the process slower. However, it has been observed that fibrinogen adsorption from plasma is dependent on the degree of dilution [33]; at plasma concentrations of 5% or less, the adsorbed fibrinogen layer is stable, while at intermediate dilutions the exchange processes noted above (for undiluted plasma) occur, and no fibrinogen adsorption occurs with concentrated plasma. Two mechanisms have been proposed to explain this peculiar behavior of plasma protein adsorption on a surface at different dilutions of the plasma—the so-called Vroman effect [30]. The first is a surface occupancy lateral interaction model, which allows an exponential decrease in the affinity constant with increasing occupancy of the surface and an interaction term for the mutual interactions of the adsorbed molecules [34]. The second is a surface denaturation model in which the surface-induced conformational change of an adsorbed protein molecule is dependent on the number and type of the neighboring molecules [35]. In this model, a protein molecule that is more labile or conformationally adaptable to the surface will displace one that is less "surface-active."

2.6 Factors Involved in Protein Adsorption

Protein adsorption is a complex multifactorial phenomenon, and a number of factors are important in determining the extent of protein adsorption, including the nature of the protein, the solution and/or process conditions, and the membrane surface chemistry (see Table 1).

The surface of a protein is often complex, with differences in characteristics such as hydrophobicity, charge, and degree of hydration, and can change with protein conformation and solution characteristics. Similarly, the solid adsorbent can exhibit considerable heterogeneity in surface composition (chemistry), surface potential, and surface topography. In addition, the behavior of both proteins and solid surfaces can depend on various solution and/or process conditions (such as pH, ionic strength, buffer composition, protein concentration, nature and concentration of other proteins, temperature, pressure, and hydrodynamics). This complexity renders the prediction of how a given protein will interact with a surface extremely difficult. Nevertheless, the following "rule-of-thumb" observations have been generated from the vast experimental literature on protein adsorption.

First, it has been generally observed that interaction between a protein and a surface increases with increasing hydrophobicity of both the protein and the surface [36]. In proteins, the hydrophobic amino acids (such as tryptophan, phenylalanine, and tyrosine) tend to be excluded from the surface of the protein, thereby minimizing their contact with water. However, restrictions due to other types of interactions and more often geometrical (or steric) considerations generally cause a fraction of the hydrophobic residues to be exposed to the aqueous solvent. The fraction of a protein's surface that is hydrophobic is therefore determined both by its composition (primary structure) and by its three-dimensional structure (secondary, tertiary, and quaternary structures). The solid surface may also contain hydrophobic regions; dehydration of the hydrophobic regions of the protein and the solid surface is entropically driven and thus promotes adsorption. In addition, desorption from hydrophobic surfaces does not usually occur (as noted in Sec. 2.4), and proteins can often be more easily removed from hydrophilic surfaces by exposure to different solution conditions. The experimental literature also reveals a stronger tendency to structural alterations in the adsorbed state with increasing protein and/or solid surface hydrophobicity; this can be explained on the basis of the large contribution of hydrophobic interactions to the overall stability of the protein in these cases. In cases where adsorption is driven by hydrophobic considerations, it follows that solution conditions that adversely affect hydrophobic interactions, such as the presence of alcohols, glycols, and surfactants, would tend to reduce protein adsorption.

Second, it has been shown that adsorption generally increases with decreasing charge on the protein and the surface [37]. It is well known that protein adsorption tends to be at a maximum at the isoelectric point (pI), the pH at which the protein has no net charge. This has been attributed to either changes in the structure of the protein molecule (e.g, albumin), the elimination of a barrier to adsorption (e.g., at like-charged surfaces), or the elimination of lateral (repulsion) interactions within the adsorbed layer. An exception to this generalized rule occurs when the protein and the surface are oppositely charged; in this case, the amount of protein adsorbed increases with increasing charge contrast. In cases where adsorption is driven by ionic considerations, it follows that solution conditions that affect electrostatic interactions, such as pH and ionic strength, would tend to affect protein adsorption. For example, increasing the ionic strength can result in electrostatic "screening" of charge interactions as well as increasing hydrophobic interactions; thus, increased ionic strength generally results in increased adsorption.

The aforementioned principles are demonstrated in Fig. 3 in the case of bovine serum albumin (BSA) adsorption to polymer latices [38]. First, Fig. 3a shows a comparison of the extent of BSA adsorption (at 25°C and 0.1 M ionic strength) to hydrophobic polystyrene latex beads versus two hydrophilic copolymer surfaces [$P(St/HEMA)_n$, a styrene/2-hydroxyethyl methacrylate copolymer, where the subscript represents the percentage of HEMA]. The amount of BSA adsorbed to hydrophobic polystyrene is higher than that in the case of the two hydrophilic surfaces, at pH greater than the pI of BSA (about 5.0). This is because in this pH range BSA adsorption is primarily mediated by hydrophobic interactions, and hence the hydro-

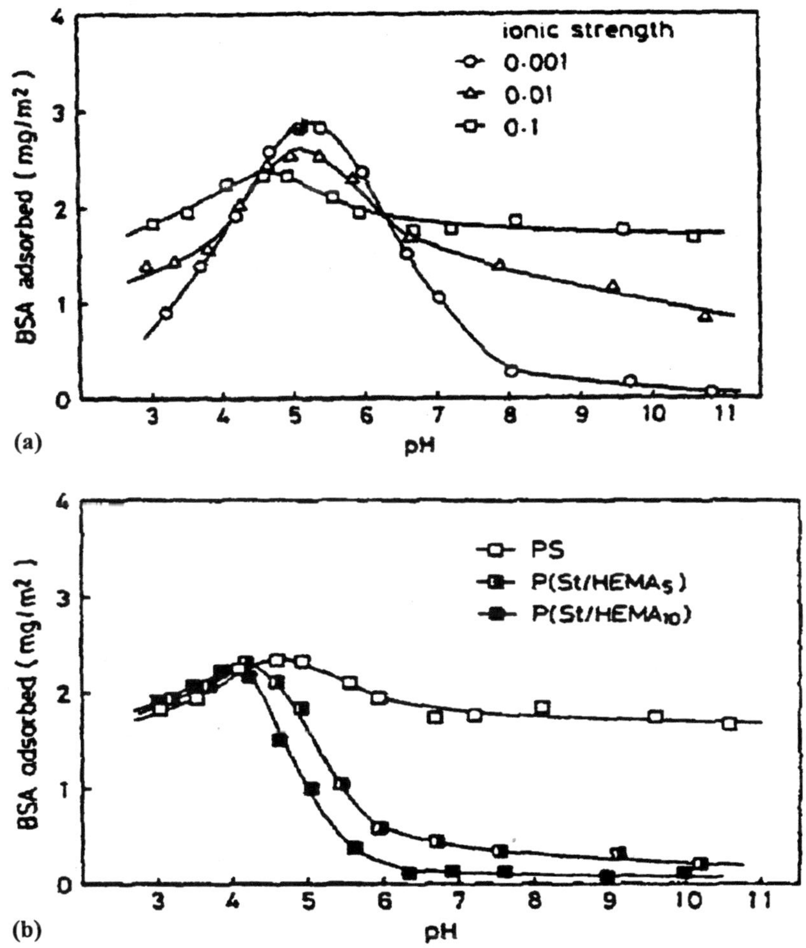

Figure 3 (a) Effect of ionic strength on the adsoption of BSA to polystyrene. (b) pH dependence of BSA adsorption to various polymer latices (25°C, ionic strength 0.1 M) (From Ref. 38.)

philic surfaces showed little protein adsorption. However, at pH values corresponding to the pI value and below, surface hydrophobicity showed little effect on the amount of protein adsorbed. This is due to the fact that at this acidic pH range, an electrostatic attraction acts between the positively charged BSA and the negatively charged surfaces. Second, the effect of pH and ionic strength on BSA adsorption to polystyrene latex beads (Fig. 3a) shows a maximum in protein adsorption at and around the p*I* of the protein. The effect of increasing ionic strength was to effectively increase the amount of protein adsorbed at all pH values except perhaps in the immediate vicinity of the isoelectric point. It appears that in this case increased ionic strength increased protein adsorption, primarily by promoting hydrophobic interactions. Charge screening, which could potentially reduce the unfavorable electrostatic interaction between the like-charged protein and the polystyrene surface at pH above the isoelectric point and reduce the favorable electrostatic attraction between the protein

Table 2 Principles of Protein Adsorption

Subject	Principle
Foothold	The minimum contact area required for initial adsorption (foothold) is very small, 100–200 Å^2.
Adsorption rates	At short times, adsorption is rapid and transport-limited. Slower rates suggest energy barriers to adsorption; faster rates indicate augmented transport (e.g., convection).
Reversibility	Protein adsorption on uncharged hydrophilic surfaces is often at least partly reversible; adsorption on hydrophobic surfaces is often irreversible.
Electric potentials	Electric potentials can lead to enhanced adsorption (unlike charges on protein and surface) or reduced adsorption (like charges on both).
Isoelectric point	Adsorption is generally maximal at a pH corresponding to the isoelectric point (pI) of the protein.
Hydrophobicity	Adsorption increases with increasing hydrophobicity of the protein and/or the surface.
Conformational rearrangements	At longer residence times, adsorbed proteins may undergo conformational rearrangements to optimize their interactions with the surface.
Extent of adsorption	The amount of protein adsorbed on a given surface is governed by many factors, including the nature of the protein and its properties, its concentration, solution conditions, membrane surface characteristics, etc.

and the surface at acidic pH (below the isoelectric point), does not appear to be significant in this case as evidenced by the increased protein adsorption below the isoelectric point. At the isoelectric point, ionic strength had no significant effect, because protein adsorption was at the maximal "monolayer" level; a closely packed monolayer of unperturbed "side-on" protein molecules yields a protein adsorption value of 2.5 mg/m^2.

Based on the vast experimental literature on the adsorption of proteins to solid surfaces, several general principles of protein adsorption have been formulated that also apply to adsorption to microporous membranes. These are summarized in Table 2.

3 PROTEIN ADSORPTION IN MICROFILTRATION APPLICATIONS

3.1 Phenomenological Aspects

Static Studies

Protein adsorption experiments with microporous membranes are sometimes carried out under "static" conditions. "Static" studies are essentially soak or immersion tests. Filter disks, typically 13 or 25 mm in diameter, are incubated in the protein solution of interest for a period of time long enough to reach steady state. At periodic intervals, the amount of protein adsorbed is determined by suitable means; it is then normalized per unit area and is plotted as a function of time. Such a study yields a curve similar to the one shown in Fig. 2a. Static systems that are not stirred generally do not reach steady state quickly; this is due to the fact that the thickness of the stagnant boundary layer through which the protein has to diffuse to reach the membrane surface is greater than that encountered in flow systems or stirred cells. In principle, the amount of protein bound can be determined by withdrawing small aliquots of the incubating solution and determining its concentration; the amount of protein bound is obtained indirectly by carrying out a mass balance, i.e., by multiplying the measured change in concentration by the volume of the incubating solution. However, the amount of protein bound is usually low, and the change in protein concentration measured, quite small. Most static studies are therefore carried out using radiolabeled protein. In this case, kinetic experiments can be carried out by incubating filter disks with the radiolabeled protein solution for varying lengths of time. Each filter disk is removed after a given exposure period and washed with buffer, and the amount of protein bound is determined directly by (γ) counting. It is also desirable to assay aliquots of the incubating solution to ensure that a mass balance can be closed. Containers with low protein binding characteristics should be used for these studies (or appropriate controls to account for any adsorption to the walls of the container must be included).

Static studies are usually of limited value for the following reasons. First, they require the use of radiolabeled proteins. This method is simple to use and extremely sensitive but may produce artifacts. The labeling process and/or the presence of the label may change the physicochemical properties of the protein and alter its adsorption properties [39,40]. Second, if the protein–radionuclide bond is not stable, the label could be released with time, leading to errors in the experimental data. Finally, static studies yield no information on the saturation volume or the dynamics of protein concentration recovery and do not account for the effects of the rate of adsorption or of process parameters such as flow rate of batch size; the data obtained using these studies therefore cannot be extrapolated to the actual process. These limitations mean that soak testing is generally useful only as a rapid and cursory indicator of whether adsorption will occur.

Dynamic Studies

The effect of protein adsorption in a microfiltration process is best determined by measuring the filter effluent concentration as a function of the volume filtered per unit area (normalized throughput) as shown schematically in Fig. 3. At the start of the filtration process, the rate of adsorption is at its highest and the protein concentration in the initial effluent the lowest. As filtration continues, the filter surface starts to saturate, and the rate of adsorption decreases, resulting in an increase in the effluent protein concentration. Once the filter surface is saturated, no further net adsorption can take place, and the effluent protein concentration approaches that of the inlet feed concentration. The dynamics of protein concentration recovery during membrane filtration—the "filter saturation curve"—is a crucial piece of information for the bioprocess engineer and is the key to successful filtration process design.

The filter saturation curve contains information regarding (1) the volume required to saturate the filter with a given protein solution and achieve complete protein concentration recovery and (2) the amount of protein bound per unit area of the filter at saturation. The saturation volume is readily obtained from the binding curve as the volume at which the effluent protein concentration equals the inlet feed concentration and generally falls in a range of 5–50 L per 10 in. filter cartridge (0.5–10 mL/cm^2). The total amount of protein bound at saturation is obtained by integrating the area between the curve and the *y* ordinate corresponding to the feed concentration (i.e., complete recovery) as shown in Fig. 4; if the area of the filter is known, this permits the calculation of the saturation protein adsorption value per unit area. For the process engineer, the amount of protein bound per unit area of the filter at saturation is not nearly as useful as the volume of material that must be processed before the filtrate protein concentration recovers to that of the feed. In most processes, a preflush of the filtration system is performed to avoid dilution of the product with either condensate accumulated from steaming or an integrity test fluid, or to perform a preprocess integrity test in the process fluid itself, or to minimize potential extractables or particulates. If the flush volume dictated by these concerns is greater than the saturation volume, then the whole issue of the protein adsorption becomes irrelevant because the filter membrane has already been saturated in the preprocess steps.

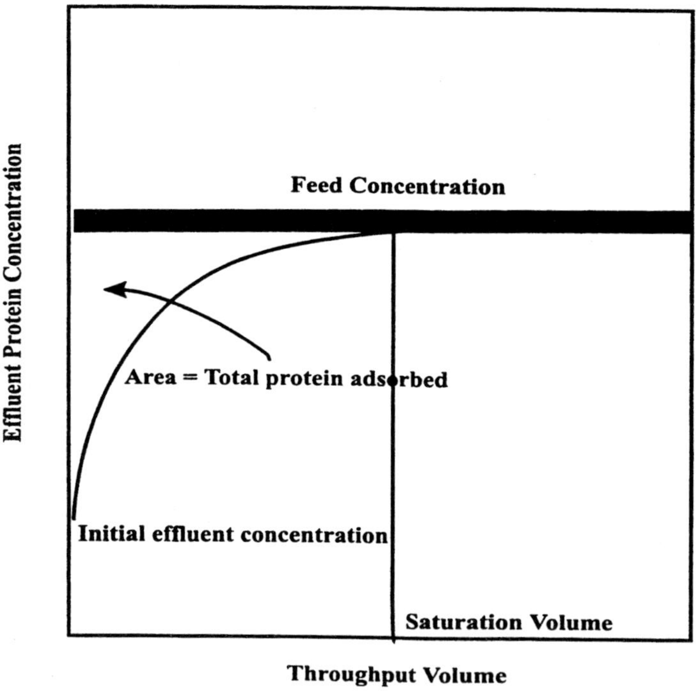

Figure 4 Typical filter binding (saturation) curve. The effluent protein concentration is plotted as a function of the throughput volume. The effluent protein concentration equals the feed concentration (within the error margin of the assay), indicating complete recovery, after the saturation volume has been processed through the filter. The initial effluent concentration is typically not equal to zero and will depend on the adsorption characteristics of the protein–membrane system in question as well as process conditions such as flow rate. The area between the feed concentration *y* ordinate and the binding curve is equal to the mass of protein adsorbed by the filter.

An important feature of the filter saturation curve is that most microporous membrane filters adsorb a comparatively small amount of protein before achieving a steady state of quantitative or complete protein recovery during the remaining filtration process. Consequently, most biotechnological/pharmaceutical processes operate under conditions where saturable binding of the protein of interest to microfiltration membranes is not and has never been a problem. Many studies dealing with protein adsorption on microporous membranes fail to point this out and therefore do the filter user a disservice by diverting attention from proper process design to a single system component (in this case, the filter). Table 3 lists the conditions under which protein adsorption to filters may be a matter of concern for the bioprocess engineer as well as conditions under which it is generally not. Adsorptive losses are not a major concern in the case of most bulk filtration processes and at most working concentrations or in cases where a preflush of the filtration system can be carried out. The conditions under which protein losses may become significant are usually limited—for example, those that involve filling small containers with a very valuable and/or very dilute product or small batch sizes or when preflushing is not feasible due to economic and/or time constraints. In such cases, it is important to design the process to limit adsorption to acceptable levels and to take this acceptable level of adsorption into account.

In most cases, the effluent protein concentration at steady state recovers completely to a value that corresponds to that of the feed solution. In some cases, however, the effluent protein concentration at steady state can plateau at a value corresponding to less than complete (100%) recovery. This type of "nonsaturable" binding can be indicative of losses associated with either sieving or multilayer adsorption mediated by protein–protein interactions. In the case of sterilizing grade filters, sieving losses are typically due to the removal of particulate- or gel-associated and/or undissolved protein. In the case of extremely "tight" filters such as virus-retentive filters, there may also be sieving losses because of the removal of high molecular weight proteins (larger than the molecular weight cutoff of the membrane). Protein losses due to sieving are essentially independent of the membrane chemistry but may depend on its removal rating. It is not advisable, however, to use this as a sole criterion for deciding if sieving-related losses are present, since coarser filters may also have less internal surface area (even though their nominal filtration surface

Table 3 Applications Where Protein Adsorption May Be of Concern in Microfiltration

Yes	No
Filling small containers/vials	Bulk filtration
Small batch size[a]	Large batch size[a]
Very dilute product	Most working concentrations
Flushing not feasible	Flushing is possible
Very valuable product	Inexpensive product

[a]Relative to filter area.

areas may be the same) and hence lower levels of protein adsorption. In situations where sieving losses are suspected, they can be confirmed by repeating the tests using material that has been freshly filtered through a filter of equivalent rating. Obviously, any undissolved protein (particles or gels) that becomes associated with the membrane as a result of its sieving action cannot be considered an adsorptive loss.

Cases where nonsaturable binding cannot be attributed to sieving may be the result of "protein deposition," primarily mediated by protein–protein interactions. There is disagreement in the literature regarding the use of the term "protein adsorption" in such cases. Some argue that the term "adsorption" strictly implies a process with partitioning of solute between a solution and a surface and therefore refers only to molecules that are in direct contact with the surface (effectively a monolayer) and use the term "protein deposition" for all additional material accumulated at the membrane surface during the process due to convection and protein–protein interactions. The primary consequence of protein deposition in microfiltration is usually membrane fouling, and only occasionally does it significantly affect protein recovery. This is due to the fact that protein deposition tends to occur at fairly high protein concentrations, where deposition of (relatively) small amounts of protein can have a large effect on membrane flux but little effect on the effluent protein concentration. Protein deposition during microfiltration (and ultrafiltration) remains a very controversial topic, with considerable disagreement over both mechanisms and rates of fouling and the overall importance of adsorption in this process. In general, recent studies have shown that protein deposition during microfiltration is caused by small amounts of aggregated and/or denatured protein that were present in the bulk protein solution [41,42]. Protein aggregation and/or denaturation can occur during the various processing operations prior to filtration, particularly when proteins are subjected to foaming, high temperature, extreme pH, and/or high shear stresses. A detailed discussion of protein fouling is beyond the scope of this chapter, but Refs. 43 and 44 provide an excellent overview of the work in this area. A number of attempts have been made also to mathematically describe the flux decline during micro- and ultrafiltration of protein solutions using particle deposition models [45–49].

3.2 Protein Adsorption and/or Recovery Studies with Microporous Membranes

Bioprocess engineers as well as those who are responsible for quality assurance and validation often desire to qualify microporous membranes on the basis of protein recovery when selecting them for use with dilute protein solutions. This has led to the publication of several studies in recent years that report on protein adsorption and/or recovery in microfiltration applications, which are discussed below. The goals of this discussion are (1) to provide a brief summary of the literature dealing with protein adsorption in microfiltration applications, thus providing experimental evidence for the phenomenological aspects discussed above in general terms, and (2) to reach general conclusions regarding both the techniques used to study the phenomenon and the phenomenon itself.

Static Studies

Pitt [50] reported on the nonspecific protein binding of representative proteins to microporous membranes composed of different polymeric materials under static conditions as well as on product recovery during sterile filtration of ^{125}I-labeled BSA to different microporous membranes. The static protocol consisted of soaking filter disks (8 mm, 0.5 cm^2 nominal area) in 1 mL of a protein solution for 18 h at ambient temperature; 1 mg/mL protein solutions containing 200 μg ^{125}I-labeled protein (and the rest being unlabeled protein) were used for these studies. Of the membranes studied, hydrophilic poly(vinylidene fluoride) (h-PVDF), hydrophilic polysulfone (h-PS), and cellulose diacetate (CDA) were found to exhibit low protein binding, on the order of less than 10 μg/cm^2 nominal area, for BSA and sheep IgG. Nylon and cellulose nitrate (CN) were found to exhibit relatively high protein binding for these two proteins, ≈190 and ≈250 μg/cm^2 nominal area, respectively. Similar results were reported for insulin and human growth hormone with h-PVDF, nylon, and PS membranes. Interestingly, no significant differences were observed between the different proteins for a given membrane, with the exception of h-PS; thus, for example, nylon adsorbed ≈200 μg/cm^2 nominal area irrespective of the actual protein studied (despite the fact that the molecular weights of the proteins vary by about two orders of magnitude from as low as 6 kDa to 160 kDa). In order to determine the amount adsorbed under filtration conditions, 4 mL of a 1 mg/mL BSA solution in phosphate-buffered saline (containing 200 μg/mL ^{125}I-labeled BSA) was filtered through a 13 mm filter disk (nominal area 0.7 cm^2) of nylon, h-PS, and h-PVDF membranes. Under these conditions, protein adsorbed in mass per unit nominal area for the h-PS and h-PVDF membranes is consistent with that observed during the static soak; in the case of nylon, however, the amount of protein adsorbed was much higher (>1000 μg/cm^2 nominal area) than indicated by the static studies.

The nylon adsorption data reported in this study are at least one order of magnitude higher than those reported by other studies discussed below [51–53]. Also, no explanation is provided for the discrepancy between the nylon adsorption data under static and filtration conditions. Both of these problems can be attributed to the use of ^{125}I-labeled proteins. Although the study reports that the adsorption of labeled proteins was shown to be "comparable" to that of the unlabeled proteins using "established procedures," no data are provided to demonstrate this. The adsorption of ^{125}I-labeled proteins can increase dramatically with age, which is generally attributed to protein denaturation caused by radiation damage, and this can even lead to precipitation of the labeled protein. No controls were performed to account for this effect. Thus, the higher adsorption seen in the filtration experiment may be the result of a combination of increased adsorptive and sieving losses (removal of precipitated protein by the filter).

This study illustrates the limitations associated with the use of data from static studies to predict process-scale performance. In this case, the static soak using 1 mL of radiolabeled protein solution and an 8 mm filter disk (nominal area 0.5 cm^2) corresponds to soaking a 10 in. filter cartridge (about 5 ft^2) in less than 10 L of the protein solution. Clearly, extrapolating the losses seen in this soak to the entire filtration process is not valid given the fact that the filter saturates after a given volume (the saturation volume) has been processed. Even in the case of the filtration experiment, the protein recoveries were determined before steady state was reached and therefore cannot be used to assess filter performance under process-scale conditions of continuous flow. It is important that laboratory tests that evaluate membrane filters for potential protein loss by adsorption during filtration be performed using throughput volumes and flow rates that are scaled down from the anticipated process filtration conditions. In addition, effluent samples to determine protein concentration recovery or protein adsorption should be taken after a suitable volume of protein solution has been passed through the filter so as to ensure that steady-state conditions have been reached.

The protein adsorption data cited above are based on the nominal (or frontal) surface area of a membrane, which does not take into account the vast internal surface area accessible to proteins. For some of the membranes studied above, this study also determined the BET surface area (after the developers of the technique —Branauer, Emmett, and Teller) using nitrogen gas adsorption/desorption isotherms [54]. There is some question as to whether BET areas are accurate representations of the area available for protein adsorption, given the fact that proteins are on average a few orders of magnitude larger than nitrogen and the minimum "foothold" for protein adsorption to occur is about 200 Å^2. The theoretical monolayer saturation of a surface for IgG can vary from about 0.27 to 1.8 $\mu g/cm^2$ BET area, depending on orientation, and that for BSA can vary from 0.25–0.90 $\mu g/cm^2$ BET area [55]. In the cases of h-PVDF and h-PS, the protein adsorption measured is about 10 and 40 ng/cm^2 BET area, respectively, indicating a surface coverage that is much less than a monolayer. In the case of nylon, the measured protein adsorption is $\approx$350 ng/cm^2 BET area for both BSA and IgG, which is consistent with monolayer surface coverage. In the case of CN, the measured protein adsorption of >2000 ng/cm^2 BET area suggests multilayer surface deposition.

Pitt [50] also studied the kinetics of protein binding to microporous membranes under static conditions as well as the effect of bulk protein concentration in the range of 0.1–10 mg/mL on the amount of protein adsorbed on typical microporous membranes (adsorption isotherm). While the former has no practical relevance under the conditions of a typical filtration operation, it is more or less consistent with the experimental literature on the kinetics of protein binding to solid surfaces discussed earlier. The study reports an equilibrium binding time for h-PVDF of 5 min, which is much less than reported by others in the literature (compare Persson et al. [51] and Bowen and Gan [60], discussed below). The equilibrium binding times for nylon and PS were reported to be on the order of 2–3 h (compare Persson et al. [51] below, where the nylon membrane saturated in less than 30 min). In terms of adsorption isotherm data, the study presents no data but claims that "adsorption isotherm of insulin, human growth hormone, BSA, and IgG show a Langmuir type adsorption which is similar to that observed for other better characterized polymeric surfaces" [50].

The controls that have to be performed when using labeled proteins to study protein adsorption are illustrated by Persson et al. [51], who studied the adsorption of ^{14}C-labeled β-lactoglobulin to four different microfiltration membranes. The protein was labeled with ^{14}C-formaldehyde through reductive alkylation. To verify that the labeling procedure had not altered the adsorptive properties of the protein, the following controls were performed. First, a dilution series with different proportions of labeled/unlabeled protein was found to display a linear relationship between the amount of labeled protein in solution and the amount of protein deposited on a membrane (nylon) under constant total protein concentration. Second, a control was also performed with β-lactoglobulin adsorption on a well-characterized surface (chromium); the amount adsorbed was consistent with the value that had been previously determined for this protein–surface combination via ellipsometry using unlabeled protein. Of the membranes tested, cellulose acetate (CA) and hydrophobic (unmodified) PVDF displayed the highest protein adsorption in general, although the CA membrane exhibited very low adsorption at the lowest protein concentration tested (0.1% or 1 mg/mL). The protein adsorption values for the hydrophobic (unmodified) PVDF membrane were 40 $\mu g/cm^2$ nominal area at 1 mg/mL and 120 $\mu g/cm^2$ nominal area at 10 mg/mL. In contrast, the hydrophilic (modified) PVDF membranes exhibited protein adsorption of <2.0 and 9 $\mu g/cm^2$ nominal area, respectively, at these concentrations. The nylon membrane tested displayed protein adsorption that was intermediate in value: 20 $\mu g/cm^2$ nominal area at 1 mg/mL and 40 $\mu g/cm^2$ nominal area at 10 mg/mL. As mentioned earlier, these values are at least an order of magnitude lower than that reported by Pitt [50], who used ^{125}I-labeled proteins.

The data presented above are consistent with one of the rules governing protein adsorption to solid surfaces described earlier: The interaction between a protein and a surface increases with increasing hydrophobicity of both the protein and the surface. The difference between the adsorption characteristics of the modified and unmodified PVDF membranes also demonstrates that it is the membrane surface chemistry that determines protein adsorption. Both PVDF membranes are made of the same base polymer, but only the surface of the hydrophilic PVDF is modified through the addition of covalently linked moieties to make it more hydrophilic.

Persson et al. [51] also concluded that the adsorption reached steady state after just a 30 min exposure to the protein solutions in the case of the hydrophobic (unmodified) PVDF, hydrophilic (modified) PVDF, and nylon membranes; the CA membranc continued to bind increasing amounts of protein even after an exposure of 2 h (compare Ref. 63). In terms of surface coverage, the protein adsorption results indicate that for CA, hydrophobic (unmodified) PVDF, and nylon membranes, a monolayer is built up on the surface only at the highest protein concentration tested (100 mg/mL); it follows, therefore, that at lower concentrations much less than a monolayer is formed. In the case of the hydrophilic (modified) PVDF membrane, much less than a monolayer is formed even at the highest concentration tested. Persson et al. suggest that the lower degree of protein adsorption in the case of the hydrophilic (modified) PVDF membrane may be due, at least in part, to its (relatively) lower porosity.

The importance of membrane surface chemistry in determining protein adsorption (under otherwise equivalent conditions) was also demonstrated by Kim et al. [56]. They showed that surface hydrophilization of an existing polyethylene microfiltration hollow-fiber membrane resulted in a reduction of nonspecific protein adsorption compared to the unmodified membrane. The introduction of 5–7 mol alcoholic hydroxyl group (per kilogram) on the surface of the membrane was sufficient to cover the entire polyethylene surface. This surface modification resulted in the reduction in the saturation capacity of the membrane for bovine γ-globulin from 7 mg/m^2 for the unmodified surface to less than 1 mg/m^2 for the modified membrane.

Dynamic Studies

This section begins with a discussion of dynamic studies that demonstrate the principle of dynamic saturation with a variety of polymeric microfiltration materials such as nylon, polyethersulfone, and hydrophilic PVDF [52,53,57,58]. A study [59] that demonstrates that similar microfiltration materials from different manufacturers exhibit slightly different adsorption characteristics is also discussed. This is followed

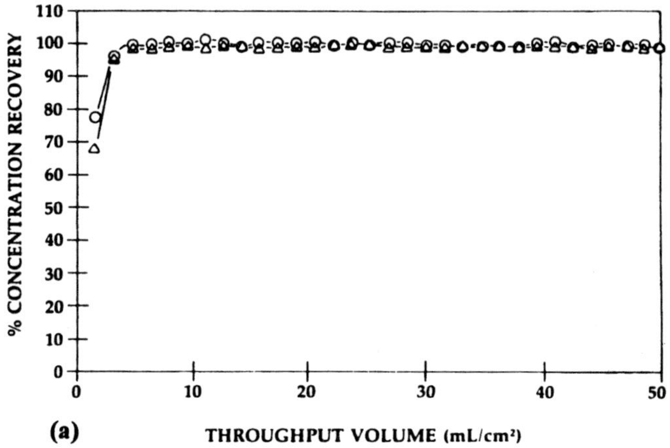

Figure 5 Recovery of (a) insulin, (b) bovine serum albumin (BSA), and (c) immunoglobulin (IgG) from membrane filters at 1 mg/mL influent concentration. (○) Hydroxyl-modified hydrophilic polyamide; (△) nylon 66; (●) hydrophilic PVDF.

by a discussion of two studies that demonstrate the effect of electrostatic and hydrophobic interactions on protein adsorption to microfiltration membranes [60,61]. Finally, a study that demonstrates the importance of testing the contribution of prefilters to the overall adsorptive loss of a filtration system and the phenomenon of nonsaturable binding that occurs with some protein systems is discussed [62]. Two of the aforementioned studies [57,62] also establish clearly that protein biological (or enzymatic) activity is not altered to any significant degree during filtration. The first study to report on the dynamics of protein recovery from process filtration systems using filter cartridges [63] is discussed in the next section.

Martin and Manteuffel [52] presented performance data for typical filter materials under simulated process-scale conditions of continuous flow and high throughput volumes. Recoveries of protein concentration were determined for three different protein solutions (insulin, BSA, and IgG) following filtration through three different microporous membranes—a hydroxyl-modified polyamide, a hydrophilic nylon, and a modified poly(vinylidene fluoride). Both the hydroxyl-modified polyamide and the modified poly(vinylidene fluoride) membranes are characterized by the manufacturers as having low protein-binding properties. Filtration studies were conducted with either 13 or 47 mm disks using working solutions of ^{125}I-labeled proteins at two different concentrations (1 mg/mL and 10 μg/mL).

Figure 5 shows the results obtained at a protein concentration of 1 mg/mL; the percent recovery, defined as counts per minute per milliliter of effluent divided by counts per minute per milliliter of influent, was plotted as a function of normalized throughput volumes (throughput per unit area). Two features are immediately apparent. First, for each of the proteins and membranes tested, steady state and hence membrane saturation is achieved rapidly. Saturation volumes were ≈5 mL/cm^2 in the case of insulin and ≈10–15 mL/cm^2 in the case of BSA and IgG. Second, the three membranes tested demonstrated essentially equal ability to recover proteins. At 1 mg/mL insulin, there was no significant difference between the nylon membrane

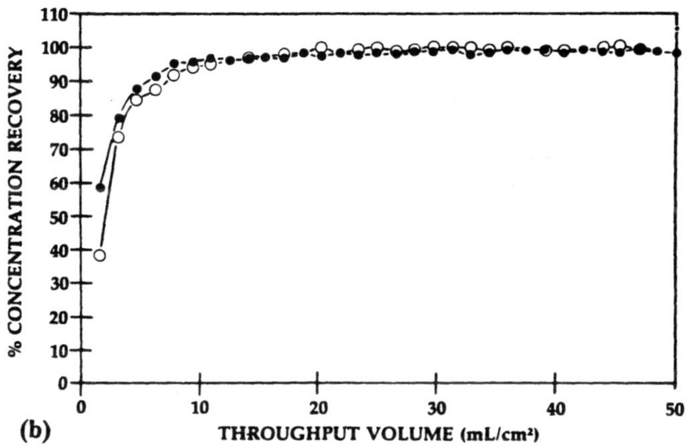

(b)

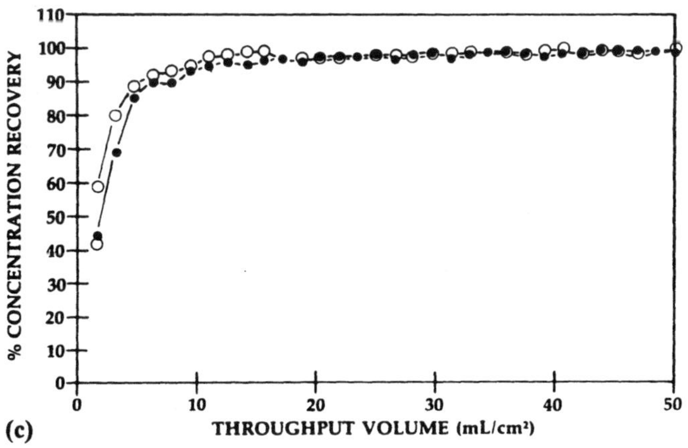

(c)

Figure 5 Continued

and the low protein binding hydroxyl-modified polyamide membrane (Fig. 5a). Similarly, at 1 mg/mL BSA or IgG, the low protein binding hydroxyl-modified polyamide membrane and the hydrophilic PVDF membrane gave identical results, except for some minor differences in the pre-steady-state portion of the curve (Figs. 5b and 5c).

Figure 6 shows the results obtained at a very dilute protein concentration of 10 μg/mL. Once again, steady state was achieved rapidly; saturation volumes were $\approx$20 mL/cm^2 in the case of insulin and $\approx$10–15 mL/cm^2 in the case of either BSA or IgG. With insulin at 10 μg/mL, the nylon membrane showed lower protein concentration recovery in the initial effluent fractions, while the behavior of the hydroxyl-modified polyamide membrane is similar to that observed at the higher protein concentration. With both BSA and IgG, there was essentially no difference between the hydroxyl-modified polyamide membrane and the hydrophilic PVDF; in addition,

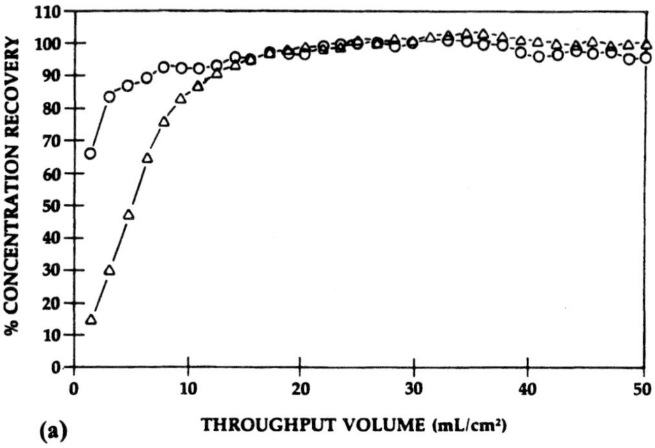

Figure 6 Recovery of (a) insulin, (b) bovine serum albumin (BSA), and (c) immunoglobulin (IgG) from membrane filters at 10 μg/mL influent concentration. Symbols as in Fig. 5.

with each of these membranes there was no difference in the protein concentration recovery characteristics at the two different protein concentrations studied.

The results presented above conclusively demonstrate that (1) protein effluent concentrations reach steady state after low throughput volumes; (2) recoveries of influent protein concentration during membrane filtration of most protein solutions (≥1 mg/mL) are extremely rapid, so the effect of individual membrane types are not distinguishable; (3) membrane filters characterized as "low protein binding" may be advantageous at very dilute concentrations (on the order of 10 μg/mL); and (4) filter performance determined either as protein bound or as effluent concentration before steady state is reached (e.g., after throughputs of less than a few milliliters per square centimeter) cannot be used to predict or determine filter performance under process-scale conditions of continuous flow and large batch sizes.

Hu et al. [53] investigated the protein adsorption characteristics of modified polyethersulfone, PVDF, and nylon membranes. One milliliter each of various protein solutions (IgG, BSA, and cytochrome c) at various concentrations (20 or 40 μg/mL) were passed through 13 mm membrane disks, and the amount of protein bound was determined by subtracting the amount of protein in the filtrate from the amount in the challenging solution using the BCA protein assay. Both modified PVDF and modified PES showed extremely low protein adsorption, typically less than 1 μg/cm^2, and the nylon membrane exhibited slightly higher levels of protein binding, 6–20 μg/cm^2 depending on the actual protein concentration. Similar results were obtained with ^{125}I-labeled IgG at total protein concentrations of up to 1 mg/mL, with the modified PVDF and modified PES binding less than 5 μg/cm^2, while the amount of nylon adsorbed was 0.4–20 μg/cm^2, depending on the protein concentration. The nylon adsorption data reported here is much lower than that reported by Pitt [50] but is consistent with other studies using nylon membranes [51,52].

Sarry and Sucker [57] reported on the adsorption and inactivation of various model proteins, particularly enzymes, on commercially available membranes under various conditions. All of the data presented, with one exception, appear to have

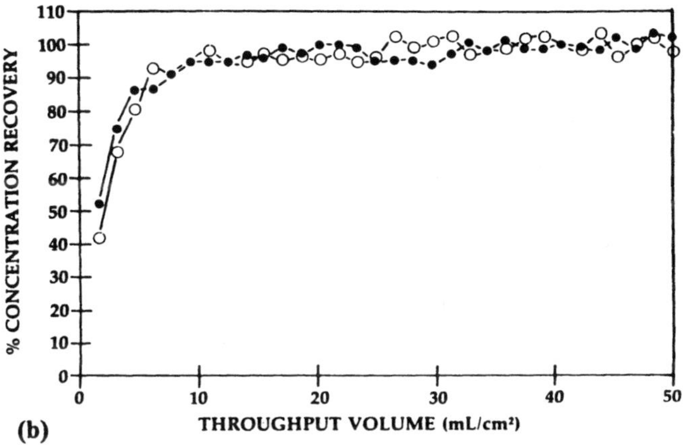

(b)

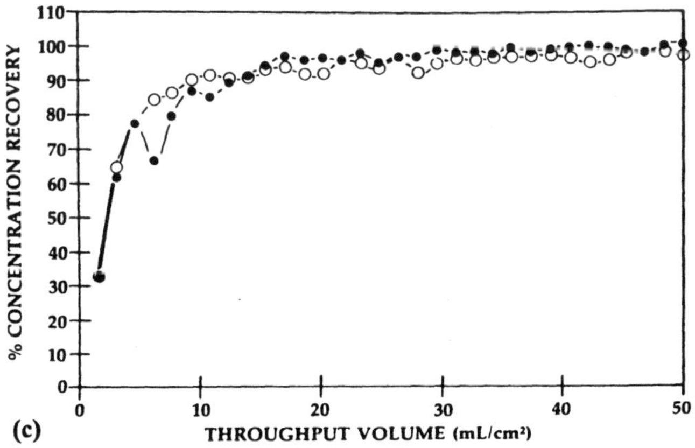

(c)

Figure 6 Continued

been gathered from static soak studies or dynamic studies where effluent concentrations or protein adsorption values are based on throughputs of less than 3 mL/cm^2; the disadvantages of both these approaches have already been discussed in detail earlier. However, the phenomenon of dynamic saturation of filter membranes, demonstrated earlier by Martin and Manteuffel [52], is also shown here in the case of maleate dehydrogenase (MW = 70,000 Da, isoelectric point 6.1–6.4) with two different filter membranes. For this dynamic study, about 20–100 mL of a 50 μg/mL maleate dehydrogenase in 0.1 M NaCl, pH 7.5, was filtered through 25 mm filter disks (effective filtration area 3.5 cm^2); recovery of protein in the filter effluent was followed by a protein assay and by monitoring the enzyme activity. For both filter membranes tested (cellulose nitrate and polysulfone), steady state is achieved rapidly, and saturation volumes were about 5 mL/cm^2 even though the cellulose nitrate membrane showed significantly lower protein concentration recovery in the initial effluent fractions than to the polysulfone membrane. The results presented thus confirm the finding of Martin and Manteuffel [52] that even at low protein concentrations, saturation of filter membranes occurs at relatively low throughput volumes. In addition, the recovery of protein concentration in the filter effluents as measured by a protein assay was essentially identical to that based on the enzymatic activity; thus, filtration through these microporous filter membranes did not adversely affect the activity of the protein. This study goes on to conclude that adsorption of proteins to microporous membranes is a complex phenomenon, dependent on the properties of the protein (such as its structure, surface charge, hydrophobicity, degree of hydration), the solution conditions (such as pH, temperature, ionic strength, and solvent composition), and the membrane surface chemistry.

Jaenchen et al. [58] studied the effect of filtration of three different proteins under various conditions using a hydroxyl-modified polyamide filter membrane. The three proteins studied had varying isoelectric points and molecular weights—BSA (MW 67,000; and pI 4.9), ferritin (MW 450,000; pI 4.4), and cytochrome c (MW 12,300; pI 10.65). Three different buffers were used for these studies to simulate the possible variation in solution conditions—100 mM potassium phosphate buffer (pH 7.0), 100 mM sodium acetate buffer (pH 5.5), and 100 mM Tris-HCl buffer (pH 8.2), with and without 100 mM NaCl. Protein solutions at 10–20 μg/mL protein concentration were pumped through 47 mm hydroxyl-modified polyamide filter membrane disks (14 cm^2 effective filtration area); effluent was collected in 1 mL fractions, and protein concentration was determined using a protein assay. To avoid dilution of the protein solution by residual buffer solution that may be present in the membrane and/or test equipment, the filter disk was used dry and the system was not preflushed.

No measurable protein loss was observed for any protein under any buffer condition; the protein concentration of the first milliliter of the effluent was essentially unchanged from that of the feed, indicating complete recovery of effluent protein concentration and membrane saturation at a throughput of much less than 1 mL/cm^2. The performance of the hydroxyl-modified polyamide membrane is much better than expected from the results of Martin and Manteuffel [52] discussed earlier but consistent with those of Brophy and Lambert [61] discussed below. The discrepancy may be due to the fact that Jaenchen et al. [58] and Brophy and Lambert [61] avoided dilution effects and, which is more important, did not use radiolabeled proteins. As has been mentioned before, the use of radiolabeled proteins can produce serious potential artifacts as the labeling procedure and the presence of the label may change the physicochemical properties of the protein and alter its adsorption properties. The filter performance measured using 47 mm disks was then verified using a filter cartridge with a larger filtration area (1.8 ft^2); no measurable adsorption was observed even at this higher surface area.

A recent report [59] compared the adsorption of BSA and IgG to hydrophilic PVDF membranes from two different filter manufacturers. Both membranes are characterized by their manufacturers as low protein binding, and therefore both were expected to saturate rapidly. Thus, the comparison was confined to the initial phase of rapid binding before saturation was achieved. Solutions of radiolabeled protein at 100 μg/mL in PBS (pH 7.0) were filtered through 13 mm disks; the filtration conditions corresponded to filtering a total volume of 10 L at a flow rate of 2 L/min through a 10 in. cartridge. Following filtration, the amount of radiolabeled protein retained by the filter was determined using a gamma counter; the disks were analyzed while still wet, and without any flushing with buffer, to simulate actual production conditions where filters may remain wet with the product at the end of the filtration run. In the case of IgG, the double-layer hydrophilic PVDF membrane from one manufacturer exhibited higher protein transmission (94% recovery) than another manufacturer's single-layer PVDF membrane (87%). On the other hand, the recovery of BSA through both filter membranes was identical (96%).

Bowen and Gan [60] reported on the adsorption of BSA to hydrophilic PVDF membranes and showed that the extent of adsorption was strongly dependent on pH. In this study, protein solutions (10 mg/mL BSA) were recycled through up to six 25 mm disks; the amount of protein adsorbed was obtained by measuring the depletion of protein in the recirculating solution. Kinetic studies showed that there is a phase of rapid adsorption followed by a slower approach to a limiting value, with the limiting value being reached on the time scale of about 30 min. In addition, the amount of protein adsorbed was shown to be a function of the pH of the solution. At pH 7.0, the authors report no detectable adsorption of protein. As the pH was decreased below 7.0, protein adsorption increased to a broad maximum of about 9 $\mu g/cm^2$ nominal surface area (calculated from the reported value of about 0.23 mg/m^2 BET area and a BET surface area of 0.19 m^2 per 25 mm disk) at a pH range that corresponded roughly to the isoelectric point of BSA (about 5.0). Below pH 4.5, there was an initial decrease in the amount adsorbed at pH 4.0 to about 5 $\mu g/cm^2$ nominal area followed by sharp increase to 15 $\mu g/cm^2$ of nominal surface area at pH 3.0.

The complex pH adsorption profile described above can be explained on the basis of a combination of electrostatic and conformational effects. The magnitude of the zeta potential of the PVDF membranes used in this study decreases from about −19.5 mV at pH 7.0 to about −17.0 mV at pH 3.0. The isoelectric point of BSA is reported to be about 4.5–5.0. At pH 7.0, both the membrane surface and the protein are negatively charged; thus, electrostatic repulsion is responsible for the low protein adsorption observed at this pH. As the pH is lowered to the isoelectric point of the protein, the amount of protein adsorbed increases due to the lowering of the adsorption energy barrier as the protein (and to a smaller extent the surface) becomes less charged. At the isoelectric point, the protein has no net charge, leading to a reduction of the adsorption electrostatic energy barrier and a maximum in protein adsorption. This observation is consistent with the general rule of thumb formulated earlier for protein adsorption: Protein adsorption tends to be at a maximum at the isoelectric point. Below the isoelectric point, the membrane and protein are oppositely charged; thus, adsorption increases with decreasing pH due to the increasing charge contrast. The local minimum in adsorption at pH 4.0, which is not consistent with the aforementioned mechanism, is believed to be related to reversible structural changes that BSA undergoes at this lower pH.

Bowen and Gan [60] also studied the effect of ionic strength on the adsorption of BSA to hydrophilic PVDF membranes at three different pH conditions (3.0, 5.0, and 6.0). No significant difference was observed in the amount of BSA adsorbed as a function of ionic strength of 0.001–0.1 M NaCl or Na_2SO_4 at any of the three pH conditions. This implies that either the simple electrostatic interpretation proposed above is incorrect or, more likely, the ionic strength variations used did not result in a significant charge-screening effect. In the case of 0.001–0.1 M $CaCl_2$, increasing ionic strength did result in increased protein adsorption, presumably due to the ability of BSA to bind calcium ions, which then act as a bridge to the charged membrane surface.

Bowen and Gan [60] also analyzed their adsorption isotherms using the standard Langmuir model and found that it did not provide a reasonable fit to the experimental data. For example, plotting the adsorption data in the ''double-reciprocal'' format (i.e., 1 divided by amount of protein adsorbed versus 1 divided by protein concentration) did not yield a straight line as predicted by the Langmuir isotherm. The protein adsorption isotherms were adequately explained by using a model that allows for two types of sites of different affinities on the membrane surface. They conclude that adsorption of BSA on hydrophilic PVDF occurs through two classes of binding sites of affinities of about 8.5×10^4 and 5.6×10^6 M^{-1}, respectively. Approximately 40% of the BSA bound to the surface at saturation is through the high affinity (5.6×10^6 M^{-1}) sites. The affinity constants reported here are on the low end of values expected for specific protein–protein interactions.

Brophy and Lambert [61] studied the adsorption of a hydrophobic peptide, insulinotropin, to polymeric sterilizing filters. Apart from demonstrating the principle of saturation of filter surfaces after relatively small volumes have been processed even with dilute protein solutions, this study also demonstrates the rule-of-thumb observation regarding the effect of hydrophobicity on protein adsorption. In this study, a 40 μg/mL solution of insulinotropin was passed through 25 mm disks composed of different polymeric materials. In the case of hydrophilic filters, such as the hydroxyl-modified polyamide, the effluent protein concentration recovered completely after processing about 3 mL; this corresponds to a normalized throughput of less than 1 mL/cm^2, which is consistent with the findings of Martin and Manteuffel [52] and Jaenchen et al. [58]. On the other hand, with a hydrophobic filter, such as unmodified PVDF, saturation was not attained even after processing 10 mL of the protein solution. This indicates that protein adsorption increases with increasing hydrophobicity of both the protein and the membrane.

Nema and Avis [62] studied the behavior of lactate dehydrogenase (LDH) during filtration through the following microporous membranes of various pore sizes: hydrophilic PVDF, cellulose mixed esters, polycarbonate, hydrophilic polysulfone, and acrylic copolymer on a nylon support. Although this study used a limited throughput (<5 mL/cm^2; the disadvantages of such tests have been discussed before), it nevertheless demonstrates (1) the importance of testing the contribution of prefilters to the overall adsorptive loss of a filtration system, (2) the retention of protein biological (or enzymatic) activity during filtration, and (3) the phenomenon of ''nonsaturable'' binding that occurs with some protein systems. All membranes used in this study except cellulose mixed esters are described by their manufacturers as ''low'' protein-binding. LDH at 22 μg/mL was filtered through 25 mm diameter filter disks at a constant rate of 2.7 mL/min until a total of 25 mL had been collected in 5 mL aliquots. Each effluent aliquot was then assayed for protein recovery using the Bradford assay, and the first 5 mL aliquot was also tested for enzyme activity. The study reports a good correlation between the protein content and protein activity in the filtrate in all cases, indicating that the protein recovered in the filtrate maintained its enzymatic activity. The hydrophilic PVDF and polycarbonate membranes showed the least loss of LDH during filtration, with close to complete recovery within the first 5 mL (about 1 mL/cm^2). The exception to this general observation was the 5.0 μm-rated hydrophilic PVDF, which showed a significantly higher protein loss than either the 0.65 or 0.2 μm-rated filters; this was attributed to the fact that this filter is the only PVDF filter tested that was cast on a support polymer. This observation stresses the importance of testing not only the final sterilizing grade filter but also any prefilter that may be present in the system (see also Datar et al. [63]). The other membranes used in the study (hydrophilic polysulfone, acrylic copolymer on nylon, and cellulose mixed esters) all exhibited higher levels of protein loss during filtration; a stable plateau value was not reached until about 15–20 mL of solution had been passed through (about 3–4 mL/cm^2).

In all cases, including the hydrophilic PVDF membranes, a stable plateau value that represented significantly less than complete (100%) recovery was attained. This type of nonsaturable binding can sometimes be indicative of losses associated with sieving (i.e., removal of particulate-associated or undissolved protein) or protein deposition. The latter is the more likely explanation in this case, given the fact that the stable plateau value was dependent on the membrane type. In protein deposition, the protein is initially adsorbed to the membrane surface; the adsorbed protein layer then can continue to adsorb more protein, primarily as a result of protein–protein interactions. Generally, the phenomenon of protein deposition is membrane-independent as observed here (i.e., it occurs irrespective of the membrane type), but its extent may depend on the membrane type. Thus, a membrane that inherently adsorbs low amounts of protein due to membrane–protein interactions (for example, the hydrophilic PVDF membrane, which adsorbs much less than a monolayer of protein; see Ref. 50) may exhibit a higher plateau value (or lower loss through the course of the filtration) because there are few adsorbed protein molecules through which additional protein adsorption can occur. In this case, the hydrophilic PVDF membranes (with the exception of the 5, μm-rated membrane) exhibit a stable plateau value of very close to 100%. On the other hand, a membrane that inherently binds a larger amount of protein due to membrane–protein interactions (such as the cellulose mixed esters in this study, which can adsorb a monolayer or more of protein under static conditions [50]) can adsorb significantly more protein onto this monolayer via additional protein–protein interactions; consequently, the stable plateau value reached will be lower (about 80% in the case of the cellulose mixed esters).

Filter Cartridge Studies

All of the studies reviewed above used small filter membrane disks to evaluate potential protein loss during microporous membrane filtration. The use of small filter membrane disks does not adequately address the overall effect of cartridge support and drainage layers or of any prefilters in the system. The first study to report on the dynamics of protein recovery from process filtration systems using filter cartridges was published by Datar et al. [63]. A dilute solution of BSA in phosphate-buffered saline (PBS, 150 mM NaCl, 10 mM Na_2PO_4, pH 7.0) was used following prefiltration through a 0.2 μm filter cartridge to remove particulates and undissolved protein; the protein concentration was 90 μg/mL (±3%) following particulate prefiltration. Several sterilizing grade filter cartridges as well as prefilter grade cartridges were included in the study. All filter cartridges were prewet with deionized water and allowed to drip drain for 15 min before being placed in their housings, and flow was maintained at 2 L/min. Upstream and downstream protein concentrations were constantly monitored during the run by measuring the UV absorbance at 280 nm using an optical flow cell and photodiode array system; protein recovery was expressed as downstream filtrate concentration as a percent of the upstream feed concentration.

Figure 7 shows the recovery of BSA at 90 μg/mL through several different 10 in. filter cartridges. Both the hydroxyl-modified polyamide and the hydrophilic PVDF membrane cartridges, characterized by their manufacturers as "low protein binding" show no discernible loss in the effluent protein concentration. This performance is considerably better than can be expected from the results of the filter membrane disk studies of Martin and Manteuffel [52] reviewed earlier; the discrepancy is more than likely the result of differences in the adsorption characteristics of unlabeled and

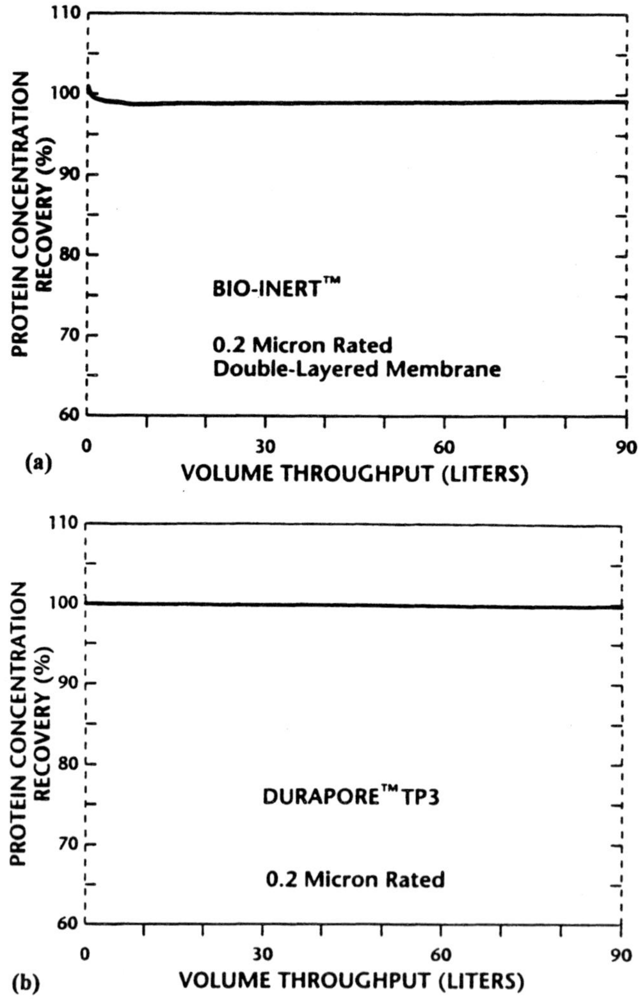

Figure 7 Recovery of bovine serum albumin (90 μg/mL) through 10 in. membrane final filter cartridges. (a) Hydroxyl-modified hydrophilic polyamide membrane cartridge. (b) Hydrophilic PVDF membrane cartridge. (c) Polysulfone membrane cartridge. (d) Cellulose acetate membrane cartridge. (From Ref. 63.)

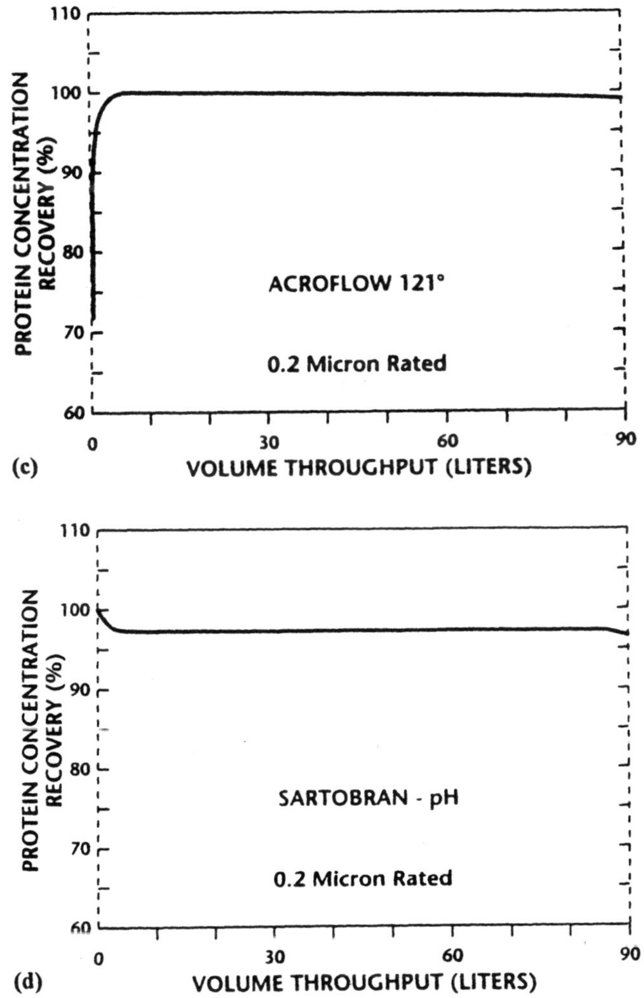

Figure 7 Continued

radiolabeled protein. The polysulfone membrane cartridge exhibited a saturation volume of less than 5 L; however, despite excellent protein recovery in the initial stages of the test, the effluent protein concentration appeared to drop slightly with increasing throughput. Finally, the cellulose acetate membrane cartridge continued to exhibit protein loss throughout the course of the filtration. This is possibly attributable to the presence of surfactant in the cellulose acetate membrane for wettability, which coincidently retards protein loss in initial throughputs; with increasing throughputs, the surfactant is extracted out from the membrane, resulting in an increase in protein binding later in the process.

Figure 8 shows the recovery of BSA at 90 μg/mL through several different 10 in. prefilter cartridges. During sterile process filtration, it is common to incorporate pleated or depth prefilters to protect the more expensive sterilizing grade filters and to enhance the economy of the filtration system. Polypropylene prefilters commonly

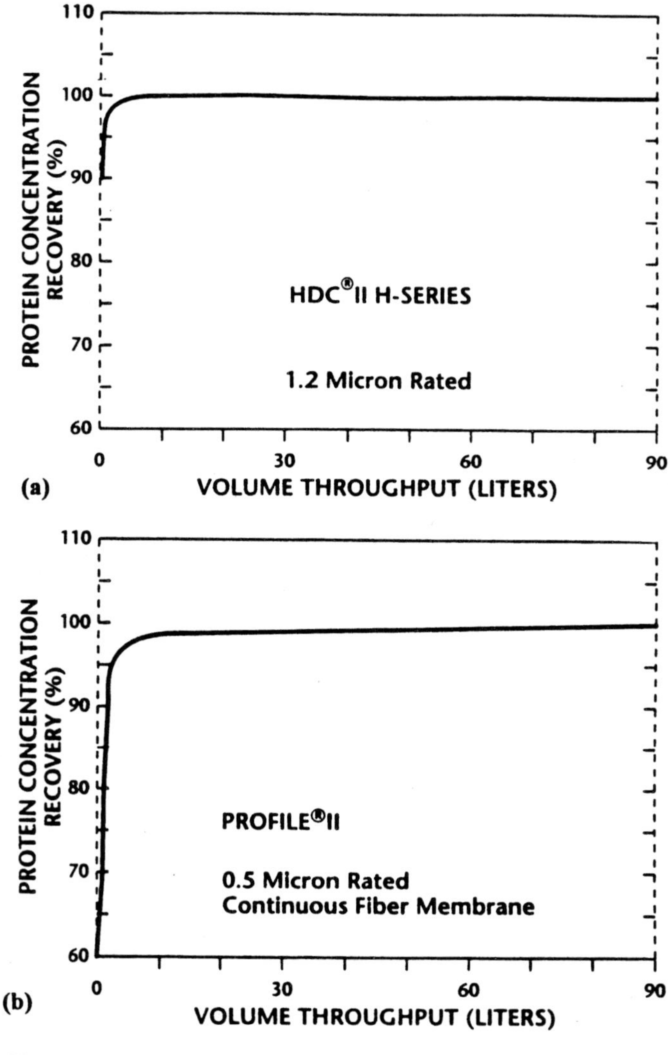

Figure 8 Recovery of bovine serum albumin (90 μg/mL) through 10 in. membrane prefilter cartridges. (a) Pleased polypropylene membrane cartridge (1.2 μm particulate rating). (b) Depth polypropylene cartridge (0.5 μm particulate rating). (c) Hydrophilic hydroxyl-modified polyamide membrane. (d) Cellulose mixed ester membrane cartridge. (From Ref. 63.)

recommended for cell and debris removal have raised concern over the potential for protein binding to the relatively hydrophobic polypropylene. Neither the pleated nor the depth polypropylene filter used in this study contributed to any significant protein loss; in both cases, saturation volumes were about 1–2 L per 10 in. cartridge. The hydroxyl-modified polyamide prefilter cartridge showed no discernible protein loss as expected from the results with the sterilizing grade filter. On the other hand, the cellulose acetate prefilter showed considerable protein loss, with recovery of effluent protein concentration not complete even after processing 90 L through a 10 in. cartridge.

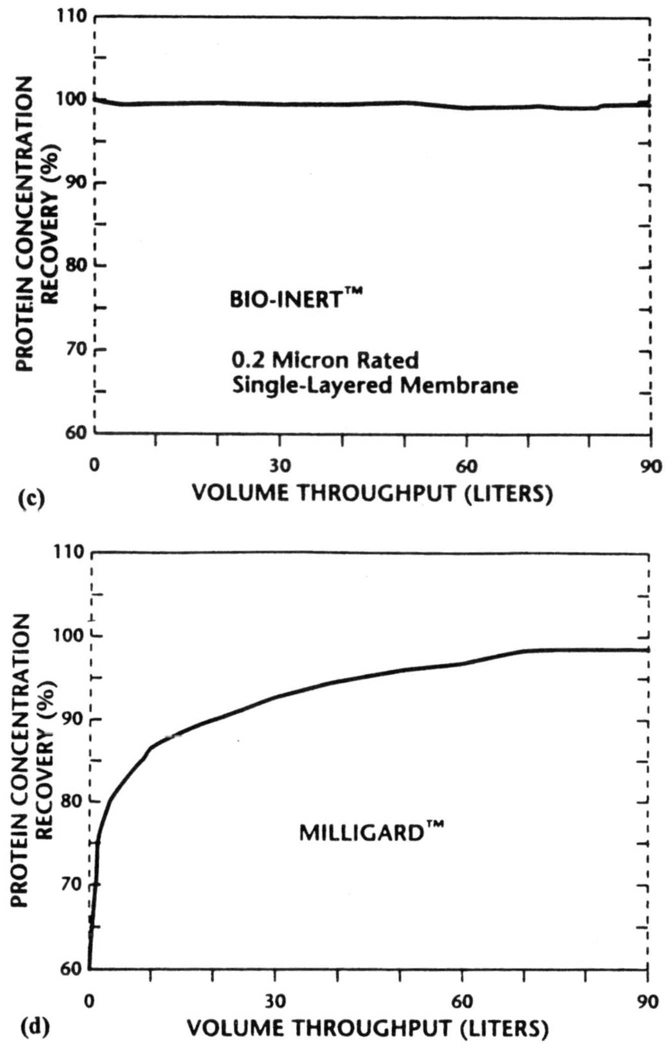

Figure 8 Continued

Figure 9 shows the recovery of BSA at 90 μg/mL through two different 10 in. prefilter–filter combinations. The hydroxyl-modified polyamide prefilter–final filter combination demonstrated high protein recoveries, as expected from the performance of the individual filter cartridges. The slightly lower protein recovery in the initial effluent fractions as well as the slightly higher saturation volume for the prefilter–filter combination compared to the final filter alone is directly related to the additional contact area for the fluid available as a result of addition of the prefilter. The results for the cellulose acetate prefilter–hydrophilic PVDF final filter combination demonstrate the importance of considering the protein adsorptive characteristics of the entire filtration system including the prefilters rather than just that of the final filters alone. In this case, the use of a low protein binding filter as the final filter did not

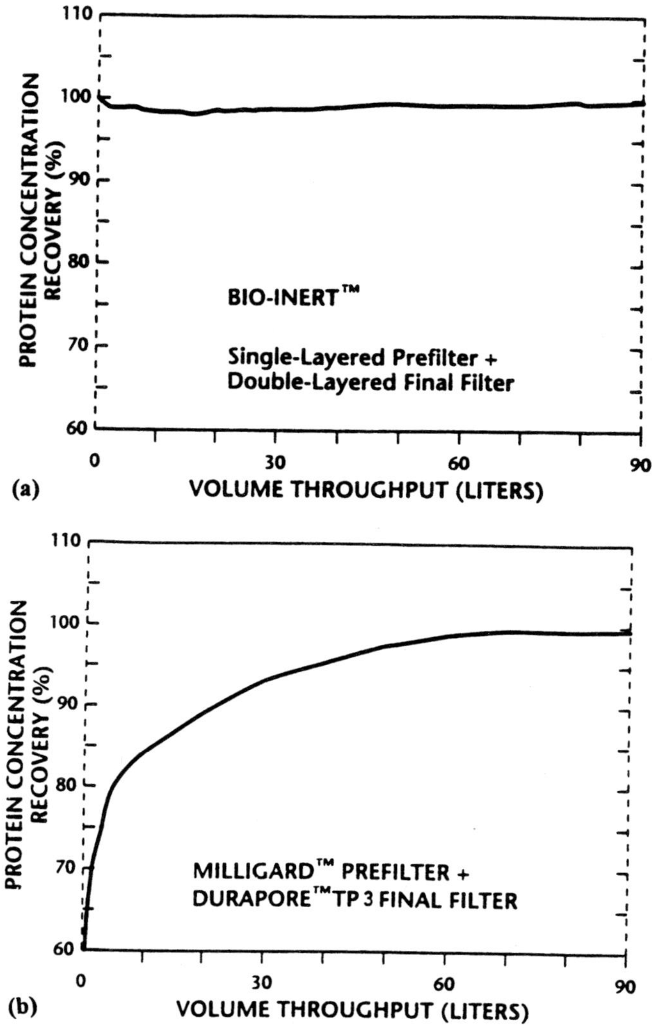

Figure 9 Recovery of bovine serum albumin (90 μg/mL) through 10 in. prefilter to final filter cartridge systems. (a) Hydrophilic hydroxyl-modified polyamide membrane system. (b) Cellulose mixed ester prefilter plus hydrophilic PVDF system. (From Ref. 63.)

succeed in reducing protein loss due to the high binding capacity of the cellulose acetate prefilter.

4 LABORATORY-SCALE DETERMINATION OF PROTEIN ADSORPTION

It is clear from the preceding discussion that adsorption of proteins to microporous membranes is a complex multifactorial phenomenon. It is dependent on the properties of the protein, the solution conditions, the process parameters, and the nature of the membrane surface. The literature of many manufacturers contains protein adsorption data, usually expressed as mass (in micrograms) of protein bound per unit area. However, such values are usually not of much use when it comes to predicting filter performance in an actual process-scale application. First, data reported apply only to the model protein used (typically, BSA and IgG) under the specific conditions (buffer composition, protein concentration, pH, temperature, etc.) used to generate the information; other proteins under different conditions could show different results, and thus the relevance of the data to a specific process is questionable. Second, experimental protocols used to generate this information are normally not reported, making it difficult to assess the data. Third, as has been mentioned earlier, protein adsorption values expressed as counts per minute per square centimeter (cpm/cm^2) or micrograms per square centimeter ($\mu g/cm^2$), do not provide the process engineer information on the saturation volume or the dynamics of protein concentration recovery and do not account for the effect of process parameters such as flow rate and batch size.

Effects of the filter on the product formulation, including adsorption and extractables, should be documented [64]. Information regarding extractables is usually readily available from the filter manufacturer. Adsorption testing, on the other hand, is frequently done by the filter user, due to its multifactorial on nature as well as the need for product-specific assays. It must be pointed out that laboratory-scale adsorption experiments carried out early in and during process development can guide efforts to mitigate adsorptive losses by proper selection of process parameters such as flow rate and formulation parameters such as pH and ionic strength [65]. Appropriately scaled-down laboratory tests using filter membrane disks can yield much of the information needed. Generally, the largest filtration area (typically 47 mm disks) that is reasonable with respect to accuracy, time, and expense should be considered. It is important to account for the presence of any nonwoven support material in the filter cartridge by including disks of these materials, if available, along with the filter membrane during the tests.

4.1 Test Conditions

The first step is to scale down the process parameters as a ratio of the production filter and test filter surface areas. Thus, the flow rate and throughput required in the lab-scale test to simulate the production-scale run are calculated using the formulas

$$\text{Test flow rate} = \text{process flow rate} \times \frac{\text{test filter area}}{\text{process filter area}} \tag{2}$$

and

$$\text{Test throughput} = \text{process batch size} \times \frac{\text{test filter area}}{\text{process filter area}} \tag{3}$$

For example, a standard filter cartridge may have an effective filtration area of 5 ft^2 (about 4650 cm^2), whereas a 47 mm disk has an effective filtration area of 0.015 ft^2 (about 14 cm^2). Thus, a process involving the filtration of 100 L of a protein solution through a standard filter cartridge at a flow rate of 1 L/min corresponds to filtering 300 mL of the solution at 3 mL/min through a 47 mm disk. It must be noted that the filter membrane becomes saturated rapidly in most cases; consequently, it may seem unnecessary to process the entire scaled-down batch volume in the test. However, it is advisable to continue the test until the entire scaled-down batch volume has been processed, especially with complex protein solutions.

4.2 Test Equipment

The test equipment should simulate the actual process to the fullest extent possible by using the same materials of construction as those anticipated for manufacturing (tubing, housing, etc). It is important to include the appropriate negative control, i.e., a "blank" run without a filter membrane, to account for any adsorption to the test equipment. It may also be desirable to include a positive control, one using a filter membrane of known high protein adsorption capacity (e.g., alcohol- and then water-wetted polyethylenetetrafluoroethane (PTFE) membrane, or cellulose mixed esters as used by Nema and Axis [62]) to ensure that both the test protocol and the protein assay procedure are capable of detecting adsorptive losses.

4.3 Prefilters

As has been established by Nema and Avis [62] and Datar et al. [63], prefilters can contribute in a significant manner to the protein adsorption capacity of a filtration system; consequently, any prefilters that are present in the process must be included in the test setup. This is easily done in the case of membrane prefilters by including the appropriate filter membrane disks in the filter holder. In the case of depth prefilters, where filter disks are not available, tests can be carried out using smaller segments (e.g., 1 in. segments) if available. It is important to keep the ratio between the prefilter and final filter areas in the test the same as that in the process, as it is not uncommon to have different filter areas at these two stages. In cases where it is logistically difficult to maintain this ratio (e.g., in cases involving depth prefilters), it may be easier to test each stage separately.

4.4 Test Protein Solution

The protein solution used for the test should also simulate the production sample as much as possible. This includes factors such as protein concentration, pH, ionic strength, buffer composition (including additives, organic solvents, stabilizers, etc.), degree of purity of the protein, and presence of protein aggregates. It is important to note that any undissolved protein present will be removed by the filters as a result of sieving. Such losses cannot be ascribed to adsorption and can be avoided by filtering the test protein solution to remove particulates prior to using it in the test. The actual mechanism of protein loss during filtration (sieving losses vs. adsorptive losses) may sometimes seem secondary to a process engineer, but it is crucial in determining the strategies that will be useful in minimizing adsorption effects. In such cases where the intent is to determine the total protein loss irrespective of mechanism, the protein solution for the test should be formulated under exactly the same conditions as the process fluid—for example, using identical mixing times. Sieving losses, if present, will show up in the saturation curve as a plateau value that is consistently below complete recovery of the effluent protein concentration.

4.5 Sampling Regime

Samples of the feed protein solution should be taken immediately before and after the test; the latter is especially important if biological activity of the protein is also being measured. Samples of the filtrate should be taken sequentially, starting with the initial effluent and including points within the intended discard volume (if known) and points out on the plateau. As has been shown by a number of studies reviewed in the preceding section, membrane saturation occurs rapidly; thus, it is important to sample more frequently in the initial stages of the test. The sample size should be the smallest volume possible still sufficient to perform the requisite protein assays. This restriction minimizes ''averaging'' effects and provides a fairly close approximation to the instantaneous protein concentration in the filtrate.

4.6 Protein Assay

Finally, the appropriate protein assays should be used to assess recovery. These include total protein assays such as the Folin–Lowry assay and its numerous modifications and the Bradford and other dye-binding assays [66]. In many cases, complete reagent kits with detailed instructions on carrying out such assays are available from several commercial sources. It is important to ensure that the assay selected can accurately determine protein content at the concentration level used in the test and that there are no interfering components in the formulation. Standard curves for such assays should be generated using known concentrations of the test protein solution in the same buffer; if this is not possible, the standard curve can be generated using a model protein (usually BSA) in the same buffer as the test solution. Another assay that can be used to determine protein recovery is UV spectrophotometry at 280 nm; this is based on the absorbance of residues such as tyrosine and tryptophan at this wavelength. This method is generally used with high purity products and requires an accurately determined extinction coefficient. Unlike the aforementioned assays, which are mass-based, activity-based assays that use a specific biological property of the protein such as its enzymatic activity or binding to antibodies can also be employed. Activity-based assays commonly used include specific enzyme assays as well as immunoassays such as ELISA (enzyme-linked immunosorbent assay). When using an activity-based assay, it is important to also include a mass-based assay in order to distinguish between loss of protein and loss of protein activity.

5 STRATEGIES TO MINIMIZE ADSORPTIVE LOSSES DURING MICROFILTRATION

Adsorption of proteins can occur whenever any solid surface comes in contact with a protein solution. Thus, contributions to adsorptive losses (or other losses) in a given process can come from many sources, including the filter. It is therefore important to first identify the source(s) of the problem instead of focusing just on the filter. When it has been established that the filter contributes significantly to protein adsorption, adsorptive losses can often be minimized using a number of different strategies, some of which are described below. It must be emphasized that these options are not mutually exclusive and that the best results are often obtained by combining two or more approaches. Initiating tests early in process development allows the bioprocess engineer to take full advantage of these options.

5.1 System Design

Adsorption saturates in a small volume relative to batch size; thus, adsorption affects only the initial filtrate. In a batch operation, where the initial filtrate is pooled with the whole filtrate, the loss is often a minimal percent of the product. Thus, designing the system so as to average the lowered concentration of the initial effluent with the bulk of the effluent that contains the expected concentration of the protein can minimize or eliminate the consequences of adsorptive losses. In a filling operation, where the initial filtrate is often discarded for other reasons, such a loss does not affect the process. If the product is expensive and a discard is not feasible, a frequently used strategy to minimize the consequence of adsorptive losses is to recirculate the product through the filter prior to the filling process. An alternative strategy is to filter into a sterile holding tank downstream of the filter prior to filling; this is, in effect, operating the filtration process in a batch mode separate from the filling mode to take advantage of the averaging phenomenon. In some filling operations, a holding tank is normally included between the filter and the filling operation to either average flow rates or prevent water hammer and can even permit downsizing of the filter system.

5.2 Optimal Filter Size

Since the amount of protein adsorbed is a function of the area available for adsorption to take place, reducing the filter system size will also reduce the magnitude of saturable adsorption. In many cases, the filter is oversized and careful testing can result in its replacement with a smaller filter without altering any other system parameters. In other cases, appropriate prefiltration will often extend final filter life and allow the use of a smaller filter. It is important to remember that the prefilter can itself contribute to adsorptive losses and therefore addition of a prefilter can be justified only when there is a reduction in the overall system size. Alternatively, the prefilter can be operated in a batch process to minimize the consequence of adsorptive losses at this stage.

Consideration should also be given to membrane cartridge area relative to flow rate and differential pressure. For example, different filter cartridge materials may have similar protein-binding characteristics on a unit area basis, but the one that has the lowest clean differential pressure and/or filter area in the cartridge format offers the most potential for minimizing adsorption effects. In such a case, it may be possible to operate the process at either a higher flow rate or with a lower area, thus minimizing adsorptive losses.

5.3 Process Fluid Composition

The solution conditions and buffer composition of the process fluid can have a large impact on adsorption; consequently, manipulation of such solvent properties as pH, ionic strength, concentration of organics, surfactants, stabilizers, and other additives (including carrier proteins such as albumin) can be used to minimize adsorptive losses [67,68]. pH and ionic strength may be expected to have an impact when adsorption is driven by electrostatic considerations, and organic solvents and surfactants when it is hydrophobic in nature. Typically, such parameters are set early in process development prior to development of the filtration system. To avoid getting locked into a formulation with unfavorable adsorption characteristics, development of the filtration system concurrently with the product formulation may be advisable.

In a recent study, Johnston [69] investigated the effect of solvent additives on the adsorption of recombinant human granulocyte colony stimulating factor (rhG-

CSF) to materials such as glass and other polymeric materials commonly used in the packaging and delivery of therapeutic proteins. The use of polymers, polyols, and surface-active agents (including nonionic and anionic surfactants) as stabilizers in protein formulations has been well established [70]; these additives may also serve to reduce adsorptive losses. Solvent additives that were tested included glycerin USP at concentrations ranging from 0.5 to 25% (v/v), Pluronic F-127 and Pluronic F-68 at concentrations ranging from 0.005 to 0.5% (w/w), and Tween 80 and Tween 20 at concentrations ranging from 0.005 to 0.5% (w/w). Of the additives tested, Tween 20 was generally found to be most efficacious in inhibiting the adsorption of rhG-CSF to PVC and glass. The one exception was Pluronic F-127 at 0.05%, which gave the best results, a twofold reduction, in the amount of rhG-CSF adsorbed on PVC. In an earlier study, Pluronic F-127 at 0.05% was found to be as effective as human serum albumin (HSA) in inhibiting adsorption of rhG-CSF to PVC [71]. Interestingly, the amount of protein adsorbed on PVC was determined to be in the range of 40–170 ng/cm^2, which is very consistent with the adsorption values per unit BET area seen for typical filter materials.

5.4 Optimal Membrane Surface Chemistry

When it has been established that the filter contributes substantially to observed adsorptive losses, changing the membrane surface chemistry may result in decreased adsorption. Such effects are often modest, but significant decreases have been observed in some cases upon switching to a low protein binding membrane. Most filter manufacturers offer a variety of low protein binding surface chemistries that may be tested to minimize adsorption. However, switching membrane chemistries based solely on filter manufacturer claims and data without actual testing under the user's process conditions is not advisable. The effect of changing filter membranes on other aspects of the process should be carefully considered along with the enhanced performance of the filter with respect to adsorption. These include changes in process parameters such as flow rate and filtration system size as well as other measures of filter performance such as extractables.

5.5 Nonsaturable Binding

If the phenomenon of nonsaturable binding occurs, an investigation into the cause is necessary in order to devise solutions. If sieving-related losses are responsible, merely changing membrane chemistry will not resolve the problem. In such a case, formulation of the protein solution needs to be reexamined in order to reduce or eliminate undissolved protein. Typically, one would expect losses from sieving with proteins that are poorly soluble and/or at high protein concentrations. Cases where nonsaturable binding cannot be attributed to sieving may be the result of protein deposition primarily mediated by protein–protein interactions. The primary consequence of protein deposition in microfiltration is usually membrane fouling, and only occasionally does it significantly affect protein recovery. Protein deposition tends to occur at fairly high protein concentrations, where (relatively) small amounts of protein are deposited that can have a large effect on membrane flux but little effect on the effluent protein concentration. In cases where it does occur, it can usually be resolved by eliminating causes of protein aggregation and/or denaturation such as foaming, extreme temperature and/or pH, and shear stress. Changing solution characteristics such as pH and ionic strength to minimize protein–protein interactions can also help [72,73]. In one case [74], BSA aggregation in bulk solution and the resultant fouling were shown to occur through the formation of intermolecular thiol disulfide linkage between BSA molecules through its free sulfhydryl residue, Cys 34. Blocking this reactive moiety by chemical modification was shown to eliminate fouling during BSA microfiltration. In addition, fouling was shown to be reduced in the presence of metal chelators such as EDTA and citrate, low pH (<7.0), and the presence of reducing agents (dithiothreitol), all of which also operate by reducing BSA aggregation.

6 SUMMARY

The phenomenon of protein adsorption is not unique to membrane filtration but affects the performance of many materials and processes in areas ranging from medicine to biochemical engineering. Based on the vast experimental literature on the adsorption of proteins to solid surfaces, several general principles of protein adsorption have been formulated that also apply to adsorption to microporous membranes; these are summarized in Table 2. An understanding of the basic principles governing protein adsorption is essential to the proper design and operation of microfiltration applications.

Most biotechnological/pharmaceutical processes operate under conditions where saturable binding of protein of interest to microfiltration membranes is not and has not been of concern. Adsorptive losses are thus not an actual problem in the case of most bulk filtration processes and at most working concentrations or in cases where a preflush of the filtration system is possible. The conditions under which protein losses may become significant are usually limited: (1) When small batches of expensive and relatively dilute protein solutions need to be sterile-filtered for maximum product recovery and (2) in vial-filling operations with such solutions, where it is important to maintain constant concentration levels in each vial and when preflushing is not feasible due to economic and/or time constraints.

Studies with microporous membranes as well as filter cartridges have shown that:

1. Membrane saturation occurs relatively rapidly, with effluent protein concentrations reaching steady state after low throughput volumes.
2. Recoveries of influent protein concentration during membrane filtration of nondilute protein solutions (≥1 mg/mL) are extremely rapid, so the effects of individual membrane types are not distinguishable.
3. Membrane filters characterized as "low protein binding" may be advantageous at very dilute concentrations (on the order of 10 μg/mL).
4. Filter performance determined either as protein bound in static soak tests or as effluent concentration in dynamic tests before steady state is reached (e.g., after throughputs of less than a few milliliters per square centimeter) cannot be used to predict or determine filter performance under process-scale conditions of continuous flow and large batch sizes.
5. Adsorption of proteins to microporous membranes is a complex phenomenon, dependent on the properties of the protein (such as its structure, surface charge, hydrophobicity, degree of hydration), the solution condi-

tions (such as pH, temperature, ionic strength, and solvent composition), and the membrane surface chemistry.

Adsorption of proteins to microporous membranes is a complex, multifactorial phenomenon. It is dependent on the properties of the protein, the solution conditions, the process parameters, and the nature of the membrane surface. It is therefore important to conduct laboratory tests to evaluate membrane filters for potential protein loss by adsorption during filtration. These can be performed using throughput volumes and flow rates that are scaled down from the anticipated process–filtration conditions. These tests yield much of the information needed by the process engineer to predict filter performance in an actual process-scale application. It is important to include the appropriate negative control, i.e., a "blank" run without a filter membrane, to account for any adsorption to the test equipment. Prefilters can contribute in a significant manner to the protein adsorption capacity of a filtration system; consequently, any prefilters that are present in the process must be included in the test setup. The protein solution sued for the test should also simulate the production sample as much as possible. These include factors such as protein concentration, pH, ionic strength, buffer composition (including additives, organic solvents, stabilizers, etc.), degree of purity of the protein, and presence of protein aggregates. Samples of the feed protein solution should be taken immediately before and after the test; the latter is especially important if biological activity of the protein is also being measured. Samples of the filtrate should be taken sequentially, starting with the initial effluent and including points within the intended discard volume (if known) and points out on the plateau. Appropriate protein assays, total protein (e.g., dye-binding assays) and/or protein activity-based assays (e.g., enzymatic activity, ELISA), should be used to assess recovery.

Adsorption of proteins can occur whenever any surface comes in contact with a protein solution. Thus, contributions to adsorptive losses (or other losses) in a given microfiltration process can come from many sources, including the filter. Many studies dealing with protein adsorption on microporous membranes fail to point this out and therefore do the filter user a disservice by diverting attention from proper process system design to a single system component (in this case, the filter). When it has been established that the filter contributes significantly to protein adsorption, adsorptive losses can often be minimized using a number of different strategies. These include proper system design, optimizing filter size, manipulating fluid composition and conditions, and evaluating "low protein–binding" membrane chemistries. These options are not mutually exclusive, and the best results are often obtained by combining two or more of these approaches. Initiating tests early in process development allows the bioprocess engineer to take full advantage of these options.

REFERENCES

1. J.-F. P. Hamel and J. B. Hunter, Modeling and applications of downstream processing, in *Downstream Processing and Bioseparation: Recovery and Purification of Biological Products*, ACS Symp. Ser. 419 (J.-F. P. Hamel, J. B. Hunter, and S. K. Sikdar, eds.), American Chemical Society, Washington, DC, 1990, pp. 1–35.
2. G. Belfort and C. A. Heath, Biotechnology processes: Membrane materials, modules, and process design, in *Membrane Processes in Separation and Purification* (J. G. Crespo and K. W. Boddeker, eds.), Kluwer Academic, Boston, 1994, pp. 9–26.

3. K. H. Oshima, T. T. Evans-Strickfaden, A. K. Highsmith, and E. W. Ades, The use of a microporous polyvinylidene fluoride (PVDF) membrane filter to separate contaminating viral particles from biologically important proteins, *Biologicals, 24*: 137–145 (1996).
4. H. Aranha-Creado, K. Oshima, S. Jafari, G. Howard, Jr., and H. Brandwein, Virus retention by a hydrophilic triple layer PVDF microporous membrane filter, *J. Pharm. Sci. Tech.*, in press (May/June 1997).
5. K. H. Oshima, T. W. Comans, A. K. Highsmith, and E. W. Ades, Removal of human immunodeficiency virus by a 0.04-μm membrane filter, *J. AIDS 8*: 64–65 (1995).
6. K. H. Oshima, A. K. Highsmith, and E. W. Ades, Removal of influenza A virus, phage T1, and PP7 from fluids with a nylon 0.04-μm membrane filter, *Environ. Toxicol. Water Qual.: Int. J., 9*: 165–170 (1994).
7. M. Wahlgren and T. Arnebrant, Protein adsorption to solid surfaces, *Trends Biotechnol. 9*(6): 201–208 (1991).
8. Y. J. Wang and M. Hanson, Parenteral formulation of proteins and peptides: Stability and stabilizers, Tech. Rep. 10, *J. Parenter. Sci. Technol. 42*: S1 (1988).
9. J. D. Andrade, Principles of protein adsorption, in *Surface and Interfacial Aspects of Biomedical Polymers*, Vol. 2, *Protein Adsorption* (J. D. Andrade, ed.), Plenum, New York, 1985, pp. 1–79.
10. T. A. Horbett, Adsorption of proteins and peptides at interfaces, in *Stability of Protein Pharmaceuticals, Part A: Chemical and Physical Pathways of Protein Degradation* (T. J. Ahern and M. C. Manning, eds.), Plenum, New York, 1992, pp. 195–214.
11. J. L. Brash, Mechanism of protein adsorption to solid surfaces, in *Biocompatible Polymers* (M. Szycher, ed.), Technomic, 1983, pp. 32–52.
12. A. G. Walton and B. Koltisko, Protein structure and kinetics of interaction with surfaces, in *Biomaterials: Interfacial Phenomena and Applications*, Adv. Chem. Ser. 199, 1982. pp. 245–264.
13. W. Norde, Adsorption of proteins from solution at the solid–liquid interface, *Adv. Colloid Interface Sci., 25*: 267–340 (1986).
14. B. W. Morrissey and C. C. Han, The conformation of gamma-globulin adsorbed on polystyrene lattices determined by quasielastic light scattering, *J. Colloid Interface Sci., 65*: 423–431 (1978).
15. B. W. Morrissey, L. E. Smith, R. R. Stromberg, and C. A. Fenstermaker, Ellipsometric investigation of the effect of potential on blood protein conformation and absorbance, *J. Colloid Interface Sci., 56*: 557–563 (1976).
16. W. J. Dillman and I. F. Miller, On the adsorption of serum proteins on polymer membranes, *J. Colloid Interface Sci., 44*: 221–241 (1973).
17. W. Norde and J. Lyklema, The adsorption of human plasma albumin and bovine pancreas ribonuclease at negatively charged polystyrene surfaces, *J. Colloid Interface Sci., 66*: 257–266 (1978).
18. E. Nyilas, T. H. Chiu, and G. A. Herzlinger, Thermodynamics of native protein/foreign surface interactions. I. Calorimetry of the human globulin/glass system, *Trans. Am. Soc. Artif. Intern. Organs, 20*: 480–490 (1974).
19. C. R. McMillin and A. G. Walton, Circular dichroism technique for study of adsorbed protein structure, *J. Colloid Interface Sci., 48*: 345–348 (1974).
20. A. G. Walton and F. C. Maenpa, Applications of fluorescence spectroscopy to the study of proteins at interfaces. *J. Colloid Interface Sci., 72*: 268–278 (1979).
21. B. M. C. Chan and J. L. Brash, Conformational change in fibrinogen desorbed from glass surfaces, *J. Colloid Interface Sci., 84*: 263–265 (1981).
22. G. K. Iwamoto, L. Winterton, R. A. Van Wagenan, J. D. Andrade, and D. Mosher, Fibronectin adsorption via TIRF, *J. Colloid Interface Sci., 112*: 447–456 (1985).
23. V. Hlady, R. A. Van Wagenan, and J. D. Andrade, Total internal reflection intrinsic fluorescence spectroscopy applied to protein adsorption, in *Surface and Interfacial Aspects*

of Biomedical Polymers, Vol. 2, *Protein Adsorption* (J. D. Andrade, ed.), Plenum, New York, 1985, pp. 81–106.

24. D. R. Lu and K. Park, Effect of surface hydrophobicity on the conformational changes of adsorbed fibrinogen, *J. Colloid Interface Sci., 144*: 271–281 (1991).
25. W. G. Pitt, D. J. Fabrizius-Homan, D. F. Mosher, and S. L. Cooper, Vitronectin adsorption on polystyrene and oxidized polystyrene, *J. Colloid Interface Sci., 129*: 231–239 (1989).
26. C. Narasimhan and C. S. Lai, Conformational changes of plasma fibronectin detected upon adsorption to solid substrates: A spin-label study, *Biochemistry, 28*: 5041–5046 (1989).
27. A. Kondo, F. Murakami, and K. Higashitani, Circular dichroism studies on conformational changes in protein molecules upon adsorption on ultrafine polystyrene particles, *Biotech. Bioeng., 40*: 889–894 (1992).
28. M. E. Soderquist and A. G. Walton, Structural changes in proteins adsorbed on polymer surfaces, *J. Colloid Interface Sci., 75*: 386–392 (1980).
29. W. Norde, F. MacRitchie, G. Nowick, and J. Lyklema, Protein adsorption at solid–liquid interfaces: Reversibility and conformation aspects, *J. Colloid Interface Sci., 112*: 447–456 (1986).
30. J. L. Brash, S. Uniyal, and B. M. C. Chan, Interactions of proteins in plasma with various foreign surfaces, *Artif. Organs 5*(Suppl.): 475–477 (1981).
31. L. Vroman, A. Adams, M. Klings, and G. Fisher, Fibrinogen, globulins, albumin and plasma at interfaces, *Adv. Chem. Ser., 145*: 255 (1975).
32. L. Vroman, A. Adams, M. Klings, G. Fisher, P. C. Munoz, and R. P. Solensky, Reactions of formed elements of blood with plasma proteins at interfaces, *Ann. N.Y. Acad. Sci., 283*: 65–76 (1977).
33. J. L. Brash and P. Ten Hove, Effect of plasma dilution on adsorption of fibrinogen to solid surfaces, *Thromb. Haemostas., 51*: 326–330 (1984).
34. J. W. Corsel, G. M. Willems, J. M. M. Kop, P. A. Cuypers, and W. Th. Hermens, The role of intrinsic binding rate and transport rate in the adsorption of prothrombin, albumin, and fibrinogen to phospholipid bilayers, *J. Colloid Interface Sci., 11*: 544–533 (1986).
35. R. D. Bagnall, J. A. D. Annis, and P. A. Arundel, Adsorption of plasma proteins, *J. Biomed. Mater. Res., 12*: 653–663 (1978).
36. W. Norde, Adsorption of proteins at solid surfaces, in *Adhesion and Adsorption of Polymer*, Vol. 2 (L.-H. Y. Lee, ed.), Plenum, New York, 1980, pp. 801–826.
37. F. MacRitchie, Proteins at interfaces, *Adv. Protein Chem., 32*: 283–326 (1978).
38. T. Suzawa and H. Shirahama, Adsorption of plasma proteins onto polymer latices, *Adv. Colloid Interface Sci., 35*: 139–172 (1991).
39. R. E. Crandall, J. Janotova, and J. D. Andrade, Effects of radioiodination and fluorescent labelling in albumin, *Prep. Biochem., 11*: 111–138 (1981).
40. H. G. W. Lensen, D. Bargeman, P. Bergueld, C. A. Smolders, and J. Feijen, HPLC to measure competitive adsorption of proteins, *J. Colloid Interface Sci., 99*: 108 (1984).
41. S. T. Kelly, W. S. Opong, and A. L. Zydney, The influence of protein aggregates on the fouling of microfiltration membranes during stirred cell filtration, *J. Membrane Sci., 80*: 175–187 (1993).
42. Y.-F. Maa and C. C. Hsu, Membrane fouling in sterile filtration of recombinant human growth hormone, *Biotech. Bioeng., 50*: 319–328 (1996).
43. A. D. Marshall, P. A. Munro, and G. Tragardh, The effect of protein fouling in microfiltration and ultrafiltration on permeate flux, protein retention, and selectivity: A literature review, *Desalination, 91*: 65–108 (1993).
44. A. L. Zydney, Membrane fouling, in *Microfiltration and Ultrafiltration: Principles and Applications* (L. J. Zeman and A. L. Zydney, eds.), Marcel Dekker, New York, 1996, pp. 397–446.

45. A. S. Chandarvarkar, Dynamics of fouling of microporous membranes by proteins, Ph.D. Thesis, Massachusetts Institute of Technology, Cambridge, MA, 1990.
46. W. R. Gowen and Q. Gan, Properties of microfiltration membranes: Flux loss during constant pressure permeation of bovine serum albumin, *Biotech. Bioeng., 38*: 688–696 (1991).
47. W. R. Gowen and Q. Gan, Properties of microfiltration membranes: The effects of adsorption and shear on the recovery of an enzyme, *Biotech. Bioeng., 40*: 491–497 (1992).
48. M. Hlavacek and F. Bouchet, Constant flowrate blocking laws and an example of their application to dead-end microfiltration of protein solutions, *J. Membrane Sci., 82*: 285–292 (1993).
49. S. T. Kelly and A. L. Zydney, Fouling mechanisms during BSA microfiltration, *J. Membrane Sci., 107*: 115–124 (1995).
50. A. M. Pitt, The nonspecific protein binding of polymeric microporous membranes, *J. Parenter. Sci. Technol. 41*(3): 110–113 (1986).
51. K. M. Persson, G. Capannelli, A. Bottino, and G. Traagardh, Porosity and protein adsorption of four polymeric microfiltration membranes, *J. Membrane Sci., 76*: 61–71 (1993).
52. J. M. Martin and R. L. Manteuffel, Protein recovery from effluents of microporous membranes, *Biopharm, Nov/Dec*: 20–25 (1988).
53. H. Hu, J. Camilleri, and W. Tamashiro, A new membrane for biopharmaceutical filtration, *Pharm. Tech., 17*:30–44 (1993).
54. L. J. Zeman, Characterization of MF/UF membranes, in *Microfiltration and Ultrafiltration: Principles and Applications* (L. J. Zeman and A. L. Zydney, eds.), Marcel Dekker, New York, 1996, pp. 180–291.
55. A. Baskin and D. J. Lyman, The interaction of plasma proteins with polymers. I. Relationship between polymer surface energy and protein adsorption/desorption, *J. Biomed. Mater. Res., 14*: 393–401 (1980).
56. M. Kim, J. Kojima, K. Saito, and S. Furusaki, Reduction of the nonselective adsorption of proteins by hydrophilization of microfiltration membranes by radiation-induced grafting, *Biotechnol. Prog., 10*: 114–120 (1994).
57. C. Sarry and H. Sucker, Adsorption of proteins on microporous membrane filter: Part II, *Pharm. Tech., 17*(1): 60–70 (1993).
58. R. Jaenchen, P. Ball, C. Rohrich, and D. Nitze, Investigations into Filtration of Protein Solutions with Pall Bio-Inert® Membranes, Pall Sci. Tech. Rep. STR PUF 16, Pall Corp., Port Washington, NY, 1992.
59. Transmission of Proteins and Preservatives through Pall Fluorodyne® II Filters, Pall Sci. Tech. Rep. STR PUF 25, Pall Corp., Port Washington, NY, 1996.
60. R. W. Bowen and Q. Gan, Properties of microfiltration membranes: Adsorption of BSA at polyvinylidene fluoride membranes, *J. Colloid Interface Sci., 144*: 254–261 (1991).
61. R. T. Brophy and W. J. Lambert, The adsorption of insulinotropin to polymeric sterilizing filters, *J. Parenteral Sci. Technol., 48*: 92–94 (1994).
62. S. Nema and K. E. Avis, Loss of LDH activity during membrane filtration, *J. Parenter. Sci. Technol., 47*: 16–21 (1993).
63. R. Datar, J. M. Martin, and R. L. Manteuffel, Dynamics of protein recovery from process filtration systems using microporous membrane filter cartridges, *J. Parenter. Sci. Technol. 46*(2): 35–42 (1992).
64. FDA Sterilization Process Validation—Recommendations for Information To Be Submitted to Human and Veterinary Applications, Food and Drug Administration, Bethesda, MD, 1993.
65. J. Detyna, Adsorption validation for aseptic filtration, *J. Validation Tech., 1*(4): 46–50 (1995).

66. A. Darbre, Analytical methods, in *Practical Protein Chemistry: A Handbook* (A. Darbre, ed.), IRL Press, 1986, pp. 227–337.
67. S. Sato, C. E. Ebert, and S. W. Kim, Prevention of insulin self-association and surface adsorption, *J. Pharm. Sci., 72*: 228–232 (1983).
68. C. H. Suelter and M. DeLuca, How to prevent losses of protein by adsorption to glass and plastic, *Anal. Biochem., 135*: 112–119 (1983).
69. T. P. Johnston, Adsorption of recombinant human granulocyte colony stimulating factor (rhC-CSF) to polyvinyl chloride, polypropylene, and glass: Effect of solvent additives, *J. Parenter. Sci. Technol., 50*(4): 238–245 (1996).
70. Y. J. Wang and M. Hanson, Parenteral formulations of proteins and peptides: Stability and stabilizers, Tech. Rep. 10, *J. Parenter. Sci. Technol., 42*: S1 (1988).
71. P. Wang, G. O. Udeani, and T. P. Johnston, Inhibition of granulocyte colony stimulating factor (G-CSF) adsorption to PVC using a nonionic surfactant, *Int. J. Pharm., 1995*: 177–182.
72. S. P. Palecek and A. L. Zydney, Hydraulic permeability of protein deposits formed during microfiltration: Effect of pH and ionic strength, *J. Membrane Sci., 95*: 71–79 (1994).
73. S. P. Palecek and A. L. Zydney, Intermolecular electrostatic interactions and their effect on flux and protein deposition during protein filtration, *Biotechnol. Prog., 10*: 207–213 (1994).
74. S. T. Kelly and A. L. Zydney, Effects of intermolecular thiol-disulfide interchange reactions on BSA fouling during microfiltration, *Biotechnol. Bioeng., 44*: 972–982 (1994).

18

Microbial Retention Testing in the Validation of Sterilizing Filtration

JEFFREY R. CARTER and RICHARD V. LEVY
Millipore Corporation, Bedford, Massachusetts

1 INTRODUCTION

The objective of this chapter is to provide the pharmaceutical manufacturer with an introduction to the microbiological aspects of verifying the performance of sterilizing grade filters, including filter qualification and validation. It should be used as a practical guide and as a review of the current literature and thinking within the industry.

A filter is qualified by the filter manufacturer as sterilizing grade on the basis of its ability to completely retain high levels of microorganisms, as demonstrated by the results of a microbial retention test. Filter manufacturers generally base their testing method on methods published by the American Society for Testing and Materials (ASTM Committee F-21, 1988) and Health Industry Manufacturers Association (HIMA, 1982) and on guidance provided the Food and Drug Administration's Guideline on Sterile Drug Products Produced by Aseptic Processing (FDA, 1987). Table 1 provides a comparison of the information contained in these documents.

Generally, there is a great deal of overlap between the first two documents, which provide substantially more procedural detail than the FDA guideline. Still, because the ASTM and HIMA methods are not specifically intended as qualification or validation tests, many critical components are missing. For example, the ASTM and HIMA documents do not provide guidance on critical issues such as the number of tests required per lot, how positive results (organisms detected in the filtrate) are handled, and qualification of membrane versus qualification of fabricated filter device. These issues are left to the discretion of the filter manufacturer, and the stringency of the standards to which the various filter vendors hold themselves serves to

Table 1 Relevant Documents Used to Define the Basic Principles Used in Microbial Retention Testing

Document	Stated purpose
HIMA, Document No.	"[To document] some methods that may be used by filter manufacturers to microbiologically evaluate sterilizing filters . . . to serve as an informative document for users of sterilizing filters in their choice of filters for their specific applications."
ASTM, Method No. F 838-83, reapproved 1988	"This test method determines the bacterial retention characteristics of membrane filters for liquid filtration using *Pseudomonas diminuta* as the challenge organism. This test may be employed to evaluate any membrane filter system used for liquid sterilization."
FDA Guideline on Sterile Drug Products Produced by Aseptic Processing, 1987	"This guideline informs interested persons on certain practices and procedures for the preparation of sterile drug products by aseptic processing that constitute acceptable means of complying with certain sections of the Current Good Manufacturing Practice (cGMP) regulations for drug products (Title 21 Code of Federal Regulations, Parts 210 and 211)."
PDA Technical Report No. 26: Sterilizing Filtration of Liquids	"To provide a systematic approach to selecting and validating the most appropriate filter for a sterilizing filtration application."

differentiate the products they market. In other words, not all sterilizing grade filters are qualified by equal or even equivalent standards. Nevertheless, the ASTM and HIMA documents provide methods to evaluate filters, independently of the many applications in which the filter can be used. As such, the principles embodied in these methods can very easily be adapted for use as a qualification test. The FDA guideline, on the other hand, focuses primarily on validating that the filter one chooses to use in a given application will provide a sterile effluent. Table 2 summarizes the differences between the methods described in each document. Very recently, the Parenteral Drug Association's (PDA) sterile filtration committee has drafted a technical report on sterilizing filtration (1997). Prompted at least in part by the FDA guideline's insufficient level of specific information to satisfy present-day filter validation needs, the PDA document is much more detail oriented. Still, the reader should recognize that until specified by regulatory authorities, the PDA document holds no legal standing.

2 BACKGROUND: MECHANISMS OF MICROBIAL RETENTION

To understand the principles and objectives for performing microbial retention tests, it is beneficial to review the mechanisms by which microporous sterilizing grade filters are thought to remove particulate matter from liquid streams. The three generally recognized classes of bacterial retention mechanisms used by microporous

Table 2 A Comparison of "Guidelines" for Performing Microbial Retention Testing of Sterilizing Grade Filters

	HIMA (1982)	**ASTM** (1983, 1988)	**FDA Guideline** (1987)	**PDA Technical Report** (1997)
Organism	*P. diminuta*	*P. diminuta*	*P. diminuta*	*B. diminuta*, bioburden second choice
Challenge level	10^7 cfu/cm^2 of effective filtration area	10^7 cfu/cm^2 of effective filtration area	$\geq 10^7$ cfu/cm^2 of effective filtration area	$\geq 10^7$ cfu/cm^2 of effective filtration area
Culturing Method	1. Saline lactose broth method 2. Frozen cell paste method 3. An equivalent method	1. Saline lactose broth method 2. Frozen cell paste method 3. An equivalent method	"Properly grown, harvested, and used"	1. Saline lactose broth method 2. Frozen cell paste method 3. An equivalent method
Challenge Volume	Not considered	Not considered	Not considered	Simulate an actual process
Challenge ΔP across membrane (disks)	30 psig	30 psig maximum	Simulate an actual process	Simulate an actual process
Challenge ΔP across membrane (devices)	Cartridge test not controlled by pressure	30 psig maximum	Simulate an actual process	Meet or exceed actual process
Challenge flow rate (disks)	Disk test not controlled by flow rate	0.5 - 1 gpm per ft^2 of filter surface area	Simulate an actual process	Meet or exceed actual process
Challenge flow rate (cartridges)	1 gpm per 0.1 m^2 of filter area	0.5 - 1 gpm per 1 ft^2 of filter surface area	Simulate an actual process	Meet or exceed actual process
Challenge vehicle	Not considered	1. Saline lactose broth 2. Sterile saline	Simulate an actual process	Simulate actual product
Methods for detecting organism passage	1. 0.45 μm analytical filter 2. Direct incubation (presence/absence test in broth medium)	0.45 μm analytical filter	Not considered	0.45 μm or 0.2 μm analytical filter
Integrity Test	Correlation to bacterial retention is presumed	Not considered	Correlate to filter performance	Must correlate to bacterial retention
Status	No longer supported by HIMA	Still available and supported	Being considered for revision	Scheduled for publication in 1997

membranes are size exclusion, adsorption, and cake filtration[1] (Lee et al., 1993). Virtually all microporous membranes used in pharmaceutical processing can employ

[1]Cake filtration refers to a situation in which a heavily loaded filter relies on the buildup of contaminant particles on the surface for the removal of subsequent particles. Sterilizing grade filters in the pharmaceutical industry are usually not subjected to such heavy particulate loads that cake filtration becomes a significant mechanism of microbial retention.

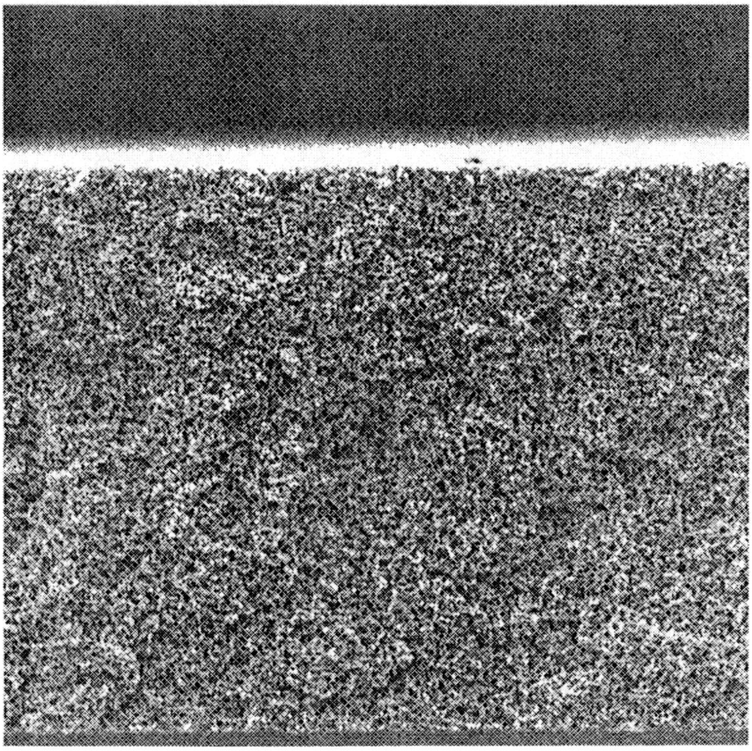

a

Figure 1 Scanning electron micrographs of (a) symmetric and (b) asymmetric microporous membranes.

any of the three retention mechanisms, to varying degrees. It has been generally claimed that the current sterilizing grade membranes rely almost exclusively on size exclusion and/or adsorptive properties.

''Size exclusion'' refers to the inability of a particle to travel through a microporous membrane simply because a critical opening in the path of the particle is prohibitively small. The particle is therefore mechanically prohibited from further movement through the filter. If this critical opening occurs at the surface of the filter, the filter is said to act by sieving. If it occurs within the depth of the filter, the filter is said to act by entrapment. Thus, size exclusion is a combination of sieving and entrapment, and in practice most sterilizing grade filters use a combination of sieving and entrapment. However, membranes can be specifically engineered, by modulating the symmetry of the porous structure, to favor either sieving or entrapment. Examples of variations in structural symmetry are shown in Fig. 1. Figure 1a is a scanning electron micrograph of a symmetric microporous membrane, and Fig. 1b is a scanning electron micrograph of an asymmetric microporous membrane. Whereas a large proportion of the critical openings is located toward the upstream surface of the symmetric membrane, the critical openings of the asymmetric membrane are generally well within its microporous structure.

Because size exclusion is a physical or mechanical removal of particles, as long as the relationship between particle size distribution and pore size distribution

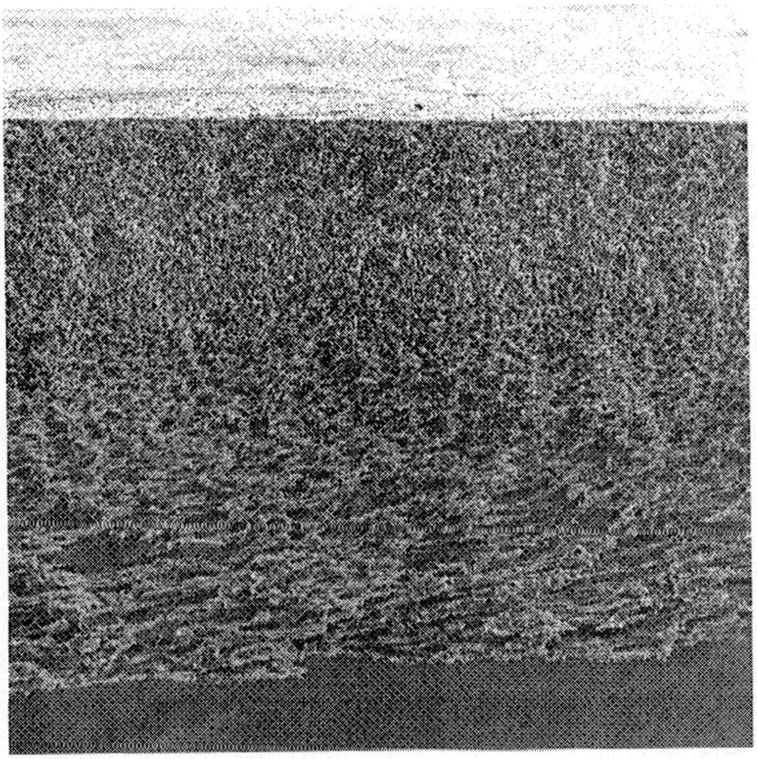

b

Figure 1 Continued

remains constant, size exclusion should remain independent of changes to any filtration parameter. Evidence to support the belief that sterilizing grade filters rely primarily on size exclusion has been presented by several authors.

Levy (1987) showed that hydrophilic poly(vinylidene fluoride) sterilizing grade membrane is fully retentive of organisms suspended in solutions of pH 6.3–8.0, 0.01% Triton X-100, 0.01 M $MgCl_2$, 0.01 M $AlCl_3$, 20% glycerol, and 5% propylene glycol, all of which were tested at applied pressures of 30 and 50 psi. These fluids and pressures were chosen for their potential for reducing the efficiency of adsorptive removal of bacteria. Perhaps the best intuitive evidence for the primary role of size exclusion is provided by the relationship between microbial retention and the bubble point, an indirect indicator of the largest pores in the filter.[2] It has been clearly documented that microbial retention efficiency increases in direct proportion to filter bubble point (Reti et al., 1979; Leahy, 1983; Levy and Leahy, 1991). Simply stated, these works show that retention efficiency is directly related to filter pore size, a strong indication of the prevalence of size exclusion.

---

[2]Bubble point, described elsewhere in this book, is the pressure required to overcome capillary forces that serve to hold a liquid within the pores of a wetted filter. Because this pressure is inversely related to capillary diameter, the largest pores will be voided of liquid first. Therefore, bubble point is an indication of the largest pores of the filter.

The second retention mechanism, absorptive removal, requires a physicochemical, noncovalent bonding or interaction between the filter medium and the particle to be removed. The efficiency of adsorptive removal is dictated primarily by the surface chemistry of the membrane and that of the organism, the physical and chemical attributes of the liquid vehicle, and the processing conditions. Organism adsorption requires a series of events that can be split into three phases: physical approach of the organism to the filter matrix, formation of a noncovalent bond, and maintenance of this bond throughout the entire filtration process. Although volumes could be written about the chemistry and physics of these interactions, what follows is a broad description of the various factors that could influence each of the three phases. Although size exclusion is the most desirable retention mechanism from a reliability point of view, some sterilizing grade filters may be specifically designed to take advantage of such adsorptive removal.

2.1 Approach

Bond formation initially requires an approach to the surface of the filter by the bacterial cell, until a critical distance is achieved. Beyond this distance, the two surfaces do not interact. This approach can be modulated by many factors. For example, the size of the pores relative to the size of the target particle will dictate the maximum distance that a particle can be separated from the wall of the filter while it is traveling through the porous structure. The tortuosity of the flow path within the filter will contribute to the likelihood that a particle can deviate from a laminar flow streamline to collide with the pore wall. The rate of flow per unit area has potential to influence particle approach. As speed increases, the residence time of the particle in the membrane matrix will decrease, which will provide less opportunity for surface–surface interaction. Higher solution viscosity will provide a hindrance to random migration (diffusion, Brownian motion, motility) of organisms, reducing random collisions with the internal membrane surface.

2.2 Noncovalent Bond Formation

The primary modes of this interaction are ionic/electrostatic interactions and hydrophobic interactions. Both are subject to modulation by the suspending medium, in that the liquid vehicle has an effect on the physicochemical surface character of both the bacterial cell and the membrane filter (Grant et al., 1988). The strength of ionic interactions is dictated by the surface charges of the bacterial cell and the membrane filter. In its most simplified form, the explanation of ionic interactions is that opposites attract. Because most bacterial cells and organic matter have a net negative charge under relatively neutral pH (e.g., Bayer and Bayer, 1994), positively charged membranes or filter media can be used to remove these particles. The strength of the interaction depends on the degree of ionization of the ionizable species and the number or density of the charges. These factors are partly intrinsic properties of the chemical groups providing the charge and are partly dictated by the liquid in which the surfaces are in contact. For example, the negative charge of a particle will tend to be neutralized as pH is lowered (e.g., Drozd and Schwartzbrod, 1996). Similarly, a high density of charged solute molecules, i.e., a high ionic strength, tends to effectively shield or counter particle charges, thus reducing surface–surface charge attraction.

Hydrophobic interactions result when it is energetically more favorable for a surface to contact another surface rather than for it to remain in contact with the aqueous vehicle. Again, the degree to which these interactions occur is dictated by fluid chemistry and by particle and membrane surface chemistries. These interactions are primarily dictated by the polarity of the suspending fluid and by the relative hydrophobicities of the particle and membrane surface.

2.3 Bond Maintenance

Once the noncovalent bond has been formed, it is critical that it be maintained throughout the entire filtration process. Alterations in both the physical and chemical conditions can lead to breakage of the bond, reentrainment of the particle, and potential passage of the particle through the filter. Pressure spikes throughout a process cause rapid changes in shear force on an adsorbed particle, a force that works against those of the adsorptive bond. Pressure spikes are common with blow-fill-seal machines, in which flow is interrupted and resumed on the order of once per second. Chemical changes that could disrupt the surface–surface interaction are analogous to those at play in various chromatographies. Ionic interactions can be disrupted by increasing the ionic strength or changing the pH of the solution. Hydrophobic interactions can be weakened or reversed by reducing the polarity of the solution, reducing the ionic strength, adding a nonpolar solute (e.g., ethanol, ethylene glycol), or adding a surfactant.

3 THE MICROBIAL RETENTION TEST

The microbial retention test is performed to measure the retention efficiency of the test filter. Its three most basic components are as follows.

A test filter. In theory, the test filter can range from flat disks in filter holders to relatively large fabricated devices such as stacked disk devices or pleated cartridges. If disk testing is meant to provide information on the performance of a filter device, it is critical that the disks be of the same membrane as that which is incorporated into the device. Not all manufacturers offer flat disks of the same membrane that is incorporated into devices.

A system to deliver the microbial (bacterial) challenge suspension to the test filter. The delivery system can range from a small reservoir plumbed to the upstream of the filter holder and filled by hand with a bacterial suspension to a large manifolded system simultaneously feeding several test filters. To simplify the design, flow is usually delivered by an upstream applied pressure source using sterile compressed gas. However, flow can be delivered by pumps and can be modulated if the test requires control over flow rate.

A system to assay the test filter effluent. The system for assaying the effluent is generally that of a membrane-based recovery system. Typically, the downstream effluent is passed through an assay membrane disk rated at 0.45 μm. This disk is placed on a solid bacteriological growth medium and incubated under appropriate conditions to favor the growth of organisms. The assay filter can be placed in line with the test filter, in which case fluid will flow through the test filter and the assay filter concurrently. Alternatively, the filtrate may be collected in a sterile reservoir and subsequently passed through an independent assay filter.

There has recently been considerable discussion concerning the appropriateness of using a 0.45 μm filter to detect organisms that have already passed through a sterilizing grade filter (Groves, 1991; Meltzer, 1993). In fact, the performance advantages of a 0.45 μm filter over that of a 0.2 or even a 0.1 μm filter for water and wastewater microbiology have been recognized for years (Sladek et al., 1975; Taylor and Geldreich, 1979). Moreover, 0.45 μm filters have been specified for bacterial recovery in standard methods of the American Public Health Association (APHA, 1992), HIMA (1982), ASTM (ASTM Committee F-21, 1988), and U.S. Pharmacopeia (1995). Essentially, the rationale for using a 0.45 μm filter (Sladek et al., 1975) is that the more open pore structure of this filter provides a more favorable environment for the trapped cells to proliferate into a colony after the filter is placed on a solid growth medium. On a 0.2 μm filter, most of the trapped organisms remain on the surface of the filter, where they are more susceptible to desiccation. Moreover, the tighter pore structure is seen as an impediment to diffusive flow of nutrients from the growth medium to the cell and of metabolic waste products away from the cell. Thus, although a 0.45 μm filter might allow passage of a small percentage of microorganisms, this percentage is smaller than the percentage of organisms that will fail to form colonies on a 0.2 μm filter due to the poorer growth environment. In fact, it has been shown that with freshly cultured *B. diminuta*, neither the perceived disadvantages of the 0.45 μm filter (bacterial passage) nor those of the 0.22 μm filter (reduced colony formation efficiency) were realized; the filters recovered the challenge organisms equally well (Carter, 1996).

Having said this, is must be emphasized that the choice of a recovery filter should be based on the performance of that filter in the particular application. The 0.45 μm filter has a very long and successful track record in the area of bacterial recovery and should be considered the more appropriate candidate in almost all cases. Nevertheless, there are situations in which a 0.22 μm filter might be the better membrane. For example, where the assay filter is used to monitor a dilute process stream, medium, or drug product known to harbor small microorganisms and the assay filter is to be immersed in liquid growth medium as part of a presence/absence test, it would be hard to argue against the use of a tighter filter. Ultimately, the choice of membranes should, in every case, be justified on the basis of performance, not on pore size rating.

Regardless of the test filter size and process complexity, every test system should have certain basic features. First, valves should be included in appropriate positions throughout the system and should not be installed if they are not necessary. Pressure gauges should be placed upstream and downstream of the test filter in order to most accurately determine a pressure differential (ΔP) across the filter. This is especially important if the assay filter is used concurrently with the test filter, for a ΔP across the assay filter must be accounted for when ΔP across the test filter is being measured. Hydrophobic vent filters should be a part of every reservoir that will require air exchange due to emptying or filling of the reservoir. In all cases, aseptic connections should be minimized.

The very nature of the microbial retention test dictates that only filters for which no test organism (*B. diminuta* or other relevant microorganism) is detected downstream are deemed sterilizing grade and that the appearance of even one bacterial colony detected on an assay filter is reason to consider the filter nonretentive. Thus, results of 0 and 1 are considered to be significantly different, and controls are required to ensure that one does not obtain either of these values illegitmately. In this context, a false positive result is the presence of colonies on the assay filter of what was truly a sterilizing grade test filter (no passage through the filter, but some recovered on the assay filter), and a false negative result is the absence of colonies on the assay filter of a defective or non-sterilizing-grade test filter.

False positives can occur via several possible sources. One should be especially suspicious of growth on assay filters if there is also growth on the agar surrounding the assay filter. Generally, this is caused by airborne bacteria, possibly the aerosolized challenge organisms, that have settled on the assay filter and the agar. A second suspicious scenario is one in which the positive results are clustered. Generally, this is caused by operator error leading to aerosolization that will potentially contaminate all of the assay filters processed after the error occurred. Other sources of false positives are improperly sterilized equipment or reagents or improperly sealed filters. The common sources of false positives are summarized in Table 3.

False negatives are defined in the context of microbial retention testing as a negative result (zero colonies on the assay filters) obtained by testing a truly nonretentive filter. It is not a simple task to gather retrospective evidence to prove or disprove the occurrence of a false negative. Therefore, rigorous preventive measures intrinsic to proper test design and validation should be in place to ensure that potential sources of false negatives have been accounted for and thereby to avoid false negatives in the first place. For example, organism viability in the test liquid vehicle should be established to prevent a retention test from being run with dead organisms.

Table 3 Sources and Prevention of False Positives in Microbial Retention Testing

Source of false positive result	Prevention/determination
Improperly sterilized assay filters or other part of the testing apparatus	Determine identity of the bacterial colonies. Review assay filter sterilization records and procedures. Prior to the test, pass sterile fluid through the system and assay the fluid for presence of contamination.
Aerosolization of the bacterial challenge suspension	Use equipment designed to minimize the occurrence. Use environmental monitoring to detect the event. Plate filters in a facility different from that in which the challenge test is performed. Provide proper operator training. Colonies on the agar as well as on the assay filter generally indicates that the entire plate was contaminated by airborne organisms.
Operator contamination	Provide proper operator training.
Nonintegral filter; damaged O-ring; improperly seated disk filter	Integrity test unit before and after retention testing. Do not perform tests on filters that do not pass the integrity test.
Nonsterilizing grade filter placed in test filter position	Check bubble point or other integrity test value to ensure that minimum specification is met.

Table 4 Sources and Prevention of False Negatives in Microbial Retention Testing

Source of false negative result	Prevention/determination
Test organism not viable in liquid vehicle.	Establish viability before proceeding with the retention test.
Test organism does not form visible colonies on assay filter.	Establish a validated protocol for detecting microorganisms on the assay filter.
Test organism not properly cultured.	Test method must be established and followed to prevent culturing of cells that are unacceptably large for this purpose. Use 0.45 μm size control to verify that organism is of suitable size compared to *B. diminuta.*
Test organism forms aggregates in liquid vehicle.	Check challenge solution for aggregation by light microscopy using wet mount preparation (hanging drop) or Gram stain.
Other microorganisms on assay filters.	Contamination on assay filter may mask presence of test microorganism.
	Determine and correct cause of contamination, and rerun test.

Similarly, one should validate a microbial recovery method to ensure that organisms passing through the test filter will be detectable. Generally, this will involve capturing the organisms on a 0.45 μm filter and then rinsing the filter with a defined volume of fluid that is effective in removing bacteriostatic activity from the filter.

With regard to the test organism, one should verify that the appropriate microorganism is being used and that it is being properly cultured according to a standard procedure. Some procedures, such as the frozen cell paste method (ASTM Committee F-21, 1988), have the potential for inducing microorganism aggregation. (The protocol itself calls for ultrasonic pretreatment of the bacterial suspension.) Aggregation may also occur when test microorganisms are introduced into certain fluids. Certainly, aggregated organisms will be removed more efficiently from the liquid stream than nonaggregated cells. The problem with cellular aggregation is acknowledged in the 1987 Guideline on Sterile Products Produced by Aseptic Processing (FDA, 1987). The common sources of false negatives are summarized in Table 4.

3.1 The Test Organism: *Brevundimonas diminuta*

The industry standard test organism for qualifying sterilizing grade filters is *Brevundimonas diminuta* [*B. diminuta*; formerly *Pseudomonas diminuta* (Segers et al., 1994)], ATCC19146. As well as any other single species, *B. diminuta* meets the requirements of a standard test organism.

Relevance

A microorganism is considered relevant if it was isolated from a raw material such as water, a purified intermediate, or final drug formulation *and* if it is considered to be at risk for passing through a sterilizing grade filter based on size or other attributes such as cell wall deficiency. *B. diminuta* was originally isolated as a contaminant in a penicillinase solution that had been filtered through a 0.45 μm filter in a pharmaceutical process (Bowman and Holdowsky, 1960) that was intended to be aseptic, and is therefore considered a relevant test organism. This bacterium, or any other microorganism, could be considered relevant.

Aggregation

If a sterilizing grade filter removes organisms via size exclusion, the most stringent test of this filter should employ a nonaggregated particle. Very small cells that become aggregated may behave as a single large particle that is relatively easy to remove from the fluid stream. When cultured according to accepted methods, *B. diminuta* exhibits very little aggregation.

Size

In a similar vein, the ideal test organism should be cultured to a very small size. To date, of the organisms we have studied, *B. diminuta* represents the smallest. (See also Sec. 4.3 and 5.1.)

Shape

It is generally accepted that for cells of any given width, those with the smaller length will represent the most stringent challenge. Thus, the most stringent challenge would be to use perfectly spherical cells. In practice, coccoid cells have a relatively large diameter compared to the width of properly cultured *B. diminuta*. They generally do not represent a microorganism that one would encounter in an aseptic processing facility (human flora not withstanding), and they generally grow as aggregated clusters or chains, which in effect negates the benefit of the coccoid shape. Properly cultured *B. diminuta* cells have a marked reduction in length-to-width ratio, changing from a true bacillary form to a coccobacillary form (Meltzer, 1987, pp. 502–503).

Ease of Culture

Brevundimonas diminuta can be cultured to relatively high densities using inexpensive and simple growth media. Presently there are two recognized methods for culturing *B. diminuta* for use in microbial retention testing of sterilizing grade filters: the saline lactose broth method and the frozen cell paste method (FDA, 1987; ASTM Committee F-21, 1988), which have been previously described. If other culturing methods are considered, nutrient-rich media, which might be used to promote shorter generation times and higher cell densities at stationary phase, typically lead to larger cellular dimensions and should be avoided. More dilute media, nutrient-poor media, or media that are antagonistic to the microorganism typically lead to longer generation times, smaller cell densities, and smaller cellular dimensions. These conditions are generally preferable for use in culturing test microorganisms to achieve "worst-case" characteristics.

Safety

As a general theme with all microbiological test organisms, operator safety dictates that the organism be nonpathogenic. This is especially true of a test that must employ large numbers of organisms, must be done on a continual basis for lot release of membranes and devices, and ideally should be capable of being carried out by individual pharmaceutical facilities wishing to characterize the performance of filters in their particular processes. *B. diminuta* is known to be nonpathogenic and can be handled safely in standard microbiological labs. There is no demonstrated health concern from *B. diminuta* when it is aerosolized, which makes it desirable for challenges conducted under pressure and for aerosol challenges of gas filters.

3.2 Challenge Level

A sterilizing grade filter is defined operationally as one that will yield a sterile effluent when challenged with a suspension of bacteria sufficient to provide 10^7 colony-forming units (CFU) per square centimeter of effective filtration area. This level was first recognized in the HIMA test method and later adopted by the ASTM and by the FDA in their 1987 Guideline on Sterile Drug Products Produced by Aseptic Processing. One should be careful not to confuse this target value with the total number of colony-forming units required to attain the target for any given filter. For example, a typical 10 in. cartridge filter containing 7000 cm^2 of membrane filter would require 7×10^{10} CFU to reach the required 10^7 CFU/cm^2.

The origin and the rationale for the 10^7 CFU/cm^2 value are somewhat obscure. Some authorities believed that there are approximately 10^7 pores/cm^2 of filter surface area of cellulosic membranes and that a challenge level of 10^7 CFU/cm^2 would, in theory, challenge every pore of the membrane. Others have claimed that this level represents a monolayer on the membrane surface or that this level is sufficiently high to challenge oversized pores in a 0.22 μm filter. Leahy and Sullivan (1978), in their seminal work on filter validation, recommended a level of 10^8 CFU/cm^2, tenfold higher than the ASTM and HIMA methods, which themselves were derived from the methods reported by Leahy and Sullivan. These authors suggested that this higher challenge level "exceeds complete coverage" of the test filter, thus providing the greatest assurance that a filter defect or oversized opening in the filter will be challenged by the test organism. More recently, others have favored even higher challenges than the 10^7 CFU/cm^2 standard, going to as much as 10^9 CFU/cm^2 (Pall Corp., 1990). Aicholtz et al. (1987) challenged sterilizing grade 10 in. cartridges with 10^{13} CFU of *B. diminuta* per cartridge (about 10^9 CFU/cm^2) and found the cartridges to be fully retentive. However, the organisms were cultured in a high-nutrient medium (tryptone soy broth), which lessens the relevance of this work to the retention of small organisms. In opposition to the use of very high challenge levels are Mouwen and Meltzer (1993). Since basic principles of fluid flow dictate that flow through restricted openings is proportional to the radii of the openings raised to the fourth power, these authors reasoned that membrane defects or areas of aberrant microporous structure, even though few in number, would be subjected to an inordinately large volume of flow and would therefore be adequately challenged at a level of 10^7 CFU/cm^2. This point of view has long been held by the majority of researchers in the field. In any case, this level of challenge organisms per unit of filter surface area is likely to continue to be recommended, even in future guidelines.

4 VERIFYING MICROBIAL RETENTION

4.1 Vendor's Qualification of Filters by Microbial Retention Testing

The microbial retention test is used by filter vendors for two primary purposes: membrane and filter device qualification and filter lot release.

Filter Qualification

The basic principle that quality is engineered into a product should apply equally to filter manufacturers and pharmaceutical drug manufacturers. The microbial retention test is used throughout the entire membrane development process to provide data on the ability of newly developed membranes to remove bacteria. The ultimate conclusion to this process is that the membrane produced by the manufacturing facility is qualified as sterilizing grade. This having been proved, the next step is to validate the manufacture of the fabricated filter device into which the qualified membrane will be incorporated. Undoubtedly, almost all filter manufacturers use a nondestructive filter integrity test (e.g., diffusion test or bubble point test) during device research and development to test for proper manufacture of the devices. In addition, some manufacturers use the microbial retention test to qualify manufacture of the fabricated device. Filter users should be able to assess the rigor with which a filter device has been qualified by reviewing the validation guide for the device, which is available from the filter manufacturer.

Filter Lot Release

The membrane and filter device manufacturing processes should be fully validated and under control. This being the case, the bacterial retention test should not be relied on to test quality into the product but should instead be used to monitor both the membrane casting and the manufacturing process from lot to lot. In this respect, the test is analogous to the USP sterility test. Because the bacterial retention test is destructive, only a small percentage of each manufacturing lot can be tested. Nevertheless, the retention test should be used for lot release of both the flat stock membrane and the final fabricated devices, for it serves as a mechanism to monitor for any gross manufacturing problems. The filter user should not assume that all filter manufacturers use the microbial retention as a lot release measure. The certificate of quality that should accompany each filter will provide information on the criteria by which the manufacturer releases the product.

Correlation of Microbial Retention Test Results to a Physical Filter Integrity Test

All filter manufacturers should have established a relationship between a recommended physical integrity test and microbial retention. These data are used by filter vendors to establish minimum integrity test specifications for their sterilizing grade filters. The pharmaceutical manufacturer is responsible for establishing minimum integrity test values for the filter when it is wetted with the pharmaceutical product to be filtered. These specifications will be used for release of the drug product, since microbially challenging each filter used in production is not practical.

When used for filter qualification and lot release, the microbial retention test is a standardized test run under conditions that are not intended to mimic any particular pharmaceutical aseptic process. Indeed, the wide range of applications in which filters are currently used makes it unfeasible for filter vendors to develop a qualification or lot release test that would mimic the "typical" filter application. Thus, the filter vendor's qualification data and standard product lot release retention test data are usually not sufficient to claim that a filter will completely remove organisms under a given set of processing conditions. These considerations dictate

Table 5 Filter Validation Recommendations and Responsibilities of the Filter User and the Filter Manufacturer[a]

Criterion	Filter user	Filter manufacturer	
		Membrane	Device
Bacterial retention–integrity test relationship data	—	Q	Q
Integrity test			
Water/solvent	V	Q/R/L	Q/R/L
Product	V		
Integrity test methodology and selection	V	R	
Microbial retention			
SLB/FP[b]	—	Q/L	Q/L
Product	V		
Microbial retention/integrity test methodology	V		R
Effects of chemical compatibility on filter integrity	V	Q	Q
Toxicity testing	—	Q	Q
Extractable	V	Q/R/L	Q/R/L
Effects of sterilization methods on filter integrity	V	Q	Q

[a]Q = qualification testing; V = validation testing, process-specific; R = recommendation for validation; L = lot-specific release criteria.
[b]SLB = saline lactose broth; FP = frozen cell paste.
Source: PDA Technical Report No. 26 (1997).

that microbial retention be verified using a test that will mimic the actual processing conditions of the product to be filter-sterilized. Table 5 summarizes the current status of both filter manufacturer and filter user responsibilities as summarized in the PDA monograph on sterile filtration (PDA, 1997).

4.2 Pharmaceutical Manufacturer's Validation of Filters by Microbial Retention Testing

As defined by the FDA (1987), validation is "establishing documented evidence which provides a high degree of assurance that a specific process will consistently produce a product meeting its predetermined specifications and quality attributes." One often-asked question concerns the need for filter users to perform microbial retention validation studies if the filter vendor has already qualified the filter as being sterilizing grade. The need for microbial retention validation is based on the fact that microbial retention efficiency cannot be absolutely predicted and is not necessarily verified by the conditions under which the filter vendor qualifies the filter. For example, it has been shown that organism retention by more open filters such as those rated at 0.45 μm is affected by changing applied pressure (Reti et al., 1979). Moreover, fluid mechanics and adsorptive mechanisms predict that changes to other physicochemical attributes of the filtration conditions could affect retention efficiency in those cases where size exclusion is not the primary mechanism of particle removal.

From a regulatory perspective, the pharmaceutical manufacturer is ultimately responsible for providing data that support the claim of microbial retention validation. However, most pharmaceutical manufacturers have neither the facilities to perform the test nor the desire to introduce even small volumes of concentrated bacterial suspensions into their facility. Therefore a microbial retention validation test is usually performed at a contract testing laboratory that has the expertise and trained personnel required to do the test. In addition, designing a validation test protocol requires an intimate understanding of how filters work, an understanding that is held by the filter vendor. For this reason, the pharmaceutical manufacturer has looked to the filter vendor for advice on how to best challenge the filters. Indeed, the bulk of microbial validation tests are performed by filter vendors. The advantage of this is that the filter user is able to tap the knowledge and understanding the vendor has of the filter. This close partnership between vendor and user is often the difference between an ill-conceived design and a successful validation. Nevertheless, the user must understand that from a regulatory point of view the user is ultimately responsible for the design and execution of the test and for reporting the results to the relevant regulatory agency. *The responsibilities of the filter vendor are limited to providing sound, scientifically founded advice to the pharmaceutical manufacturer, performing the test, and providing the documentation required after the test is completed.* Therefore, the filter user must take steps to ensure that the contract facility is operating in a manner consistent with the generation of valid and defensible data. Often this is accomplished by an audit of the test facility and occasionally by eyewitness viewing of the test as it is being run.

4.3 Design of the Microbial Validation Test

Despite its vintage and statements from the FDA on its inadequacy, the 1987 guideline (FDA, 1987) is still the document to which people turn for guidance on microbial retention validation test design. However, the PDA Technical Report on sterile filtration (PDA, 1997) addresses many of the technical details of microbial retention testing.

In practice, designing the microbial validation test that will best provide documented evidence that the sterile filtration process will indeed yield a product that meets the definition of being bacteria-free is technically complicated. For this reason, it is beneficial for the drug manufacturer to understand, and agree with, the basic scientific tenets or premises on which the validity of the microbial retention testing is based. We have developed a short list of such premises that should be considered when designing and evaluating a microbial retention test protocol. These appear to be consistent with most microbial retention testing programs offered by filtration companies regardless of the marketing inferences of differences among the programs.

1. A model or relevant microorganism is an appropriate indicator microorganism to replace natural bioburden and can be used as an equivalent or more stringent challenge relative to natural bioburden organisms.
2. *B. diminuta* can be used as such an appropriate model or relevant organism.

3. *B. diminuta* grown in saline lactose broth or by the frozen cell paste method provides an appropriately rigorous challenge.
4. The challenge level that 10^7 CFU/cm^2 of filter surface area provides is sufficiently rigorous.
5. It is generally not necessary to culture the challenge microorganism in the actual pharmaceutical product.
6. Flat stock membrane sterilization performance is an appropriate predictor of fabricated device sterilization performance. For this to be true, the filter manufacturer must validate that none of the fabrication steps has had an impact on filter integrity.
7. The best retention test is one in which the organism optimally, should be suspended in the pharmaceutical formulation.
8. At least three lots of filter material, representative of that used in standard production, should be tested for each product.
9. Filters used in the study should be representative of those that will be used in the sterile filtration of the pharmaceutical formulation.
10. In the case where a drug product is toxic to the test microorganism and no alternative microorganism is available, it is appropriate to expose the test filters to the test solution, rinse out the toxic solution, and follow that rinse with a *B. diminuta* challenge in a vehicle that is nontoxic to the test microorganism.
11. A 0.45 μm membrane is an appropriate microorganism size control and positive control.
12. The entire solution that passed through the test filter should be analyzed for the presence of the test microorganism.
13. It is acceptable to use a 0.45 μm filter to analyze the filter effluent for the test microorganism.
14. There are situations in which it is valid to interpolate between extremes of one or more process or product characteristics, thus obviating the need to perform retention tests on all products between those extremes.
15. Scale-down tests are generally appropriate to use in validation of the sterilizing filter's performance.
16. A membrane filter's manufacturing process must be well controlled in order to consistently produce filter material equivalent to those used during the validation.

During the process of designing the test protocol, several questions must be addressed. Some will be simple to answer and others will be difficult, generally due to the need to compromise between two mutually exclusive aspects of the test that are both considered important. Because the FDA guideline and PDA monographs are not able to provide the detail relevant to everyone's process, there will be times when judgment calls will have to be made. In these cases, it can be helpful to receive input from appropriate regulatory personnel. Some of the more common test design questions, as well as examples of compromise situations, are discussed below. Figure 2 summarizes the pathways one may take in conducting a microbial retention validation study. These steps are discussed below.

After choosing a sterilizing grade filter (Fig. 2, steps 1 and 2) that meets the application need, test to determine the extractables level and the physical integrity

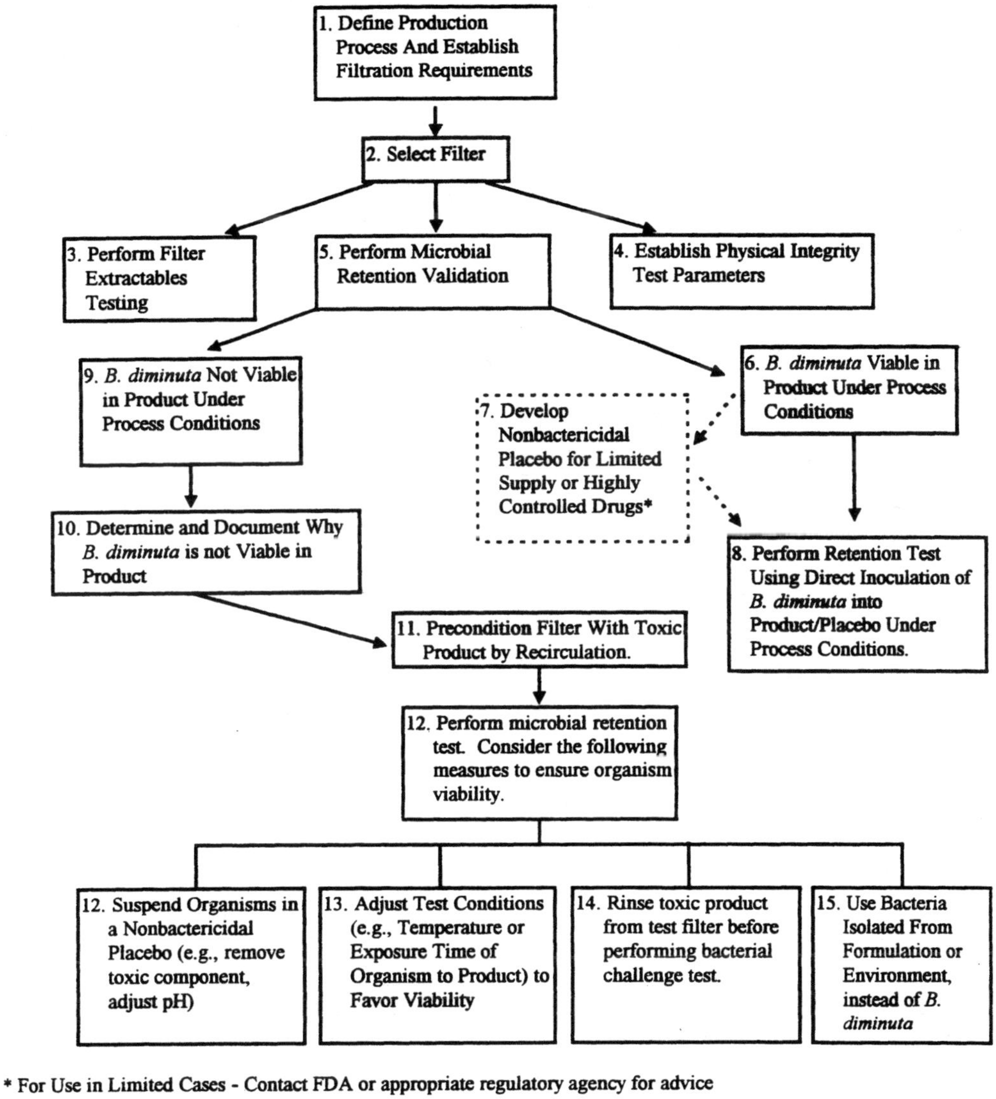

Figure 2 PDA Task Force decision tree for microbial retention testing. (After PDA, 1997.)

test parameters (acceptance criteria) and to validate the microbial retention, taking into consideration the drug product attributes (physicochemical properties) and process conditions (Fig. 2, step 5).

Choice of Test Organism and Viability Studies

Sterilization validation requires the use of a biological indicator (BI) organism. In moist heat sterilization, spores of *Bacillus stearothermophilus*, *Bacillus coagulans*, *Bacillus subtilis*, and *Clostridium sporogenes* are considered acceptable, although the former is considered most heat-resistant. In filtration validation, the FDA guideline states that *B. diminuta* [formerly named *Pseudomonas diminuta* (Segers et al., 1994)], when properly cultured, is generally an acceptable organism because of its small size.

The BI is taken to represent the worst-case microorganism, the one most resistant to the particular form of sterilization. This being true, the sterilization process characterized with the BI is expected to perform at a level greater than or equal to its performance in validation trials. However, before accepting this premise at face value, one must be aware of the unavoidable differences between BIs and native organisms. In the context of aseptic processing, one of the most important characteristics is cell size. Thus, the guideline also states that it is "important to assure that actual influent bioburden does not contain microorganisms of a size and/or concentration that would reduce the targeted high level of filtrate sterility assurance," leaving open the inference that one should perform validation tests with a bioburden organism if it is shown to be smaller than *B. diminuta*. In our experience, bioburden testing is very rarely performed.

The most common issue with choosing a test microorganism concerns viability: Will the microorganism remain viable and recoverable when exposed to product under actual process conditions, particularly exposure time? The choice of test organism often requires making a compromise between organism size and organism viability. For example, if *B. diminuta* is shown to have a moderate reduction in viability upon exposure to the test product, one might need to weigh the relative merits of testing with *B. diminuta* or with a more resistant, but larger, bioburden organism. Alternatively, it might be most appropriate to modify the actual product to alleviate the toxicity problem or to run a test that does not require introduction of the organism into the test solution (as will be discussed later).

Culture Maintenance

Brevundimonas diminuta is readily available from the American Type Culture Collection in Rockville, Maryland. The strain is numbered ATCC 19146. Other sources must be traceable to the original strain isolated by Bowman and Holdowsky (1960). After reconstitution, the culture can be maintained for several months on refrigerated agar slants. These slants must be shown to produce viable cells biochemically identical to the Bowman strain.

Choice of Culture Conditions

As discussed earlier in this chapter, there are two recognized culture methods: saline lactose and frozen cell paste. Alternative media and culture methods may be equally acceptable, provided they can be shown to produce single monodisperse cells and that they allow for the production of the minimum desired challenge load per filter. The size and degree of aggregation should also be verified and documented.

Choice of Effective Challenge Level

The FDA guideline states that a challenge level of at least 10^7 organisms per square centimeter of filtration area is acceptable, leading one to infer that a challenge level below this number is not acceptable. Challenging at this level should be considered the rule, even when low bioburden levels can be demonstrated in the process and environment.

Nevertheless, there may be defensible situations in which it is legitimate to consider an effective challenge level below 10^7 CFU/cm^2. For example, a product that leads to a 100-fold reduction in *B. diminuta* viability over the time of the test could be spiked with enough organisms to give a calculated challenge level of 10^8 CFU/cm^2, which would yield a final effective challenge level of 10^6 CFU/cm^2. The disadvantages of falling below the standard challenge level (and missing the traditional level of challenge used to define a sterilizing grade filter) would have to be balanced by the potential disadvantages of needing to alter the drug formulation, reduce the duration of the test, or use a different organism that is inferior to *B. diminuta*.

Choice of Test Solution

Ideally, the test vehicle would be the actual product that one is processing (Fig. 2, steps 6 and 8). However, there are several reasons that this ideal might not be realized. A limited supply of the product or, more often, of the active ingredient may require modification of the product, i.e., removal or replacement of the active ingredient (Fig. 2, step 7). Federal shipping regulations prohibit transport of controlled substances to facilities not authorized to receive them. Thus, some contract facilities may not be able to receive or work with this kind of product. After testing, the controlled substance will need to be sent back to the drug manufacturer or destroyed.

Toxicity of the product toward the test organism might necessitate modification of the process and/or product. The former involves reducing the processing time (exposure of the product to the microorganism) or temperature (Fig. 2, step 14). The latter involves removing or reducing the concentration of an active ingredient or preservative, adjusting the pH, or developing a nonbacteriocidal placebo that mimics as many of the product characteristics as possible (Fig. 2, step 13).

There are several issues surrounding modifications to the test solution. First, it is not always evident what property of the solution should actually be changed or to what extent the product should be changed to make the product usable in the test. If the active ingredient must be removed, what would constitute a legitimate substitution of that active? If the actual solution is toxic, should the toxic ingredient be eliminated, or should it be reduced in concentration? Is it even chemically or pharmacologically possible to modify the solution without, for example, encountering a problem with solubility of the ingredients? Finally, how drastically can one change a test solution before the changes render it completely nonrepresentative of the test solution? Due to the wide diversity of pharmaceutical formulations, the methods used in this process have not been elaborated. Regulatory agencies and filter manufacturers may be able to provide some technical direction in this regard, but it is the pharmaceutical manufacturer, with his unique understanding of his product who must ultimately provide a rationale for this choice.

When all attempts to modify the product or the process prove not to be appropriate, the final alternative is that of a recirculation test (see Fig. 2, step 6e). In this procedure, which is very time- and resource-intensive, the product is circulated through the test filter under process conditions. Following a validated rinsing procedure, the filter is challenged with *B. diminuta* suspended in saline lactose broth or buffer, again under process conditions. This type of test effectively doubles the time required to conduct the test and requires extensive viability determinations to ensure that product residuals in the test and/or assay filters do not create false negative test results.

Test Scale and the Choice Between Flat Stock Membrane and Fabricated Device

Ideally, the validation test should be an exact replica of the actual filtration process that the product will undergo and should be performed in the actual facility in which production will occur. There are several obvious practical and economic reasons why this ideal is rarely, if ever, achieved. For the reasons mentioned below, as well as others, the validation test is almost always a scaled-down version of the actual process.

1. Desire not to introduce high levels of *B. diminuta* into the processing facility
2. Impracticality of analyzing very large volumes for the presence of very small numbers of organisms
3. Cost associated with use of the production facility for other than product manufacture
4. Prohibitively high cost of product
5. Lack of trained personnel to run the test at full scale

The decision to scale the test down invariably leads one to choose between a flat disk and a fabricated device that is smaller than the actual production device. The debate surrounding this issue focuses primarily on the concern that cartridge fabrication can lead to structural damage in the membrane that would not be apparent in the flat stock membrane. Similarly, there is concern that the membrane might not be properly sealed in the device at the seam or at the cartridge end caps. This could lead to organism passage *around* the membrane as opposed to *through* the membrane. Finally, it is often not possible to scale process parameters such as flow rate or pressure differential linearly from device to disk. In any case, the validation test could be seen as not adequately simulating the processing conditions, such as pressure differential and flow rate.

This issue begs the more philosophical question regarding the purpose of the microbial retention validation test. If the test is to assay for filter or device integrity or for compatibility between product and filter, then there can be little question that the fabricated device is the legitimate choice. However, one must remember that this is a microbial retention test and not a filter integrity test or filter compatibility test. If one has not gathered proper documentation to show that filter integrity and compatibility can be ensured in production, then one probably should not be running the microbial retention test. This should not be construed to mean that fabricated device testing is not appropriate, but rather that flat stock testing is often sufficient for validating microbial retention.

Two practical considerations in this choice are (1) the volume requirements and (2) the differences between flat sheet filter membrane and the membrane incorporated into fabricated devices. With regard to volume requirements, it is usually desirable to scale a process linearly with respect to volume per square centimeter of filtration area. At high volume-to-surface area ratios, the volume of drug product required is often too expensive to consider, too impractical to ship to the testing facility, or too difficult for the testing facility to handle. Conversely, testing even moderate volumes could be prohibitive if the product is in short supply. In these cases, economics will dictate that flat stock membrane be used or that the volume-to-surface area scaling factor be reduced.

As discussed previously, one should verify that the membrane incorporated into the device used in product processing is identical to the flat stock membrane used in the validation test. In this vein, it is not sufficient to verify the identity of polymer type and the pore size rating between the flat stock membrane and the device membrane. One should require formal verification from the supplier that the flat stock membrane is the actual membrane that is used in device manufacturing.

Establishment of Process Requirements

For any testing procedure, the test conditions should simulate processing conditions as closely as possible. Typically, in filtration processes where the flow rate is controlled, the flow rate is scaled down to an equivalent flow rate based on the full-scale product volume per unit surface area of the true-scale filter device. Pressures should be recorded for historical purposes; the recorded pressures may not match those seen in actual production.

If the filtration is regulated by pressure, the challenge pressure should be maintained at the processing pressure. This may prove difficult in scaled-down processing using disk filters. Trial runs should be conducted to determine how well the scaled-down process is likely to simulate actual process conditions.

5 ISSUES IN FILTER VALIDATION

A recent stimulus to the revision process (Meltzer, 1993) discusses many current issues in filter validation. This paper addresses the current climate, conditions affecting retention, assumptions inherent in actual validations, recovery methods, differential pressure, challenge densities, pore size distributions, and pore size designations. However, several other issues are not addressed in it and are covered in this section.

5.1 Bioburden

Bacteria are normal inhabitants of raw materials used to manufacture pharmaceuticals. They may be present as viable vegetative cells or in a desiccated, quiescent state. Since these bacteria may have the ability to survive and reproduce in these materials, they should be identified, characterized, and quantified as an aid to evaluating the probability of these microorganisms penetrating downstream filters and challenging final sterilizing filters. This step provides an estimate of the total load the sterilizing grade filter may experience during the sterile filtration. Clearly, high bioburden loads should be reduced prior to final filtration. This process will also provide candidates for the microbial retention validation studies.

It is well recognized that bacterial cells become smaller under nutrient-limited growth conditions [e.g., Givskov et al. (1994)]. For this reason, many people have suspected that water systems are breeding grounds for organisms, generally *Pseudomonas* species, that could pass through sterilizing grade filters. In another vein, it is also well recognized that cells introduced into very high osmolarity solutions are susceptible to a reduction in cell volume (Stock et al., 1977; Koch, 1984; Csonka and Hanson, 1991). Several investigators have addressed the issue of small, generally waterborne, bacteria penetrating 0.2 μm rated filters (Wallhäusser, 1979; Howard and Duberstein, 1980; Johnston, 1985). As in the case of grow-through (described below), cases of demonstrated passage through sterilizing grade filters have been limited. In the only documented, laboratory-confirmed passage of a microorganism through a sterilizing grade filter, Anderson et al. (1985) reported that a strain of *Pseudomonas pickettii* penetrated a 0.2 μm nylon membrane filtration system and subsequently contaminated a commercial respiratory therapy solution. In this case, a water holding tank held at 82°C was bypassed, which allowed these bacteria to pass downstream in large numbers. Thus, a heat inactivation step could have eliminated or reduced numbers of these bacteria in the product prior to filtration.

A second report of bacterial passage through sterilizing grade filters gains credibility simply because the authors represent the manufacturer of filters used in the study (Howard and Duberstein, 1980). In this study, both 0.2 μm nylon and 0.22 μm cellulose acetate membrane disks are shown to pass a number of species of organisms indigenous to well water. Nylon cartridges were also reported to pass these water organisms while at the same time retaining all of the high levels of *B. diminuta* spiked into the water. Cellulose acetate membranes were not tested. A third report claims to provide data that 0.2 μm sterilizing grade filters from the "four most important filter manufacturers" all pass *B. diminuta* (Wallhäusser, 1979). Unfortunately, the methods used for performing the challenge tests and for detecting organisms in the filtrate are not provided in the report. The reader is therefore left without the means to make an informed evaluation of the study.

There has recently been discussion concerning anecdotal references to occurrences in which sterilizing grade filters have been suspected of passing organisms. At the Parenteral Drug Association's (PDA) special scientific forum of 1995 entitled Validation of Microbial Retention of Sterilizing Filters, representatives of two major filter vendors and of the FDA related instances of filter failures that most likely involved passage of organisms through the filter matrix. One filter manufacturer reported filter failures, at a contract pharmaceutical manufacturer, in which *B. diminuta* and *Pseudomonas pickettii* were reported to have passed through 0.2 μm filters. Apparently these were confirmed by the filter manufacturer, who conducted retention tests with the same organisms. No other details have been forthcoming. A second filter manufacturer reported that *B. diminuta*, when suspended in concentrated sodium chloride, seemingly passed through a 0.22 μm filter. The vendor was unable to repeat the failure upon retest. Documentation of these cases has not generally been published and remains unavailable for public review, usually due to confidentiality limitations. This situation makes it very difficult for both the pharmaceutical industry and the filter vendors to ascertain both the validity of these anecdotal reports and the details of the situations in which the observations were made.

We have examined a number of bacteria purported to have passed through 0.22 μm filters. These are summarized in Table 6. These bacteria were cultured in various media and also in the solution in which they were originally isolated. Table 6 also reports the size in the milieu in which they grew to be the smallest, as determined by scanning electron microscopy analysis. The bacteria listed in this table were shown to be retained by 0.22 μm hydrophilized poly(vinylidene fluoride) membrane. Although it is recognized that smaller organisms could exist in some environments, their occurrence has been, in our experience, very rare. Moreover, culturing limitations make it very difficult to propagate small native organisms in a manner that preserves their physical and physiological attributes.

Table 6 Sizes of Microorganisms Isolated from Process Streams, Drug Products, or Media

Organism	Source reference	Growth medium	Length (μm)	Width (μm)
Brevundimonas diminuta	ATCC 19146	SLB	0.68	0.31
Pseudomonas cepacia	ATCC 35254	DI H2O	1.11	0.46
P. cepacia	ATCC 25416	SLB	1.15	0.42
P. cepacia	Process isolate	Saline	1.00	0.43
P. fluorescens	Process isolate	SLB	0.90	0.53
P. fluorescens	Process isolate	SLB	1.17	0.46
P. fluorescens	Process isolate	DI H2O	1.02	0.22
P. luteola	Process isolate	SLB	0.72	0.39
P. luteola	Process isolate	DI H2O	0.86	0.33
P. maltophilia	Process isolate	DI H2O	0.88	0.44
P. maltophilia	Process isolate	Product	1.40	0.52
P. pickettii	CDC-Anderson	DI-H2O	1.37	0.48
P. pseudoalcaligenes	Process isolate	RPMI	1.06	0.32
P. stutzeri	Process isolate	SLB	1.22	0.50
P. testoseroni	Process isolate	SLB	0.99	0.38
Xanthamonas maltophilia	Process isolate	DI H2O	1.28	0.37
Bacillus cereus	Process isolate	Media fill	1.19	0.36

5.2 Filter Penetration, Grow-Through, and Blow-Through

Microporous membrane filters have been demonstrated to allow, over extended periods of time, the penetration of bacteria through the filter and into the effluent (Wallhäusser, 1983; Leahy and Gabler, 1984; Simonetti and Schroeder, 1984; Peterson and Hankner, 1985). Filter penetration is simply a term used to describe the depth to which a target particle will travel through the filter before it is removed from the fluid stream. In fact, sterilizing filters, as a rule, allow some penetration into the depths of the filter. This is clearly consistent with both size exclusion and adsorptive removal mechanisms.

The term ''grow-through'' describes a theoretical phenomenon in which organisms, initially trapped by a filter, will multiply on and in the filter. In the process of multiplying, the organisms pass deeper and deeper into the filter matrix until they eventually emerge downstream of the filter. The term ''blow-through'' describes a phenomenon in which organisms initially trapped on a filter are subsequently hydraulically forced through the matrix of the filter, due to an increase in pressure differential, and eventually pass through the entire thickness of the filter to contaminate the fluid being filter-sterilized. Both phenomena are hypotheses and have never been rigorously demonstrated to be real events in pharmaceutical process. Although there are reports of such occurrences, the complexity of the phenomena, coupled with the difficulties in experimentally repeating these presumptive occurrences, make prophylactic measures all the more important. Perhaps as increasingly greater attention is paid to GMP, aseptic manipulations, process system sterilization, and barrier technology, the frequency of occurrence of these purported events may decrease further.

Nervertheless, the reliability of sterile filtrations can only be increased by limiting the process time. Filter manufacturers recommend that aseptic processing be completed within a preestablished period of time based on their experience with that membrane or fabricated device. Most manufacturers have conducted retention tests over extended times, and data generally suggest that filters should retain bacteria the size of *B. diminuta* in excess of 48 h. Limiting the filtration to a time less than that which is recommended by the manufacturer provides increased assurance that grow-through or blow-through, if they are real phenomena, will not occur. This subject has been reviewed by Christian and Meltzer (1986).

5.3 L Forms and Bacterial Passage Through Filters

The nature of L-form bacteria and their significance in pharmaceutical processing have been summarized by Thomas et al. (1991). In this paper, the authors report that L forms, generated from water-derived *Pseudomonas aeruginosa*, are able to penetrate nonintegral 0.45 μm membranes from three filter manufacturers. The definition of "nonintegral" undoubtedly relates to their passage, since no physical integrity test measurements were performed on the membranes. All were assumed to be initially integral. However, this passage should be of no surprise as these cells are undoubtedly smaller than the *Serratia marcescens* that is used to standardize these filters. The testing of 0.22 μm filters would have better demonstrated the relative significance of L forms to sterile filtration.

Hargreaves (1993) reported that the Medicines Control Agency had encountered a number of cases in the United Kingdom where there was a high probability that microorganisms passed through sterilizing grade filters. L forms were deemed to be the most likely cause. On a worldwide basis, approximately 70 cases of breakthrough were suspected. These cases are, of course, difficult to confirm for reasons discussed in Sec. 5.1 and 5.2. Moreover, it is well known that changes occur in microorganisms when they are subcultured. In this context, unstable L forms could revert to a normal cell-walled state on laboratory growth media. Hargreaves postulated (in the absence of scientific data) two possible mechanisms: When breakthrough occurs in a short time frame, L forms are probably present in the water system, and when breakthrough occurs after an extended time, L forms are probably forming on or in the filter.

L forms are most likely to be present in animal-derived products such as animal sera. Haycock et al. (1994) reported that viable L-form bacteria were present in 60 animal sera from several commercial suppliers and that L-form growth could occur in neat sera or sera-supplemented media, in prefiltered (0.2 and 0.04 μm) sera, and in heat-inactivated (2 h, 60°C) and refiltered (0.2 and 0.1 μm) sera. They reported that ultrafiltration, with 300,000 molecular weight cutoff membranes, appeared to eliminate contamination. By contrast, eliminating these bacteria from cell lines may prove difficult.

5.4 "Absolute" Filter Sterilization

Debate over the meaning of "sterility" in production of parenteral products and products intended for other methods of administration has continued over many years in the published literature. Sterility is defined as an absolute negative state: the complete absence of all life forms. Using empirically derived data, it is simply not possible to gain absolute proof of the existence of a negative situation. It is precisely for this reason that the term ''sterility assurance'' exists. Although there are debates concerning the true meaning of the term ''sterility'' [most recently, Sharp (1995) summarized the current thinking on the subject, which will not be debated here], most definitions talk about the probability of reaching the absolute state of sterility. Thus, an acceptable sterility assurance for terminal sterilization is considered 10^{-6}. Taking the USP definition

> [It is] generally accepted that . . . injectable articles or . . . devices purporting to be sterile . . . [when autoclaved] attain a 10^{-6} microbial survivor probability, i.e., assurance of less than one chance in a million that viable organisms are present in the sterilized article or dosage form (USP XXI).

Very heat-tolerant solutions, overkill sterilization cycles providing a sterility assurance orders of magnitude lower than 10^{-6} are often employed. The important point is that although numbers of 10^{-6} and lower are extremely small, they do not represent zero probability of organism survival. In other words, in theory, absolute sterility assurance is not achievable.

The same logic can be applied to filtration. As discussed, most sterilizing grade filters are intended to rely primarily on size exclusion to remove organisms from fluid streams. The reliability of these filters is due primarily to the relationship between the filter's pore size distribution and the test organism's size distribution. Assuming that size exclusion is the overriding mechanism of removal, the successful use of the filter is due in large measure to the very small overlap between the two size distributions. If we take the typical example of a sterilizing grade filter that repeatedly yields a filtrate free of detectable challenge organisms when challenged with *B. diminuta* at 10^7 CFU/cm^2, it is not difficult to convince oneself that the two size distributions are indeed very far apart. The key question at this point is: Do the pore size distribution and the organism size distribution overlap, or is the smallest organism larger than the largest pore?

Certainly there is compelling reason to believe that neither of the two distributions continues on indefinitely. Rather, there are most likely discrete minima and maxima for both distributions. Nevertheless, both pore sizes and bacterial cell sizes are difficult to measure with great confidence. Therefore, the argument invariably ends with the rhetorical question: If there were pores large enough to allow bacterial passage, what is the probability that we would always see sterile filtrates? Seemingly, the only defensible position is that an overlap in the two size distributions could exist but is small enough not to be detected by the standard bacterial retention test.

Based on this size distribution discussion, it is evident that sterility assurance afforded by filtration is organism size dependent. Therefore, the term ''absolute'' must be taken in context, since it is relative to the particles being targeted for removal by the filter. Even if one could claim absolute removal of a given organism by a given filter, that same filter might not be effective in removing a smaller organism. From a practical point of view, this means that the filter user must know what organism (BI) was used in the manufacturer's qualification of a given filter and not expect that filter to be effective against other, perhaps smaller, organisms. Thus, today's sterilizing grade filters with ratings of 0.2 μm generally are not used or recommended as the final filter in applications that require the complete removal of organisms, such as mycoplasma, that are smaller than *B. diminuta*.

REFERENCES

Aicholtz, P., R. Wilkins, and R. Gabler. (1987). Sterile filtration under conditions of high pressure and bacterial challenge levels, *J. Parenter. Drug Assoc. 41*:117–120.

APHA. (1992). Membrane filter technique for members of the coliform group in *Standard Methods for the Examination of Water and Wastewater* (A. E. Greenberg, L. S. Clesceri, and A. D. Eaton, eds.), American Public Health Association, Washington, DC, pp. 9-54–9-55.

Anderson, R. L., L. A. Bland, M. S. Favero, M. M. McNeil, B. J. Davis, D. C. Mackel, and C. R. Gravelle. (1985). Factors associated with *Pseudomonas pickettii* intrinsic contamination of commercial respiratory therapy solutions marketed as sterile, *Appl. Environ. Microbiol. 50*:1343–1348.

ASTM Committee F-21. (1988). Standard test methods for determining bacterial retention of membrane filters utilized for liquid filtration, *Annual Book of ASTM Standards*, American Society for Testing and Materials, Philadelphia, pp. 790–795.

Bayer, M. E., and M. H. Bayer. (1994). Biophysical and structural aspects of the bacterial capsule, *ASM News, 60*:192–198.

Bowman, F. W., and S. Holdowsky. (1960). Production and control of a stable penicillinase, *Antibiot. Chemother., 8*:508.

Bowman, F. W., Calhoun, M. P., and White, M. (1967). Microbiological methods for quality control of membrane filters, *J. Pharm. Sci., 56*:222–225.

Carter, J. R. (1996). Evaluation of recovery filters for use in bacterial retention testing of sterilizing-grade filters, *PDA J. Pharm. Sci. Technol., 50*:147–153.

FDA. (1987). Guideline on Sterile Drug Products Produced by Aseptic Processing, Center for Drugs and Biologics and Office of Regulatory Affairs. Food and Drug Administration, Rockville, MD.

Christian, D. A., and T. H. Meltzer. (1986). The penetration of membranes by organism grow-through and its related problems, *Ultrapure Water, 3*:30–44.

Csonka, L. N., and A. D. Hanson. (1991). Prokaryotic osmoregulation: Genetics and physiology, *Annu. Rev. Microbiol., 45*:569–606.

Drozd, C., and J. Schwartzbrod. (1996). Hydrophobic and electrostatic cell surface properties of *Cryptosporidium parvum, Appl. Environ. Microbiol., 62*:1227–1232.

Givskov, M., L. Eberl, S. Møller, L. K. Poulson, and S. Molin. (1994). Responses to nutrient starvation in *Pseudomonas putida* KY2442: Analysis of general cross-protection, cell shape, and macromolecular content, *J. Bacteriol., 176*:7–14.

Grant, D. C., B. Y. H. Liu, W. G. Fisher, and R. A. Bowling. (1988). *Particle capture mechanisms in gases and liquids: An analysis of operative mechanisms*, Proceedings of the 34th Annual Meeting of the Institute of Environmental Sciences.

Groves, M. J. (1991). Letters to the Editor, *Pharm. Tech., 51*:18.

Hargreaves, P. (1993). Paul Hargreaves speaks out on pharmaceutical manufacturing, *PDA Letter 29*:10–13.

Haycock, J. W., K. E. Joho, J. C. Galyon, and R. L. Moses. (1994). Bacterial L forms are omnipresent in ''sterile'' tissue culture sera.

HIMA. (1982). Microbial evaluation of filters for sterilizing liquids, Health Industry Manufacturers Association. Washington, DC Document 3, Vol. 4.

Howard, J. G., and R. Duberstein. (1980). A case of penetration of 0.2-μm rated membrane filters by bacteria, *J. Parenter. Drug Assoc. 34*:95–102.

Johnston, E. B. (1985). Microbiological controls in the manufacture of respiratory therapy solutions, *Pharm. Manuf., 2*:29–32.
Koch, A. L. (1984). Shrinkage of growing *Escherichia coli* cells by osmotic challenge, *J. Bacteriol., 159*:919–924.
Leahy, T. J. (1983). Validation of bacterial retention by membrane filtration: A proposed approach for determining sterility assurance, Ph.D. Thesis. Graduate School of The University of Massachusetts, Amherst, MA, p. 303.
Leahy, T. J., and R. Gabler. (1984). Sterile filtration of gases by membrane filters, *J. Biotechnol. Bioeng., 26*:836–843.
Leahy, T. J., and M. J. Sullivan. (1978). Validation of bacterial-retention capabilities of membrane filters, *Pharm. Technol., 2*:65–75.
Lee, J.-K., B. Y. H. Liu, and K. L. Rubow. (1993). Latex sphere retention by microporous membranes in liquid filtration, *J. Inst. Environ. Sci., 36*:26–36.
Levy, R. V. (1987). The effect of pH, viscosity, and additives on the bacterial retention of membrane filters challenged with *Pseudomonas diminuta*, American Society for Testing and Materials, Philadelphia.
Levy, R. V., and T. J. Leahy. (1991). Sterilization filtration, in *Disinfection, Sterilization, and Preservation* (S. S. Block, ed.), Lea & Febiger, Philadelphia, pp. 527–551.
Meltzer, T. H. (1987). *Filtration in the Pharmaceutical Industry*, Marcel Dekker, New York.
Meltzer, T. H. (1993). Some unaddressed issues in filter validation, *Pharmacop. Forum, 19*: 5040–5045.
Mouwen, H. C., and T. H. Meltzer. (1993). Sterilizing filters: Pore-size distribution and the $1 \times 10^7/cm^2$ challenge, *Pharm. Technol., 17*:28–32.
Pall Corp. (1980). Validation Guide for Pall 0.2 μm Ultipor® and N_{66} Posidyne Membrane Cartridges, Pub. TR-680b, Pall Ultrafine Filtration Co., Pall Corp., East Hills, NY.
PDA Sterile Filtration Committee. (1977). PDA Technical Report No. 26: Sterilizing filtration of liquids, Parenteral Drug Association, Bethesda, MD. 52 pages.
Peterson, A. J., and D. O. Hankner. (1985). Assessment of long-term bacterial retention, *Med. Device Diagn. Ind.,* 150–155.
Reti, A. R., T. Leahy, and P. M. Meier. (1979). The retention mechanism of sterilizing and other submicron high efficiency filter structures, *Second World Filtration Congress*, London, pp. 427–435.
Segers, P., M. Vancanneyt, B. Pot, U. Torck, B. Hoste, D. Dewettinck, E. Falsen, K. Kersters, and P. De Vos. (1994). Classification of *Pseudomonas diminuta* Leifson and Hugh 1954 and *Pseudomonas vesicularis* Büsing, Doll, and Freytag 1953 in *Brevundimonas* gen. nov. as *Brevundimonas diminuta* comb. nov. and *Brevundimonas vesicularis* comb. nov., respectively, *Int. J. Syst. Bacteriol., 44*:499–510.
Sharp, J. (1995). What do we mean by "sterility"? *PDA J. Pharm. Sci. Technol. 49*:90–92.
Simonetti, J. A., and H. G. Schroeder. (1984). Evaluation of bacterial grow through, *J. Environ. Sci. 10*:27–32.
Sladek, K. J., R. V. Suslavich, B. I. John, and F. W. Dawson. (1975). Optimum membrane structures for growth of coliform and fecal coliform organisms, *Appl. Microbiol., 30*: 685–689.
Stock, J. B., B. Rauch, and S. Roseman. (1977). Periplasmic space in *Salmonella typhimurium* and *Escherichia coli, J. Biol. Chem., 252*:7850–7861.
Taylor, R. H., and E. E. Geldreich. (1979). A new membrane filter procedure for bacterial counts in potable water and swimming pool samples, *J. Am. Water Works Assoc., 71*: 402–405.
Thomas, A. J., H. H. Durrheim, M. Alport, and P. Evers. (1991). Detection of L-forms of *Pseudomonas aeruginosa* during microbiological validation of filters, *Pharm. Technol., 15*:74–80.

The United States Pharmacopeial Convention. (1995). Sterility tests, *U.S. Pharmacop.* Vol. 23, Rockville, MD.

Wallhäusser, K. H. (1979). Is the removal of microorganisms by filtration really a sterilization method?, *J. Parenter. Drug Assoc., 33*:156–170.

Wallhäusser, K. H. (1983). Durchwachs- und durchblaseffekte bei langzeit-sterilifiltrationsprozessen (English: Grow-through and blow-through effects in long-term sterile filtration processes), *Pharm. Ind., 45*:527–531.

19

Limulus Amebocyte Lysate Assays and Filter Applications

MARILYN J. GOULD
Associates of Cape Cod, Inc., Falmouth, Massachusetts

1 INTRODUCTION

Lipopolysaccharide (LPS), the biochemically purified endotoxic or pyrogenic structural molecule unique to the gram-negative bacterial cell wall, is easily detected and quantified using an in vitro assay referred to as the limulus amebocyte lysate or LAL test. LAL is a very sensitive reagent made from the soluble protein extract or lysate of horseshoe crab (genus *Limulus*) blood cells (amebocytes).

Endotoxins from gram-negative bacteria (classified on the basis of their cell wall structure) are the most common contaminants of water systems and biologically derived materials and are resistant to most methods of sterilization. Very low concentrations of endotoxins or LPS are toxic in vivo in blood or cerebral spinal fluid (FDA, 1987) and may affect the growth and function of vertebrate cells in vitro (Gould, 1984). Because LPS is a potential toxic contaminant of pharmaceuticals, its detection in finished products and its control or removal from parenteral and medical devices is especially important to the pharmaceutical industry.

Applications for the LAL test also extend beyond those of the pharmaceutical industry because LAL detects LPS in a variety of backgrounds. LPS is detected when it is part of the bacterial cell or when it is "free" in solution as the result of bacterial growth, bacterial cell lysis, or chemical extraction. This means that the LAL test can be used to indicate both present and past contamination by the ubiquitous gram-negative bacteria, a group of organisms known for their ability to grow in the harshest environments.

Numerous papers address the structure, function, and bioactivity of lipopolysaccharides and the development and various applications of the LAL test. References are included here to provide initial sources of more information or as they pertain to specific topics, but the list is not meant to be exhaustive. The reader is encouraged to review these topics in more depth, especially if the LAL test is to be applied under conditions that have not been defined previously.

2 LIPOPOLYSACCHARIDES

The lipopolysaccharide molecule is an amphiphile. It has a hydrophilic polysaccharide attached to a hydrophobic lipid moiety. Molecules vary in molecular weight from a few thousand to roughly 25,000 but are rarely found as unimolecular entities. Because of their amphiphilic nature, LPS molecules spontaneously aggregate in water to form membranes and vesicles. These particles reach molecular weights in the millions (Gould et al. 1991).

Lipid A is the smallest portion of the molecule that is endotoxic and reacts with LAL (Kotani and Takada, 1990). It has a hydrophilic backbone composed of two sugars and a hydrophobic region composed of nonhydroxylated and hydroxylated fatty acids (Rietschel et al., 1992; Takayama and Qureshi, 1992).

Lipid A has a negative charge that is neutralized in the cell membrane by cations, polyamines, and proteins with positive charges. In order to achieve stable and highly aggregated states, the charge on the LPS has to be neutralized. Purified endotoxins retain a mixture of cations that depends on the composition of the bacterial growth medium and on the method of purification (Coughlin et al., 1983b). The resultant bioactivity of the various salt forms of purified LPS or lipid A and their physicochemical behavior has been elucidated (Coughlin et al., 1983a; Galanos et al., 1979a).

Aggregate size and stability are also a function of the polysaccharide chain length (Lüderitz et al., 1986; Peterson and McGroarty, 1986). The differences in molecular weight among the LPS molecules even in a single bacterial cell are attributed to the heterogeneity of polysaccharide chain lengths (Hitchcock and Brown, 1983). Some types of bacteria make only short-chain oligosaccharides as opposed to polysaccharides. This purified endotoxin is called a lipooligosaccharide (LOS) and is extremely reactive on a weight basis (Rietschel et al., 1992).

Because of the nature of the LPS and the factors that influence its activity, chemical manipulation of solutions or surfaces contaminated with endotoxins may alter its structure and therefore its biological activity, including its reactivity with LAL. For example, mild acid hydrolysis (0.02 N sodium acetate buffer, pH 4.5, for 60 min at 100°C) will yield a precipitable lipid A, free of the polysaccharide (core and O-antigen) but still toxic in a solubilized form (Rietschel et al., 1992). Acid hydrolysis of LPS with 0.1 N HC1 for 15–30 min at 100°C yields a form of LPS that lacks the 1-position phosphate (Rietschel et al., 1992) and is no longer pyrogenic but retains its ability to cause tumor regression (monophosphoryl lipid A). Treatment with 0.2 N NaOH for 1 h at 100°C liberates ester-bound fatty acids from lipid A, which alters the lipid A sufficiently to achieve true chemical depyrogenation. Treatment with highly oxidizing agents will also liberate fatty acids (Gould and Novitsky, 1985). Other treatments with acids, bases, salt solutions, or oxidizing agents, especially at temperatures less than 100°C, may alter the structure of endotoxins in ways that are not clearly defined, but an altered structure invariably means altered activity.

The heterogeneity of endotoxins affects the strategies applied to their removal from surfaces and solutions. All endotoxins have some nonspecific affinity for surfaces via hydrophobic or ionic interactions. Depending on the strengths of those interactions, only those molecules or aggregates with greater affinity for the solute are going to rinse off a surface into that solute, and the rest will remain on that surface. Of those remaining after a water rinse, another fraction may rinse off in a saline solution, and another fraction only in solutions with a high or low pH. Surfactants and compounds with lipid-solubilizing capacities such as albumin will often solubilize endotoxins that will not be released with other compounds (Twohy and Duran, 1986). I have not been able to show convincingly that any one solution is capable of removing all surface-bound endotoxins, but once endotoxin has been removed with any one solution chemistry, subsequent further rinsing with the same solution does not release more (Gould, unpublished data). Therefore, prerinsing the purification or separation media with product will effectively "depyrogenate" the media because any remaining endotoxin is unlikely to get into subsequent product unless some physical or chemical condition is changed.

3 ENDOTOXINS AS STANDARDS FOR THE LAL TEST

The term "endotoxin" was coined by Pfeiffer to distinguish a toxin that seemed to be an "integral part of the bacterial body" from the endotoxin elaborated by the cholera bacilli (Westphal, 1993). The term is still in use today. It is used indiscriminately to refer to the naturally occurring wall fragments, to incompletely purified preparations of LPS that retain proteins and other components normally associated with LPS in the bacterial membrane, and to purified LPS preparations.

3.1 Methods of Purification

Several common methods to purify endotoxins are described in the literature. These include the classic trichloroacetic acid (TCA) extraction of Boivin et al. (1933), which results in LPS still associated with membrane proteins; Westphal and Jann's (1965) phenol extraction, which results in recovery of high molecular weight LPS free of proteins; the phenol–chloroform–petroleum ether (PCP) extraction developed by Galanos et al. (1969) for recovery of low molecular weight or R-form LPS; and a phenol extraction followed ultimately by electrodialysis to remove cations and enable manufacture of a highly purified uniform salt (Galanos et al., 1979b).

3.2 Reference Endotoxins

The endotoxin preparation that is the reference standard for the USP bacterial endotoxins test (USP, 1995a) is referred to as an RSE (reference standard endotoxin); it is a Westphal extracted preparation of endotoxin from cells of *Escherichia coli* O113 that is colyophilized with lactose and polyethylene glycol. The latest lot, designated lot G by USP and EC-6 by FDA, is a sublot of a large number of vials prepared at the National Institute for Biological Standards and Control (NIBSC) in the United Kingdom. Two other sublots were pooled, and the second international standard (IS) was taken from these pooled sublots. The biological activity of lot G/FDA EC-6 and that of the second IS as measured by LAL are equivalent; 10,000 EU per vial = 10,000 IU per vial, where EU stands for endotoxin unit (a U.S. designation for LPS activity) and IU stands for international unit (a European designation for activity). The recent acceptance of this standard by the Expert Committee on Biological Standardization, World Health Organization, as the international standard has very important consequences for companies releasing product in the United States or Europe because it enables all laboratories to perform tests calibrated against the same reference.

Other purified endotoxins may be calibrated against the RSE (see potency determination below) and used to control the LAL test. These secondary standards are referred to as a control standard endotoxins (CSEs).

3.3 Relative Activity of Endotoxins

Since it is the amount of lipid A and its functional activity as determined by its bacterial source that correlate with biological activity, activity cannot be compared between different endotoxin preparations on a weight basis. Endotoxin units, EUs or IUs, express the relative pyrogenic activity of an LPS preparation or unknown when tested with LAL. Originally defined for the Food and Drug Administration's endotoxin standard EC-2, the EU made it possible to compare any endotoxin preparation to the well-characterized standard in order to anticipate the preparation's pyrogenic potential. Once the activity of the preparation was standardized, it could be used instead of the RSE as the control standard in the LAL test. In the same way, the amount of endotoxin in an unknown must be expressed in endotoxin units per milliliter (EU/mL) so results, standardized to the activity of a known RSE, can be compared.

The LAL test has been approved by the U.S. FDA for 20 years now as the release test for medical devices and began replacing the rabbit pyrogen test in USP monographs in 1983. Today, the LAL test for gram-negative bacterial endotoxins has succeeded in replacing the rabbit pyrogen test in the majority of monographs, and most comparisons between the two have shown that the LAL test is an excellent predictor of pyrogenicity.

4 LIMULUS AMEBOCYTE LYSATE

The LAL reaction is an enzyme activation cascade that results in cleavage of a protein substrate. Under the right ionic conditions, the insoluble cleavage product coalesces with others to form a gel. As the pre-gel matrix grows, the particles become visible and the test solution becomes turbid. If an artificial, chromogenic, substrate is added to the reaction mixture, a chromophore will be cleaved that will cause the test solution to become colored. These three types of end points—gelation, turbidity, and intensity of color—define the three standard LAL test methods.

The LAL test is used worldwide as an end product release test for regulated products, and standard procedures are described in the various pharmacopoeias. In the United States, the manufacture of LAL reagent and the performance of LAL tests on pharmaceutical products are regulated by the Food and Drug Administration (FDA). The bacterial endotoxins test is the official method described in the U.S. Pharmacopeia (USP, 1995a). The test is modified with respect to assay validation and for routine release of end products by FDA in a guideline published in 1987 (FDA, 1987). This guideline, currently under revision (H. D. Hochstein, Center for Biologics Evaluation and Research of the FDA, personal communication), also describes the alternative methods, turbidimetric and chromogenic, that are not part of the pharmacopeial test. An FDA interim guidance publication (FDA, 1991) expands on the kinetic methodologies.

These documents, taken with the manufacturers' product inserts, provide the information necessary to perform LAL tests that would be acceptable to release product in the United States. The instructions for use are not exactly alike between manufacturers. Minor differences in the recommended test procedures and types of materials may be important for the success of the test, so it is important to follow the procedure described by the manufacturer of the LAL being used.

4.1 Gel-Clot Method

The gel-clot reagent was the first LAL reagent licensed, and the gel-clot method is still used for the majority of LAL tests. Equal volumes of sample and solubilized LAL are mixed in a 10 × 75 mm glass reaction tube. The mixture is incubated for 1 h at 37°C. At the end of the incubation period, tests are read one at a time by removing an individual tube from the incubator (from a rack in a water bath or from a well in a dry-block heater) and inverting it in one smooth motion through 180°. If a gel has formed during the incubation and remains intact on inversion, then the test is positive, and the amount of endotoxin in the tube is greater than or equal to the labeled sensitivity of the LAL reagent. Any other state of the reaction mixture at the end of the incubation period constitutes a negative test.

Flocculant or "snowflake" precipitation is indicative of the presence of endotoxin in the reaction mixture but in an amount that is less than the sensitivity (see Sec. 4.2). It is useful to note this precipitation when reading the test. If it occurs in the negative controls, it often means that the water source is contaminated with a low level of endotoxin. If low levels of endotoxin are added to the reagent when it is solubilized, the LAL reaction is initiated in the vial and the assay will appear to be more sensitive than it should be when standards are tested. Higher levels of endotoxin in the reagent will cause all the tests to be positive, including the negative control. If the gel matrix has started to form in the vial and is disrupted to set up the test, none of the tests will clot because the disrupted matrix will not gel again.

The sensitivity of the gel-clot method is limited by the time and temperature of incubation. The most sensitive reagent, defined by the 1 h incubation at 37°C, is able to detect as little as 0.03 EU/mL. The U.S. reference endotoxin is always used to establish the sensitivity of licensed reagents.

4.2 Turbidimetric Methods

As the LAL reaction progresses toward gelation, the reaction mixture becomes turbid. Those samples with greater concentrations of endotoxin become turbid more rapidly. Optical density, used as a measure of turbidity, may be read at the beginning of incubation and again at a given point in time after onset of incubation, in every sample. A standard curve may be drawn by plotting optical density (OD) against endotoxin concentration. This method of performing a turbidimetric assay is called an end-point method because samples are read at the end of a predetermined period of time.

The first descriptions of a turbidimetric method were given by Levin and Bang (1968). They performed what is termed a kinetic turbidimetric method because they took frequent OD readings in the same sample, and they showed that the samples with the greater endotoxin concentrations had greater rates of increase in turbidity than those with less endotoxin. Today, incubating spectrophotometers have been developed that will read OD values from multiple wells and read each sample multiple times, each reading made within seconds of the previous one. These values are transferred to a computer for storage and analysis. Calculations are performed, and the system returns endotoxin concentrations to the operator.

Kinetic methods lend themselves to screening samples that vary over a wide range of endotoxin concentrations, typically four to five orders of magnitude. The tests are performed by mixing solubilized LAL reagent and sample in whatever ratio is recommended by the manufacturer for the type of reaction vessel being used. Data are collected, and a standard curve is constructed by plotting the logarithm of the onset time against that of the endotoxin concentration. Onset time is the time at which the optical density reaches a predetermined value and is an indicator of the rate of the reaction. The standard curve has a negative slope because the onset time is fastest (lowest numerical value) for the greatest concentration of endotoxin.

Because turbidity can be detected before a reaction mixture clots, a given endotoxin concentration will yield a turbidimetric result sooner than it will yield a gel-clot result. Very low concentrations of endotoxin can be measured within a reasonable incubation time by turbidimetric means that would not be likely to cause a clot for several hours. The kinetic turbidimetric assay may be as sensitive as 0.001 EU/mL in a test that incubates for approximately 90 min.

The sensitivity of turbidimetric reagents, unlike that of the gel-clot reagents, is not determined by the manufacturer. The sensitivity is defined to be the lowest concentration used to construct the standard curve, so the analyst defines it and can change it to accommodate the interference characteristics of the sample and its endotoxin limit.

4.3 Chromogenic Methods

In 1977, Japanese investigators reported using synthetic or artificial substrates in the LAL assay (Nakamura et al., 1977). These substrates comprised a chromophore attached to a smaller number of amino acids in a structural sequence that mimicked the cleavage site of coagulogen, the naturally occurring LAL substrate. When activated clotting enzyme cleaved synthetic substrate, the chromophore was released. Thus, the amount of absorbance measured in the reaction mixture at any time was a function of the amount of chromophore released, which was in turn a function of the concentration of endotoxin in the sample.

As with the turbidimetric assay, the chromogenic assay may be performed using either an end-point or kinetic protocol, and the data are plotted and analyzed in the same way as for the turbidimetric method. Variants to the end-point method include use of diazotization chemistry to transform the typical yellow of the cleaved *para*-nitroanaline (pNA) chromophore to a magenta. This is a useful step when performing the LAL test on samples that are already yellow.

The sensitivity of the chromogenic method is the least concentration of endotoxin included in the standard curve. The greatest sensitivity claimed for this method is 0.005 EU/mL.

4.4 Differences Between LAL Reagents

The formulations of currently available commercial LAL reagents differ from one manufacturer to another. These differences mean that some substances containing endotoxin will interfere with the sensitivity of one manufacturer's test more than with the sensitivity of another's (Twohy et al., 1983). Formulations may differ in their capacity to disaggregate or solubilize LPS particles to make a lipid A more accessible to LAL enzyme(s). Some formulations may stabilize the pH of reaction mixtures within the optimum range more efficiently or have components that adsorb LPS in such a way that lipid A regions are exposed.

4.5 β-Glucans

The LAL test was originally thought to be highly specific for lipopolysaccharides, but more recently it has been found to be sensitive to the presence of certain types of β-glucans, also referred to as LAL-reactive material or LRM (Kakinuma et al., 1981; Pearson et al., 1987; Roslansky and Novitsky, 1991). Factor G, an enzyme that is present in LAL, is activated by β-1,3-glucans or by β-1,4-glucans. The β-1,3-glucans are components of fungal and algal cell walls; the β-1,4-glucans are common extractables from cellulosic materials. Formulations of LAL reagent differ in the level of sensitivity they have to the β-glucans; some are very sensitive, and others are practically insensitive. Endotoxins and β-glucans often act synergistically in an LAL test, so alterations to formulations that reduce sensitivity to the β-glucans may also reduce sensitivity to certain LPS structures (Roslansky and Novitsky, 1991).

Pharmaceutical products are rarely contaminated with β-glucans. Unless the product is derived from fungal or algal culture, these organisms and therefore the β-glucans are not found as contaminants in a facility that maintains good manufacturing practices. The most common source of cellulosic extractables is cellulosic filter media, but not all such media shed these polysaccharides. For example, chemically produced non-naturally derived cellulose acetate membranes are free of β-1,4-glucans. Filtrates that yield positive LAL tests indicate contaminated filter media whether the source is endotoxin or β-glucans. If the tests are negative, then β-glucans are not an issue. It is usually possible to exclude filter media suspected of excreting β-glucans from production processes. When it is not possible to change the type of filter medium, it is usually possible to rinse the medium before use to reduce the level of contamination.

A phenomenon noted in my laboratory and conveyed by others who have also looked at cellulosic materials is something referred to as "rebound." If a cellulosic substrate is rinsed until the effluent no longer causes a positive LAL test, stored for several hours under conditions that prevent bacterial growth, and then rinsed again with the same type of rinse solution as before, the second effluent will be positive or rebound if the original source of the LAL reactivity was LRM. The second effluent will be negative if the original source was endotoxin. Therefore, less LRM is likely to contaminate a product if the filter is rinsed with product and used immediately.

5 ANCILLARY LAL REAGENTS

The manufacturers of LAL reagents may supply ancillary reagents either separately or as kits. Ancillary reagents and materials that are required to perform the test are listed in the product insert or instructions for use.

To perform a satisfactory LAL test, one must have LAL reagent, an endotoxin control (CSE or RSE), and a source of water that has less endotoxin than is detectable by the type of LAL method used. Equipment includes reaction vessels (glass tubes or plastic microplates), a mixing device, dilution tubes, storage containers, pipetes and other such transfer devices, and closures. Equipment materials should not adsorb endotoxin or leach substances that interfere with the test.

Materials that come in contact with the sample or any of the reagents should be rendered, or shown to already be, free of detectable endotoxin and free of substances (extractables) that interfere with the LAL test. Materials that are labeled ''sterile'' may not be suitable for use, while and, on the other hand, materials that have not been sterilized may be perfectly acceptable. Materials labeled ''nonpyrogenic'' may still contain enough endotoxin to affect an LAL test even though they do not contain enough endotoxin to be considered pyrogenic. Medical devices are nonpyrogenic if the average amount of endotoxin detected per unit from a pooled sample is less than 20 EU (USP, 1995b; FDA, 1987). Polypropylene plastics have been particularly subject to endotoxin adsorption and to leaching of interfering substances (Novitsky et al., 1986).

6 ERROR OF THE LAL TEST

The error of the test currently depends on the method. Quantitation by the gel-clot method is performed by titrating the endotoxin to an end point (last positive test in a series of increasing dilutions of sample), so the error is plus or minus a dilution. The gel-clot assay is generally performed on serial twofold dilutions, so the commonly expressed error for the test is plus or minus twofold or 50–200% of the measured value.

The so-called quantitative assays, the turbidimetric and chromogenic LAL assays, are also performed on serial dilutions, but the measured response (optical density or onset time) of the unknown is taken from a standard curve derived from the responses of known endotoxin concentrations. It is possible to narrow the observed range of the error to something that approaches the ability of the LAL reagent to discriminate concentrations, i.e., reduce technician error to a minimum, but in reality manufacturers and the FDA recommend that the error of these tests be maintained within 25% for end-point assays and 50% for kinetic assays (FDA, 1991). Most recently, the Japanese Ministry of Health and Welfare has taken responsibility for writing a version of the bacterial endotoxins test in an effort to promote international harmonization. They propose a 50–200% error around the recovered value for kinetic methods in which endotoxins are quantified using a log–log relationship. Thus, in practice, there may be little real difference in the error of the LAL test no matter what method is used, and it is misleading to refer to the gel-clot method as qualitative and to the turbidimetric and chromogenic methods as quantitative.

7 CONFIRMATION THAT THE TEST WORKS PROPERLY

It is very important to confirm that the test is working satisfactorily within one's own laboratory by the use of controls, and this is addressed by the U.S. Pharmacopeial Convention and the FDA in the appropriate references. The sensitivity of the gel-clot lot should be obtained within the error of the test. The sensitivity of the turbidimetric and chromogenic methods must be demonstrated by achieving a linear relationship over a given range of endotoxin concentrations that is also sufficient to distinguish the concentrations from each other within the error of the test. The definition of linearity is an issue for the kinetic methods. Over broad ranges of endotoxin concentrations, it is very apparent that the points on the standard curve more closely resemble a curved line than a straight line. The log–log representation cannot eliminate the curvature completely, but linearity, as defined, is met if the absolute value of the correlation coefficient is less than or equal to 0.980, a relatively easy specification to obtain.

On close inspection of the data plotted as optical density versus time of incubation, it is obvious that as the concentration of endotoxin being assayed increases, the difference in time between the concentrations narrows until the ability to measure accurately at very short intervals of time becomes the limiting factor. So, even though linearity is confirmed, more precise measurements are made by working with lower concentrations of endotoxin and by limiting the range, two conditions that also virtually eliminate curvature as an issue.

8 SOFTWARE

Software used to analyze the data obtained by the kinetic methods should be well understood. Software manufacturers, whether the LAL manufacturer or otherwise, have chosen ways to deal mathematically with the inherent kinetics of the LAL reaction. Questions may arise about how onset times are determined, how regressions are calculated to obtain standard curve parameters, whether or not threshold OD values should be varied during analysis, and how parameters that were used to validate products can be identified and stored, if necessary, to use for routine product release.

9 INSTRUMENTATION

More elaborate instrumentation is necessary for turbidimetric and chromogenic methods to incubate the samples during the reaction period and to read and record the OD values either directly to paper or to a computer so they are available for analysis. Computers are used to collect and store the variables of time and OD, perform the calculations to return the parameters of the standard curve, and calculate the concentrations of endotoxin in the unknowns.

Incubators are important to the performance of the LAL test. The LAL reaction is enzymatic; therefore, the rate of the reaction varies with the temperature of incubation. The test requires that multiple samples be incubated in the same device, so all reaction mixtures have to be maintained at the same temperature for the results of one test to be related to those of another. Incubators that accept tubes are relatively easy to validate with respect to the temperature in individual reaction mixtures. Microplate incubators are generally more difficult and sometimes impossible to monitor because thermistors are difficult to place or cannot be placed in individual reaction wells. The ultimate test for these systems is to perform the LAL assay on one concentration of endotoxin in all tubes or wells. By using standard parameters obtained from a previous test, concentrations may be assigned to the tests in each well. The results are assessed two ways in my laboratory. First, the concentration in each well is expected to be within 25% of the mean concentration recovered for all wells;

second, even when all wells pass the 25% test, there is no tendency for concentrations to increase or decrease from one side of the plate to the other or from the center of the plate to the edges.

10 POTENCY AND RELATED ISSUES

The method used to determine the potency (EU/ng) of an LPS is described in both the USP bacterial endotoxins test (USP, 1995a) and the 1987 FDA guideline (FDA, 1987). The reference endotoxin is diluted and assayed in parallel with dilutions of the endotoxin preparation to be standardized. The sensitivity of the LAL expressed in endotoxin units per milliliter of reference endotoxin is equivalent to the sensitivity of the LAL expressed in units of mass per milliliter of the test preparation. The potency is the RSE sensitivity divided by the CSE sensitivity, generally expressed as endotoxin units per nanogram. As long as the activity of the RSE and CSE remain the same or are affected to the same extent by the solubilizing agent, the potency should remain the same. In general, the relative potencies do remain the same, a satisfying situation, because it is the basis of being able to use the LAL test to quantify endotoxins.

One of the more subtle issues to bear in mind during experimentation with endotoxins is the issue of enhancement and inhibition of the LAL test by the test solution. Enhancement is defined as the recovery of more endotoxin than expected; inhibition is the recovery of less endotoxin than expected. No matter which method is used, the initial qualification of the LAL test method, or of the technician performing the LAL test, is performed on endotoxin suspended in water. Manufacturers label gel-clot formulations with the sensitivity determined by measuring endotoxin concentrations in water, and they characterize the turbidimetric and chromogenic methods using endotoxin in water. When endotoxin is suspended in solutions other than pure water, it may assume a configuration that is more or less reactive in a biological assay, including the LAL test. The level of enhancement or inhibition that results can be thought of as a change in potency between the endotoxin in water and the endotoxin in the test solution. Enhancement or inhibition may be overcome by sufficient dilution with water to ensure that the endotoxin is, in fact, in water and no longer influenced by the test solution.

The presence of enhancement or inhibition is demonstrated by performing the LAL test in parallel on endotoxin concentrations prepared in pure water and on endotoxin concentrations prepared in the test solution. Using the gel-clot method, one shows that the sensitivity of the LAL to endotoxin in the test sample is the same as in water, i.e., the labeled sensitivity of the LAL is recovered in each test. To perform this test by the gel-clot method, the sample cannot contain detectable endotoxin because the test cannot quantify less than the concentration that causes a clot to form. The inhibition/enhancement test can be performed on samples that already contain measurable endotoxin only with the turbidimetric and chromogenic methods, with which endotoxin may be quantified by reference to a standard curve. The recovered additional or "spiked" endotoxin is distinguished from the endogenous endotoxin by subtracting the amount recovered in the sample from the amount recovered in the spiked sample.

If kinetic methods are used and several concentrations of endotoxin have been used to spike the sample, two standard curves are generated: the standard curve in water and the standard curve prepared in a single concentration of sample. These two curves on a log–log plot should have identical slopes, showing that the endotoxin activity dilutes in the same way for both preparations. If there is no enhancement or inhibition, the lines will overlie each other. If there is either enhancement or inhibition, then the vertical distance between the two lines is a measure of the difference in activity. If the slopes are not identical, then one line will cross the other, indicating that the sample enhances the activity of the endotoxin relative to water on one side of the crossover point and inhibits it on the other side. When the slopes are not identical, the concentration of endotoxin in the sample cannot be calculated by comparison to the activity of concentrations in water. The sample must be diluted further to a concentration that more closely resembles water and the test repeated (Remillard et al., 1987).

Obviously, the usefulness of dilution is limited for many experimental applications because the activity of the endotoxin is of interest only in the more concentrated sample. In these situations, there are two choices. If the sample can be rendered free of detectable endotoxin, the standard curve is prepared by making dilutions of RSE (or CSE that has been calibrated in the sample against RSE) in sample that is free of endogenous endotoxin. This "product standard curve" can then be used to quantify endotoxin in the unknown. The parameters of the standard curve should be shown to be constant between several samples before one sample is used to prepare standard curves for other unknown samples. One application for which it is inappropriate to use one sample to prepare standard curves is in the measurement of endotoxin in blood, because activity of endotoxin detected by LAL is a function of the neutralizing capacity of the individual source of the blood as well as the amount of endotoxin in the sample (Warren et al., 1985; Novitsky, 1994).

The second method used to measure endotoxin in a sample concentration that otherwise interferes with the LAL test is to remove the endotoxin from the sample and restore it to a water solution before performing the assay. This has the advantage of putting the endotoxin in the same background, and presumably in the same active configuration, so that concentrations obtained for endotoxin from the different types of samples can be compared to the activity of the standard endotoxin in water. Most methods that may be devised to quantitatively transfer endotoxin in low concentrations from one type of solution to another do not work. The greatest impediment to these procedures is the tendency of endotoxin to adsorb, and always to some degree adsorb irreversibly, to surfaces. This occurs when solutions are evaporated and the residue is resolubilized in water or when solutions are filtered and the material is resuspended in solution.

11 REMOVAL OF LAL BY FILTRATION

There are very few filtration materials that do not adsorb endotoxin; therefore, most are useless for recovering small concentrations of endotoxin. One commercially available ultrafiltration system that does work is specifically advertised to enable the user to remove low molecular weight interfering factors from LAL samples while retaining the higher molecular weight endotoxins in the retentate. It is basically a diafiltration system that replaces the sample solute with water; the sample (retentate) can be adjusted to the original volume at the end of the process and assayed directly. As long as the ultrafilter remains wet, endotoxins do not bind; and as long as the endotoxins are maintained in high molecular weight structures so that they are retained, they will be recovered completely in the assay.

This method works only if endotoxin can be retained in a high molecular weight form and if the solute is of a low enough molecular weight to be removed. If the solute causes endotoxin to disaggregate, the endotoxin will be lost with the low molecular weight substances in the filtrate.

This diafiltration method is extremely valuable if products that are insoluble in water are soluble in another solvent that is compatible with the filtration membrane and cartridge. Product can be solubilized in the solvent and diafiltered with the solvent to remove the low molecular weight product and retain the high molecular weight endotoxin. Once product is removed, the solvent can be replaced with water and the retained endotoxin tested.

This method has also been used in my laboratory to concentrate the endotoxin in samples. Some medical devices, for example, are so large that the rinse volume necessary to extract the contaminating endotoxin dilutes the endotoxin beyond the limit of detection (USP, 1995b; FDA, 1987). If the system is modified to ultrafilter several known volumes of sample, the retentate represents a concentration of the extraction volume and of the endotoxin, so an LAL test can be used.

Filtration is often used in a production process to remove endotoxin (depyrogenate). While there are some general considerations useful in choosing the type of filter medium and size or molecular weight cutoff, the only ultimate way to be assured that the filtration works is to use it successfully.

Sterilizing filters will not exclude passage of endotoxins on the basis of size but are successfully used to nonspecifically adsorb endotoxins. These filters "work" until the surfaces are saturated with endotoxin; therefore their use requires monitoring to ensure that endotoxins do not "break through." Positively charged filters often are more efficient at adsorbing negatively charged endotoxins. Adsorption, whether facilitated by surface hydrophobicity or by charge, works most efficiently when the nature of the solute promotes adsorption and does not block it. Water and saline solutions generally facilitate adsorption.

Ultrafilters retain endotoxins as long as the endotoxins are large enough to be excluded by the pores of the membrane. If the molecular weights of product and endotoxin are different enough for one to be retained, then ultrafiltration can be used to separate the endotoxin from the product. Ultrafilters rated to retain particles that have molecular weights of 100,000 or greater will be perfectly adequate to remove endotoxin from water where endotoxins are expected to be in highly aggregated states. On the other hand, if the solute disaggregates endotoxins, then smaller pore diameters will be required to retain the endotoxin (Sweadner et al., 1977). If the product itself adsorbs endotoxin, then filtration will not separate them.

The aggregate state of the endotoxin is not always known before filtration is attempted. Some solutes seem to have somewhat surprising effects; for example, Tris ion competes with other cations for specific cation-binding sites on the LPS molecule and apparently facilitates solubilization (disaggregation) of the bacterial outer membrane (Schindler and Osborn, 1979). Consequently, it is relatively difficult to remove endotoxins from Tris buffers by ultrafiltration.

12 CONCLUSION

The LAL test has been developed and works very well to estimate the concentrations of gram-negative bacterial endotoxins in samples. The test is used to monitor production processes and release finished product. It is used to measure the efficiency of endotoxin removal by depyrogenation methods. It is used to help elucidate the biological activity of endotoxins as they are moved from one chemical environment to another. It can be used to detect inadvertent changes to formulations, especially changes introduced by β-glucan contamination, by responding with an uncharacteristic inhibition/enhancement pattern. In fact, LAL is a very useful tool with broad applications for the technician who takes the time to understand both endotoxins and LAL methodology.

REFERENCES

Boivin, A., J. Mesrobeanu, and L. Mesrobeanu. (1933). Extraction d'un complexe toxic et antigenic a partir du bacille d'aertrycke, *Compt. Rend. Soc. Biol.*, *114*:307–310.

Coughlin, R. T., A. Haug, and E. J. McGroarty. (1983a). Physical properties of defined lipopolysaccharide salts, *Biochemistry*, *22*:2007–2013.

Coughlin, R. T., S. Tonsager, and E. J. McGroarty. (1983b). Quantitation of metal cations bound to membranes and extracted lipopolysaccharide of *Escherichia coli*, *Biochemistry*, *22*:2002–2007.

FDA. (1987). Guideline on Validation of the Limulus Amebocytc Lysate Test as an End-Product Test for Human and Animal Parenteral Drugs, Biological Products, and Medical Devices, Docket #79D0465 U.S. Department of Health and Human Services, Food and Drug Administration, Rockville, MD.

FDA. (1991). Interim Guidance for Human and Veterinary Drug Products and Biologicals. Kinetic LAL Techniques, U.S. Department of Health and Human Services, Food and Drug Administration, Rockville, MD.

Galanos, C., M. A. Freudenberg, O. Lüderitz, E. T. Rietschel, and O. Westphal. (1979a). Chemical, physicochemical and biological properties of bacterial lipopolysaccharides, in *Biomedical Applications of the Horseshoe Crab (Limulidae)*, Prog. Clin. Biol. Res., Vol. 29 (E. Cohen, ed.), Alan R. Liss, New York, pp. 321–332.

Galanos, C., O. Lüderitz, and O. Westphal. (1969). A new method for the extraction of R lipopolysaccharides, *Eur. J. Biochem.*, *9*:245–249.

Galanos, C., O. Lüderitz, and O. Westphal. (1979b). Preparation and properties of a standardized lipopolysaccharide from *Salmonella abortus equi* (Novo-Pyrexal), *Zbl. Bakt. Hyg. I. Abt. Orig. A*, *243*:226–244.

Goldman, R. C., and L. Leive. (1980). Heterogeneity of antigenic-side-chain lengths in lipopolysaccharide from *Escherichia coli* O111 and *Salmonella typhimurium* LT2, *Eur. J. Biochem.*, *107*:145–153.

Gould, M. C. (1984). Endotoxin in vertebrate cell culture: Its measurement and significance, in *Uses and Standardization of Vertebrate Cell Cultures*, In Vitro Monograph No. 5 (M. K. Patterson, Jr., ed.), Tissue Culture Association, Gaithersburg, MD, pp. 125–136.

Gould, M. J., and T. J. Novitsky. (1985). Depyrogenation of hydrogen peroxide, in *Depyrogenation*, Tech. Rep. 7, Parenteral Drug Association, Philadelphia, pp. 84–92.

Gould, M. J., M. E. Dawson, and T. J. Novitsky. (1991). A review of the particulate nature of lipopolysaccharide and its measurement by the *Limulus* amebocyte lysate test, *Particle Sci. Technol.*, *9*:55–59.

Kakinuma, A., T. Asano, H. Torii, and Y. Sugino. (1981). Gelation of Limulus amebocyte lysate by an antitumor (1 → 3)-β-D-glucan, *Biochem. Biophys. Res. Commun.*, *101*(2): 434–439.

Kotani, S., and H. Takada. (1990). Structural requirements of lipid A for endotoxicity and other biological activities —an overview, *Adv. Exp. Med. Biol.*, *256*:13–43.

Levin, J., and F. B. Bang. (1968). Clottable protein in *Limulus*: Its localization and kinetics of its coagulation by endotoxin, *Thromb. Diath. Haemorrh.*, *19*:186–197.

Lüderitz, O., C. Galanos, E. Th. Rietschel, and O. Westphal. (1986). Lipid A: Relationships of chemical structure and biological activity, in *Immunobiology and Immunopharma-*

cology of Bacterial Endotoxins (A. Szentivanyi, H. Friedman, and A. Nowotny, eds.), Plenum, New York, pp. 65–74.

Nakamura, S., T. Morita, S. Iwanaga, M. Niwa, and K. Takahashi. (1977). A sensitive substrate for the clotting enzyme in horseshoe crab hemocytes, *J. Biochem.*, *81*:1567–1569.

Novitsky, T. J., J. Schmidt-Gengenbach, and J. F. Remillard. (1986). Factors affecting the recovery of endotoxin adsorbed to container surfaces, *J. Parenter. Sci. Technol.*, *40*: 284–286.

Novitsky, T. J. (1994). Limulus amebocyte lysate (LAL) detection of endotoxin in human blood, *J. Endotoxin Res.*, *1*:253–263.

Pearson, F. C., R. Caruana, J. Burkart, D. V. Katz, D. Chenoweth, J. Dubczak, J. Bohon, and M. Weary. (1987). The use of Limulus amebocyte lysate to monitor hemodialyzer-associated soluble cellulosic material (LAL-reactive material), in *Detection of Bacterial Endotoxins with the Limulus Amebocyte Lysate Test* (S. W. Watson, J. Levin, and T. J. Novitsky, eds.), Alan R. Liss, New York, pp. 211–222.

Peterson, A. A., and E. J. McGroarty. (1986). Physical properties of short-chain and long-chain fractions of lipopolysaccharide, in *Immunobiology and Immunopharmacology of Bacterial Endotoxins* (A. Szentivanyi, H. Friedman, and A. Nowotny, eds.), Plenum, New York, 83–87.

Remillard, J. F., M. C. Gould, P. F. Roslansky, and T. J. Novitsky. (1987). Quantitation of endotoxin in products using the Limulus amebocyte lysate kinetic turbidimetric assay, in *Detection of Bacterial Endotoxins with the Limulus Amaebocyte Lysate Test* (S. W. Watson, J. Levin, and T. J. Novitsky, eds.), Alan R. Liss, New York, pp. 197–210.

Rietschel, E. Th., L. Brade, B. Lindner, and U. Zahringer. (1992). Biochemistry of lipopolysaccharides, in *Bacterial Endotoxic Lipopolysaccharides*, Mol. Biochem. Cell. Biol., Vol. 1 (D. C. Morrison and J. L. Ryan, eds.), CRC Press, Ann Arbor, MI, pp. 3–41.

Roslansky, P. F., and T. J. Novitsky. (1991). Sensitivity of limulus amebocyte lysate (LAL) to LAL-reactive glucans, *J. Clin. Microbiol.*, *29*:2477–2483.

Schindler, M., and M. J. Osborn. (1979). Interaction of divalent cations and polymyxin B with lipopolysaccharide, *Biochem.*, *18*:4425–4430.

Sweadner, K. J., M. Forte, and L. L. Nelsen. (1977). Filtration removal of endotoxin (pyrogens) in solution in different states of aggregation, *Appl. Environ. Microbiol.*, *34*:382–385.

Takayama, K., and N. Qureshi. (1992). Chemical structure of lipid A, in *Bacterial Endotoxic Lipopolysaccharides*, Mol. Biochem. Cell. Biol. Vol. 1 (D. C. Morrison and J. L. Ryan, eds.), CRC Press, Ann Arbor, MI, pp. 43–65.

Twohy, C. W., and A. P. Duran. (1986). Extraction of bacterial endotoxin from medical devices, *J. Parenter. Sci. Technol.*, *40*:287–291.

Twohy, C. W., M. L. Nierman, A. P. Duran, and T. E. Munson. (1983). Comparison of Limulus amebocyte lysates from different manufacturers, *J. Parenter. Sci. Technol.*, *37*:93–96.

USP. (1995a). The United States Pharmacopeial Convention, Bacterial Endotoxins Test, *United States Pharmacopeia*, Revision 23, pp. 1696–1697.

USP. (1995b). The United States Pharmacopeial Convention, Transfusion and Infusion Assemblies and Similar Medical Devices, *United States Pharmacopeia*, Revision 23, First Suppl., Mack Printing Company, Easton, PA, p. 2523.

Warren, H. S., T. J. Novitsky, P. A. Ketchum, P. F. Roslansky, S. Kania, and G. R. Siber. (1985). Neutralization of bacterial lipopolysaccharides by human plasma, *J. Clin. Microbiol.*, *22*:590–595.

Westphal, O. (1993). An old-timer's reflections on endotoxin, in *Bacterial Endotoxin: Recognition and Effector Mechanisms* (J. Levin, C. R. Alving, R. S. Mumford, and P. L. Stütz, eds.), Elsevier, Amsterdam, The Netherlands, pp. 17–36.

Westphal, O., and K. Jann. (1965). Bacterial lipopolysaccharides. Extraction with phenol-water and further applications of the procedure, in *Methods in Carbohydrate Chemistry* (R. L. Whistler, ed.), Academic, New York, pp. 83–91.

20

Filtration and the Removal of Viruses from Biopharmaceuticals

RICHARD V. LEVY, MICHAEL W. PHILLIPS, and HERBERT LUTZ
Millipore Corporation, Bedford, Massachusetts

1 THE PROBLEM: VIRUSES IN BIOPHARMACEUTICALS

Many biotherapeutic proteins of commercial interest are obtained from human or animal tissue extraction processes or, more recently, from continuously cultured, transformed mammalian cells and transgenic mammals. Although these protein-based drugs have proven to be very effective, there exists a potential risk that endogenous viruses or virus-like particles will be transmitted to human beings. Concerns exist that some of these contaminants may be infectious or cause oncogenic events in humans (Lubiniecki, 1988; Petricciani, 1985). This risk has led both producers and regulatory agencies to address issues of product safety as it relates to virus transmission (Builder et al., 1989; USFDA, 1996; Eshkol et al., 1988).

One strategy for ensuring that biotherapeutics are free of viral contaminants is to prevent viral entry from raw materials in the production process. However, it has become evident that the detection limit of modern viral assays is not sufficient to guarantee the absence of both known and unknown viral contaminants. In fact, many existing virus assays lack the sensitivity to even detect virus titers that may be of medical concern. For example, some retroviral assays have been reported to have a detection limit of about 100 particles/mL (Builder et al., 1989), especially when chemical inactivation agents are employed. Additionally, in contrast to many bacterial assays, no generic viral assay exists that is capable of determining total virus titer in all applications (DiLeo et al., 1992). For these reasons, the use of strategies relying solely on assays for detecting virus titer within incoming raw materials and/or the final product do not completely allay the fear of virus transmission.

Consequently, producers of biotherapeutic drugs have adapted a manufacturing control strategy for minimizing the potential of viral transmission. This strategy, used in conjunction with incoming raw material and final product virus testing, consists of two parts: (1) cell line characterization both before and after representative production and (2) the use of downstream purification operations that are validated for their ability to remove and inactivate virus (DiLeo et al., 1992). Filtration, an ever-increasingly important component of this control strategy, is the subject of this chapter.

1.1 Viral Contaminations

In recent history, there have been documented cases of individuals inoculated with biotherapeutics contaminated with virus. Specific instances include yellow fever virus vaccine contaminated by avian leukosis virus and/or hepatitis B virus, poliovirus vaccine contaminated with SV40, and adenovirus vaccines contaminated with SV40 (CPMP, 1991a).

Blood-derived products have also been suspected or directly implicated in viral infections. For instance, in 1994, several cases of hepatitis C virus (HCV) infection in the United States were directly linked to an IgG product (*Wall Street Journal*, 1994). In 1996, Factor VIII, a blood-clotting factor used in the treatment of hemophilia A, was found to be contaminated with hepatitis A virus (HAV). The same strain of HAV was found in the final drug product and in two patients who were administered the product. The two proven cases of HAV transmissions are the first known occurrences of hepatitis A associated with clotting factor medications in the United States. Factor IX, a blood-clotting factor used in the treatment of hemophilia B, was derived from the same pool of plasma and may also have been contaminated (Altman, 1996). Also in 1996, China banned a widely distributed blood product found to be tainted with AIDS antibodies. Fortunately, there were no reports of HIV transmission to patients using the tainted products.

Additional concerns exist relative to the transmission of parvovirus and prions. In 1995, it was reported that a cell reactor was contaminated with minute virus of mice (MVM), a parvovirus with an approximate diameter of 22 nm. Although the virus was able to reproduce within the bioreactor, no final product was contaminated. The origin of the MVM virus was never confirmed, but it was suspected that a GMP failure led to the introduction (Garnick, 1995).

Prions, the proposed agents responsible for transmissible spongiform encephalopathies (TSEs), have recently been suspected in plasma pools used in the production of plasma derivatives due to plasma donors being diagnosed with Creutzfeldt–Jacob Disease (CJD). In 1994, the Ministry of Health and Welfare (Tokyo, Japan) ordered a U.S. pharmaceutical company to recall Japanese market products (human serum albumin) containing blood collected from a patient infected with Creutzfeldt–Jacob disease (CJD) (Kyodo News International, 1994). In 1995, the Canadian Red Cross recalled albumin, IVIG and Factor-I worth an estimated $10 million because of suspected CJD contamination (Infectious Disease Weekly, Aug. 7, 1995). In 1996, several manufacturers were also forced to withdraw roughly 500 lots of human albumin products due to the possibility of transmission of CJD (FDA Web site). Prion contamination of serum containing fermentor growth media, transgenic expression systems, and final formulation excipients (e.g., plasma derived albumin) are also of concern to the biotechnology industries.

1.2 Regulatory Perspective

Regulatory authorities generally recommend that protein purification processes achieve an overall cumulative viral clearance factor of at least 12 logs (orders of magnitude reduction). Conventionally, such viral clearance has been achieved by a combination of techniques such as solvent-detergent, pH and heat inactivation, and chromatographic removal. These techniques are all effective to a degree but suffer from certain drawbacks. For instance, although very effective against lipid-coated (enveloped) viruses, solvent-detergent treatment is not effective against nonenveloped viruses such as hepatitis A virus.

Physical inactivation methods—heat, chemical, ultraviolet or gamma irradiation—can denature sensitive proteins and may leave inactivated viral particles in solution. This can lead to antigenic problems as well as requiring the removal of chemical agents or denatured proteins. Affinity and/or ion-exchange chromatographic techniques are not considered sufficiently robust in use for viral clearance (that is, able to work under a variety of conditions).

In 1989, the European Union was the first to provide written guidance on viral clearance on biopharmaceutical manufacturers. The published document was written by the Committee for Proprietary Medicinal Products (CPMP, 1991a). Further details were provided for human blood and plasma-derived products (CPMP, 1991b). These documents became the corner-stones for future guidance documents.

In 1993, the U.S. FDA's Center for Biologics Evaluation and Research (CBER) issued a general framework for conducting process evaluation studies. In 1994, CBER issued a revision to its "Draft Points to Consider (PTC) in the Manufacture and Testing of Monoclonal Antibody Products for Human Use" (FDA, 1994). This was the first attempt by the FDA to provide guidance in the area of viral clearance and validation. Salient points from this document include: "Validation that retroviruses are removed or inactivated by the purification scheme is ultimately required" and "it is recommended that all purification schemes use one or more *robust* virus removal or inactivation steps." Robust steps are defined as those that work well under a variety of conditions (for instance, pH or ionic strength of column buffers with a variety of monoclonal antibodies). As seen in Table 1, taken from this guideline, robust steps include low pH, heat, solvent-detergent inactivation, and filtration.

Recent monographs from regulatory authorities have reflected concerns related to several occurrences of viral contaminants (HAV, HBV, HCV, and HIV) present in

Table 1 Ranges of Retroviral Removal (Expression in Logs)

Inactivation/removal step	Robust	Reported viral LRV[a]
pH	Yes	3–4
Heat	Yes	4
Solvent/detergent	Yes	5
Filtration	Yes	4–8
Detergent	No	4
Affinity/ion exchange	No	1–5

[a]LRV = log reduction value. See Sec. 5.1.
Source: FDA (1994).

plasma-derived products. In June 1994, the CPMP decided that new measures were required to reduce the risk of transmission of infective agents from medicinal products derived from human blood or plasma.

> For all presently authorized blood-derived medicinal products, an appropriate validation with respect to non-enveloped viruses is necessary. Therefore, marketing authorization holders will be requested to develop and validate additional virus elimination and inactivation steps as a matter of urgency in order to improve safety. (CPMP, 1994)

In May and August of 1994, the Paul Erlich Institute (PEI) issued documents raising the ante on virus removal in plasma-derived products. These documents set minimum standards for the removal of both enveloped and nonenveloped viruses. Their recommendations are summarized in Table 2. These recommendations reflected the need to provide adequate inactivation or reduction of nonenveloped viruses that were not inactivated by traditional solvent-detergent treatments.

In 1995, the CPMP of the European Union issued two documents. The first document provided a framework for designing viral validation studies and demonstrated that viral clearance steps were effective based on scaled-down studies. Although the various sections have been frequently presented in public forums, the main points may be summarized as follows:

Selection of viruses: use relevant and models
Evaluation of production steps likely to removal or inactivate viruses
Scale-down of purification processes
Evaluation of toxic effects of product and buffers on virus assays
Validation of virus assays
Statistical accuracy of assays

This document was updated in 1996 (CPMP, 1996a). The second CPMP document, first issued in 1995 was also updated in 1996 (CPMP, 1996b). These documents continue to be extremely useful when designing viral validation studies.

The International Conference on Harmonization (ICH-3) gave rise to a draft ICH guidance document on quality of biotechnology products (ICH, 1996). As an ICH document, the guidance document was prepared by an expert working group with representatives from the United States, the European Union, and Japan and their respective pharmaceutical manufacturing associations. This viral guideline covers only bankable cell lines (primary cell cultures) and cells of human origin, including hybridomas grown in vivo as ascites. It does not cover live vaccines, in vivo cell cultures, microorganisms, blood, or blood derivatives. The document serves as an international framework for evaluating and ensuring the viral safety of biotechnology

Table 2 Paul Erlich Institute Recommendations for Viral Clearance from Plasma-Derived Products

Virus classification	Total required reduction factor (minimum)	Number of steps required with 4 log reduction
Nonenveloped	6 logs	1
Enveloped	10 logs	2

products and provides a recommended approach for testing drug products for the presence of viruses and for conducting process validation. In May 1996, the FDA draft guideline on viral safety evaluation of biotechnology products derived from cell lines of human or animal origin (FDA, 1996) was published in the *Federal Register*. As has become standard practice, this graft guidance document is the FDA version of the above-mentioned ICH document.

These guidance documents provide an increasingly consistent framework for approaching the validation of viral clearance from biopharmaceuticals. A summary of worldwide regulatory trends is as follows:

Ever-increasing attention to design and scaling of validation studies
Reliance on and assessment of independent removal and inactivation steps in each process (both required in one purification process)
Increasing attention to plasma-derived products, including albumin
Concern regarding contamination of biopharmaceuticals with prions
Ongoing assessment of starting materials and purified bulk (fermentors) for known and adventitious viruses
Worldwide harmonization of scientifically based technical procedures and standard requirements for drug development

2 THE SOLUTION: A VIRAL CLEARANCE STRATEGY

Purification process validation studies provide assurance that the manufacturing process will remove or inactivate those viruses that may be present in starting materials (endogenous viruses), viruses used in the manufacturing process, unidentified viral contaminants, and viral contaminants present in concentrations below the limits of detection. With regard to the downstream purification operations, a goal was establishd to incorporate methods that could be demonstrated to clear model viruses across the recovery process by a cumulative 12 orders of magnitude (Builder et al., 1989), a value calculated to result in less than one infectious particle per 10^6 doses. Specific physical removal and inactivation operations in the downstream purification process are validated for viral clearance (Pocchiari et al., 1988; Bechtel et al., 1988). The clearance factors associated with those operations that are based on different physical principles, such as size exclusion and thermal inactivation, are cumulative (add the logs of the clearance factors) and are counted in the overall clearance factor of the entire purification process. This overall strategy of control, monitoring, and clearance has proven effective in providing security against virus transmission.

Several inactivation operations, based on heat or chemical treatment, are practiced worldwide today. Among these are thermal inactivation, tri(*n*-butyl) phosphate/sodium cholate treatment (Horowitz et al., 1985), treatment with urea or other denaturants (Pocchiari et al., 1988; Microbiological Associates, 1988), and β-propiolactone/ultraviolet light exposure (Prince et al., 1984). These techniques have achieved validated viral clearance ranging from 10^3 to 10^6. Their efficacy may vary with, or depend on, the type of virus. However, these inactivation techniques may also degrade the product protein. In these instances, stabilization procedures may be required to minimize protein losses. In any case, the removal of the inactivation agent must be validated.

If no other viral clearance steps are incorporated in the purification process, inactivated viral particles and their nucleic acids may remain in the solution. To remove such contaminants, physical separation techniques have been introduced. These techniques have usually been limited to chromatography and membrane filtration (Builder et al., 1989; Pocchiari et al., 1988; Microbiological Associates, 1988). Chromatographic operations, primarily ion-exchange and gel permeation chromatography, are widely used and have demonstrated significant clearance factors. However, it is recognized that the specific characteristics of the product, along with all the other process conditions used to define the chromatographic step, will determine the degree of removal of a specific virus from a specific protein. Unlike chromatographic processes, membrane filtration is considered a robust technique for the removal of viral contaminants. Membrane filtration, a process that typically removes viral contaminants via a sieving, or size-based, mechanism is the focus of the remainder of this chapter.

3 VIRUS REMOVAL FILTRATION TECHNOLOGIES

A virus filtration system includes the filter medium, module design, system design, operating conditions, and system standard operating procedures (SOPs). Virus filter media are generally cast polymeric membranes. Module types include pleated cartridge, hollow-fiber, both open-channel and screened channel plate-and-frame, and spirals. Two standard modes of operation include normal flow filtration (NFF; also called dead-ended, single-pass, and direct flow filtration) and tangential flow filtration (TFF; also called crossflow filtration).

3.1 Modes of Operation

Normal Flow Filtration

Normal flow filtration (NFF) involves passing the challenge fluid directly through the membrane so that the direction of flow is perpendicular to the plane of the filter medium, coincident with a vector normal to the plane of the filter medium. The fluid that has passed through the filter medium (called the filtrate or permeate) is collected as product. NFF modules include both cartridges and TFF modules run in the NFF mode. NFF system operation can involve the following sequence of operations: loading the sterilizer filter modules within their housings, flushing, pre-use integrity testing, flushing, sanitization, buffer flushing, challenge fluid processing, product recovery flushing, cleaning, post-use integrity testing, and module removal. Fluid processing is performed using either constant pressure or constant flow operating conditions. Figure 1 depicts the typical characteristics of normal flow filtration in a cartridge filter.

Several mechanisms can play a role in changing the permeability and retention characteristics of the filter during processing. First, protein products or other components in the fluid can adsorb to the surfaces on top of and within the filter medium, constricting the internal pores. Adsorption will reduce the hydraulic permeability and increase the retention of larger components. Second, any partially retained particles will accumulate as a cake on top of or within the filter medium. Particle capture will reduce the hydraulic permeability as described by various blocking models associated with pore blockage, surface cakes, or cake formation within the filter medium (Grace

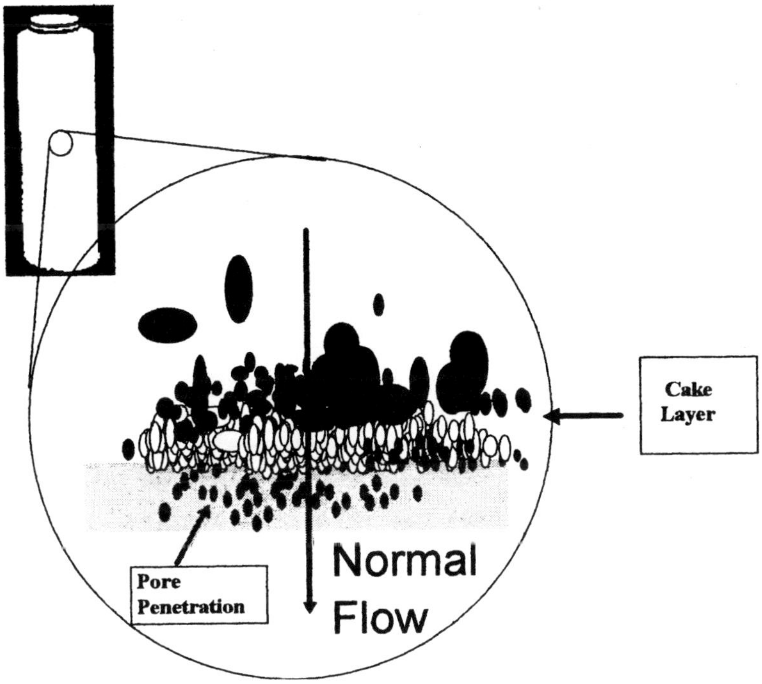

Figure 1 Schematic of normal flow filtration (NFF) in a filter cartridge.

1956). The effect of particle capture on further particle retention is more complex. As described by Grant (1988), preferential plugging of smaller pores of the filter medium diverts flow to larger pores, resulting in an increase in particle passage. Formation of a cake layer (protein and/or virus) that covers all of the pores on the top surface of the membrane will serve as a secondary filter medium. This phenomenon generally leads to a decrease in particle passage. These two opposing effects typically occur in sequence, with an initial increase in passage followed by a drop in passage.

Thirdly, any partially retained dissolved components such as proteins will accumulate above the retention layer of the filter medium in a region of high concentration referred to as the polarization layer (Blatt et al., 1970). The presence of this layer causes an osmotic pressure effect that leads to a reduction in the hydraulic driving force for flow through the filter (Nabetani et al., 1990). This region of increased concentration can also lead to a change in passage of the soluble species (Opong and Zydney, 1991; Deen, 1987) or cause protein precipitation. These effects may cause a change in flow or a pressure drop through the filter medium and a change in the passage of the different components in the challenge solution during the course of processing.

Tangential Flow Filtration

Tangential flow filtration (TFF) involves passing some portion of the challenge fluid across the surface of the filter medium, in a direction tangent to the plane of the filter medium, while passing the remaining fluid through the filter. The fluid flowing

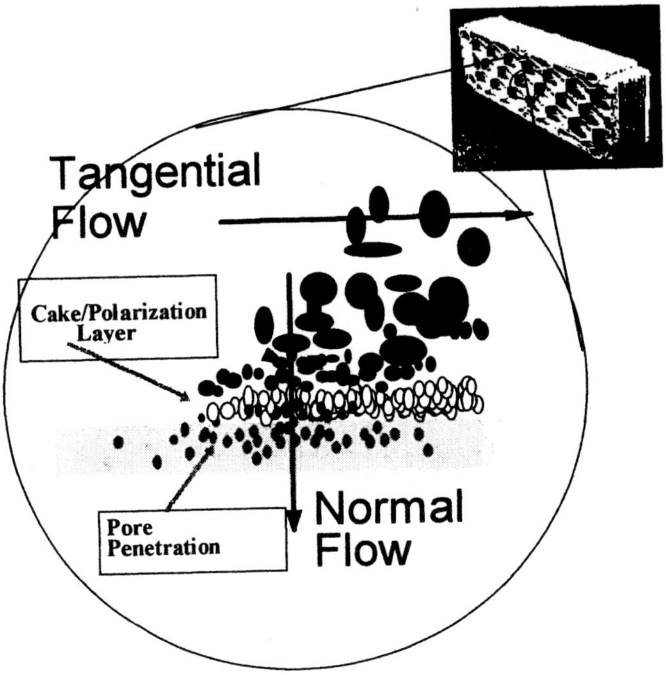

Figure 2 Schematic of a tangential flow filtration (TFF) device.

tangentially across the filter surface, or retentate, is recycled back to a feed tank. TFF system operation involves the same operating steps as NFF operation and in certain instances a diafiltration step. Fluid processing is performed using either constant pressure or constant flow operating conditions. The TFF system has more components than the NFF system, including the retentate line with valve, a feed pump, a heat exchanger for removing feed pump heat, and associated monitoring and control components. Figure 2 is a schematic of the processes occurring in a membrane operated in a tangential flow filtration device.

Tangential flow serves to limit the accumulation of retained suspended particulates and dissolved components on the surface of the membrane through a variety of mechanisms (Belfort et al., 1994). This effect reduces filter plugging, maintaining high hydraulic permeability and component passage throughout the course of processing. In particular, the presence of trace high molecular weight contaminants in the feedstock that build up on the membrane surface is mitigated by the effect of tangential flow. In the case of NFF, these components would continue to accumulate on the membrane surface.

Pros and Cons of NFF vs. TFF

The NFF system has fewer components than the TFF system and is generally considered both easier to operate and lower in capital costs for comparable membrane area. However, depending on the nature and amount of components present in the feedstock, NFF systems may require much larger membrane areas if the filter medium rapidly plugs. The need for large NFF system areas and the increasing use of automated TFF systems can make TFF the preferred mode of operation. NFF systems may also show variable performance over the course of processing and exhibit variability with different feedstocks if the permeability and component passages change appreciably with plugging. The consistency of TFF system operation over the course of fluid processing and its ability to process different feedstocks without plugging make it a more robust manufacturing process.

3.2 Commercial Products

Conventional Ultrafilters

Ultrafiltration membranes are used in virus removal applications assuming a sieving, size-based mechanism of removal. However, experimental evidence indicates that these membranes are unable to discriminate between viruses of different sizes, as would be expected with a sieving mechanism. In one study by Bechtel et al. (1988), a membrane system was challenged with three widely different viruses: encephalomyocarditis virus (EMC, 25–30 nm diameter), Sindbis virus (50–70 nm diameter), and vesicular stomatitis virus (VSV, 70–100 nm diameter). In all three cases, a 3.3–3.5 log removal was reported, independent of virus diameter. This observation illustrates the most significant limitation of conventional membranes: their inability to discriminate between viruses of different sizes. Ultimately, this limitation may result in membrane processes with less predictable performance.

The reason conventional ultrafiltration membranes lack the ability to discriminate between viruses of different sizes is clear. In addition to the inherent pore size distribution of the active skin, conventional ultrafiltration membranes are susceptible to large pore mechanical defects that result from imperfections in the active skin located above a ''finger void'' that is too close to the upper surface of the membrane. This type of behavior is depicted in Fig. 3. In this scanning electron micrograph, a ''finger void'' comes very close to the surface, which may result in a pore much larger than those in the skin matrix.

The observed retention of proteins by conventional ultrafiltration membranes is based on the average retention of protein molecules across the entire membrane surface, including large pores and imperfections discussed above. However, the presence of even a small number of pores or defects large enough to pass virus particles has a profound effect on the membrane's ability to reproducibly provide high virus clearance. To quantify the magnitude of this effect, a calculation was performed in which a membrane was modeled as consisting of pores of only two sizes (see Fig. 4). The majority of pores are 10 nm in diameter, large enough to pass human serum albumin but small enough to retain a 30 nm virus particle. The large pores, which occur at much lower frequency, are 60 nm in diameter, large enough to freely pass the 30 nm virus particles. The fraction of the total volumetric flow rate through the large pores relative to the total flow and the corresponding virus log reduction value are computed as a function of the surface number density of the large pores. Using this simplified conceptual model, it is not until the large pore density is below 1 in 10^6 that the virus clearance factor can exceed 3 logs. Also, the larger in diameter these large pores are, the less capable the membrane is of discriminating between particles of different sizes. It is this phenomenon that helps explain the performance of commercially available ultrafiltration membranes in virus removal applications.

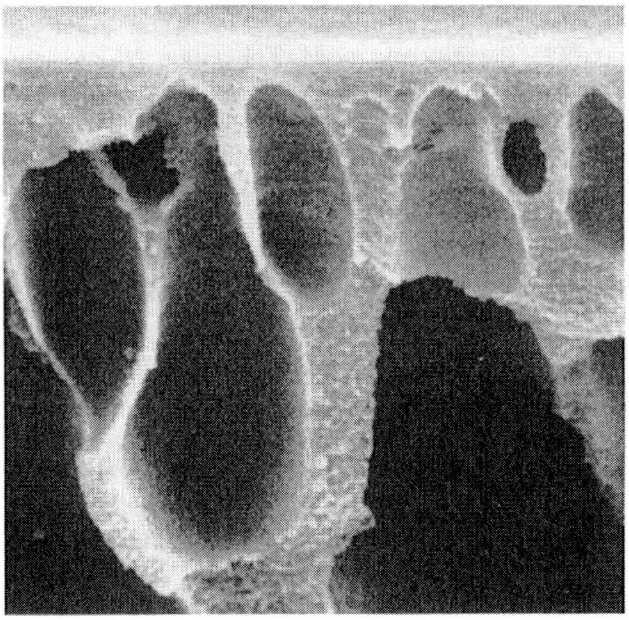

Figure 3 Scanning electron microscopic image of an ultrafiltration membrane.

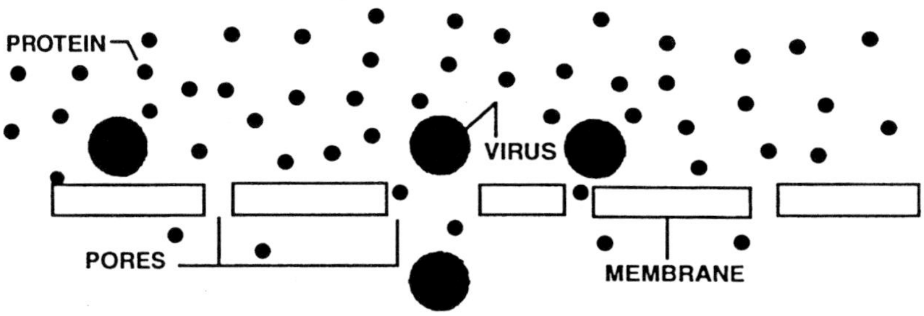

Large pore number density	Large pores (% total area)	Percent flow through large pores	LRV
1 in 10^3	3.48	58	0.25
1 in 10^4	0.36	11	0.94
1 in 10^5	3.6×10^{-2}	1.3	1.8
1 in 10^6	3.6×10^{-3}	0.1	3
1 in 10^7	3.6×10^{-4}	0.01	4
1 in 10^8	3.6×10^{-5}	0.001	5
1 in 10^9	3.6×10^{-6}	0.0001	6

Figure 4 The contribution of large pores to the fluid flow distribution and particle log reduction for a simplified membrane. The model consists of 10 nm diameter small pores and 60 nm diameter large pores. The model challenge solution contains HSA (7 nm diameter) and ϕX-174 (28 nm diameter) at 1×10^7 PFU/mL. [From DiLeo et al. (1992).]

Table 3 Validation Data for Two YM-100 Modules Configured in Series

Virus	PPV	EMC	HAV	SIN	VSV	HIV	Vàccina
Size (nm)	18–24	25–30	25–30	60–70	70 × 175	80–120	200–300
LRV	5.1, > 7.2	>7.8	>7.1	>7.5	>7.1	>7.4	>7.3

The preferred membrane structure in these applications would have a narrower pore distribution and no large pore defects.

The attribution of low log reduction values to membrane defects is consistent with detailed pore modeling using a log-normal size distribution (Urase et al., 1994). The log-normal distribution has been shown to correlate well over most of the pore size range, but the presence of large defects in the tail of the distribution invariably dominates the retention properties. Data on the retention of viruses over a range of average membrane pore sizes ranging from microporous to reverse osmosis (Urase et al., 1996) indicate that virus retention does not increase with nominal pore size but reaches some limit that can be associated with a nominal level of defects.

Millipore PTHK (Pocchiari et al., 1988; Bechtel et al., 1988) polyethersulfone membrane and Amicon YM-100 (Feldman et al., 1995) regenerated cellulose ultrafiltration membranes with nominal 100 kDa protein retention ratings have been shown to deliver a 2–3.5 log removal with viruses that range in size from 40 to 100 nm. Validation data for a YM-100 membrane employed with two spiral configuration modules in series are shown in Table 3. The Pall 0.04 μm Nylon N_{66} membrane has been reported to remove 3.7 logs of reovirus-3 from fetal calf serum.

The Pall Filtron Omega VR filter module consists of a strongly hydrophilic polyethersulfone membrane in a polyurethane ultrafiltration cassette format with a turbulence-promoting feed channel screen. Module membrane areas range from 0.1 to 2.5 m^2 with a membrane molecular mass rating of 100 or 300 kDa. These ratings refer to the kilodalton protein molecular mass that is fully retained by the membrane. These modules are operated in the TFF mode. Virus retention data are shown in Table 4 (Walter et al., 1992; *Genetic Engineering News*, 1996).

Table 4 Omega VR Filter Module Virus Retention Performance Data

	Virus		
Property	PPV	Reo-3	PI-3
Size (nm)	20	60–80	150–300
Envelope	No	No	Yes
TFF LRV w/MAb			
Omega 100	4.5		
Omega 200		>5.9	>6.8
Omega 300		2.8	4.4

The Sartorius group assayed two different ultrafiltration cassettes that consist of polysulfone in a silicon frame. The cassettes have a filtration area of 0.1 m^2 with a molecular cutoff of 100 and 300 kDa. The tests were performed by Microbiological Associates Ltd. The cassettes were used in the TFF mode, and the medium used was Dulbecco's Modified Eagle Medium (DMEM). The results obtained are given in Table 5.

Asahi Planova

The Asahi Planova filter module consists of a polycarbonate housing and a polyurethane sealant containing an assembly of hollow fibers with 400 μm diameter and a 35 μm wall diameter. Module membrane areas range from 0.001 to 1.0 m^2 with filter ratings of 15N, 35N, and 75N. These ratings correspond to mean pore size diameters of 15, 35, and 75 nm, respectively, as estimated from membrane permeability. The hollow fiber is a Bemberg microporous membrane (BMM) spun from a cuprammonium cellulose solution. The modules are operated in NFF or TFF modes at constant transmembrane pressure. The filter modules are subjected to a destructive post-use integrity test consisting of a gold particle suspension challenge (Hirasaki et al., 1994).

Protein passage and virus retention performance data on these modules are shown in Table 6 (Satoh, 1996). For a more complete description of the virus abbreviations used, see Table 10. In reference to Table 6, DMEM indicates Dulbecco's Modified Eagle Medium and DMEM-10 indicates this medium with 10% fetal calf serum added. Typical operation involves the use of two molecules in series as designated under the row "filter rating" by 35N + 15N. When the first filter has a higher rating (larger pore size), it acts as a prefilter to remove large components that could plug the tighter second filter and prevent passage of product protein. For two modules with the same rating in series, the modules act together to increase the overall virus retention.

The 15N module is retentive of small viruses down to 4 logs of 18–24 nm parvovirus. The 35N module is not retentive of the small viruses (only 0.6 log of 18–24 nm PPV) but will retain 4 logs of the 30–60 nm hepatitis C virus. The 75N module is more open and appears to be retentive of only large viruses (>5 logs of 80–120 nm HIV-1). It has been reported that virus and gold particle retention decline with increasing protein concentrations and with increasing process volumes when operated in the NFF mode (Hirasaki et al., 1994). This suggests that high protein

Table 5 Microsart Ultrafilter Cassettes Retention Performance Data

	Virus		
Property	SV-40	Reo	MuLV
Size (nm)	45–60	75–80	80–100
TFF LRV[a]			
Microsart 100	>6.42	>7.06	>5.82
Microsart 300	2.55	4.84	5.76

[a]See Sec. 5.1.

Table 6 Asahi Filter Cartridge Virus Retention Performance Data

	Product									
Property	FBS DMEM[a]	FBS DMEM[a]	FBS DMEM[a]	FVIII	PPSB	IVIG	FIX	PCC	MAb	MAb
Filter rating	15N	35N	75N	35N	35N	75N + 35N	15N + 15N	15N + 15N	15N + 15N	35N
Feed concn	100 g/L	100 g/L	100 g/L	101 U/mL	10 g/L	30 g/L	5 g/L		10–12 g/L	.3–2 g/L
LMH Flux				50–60		55			9.6–15.9	36–108
Loading (L/m^2)	3	3	3	30	30	200	20		10–30	2.5–37
Recovery				95%	>90%	>90%	>90%		84–92%	92%
LRV										
PPV	4.0	0.6	0.3			<0.4	4.4			
CPV								>5.1*		
Polio	5.0	0.2	0.1	0.9	0.3		>5.7		>7.6	0.7
EMC				0.6			>5.3	>7.3*		
HAV								>6.0*		
HCV	>4.0	4.0	1.5							
HBV		6.0	1.9		4.3					
JEV	>7.0	5.5	1.8				>5.8			
SV-40	>7.0	6.5							>7.0	>7.4
BVDV					3.8	>6.4		>5.9*		
SIN	>8.0	>8.0	0.1	>6.0						
Reo-3						>6.6				
ADV				>4.2						
HIV		>6.0	>6.0		>7.3	>4.8		>7.0*		
HSV		>5.0	>5.0	>5.0	>7.2					
PRV						>7.1		>6.2*	>7.8	>7.8
CMV		>6.0		>4.9	>7.3					

[a]DMEM = Dulbecco's Modified Eagle Medium.
[b]Log reduction value; see Sec. 5.1.
*Refers to the combined LRV of 2 modules in series.

concentrations and large process volumes represent a worst-case condition for retention.

Pall Ultipor

The Pall Ultipor[tm] VF DV50 filter cartridge consists of three layers of hydrophillic polyvinylidine difluoride membrane on nonwoven polyester support in a pleated cartridge with a polypropylene core. Cartridge membrane areas range from 0.075 to 1.63 m^2 with a claimed 6 LRV retention of viruses whose diameters are >50 nm. The membrane is a skinless microporous structure. These cartridges are operated in the NFF mode with a recommended constant pressure differential operation of 3–30 psid. The filter cartridges are subjected to a nondestructive pre-use integrity test consisting of a forward airflow in a 30% IPA solution at 85 psi.

Virus retention performance data and protein challenge data for these modules are shown in Tables 7 and 8, respectively (Oshima et al., 1996). The DV50 is not retentive of small viruses, with only a 1.3–1.4 log removal of 30 nm poliovirus. The membrane will remove 7.4–7.5 logs of the larger 53 nm PR772 bacteriophage. Viral spikes in water show greater retention than in buffer or a protein buffer solution, indicating an effect of viral aggregation. This suggests that a worst-case retention is seen in high protein concentration solutions.

Millipore Viresolve

The Millipore Viresolve membrane filter module consists of single layers of hydrophilic polyvinylidine difluoride membrane in a TFF open-channel module. Module membrane areas range from 0.001 to 2.0 m^2 with filter ratings of V70 and V180. These ratings refer to the kilodalton molecular mass of proteins that are able to freely pass through each membrane type. The membrane is a skinned composite structure. These modules are operated in the TFF mode with a recommended constant permeate flow operation. The membrane and filter modules are subjected to a nondestructive liquid porosimetric integrity test (Phillips and DiLeo, 1996).

Virus retention appears to increase in the presence of protein as shown in Table 9. Additional data indicate that viral retention appears to increase during processing (Millipore Corporation, 1995). This result suggests that initial conditions in buffer or dilute protein represent a worst-case condition for retention.

Table 7 Pall Ultipor™ DV50 Filter Cartridge Virus Retention Performance Data

	Virus				
Property	PP7	Polio-2	PR772	Influenza A	T1
Size (nm)	25	28–30	53	80–120	50 × 150
Envelope	No	No	No	Yes	No
Disk LRV					
Water	7.3	4.5	NA	NA	>8.9
DMEM	0.3	2.7	NA	NA	>8.8
DMEM-10	0.4	1.3	NA	>6.3	>8.9
Cartridge LRV					
DMEM-10	5.9–6.2	1.3–1.4	7.4–7.5	>5	6.6–7.6

Table 8 Pall Ultipor™ DV50 Filter Cartridge Protein Performance Data

Property	Product					
	BSA		IgG		FIX	FX
Concentration	20 mg/L,	50 g/L	14 mg/L,	30 g/L	55 U/mL	54–62 g/L
Passage	98%	98%	98%	98%	100%	
Recovery	NA	89%	NA	95%		

The V70 module retains the small 25–30 nm poliovirus by 3.5 logs in buffer. The more open V180 membrane retains only 2.5 logs of poliovirus in buffer but will retain 5.4 logs of 54 nm Sindbis virus. In the presence of protein, V70 membrane will retain 5.2 logs of the small 18–24 nm Canine Parvo Virus. In the presence of protein, the more open V180 membrane retains over 3 logs of the small 18–24 nm canine parvovirus and over 5 logs of 25–30 nm hepatitis A virus.

3.3 Conclusions

Filtration has become an important technology in the removal of viruses from biotherapeutic materials. There are many filters available, each with its own strengths and weaknesses. The decision about which filter to use should be based on the nature of the application (product and process) and the performance of the filter as dem-

Table 9 Millipore™ 70 and 180 Filter Device Performance Data

Product	PBS	HSA	PBS	FIX	IgG	Hb
Filter rating	V70	V70	V180	V70	V180	V70
Concentration		0.65 g/L		30 IU/mL	50 g/L	30 g/L
Passage				50–75%	>80%	80%
Recovery				>90%	95%	97%
Loading				4.3 IU/m^2	750 g/m^2	450 g/m^2
LRV						
CPV				5.2	3.1–3.5	
Polio	3.5	4.0	2.5	3.5		3.3
HAV					>5.0	
SV-40	5.7	>5.7		5.7		
BVDV					4.1–6.2	>5.3
SIN	7.4	>8.2	5.4	7.4		
Reo-3	7.2	>7.6	6.1	7.2		
PSR				>5.5		
VSV				>7.5		
MuLV		>6.8	>3.3			
HIV-1					>5.2	>4.1
HSV						>5.4
PRV					>6.0	

onstrated in both qualification and validation studies. Applications and validation are the focus of the next two sections.

However, it is important to point out that viral filtration, while capable of removing most bacteria and mycoplasma, should not be used as a replacement for the final, 0.22 μm filter prior to filling. Typically, these filters have only been validated for virus removal and may not have a claim for *Brevundimonas diminuta* as recommended by the aseptic processing guidelines (FDA, 1987a).

4 VIRUS REMOVAL APPLICATIONS

4.1 Recombinant Therapeutics

Recombinant therapeutics can be expressed by recombinant mammalian, bacterial, or yeast cells in fermentors, within ascites fluid, or within fluids from transgenic mammals. These proteins are then clarified and purified in a processing train. Monoclonal antibodies (MAbs), with a molecular mass of around 160 kDa, form a large class of these proteins. Cytokines and other recombinant proteins such as growth hormones are smaller and more diverse in molecular weight. Many protein products originally obtained from human plasma are now being expressed in recombinant form as well. Recombinant protein products tend to be present in low concentrations and are highly uniform in composition. For these reasons, recombinant protein products are relatively easy to filter. When used as therapeutic agents, regulatory guidelines for viral reduction apply to the mammalian expression systems.

Protein purification steps designed to remove such impurities as particulates, extraneous proteins, DNA, endotoxin, and multimers will frequently show a viral clearance capability as well. These steps typically involve a variety of chromatographic operations. When total removal of all the model viruses is insufficient to meet product safety requirements using the normal purification train, an extra dedicated step such as filtration is required. As seen in Fig. 5, virus filtration is generally performed on a purified solution and is generally located toward the end of the downstream purification train. In this manner, the size of the required filter system will be minimized. This process will provide the necessary additional viral clearance. It may also remove large protein impurities such as protein aggregates and other large molecular weight species.

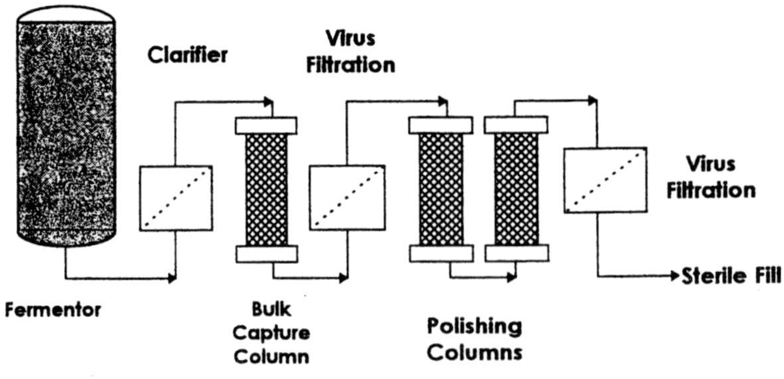

Figure 5 Process flow diagram showing possible placement of virus removal steps.

4.2 Blood Plasma Proteins

Blood plasma proteins are a large class of therapeutic products that have demonstrated viral contamination. Major protein products of interest include gamma globulins, serum albumin, and clotting factors VIII and IX. IgIV is composed of polyclonal gamma globulins of around 160 kDa. Clotting factor VIII is a large molecular weight protein of comparable size to small viruses, and clotting factor IX is around 70 kDa. Human serum albumin, at 67 kDa, is present in the highest concentrations in plasma. Additional proteins that have been prepared in small volumes from plasma include thrombin, antithrombin III, prothrombin complexes containing multiple clotting factors, and α-protease inhibitor.

Pooled plasma source material is known to contain a variety of viruses including HIV, parvovirus, and a number of hepatitis strains. The plasma protein products are generally produced from human plasma by variants on the Cohn fractionation process (Cohn et al., 1946). This process employs increasing concentrations of ethanol at low temperatures and decreasing pH to selectivity precipitate first the large molecule products such as fibrinogen and Factor VIII, then successfully smaller proteins down to serum albumin. The fractionation process also tends to preferentially precipitate viruses within the large molecule protein products, rendering factor VIII concentrated in viruses and albumin relatively free of viral contamination.

Plasma products are subjected to filtration, heat, and solvent detergent treatment for virus removal or inactivation. Filtration is most effective on the smaller proteins and has not been applied to Factor VIII to any significant degree. The high protein concentrations of 10–200 g/L found in plasma processing operations can be difficult to filter due to aggregation and concentration polarization. In addition, the presence of small amounts of impurities can quickly plug filters, thereby inhibiting product passage.

Therapeutic products whose preparation includes virus filtration steps currently licensed for sale include Factor IX (Jernberg et al., 1996; Feldman et al., 1995; Hoffer et al., 1995; Burnouf-Radosevich et al., 1994), Prothrombin Complex (Ristol, 1997) and IgG (Van Holten et al., 1995).

4.3 Blood Substitutes

A growing area of application is the variety of modified hemoglobin products designed as red blood substitutes. These products are derived from human, mammalian, or recombinant bacterial sources. The possibility of source contamination and large dosage of these products require a viral clearance processing step. Purified hemoglobin tends to filter rather easily.

4.4 Serum

Mammalian serum is presently used in a wide variety of cell fermentations, although its use in production is predicted to diminish. This serum is a potential source of bioreactor contamination where trace amounts of virus could multiply in cell hosts. This risk is mitigated by the use of segregated groups of animals that are continuously monitored, screening assays, and the use of filtration and gamma radiation treatment. Gamma radiation can denature serum proteins vital to cell growth and product expression. Filtration requires passing the complex mixture of these vital serum proteins while retaining virus particles.

4.5 Virus Barrier Applications

Virus removal technology can be used to protect a mammalian cell fermentor from viral contamination. Fermentation media, nutritive or buffer additives, and gases introduced into the fermentor represent potential sources of contamination. Viruses can multiply within the fermentor and require the production to be scrapped. This is expensive in terms of production costs and lost sales. Virus removal filters placed around the fermentor are termed the virus barrier. There are at present no regulatory agency comments on this approach.

5 FILTER VALIDATION

5.1 Integrity Testing

A key advantage associated with properly engineered virus-removing membranes is that virus removal is based on a size-exclusion mechanism independent of virus type or surface character. For this reason, the filtration process can provide for a reproducible, predictable, and validatable removal of virus particles from biopharmaceuticals. To ensure that virus removal is consistent with validation studies, membrane integrity should be monitored both pre- and post-use (Grun et al., 1992). Currently, the integrity of virus removal membranes is measured by a particle challenge test (dextran, PVP, colloidal gold), an air porosimetry test (bubble point or air diffusion), or a liquid porosimetry test (CorrTest). The details of each of these tests, including advantages and limitations, are described below.

Particle Challenge Tests

The performance of virus-retentive membranes is based on their ability to efficiently retain viruses or virus-like particles. The ability of a membrane sample to retain viruses of a certain size is normally expressed in terms of a log reduction value (LRV), defined as

$$\mathrm{LRV} = \log\left(\frac{c_\mathrm{f}}{c_\mathrm{p}}\right) \tag{1}$$

where c_f and c_p are the virus concentrations within the feed and permeate streams, respectively. Integrity tests capable of accurately correlating and predicting virus passage must be based on physical principles capable of nondestructively approximating this concentration ratio.

The most straightforward approach for approximating this concentration ratio is to perform an actual particle challenge experiment with an appropriately sized particle and measure the resulting feed and permeate particle concentrations. Provided a statistically valid relationship exists, the virus reduction properties of the membrane sample can be predicted from the particle challenge experiment. Similarly, the ability of the membrane sample to retain either larger or smaller virus particles can be approximated by varying the particle size within the challenge solution. This methodology forms the basis of the dextran rejection test, the PVP challenge test (Feldman et al., 1995), and the gold colloidal challenge test (Hirasaki et al., 1994).

There are several advantages associated with particle challenge tests for integrity testing virus retentive membranes. First and foremost, particle challenge tests provide for a direct measure of the concentration ratio defined by Eq. (1). Because of this fact, interpretation of results obtained from particle challenge integrity tests is intuitively straightforward. Higher levels of particle retention translate directly into higher levels of virus retention. Second, particle challenge tests are based on a sound and easily understood theoretical framework. Again, this quality underlies the intuitive nature of particle challenge tests. Finally, particle challenge integrity tests are relatively easy to perform, and results can be obtained within a short time.

However, there are several practical limitations associated with particle challenge tests. First, the results are highly dependent on the solution conditions (solute concentrations, temperature, and pH) and system hydrodynamics (transmembrane pressure, feed velocity, membrane permeability, module geometry). Unless tightly controlled or automated, variations in these variables can lead to irreproducible results. Second, the retention of particles by virus-retentive membranes may be controlled by factors other than sieving, such as concentration polarization and membrane fouling (Kim et al., 1994). Although these effects can be either minimized or controlled in tangential flow filtration systems, dead-ended systems may be prone to variations caused by them. Third, current detection systems are capable of detecting only extremely high concentrations of nanometer-sized particles. For example, the fluorescence detection limit for a commercially available 14 nm fluorescently labeled particle is on the order of 10^{11} particles/mL. By necessity, a membrane capable of 2 log removal of 14 nm particles must be challenged with a feed concentration of greater than 10^{13} particles/mL. At these concentrations, particle aggregation, membrane fouling, and concentration polarization may actually change the membrane's primary retention mechanism, essentially masking the effect of subtle differences in membrane pore size distributions. Finally, the test is inherently destructive, relegating its usefulness for integrity testing virus-retentive membranes to a post-use integrity test. This fact may have certain implications concerning the reliability of integrity testing previously integrity tested membranes or modules.

Porosimetry Tests

A second approach for approximating the concentration ratio given as Eq. (1) is to relate the individual virus concentrations to independently measured physical parameters. For virus-retentive membranes with a virus retention based on a sieving mechanism, this is a relatively straightforward analysis. Assuming rigid, spherical virus particles of diameter d_s and neglecting hydrodynamic forces, which normally oppose the unhindered transport of virus particles through membrane pores, the permeate virus concentration can be approximated as

$$c_p \approx c_f \left(\frac{Q_{ds}}{Q_{tot}}\right) \tag{2}$$

where Q_{tot} is the total amount of flow through the membrane sample under a given set of operating conditions and Q_{ds} represents the amount of flow through those membrane pores equal in size to or larger than d_s, the virus particle diameter. Therefore, the ratio of flow rates given in Eq. (2) actually represents the percentage of total flow through the membrane pores equal in size to or greater than the virus of interest. Substituting (2) into Eq. (1), the membrane log reduction value can be approximated as

$$\mathrm{LRV} \approx \log\left(\frac{Q_{\mathrm{tot}}}{Q_{\mathrm{ds}}}\right) \tag{3}$$

Thus, approximating the membrane LRV has been reduced to measuring a ratio of flow rates, variables that are uniquely dependent on the specific pore size distribution of the given membrane sample. The determination of Q_{tot} can be accomplished by conducting a water permeability measurement. The estimation of Q_{ds}, however, requires the selective intrusion of those pores accessible to the virus particles.

Bubble Point and Air Diffusion Tests

The most familiar means for selectively intruding pores of a given size is through a technology known as air porosimetry. The most widely known variations of air porosimetry include the bubble point and air diffusion tests (Emory, 1989a, 1989b). In the bubble point test, a thoroughly wetted membrane is placed into a housing and contacted with air. The upstream air pressure is then gradually increased, eventually resulting in the selective intrusion of air through the larger pores and the subsequent formation of air bubbles downstream of the membrane. Assuming cylindrical pores, the pore diameter corresponding to the pressure at which these bubbles are first observed (the bubble point) can be approximated by the capillary equation, given by

$$P = \frac{4K\gamma \cos\theta}{d_{\mathrm{p}}} \tag{4}$$

where P is the transpore pressure drop, d_{p} is the pore diameter intruded, θ is the contact angle, K represents a shape correction factor, and γ is the air/liquid surface tension. Since capillary forces dictate that the largest pores are those first intruded with air, the bubble point test can be considered a measure of the largest pore present in a given membrane sample.

In the air diffusion test (sometimes called the forward flow, pressure hold, or pressure decay test depending on the specific gas flow measurement technique used), the membrane is again wetted and contacted with air. The air pressure is increased to some prescribed value below the bubble point of an integral membrane. The total amount of airflow through the wetted membrane due to both diffusion and convection is measured, and the resulting value is compared to a preestablished specification. Airflow values greater than the specification indicate the presence of large pores or defects that were intruded at the test pressure, indicating a nonintegral filter. Provided a statistically valid relationship exists and assuming that an appropriate transmembrane pressure is employed, the virus retention properties of a membrane sample may be predicted from either the bubble point or air diffusion test.

The advantages of bubble point and air diffusion tests for determining the integrity of virus retention membranes are numerous. First, they are the most common and preferred integrity tests for testing bacterial-retentive membranes. Consequently, the extension of these technologies into the domain of virus-retentive membranes is quite natural. Second, air porosimetric tests are an indirect measure of the largest pores present in the virus-retentive membranes. Therefore, interpretation of results obtained from standard bubble point and air diffusion tests are relatively straightforward. All other things being equal, the more virus-retentive membranes have higher bubble points and lower air diffusion values. Third, bubble point and air diffusion tests are nondestructive integrity tests. Therefore, these tests can be used both pre- and post-use to verify membrane integrity. Finally, air porosimetry tests are rapid, easy to perform, and amenable to manufacturing environments.

However, a major problem exists with traditional bubble point and air diffusion integrity tests as they pertain to the evaluation of virus-retentive membranes. Due to the extremely large surface tension at the air/liquid interface [see Eq. (4)], the pressures required to observe the bubble points for these membranes can be in excess of 300 psi. Experimental data have shown that the water bubble point of Viresolve membranes capable of 3 log removal of 30 nm diameter viruses is in excess of 500 psi (35 bar) (Phillips, 1996a). Although the air/liquid surface tension can be significantly decreased by using alternative wetting fluids (isopropyl alcohol has a surface tension approximately one-third the surface tension of water), the bubble points of highly retentive membranes are still in excess of 200 psi. Many virus-retentive membranes compress when subjected to pressures in this range, leading to erroneous results. Additionally, pressure in this range are both impractical and potentially dangerous.

Liquid Porosimetry

Another means of selectively intruding pores of a given size is through a technique called liquid porosimetry (Munari et al., 1989; Gekas et al., 1990). In liquid porosimetry, the air/liquid interface encountered in bubble point and air diffusion tests is replaced with the interface between two immiscible fluids. First, a membrane sample thoroughly wetted with one of two immiscible fluids is placed into a housing and contacted with the second immiscible fluid. The upstream pressure is then gradually increased, eventually resulting in the selective intrusion of the second immiscible fluid through the larger pores. The total amount of liquid flow through the wetted membrane at a prescribed transmembrane pressure is measured, and the resulting value is compared to a preestablished specification to determine the integrity of the membrane sample. Provided a statistically valid relationship exists, the virus-retention properties of a membrane sample can be predicted from the liquid porosimetric results. An example of a liquid porosimetric integrity test is the CorrTest (DiLeo and Phillips, 1994; Phillips and DiLeo, 1996).

The advantages of liquid porosimetric tests for determining the integrity of virus-retentive membranes are numerous (Phillips and DiLeo, 1996). First, as can be seen from the descriptions above, the methodologies for conducting liquid porosimetric tests are identical to the methods employed for conducting the universally accepted bubble point and air diffusion tests. Consequently, the interpretation of integrity test data obtained from liquid porosimetric tests is relatively straightforward. Second, the interfacial tensions associated with many pairs of immiscible liquids are extremely small, resulting in low transmembrane pressures necessary to selectively intrude nanometer-sized pores. For example, assuming an ideal cylindrical pore ($K = 0$), a contact angle of 0 ($\theta = 0$), and a liquid/liquid interfacial tension of 0.5 dyn/cm (typical of many pairs of immiscible fluids), the pressure required to intrude a 20 nm pore is on the order of 1 bar (14.5 psi). In contrast, the air/water surface tension is approximately 72.8 dyn/cm. In this instance, the pressure required to intrude the same 20 nm pore is on the order of 145 bar (2110 psi). Third, since the two liquid phases are completely immiscible, there is no background diffusional flow to contend with, resulting in a highly sensitive membrane characterization technique (Wienk et al., 1994). Finally, the membrane is tested in a wetted state, thereby more closely approximating typical operating conditions for virus removal.

The disadvantages associated with liquid porosimetric tests generally concern ease-of-use considerations. Since liquid porosimetric tests are more sensitive than bubble point and air diffusion integrity tests for detecting subtle variations in membrane pore size distribution, measurement errors become magnified. For example, a 1 psi error in measuring the transmembrane pressure is insignificant in air porosimetric tests in which the membrane bubble point often exceeds 200 psi. However, this 1 psi error can have a tremendous impact on the results obtained with liquid porosimetric tests where nanometer-sized pores are often intruded at pressures of less than 20 psi. Consequently, proper precautions must be exercised when conducting liquid porosimetric tests. In addition, since the liquid porosimetry technology is relatively new compared to bubble point and air diffusion integrity tests, automated integrity testers have yet to be developed. The introduction of automatic testers for liquid porosimetric tests would greatly increase the ease-of-use characteristics of this technology.

5.2 Viral Spiking Studies

As in the verification of the ability of microporous membranes to remove bacterial cells, such as *Brevundimonas diminuta* ATTC 19146, viral removal systems are qualified by the filter manufacturer and validated by the filter user using relevant or model viruses. Although *B. diminuta* was selected as an industry standard and worse-case model for other bacteria that may occur in process streams, no single virus has been agreed upon as a worst-case challenge for viral validation studies. Thus viral validation studies typically employ a small panel of viruses selected from a larger list (see Table 10).

This short list is first populated by viruses that represent relevant or suspected contaminants. To round out the panel of viruses, other viruses known to contaminate similar products or model viruses with characteristics similar to known contaminants are selected. The panel is then expanded to include viruses with differing characteristics (small vs. large, enveloped vs. nonenveloped, etc.). In principle, the expanded panel is necessary because viruses appear to be more dissimilar than similar in a variety of characteristics that may affect removal efficiency. The most visible differences that could be hypothesized to influence removal by filtration are virus size and exterior surface characteristics. The number of viruses used in these studies is frequently increased as one proceeds toward clinical trials and approval.

Several papers have discussed the subject of viral clearance and process validation, including Grun et al. (1992), White et al. (1991), and White and Woodward (1995). To summarize, the objectives of virus removal validation are severalfold:

1. To verify that the process can remove known relevant viruses beyond the level of detection
2. To verify that the process can remove model viruses beyond the level of detection
3. To provide a quantitative assessment of the overall process to remove viruses

Table 10 Characteristics of Relevant and Model Viruses Used in Filter Validation Studies

Model and relevant virus								
Acronym	Name	Size (nm)	Natural host	Envelope	Shape	Genome	Family	Physicochem resistance
φX-174	φX174	28	Bacteria	No	Icosahedral	SS-DNA	Micro	Medium
PP7	PP7	25	Bacteria	No	Icosahedral	SS-RNA	Levi	Medium
φ-6	φ-6	78	Bacteria	Yes	Icosahedral	SS-RNA	Cysto	Low
PR772	PR772	53	Bacteria	No	Icosahedral	SS-DNA	Tecti	Medium
T1	T1	50 × 150	Bacteria		Icosahedral	DS-DNA	Sypho	Low
CPV	Canine parvovirus	18–24	Mammals	No	Icosahedral	SS-DNA	Parvo	Very high
PPV	Porcine parvovirus	18–24	Mammals	No	Icosahedral	SS-DNA	Parvo	Very high
MVM	Minute virus of mice	18–26	Mouse	No	Icosahedral	SS-DNA	Parvo	Very high
B19	Human parvo	18–26	Human	No	Icosahedral	SS-RNA	Parvo	Very high
Polio-I	Poliovirus sabin 1	25–30	Human	No	Icosahedral	SS-RNA	Picorna	Medium
EMC	Encephalomyocarditis	25–30	Mouse	No	Icosahedral	SS-RNA	Picorna	Medium
HAV	Hepatitis A	25–30	Human	No	Icosahedral	SS-RNA	Picorna	High
HCV	Hepatitis C	30–60	Mammals	Yes		RNA	Flavi	High
HBV	Hepatitis B	42	Mammals	Yes	Icosahedral	DS-DNA	Hepadna	High
SV-40	Simian virus 40	40–50	Monkey	No	Icosahedral	DS-DNA	Papova	Very high
BVDV	Bovine viral diarrhea virus	50–70	Bovine	Yes	Pleospherical	RNA	Flavi	Low
SIN	Sindbis	50–70	Human	Yes	Spherical	SS-RNA	Toga	Low
REO-3	Reovirus-3	60–80	Mammals	No	Spherical	DS-RNA	Reo	Medium
ADV	Adenovirus	70–90	Mammals	No	Icosahedral	SS-DNA	Adeno	Medium
VSV	Vesicular stomatitis virus	70 × 175	Bovine	Yes	Bullet	SS-RNA	Rhabdo	Low
eMuLV	Murine leukemia virus	80–110	Mouse	Yes	Spherical	SS-RNA	Retro	Low
XMuLV	Xenotropic murine leukemia virus	80–110	Mammals	No	Spherical	SS-RNA	Retro	Low
HTLV	Human T-cell leukemia virus	100	Mammals	Yes	Spherical	SS-RNA	Retro	Low
HIV-4	Human immunodeficiency virus	80–120	Mammals	Yes	Spherical	SS-RNA	Retro	Low
HIV-1	Human immunodeficiency virus	80–120	Mammals	Yes	Spherical	SS-RNA	Retro	Low
HIV-2	Human immunodeficiency virus	80–120	Mammals	Yes	Spherical	SS-RNA	Retro	Low
INFA	Influenza A	80–120	Mammals	Yes	Helical	SS-RNA	Orthomyxo	Medium
HSV	Herpes simplex virus	120–150	Mammals	Yes	Spherical	DS-DNA	Herpes	Medium
PRV	Pseudorabies virus	120–200	Swine	Yes	Spherical	DS-DNA	Herpes	Medium
EBV	Epstein Barr virus	120–200	Human	Yes	Spherical	DS-DNA	Herpes	Medium
CMV	Cytomegalovirus	150–200	Mammals	Yes	Spherical	DS-DNA	Herpes	Medium
PI-3	Parainfluenza virus	150–300	Mammals	Yes	Pleospherical	SS-RNA	Paramyxo	Low
Vaccinia	Vaccinia	200–300	Mammals	Yes	Brick-shaped	DS-DNA	Pox	Medium

What the validation study cannot do is ensure that even unknown viruses will be removed by the process. The removal of these unknown viruses can be supported by selecting a technology whose removal mechanism(s) can be expected to operate over a wide range of operating parameters.

Another important consideration, from a regulatory point of view, is that scaled-down spiking studies include a rationale that supports the concept that a scaled-down validation system is equivalent to the full-scale process. The design of viral validation studies must provide for accurate modeling of the process and assess overall clearance or validate specific steps in the process. From the analytical side, key limitations include viral culturing methods and filter levels, cytoxicity of buffers, and limits of detection for viral assays.

Model vs. Relevant Viruses

Viruses used in filter validation studies should be chosen (1) for their relevance to or ability to survive or be propagated in the raw materials, cell lines, or purified bulk being filtered or (2) to represent a wide range of physicochemical properties so as to challenge the filtration system as rigorously as possible. The latter battery of viruses give some assurance that even unknown viruses may be eliminated. Relevant viruses are those likely to be present or those most likely to enter from the environment. Model viruses are used when assay systems are not available for known, relevant viruses or to complete the test battery with respect to physicochemical properties.

Table 10 summarizes meaningful parameters that may play a role in the decision about which viruses to use in the viral spiking studies. The table includes relevant, model, and "bacteriophage" models that have been used by filter manufacturers in lieu of pathogenic or mammalian viruses. Some bacteriophage models have been shown to be comparable to mammalian viruses in terms of relative removal. Size, shape, and envelope are considered to be the most important parameters when filtration is the removal method being evaluated. In cases where two viruses of similar phylogenetic origin, size, or surface properties (presence or absence of an envelope) are proposed for testing, the strain that is most resistant to removal or inactivation should be chosen.

In all cases, the highest titers available should be used to maximize the possibility of detection downstream of the filter. Further information on the selection of appropriate spiking viruses should be obtained through consultation with the appropriate regulatory documents and/or regulatory agencies.

5.3 Reuse and Cleaning

Although the cleaning and reuse of chromatographic columns is well documented, virus-retentive filters have not been routinely reused. In fact, the cleaning and subsequent reuse of virus-retentive filters has been discouraged. Critical considerations include the fact that these filters, unlike chromatographic methods, are dedicated to the collection of viral particles. Current cleaning regimes, although used for chromatographic columns with some confidence, have been reported to provide inadequate inactivation of viruses.

Ultimately, it is the responsibility of the drug manufacturers to both validate the cleaning of viral filters and provide evidence that the cleaning/sterilization regime is adequate. The nagging question of unknown viruses confounds the decision of reuse. To date, no procedures have been published on the validation of virus removal filters for reuse.

6 ECONOMICS

The cost of implementing a virus filtration step includes up-front regulatory submission costs, system capital costs, and operating costs. To the extent that speed to market to capture market share dominates the economics, it is critical to have a complete validation package for submission to regulatory authorities that will not cause delays in approval. Although the cost of a virus removal system may be as high as several hundred thousand dollars, the amortization of this capital cost over many production lots tends to make it a small overall component.

Product yield and filter costs tend to dominate the economics (due to single-use operation). Other costs that can play a role include buffer costs associated with diluting the feed or washing the product through the filter, product quality assays, and costs associated with reconcentrating any diluted product (e.g., an ultrafiltration system following the virus filtration step). For large filter area systems or complex operations, labor costs can also play a role. It should be noted that the virus filtration step will not only remove viruses but may also have the economic benefit of removing large protein impurities as well.

For small volume–high value products such as recombinant proteins or Factor IX, the processing costs are typically not a significant factor and up-front validation issues are of greatest concern. For large volume products that tend to be more of a commodity, such as hemoglobin, the processing costs can be a significant factor in the decision to implement a virus filtration step.

REFERENCES

Altman, L. K. (1996). Hepatitis virus passed to hemophiliacs by clotting compound. *New York Times* News Service, Jan. 1, 1996.

Bechtel, M. K., A. Bagdasarian, W. P. Olson, and T. N. Estep. (1988). Virus removal or inactivation in hemoglobin solutions by ultrafiltration or detergent/solvent treatment, *Biomater. Art. Cells, Art. Orig.*, *16*:123–128.

Belfort, G., R. H. Davis, and A. L. Zydney. (1994). The behavior of suspensions and macromolecular solutions in crossflow microfiltration, *J. Membrane Sci.*, *96*:1–58.

Blatt, W. F., A. Dravid, A. S. Michaels, and L. Nelson. (1970). Solute polarization and cake formation in membrane ultrafiltration: Causes, consequences, and control technique, in *Membrane Science and Technology*, Vol. 47 (J. E. Flynn, ed.), Plenum, New York, Chap. 4.

Builder, S., R. van Reis, N. Paoni, and J. Ogez. (1989). Process development and regulatory approval of tissue-type plasminogen activator, in *Advances in Animal Cell Biology and Technology for Bioprocesses* (R. E. Spier, J. B. Griffiths, J. Stephenne, and P. J. Crooy, eds.), Butterworths, Stoneham, MA, pp. 452–646.

Burnouf-Radosevich, M., P. Appourchaux, J. J. Huart, and T. Burnouf. (1994). Nanofiltration, a new specific virus elimination method applied to high-purity factor IX and factor XI concentrates, *Vox Sang.*, *67*:132–138.

Cohn, E. J., L. E. Strong, W. L. Hughes, Jr., D. J. Mulford, J. N. Ashworth, M. Melin, and H. L. Taylor. (1946). Separation into fractions of proteins and lipoprotein components, *J. Am. Chem. Soc.*, *68*:459–475.

CPMP (Committee for Proprietary Medicinal Products). (1991a). Note for guidance: Validation of virus removal and inactivation procedures, CPMP/III/8115/89, *Biologicals*, *19*: 247–251.

CPMP. (1991b). Note for guidance: Guidelines for medicinal products derived from human blood and plasma. CPMP/III/8379/89, *Biologicals*, *20*:159–164.

CPMP. (1996a). Note for guidance on virus validation studies: The design, contribution and interpretation of studies validating the inactivation and removal of viruses, CPMP/BWP/ 268/95, p. 13.

CPMP. (1996b). Note for guidance on plasma derived medicinal products, CPMP/BWP/269/ 95, p. 17.

D'Arcy, P. F., and D. W. G. Harron. (1996). Quality of biotechnology products: Viral safety evaluation of biotechnology products derived from cell lines of human or animal origin, Proceedings of the Third International Conference on Harmonization, Yokohama, 1995, pp. 161–176.

Deen, W. M. (1987). Hindered transport of large molecules in liquid-filled pores, *AIChE J.*, *33*:1409–1425.

Degen, P. J., I. P. Sipsas, G. C. Rapisarda, and J. A. Gregg. (1995). Polyvinylidene fluoride membrane for filtering viruses, U.K. Patent 2,285,010 (June 28).

DiLeo, A. J., and M. W. Phillips. (1994). Integrity test for membranes, U.S. Patent 5,282,380.

DiLeo, A. J., A. E. Allegrezza, and E. T. Burke. (1992). Membrane, process and system for isolating virus from solution. U.S. Patent 5,017,292 (May 21).

DiLeo, A. J., D. A. Vacante, and E. F. Dean. (1993a). Size exclusion removal of model mammalian viruses using a unique membrane system, Part I: Membrane qualification, *Biologicals*, *21*:275–286.

DiLeo, A. J., D. A. Vacante, and E. F. Dean. (1993b). Size exclusion removal of model mammalian viruses using a unique membrane system, Part II: Module qualification and process simulation, *Biologicals*, *21*:287–296.

Emory, S. F. (1989a). Principles of integrity-testing hydrophilic microporous membrane filters. Part I, *Pharm. Tech.*, *13*(9):68–77.

Emory, S. F. (1989b). Principles of integrity-testing hydrophilic microporous membrane filters. Part II, *Pharm. Tech.*, *13*(10):36–46.

Eshkol, A., F. Maillard, and G. Stiles. (1988). Purification of biological fluid by filtration through ultrafiltration membrane, Eur. Patent EP030737A2.

FDA. (1985). Points to Consider in the Production and Testing of New Drugs and Biologicals by Recombinant DNA Technology, Office of Biologicals Research and Review.

FDA. (1987a). Guideline on Sterile Drug Products Produced by Aseptic Processing, Center for Drugs and Biologics and Office of Regulatory Affairs, Rockville, MD.

FDA. (1987b). Points to Consider in the Characterization of Cell Lines Used to Produce Biologicals, Office of Biologics Research and Review.

FDA. (1994). Draft Points to Consider (PTC) in the Manufacture and Testing of Monoclonal Antibody Products for Human Use, Center for Biologics Evaluation and Research (CBER).

FDA. (1996). Draft Guideline on Viral Safety Evaluation of Biotechnology Products Derived from Cell Lines of Human or Animal Origin, *Fed. Reg.*, *61*(92):21881–21891 (May 10, 1996).

Feldman, F., S. Chandra, and C. Huang. (1995). Improved safety from plasma derivatives: Purification and viral elimination characteristics of mononine, *Acta Haematol.*, *94*:25–34.

Garnick, R. L. (1996). Experience with viral contamination in cell culture, in, Viral Safety and Evaluation of Viral Clearance from Biopharmaceutical Products (F. Brown and A. S. Lubiniecki, eds.), Dev. Biol. Stand., Basel, Korger, Vol. 85, p. 49–56.

Gekas, V., G. Tragardh, G. Capennelli, and A. Bottino. (1990). Correlation of direct porosimetric data and performance of ultrafiltration membranes, *Proc. Biochem. Int.*, August, pp. 111–116.

Genetic Engineering News. (1996). Advances in blood filtration methods improve supply safety, Oct. 1, p. 8.

Grace, H. P. (1956). Structure and performance of filter media, *AIChE J.*, *2*:307–336.

Grant, D. C. (1988). Sieving capture of particles by microporous membrane filtration media, M.S. Thesis, University of Minnesota, Minneapolis, MN.

Grun, J. B., E. M. White, and A. F. Sito. (1992). Viral removal inactivation by purification of biopharmaceuticals, *BioPharm.*, *5*(9):22–30.

Hirasaki, T., T. Noda, H. Nakano, Y. Ishizaki, S. Manabe, and N. Yamamoto. (1994). Mechanism of removing Japanese encephalitis virus (JEV) and gold particles using cuprammonium regenerated cellulose hollow fiber (i-BMM or BMM) from aqueous solution containing protein, *Polym. J.*, *26*:1244–1256.

Hoffer, L., H. Schwinn, L. Biesert, and D. Josic. (1995). Improved virus safety and purity of a chromatographically produced Factor IX concentrate by nanofiltration, *J. Chromatog.*, *669*:187–196.

Horowitz, B., M. E. Wiebe, A. Lippin, and M. H. Stryker. (1985). Inactivation of viruses in labile blood derivatives, *Transfusion*, *25*:516–522.

Infectious Disease Weekly. (1995). Blood Banking Canadian Red Cross Recalls Blood Tainted with CJD, Aug. 7, 1985, Charles Henderson Publisher, ISSN#1065–1073.

Jernberg, M., E. Ohlsson, S. Winge, L. Westman, and B. Eriksson. (1996). Removal of viruses from Factor IX solutions by Viresolve 70 filtration, XXII International Congress of the World Federation of Haemophilia, Dublin, Ireland, June 23–28.

Kim, K. J., A. G. Fane, R. Ben Aim, M. G. Liu, G. Jonsson, I. C. Tessaro, A. P. Broek, and D. Bargeman. (1994). A comparative study of techniques used for porous membrane characterization: Pore characterization, *J. Membrane Sci.*, *87*:35–46.

Kyodo News International (1994). U.S. Medicine Manufacturer Ordered to Recall Blood Product, File: kl121095.100, Nov. 21.

Lubiniecki, A. L., and L. H. May. (1984). Cell bank characterization for recombinant DNA mammalian cell lines, *Develop. Biol. Stand.*, *60*:141–146.

Lubiniecki, A. S. (1988). Safety of recombinant biologics: Issues and emerging answers, in *Animal Cell Biotechnology*, Vol. 3 (R. E. Spier and J. B. Griffiths, eds.), Academic, London, pp. 3–12.

Manabe, S., and M. Santani. (1989). Porous hollow fiber membrane and a method for the removal of a virus by using same, U.S. Patent 4,808,315 (Feb. 28).

Microbiological Associates, Inc. (1988). Evaluation of removal of simian virus 40 from human growth hormone by PTKH membrane purification process, in *Validation of Ares Serono Pharmaceutical Production*, Vol. 1, Ares-Serono S.A., Switzerland, p. 41.

Millipore Corporation. (1995). *Viresolve Validation Guide*, Literature No. VG024 Rev. 1, 11/95, Millipore Corp., Bedford, MA.

Munari, S., A. Bottino, P. Moretti, G. Capennelli, and I. Becchi. (1989). Permoporometric study on ultrafiltration membranes, *J. Membrane Sci.*, *41*:69–86.

Nabetani, H., M. Nakajima, A. Watanabe, S. Nakao, and S. Kimura. (1990). Effects of osmotic pressure and adsorption on ultrafiltration of ovalbumin, *AIChE J.*, *36*:907–915.

Opong, W. S., and A. L. Zydney. (1991). Diffuse and convective protein transport through asymmetric membranes, *AIChE J.*, *37*:1497–1510.

Oshima, K. H., T. T. Evans-Strickfaden, A. K. Highsmith, and E. W. Ades. (1996). The use of a microporous polyvinylidene fluoride (PVDF) membrane filter to separate contaminating viral particles from biologically important proteins, *Biologicals*, *24*:137–145.

Petricianni, J. C. (1985). Regulatory considerations for products derived from the new biotechnology, *Pharm. Manuf.*, *5*:31–34.

Phillips, M. W. (1996). Integrity testing virus-retentive membranes, Presented at the PDA's Fourth Annual International Congress, Vienna, Austria.

Phillips, M. W., and A. J. DiLeo. (1996). A validatible porosimetric technique for verifying the integrity of virus-retentive membranes, *Biologicals*, *24*(3):243–253.

Pocchiari, M., G. Macchi, S. Peano, and A. Conz. (1989). Can potential hazard of Creutzfeldt–Jacob disease infectivity be reduced in the production of human growth hormone?, *Arch. Virol.*, *98*:131–135.

Prince, A. M., W. Stephen, and B. Brotman. (1984). Beta-propiolactone/UV irradiation: A review of its effectiveness, *Rev. Infect. Dis.*, *5*:92–107.

Satoh, S. (1996). Presented at the International Conference on the Virological Safety of Plasma Derivatives, CBER-USFDA, NHLBI, CDC, WHO, IABS, Bethesda, MD, Nov. 20–22.

Urase, T., K. Yamamoto, and S. Ohgaki. (1994). Effect of pore size distribution of ultrafiltration membranes on virus rejection in crossflow conditions, *Water Sci. Technol.*, *30*: 199–208.

Urase, T., K. Yamamoto, and S. Ohgaki. (1996). Effect of pore structure of membranes and module configuration on virus retention, *J. Membrane Sci.*, *115*:21–29.

Van Holten, R. W., S. Riester, T. M. Setcavage, R. Levy, M. Carroll, G. Oulundsen, and V. Pizzi. (1995). Incorporation of a viral clearance step into a modified Cohn fractionation, Presented at the American Association of Blood Banks Annual Meeting, November, New Orleans, LA.

Wall Street Journal. (1994). Baxter product, hepatitis case may be linked, *Wall Street Journal*, 3 Star, Eastern Edition, July 22, p. B7.

Walter, J., W. Werz, and W. Berthold. (1992). Virus removal and inactivation, *Biotech. Forum Eur.*, *9*:560–564.

White, E. M., J. B. Grun, C.-S. Sun, and A. F. Sito. (1991). Process validation for virus removal and inactivation, *BioPharm.*, *4*(5):34–39.

White, E. M., and R. S. Woodard. (1995). Recent issues raised in the evaluation of virus removal and inactivation, *Genet. Eng. News*, *15*(10):6.

Wiebe, M., F. Becker, L. Lazar, L. May, B. Casto, M. Semense, C. Fautz, C. Garnick, C. Miller, G. Masover, D. Bergmann, and A. S. Lubiniecki. (1989). A multifaceted approach to assure that recombinant tPA is free of adventitious virus, in *Advances in Animal Cell Biology and Technology for Bioprocessers* (R. E. Spier, J. B. Griffiths, J. Stephenne, and P. J. Crooy, eds.), Butterworths, Stoneham, MA, pp. 68–71.

Wienk, M., B. Folkers, Th. van den Boomgaard, and C. A. Smolders. (1994). Critical factors in the determination of the pore size distribution of ultrafiltration membranes using the liquid displacement method, *Separ.-Sci. Technol.*, *29*(11):1433–1440.

21

Aspects of Air and Gas Filtration in the Biopharmaceutical Industry

MAIK W. JORNITZ
Sartorius AG, Göttingen, Germany

1 INTRODUCTION

The filtration of gases and air finds a wide spectrum of use in various industries in applications with specific requirements and demands on the filtration system. This chapter concentrates on the requirements of air filtration in the pharmaceutical and biotechnological industries, excluding the filtration of air via cleanroom filters such as HEPA and ULPA filters. Various specific aspects are viewed from a practical side, including design criteria and applications. The main applications in the pharmaceutical industry are the filtration of compressed gases or air and sterile venting.

Compressed gas and air filtration is predominantly found in the fermentation industry and the filtration of service gases, for example for blow–fill–seal machines and pneumatically actuated valves. Fermentors can have a volume of 150 m^3, vented with a 1:1 ratio of air volume to fermentor medium volume per minute, which is equivalent to 9000 m^3 of air per hour, not an unusual amount. With a service lifetime of over a year, such filters have to sterilize a total air volume of around 50×10^6–60×10^6 m^3. Moreover, in such applications design criteria are of fundamental importance; when inefficient the running costs of these plants can be tremendous, understandable considering the air volume required per annum. The gas volumes required for service gases are far smaller, but their quality is nonetheless extremely critical because the filtered air comes in contact with the final container or even the product.

Venting applications are manifold and mainly highly critical, because again the air or gas can come in direct contact with the product. This is predominantly the case in vent filter systems on product and water storage tanks, autoclaves, and freeze dryers. The right sizing of these filter systems is of great importance, for an inadequate system could have disastrous consequences.

Biopharmaceutical applications require not only highest security of the filter device and quality standards, but also exceptionally high performance criteria in regard to flow rates, service life, and mechanical and thermal stability. An air or gas filtration system is a complex system that needs to function optimally from the intake of the air to the exhaust from the plant. Every step in an air filtration system must be designed to specific requirements to achieve the highest performance levels with the lowest possible running costs.

2 CONTAMINANTS

A wide range of contaminants can be found in air and even in bottled nitrogen. The main contaminants are particles of diverse sizes originating from natural sources and introduced by the compressors. These natural particle contaminations can range from 100 to 800 million particles per cubic meter of air, and 90% of them are smaller than 0.5 μm (Straus-Zunker, 1996). In addition to particles, there are a wide variety of yeast (≈5 μm), fungi (2.5–14 μm), spores, bacteria (<0.2 to 30 μm), and phage and viruses (0.02–0.2 μm) (Chemie Technik, 1987; Inman, 1993). The latter in particular must be removed from the air stream to avoid infections of fermentors or assure the final product quality, for example in the processing of blood products. Iron oxide, oil and oil vapor, and water are further contaminants that need to be removed to protect the final filtration system.

Certainly the contaminants present and their concentrations will depend on the environment surrounding the facilities. Humidity, dust, and microorganism levels differ in the individual locations and also vary on a seasonal basis. For example, the average dust concentration of city air is 0.2 mg/m^3 but can rise to >100/m^3. Therefore, the pretreatment of the air inlet needs to be adjusted to individual requirements and purposes. It is advisable to design the system to an expected worst-case situation. The particle load must be greatly reduced directly at the inlet to the compressors; otherwise the compressor may become obstructed or damaged. This is usually done by appropriate cloth or paper air intake filters (Mohrig, 1988). These filters must be maintained on a regular basis, sometimes weekly, to avoid pressure losses from filter blocking.

Coalescing filters, used after the compressor, play a very important role in reducing the particle and bioburden level in the first stage and if necessary separating oil and condensate (Kronsbein, 1989). Dryers will create appropriate water vapor levels for individual applications. It is important that the water vapor level be kept low to avoid any condensation of water, which could result in corrosion (Sitter, 1994). Oil vapor can be removed only by adsorptive filter units such as activated carbon filters. It is advisable to use a coarse depth filter after the activated carbon element to capture any particles that are shed. These pretreatment stages are described in detail in Chapter 25. Sterilizing grade hydrophobic membrane final filters are used to completely remove particulate and microbial contaminants.

A common contaminant coming from the plant is iron oxide, which is found when lower grade stainless steel or even cast iron is used as piping material or low quality water is supplied to the steam generator. Condensation, which may form when there is insufficient pretreatment in the drying step or high temperature gradients between parts of the plant, can trigger corrosion of the piping. In older large-scale fermentation plants one often witnesses cast iron piping, which corrodes easily,

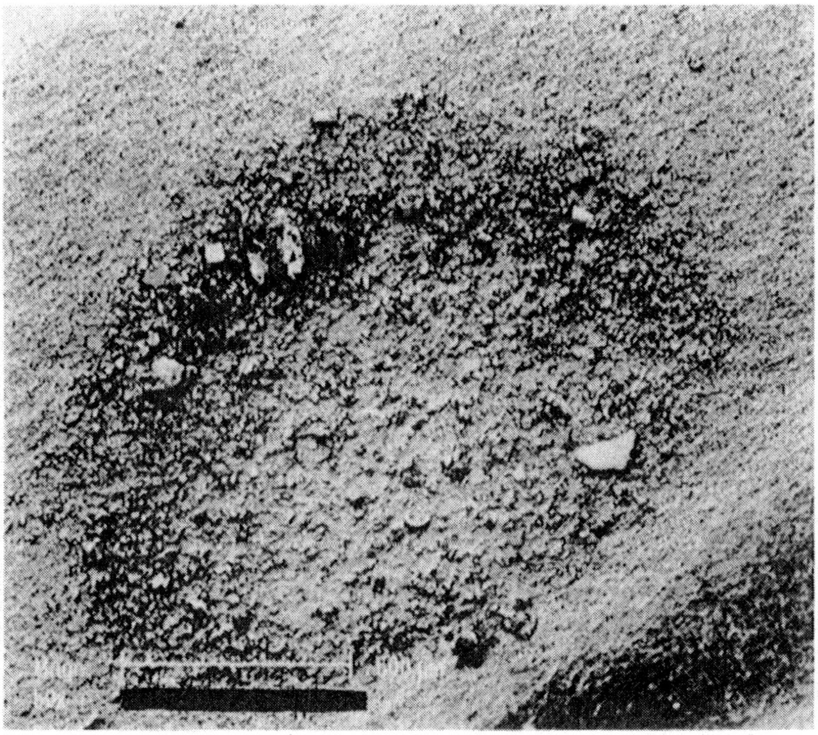

Figure 1 Scanning electron micrograph of oil contamination on an air filter membrane.

particularly when steam is transferred through it. Iron oxide is the main contaminant that blocks sterilizing grade filter cartridges and when encountered should be treated with a prefiltration step to prolong the service life of the more expensive membrane filter.

In fermentor and bioreactor offgas filtration, the amounts and kinds of contaminants can be even more detrimental to the filtration system (Orchard, 1991; Jaenchen, 1988). There foaming can be a major hazard for sterilizing grade filters, which can block rapidly when they come in contact with biomass foam. Usually the offgas air is saturated with water, which can lead to waterlogging of the filter system due to the formation of condensate on the filter membrane. The air at this point has a higher viscosity, and it is unavoidable that biological contaminants such as cell debris, microorganisms, and proteins will be carried in the airstream. Sufficient pretreatment is necessary to prevent premature blocking of the sterilizing grade membrane filters. The individual pretreatment steps are discussed in Sec. 14.

3 HYDROPHOBICITY

High hydrophobicity is essential for the membranes and fleeces used in air and vent filter cartridges. If their hydrophobicity is low, the membrane matrix may wet out with condensate and the bubble point will then have to be overcome to achieve an airflow. In this case the differential pressure would be so high that either a tank could implode or production processes could be disrupted.

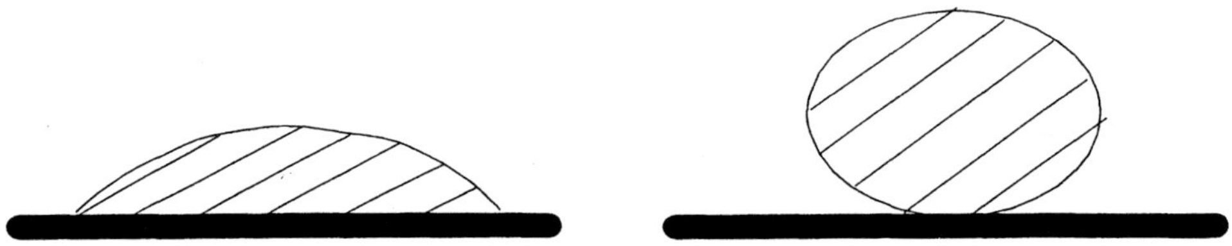

Adhesion Force > Cohesion Force — Adhesion Force < Cohesion Force

Hydrophilic — Highly hydrophobic

Figure 2 Typical droplet shape of liquids on (left) hydrophilic and (right) hydrophobic surfaces.

Hydrophobicity means that the cohesive forces between the water molecules are greater than the adhesive forces between the water and the other liquid or solid (e.g., oil/water, or PTFE/water). No wetting or mixing occurs. Thus hydrophobicity is based on high cohesive forces. The higher the cohesive force, the higher the hydrophobicity. If there is no attraction between the membrane material and the water molecules, water will be repelled.

The measurement of the hydrophobicity of a membrane filter is the water penetration point. Water is flowed onto the upstream side of the filter, and the pressure is increased to the point at which water breaks through the membrane; at this point the pressure force has overcome the cohesive forces. The higher the water penetration point, the higher the hydrophobicity.

Most vent filters contain highly hydrophobic polytetrafluoroethylene (PTFE) membranes and polypropylene (PP) fleeces. In some instances other membrane materials are used, for example polyvinylidene fluoride (PVDF) and polypropylene (PP), but these are not recommended for use as vent filter membranes because they are not sufficiently hydrophobic (Zind, 1990). The differences are illustrated in Figure 3.

A high hydrophobicity reduces the danger of waterlogging because the water will run down the filter matrix and drainage fleece. This is especially important for such applications as venting of water-for-injection (WFI) tanks and offgas filtration; moreover, a high hydrophobicity is the basic requirement when using the water intrusion integrity test (described in Sec. 10).

Often, after steam sterilization, when vent filters do not immediately experience a drying airflow, less hydrophobic filter membranes trap condensate within their matrix that partly or completely blocks the filter. This can be especially severe with non-vacuum-resistant tanks, where the condensation vacuum after steam sterilization has to be compensated for by supplying sterile air via the air filter. When the filter matrix is waterlogged and no protective devices such as burst disks or pressure release valves are installed, an implosion of the tank is possible. In some instances it is advisable to use steam-jacketed or heat-traced housings to avoid extensive condensation on the filter unit. In large volume fermentation, waterlogging causes pressure surges and additional running costs, as well as shutdown periods, which also raise cost levels, PTFE membrane materials, due to their high hydrophobicity, reduce

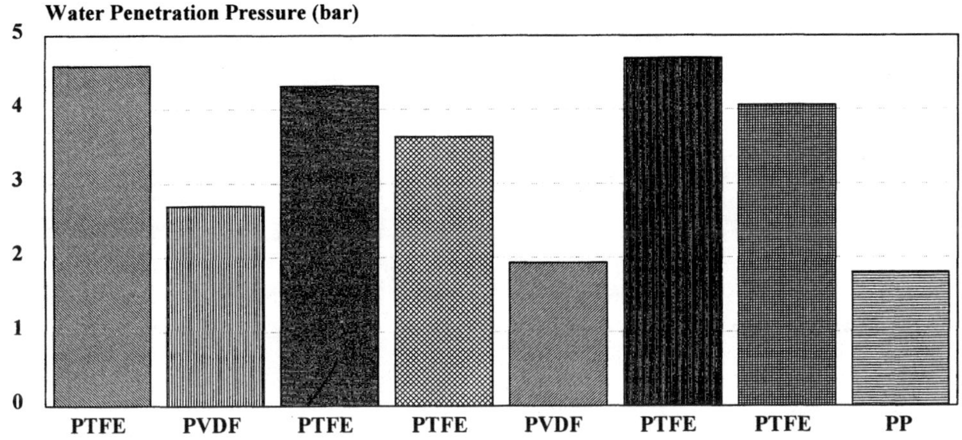

Figure 3 Differences in hydrophobicity of several hydrophobic membrane filter cartridges. (Commercially available 0.2 μm membrane filter elements; height 10 in., temperature 20°C.)

the effect of condensate blockage, especially when the prefilter fleeces and construction of the filter element are optimized.

The time required by a filter membrane to recover to its initial airflow is called blowdown time. This time should be as short as possible to reduce plant shutdown time and the risk of restricted airflow during venting applications. Blowdown time also depends on the hydrophobicity of the filter membrane. Figure 4 shows the blowdown time for PTFE and PVDF sterilizing grade filters. The difference in the length of time needed to cover the initial flow rate is obvious. The reason is the lower hydrophobicity of the PVDF membrane material.

In addition, water that collects in the membrane matrix of less hydrophobic membrane materials can promote the growth of microorganisms. Even water in adequate prefilter fleeces or badly constructed filter cartridges will increase the chance

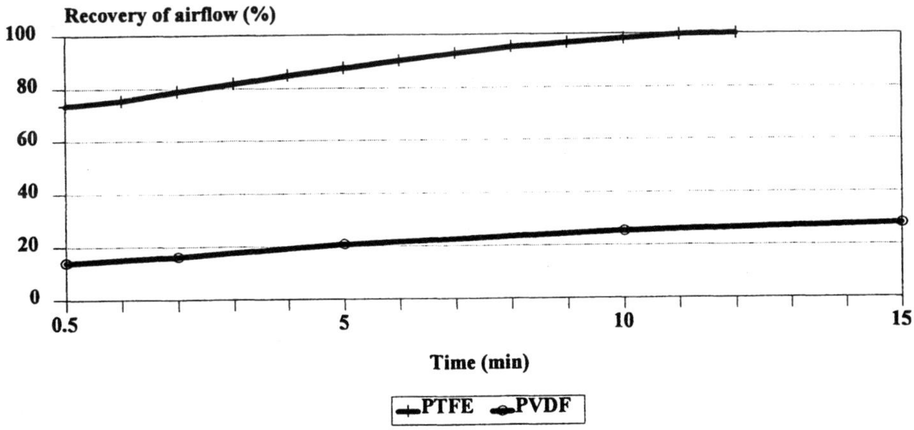

Figure 4 Differences in blowdown time due to membrane materials. (Two airflows measured at Δp = 200 mbar.)

of microorganism growth. Water retention therefore needs to be avoided, due to the increased risk of microbial contamination and cross contamination. This risk is highly likely at applications such as exhaust gas filtration, where microorganisms can be carried over from a fermentor, bioreactor, or service gas filter that is not steam sterilized on a routine basis (Meltzer, 1996; Rowe et al., 1996).

It is evident that high membrane hydrophobicity is necessary to ensure the performance of sterilizing grade 0.2 μm filter units and meet the security levels set by the regulatory agencies and the industry (Keating et al., 1992). Therefore, most commercially available sterilizing grade air filter cartridges are membrane filter cartridges with PTFE membranes.

4 AIR FILTER MEMBRANE MATERIALS

The three membrane materials most commonly used for sterilizing grade air filters are polypropylene (PP), polyvinylidine fluoride (PVDF), and polytetrafluoroethylene (PTFE). Because of their chemical structure (Fig. 5), these materials have properties that play an important role in meeting the requirements of air filtration systems.

PTFE is certainly the most hydrophobic material, the benefits of which were discussed in the previous section. It has no water adsorption and has the best thermal and mechanical strength of the three materials (Meltzer et al., 1994; Zind, 1990). PTFE membranes are produced by a stretching process under specific temperature conditions. The process is described in Chapter 2. The result is a highly porous (Fig. 6) but also mechanically resistant filter membrane. Due to the stretching process, the membrane experiences a certain amount of mechanical and thermal stress, which gives it stability.

This aspect is highly important, due to the fact that changes in the properties of the filter membrane that occur during plant procedures can have dramatic results. For example, a reduction in hydrophobicity or shrinkage of the membrane can reduce the flow rate drastically. In one specific case, it was reported that a PVDF sterilizing grade filter experienced a reduction of up to 20% of its initial flow rate after repeated steam sterilization. This would mean that the system needs to be sized with a higher security margin to avoid damage or failure. Figure 7 compares the changes in penetration point and flow rate experienced by three membrane materials that were steam sterilized.

Other materials show specifically their weakness with steam sterilization. Polypropylene, which has a low maximum short-term temperature resistance, starts flowing and becomes soft in the region of usual steam temperature. This is especially critical with thin filter membrane materials.

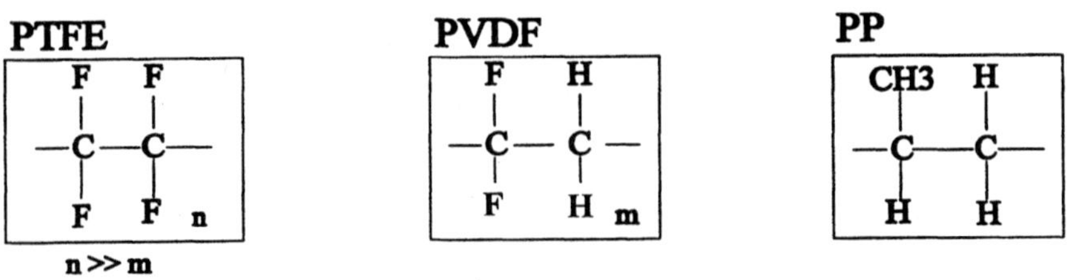

Figure 5 Chemical structures of three air filter membrane materials.

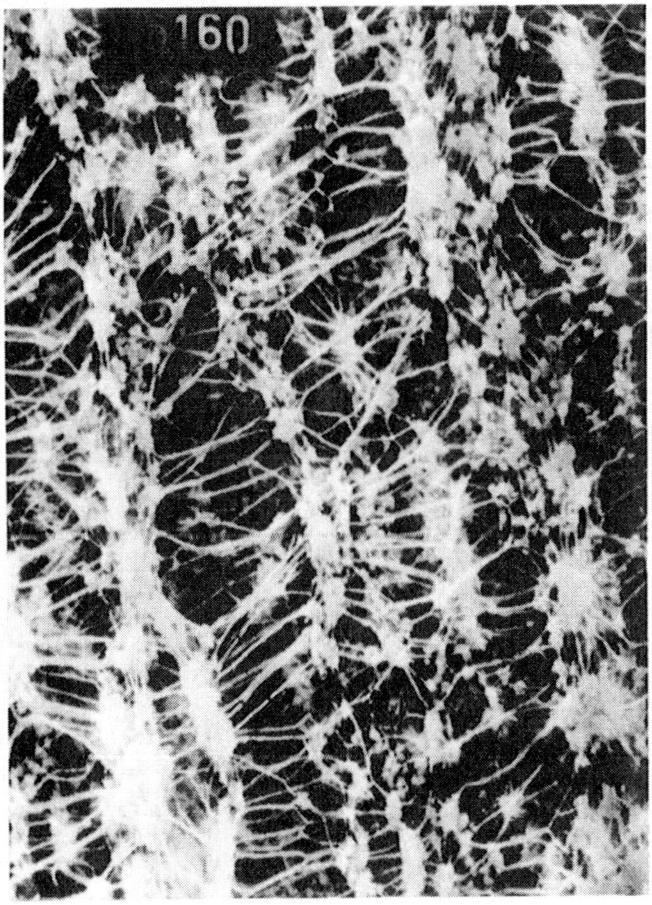

Figure 6 Scanning electron micrograph of a PTFE air filter membrane.

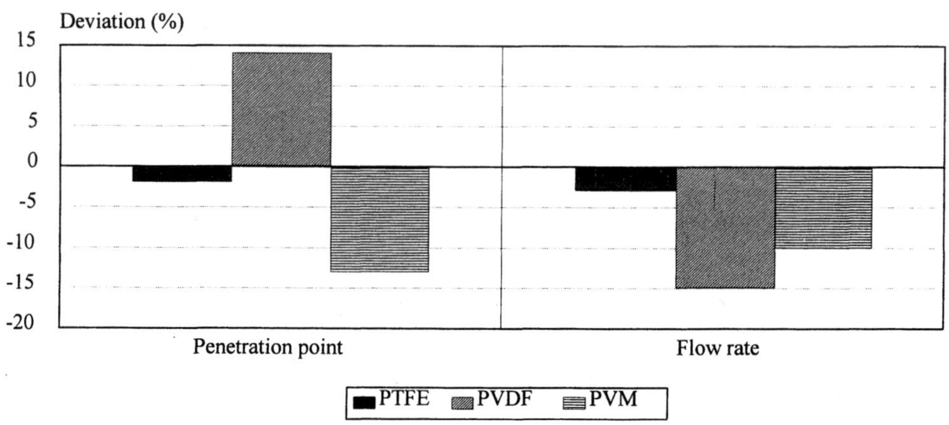

Figure 7 Deviation of the flow rate and water penetration point of three air filter membranes after steam sterilization. (25 steaming cycles; 134°C; 30 min.)

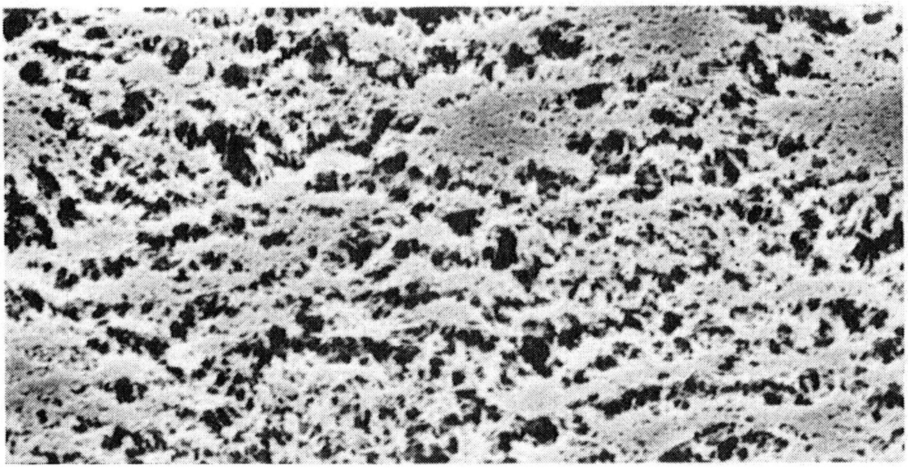

Figure 8 Scanning electron micrograph of a polypropylene air filter membrane.

PVDF also has a low short-term temperature resistance, 10°C higher than PP, but again for a thin membrane this physical property reflects an extremely negative factor of membrane shrinkage during steam sterilization that results in lower airflow rates after repeated steaming. Membrane shrinkage can stretch the membrane to such a degree that flaws and microleaks occur, especially in the area of end cap welding.

Polypropylene and PVDF can both be affected by long-term degradation, i.e., disintegration of the filter membrane to a powder. This is due to the loss of stabilizers when the filter cartridges are repeatedly steam sterilized over a long period of time,

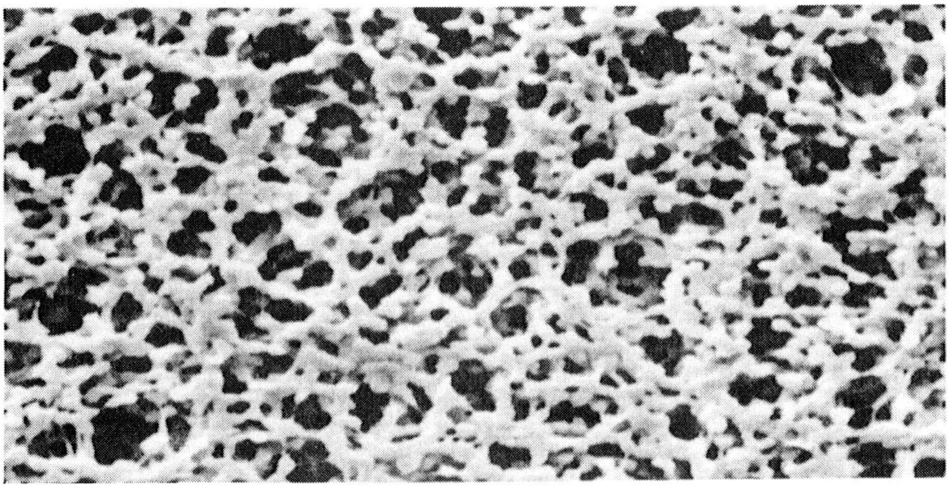

Figure 9 Scanning electron micrograph of a PVDF air filter membrane.

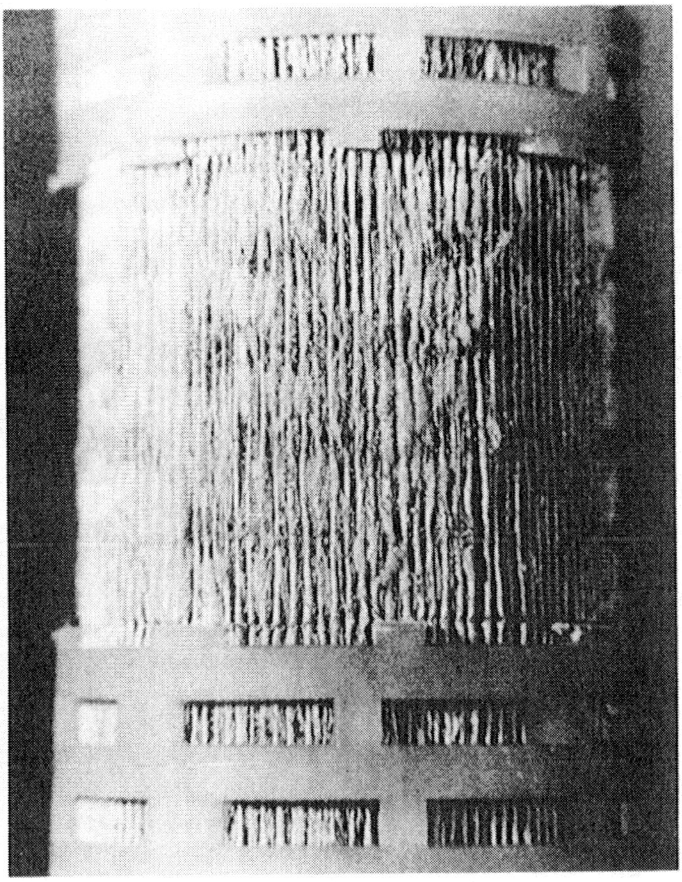

Figure 10 Sterilizing grade filter with oxidized polypropylene prefilter fleece.

for example in large-scale fermentation applications, where the usual lifetime of air filter cartridges can be up to 2 years.

Support fleeces can also be affected by oxidation, especially when the temperature of the supplied air is higher than 80°C, which is not unusual in large-scale fermentation. Such higher air temperatures are found in plants that used to use glass fiber towers. The higher air temperatures were required to avoid condensate in the filter matrix of the towers (Fay, 1995). Such elevated temperatures plus repeated steaming initiate an oxidative breaking up of the polypropylene support fleeces, as shown in Fig. 10. This effect can be seen after a period of about 6 months. At that point the PP starts to become brittle and disintegrates.

Some filter manufacturers reacted to this by introducing heat-resistant support fleeces, which are stable at high temperatures in long-term use. In certain applications where hot, dry air must be filtered, for example for melt-blow processes, full PTFE filter cartridges are used because of their temperature resistance. These filters are extremely expensive.

5 SEPARATION MECHANISMS IN AIR AND GAS FILTRATION

In liquid filtration the main separation mechanism is sieve retention; that is, particles larger than the largest pore of the filter membrane are retained. Another mechanism is adsorptive capture of the particles or microorganisms by adsorptive membrane materials such as nylon or depth filter material such as glass fiber. Both mechanisms are also valid for air and gas filtration in addition to having other effects described in the following sections, which result mainly from the physical attributes of air, especially its low viscosity.

In addition to sieve retention (also called direct interception and capture), there are other main separation mechanisms particular to air filtration that influence the quality of the filtrate and the efficiency of the filter. These are mainly known as diffusive interception, interception, and impaction (Lathrache, 1991; Kronsbein, 1989; Grant, 1988; Blakie, 1987; Meltzer, 1987). There is also the mechanism of gravitational settling, which is effective at low velocities and bigger particle sizes, usually >1 μm, depending on particle mass.

Sieving or Direct Interception. As illustrated in Fig. 11, in sieve retention a particle is separated from the main airflow because of its size, which is bigger than the pores of the filter membrane itself. For hydrophobic membrane filters the average particle size is >0.2 μm.

Diffusive Interception. Particles of small sizes (<0.3 μm) have a Brownian motion; that is, they move about randomly due to collisions with gas molecules and the low viscosity of the air. Eventually they collide with the filter material and become captured (Fig. 12). Once captured, van der Waals forces or covalent or ionic bonds (depending on the particle material) keep the particles on the filter material. They are not released again, even at pressure pulsations, because the bonding forces are up to 1000 times higher than the mass of the particle. The diffusion parameter, D, can be expressed as

$$D = \frac{1}{v d_{\mathrm{f}}} \left(\frac{CkT}{3N_{\mathrm{y}} d_{\mathrm{p}}} \right) \tag{1}$$

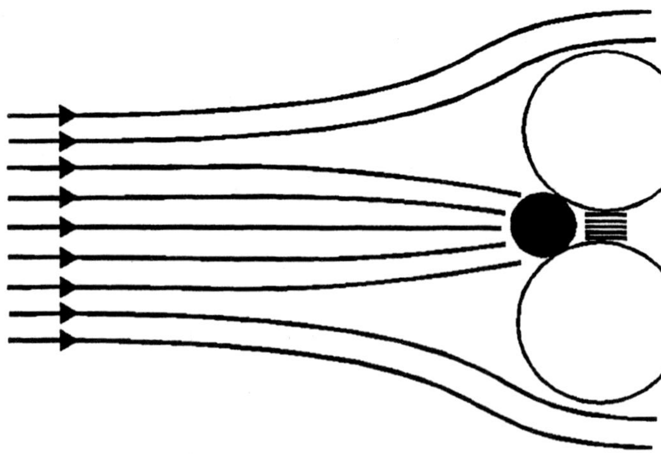

Figure 11 Schematic of sieve retention mechanism.

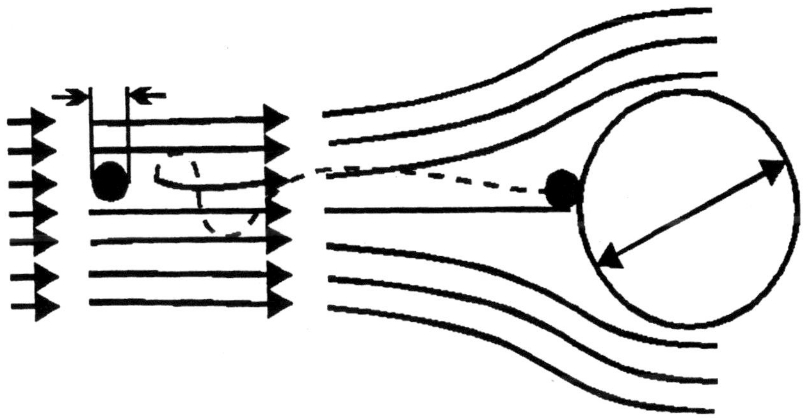

Figure 12 Schematic of diffusional interception.

where

C = Cunningham correction factor
k = Boltzmann constant
T = absolute temperature of the air in kelvin
N_y = viscosity of air
d_p = particle diameter
v = velocity of air
d_f = fiber diameter

and the term in parentheses on the right is known as the diffusion coefficient.

As Eq. (1) shows, to achieve the highest effect of retention the velocity has to be low to get the highest residence time within the filter matrix; the higher the velocity, the lower the retention effectiveness at small particle sizes. Also the humidity needs to be low; otherwise the particles will be surrounded by moisture and lose their ability to move around freely. The same is true of the viscosity of the air, which will be influenced by the humidity.

Inertial Impaction. When particles with a higher mass or bigger size are not able follow the air streamline, which suddenly diverts around the filter matrix, they hit the filter matrix. This inertial impaction is illustrated in Fig. 13. This separation mechanism is most effective with bigger particles (>1 μm), higher particle density, and high velocities. Higher viscosity of air due to higher humidity can again influence this separation mechanism negatively. The inertia parameter, My, can be expressed as

$$\text{My} = \frac{C\rho v d_p^2}{18 N_y d_f} \qquad (2)$$

where

C = Cunningham correction factor
ρ = density of the particle
v = velocity of air

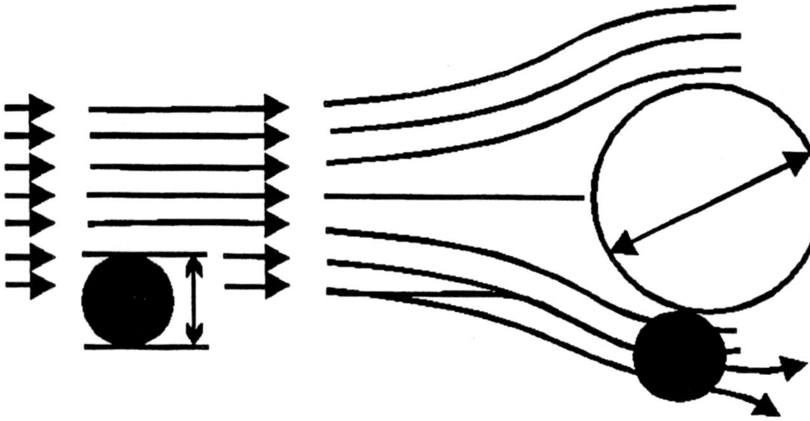

Figure 13 Schematic of inertial impaction.

d_p = particle diameter
N_y = viscosity of air
d_f = fiber diameter

Interception. When the location of the streamline and the size of the particle result in contact between the particle and the filter material, the particle is captured by interception (Fig. 14). The particle radius here is bigger than or equal to the distance between the streamline and the filter matrix. The particles stay in their streamline, which means that they are usually particles of smaller sizes and lower mass. The characteristic value, R, for the interception is

$$R = \frac{r}{r_f} = \frac{d_p}{d_f} \tag{3}$$

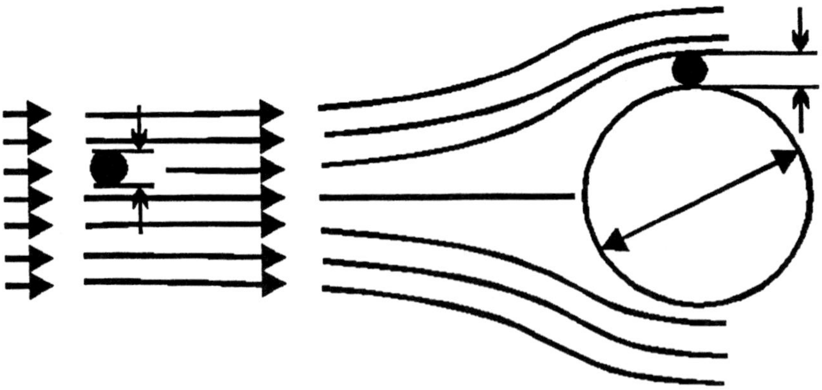

Figure 14 Interception.

where

r = particle radius
r_f = fiber radius
d_p = particle diameter
d_f = fiber diameter

Gravitational Settling. The gravitational settling mechanism (Fig. 15) is not the most influential, but it still separates particles from the airstream, especially dense particles traveling at low velocities. Usually the particles are >1 μm in size. The particles leave the air streamline due to gravity forces and collide with the filter matrix. Once attached to the filter material, they are not released. As expressed in Eq. (4), the gravitational settling mechanism is highly influenced by the viscosity and velocity of the air. The settling parameter G can be calculated as

$$G = \frac{u}{v} = \frac{c\rho g d_p^2}{18 N_y v} \qquad (4)$$

where

u = settling velocity of the particle
v = air velocity
C = Cunningham correction factor
ρ = density of the particle
g = gravitational constant
d_p = particle diameter
N_y = viscosity of air

Electrostatic Capture. The retention mechanism of electrostatic capture is the most effective one for filters such as HEPA (high efficiency particulate air) and ULPA (ultralow penetration air) cleanroom ceiling filter materials, which

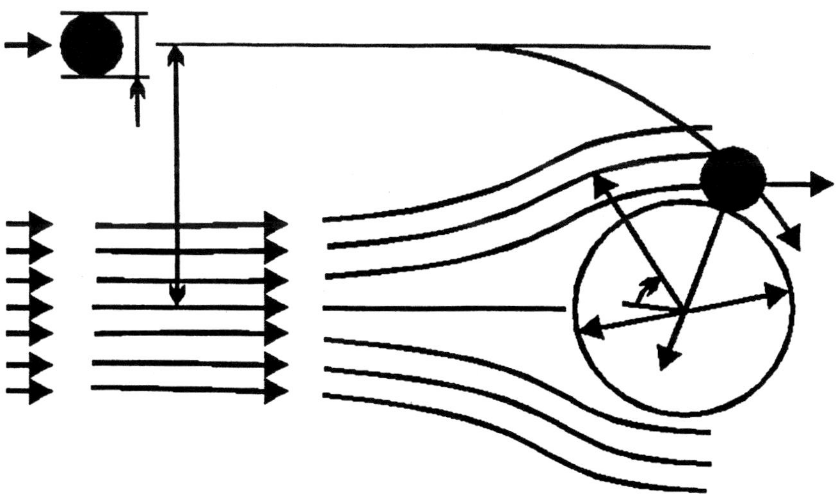

Figure 15 Gravitational settling.

are usually packed glass fiber filter materials (Ziemer, 1987). These filters rely on their electrostatic capacities and capture particles of opposite charge. The effectiveness of such filters depends on two major parameters, the humidity of the air and the velocity. The humidity needs to be low because the electrostatic charges are highest when the air is dry. Also there is no danger of condensate buildup within the filter matrix, which could lead to premature blockage of the filter and the danger of microorganism growth within the condensate layer. The velocity varies from 5 to 30 cm/s, which is highly important for the separation efficiency, to create a long enough contact time for the particles to be separated (Grant, 1988; Ziemer, 1987).

The individual separation mechanisms are most effective under specific conditions but especially at specific particle dimensions. The diffusive interception mechanism works most effectively at very small particle sizes; therefore the retentive effectiveness decreases with increasing particle size. In contrast, the retentive efficiency of interception and impaction increases with particle size and is therefore less with smaller particles. Thus the retention graph of these mechanisms will cross over at a point of lowest retention, which is called the most penetrating particle size (MPPS). At this specific point the air filter has its highest penetration rate but it will not reach 100% penetration (Fig. 16).

The position of the most penetrating particle size depends very much on the air velocity through the filter. When the airflow rate is high, the contact time within the filter is low, and the retentive capacity of the diffusion mechanism no longer works as well as at low velocities. The Brownian movement of the particles is also

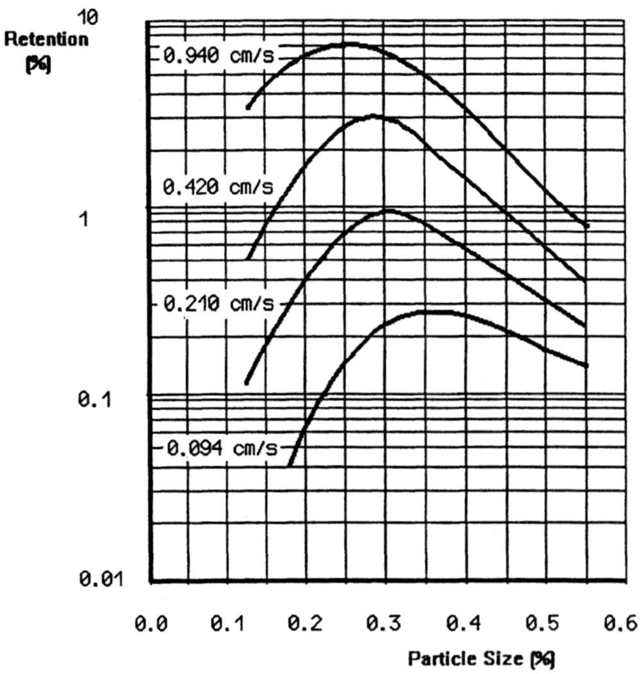

Figure 16 Shift of the retention graph at higher velocities.

influenced by the air velocity. Therefore the MPPS shifts to smaller particles. Direct interception and impaction are not influenced to such an extent by the velocity (Liu et al., 1985; Grant, 1988). Nevertheless, to achieve optimal retention, the design velocity needs to be viewed appropriately and the system needs to be sized accordingly.

Common sterilizing grade air filter cartridge membranes used in the biopharmaceutical industry are constructed of materials such as PTFE or PVDF. These membranes have a thickness of around 60–100 μm, are highly hydrophobic, and have a defined pore structure. They are challenged with various tests to determine their separation efficiency, such as Arizona fine test dust or, for the measurement of very small particles, a condensation nucleus counter (CNC) is used. The separation efficiency is usually determined at around 0.01–0.02 μm for a 0.2 μm membrane filter, depending on the velocity and humidity of the air. It is therefore understandable that 0.2 μm rated hydrophobic membrane filters are able to retain even particles as small as viruses, depending on the process parameters.

6 AIR VELOCITY

When designing an air filtration system, often the velocity of the air stream is not considered and put into the equation. Yet this factor has a major influence on running costs of the plant, the working environment, and the separation mechanisms.

Often filter systems are designed too small in terms of the effective area of the inner core of the filter cartridge system or the piping of the filter housing. This creates an immediate high velocity and high pressure loss; therefore running costs soon exceed the initial investment cost savings (see Fig. 17).

High velocities through pipes and filter cartridge systems also create an exceedingly high noise level. Legal borders of specific reinforcement laws for protection of workers, such as Germany's Arb.St.Vo.par.15 and Betr.Verf.par.89ff, need to be followed. Exposure of workers to noise levels below 85 dB are permissible in the long term. Figure 18 shows that a level of 85 dB is achieved easily with small

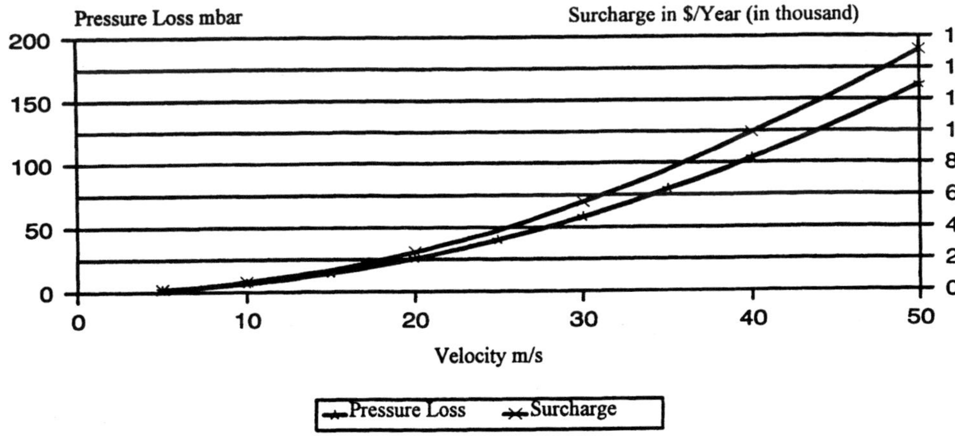

Figure 17 Surcharge costs due to pressure losses. ($0.08/kWh; 6000 operating hours per year.)

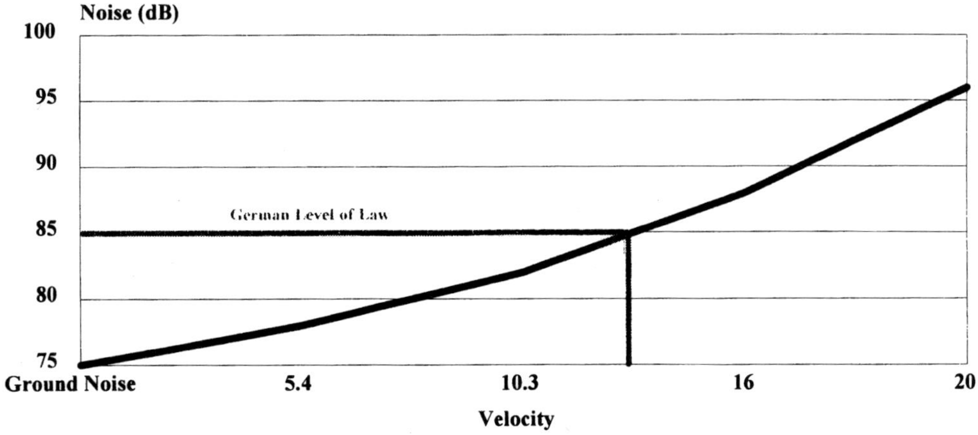

Figure 18 Noise level due to airflow velocity through a 28 mm adapter. The German maximum legal noise level is 85 dB.

inner core diameters, and therefore to achieve the right airflow rate, the inner core or pipe diameter has to be enlarged. The system must be sized appropriately.

Experience shows that most adequately sized filter systems use multiplace round filter cartridges with a height of 20 in. It does not make sense to use a height of 30 in. The filtration area of a 30 in. filter cartridge is greater, but the restriction in airflow with these systems is not the effective filtration area but the inner core and adapter area. The flow rate of a 30 in. cartridge is insignificantly higher than that of a 20 in. cartridge. It makes more sense to use a housing that accommodates more 20 in. cartridges than to extend the height of the cartridge. This fact becomes evident in the flowchart of Fig. 19.

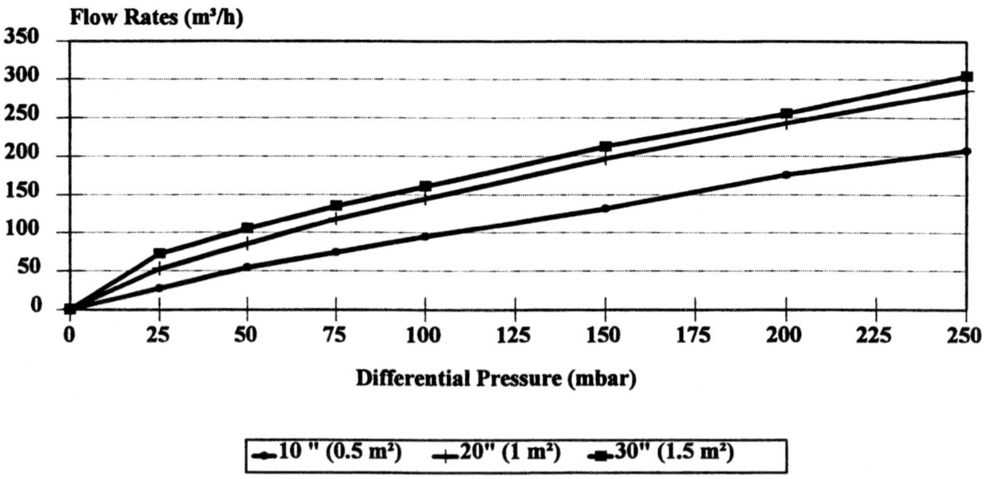

Figure 19 Comparison of airflow rates of filter cartridge of different heights. (Atmospheric pressure; 0.2 μm double-bayonet adapter.) Top to bottom: 30 in. (1.5 m^2); 20 in. (1 m^2); 10 in. (0.5 m^2).

Velocity very much influences the penetration of submicrometer particles through a filter. If the flow rate increases, the penetration of smaller particles increases due to the fact that the separation mechanism of diffusion (Brownian motion) will not be as effective as at a lower velocity. At high flow rates the contact time within the filter is shortened; therefore, the probability of particle–filter contact becomes less. Capture by interception is not influenced by airflow velocity (Fuchs, 1964).

Nowadays design criteria usually include a pipe airflow velocity of $\approx$10 m/s and airflow velocity through the filter medium around 0.01–0.05 m/s for sterilizing grade membrane filters. The velocity over the filter medium needs to be lower to ensure a certain contact time and therefore finer retention. The restrictive area of a filter system is always the pipe, inner core, or adapter diameter. At these points the velocity increases and pressure losses occur.

7 AIR FILTER HOUSINGS

It is important to have not only the right filter cartridge construction but also a well-constructed filter housing suitable for the requirements of air filtration, mainly in terms of lowest possible pressure losses and condensate chambers, and polishing to avoid microbial growth on the stainless steel surface. If microbial growth occurs on the housing, especially when the system is not steam sterilized on a regular basis, the sterilizing grade filter could be challenged by an increasing bioburden. The housings have to be well engineered; i.e., certain requirements have to met:

- The correct pipe diameter to avoid pressure losses
- A condensate chamber to collect condensate, which could otherwise flood and block the filter cartridge
- Common connectors on the inlet and outlet sides as well as the condensate drain and venting/gauge connection to ease installation requirements
- A housing system that can be scaled from small scale to multiplace cartridge housings
- A high quality stainless steel such as AISI 316 L
- Polished surface and weld (certain standards call for a surface roughness of Ra <0.5 μm)
- Housings that comply with common pressure vessel regulations and have been tested and certified to do so

Most of the available compressed gas housings fulfill these requirements and are fitted with standard cartridge adapter recesses such as the common double-bayonet, double O-ring adapter. These features allow the user to switch filter types if necessary. Most housings are constructed to include condensate chambers and valves to easily drain condensate from the housing. The standard stainless steel nowadays is AISI 316 L with electropolished surfaces. All housings are available from smaller dimensions, i.e., to fit small-scale filter cartridges of 300 cm^2 filtration area, to large-scale multiplace housings such as the one diagrammed in Fig. 20. The largest I have seen so far was a 96-round 30-in. high sterilizing grade filter housing.

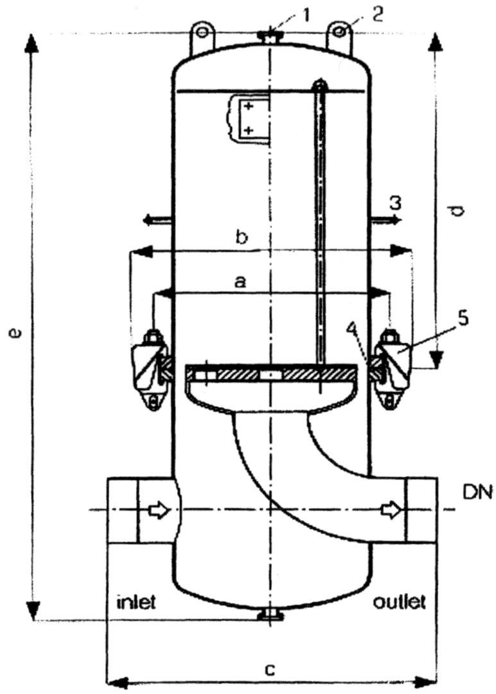

Figure 20 Typical compressed gas multiplace cartridge housing.

Tank venting housings are sometimes constructed differently (see Fig. 21). These housings are used to avoid any mechanical damage of the filter cartridge and are fitted on top of storage tanks. The filtrate side of the housing is connected to the tank. The upstream side of the housing is open to the atmosphere through recesses or holes in the baseplate. Recesses are also found in the housing bell to create air circulation in the housing to dry off any condensate droplets on the housing wall or the filter cartridge itself. The stainless steel and surface polish quality are the same as for compressed gas housings. Tank venting housings are usually employed in applications that do not require steam sterilization and integrity testing, as they do not have the inlet pipes and valves necessary for those operations.

8 PREFILTRATION

Usually, protective prefiltration, which prevents premature clogging of sterilizing grade filters, is not required in air filtration because of the thorough pretreatment of the air by air intake and coalescing filters and dryers after the compressors. As always, however, there are some exceptions where prefilters are needed to ensure the performance of the sterile filter (Orchard, 1991). These instances are mainly found in older plants with old pipes in which either coarse rust particles flake off the walls of the piping or brittle sealing material (from connections or valves) contaminates the air stream. Cast iron pipes and inferior quality stainless steel are often used, which can lead to corrosion. In such plants the investment costs are

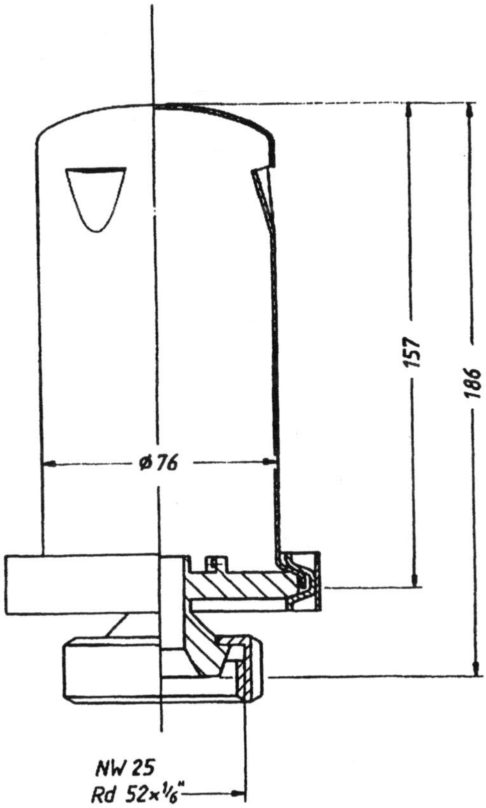

Figure 21 Typical tank venting housing.

reduced, but very soon these savings are overcome by exceptionally high running costs, such as those incurred by the need for frequent changes of filter cartridges. Steam generators supplied with low quality water add iron oxide to the system. In these instances it is more economical to use a prefilter to protect the more costly final filter.

The main application for a prefiltration is offgas filtration, where a high moisture aerosol content can carry particles such as cell debris as well as foaming fermentation broth, which upon reaching the final filter blocks it instantly. Also, due to the higher temperatures and enrichment of the offgas with moisture, condensation will occur when the air reaches the colder filter and reduce the effective filtration area. All these applications require prefiltration to protect the more expensive final filter.

There are several types of prefilters—stainless steel mesh or sintered filter cartridges and depth filter cartridges constructed of polypropylene (Fig. 23), cellulose, or borosilicate fibrous fleeces.

Stainless steel AISI 304 or 316 L filters with nominal retention rates of 3 and 1 μm are commonly used for the filtration of the steam supplied to the plant. These filters are very efficient in removing any particles and iron oxide generated by corrosion. Installed in AISI 304 industrial type housings, they may perform with high

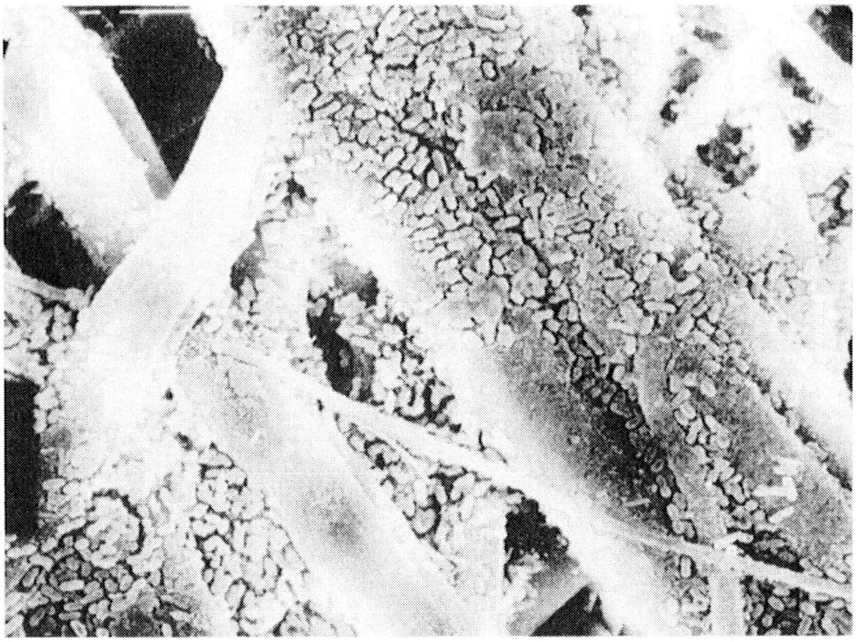

Figure 22 Microorganism contamination on a prefilter fleece.

efficiency over very long service lives. Certainly, maintenance should be carried out on a regular basis; usually an experience level is documented that indicates when the filters need to be exchanged to avoid buildup of pressure and low flow rates due to blockage. Some filter manufacturers even offer to regenerate iron oxide–contaminated stainless steel filter cartridges for their clients. This regeneration is usually done with acids or special cleaning solutions under high flow rate and pressure conditions or with ultrasonic baths.

Polymeric depth filter cartridges with nominal retention ratings of 0.3–5 μm are usually used directly in front of the sterilizing grade membrane filter. Sometimes, according to the application, these depth filters are also used for venting purposes, when absolute sterility is not required or the medium to be protected is not conducive to microbial growth. In either case, it is highly important that the prefilter material be hydrophobic to ensure that condensate will not block the filter matrix; i.e., it must not become waterlogged. Otherwise the pressure loss over the filter will be extremely high, because the bubble point needs to be achieved to force any liquid out of the filter matrix. With some tighter, less hydrophobic (cellulosic) prefilter materials, the bubble point can be as high as 500 mbar. This can have disastrous consequences. In one reported instance, when this type of filter was used as a vent filter for a non-vacuum-resistant tank, the tank imploded. Besides the danger of waterlogging, microbiological growth can be promoted by the moisture entrapped in the filter's matrix. This would result in a higher bioburden in front of the final membrane filter and, in tank venting use, the danger of grow-through and contamination of the filtrate side.

The construction of prefilters is highly important. Pleat construction that is too tight will entrap condensate between the pleats and lead to waterlogging. The airflow

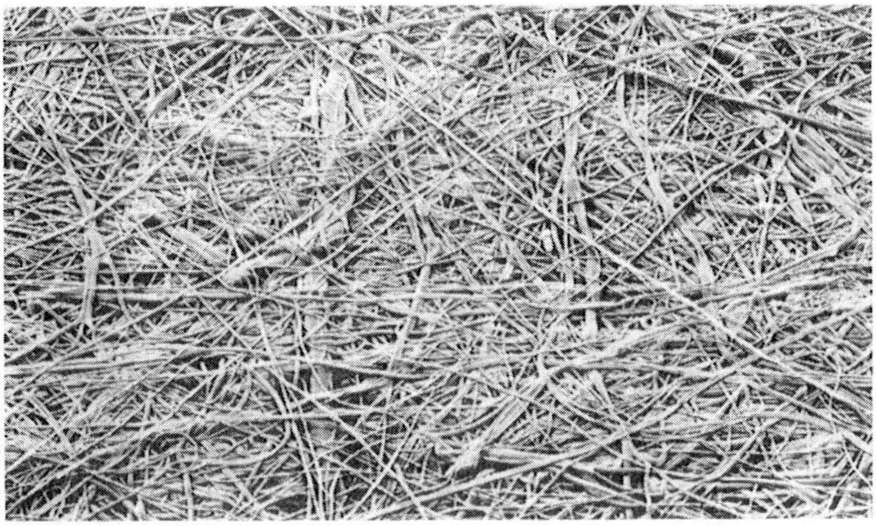

Figure 23 Scanning electron micrograph of a polypropylene prefilter matrix.

will be highly restricted, leading to higher differential pressure demand and reactor backpressure. The effective filtration area needed to ensure a high dirt load capacity will be reduced. The use of several different materials can cause problems due to different coefficients of heat expansion during steam sterilization. The core and adapter diameter must be big enough to avoid pressure losses due to high velocities. The need for high hydrophobicities and optimized filter cartridge construction is discussed at length in Sec. 9.

Prefilters need to have a high dirt load capacity, sometimes even need to break foam, to protect the sterilizing grade filter; otherwise the plant procedures will be disrupted or even brought to a halt. To achieve a high dirt load capacity, several manufacturers use fleeces of different retention values in their cartridges, i.e., the outermost fleece has a coarser retention rating than the innermost. With this type of construction the whole depth of the filter matrix is used, besides the effect of fractionate retention, which usually prolongs the lifetime of a filtration system anyway. Moreover, this type of construction allows high flow rates at low pressure losses due to the high pore volume on the upstream side.

The usual prefiltration system is of the same size as the sterilizing grade filter system. The size is usually determined by the flow rate required through the sterilizing grade filter system. Sizing of these filter systems is discussed in Chapter 12. When the size of the sterilizing grade system is known, the same size is used for the prefiltration system in order to avoid high pressure losses. The differential pressure over the prefiltration system is usually lower than that over the sterilizing grade filter owing to the higher void volume. On the other hand, the main restrictive area of flow in air filtration is the inner core and adapter area, which must therefore be big enough, otherwise high velocities will create high pressure losses. It is always advisable to calculate the airflow velocity by determining the total cartridge adapter area and dividing it by the required volume flow. Design criteria often stipulate a maximum pipe velocity of 10 m/s, and this maximum is also valid for the cartridge adapter. Certainly the air velocity over the filter material is far lower due to the higher filtration area. The commonly used double-bayonet adapter has an area of 25–27 cm^2, and the filtration area of the filter cartridge can then vary from 8000 cm^2 for a 10 in. element to 24,000 cm^2 for a 30 in. element.

9 STERILIZING GRADE FILTERS

In the past, glass fiber packed towers were used to "sterilize" the air supplied to plant processes. Due to insecurities in their performance and the space needed by these towers, sterilizing grade membrane filters were developed. These membrane filters are usually built in a filter cartridge format in different sizes and effective filtration areas. Commonly, a hydrophobic membrane placed between supporting fleeces is pleated and seam-welded to a cylinder (Fig. 24). The membrane materials used are thoroughly described in Sec. 4. This cylinder is then backed up by either a polypropylene or stainless steel inner core and an outer support cage. Finally, end caps and adapters are welded onto the ends of the cartridge cylinder to securely bind the outer support, filter material, and end cap together. The end caps prevent any bypass of contaminants, and the adapters allow a secure installation of the cartridge into the appropriate filter housing.

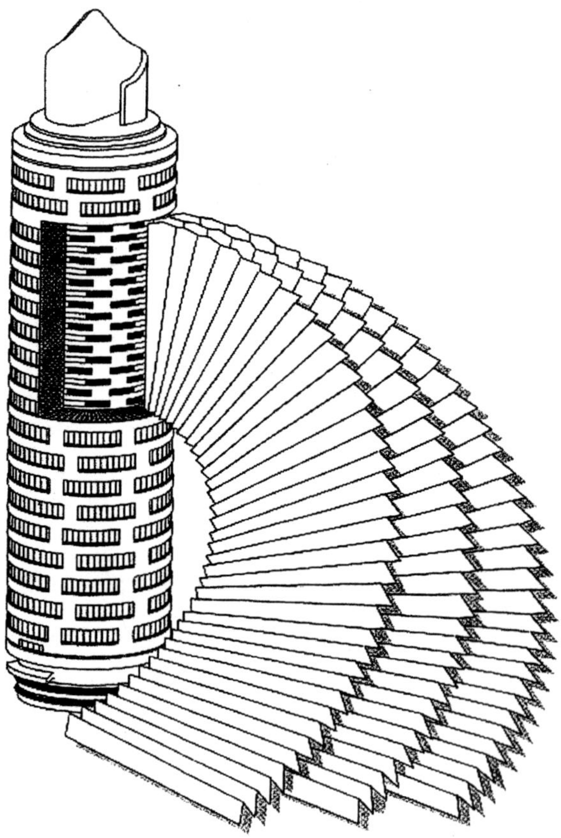

Figure 24 Filter cartridge construction with pleated fleeces and the filter membrane.

Sterilizing grade membrane filters are usually the last barrier between an unsterile atmosphere and the sterile product or equipment. The demands and requirements on these filters are therefore high and manifold (Keating et al., 1992; Meltzer, 1987). The main requirements are the following:

1. The filter must retain microorganisms, even under conditions of high moisture or high air humidity.
2. The filter must have a high thermal and mechanical resistance over a long term at rigorous conditions.
3. The filter must be repeatedly steam sterilizable even at elevated steam temperatures (134°C).
4. The filter must allow high airflow rates at low differential pressures.
5. The filter membrane must have a high hydrophobicity to avoid blockage by condensate.
6. The filter must have an optimal construction for highest performance and security over long periods of time.
7. The filter must be nonfiber-releasing.
8. The filter must be integrity testable.
9. The filter must be easy to install and maintain.
10. The filter must fulfill all regulatory issues and be supported by validation documentation.

Viewing this list of requirements it is not surprising that the development of air filter units progressed rapidly over the last few years. Filter manufacturers continuously optimized their range of filter elements to meet the growing demands of the pharmaceutical and biotech industries. The filter cartridge construction and materials must be considered carefully. Often the complexity of the parameters makes a filter cartridge comparable to a fine-tuned recipe. If one of the construction parameters is not optimal, if one of the ingredients is too plentiful, the system or products will not be satisfactory. Therefore, tests are made and results documented to find the optimal choice and balance of properties that influence the performance of the filter. The same is valid for liquid filter cartridges for complex pharmaceutical processes.

Table 1 lists some essential parameters that are considered in such tests. It shows that specific parameters can influence others in a positive or negative way. For example, the hydrophobicity, represented by the height of the water penetration

Table 1 Comparison of Parameters

	Membrane material					
Parameter	PTFE	PVDF	PTFE	PTFE	PTFE	PVDF
Filtration area[a] (m^2)	0.75	0.7	0.65	0.85	0.72	0.66
Flow rate at 100 mbar[a] (scbm/h)	146	78	140	169	110	108
WPP[b] (bar)	4.6	1.9	3.6	4.3	4.7	2.2
Number of pleats	142	130	120	184	158	129

[a]10 in. filters.
[b]WPP = water penetration point, measurement of hydrophobicity.

point, depends on the choice of membrane material. PTFE membranes usually have a higher hydrophobicity than PVDF membranes, and therefore the blowdown time, the time to recover the initial airflow rate after steaming, for example, is lower. In Sec. 3, the necessity of a high hydrophobicity is described. The blowdown time also depends on pleat density, of the number of pleats, in the filter cartridge. A larger effective filtration area does not necessarily mean a higher airflow rate, especially when the air is moist or after steam sterilization. The reason for this is that a higher effective filtration area in a cartridge format requires a higher pleat density. High pleat densities make waterlogging and condensate blockage more likely, owing to capillary action between the pleats.

Curves illustrating this phenomenon can be seen in Fig. 25. The two filter cartridges containing PTFE membranes have different blowdown times because the pleat density is higher in filter cartridge B than in cartridge A. The condensate trapped between the membranes in cartridge B blocks the filter for a longer period of time. This can have disastrous consequences in the venting of non-vacuum-resistant tanks.

A pleat density that is too tight affects the service life of a sterilizing grade membrane filter. If the pleat density is too tight, the effective filtration area cannot all be used. The separation of particles and contaminants occurs on the outside tip of the pleating and not over the entire filtration area. Experience has shown that plants with iron oxide contamination from their steam lines or piping have to change filter cartridges more frequently when the filter has a high pleat density. The iron oxide does not cover the entire filter membrane, only the outside of the filter.

The quality of the support fleece is also important. If the support or prefilter fleece has a high density, is very soft, or has very fine fibers, the condensate will be trapped in the fiber matrix. Again waterlogging and reduced flow rates will be the result. On the other hand, if the fleeces are too coarse, the fiber matrix can press against the membrane, especially at the pleat tip, and distort the membrane matrix.

To achieve high airflow rates with membrane filter cartridges, filter manufacturers optimized the inner core and adapter diameter. Too small a diameter can result in high velocities and therefore high pressure losses. Nowadays inner core and adap-

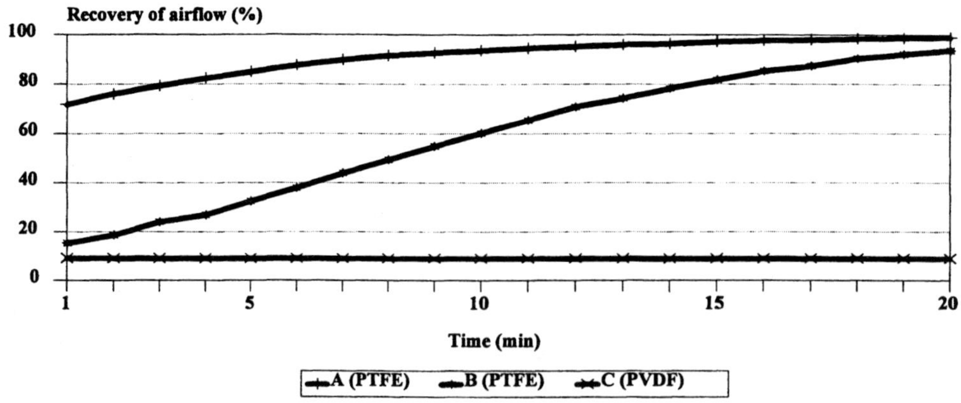

Figure 25 Measurement of the blowdown time of (A,B) PTFE and (C) PVDF filter cartridges. Measured at a differential pressure of 200 mbar after steam sterilization.

ter diameters are standardized at ≈35 mm. In Sec. 6 the influence of air velocity and the resulting pressure losses is discussed. Another relevant factor is the void volume of the pore structure of the different membrane materials. In practice, PTFE with a void volume of around 85% has found the highest acceptance due to the high flow rates achieved.

Most filter manufacturers supply validation guides with their air filter cartridges. These validation guides document HIMA bacterial challenge test correlations to nondestructive tests such as the diffusion, bubble point, pressure hold, and water intrusion tests. Results of the various required USP tests, e.g., Plastic Class VI, particulate matter, or conductivity tests, are also documented. In general, flow rates are quoted, which can be used to size systems, as well as all necessary technical data, including sizes, effective filtration areas, and maximum allowable differential pressures at different temperatures. These guides are important documents and help one to fulfill process parameters and support further on-site validation work. Users of sterilizing grade filter cartridges, especially quality control departments, should always request these documents if they are not automatically supplied.

Sizing of these filter systems is commonly divided into two specific areas of attention; compressed air filtration and tank venting. Compressed air filter systems are easily sized, bearing in mind some specific parameters such as airflow velocity and pressure drops. A high level of attention and professional expertise are required in the sizing of vent filter systems used for non-vacuum-resistant tanks that are steam-sterilized. A wrongly sized sterile filter could result in a collapsed tank. Specific calculations and formulas for sizing air filter systems are given in Chap. 12, but it is still recommended that a filter user contact the technical service department of the filter manufacturer.

Another important factor that influences the effectiveness of sterilizing grade filters is the O-ring material. Bypass situations are often experienced if the O-rings used to seal the filter element in the filter housing are chosen from polymeric materials that do not fit the stringent requirements of the applications. In O-ring material tests, different materials, like silicone, EPDM, and Viton, were tested in terms of recovery and heatset rate after steam sterilization. Such tests have shown that silicone O-rings seem to be the material of choice because of their excellent rate of recovery to their original shape. Other materials, like EPDM, have a high heatset ratio and do not regain their original O shape but remain oval. This oval shape is created by the influence of high temperatures at steam sterilization and the compression of the O-ring between the cartridge adapter and the housing recess. The tolerances of the cartridge adapter and housing recess are designed to compensate for a certain shrinkage of the material; therefore the possibility of bypass is avoided. Nevertheless, when the O-ring does not recover after steam sterilization and experiences a heatset, the deformation can be too high and the sealing starts to become slack. At this point bypass can occur, leading to contamination of the sterile side.

Besides the O-ring material itself, it is also highly important to choose O-rings with the right Shore hardness. If the O-ring material is too hard, the O-ring could be damaged when the cartridge is installed or it will not have the flexibility needed for it to press against the adapter walls. If the material is too soft, it may become distorted when the cartridge is installed. The O-ring would then not be placed properly, which could again lead to bypasses. It is therefore recommended to choose O-ring materials, such as silicone, with a Shore hardness of 60–70 and to inspect the

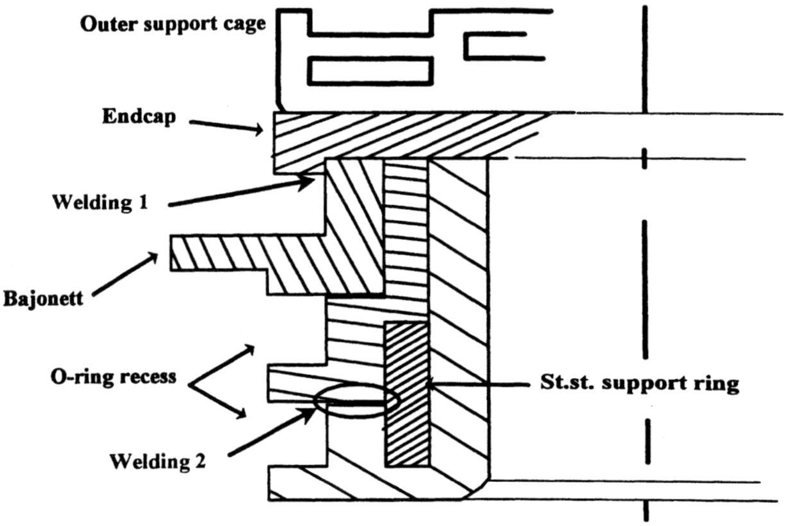

Figure 26 Schematic of the cross section of a two-piece cartridge adapter. If weld 2 breaks open, the adapter becomes distorted and the O-ring no longer has a secure fit.

cartridge O-rings on a regular basis if the system is repeatedly steam-sterilized. Some large-scale fermentation plants check the O-rings every 3 months, and some pharmaceutical companies replace the O-rings every month.

The construction of the cartridge adapter is an issue that caused problems in the past. Some users experienced major problems with a specific cartridge adapter. This double-bayonet, double O-ring lock-in type of adapter was not molded in one piece but was welded together at the critical point at the lower O-ring recess, as shown in Fig. 26. When this weld is stressed due to heat expansion of the stainless steel support ring, it breaks open. Condensate then penetrates into the space between the support ring and the plastic of the adapter. This happens even if the fracture is very fine. During the next steaming cycle, the expansion of the support ring, but especially the evaporating water, cause such mechanical stress that the adapter becomes distorted. Usually the lower edge of the adapter bends down and a wide gap is created at the weld designated welding 2 in Fig. 26. At this point the lower O-ring is no longer held in place and the risk of bypass increases dramatically. To avoid this risk, most filter manufacturers use one-piece molded adapters with support rings of, for example, polysulfone rather than stainless steel.

10 INTEGRITY TESTING

Due to the fact that most air filters are the last barrier between the atmospheric and sterile environments, they must perform at the highest assurance levels. To test their performance, various integrity test methods can be used. Most commonly the diffusive flow and bubble point measurements, as described in Chapter 11, are performed. To do so the hydrophobic air filters need to be wetted by liquids with low surface tension, usually solvent–water mixtures of isopropanol and water 60/40% or tertiary butanol and water 25/75%. The maximum allowable diffusive flow and/or minimum required bubble point for the individual filter types and wetting media are correlated directly to the HIMA bacterial challenge test, which is the most stringent test for a hydrophobic air filter. Such correlations can be found in the validation guides and user leaflets of the filter manufacturers. After the diffusive flow or bubble point test, the solvent must be removed from the filter matrix, for otherwise it will contaminate the downstream side and reduce the hydrophobicity of the filter. This can be done in several ways, including flushing with water or air, drying the filter element, or steaming. However the solvent is removed, the user has to ensure that there is no solvent residue within the filter matrix that could influence the performance of the filter element. The drying procedure needs to be well documented, and evidence has to be given that the solvent was effectively removed.

This lengthy procedure to integrity testing sterilizing grade filters often resulted in avoiding integrity tests and exchanging the filters on a regular basis, based on experience data, which can be rather unreliable. Other operating procedures called for an integrity test, typically done off-site before steam sterilization of the filter. Both procedures created insecurities, because the thermal and mechanical stress to the filter during the steam sterilization period was not considered. Experience has shown that air filter cartridges, that fail integrity tests usually do so after steam sterilization and not during production processes. Therefore the recommended procedure is to integrity test the filter element in place after it has been steam-sterilized.

The diffusive flow and bubble point tests can be performed in place, as well as aerosol challenge tests, like the sodium flame, uranin, or oil-based tests (Johnston et al., 1995). The disadvantages are that all tests cause a contamination of the filter, and the diffusive flow and bubble point tests also lead to contamination of the downstream side. All mentioned tests can be performed only when either additional piping and valves are installed on the downstream side or there are sensors for the detection of the aerosol, which means that manipulation of the downstream side is unavoidable.

In addition, the described tests are usually performed before the steam sterilizing cycle, which is not an optimal solution due to the factors discussed above. The steam sterilization needs to be done after the integrity tests because the steam is required to drive the contaminant out of the filter matrix.

Additionally, using an oil aerosol challenge test, one has to ensure that a sufficient concentration of the aerosol is spread over the entire effective filtration area; otherwise flaws may not be detected. Therefore it is essential to describe and document the test procedure, especially the test parameters such as flow rates, dosage of the aerosol, pressure conditions, and temperatures, to obtain a properly validated and reliable integrity test procedure. The benefits of using aerosol challenge tests as integrity tests is the speed with which they can be performed. Some manufacturers state that the test requires only 20 s to 5 min, depending on the system size, to obtain a result. Besides, according to the same filter manufacturer, the test is performed at an aerosol particle size that conforms with the most particle penetration size (MPPS) of their filters at around 0.2–0.3 μm, but this does not agree with findings of other sources (Grant, 1988). Johnston et al. (1995) used such an aerosol challenge test system and correlated its efficiency to three test organism aerosols, *Bacillus subtilis* var. *niger*, *Pseudomonas diminuta*, and MS-2 coliphage.

To avoid wetting of hydrophobic air filters and contamination by solvent residues, which could be left in the filter matrix after integrity testing, the trend is to use a water-based integrity test, which is usually called a water intrusion test but is also referred to as a water flow integrity test (Dosmar et al., 1992; Tarry et al., 1993; Meltzer et al., 1994; Jornitz et al., 1994; Tingley et al., 1995). Disputed by Jaenchen and Malsy (1993), it is now common practice and accepted by the industry and regulatory bodies. The water intrusion test uses the hydrophobicity of the air filter membrane material as its basis. The hydrophobicity of the usually used ePTFE is so high that the pressure needed to overcome the hydrophobic forces and force water through the membrane is ≈4–4.5 bar. This pressure and the point at which water penetrates a hydrophobic filter membrane is called the water penetration point and is comparable to the bubble point except that water is not forced from the largest pore but into and through the largest pore.

When the test pressure is reduced to a certain value, usually to ≈2.5 bar, water is intruding into but not penetrating the membrane, i.e., it does not come to a free water flow, when the membrane is integral. Therefore the test is performed by filling the upstream side of the air filter housing with water and applying a test pressure of 2.5 bar to the water column. This is commonly done by an automatic integrity test machine to achieve the highest sensitivity and reliability, as shown in Fig. 27. Such machines are described in Chapter 11. The integrity tester also measures the upstream air volume above the water column. When the water intrudes into the largest pores, the water level drops, and with this the air volume expands and the test pressure drops. The pressure drop is measured by the integrity tester and converted into an intrusion value in milliliters per minute. The measured intrusion is compared to a maximum allowable intrusion value that is correlated to the HIMA bacterial challenge test. After the test the water is drained from the housing and normal plant procedures are started. When the water intrusion test is performed on freeze-dryer vent filters, the vent filter must be dried before starting the freeze-drying process; otherwise the drying process will be contaminated with excessive humidity from the vent filter. After a comparison of drying procedures, Cappia et al. came to the conclusion that the use of a bypassing vacuum is the fastest and most thorough method.

The advantages of the water intrusion or water flow integrity test are described in several articles and the literature of filter manufacturers as

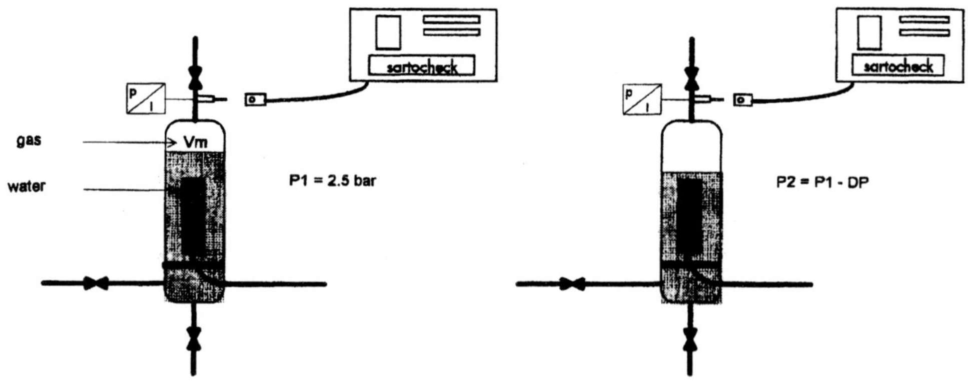

$$\text{WIT} = \frac{\text{DP} \times \text{Vm}}{\text{Po} \times \text{t}}$$

Figure 27 Water intrusion test setup and formula.

1. Due to the high test pressure, which is in the range of the water penetration pressure of 0.45 μm pore sized filters, the test is highly sensitive.
2. Contamination is avoided.
3. Not only the integrity of the filters is tested, but also its validated hydrophobicity, i.e., any contaminants on the membrane can be discovered.
4. The test can be performed in place after steam sterilization.
5. The test time is short because there is not need to flush off contaminants.

Some filter manufacturers now offer semiautomatic and fully automatic intrusion test systems that are especially useful for freeze-dry, autoclave, and blow–fill–seal systems.

11 AEROSOL BACTERIAL CHALLENGE AND PHAGENE TESTS

Integrity test data for sterilizing grade filters, such as maximum allowable diffusion, water intrusion, or minimum allowable bubble point, are correlated to the HIMA bacterial challenge test (HIMA, 1982) to test the efficiency and safety of these filters.

Filters previously wetted with a solvent–water mixture are challenged with a water–nutrient–microorganism solution (as quoted in the standard ATCC 19146), with a microorganism challenge of 10^7 organisms per square centimeter of filtration area. This test is widely accepted within the industry and even more appreciated than the aerosol or phagene challenge test because it is more stringent, as the separation mechanisms such as diffusion and inertial impaction are not at work. The only active separation mechanisms are those of sieve retention and adsorption by hydrophobic interactions.

Nevertheless some questions regarding the validity of a liquid challenge test in comparison to an aerosol challenge test became important when HIV virus issues appeared, especially in blood banks. Therefore filter manufacturers reacted by creating a number of aerosol challenge tests, all with the positive result of 100% retention of the challenge organism or particle. Unfortunately, these tests were performed using the "house standards" of these manufacturers because there was no common standard to describe the proper test setup, conditions, challenge organism, and level. Standards should be created to achieve consistent results with available sterilizing grade filters.

In simple terms, the air filter cartridge is challenged by a bacterial or phagene aerosol (spray), which should mimic the real world of microorganisms or viruses in an air supply, for example, the air supply to a fermentor. The challenge and the filter's success in retaining the challenge organisms depends on several parameters: temperature, humidity, air velocity, organism concentration, viability of the organisms, pretreatment of the filter, and the effectiveness of the sampling.

A typical aerosol challenge setup is illustrated in Fig. 28. Further descriptions of aerosol challenge tests are given by Johnston et al. (1995), Kastelein et al. (1991), Tuijenburg et al. (1987), and Meltzer (1987), who list several aerosol challenge test systems, which confirms that there is no standard in sight. The outcome of the different challenge test methods can vary immensely from filter to filter, and therefore there should be a move toward a standard challenge test that would be used by all filter vendors.

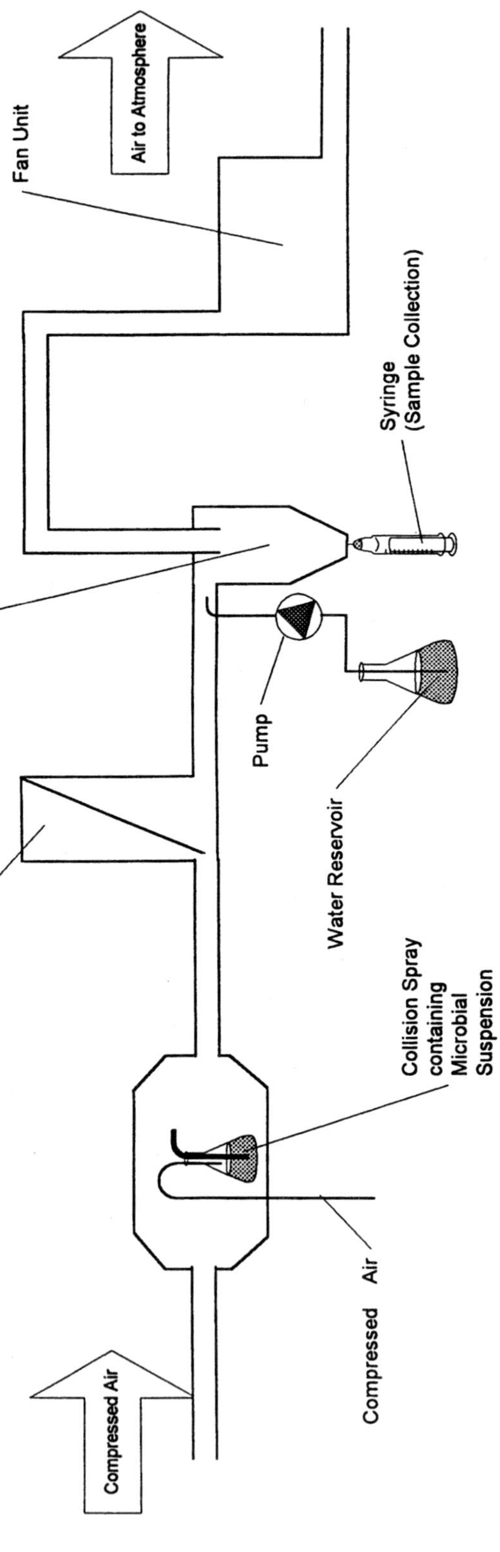

Figure 28 A typical aerosol challenge test setup.

Obviously, it is quite complicated to find the most stringent challenge test parameters to create a valid test. Challenge tests can vary widely from the actual process parameters used in the industry and lose their validity. This fact is underlined by findings in the industry, especially in dairy and large volume fermentation applications, where phage infections have been experienced even when supposedly phage-tight air filters were in use. Some of these clients used air filters of three different manufacturers, all claiming 100% phage/virus removal to their own standards.

To overcome these problems, an aerosol challenge test procedure needs to be established that is comparable to the HIMA document. The challenge test needs to be carried out at worst-case parameters but still be practical, i.e., according to plant procedures of the specific industries.

12 VALIDATION OF AIR FILTERS

Validation and qualification of the air filter or air filter system requires the highest attention not only when a new system is installed but also when filter types are changed. The main items that need to be checked when a new system is installed are usually performance criteria as described by 21 CFR 211.220 or Articles 8 and 10: 91/356/EEC. The filter system has to be able to cope with the required flow rates at specified differential pressures. Commonly the filter user specifies the maximum required flow rates to vent fermentors at the highest oxygen consumption of the organisms within the fermentation process; with tank venting systems, rapid condensation vacuums need to be overcome; with blow–fill–seal machines, minimum flow rates and pressures need to be achieved to mold the containers; and so on. The flow rates required depend on differential pressures and pressure losses within the air system. Therefore, clean differential pressures and maximum allowable differential pressures must both be specified when the filter needs to be changed and to control the air system. The required flow rates must also be achieved under conditions such as excess humidity or after steam sterilization. If the filter cartridges are challenged with an excess of moisture, the flow rate must be able to recover quickly if it is influenced to any degree whatsoever by the condensate. It is essential in the qualification stage to determine whether or not the filter system meets the stated requirements. Logically such qualification should be thoroughly documented for inspection purposes. The same is true when an existing filter is replaced by another type, as described in the EC GMP guide, Section 5.23.

As in all validation processes, these qualification steps are known as installation qualification (IQ), operation qualification (OQ), and performance qualification (PQ). In addition to these qualification steps, a new air system will undergo design qualification (DQ) and equipment qualification (EQ).

Focusing on PQ, the main items that need to be tested are

1. Steam sterilization cycles at process conditions
2. Blowdown time after steaming at process conditions or water-based integrity testing
3. Flow rates at specified differential pressures
4. O-ring seating after multiple steaming cycles
5. Integrity test performance and consistency
6. Thermal and mechanical compatibility at process conditions

Standard operating procedures (SOPs), which are part of the validation documentation need to specify maintenance cycles and procedures, are described, for example, in the cGMP for Medicinal Products, Annex 1, Section 30. Maintenance procedures should describe all the specific filter locations and the type of air filter installed at each location. Every validation should be carried out with at least two different types of sterilizing air filters to have an alternative if one is required. It would be foolish to rely on one specific type because of possible unavailability or other purchasing reasons. In addition to thorough written SOPs, staff training should be carried out on a regular basis, especially with respect to maintenance of the filters, i.e., integrity testing, systematic O-ring and cartridge inspection, and filter replacement. Training should also cover air filter installation, steaming at maximum allowable differential pressures, and blowdown pressures. This can be done either by in-house personnel or by outside sources like the filter manufacturers' support services. Sufficient training can prolong the service life of the filter and avoid detrimental situations in the production process. The main reasons for flaws and damage of filter systems have been identified as insufficient descriptions in an SOP and lack of training.

One main aspect of validation work and continuous process control is integrity testing. Several regulatory guidelines describe the need for integrity testing: "Guideline on Sterile Drug Products Produced by Aseptic Processing" (1987), the FDA "Guide to Inspections of High Purity Water Systems" and "Guide to Inspection of Lyophilization of Parenterals" (both July 1993), GMP Document No. 212.72, and ISO/TC 198. If integrity testing is not done, regulatory approval can be denied. These guidelines and recommendations are valid for a variety of applications, whether for water and product tank venting, lyophilizers, or autoclaves. Common sense will dictate the appropriate measures to be taken to evaluate the performance of the air filter by using an integrity test, on a routine basis if not after every batch cycle. Especially after steaming, an integrity test of the filter creates the highest assurance level.

As described in the FDA's guideline on sterile drug products produced by aseptic processing, "Compressed gas should be free from demonstrable oil vapor." The same guideline also states that critical vent filters, where the air comes into contact with the product, should be bacteria-retentive. These filters should be dry, either because they have been heat-dried or because the filter material is hydrophobic. These quotations certainly give the user hints on what air quality is required by the regulatory bodies and what kind of filter is expected in critical applications.

13 FERMENTOR INLET AIR

Air volume requirements vary during the different stages of fermentation, and therefore the filter systems used in large volume fermentation are of different sizes. For example, filter systems used for seed fermentors are usually single-round 10 or 20 in. filter cartridges, whereas filter systems for large-scale fermentation can be as large as 96-round 30 in., depending on the product and fermentor volume. These filter systems need to cope with up to 15×10^6 m^3 of air per year and have to sterilize the air intake reliably to avoid infections of the fermentor contents or cross contamination. Besides such filter systems are used on a long-term basis and could be used for over a year; that is, they require high mechanical and thermal stability. Chapter 25 describes the application of fermentor inlet air in detail.

In the past most large-scale fermentation facilities used glass fiber packed towers to sterilize the inlet air. The performance of such towers was not sufficient when specific criteria were not observed, and infections of the fermentor volume occurred once too often. The air supplied to such towers usually had a high temperature to avoid condensation within the packed tower. Condensate could block the tower and greatly reduce the airflow, and microbial growth was promoted. The space required by such towers was immense and the maintenance difficult. Packing the tower offered an additional danger to the staff due to the fibrous material and involved long downtime periods. Particle shedding from the fibrous material was unavoidable, and the filters could not be integrity tested sufficiently. The flow through the towers was restricted to the required low face velocity and the needed contact time.

Nowadays sterilizing grade membrane filters are usually used in the fermentation industry because they meet high security standards. These filters withstand sterilizing cycles of up to 200 cycles at temperatures up to 134°C. Filter manufacturers have optimized membrane filter cartridges to create high flow rates at very low differential pressures. Membrane materials were chosen to achieve high pore volumes, hydrophobicity, and sterile filtration capability. Construction of the filter cartridges was optimized to avoid waterlogging and high airflow velocities and the resulting pressure losses.

Fermentation can last up to 10 days; therefore, high security is required. It would be disastrous in terms of the product intake costs and running costs if a large-scale fermentor became infected after several days of fermentation.

14 OFFGAS FILTRATION

Offgas filtration is a major concern and requirement, especially in the biotech industry with recombinant products. In the past most fermentation sites did not use any exhaust filter system, because the head pressure in the fermentor eliminated the risk of contamination from the offgas side. Due to new restrictions and increased environmental awareness, more and more facilities employ exhaust filter systems. The main aim is not to protect the fermentor content, but rather to prevent microbial contamination of the environment. For this reason various separation methods were evaluated, for example cyclones in combination with depth filters or heat. Neither of these methods created the assurance level needed, and besides, one is very costly; therefore the use of a membrane filter system became common practice.

The filtration of exhaust gases creates some major problems due to the moisture content of the gas. The gas is usually warm and is saturated with moisture due to contact with the fermentation medium. When the exhaust gas cools, a large amount of condensate forms that could block the sterilizing grade filter and increase the pressure drop over the filter. An increase in pressure drop means an immediate rise in the head pressure of the fermentor, which must be avoided. Particles and microbial contamination carried over from the fermentor into the exhaust stream could also block the filter device. The retentive ability of such a filter needs to be high; otherwise organisms will penetrate the filter element. In some instances the microbial loading can be up to 10^{11} organisms in a 7-day fermentation (Orchard, 1991). Often, when the fermentor runs at the highest rate, the fermentor broth foams, which can blind the filter.

Heating by steam and electrical tracing of the filter housings or piping will avoid condensation because the system temperature is held above the dew point of the air (Jaenchen, 1988; Keay, 1991; Orchard, 1991). If condensation occurs, the filter needs to be able to achieve the required flow rates due its hydrophobicity. Condensate will be repelled and drained from the system. To ensure that the filter will not degrade in performance due to foam reaching the membrane, either antifoam agents or mechanical foam breakers like demisters and baffles or cyclones can be used. Antifoam agents can have the disadvantage of rapidly fouling downstream processing filter devices, and the antifoam agent must be sterile filtered. Mechanical foam breakers and cyclones (Hoffmann et al., 1995) avoid these disadvantages but usually work effectively only at specific airflow rates that vary from phase to phase of the fermentation process. Fine aerosol carried over from demisters or cyclones can be separated by tight depth filter cartridges containing polypropylene fleeces.

These filters are sufficiently protective of the costly sterilizing grade filter due to their high dirt load capacity and a certain hydrophobicity, which prevents blocking of the depth filter fleeces. The void volume of these filters is very high; therefore the pressure losses are minimal. Particles and microbial contamination are greatly reduced, and the lifetime of the sterilizing grade filter is prolonged.

15 TANK VENTING

Every pharmaceutical application uses tanks and containers for a wide variety of purposes—for example, storage tanks for intermediate or final products, water storage tanks, transport vessels, and mixing tanks. Some tank venting applications require only a depth filter because the product or medium stored in the tank does not support the growth of microorganisms. Nevertheless, most tank venting applications have in common that the air supplied to the tank must be sterile and free of contaminants, which is usually achieved by using a sterilizing grade, hydrophobic membrane filter.

When liquid is drawn from the tank or added to the tank, the air must be vented into or from the tank. Open to the atmosphere, the air needs to be filtered through a sterilizing grade vent filter to avoid contamination, which could spoil the product stored in the tank. Often the product fed into the tank is sterile-filtered and the tank is steam-sterilized; therefore, the vent filter needs to perform with the highest security to ensure sterility. The filter needs to be and remain hydrophobic to avoid any condensate blockage and microbial growth on or within the filter matrix, especially when the vent filter is used over a long period of time without steam sterilization. This is often the case on water storage tanks, which hold water of lower quality than water for injection, which is stored at $\approx$80°C. The water temperature of water for injection avoids or restricts microbial growth but has the side effect of a high rate of condensation due to the high humidity of the air overlaying the hot water. Condensation of water on the filter cartridge can be avoided by using a heat-jacketed filter housing, preferably an electric heater. When a heat-jacketed housing is used, the filter cartridge must be visually checked on a routine basis (some manufacturers check about every 3 months) to see whether parts of the filter have been damaged by oxidation.

Non-vacuum-resistant tanks that are stream-sterilized need to be equipped with an appropriately sized vent filter system to overcome the condensation vacuum created by the collapsing steam when the tank cools down (Cole, 1977; Meltzer, 1987). If the filter system is not correctly sized or the vent filter blocks due to low hydrophobicity, the created vacuum could cause an implosion of the tank. Therefore such vent filter systems are sized by experienced and trained professionals. The sizing of such systems is described in Chapter 12.

The volume of some tanks is too vast to use a static vent filter system, at that point compressed air is pushed via a sterilizing filter into the tank to break the vacuum in the tank. Implosion of the tank can also be avoided by using burst disks or pressure relief valves, which break or open when the vacuum in the tank reaches the design limit, allowing unfiltered air to rush into the tank and breaks the increasing vacuum.

Vent filters on tanks and vessels are often steam-sterilized from the reverse flow direction. In this instance the differential pressure over the filter device during steaming must be operated carefully. Most filter manufacturers allow a maximum differential of 0.2–0.5 bar at ≈134°C steam temperature. Steaming in the reverse direction is usually more stressful to the filter construction. It is therefore advisable to integrity test the filter system after steam sterilization.

16 AUTOCLAVE AND LYOPHILIZER VENT FILTERS

In the past the vent filters used for autoclaves and lyophilizers were depth filter cartridges, sometimes even coalescing filters. Due to stringent quality standards and demands of the regulatory agencies, these filters were replaced by sterilizing grade membrane filters. When the vacuum created in these machines is broken, the air vented into the chambers can come in direct contact with the product. Therefore, it is of great importance that these filters meet regulatory requirements.

The primary concern is the sterile filtration ability of the filters. Several sterilizing grade, 0.2 μm rated membrane filters available in the market meet requirements in this respect. These filters are usually correlated to challenge tests such as the HIMA bacterial challenge test (HIMA, 1982) or aerosol challenge tests performed by the individual filter manufacturers or independent institutes. Having the ability to create a sterile filtrate does not mean that the individual filter will be the right choice for a particular application. Another important consideration is the hydrophobicity of the filter membrane and the cartridge construction, as pointed out in Sec. 9. If the hydrophobicity of the membrane material is insufficient, the pore structure may become blocked by condensate after steam sterilization. At this point the vacuum in the chamber cannot be broken and the filter must be bypassed, which means that the chamber becomes unsterile and the complete process must be repeated.

It goes without saying that hydrophobicity is of major importance, yet in the field some filter users still have major problems with filters of low hydrophobicity. Some users were even advised to use hydrophilic sterilizing grade filters to overcome the use of wetting media like solvent–water mixtures and to use water to integrity test the hydrophilic filters. To create an airflow through this type of filter the bubble point must be exceeded even when heat-jacketed housings are in use. This causes not only poor security but also process failures. The construction of the filter cartridge needs to be optimized so that condensate can drain into the condensate chamber. The filter system used in these units is usually large to accommodate the amount of condensation and the low differential pressures, down to 10 mbar, especially close to the end of the venting process.

These filters must withstand a high number of steaming cycles. Some large volume hospital sterilizers are used as many as five times a day, in which case the filter is steam-sterilized up to five times a day. Certainly these filters are not changed that often. The number of steaming cycles can be as high as 250.

In the past filters were either discarded without testing after a certain period of time or tested off-line before steam sterilization. These days, filter manufacturers offer integrity test methods that can be used with the filter in place even after steam sterilization. These tests methods accommodate either the common solvent–water mixture to integrity test the filter via the diffusion or bubble point test or just water for the water intrusion test (both integrity test methods are discussed in detail in Sec. 10. Moreover, manufacturers of autoclaves and lyophilizers have started to incorporate fully automatic integrity tests methods in their equipment or advise their clients to install additional test equipment.

17 FILTRATION OF SERVICE GASES

Service gases are usually air and nitrogen used for pneumatically actuated valves and switches, tank head pressures, transfer gases, drying purposes, and filling machines. These gases must be sterile because they are commonly supplied into cleanroom or sterile areas and come in contact with the product or the container, e.g., vials, flasks, bottles, and tanks. Unfortunately, often these filters are overlooked because there are so many in a standard pharmaceutical facility and they are sometimes not easily accessible or not obvious. This usually means that these filters are not integrity tested on a routine basis or are not replaced for a long period of time. Due to the more stringent requirements of the regulatory bodies, user awareness of these filter units has increased and maintenance and quality assurance departments usually enforce checks on a regular basis.

With some exceptions, installed service gas filters are either not easily accessible or in piping that is not steam-sterilized. One major exception are blow–fill–seal filling machines. These filling machines mold, sterile-fill, and seal the required containers. The need for a large amount of sterile air for extrusion, cooling, and overlaying purposes is obvious. Often the filling machines are equipped with up to four air filtration units that perform different functions. It is important here that the air come into direct contact with the plastic container and be introduced into the filling area (Wilson, 1994). Therefore emphasis is placed on routine steam sterilization and integrity testing of the filters.

Integrity testing of such filters used to be done off-line, so the solvent–water mixture used to wet the hydrophobic filter and performing the diffusion or bubble point would test not contaminate the process. Tested off-line, the filter was then flushed and dried, installed, and steam-sterilized. This created an insecurity, because there was no assurance that the filter was integral after steam sterilization. Nowadays water-based tests like the water intrusion or water flow integrity test are used to integrity test the filters in place after steam sterilization. As with the autoclave and lyophilizer vent filters, the filter elements can be tested fully automatically on a routine basis, preferably after every sterilization cycle.

REFERENCES

Blakie, E. W. (1987). Theory and practice of compressed air filtration and sterilization in the production of antibiotics, in *Filtration in the Pharmaceutical Industry* (T. H. Meltzer, ed.), Marcel Dekker, New York, Vol. 19, pp. 941–979.

Chem. Tech., *16*(7):50–52.

Cole, J. C. (1977). Consideration in applications of bacteria retentive air vent filters, *Pharm. Tech.*, *1*:49–53.

Dosmar, M., P. Wolber, K. Bracht, H. Tröger, and P. Waibel. (1992). The water pressure integrity test, *J. Parenter. Sci. Technol.*, *46*(4):102–106.

Dosmar, M., P. Wolber, K. Bracht, H. Tröger, and P. Waibel. (1993). A new in-place integrity test for hydrophobic membrane filters, *Filtr. Separ.*, June, 1993, pp. 305–309.

Fay, T. (1995). Process air: Breathing life into process plants, *Chem. Eng.*, February, pp. 86–93.

Feldman, K. H., W. Mohrig, and A. G. Stapel. (1985). *Druckluftverteilung in der Praxis*, Resch Verlag KG, München.

Fuchs, N. A. (1964). *Mechanics of Aerosols*, by C. N. Davies, Macmillan, New York.

Grant, D. C. (1988). Generation and maintenance of process gases with extremely low particle levels, *TSI J. Particle Instrum.*, *3*(1):3–11.

HIMA. (1982). Document No. 3, Vol. 4, Health Industry Manufacturers Association, April.

Hoffmann, A. C., R. de Jonge, H. Arends, and C. Hanrats. (1995). Evidence of the "natural vortex length" and its effect on the separation efficiency of gas cyclones, *Filt. Separ.* September, pp. 799–804.

Inman, F. N. (1993). Microbial contamination control in antibiotic manufacture, *Filtr. Separ.*, Sept./Oct., pp. 543–549.

Jaenchen, R. (1988). Verfahrenstechnisch relevante Parameter in der Fermenter–Abluftfiltration, *CAV*.

Jaenchen, R., and J. Malsy. (1993). Analysis of water penetration through hydrophobic filters as a method for integrity testing, Pall Sci. Tech. Rep. SD1427, Pall Corp., Glen Cove, NY.

Johnston, S., S. R. Parks, A. M. Bennett, and J. E. Benbough. (1995). Integrity testing air sterilizing filters: A comparison of aerosol challenge with airborne microbiological challenge methods, *Pharm. Tech. Eur.*, April 1995, pp. 16–25.

Kastelein, J., M. T. Logtenberg, and P. G. M. Hesselink. (1991). Test methodology for membrane gas filters by TBAC testing, *BFE*, *8*(7/8):403–405.

Keating, P., R. Levy, M. Payne, S. Proulx, P. Rowe, and S. Pearl. (1992). Performance testing of membrane based filters used in the filtration of industrial fermentation air, *Pharm. Tech. Inter.*, March 1992, pp. 46–58.

Keay, D. (1991). Gas sterilization by filtration, *Proc. Ind. J.*, June, pp. 25–29.

Kronsbein, D. G. (1989). Filter für die Druckluftaufbereitung, *F & S Filtrieren Separ.*, *3*(1): 4–10.

Lathrache, R. (1991). Luftfiltration mit Faserschichten (Teil 1), *Reinraumtechnik, 1/91*:26–34.

Liu, B. Y. H., K. L. Rubow, and D. Y. H. Pui. (1985). Performance of HEPA and ULPA Filters, 31st Annual Meeting of the Institute of Environmental Science.

Meltzer, T. H. (1987). *Filtration in the Pharmaceutical Industry*, Marcel Dekker, New York.

Meltzer, T. H. (1996). *Pharmaceutical Water Systems*, Tall Oaks Publishing, Littleton, CO.

Meltzer, T. H., M. W. Jornitz, and P. J. Waibel. (1994). The hydrophobic air filter and the water intrusion test, *Pharm. Tech.*, *18*(9):76–87.

Mohrig, W. (1988). *Druckluft Praxis, Erzeugen–Aufarbeiten–Verteilen–Anwenden*, Resch Verlag KG, München.

Orchard, T. (1991). Containment of fermenter exhaust gases by filtration, *Chem. Eng.*, March, pp. 17–20.

Rowe, P., S. Tingley, and S. Walker. (1996). Hydrophobic membrane filters: An effective means of controlling biocontamination, *Pharm. Eng.*, January/February, pp. 44–52.

Sitter, F. M. (1994). Choose the proper compressed air drying equipment, *Chem. Eng. Prog.*, pp. 59–65.

Steere, W. C., L. A. Scheer, and M. Hubbert. (1996). Sensitivity Consideration in Hydrophobic Filter Integrity Testing, ASTM STP 1260, J. K. Shillenn, ed., Philadelphia.

Straus-Zunker, W. (1996). *Filtern und Trocknen*, Zander Aufbereitungstechnik GmbH, Essen.

Tarry, S. W., J. Henricksen, M. Prashad, and H. Troeger. (1993). Integrity testing of ePTFE membrane filter vents, *Ultrapure Water*, *10*(8):23–30.

Tingley, S., S. Emory, S. Walker, and Y. S. Saburo. (1994). Water flow integrity testing: A viable and validatable alternative to alcohol testing, PDA Asia Conf., Tokyo, 1994.

Tuijnenberg Muijs, G., P. A. van Hemert, E. H. Houwink, H. L. M. Lelieveld, W. F. M. Rijnierse, G. Wies, and J. J. W. Zeegers. (1987). Assessment of microbiological contamination of air and surfaces, 4th European Congress of Biotechnology, Amsterdam.

Waibel, P. J., M. W. Jornitz, and T. H. Meltzer. (1994). The filter integrity test correlations, *Ultrapure Water*, October 1994, pp. 59–64.

Wilson, D. A. (1994). The pharmaceutical blow fill seal process, R^3 Nordic Symposium, Oslo.

Ziemer, W. (1987). Qualitätskriterium für Schwebstoffilter in der Reinraumtechnik, *Reinraumtechnik*, *3*(1):29–33.

Zind, M. (1990). Warum PTFE-Membranen, *BioTec*, November, pp. 12–16.

22

Air Filtration Applications in the Pharmaceutical Industry

HOLLY HAUGHNEY
Pall Corporation, Port Washington, New York

1 INTRODUCTION

A number of applications exist for air (or gas) filtration in the pharmaceutical industry. The filtration required can be to the 0.2 μm (sterilizing) level or to a coarser filtration level for particulate removal. Some air applications for which sterile filtration is employed are fermentor inlet air, fermentor vent gas, vents on water-for-injection tanks, and vacuum break filters during lyophilization. Coarser filtration can be employed for particulate removal in which the coarse filter acts as a prefilter to the sterilizing grade filter. Other applications employ coalescers as prefilters for the removal of liquid droplets such as oil or water.

This chapter provides information on air filtration applications in the pharmaceutical industry. Section 2 describes the types of air filters used in the industry, Sec. 3 discusses qualification tests for membrane filters, Sec. 4 describes specific air (or gas) filtration applications, and Sec. 5 contains recommendations and considerations for the proper use of membrane filters in the various applications.

2 DESCRIPTION OF AIR FILTERS

Historically, packed towers were the first air filters used by the industry for air sterilization. This section provides a general description of packed towers as well as membrane filters for air filtration.

The removal efficiency of filtration media used in packed towers or membrane filters is dependent on one or more of the following mechanisms: (1) direct interception by the fibers, (2) inertial impaction, (3) Brownian motion or diffusional interception, and (4) electrostatic attraction between the fibers and particles (Bruckshaw, 1973); see also Chapter 10).

2.1 Packed Towers

Description of Packed Towers

Packed towers used to filter fermentation air consist of beds or pads of paper, cotton wool, glass wool, or mineral slag wool. The diameter of the fibrous material is between 0.5 and 15 μm, and the space between the fibers can by many times as large.

Figure 1 illustrates a design of a packed tower air filter (Stanbury and Whitaker, 1984). The filter consists of a steel structure filled with loose fibrous packing. The air inlet is on the bottom, and the outlet is on the top of the filter. The packing is supported by a grid or perforated plate. When it is placed in the tower it is necessary to ensure that the packing density is appropriate for the application. Proper packing will preclude movement of the fibers during use. A repositioning of fibers can lead to channeling of air, which causes the packed tower to be inefficient because only a portion of the bed will be acting as a filter. Fiber movement can also lead to the dislodging of trapped microorganisms.

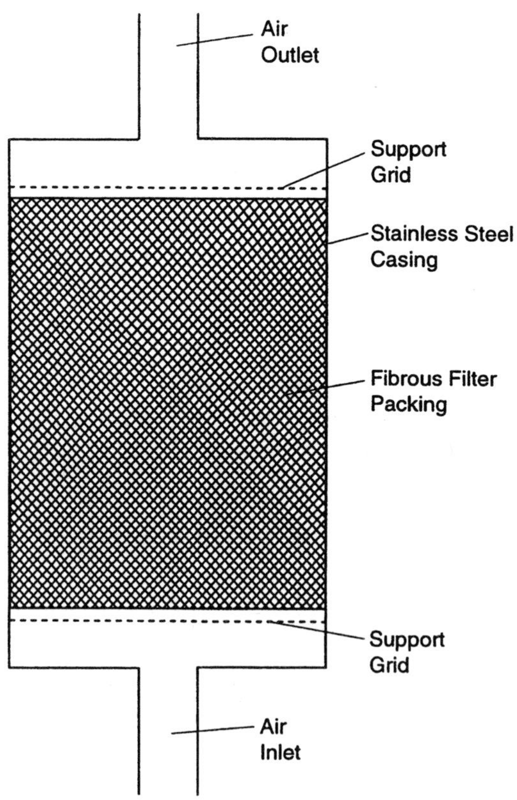

Figure 1 Packed tower design.

Once the filter has been correctly packed with fibrous material, a support grid or plate is fitted to the top of the bed to ensure that the bed remains compressed. After the first steam sterilization of a packed tower air filter, the packing will tend to settle further. It is recommended that additional fibers be added to the bed after the first steam sterilization to maintain the correct packing density.

Bonded fiber mats have been developed to use in place of loose fibers. Some are bonded with resins and must be tested to determine if they are compatible with steam sterilization. When mats are used, it is necessary to have a good seal between the mat and the tower wall so that channeling does not occur. Fiber pads often contain mineral wool with an average fiber diameter of 4–5 μm.

Thin sheets of small diameter fibers can also be used in packed towers. The sheets are placed on top of each other with a mesh or grid in between for support. The edges of the sheets are sealed between flanges.

Sterilization of Packed Tower Air Filters

Prior to using a packed tower for the sterilization of fermentor inlet air, the filter itself must be sterilized. There are two techniques that can be employed: steam sterilization and dry heat sterilization (Richards, 1968).

Passing steam at a pressure of 15 psig through a packed tower for 2 h should be adequate for sterilization. The presence of air in the packed tower during the sterilization can prevent complete sterilization of the packing. A drain at the bottom of the packed tower is needed to purge the steam and to drain any residual condensate from the filter. It is necessary to remove condensate from the bed because wetted fibers are less efficient for microorganism removal and may also decrease the retention efficiency of the packed tower well below its design value, particularly if channeling through the wetted media occurs.

Some fiber material, as well as material used to bond fibers, can be degraded by steam sterilization. An alternative to steam sterilization is dry heat sterilization, which will avoid the possibility of steam degradation and fiber wetting. This can be accomplished by using a heating device at the inlet of the tower and passing air at a temperature of 160–200°C through the bed for 2 h. During dry heat sterilization, the filter is isolated from the rest of the process. Fiber material can be stable up to 800°C; thus there is no chance of damage to the bed from this sterilization technique.

Operating Considerations for Air Sterilization by a Packed Tower

The microorganism retention efficiency of packed towers is dependent on the inlet velocity of the air. The relationship between air velocity and filtration efficiency has been determined experimentally in a number of studies (Fuchs, 1964). In the example shown in Fig. 2 (Fuchs, 1964), the particle retention efficiency may change by a factor of 10 as a result of a relatively small change in the inlet air velocity. The results also show that the most difficult particles to remove are in the size range of small microorganisms. Therefore it is quite possible to encounter airflow conditions in a packed tower that can reduce the statistical probability of complete retention of all microorganisms.

The hydrophilic nature of the fibrous material used in packed towers (e.g., glass wool) contributes to a reduction in their microorganism removal efficiency. Water

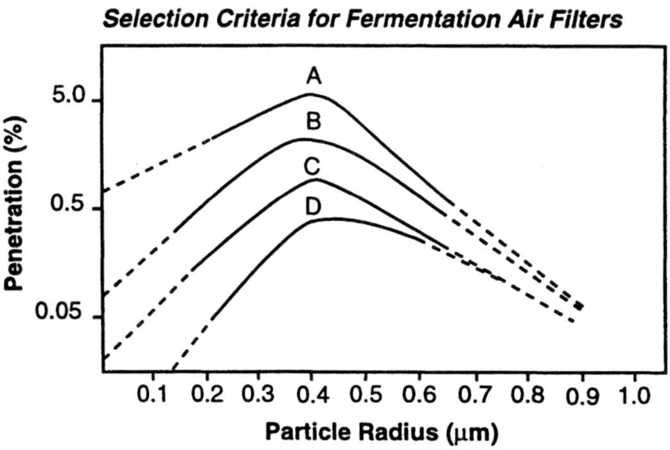

Mechanisms of aerosol filtration. Percent penetration of dioctyl phthalate particles through a resin impregnated glass fiber filter is plotted as a function of particle radius and incident air velocity (cm s^1). A.0.94: B.042: C.021: D.0.094

Figure 2 Particle retention efficiency (Fuchs, 1964).

vapor enters the system with the air discharge of the compressor. The air and water vapor mixture is initially at an elevated temperature. As the gas stream is cooled, water droplets may condense and wet the hydrophilic glass fibers. The wetted fibers are less efficient for microorganism removal and may decrease the retention efficiency of the packed tower well below its design value, particularly if channeling through the wetted media occurs. Also, organic components present in the compressor exhaust can provide a nutrient source for the retained microorganisms and increase the possibility of bacterial growth and eventual penetration through the depth filter medium. Although a number of approaches have been tried to overcome the wetting problem, such as heat tracing to maintain an elevated temperature, they are expensive to operate and have not consistently resolved the problem. The pressure differential across the tower may also increase significantly with wetting.

Although it is obvious that operating deviations such as these do reduce the reliability of a packed tower for air sterilization, there is no quantitative procedure to determine if the filtration efficiency is adequate to ensure the sterility of the air. The lack of such a quantitative procedure adds an element of uncertainty that affects both the operation and maintenance decisions. Skilled operators are necessary to monitor the packed tower to ensure that it is packed and operating efficiently. The actual source of contamination of a production batch is often difficult to identify, and the air filtration system is always suspect when there is a contamination outbreak. Without a technique for testing its efficiency, it is difficult to ascertain whether the packed tower is the cause of the contamination.

Design of Fibrous Air Filters

In order to model a fibrous air filter, several assumptions must be made. It is assumed that (1) once a particle is trapped by a fiber, it will remain trapped; (2) at a particular depth across the filter, the particle concentration does not vary; and (3) the removal efficiency at a given depth is equivalent across the filter.

The following equation describes how the concentration of particles varies with the depth position in the filter (Richards, 1968):

$$\frac{dN}{dt} = -Kx \tag{1}$$

where N = particle concentration, x = depth, and K = a constant.

Solving Eq. (1) between a depth of 0 and x and a particle concentration of N_0 particles entering the filter and a particle concentration of N particles leaving the filter yields

$$\ln\left(\frac{N}{N_0}\right) = -Kx \tag{2}$$

The relationship between depth and the logarithm of the ratio of particles removed to particles incident is known as the log–penetration relationship (Richards, 1968). This relationship has been used in sizing depth filters.

The constant K in Eq. (2) will vary with the type of packing and is dependent on linear velocity through the packed bed. If the relationship between the constant K and linear velocity through the bed is known, Eq. (2) can be used to size a packed bed for a given log reduction of particles.

Another consideration for the design of a packed bed is the pressure drop across the bed. Typically, the ΔP is linear with the linear air velocity for a given depth (Richards, 1968). The pressure drop across the packed tower can be dependent on the type of medium, the packing density, the air density, and the linear air velocity through the filter.

An example of an equation for the pressure drop across the packed bed is given in Richards (1968):

$$\Delta P = \frac{2\rho v^2 axC}{\pi D_f} \tag{3}$$

where

ΔP = pressure drop
n = linear air velocity
a = ratio of filter density over fiber density
x = filter bed depth
C = drag coefficient
D_f = fiber diameter
ρ = air density

The above relationship indicates that the pressure drop is proportional to the square of the linear air velocity. At relatively low linear air velocities (2–3 ft/s), the relationship is linear.

2.2 Membrane Filter Cartridges (Haughney, 1995; Martin et al., 1994)

Membrane filters can have absolute or nominal ratings. A nominal rating is an arbitrary micrometer value assigned by the manufacturer that is based on the removal of some percentage of all particles of a given size or larger. Nominal rating standards are arbitrary, and a comparison of nominally rated filters is very difficult. Nominal ratings can be misleading because the filter can pass particles larger than the rating indicates.

An absolute pore rating can be defined as the diameter of the largest spherical particle that will pass through a filter under specified conditions. It is an indication of the largest pore opening in the filter elements. The rating should be determined under carefully controlled conditions using industry-accepted reference standards. These include silica suspensions, latex beads, or microbial organisms.

Membrane filter cartridges are available in either prefilter (particulate contaminant rating) or sterilizing filter (bacterial contaminant rating) configurations. Prefilters in air service can be used for particulate removal or aerosol removal. Prefilters are positioned upstream of the final (sterilizing) filters to protect the final filter from premature plugging, thereby prolonging the life of the final filter.

Sterilizing Grade Membrane Filters for Air Service

Membrane filters used for fermentor and bioreactor sterile inlet air and exhaust gas vents, sterile pressure gas, sterile nitrogen blankets, storage tank sterile vents, formulation tank sterile vents, and sterile air for aseptic packaging usually contain a membrane made of hydrophobic materials such as PVDF (polyvinylidene fluoride) or PTFE (polytetrafluoroethylene).

Hydrophobic membrane filters are desired in sterile gas filtration applications because they do not spontaneously wet with water. When a hydrophilic filter is wetted with water, it will not pass air until the water-wet bubble point of the filter is exceeded; this water-wet bubble point can be greater than 50 psi. The inherent hydrophobicity of membrane filters used for fermentor air sterilization enables these filters to remove bacteria completely from inlet air even when exposed to moisture (Bruno and Szabo, 1983). The filter cartridge is expected to remove bacteria and bacteriophages from air streams with 100% efficiency.

Membrane filters are available in a variety of shapes and sizes. The most typical configuration for pharmaceutical air applications are 10 in. elements. A membrane filter is illustrated in Fig. 3.

Membrane filter elements may be integrity tested to ensure that the air that exits the membrane is sterile. The integrity tests have been correlated with bacteria removal efficiency by direct microbial challenge testing. This is further described in Chapter 11.

Sterilization of Membrane Filters

Hydrophobic membrane process filter cartridges can be subjected to multiple sterilization cycles and must be designed to be repeatedly steam sterilized in either direction of flow or repeatedly autoclaved. The vendor should provide information on filter cartridge sterilization procedures and operating data on process limitations (time and temperature). These filters should be capable of withstanding multiple in situ steam sterilizations. If needed, membrane filters can be autoclaved and aseptically installed into the process application.

Hydrophobic membrane filters are usually in situ steam-sterilized for a minimum of 30 min of exposure time (some processes may require longer) at a temperature of at least 121°C. Since the filters are hydrophobic, drying time is usually not

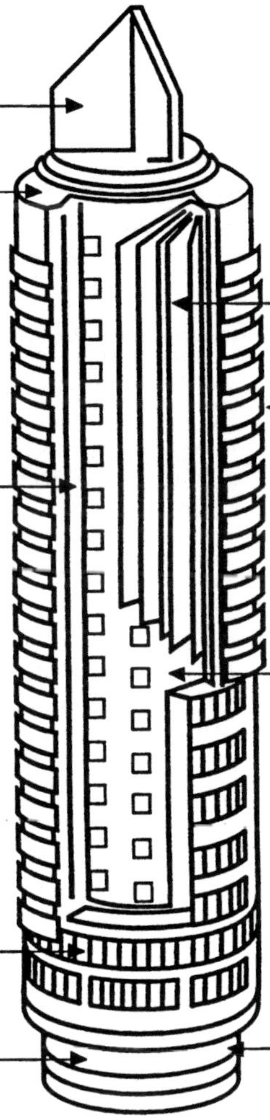

Figure 3 Membrane filter (Haughney, 1995).

required. It is necessary for membrane filters as well as for packed towers to drain the entrained condensate on the inlet side of the filter. A membrane filter housing can be isolated under pressure at the end of an aeration period and therefore does not require sterilization for each cycle.

2.3 Prefilters

For some applications it is necessary to use a prefilter to remove particulate material or liquid aerosols. It is often desirable to employ a prefilter to protect the sterilizing grade filter. Typically, the use of a prefilter will reduce the overall filtration economics.

Membrane filters composed of materials such as polypropylene or cellulose can be used effectively to remove particulate material from an air stream. The filter micrometer ratings range from ≈ 1 to ≈ 100 μm. The appropriate filter can be selected for the particulate contaminant removal.

Porous Stainless Steel Filters

A porous stainless steel medium is made by sintering small particles of stainless steel or other high alloy powder together to form a porous metal medium. Porous stainless steel can be formed as a flat sheet or, when used in filter elements, preferably as a seamless cylinder. This special manufacturing process produces a high dirt capacity medium that is temperature- and corrosion-resistant. The recommended alloy is type 316LB, which has a higher silicon content than type 316L and provides a stronger, more ductile product with better flow properties.

Standard porous stainless steel filters are $2^3/_8$ in. O.D., with a type 304 or 316 stainless steel flat blind end cap at one end and 1 or $1^1/_2$ in. NPT connection at the other or with industrial style flat gasket open end caps welded at each end. Elements have absolute ratings of 0.4–11 μm in gas service applications. Porous stainless steel filter cartridges are chemically or mechanically cleanable, offering economy of reuse.

Porous stainless steel filters find applications in the filtration of steam and for air sparging.

Resin-Free Cellulose Pleated Filter Cartridges

Resin-free pleated cellulose filter cartridges are applicable as prefilters for inlet air for fermentors and bioreactors. These filter cartridges are constructed of pure cellulose media without resin binders, which is pleated into a high area cylinder. The longitudinal side seal of the process filter cartridge is a polypropylene approved by the FDA for food contact use.

Cellulose media cartridges are assembled with hardware components consisting of a perforated inner support core, an outer support cage, and end caps melt-sealed to embed the medium in the plastic. All hardware components should be of pure polypropylene, without filler or reinforcement, to ensure a minimum of soluble extractables.

Polypropylene Pleated Filter Cartridges

Polypropylene pleated depth filters are applicable as prefilters for the prefiltration of exhaust gases. These process filter cartridges are also constructed using nonmigrating continuous strands of nonwoven polypropylene filaments. The medium should have a constant pore size section (downstream) for absolute rated filtration and a continuously graded upstream section for effective prefiltration.

The thin sheet of polypropylene is pleated and formed into a cylinder with a longitudinal side seal of melt seal polypropylene. The cylinder is then melt-sealed to injection-molded polypropylene end caps to ensure that fluid bypass is prevented. Polypropylene hardware components consisting of an inner support core and an external protective outer cage are incorporated.

Liquid Aerosol Removal

A coalescer can be used for the removal of liquid aerosols containing water or oil droplets. This is desirable as a prefiltration for a sterilizing air filter because the liquid aerosol could prevent the flow of air through the filter.

Coalescers operate efficiently if they are able to separate the liquid and the gas in the liquid aerosol. The three basic steps that are required are

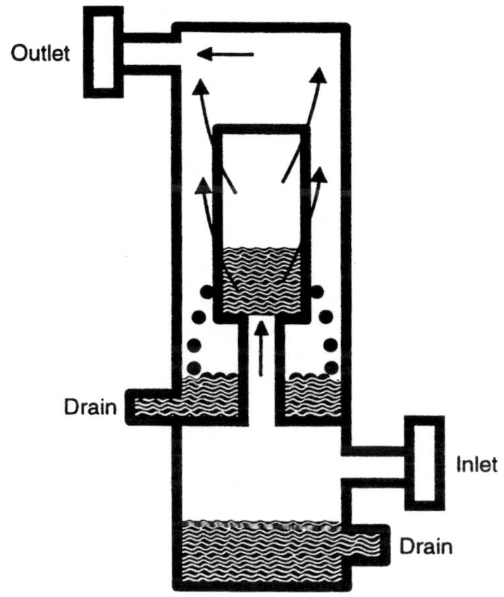

Figure 4 Liquid–gas coalescer.

1. Aerosol capture
2. Unloading or draining of the liquid
3. Separation of the liquid and gas

Figure 4 is an illustration of a liquid–gas coalescer. The coalescer in Fig. 4 has a gravity separator, which allows for the removal of large liquid aerosols (typically >300 μm). The coalescer flow direction is outward to prevent reentrainment. The liquid is captured through the coalescence of fine aerosols (0.1–300 μm) to large droplets (1–2 mm).

The coalescence of the droplets is illustrated in Fig. 5. The large droplets flow downward from a drainage layer. The separation is completed when the liquid is drained from the system. The air leaves the system from the top of the assembly.

3 QUALIFICATION TESTS FOR MEMBRANE FILTERS (Haughney, 1995)

3.1 Sterilizing Grade Membrane Filters

Organism Retention Tests (Pall, 1994)

Microorganism retention tests can be conducted to verify that membrane filters produce sterile air. Liquid challenge tests with *Brevundimonas* (*Pseudomonas*) *diminuta*

(ATCC 19146), measuring 0.3 × 0.6–0.8 μm, is a standard challenge test for the validation of sterilizing grade filters (0.2 μm) in the pharmaceutical industry. Aerosol challenge tests with *B. diminuta* should approximate extreme airflow conditions. Aerosol challenges with T_1 bacteriophage (0.05 × 0.1 μm) can provide a test of a filter's retention efficiency for extremely small organisms, so small that the bacteriophage in a liquid suspension will penetrate a 0.2 μm sterilizing grade filter.

The retention efficiency of a given filter is less when a liquid challenge is used than when an aerosol challenge is used. Thus, a liquid challenge test is a more stringent test of a filter's retention capability. A liquid challenge test can also provide retention information for process conditions such as extreme moisture after sterilization or air entrained with water drops.

The liquid test involves challenging a test filter with a known quantity of *B. diminuta*, no less than 1×10^7 organisms per square centimeter of filter area. The challenge sample is passed through the filter suspended in sterile water at a defined flow rate and for a defined time. All of the effluent from the test filter is passed through an analysis membrane. After the challenge is completed, the system is flushed for 5–10 min with sterile water. The analysis membranes are removed and placed on Mueller Hinton agar at 32°C for 48 h. After incubation, the plate is examined for the presence or absence of microbial colonies. Figure 6 illustrates a liquid bacterial challenge test stand.

The aerosol challenge test system can consist of a nebulizer loaded with the challenge microorganism suspension, a separate line for dry air makeup, and split stream impingers to sample the aerosol challenge with and without the test filter. A schematic of a test stand that can be used for the aerosol challenge procedure described is given in Fig. 7.

During the aerosol challenge, an aerosol is generated with a nebulizer. The aerosol is introduced into the test filter at a given flow rate. The filter effluent is collected in dual liquid impingers. Controls are performed simultaneously via a split

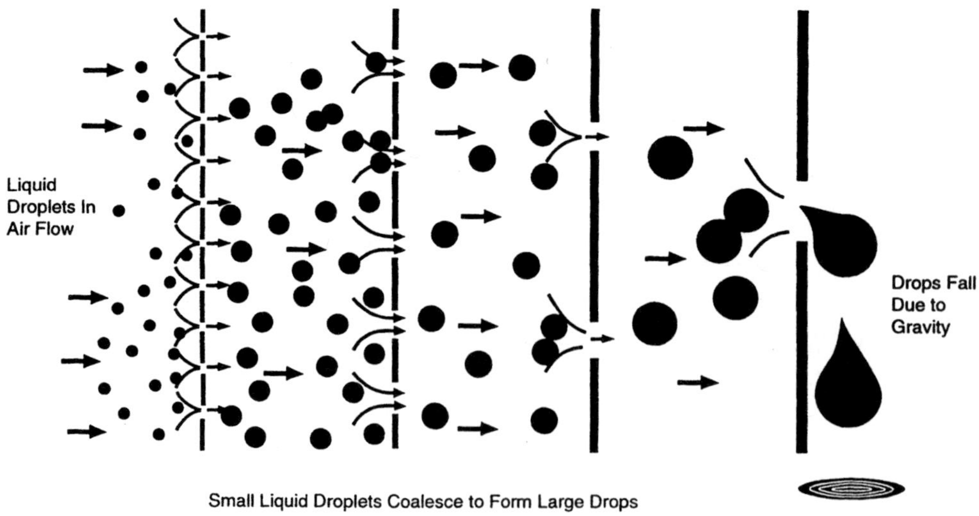

Figure 5 Coalescence of droplets.

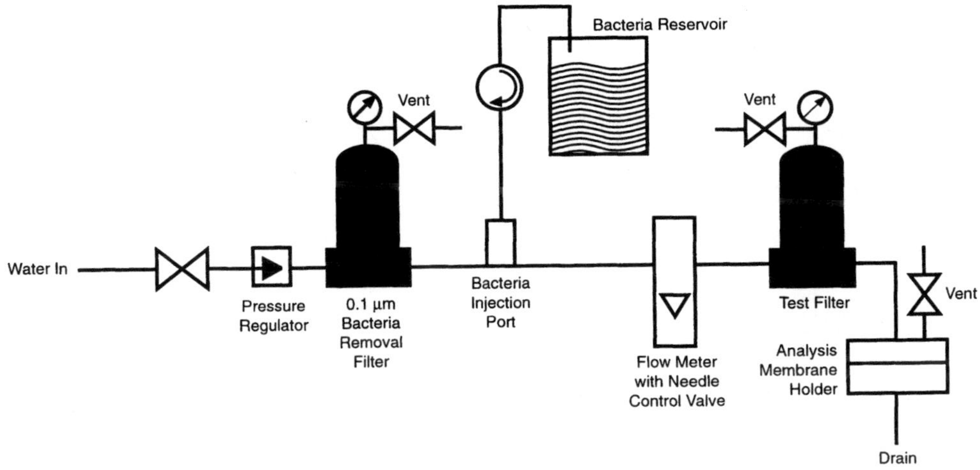

Figure 6 Liquid bacterial challenge test stand (Haughney, 1995).

stream by using a two-channel timer to direct airflow, on an alternating basis, from the test side filter impingers to the unfiltered control side impingers for recovery.

The impingers contain sterile buffer, and after the challenge is completed the buffer can be analyzed for the test organism. If *B. diminuta* is the test organism, then the buffer is analyzed by putting the buffer solutions through an analysis mem-

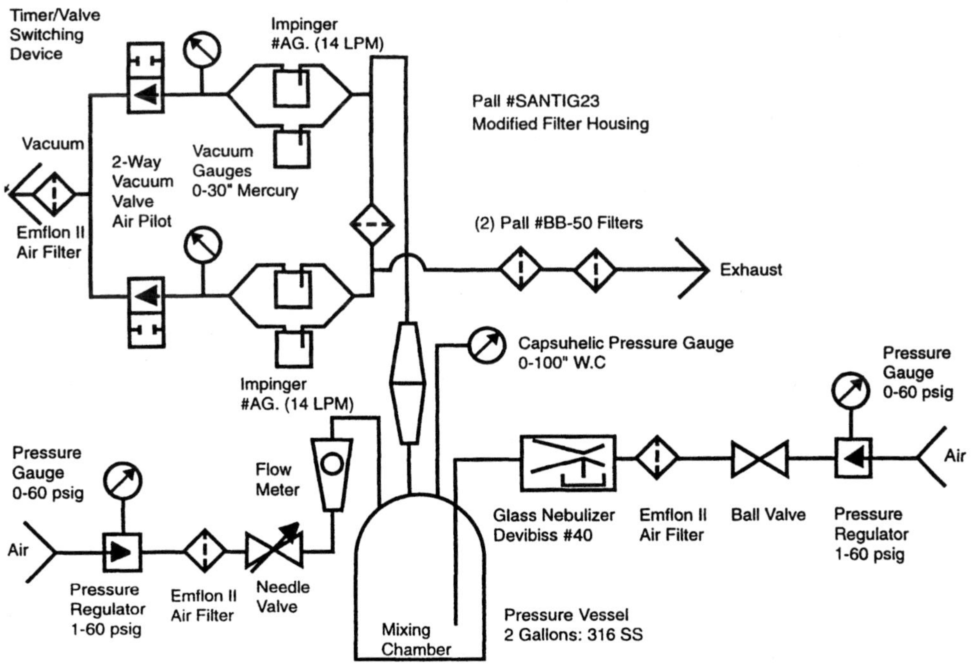

Figure 7 Aerosol challenge test stand. (Courtesy of Pall Corporation).

brane and placing the membrane on Mueller Hinton agar for 48 h before titering. If T_1 bacteriophage is the test organism, then samples of the buffer are diluted with nutrient broth and mixed with liquid nutrient agar (1.5% agar concentration; 48°C) and *E. coli* in the log phase of growth. After vortex mixing of all three components, the mix is poured over nutrient agar plates and incubated for 3–5 h at 35°C so that the plaques can be counted.

Dioctylphthalate Test

The dioctylphthalate (DOP) aerosol test has seen extensive use in measuring the efficiency of filters used to provide air to clean rooms and for similar applications. The commercially available equipment operates at 4 cfm and cannot detect fractional penetration by 0.3 μm droplets of 10^{-6} (0.0001%). In microbiological terminology, the method, at 4 cfm, is able to measure titer reduction (defined as the ratio of upstream to downstream colony-forming units) of 10^6. It cannot, for example, distinguish between two filters having respective titer reduction of 10^8 and 10^6.

A typical airflow for a fermentor air filter, such as a sterilizing grade membrane filter, is about 50–100 scfm per 10 in. module. To test a single module at 50 scfm, for example, the DOP method requires a 12.5-fold dilution with air, reducing the sensitivity to a titer reduction of 8×10^4. To test in situ at a 1000 cfm rate reduces sensitivity further to 4×10^3. A titer reduction of 10^4 corresponds to a removal efficiency of 99.99%. Higher efficiencies, such as 99.999% (or a titer reduction of 10^5) or 99.9999% (or a titer reduction of 10^6), cannot be distinguished by the DOP test.

The bacterial content of the compressed air incident on a filter could range from 10 to 10^4 per cubic foot, depending on the cleanliness of the system. Assuming a level of 10^2 organisms/ft^3, a single 10 in. module run at 50 scfm for 180 h would have approximately 5.4×10^7 bacteria incident on it. A filter able to meet the DOP test sensitivity of 8×10^4 (~99.998%) could theoretically pass 6.8×10^2 bacteria during the 180 h period (one very 15 min).

By contrast, bacterial challenge and its relationship to the forward flow or diffusion test provide reliable and convenient means to test the removal capability of a sterilizing grade filter. It is the method on which most filter manufacturer's validation data are based. As an example, a membrane filter aerosol challenge data for *B. diminuta* [challenge: $(1.2–3.6) \times 10^{10}$ total organisms at 50 scfm per 10 in. filter cartridge] and for T_1 bacteriophage (challenge: 1.7×10^8 to 1.6×10^{10} total T_1 phage at 50 scfm per 10 in. filter cartridge) demonstrate the absolute retention ability of the filters for these challenge organisms. The filters have also been shown to retain *B. diminuta* during a liquid challenge at 10^8 organisms per square centimeter of filter area or a titer reduction of $>10^{12}$ for a 10 in. filter cartridge.

For a filter cartridge to pass an aerosol challenge, all incident organisms must be retained. The test reliability is such that a single organism downstream can be detected. Thus, using the aerosol challenge tests, a titer reduction of $>10^{10}$ for *B. diminuta* (size: 0.3 μm × 0.8 μm) and a titer reduction of $>10^8$ for T_1 bacteriophage (size: 0.05 μm × 0.1 μm) can be demonstrated. A DOP test, under the same conditions, would only be able to demonstrate a titer reduction of 8×10^4 (efficiency of 99.998%) because of its limited sensitivity.

Furthermore, frequent DOP testing of a membrane filter cartridge may reduce the service life of the filter. An accumulation of the DOP oil droplets generated during the test can be deposited on the filter, accumulate as an oil film, and block the pores of the media.

Integrity Tests for Membrane Filter Cartridges

During the sterilization of fermentor air, it is necessary to achieve the highest possible assurance of filter integrity and removal efficiency. The installation of integrity-testable filters and the performance of routine integrity testing by the user are essential to demonstrate that the system is performing to specification. Tests that qualify the retention characteristics of a membrane filter can be defined as destructive or nondestructive tests.

Destructive tests are performed using an appropriate contaminant to meet a specific claim for retention of the contaminant. The test procedure must be sensitive enough to detect the passage of contaminants of interest. For sterilizing grade 0.2 μm membrane filters, the industry standard test organism (i.e., contaminant) is *Brevundimonas (Pseudomonas) diminuta* (ATCC 19146). The organism and minimum challenge level (10^7 cfu/cm^2 filter area) are specified in the ASTM standard F383-83 and referenced in the FDA guideline on sterile drug process produced by aseptic processing (ASTM, 1983; FDA, 1987).

Since most filter users would not want to perform a destructive test in a process environment, nondestructive tests related to the retention results of the destructive test are used instead. From the relationship developed between a nondestructive and a destructive test, membrane filter performance can be safely and conveniently verified in the production environment. The relationship between a nondestructive integrity test and the assurance of bacterial retention constitutes a filter validation study and is extremely important for microbe-retentive filters used in critical fluid processes. A full discussion of nondestructive tests for air membrane filters is included in Chapter 21.

3.2 Tests for Prefilters

Particulate Tests

Many filter manufacturers use a nominal micrometer rating for removal efficiency. This is defined by the American National Standards Institute (ANSI) as an "arbitrary micrometer value indicated by the filter manufacturer. Due to lack of reproducibility this rating is deprecated." An alternative method for rating filters is the Oklahoma State University (OSU) F-2 test. This rating method (ISO 4572, ANSI B93.31) has received wide acceptance for use on lubricating and hydraulic fluids.

The OSU test is based on continuous on-line particle counts of different particle sizes in both the influent and the effluent. The beta ratio at a specific particle size is defined as β_X: the number of particles of a given size (X) and larger in the influent, divided by the number of particles of the same size (X) and larger in the effluent, where X is the particle size in micrometers. The percent removal efficiency can be calculated from the beta value. The percent removal efficiency is $[(\beta_X - 1)/\beta_X] \times 100$ (Uberoi, 1992).

As an example, some prefilters are given a micrometer rating that corresponds to a 100% removal efficiency or the value in micrometers at which the OSU F-2 Test gives a beta value of >5000.

Aerosol Removal Tests

The use of the DOP test for evaluation of coalescer elements is not recommended. A coalescer effects a separation of liquid and gas by first capturing the aerosol, then unloading or draining the liquid, and finally separating the liquid and gas. For example, in coalescers, the separation occurs by gravity. The DOP test relates to capture characteristics only. Coalescer performance can be degraded by reentrainment of the discontinuous (or liquid) phase due to poor drainage, a situation that the DOP test does not address.

Another limitation of the DOP test is that the test is performed using only one liquid aerosol size, 0.3 μm. The DOP test assumes that at ambient conditions the most penetrating particle size, i.e., the particle size at which the efficiency of the filter medium for particle removal is at its minimum, is 0.3 μm. This is typically true for HEPA filters, for which the DOP test was designed. The most penetrating particle size is often smaller; it may range from 0.08 to 0.3 μm.

It is important to note that the most penetrating particle size is not necessarily the smallest particle. Smaller particles tend to be captured by diffusional interception or Brownian motion, whereas larger particles tend to be captured by inertial impaction or direct interception. Between these capture mechanisms for large and small particles there is a particle size range for which no mechanism dominates. In this range exists the most penetrating particle size.

The most penetrating particle size is dependent on the operating conditions, including filter surface area, gas flow rate, differential pressure, and humidity. Thus, a 0.3 μm liquid aerosol challenge, such as the DOP test, does not stimulate actual field conditions where the filter will be exposed to a wide range of aerosol sizes and where the operating conditions are not ambient. If the conditions are not ambient, the most penetrating particle size may not be 0.3 μm. It is preferable to use a coalescer performance test that employs an aerosol representative of actual systems and considers the three factors (aerosol capture, medium drainage, and downstream separation) of importance for proper operation. [An example of such a procedure is found in Williamson et al. (1988).]

4 AIR FILTRATION APPLICATIONS (Haughney 1995; Martin et al., 1994)

During the processing of a pharmaceutical product, the two basic processing categories are (1) fermentation and (2) downstream processing, including final purification. For each of these steps, sterilizing grade 0.2 μm hydrophobic membrane filters can be required for processing air (or gas) streams. For example, sterilizing grade 0.2 μm hydrophobic membrane filters are used during

1. Fermentation—for the sterilization of fermentation inlet air as well as for the filtration of fermentation exhaust gas
2. Downstream processing—as sterile tank vents
3. Final purification—for vacuum breaking in processes such as lyophilization

As discussed earlier, hydrophobic membrane filters are desired in sterile gas filtration applications because hydrophobic filters do not spontaneously wet with water.

Sterile air filtration applications discussed in this section include fermentor inlet air filtration, exhaust gas (vent) filtration, high temperature air filtration, and lyophilizer vacuum break filtration. Special attention is given to the specific requirements for a sterilizing filter used for these applications.

4.1 Fermentation Air Filtration Applications

During a fermentation process, a specific type of cell (yeast, bacterial, or mammalian) is grown to provide a desired product. Products can include cells, antibiotics, amino acids, or recombinant proteins. There can be a variety of sizes for the fermentor, ranging from very small (100 L or less) for cell culture to very large scale for antibiotic production (100,000 L). In these applications there is often the need to maintain sterility in both liquid and gas (air or nitrogen) feeds to support the growth of the desired cells.

Air filtration applications for fermentation are shown in Table 1 and illustrated in Fig. 8.

Prefiltration of Fermentation Air

Compressors are used to generate airflow for the manufacturing facility. There are two types of compressors: oil-free and oil-lubricated. In older facilities where oil-lubricated air compressors are commonly used, prefiltration of inlet air is necessary

Table 1 Filter Recommendations for Fermentation Air Applications

Application	Filter type	Micrometer rating	Typical gas flow rate per 10 in. module (scfm)
Prefiltration of air to sterilizing filter for particulate removal	Cellulosic or polypropylene pleated	8.0	75
Prefiltration of air to sterilizing filter for oil droplet removal (coalescer)	Coalescer	0.3	200–400
Sterile filtration of air for fermentor	Hydrophobic membrane	0.2	75–100
Sparging	Porous stainless steel	3.0	
Prefiltration of exhaust gas from fermentor	Polypropylene pleated	1.2	40
Sterile filtration of exhaust gas from fermentor	Hydrophobic membrane	0.2	40
Tank venting	Hydrophobic membrane	0.2	75–100
Steam for cleaning and sterilizing	Porous stainless steel	30 psig saturated steam (130 lb/h)	

Source: Martin et al., 1994.

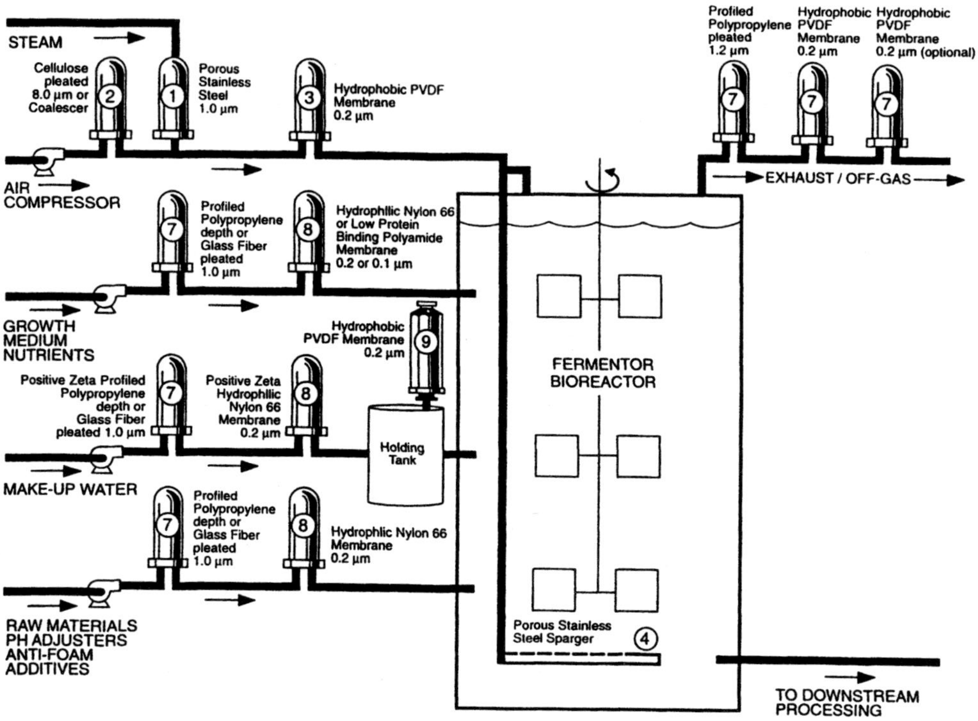

Figure 8 Fermentation air applications. (Courtesy of Pall Corporation.)

to remove oil droplets. A coalescing filter can remove >99.9% of oil and water droplets in the 0.01–0.5 μm range and larger. It also acts as an excellent prefilter for the hydrophobic membrane pleated filters that are commonly used for sterilizing the inlet air to the fermentor.

For oil-free compressors, a prefilter acts to remove dirt from the air system, extending the service life of the final filter. For use with fermentation air, a cellulose pleated filter with an absolute rating of 8.0 μm is normally the filter of choice. Alternatively, polypropylene (2.5 μm rated) pleated filters also serve as excellent prefilters for this application.

Sterile Air Filtration for Pilot and Production Fermentors and Feed Tanks

One of the largest applications for sterile air filtration is the sterile air used for an aerobic fermentor during a typical production cycle. Typically, one volume of air is used per volume of broth per minute. Thus, for a 10,000 L fermentor on line for 48 h, a total of 1.01×10^6 ft^3 of air must be sterilized.

The contaminants present in compressed air can include dust, lubricating oil, hydrocarbons, water, rust, and microorganisms including molds, bacteria, and viruses. Microorganisms in air are often associated with carrier particles such as dust. Water and oil can be present as bulk liquid, a vapor, or an aerosol. The air distribution system can give rise to contaminants such as rust and water. The concentration and size distribution of particles in compressed air are variable. The size range is generally 0.001–30 μm, with a concentration of 10^{-2}–10^{-4} g/m^3 (Richards, 1968; Bruckshaw, 1973).

Bacteria and bacteriophages, when present in air feeds, can enter fermentation tanks or bioreactors and contaminate the product. Bacteriophages or other viruses can destroy the producing cells and reduce yields.

The process requirements to supply sterile air are quite restrictive. The air sterilization process must (1) process a large volume of compressed air, (2) provide a high degree of reliability, and (3) operate economically. Several methods have been considered for the sterilization of fermentor inlet air. These include filtration, heat, irradiation, washing with sterilizing chemicals, and electrostatic precipitation. Washing and electrostatic precipitation are not effective for the removal of microorganisms. Heat and irradiation are not economical. Filtration is the only technique that meets all the requirements for sterilizing fermentor inlet air.

An early filtration approach, packed towers were once employed widely in the industry. Since the early 1980s, filtration technology has advanced (Conway, 1984a) and there has been an ongoing trend to replace depth filters with hydrophobic membrane cartridge filters [e.g., Hoffmann-La Roche (Perkowski, 1983) and E. R. Squibb and Sons (Bruno and Szabo, 1983)].

The recommended filters for sterilization of air feeds to fermentors and bioreactors are the hydrophobic membrane pleated filters. The hydrophobic (water-repelling) nature of these membranes can provide for the removal of bacteria and bacteriophages with 100% efficiency under moist or dry operating conditions. This is an important advantage over fiberglass towers and cartridges. Filters for sterile air feeds should have a 0.2 μm absolute bacterial rating in liquids and a 0.01 μm particulate rating in air service.

Some fermentations may require the filtration of fermentor air at an elevated temperature. If an application uses hot air and a longer service life is desired, then a filter that can withstand the elevated temperature is required. High temperature filters can be used in continuous service at temperatures up to 120°C. These filters have a 0.2 μm microbial rating in liquid service and a particulate removal rating of 0.01 μm in gas service. The filter membrane is made of inherently hydrophobic PTFE, and the cage, core, and end caps are specifically designed for high temperature applications.

Sparging

Sparging acts to disperse air evenly in the fermentor or bioreactor that contains the growth media and product. The product of choice for this application is porous stainless steel sparging elements, which can provide an exceptionally uniform and fine aeration gas dispersion. These elements are fabricated with one face of porous metal and one face of solid metal. If both surfaces of the sparging elements were porous, bubbles from the under surface could coalesce with bubbles from the top surface.

Porous stainless steel sparging elements should be positioned horizontally in the fermentation tank, with the porous stainless steel facing upward. Fine grades of porous stainless steel (e.g., 3.0 μm absolute liquid rated) are ideal even for shear-sensitive mammalian cell cultures because of their high gas transfer and low shear aeration capability. Elements are typically available in standard and custom designs.

Exhaust Air/Offgas Filtration

The purpose of a vent filter on a sterile fermentation tank is twofold: to prevent contamination of the tank and to contain the material inside the tank. Prevention of contamination in the tank is desirable for processes that involve long fermentation cycles or require a sensitive fermentation medium (e.g., tissue culture medium). Genetic engineering techniques and the fermentation of pathogenic organisms (such as organisms used for the manufacture of vaccines) have made it necessary to protect the environment and prevent the escape of microorganisms from the fermentation tank. The exhaust filtration system for a recombinant or mammalian cell fermentor/bioreactor must yield sterile air to the environment and provide a sterile barrier to prevent the ingress of contaminants. Additionally it must be steam sterilizable in situ and typically has a clean differential pressure less than 1 psid.

The removal efficiencies for simple depth filters (as described above) are typically poor under wet or variable flow conditions. Therefore, membrane filters are recommended for vent filtration applications.

The fermentor or bioreactor exhaust gas line can be contaminated with microorganisms or cells, growth medium components expelled from the fermentor/bioreactor as droplets or as solid particles, and aerosol condensate droplets formed during cooling of the gas in the exhaust system. These aerosol droplets, when present, can potentially block the final filter and must be removed prior to reaching the final filter. Mechanical separation devices such as cyclones, condensers, and demisters may not achieve effective aerosol removal below 5 μm (Porter, 1973). Removal efficiencies and pressure drops also vary significantly with the flow rate in such equipment. Studies have shown that aerosols in exhaust lines are predominantly in the very fine (1–5 μm) range (Jaenchen and Dellweg, 1989).

Which contaminants are present will depend on the fermentation conditions, the growth medium, and the design of the exhaust has system. The basic requirements for a vent filter are the ability to provide sterility, a low pressure drop, and the capability of being in situ steam-sterilized.

The recommended exhaust filtration system design entails two stages, using a polypropylene pleated depth filter cartridge as a prefilter and a 0.2 μm absolute rated hydrophobic membrane pleated filter cartridge. The purpose of the prefilter (typically 1.2 μm absolute rated) is to remove aerosolized particles and liquid droplets containing cells and/or growth media from the fermentation offgas or exhaust air. This serves to extend the service life of the final sterilizing filter. If the medium contains only fully dissolved components, such as with a sterile filtered cell culture medium, and if the fermentation is run at low temperatures (<30°C) and low aeration rate (1–1.5 VVM), the prefilter may be optional.

Like the final sterilizing filter, the pleated polypropylene prefilter should be able to be repeatedly steam-sterilized. An additional benefit of the prefilter is to retard "foam-outs" from reaching the final sterilizing filter.

Sterilizing grade 0.2 μm absolute rated hydrophobic membrane pleated final filters with PVDF or PTFE membranes can prevent organisms from entering or leaving the controlled reaction zone, even in the presence of water droplets and saturated gas (Conway, 1984b, Bruno and Szabo, 1983). Steam sterilizability and integrity test values correlated to microbial retention studies under "worst-case" liquid challenge conditions provide the highest degree of assurance of performance. Redundant systems using a second 0.2 μm rated sterilizing filter in series are recommended for high risk recombinant organisms.

Condensate control is usually the most critical consideration for this application. In cases in which condensate accumulates and when the fermentor is operated with overpressure in the fermentor head, the amount of condensate accumulation can be reduced if a pressure control valve is placed at the fermentor exit upstream of the exhaust gas filter. An alternative technique for the prevention of condensate accumulation is to use a heating section in the exhaust gas pipe upstream of the filter installation. This can be also be accomplished by specifying steam jacketing on exhaust filter housings. In this case the exhaust gas temperature at the terminal filter must lie above the temperature of the exhaust gas at the fermentor exit. The heater must be properly sized according to the process parameters.

4.2 Test Case for Fermentation Air: Economic Analysis for Packed Towers versus Membrane Filters

The analysis that follows is based on representative experience and costs at several field installations and therefore presents a composite picture. The model presented may be used to evaluate the expected performance at a specific installation by appropriately weighing each component. For this test case, the hydrophobic membrane filter used in the analysis is a Pall PVDF Emflon® II (Emflon II is a registered trademark of Pall Corporation) sterilizing grade membrane filter (Pall, 1989).

Contamination Control

The increase in productivity that can be achieved by reducing the contamination loss rate is a major component that must be quantified. First, the cost of the contaminated batches must be considered. The basis of the calculation will depend not only on the actual production requirements but also on several other related factors specific to the application. In a low capacity utilization case, the cost may be limited to overhead, labor, and materials. This is the "fermentation direct cost" figure that would typically be computed and reported by a production department.

For the more typical case, additional charges must be made for the loss of downstream production. However, in the case of full production or a new product introduction, the true cost of a fermentor loss is more accurately reflected by the full market value of the product. This is particularly true in the pharmaceutical and biotechnology fields, where the actual production costs may represent only a small fraction of the market value. In this situation, the corporate analyst would include a large "product value multiplier" (batch market value ÷ batch manufacturing cost) in the plant operating cost in order to accurately assess the change in productivity.

The contamination history of a particular facility must also be included. The loss rate due to contamination can be divided into two categories: the total loss rate experienced by the production plant and the fraction of that loss associated with the sterile air system.

The overall contamination rate is generally recorded by plant personnel and may be typically 3–10% for an antibiotic fermentation. The fraction associated with the air system is not usually determined because, as mentioned above, the source of contamination is often not identified in a production facility. However, independent evaluations have been conducted and published. In one study (Bruno and Szabo, 1983), existing packed towers were replaced with cartridge filters and the contamination rate was compared to that of a control group of production fermentors (1200 scfm at 22 psig). After a 6 month evaluation, the contamination rate was 50% lower in the fermentors equipped with cartridge filters. Similar evaluations were conducted in germinators; the contamination rate was reduced by 78% for the germinators that had been retrofitted with cartridges. Similar results have been reported informally by other groups. The contamination loss rate may be estimated based on a contamination rate reduction factor of 0.5.

This approach may be used to quantify the cost of contaminated batches associated with the use of packed glass wool towers. This cost can be recovered when the towers are replaced with Pall Emflon II filter cartridges. Since there is an extraordinary range in fermentation processes, example calculations for a range of parameters are shown in Table 2. The method may be used to directly estimate the expense of contaminated batches for a particular installation.

Energy Costs

At the same inlet airflow rate, Pall Emflon II cartridge filters operate at a significantly lower differential pressure than packed glass wool towers. Therefore, the energy operating expenses are significantly lower for the cartridge filters. The energy operating expenses at a specific location can be computed using Fig. 9.

Typically, a cartridge filtration system is sized so that the pressure differential across the filter housing is approximately 1–2 psi when new cartridges are installed. This clean pressure differential does not usually change significantly during the service life of a particular set of filters. With fiberglass packed towers, however, the pressure differential across the tower is quite dependent on the operation conditions. The initial pressure drop is influenced by the quality of the column packing by the maintenance operator. In addition, the pressure differential increases rapidly when hydrophilic fibers become wetted. The overall range for the pressure differential across the tower may be 5–20 psi; a normal operating range is 7–10 psi.

In the example below, an operating energy cost calculation is shown for the following operating conditions:

Airflow rate	1200 scfm
Discharge pressure	25 psig
Equipment air utilization	80%

	Pressure differential	*K* factor
Emflon II cartridge filter	2 psid	45
Glass tower	8 psid	180

Table 2 Contamination Costs Recovered by Emflon II Cartridge Filters

Case	Fermentation direct cost[a] ($)	Product value multiplier	Batches per year	Overall contamination rate	Contamination rate reduction factor	Reduction in contamination cost ($)
A	25,000	2	2	2	0.5	50,000
B	10,000	10	10	10	0.5	45,000
C	8,000	1.5	1.5	1.5	0.5	13,500

[a]Includes material, direct labor, and overhead.

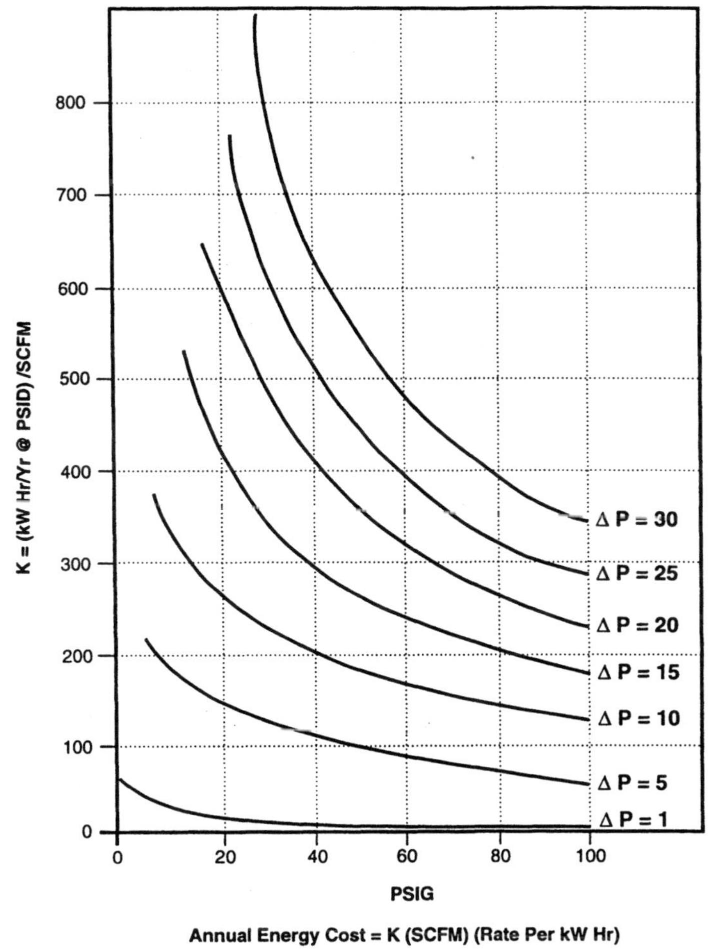

Figure 9 Annual energy consumption due to pressure drop *K* vs. psig.

$$\text{Operating energy cost} = K \text{ factor} \times \text{airflow rate} \times \text{equipment utilization rate} \times \text{energy rate}$$

The discharge pressure and the pressure differential are used with Fig. 9 to determine the *K* factor. The annual operating energy cost is tabulated below for the packed tower compared with the Emflon II cartridge filter.

	Energy cost	
	\$0.06 kW/h	\$0.12 kW/h
Packed tower	\$10,368	\$20,376
Emflon II cartridge filter	\$ 2,592	\$ 5,184
Net saving	\$ 7,776	\$15,552

The requirement that glass wool media be kept dry imposes an additional energy expense. Heat must be supplied to the system to maintain the air temperature above the dew point. Typically, this heat is added by the use of electrically heated resistance tape or steam tracers.

The energy cost is not usually computed but may be significant. Since it is dependent on site specific factors (pipe run length, quality of insulation, etc.), it must be calculated for each location. For the case of electrical resistance tape, a cost can be readily estimated from the total power consumption of the tape and the annual aeration hours. This formula is included in the Appendix.

Maintenance Costs

There are virtually no maintenance costs associated with cartridge filters. The cartridges can be installed by one operator in less than 1 h. The typical service life of a set of cartridges is 12–15 months; the cartridges can be integrity tested periodically during this time.

On the other hand, there are significant labor and time costs incurred during the maintenance of glass wool packed columns. The replacement of the packing is a cumbersome task because of the equipment and required handling procedures. The frequency of change-out depends on the utilization rate, and, under normal conditions, three or four replacements per year may be required. However, the packing may be changed more frequently if an unusually high contamination level is experienced.

The high maintenance costs are due to the large size of the packed tower compared to the cartridge filter housing. A typical tower for a 1200 scfm air service may be 2 ft in diameter and 6 ft in height. Trained operators and special equipment are usually necessary to service the equipment. Typically, two operators may require a full working day to complete the task. The job may proceed at a faster rate with closer supervision but, because of the additional labor, that will not reduce the cost. The estimate of this maintenance cost is dependent on the charge time for the operators.

Charge time[a] (hr)	Annual change-out cost
\$25	\$1600
\$40	\$2560

[a]Direct labor and overhead.

This is the labor charge only and does not include the cost of the packing material. The glass wool typically costs approximately \$3/lb. The total material cost to pack a tower 2 ft in diameter and 6 ft in length at a packing density of 6.7 lb/ft^3 is \$378.

Although the maintenance expense of these towers is significant, the direct and indirect costs of handling large quantities of fiberglass are beginning to increase rapidly. It has been noted that safety and handling advisories are now included with some types of material. There has been increasing, but not yet proven, concern that this material may be related to respiratory ailments. Any health complaint related to handling this material, whether valid or frivolous, will immediately increase the direct cost of glass wool tower maintenance. These complaints will also require additional management effort at both the production and corporate level and perhaps lead to higher health benefit costs.

Equipment Productivity Expenses

In addition to reduced direct labor maintenance costs, there are several other production advantages that result from the decreased maintenance requirements of cartridge filters.

Frequent Change-Out

Equipment downtime that is directly attributed to the packed tower sterile air filtration system is eliminated. In many cases, downtime due to the packed glass tower occurs between planned maintenance shutdown times (possibly during production). This nonscheduled downtime reduces the productivity of the production fermentor. The change-out of the glass wool medium may fall into this category (particularly during periods of contamination) and may account for as many as four lost production days per year.

This factor alone may account for the equivalent of a 1% yield improvement when a cartridge filter is used instead of a packed tower. Such a figure should be viewed in the proper perspective. At a typical facility containing 25 production units, the increase in production is equivalent to 25% of the output of an additional installed and instrumented fermentor. The addition of such a unit in an existing facility is quite expensive and often not practical.

Sterilization Cycle Time

At some installations, the sterilization time required for the existing packed tower may exceed the preparation time required for the other components and result in a process delay. Typically, 4 h of steam exposure is allowed for the tower system. At the conclusion of the steaming cycle, the hydrophilic glass fibers are wet and an additional period (≈5–6 h) may be required to adequately dry the media. In practice, an interruption in the sterilization cycle may delay the start of the production batch. Such lost production time is usually not recorded but should be viewed as reduced productivity. This is estimated to be 3–6 h/cycle.

The cartridge filters can be in situ steam-sterilized in 30 min of exposure and, since they are hydrophobic, do not require additional drying time. Therefore, it is unlikely that the sterilization cycle of the filter cartridges will ever delay the initiation of the fermentation cycle, and such production time will be recovered. Since the vessel housing can be isolated under pressure at the conclusion of the aeration period, the unit does not require sterilization for each cycle. Emflon II filters can be steam-sterilized in situ at 142°C for up to 165 cumulative hours.

Reduced Aeration Rate

The productivity of a unit may be increased further if the rate of airflow to the unit can be increased. In many fermentations, the oxygen transfer from the gas to the broth is the limiting step. Equipment restrictions in the compressor area can limit the rate of airflow to the production unit. This condition is often reflected in very strong concern expressed by the production staff about the pressure differential across the packed towers. With such a limitation, an operating condition may arise in which the peak airflow to the fermentor may have to be slightly reduced to remain within the range of the compressor equipment. The cartridge filters, since they have a consistently low differential pressure at the same airflow condition, overcome this problem and essentially increase the available airflow to the fermentor. Following this same line of reasoning, the use of Emflon II cartridges may, in fact, allow the system to operate at a slightly increased peak airflow rate to improve the oxygen mass transfer and reduce the overall aeration time.

The economic benefit of even a small change in the aeration rate should not be underestimated. The consequence of a small increase (i.e., from 1150 to 1200 scfm, a 4.3% increase) is considered in the following example.

For a production cycle in which the unit is operated at a full aeration rate for 75% of the cycle (the balance of the time may be allocated to harvest or reduced aeration conditions), the effect of a 4% increase on the capacity of the unit is calculated as follows.

$$\text{Fractional reduction in aeration cycle time} = 0.75 \times 0.043 = 0.032$$

$$\text{Productivity factor (\% increase)} = 3\%$$

The economic benefits of productivity increase from these three sources can be quantitatively estimated by using the cost data developed to determine the contamination costs shown earlier in Table 2. Input data for the three cases presented are reproduced in Table 3. The value of productivity increases is computed according to the formula shown in the Appendix, Section A.4.

At installations in which the air compressor equipment is operating near full capacity, a large productivity increase may be obtained as a result of the conversion of a glass packed tower to the Emflon II cartridge filters. This condition, of course, does not occur at all facilities. An in-plant test with a production unit can be easily performed to determine the effect for a particular fermentation product. The results of a plant test will allow a quantitative estimate of the benefit.

Emflon II Cartridge Filter Costs

The expense incurred in the conversion to Emflon II cartridge filters should be allocated between the costs for (1) the appropriately sized filters and housing and (2) additional improvements to the air delivery system. For example, a system that sterilizes air at a rate of 1500 scfm would require five 30 in. Emflon II elements. As noted, cartridge filters have a typical service life of 12–18 months; therefore the operating costs will be well below those incurred with the fiberglass packed tower filtration system.

Table 3 Equipment Productivity Increase Gained by Use of Emflon II Cartridge Filters

Case	Fermentation direct cost[a] ($)	Product value multiplier	Batches per year	Productivity factor (% increase)	Contamination rate reduction factor	Value of additional product ($)
A	25,000	2	20	6	0.5	60,000
B	10,000	10	30	2	0.5	60,000
C	8,000	1.5	45	3	0.5	16,200

[a]Includes material, direct labor, and overhead.

Emflon II elements would be installed in an high airflow filter housing. These fermentation air filter housings are ASME code stamped and feature sumps designed for easy drainage of condensate and large inlet/outlet connections designed to minimize housing pressure differential and maximize airflow. Construction material is 316L stainless steel.

For this type of equipment, the installation cost can be estimated separately or figured as a factor of the housing purchase cost. This cost must be adjusted to reflect the expected payback period (typically 2–5 years) and capital expenditure tax benefits.

Air Delivery System Improvements

The specific changes required during the retrofit process to convert from fiberglass packed towers to filter cartridges are dependent on the condition of the existing facility. The upstream requirement to operate cartridge filters is the absence of condensate water and fine particulate material from the feed stream. Since condensate water is a more critical problem for the hydrophilic glass wool media than for the hydrophobic cartridges, the existing approach (such as a coalescer or cyclone) may be sufficient. In some installations, a coalescer alone has been shown to be adequate to remove fine particulate material without requiring a separate prefilter. In dry air systems that use oil-free compressors, a coalescer is typically not required. In such cases, a dedicated air particulate prefilter upstream of the filter cartridges has also been used.

There must also be provision made to eliminate the generation of particulate contaminants in the region between the prefilter and the final filter. Stainless steel piping is recommended for this application. An evaluation of the existing system should be made to determine the best approach to minimize the extent of contamination that may reach the final Emflon II filters.

Conclusions for Test Case

Fermentation processes on a commercial scale vary widely with respect to costs, production requirements, and economic value. The conversion of fiberglass packed towers to filter cartridges can generate significant direct operating cost savings. These savings are based partly on the filter advantages of 100% microbial retention under both dry and moist air operating conditions and integrity testability to ensure that all cartridges are intact. The retention efficiency of the glass wool packed towers changes with operating conditions, and wetting of the media is a particular problem. In addition, there is no test method to determine the actual performance of the tower. As a direct consequence of this difference, the use of cartridges will result in a lower contamination rate and more efficient utilization of technical and staff personnel during contamination-prone operation periods.

The costs recovered by reducing the contamination rate due to air filtration alone were computed. The input data were fermentation direct cost, product value multiplier, production frequency, and overall contamination rate. The results show that the recovered costs can be very significant for high value products. Even for low value products, the savings may exceed the cost of the cartridge filters on an annual basis.

Additional savings are incurred with conversion to cartridge filters due to lower pressure differential and consequent lower energy costs, along with ease of change-out and safety. At typical operating conditions, the energy saving alone may account for up to four times the cost of the cartridges. Additionally, the energy expense of adding heat to keep the glass media dry and above the dew point is eliminated when fiberglass packed towers are replaced with cartridges.

Plant productivity can be increased by elimination of lost batches, reduced downtime, and increased yields. Cartridges require essentially no maintenance during their service life. The tower media must be replaced periodically during a year using special equipment and trained operators. This cost alone is estimated to be equal to 70–90% of the total cost of the cartridges. The cost of installation and operation of the cartridge filters would be easily covered by these savings. Where depreciation is over only a 2 year period, savings in subsequent years can be anticipated to be even greater.

Summary of Economic Formulas

A summary of the economic formulas developed in the report are presented in a general form in the Appendix. Operating data from a specific location may be used in these formulas to estimate the benefit of replacing glass wool packed towers with cartridges.

4.3 Downstream Processing Air Filter Applications

Starting with the cells and conditioned broth medium from the fermentor or bioreactor, the objective of downstream processing is to produce a highly purified, biologically active protein product free of contaminants such as endotoxins, bacteria, particles, or other biologically active molecules. This phase of bioprocessing typically comprises a series of unit operations including cell and cell debris separation, fluid clarification and polishing, concentration and purification, and membrane filtration sterilization of the purified product.

Cartridge filters are used in many stages of downstream processing for the filtration of both the harvest fluid and product intermediates as well as the filtration of air and gases required throughout the process. Air filtration applications include vacuum break filters for lyophilizers, sterile nitrogen blankets, tank vents, and sterile air for container cleaning. The recommended filters for these applications are listed in Table 4.

Filtration of Air, Gases, and Venting Applications

Absolute rated cartridge filters eliminate contaminants and impurities from air, nitrogen, and other gases used in downstream processing to prevent contamination of

Table 4 Filter Recommendations for Downstream Processing Air Applications

Application	Filter type	Micrometer rating	Typical gas flow rate per 10 in. module (scfm)
Sterile nitrogen blanket	Hydrophobic membrane	0.2	75–100
Tank venting	Hydrophobic membrane	0.2	75–100
Vacuum break	Hydrophobic membrane	0.2	75–100
Sterile air for container and closure cleaning	Hydrophobic membrane	0.2	75–100

Source: Martin et al., 1994.

product and further protect concentration and purification equipment. Vent filtration ensures containment and freedom from product contamination during fluid transfer operations and protects processing equipment during sterilization cycles.

In fermentation, cartridge filters are used to maintain the sterility of the makeup water, feeds, additives, and media in holding tanks and in fermentor/bioreactor exhaust. Cartridge filters are typically used in downstream processing for the filtration of air, gases, and venting applications when it is necessary to vent tanks during fluid transfers, pressurize tanks using inert gases such as nitrogen and argon, and protect vacuum lines, sterile vent holding tanks, and lyophilizers, as well as for gas purging, blanketing, drying, and when sterilizing equipment by in situ steaming or autoclaving.

The recommended filters for nonsterile particulate removal are polypropylene pleated filters. Hydrophobic membrane pleated filters such as polyvinylidene fluoride (PVDF) or polytetrafluoroethylene (PTFE) are recommended for aseptic processing. The absolute removal rating for the latter filters should be 0.2 μm determined under liquid flow conditions.

Figures 10–12 illustrate steps that can be required in downstream processing applications.

Figure 10 illustrates a cell and cell debris separation and clarification process, which is divided into a primary separation, secondary separation, and a cell concentration.

1. During primary separation, a cyclone can be used for particle removal; a sterilizing air filter can be used as a vent on the cyclone.
2. A variety of holding and receiving tanks can be employed during the separation and clarification process; these tanks can be fitted with sterile vent filters.
3. During secondary separation, a nitrogen blanket may be needed; the nitrogen gas can be sterile filtered with a hydrophobic filter.

Figure 11 illustrates a general process for concentration and purification of clarified harvest fluid. Applications for air filtration include (1) vent filters for solvent or buffer tanks and (2) vent filters for holding or buffer tanks needed for ultrafiltration and chromatography.

The final pharmaceutical product often needs to be packaged. Figure 12 shows a generalized filling operation.

1. A sterile nitrogen blanket and thus a sterilizing grade hydrophobic filter may be needed.
2. Sterile air or nitrogen may be needed for container cleaning.
3. A vent filter can be used on holding tanks.

Vacuum Break Filters

Sterilizing grade filters are employed in freeze-dryer installations to filter the gases used to maintain the chamber pressure and to break vacuum during operation and in sterilizers. As an example, the operation steps required for a sterilizing filter used in a lyophilizer as a vacuum break are described below. The system is illustrated in Fig. 13.

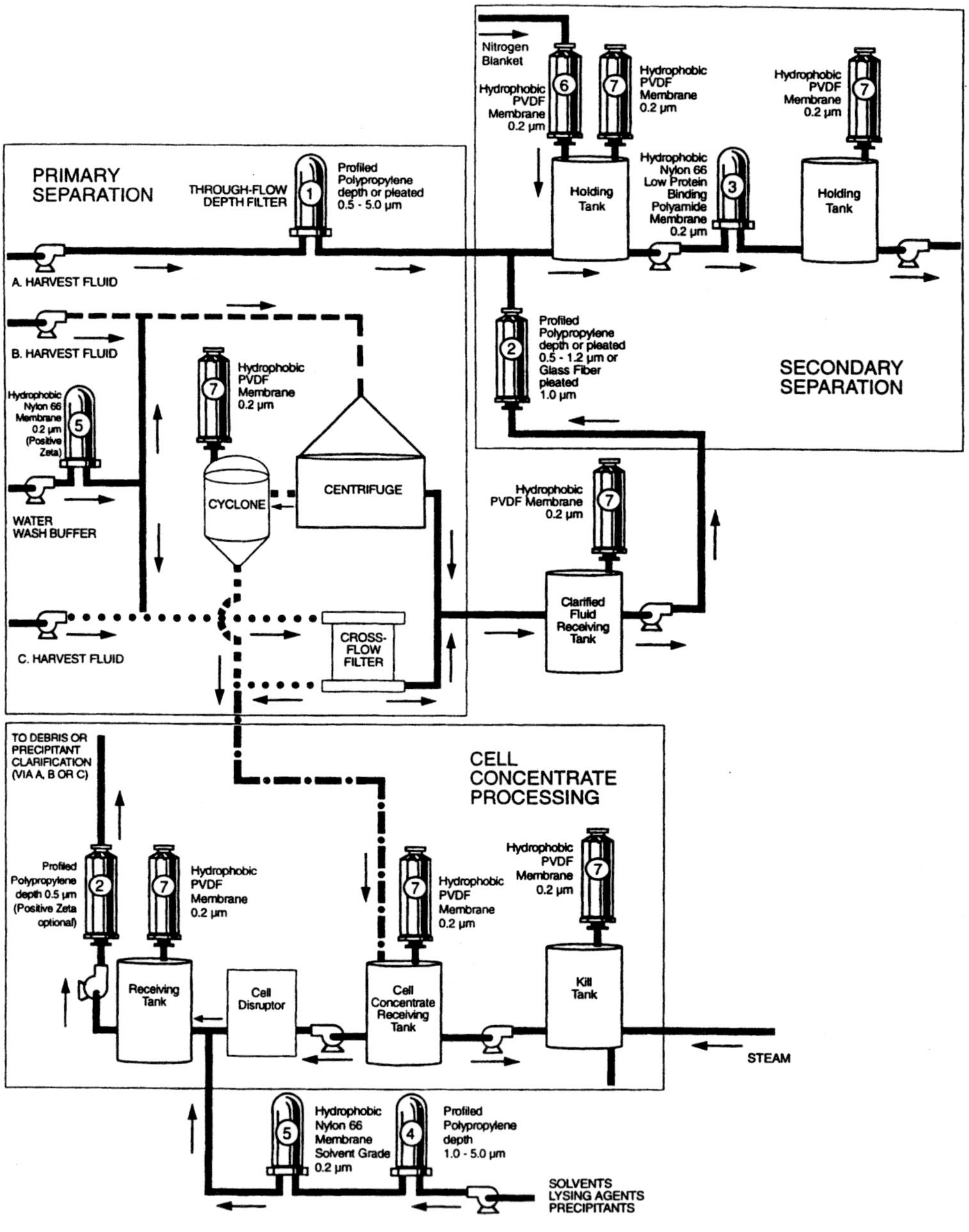

Figure 10 Air filtration applications in cell and cell debris clarification and purification processes. (Courtesy of Pall Corporation.)

1. In situ steam sterilization. The filter assembly and the receiving vessel and vent filter attached to the vessel are steam sterilized in situ.
2. Cooling. After the sterilization, the steam is shut off and air or nitrogen is immediately added to the system. Air or nitrogen gas is used to prevent a collapse (reverse pressurization; see below) and to cool the system and filter.

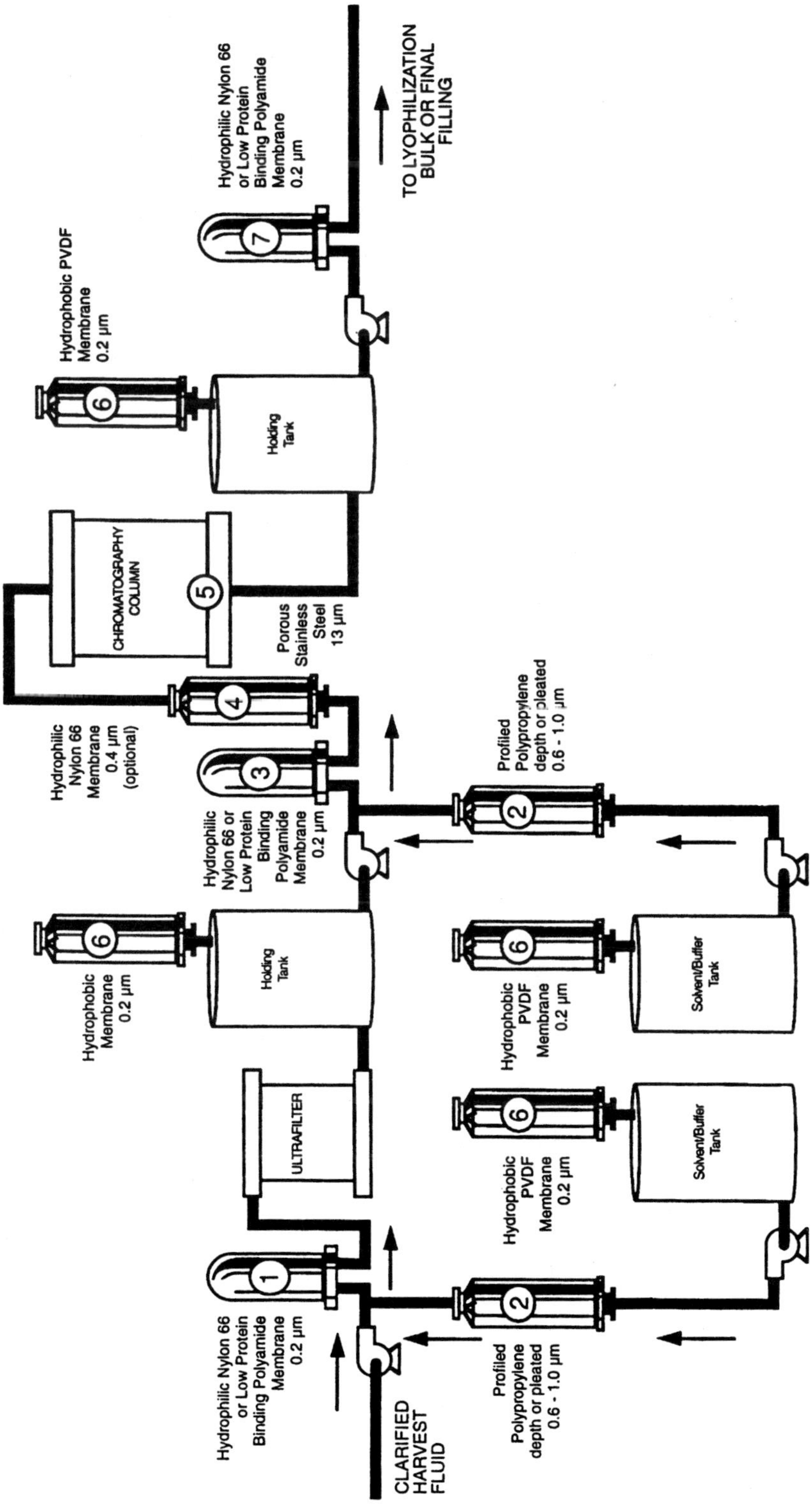

Figure 11 Air applications in the concentration and purification of clarified harvest fluid. (Courtesy of Pall Corporation.)

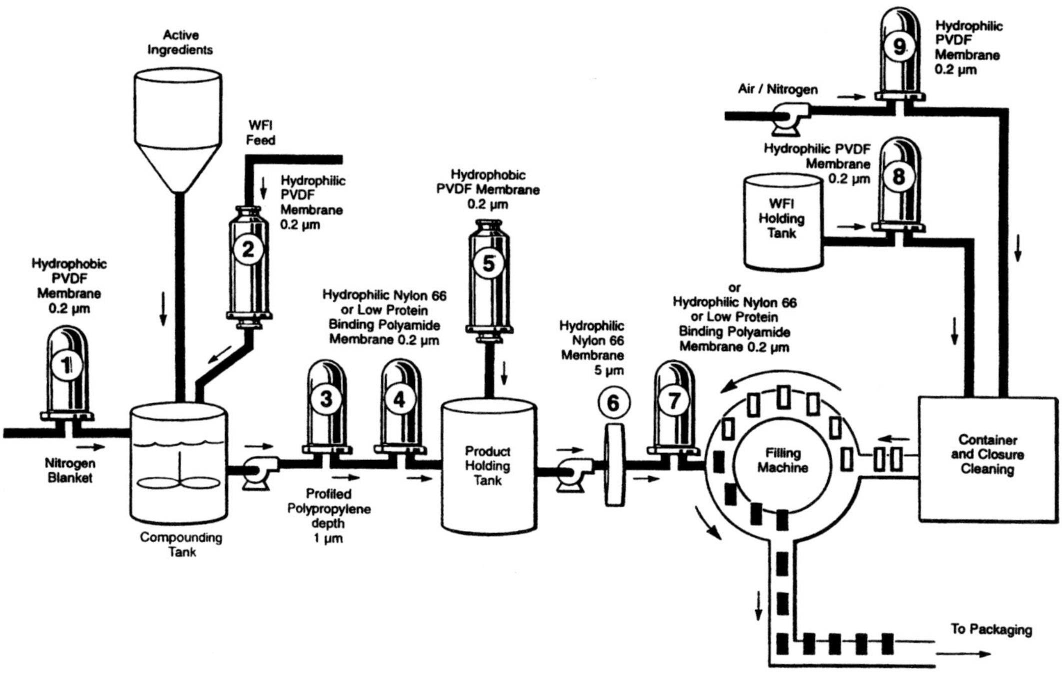

Figure 12 Air filtration applications in a filling process. (Courtesy of Pall Corporation.)

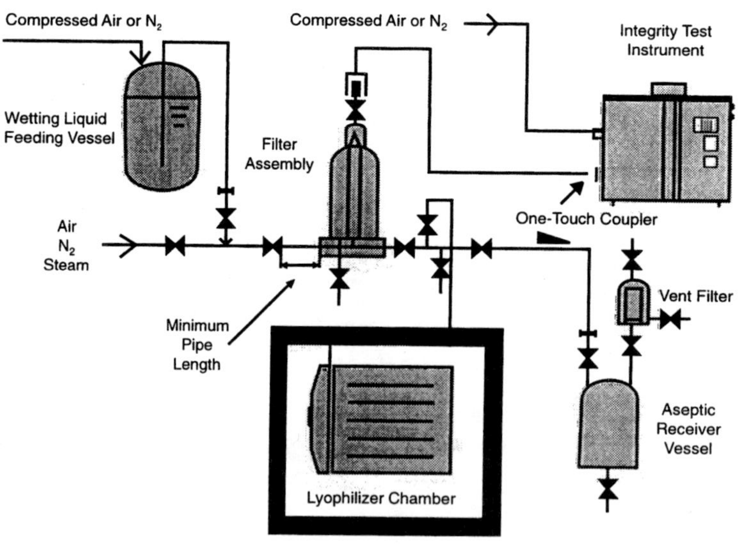

Figure 13 Air filtration applications in a vacuum break application (lyophilizer).

3. Addition of integrity test fluid. The wetting fluid for a forward flow integrity test, which is typically an alcohol–water solution, is placed in the wetting solution feed vessel. Compressed air or nitrogen pressure can be used to flow liquid through the filter cartridge to wet the membrane for an integrity test. The wetting fluid is collected in a receiving vessel. Alternatively, water could be introduced on the upstream side for the performance of a water intrusion test.
4. Integrity test. An filter integrity test instrument is connected for the performance of the integrity test. The use of an automated instrument allows for remote operation. If the filter fails the integrity test, then the filter should be changed.
5. Drying. After the test, the membrane filter is dried to remove the wetting fluid (or water if an intrusion test has been employed). Compressed air or nitrogen can be used.
6. Lyophilization. At this point the system is ready for the lyophilization operation.

Blow–Fill–Seal

Blow–fill–seal equipment can be used for the aseptic filling of pharmaceutical products. The container is formed and sealed aseptically. Air filtration is required to ensure sterility in this unit operation. A typical arrangement is illustrated in Fig. 14.

For buffer tank air, hydrophobic membrane filters are used to supply sterile air to a buffer tank on the blow–fill–seal machine. This blanket air is used to drive the sterile solution through a pneumatically controlled dosing system. The air used in the buffer tank is referred to as the gas cushion or buffer tank air. Hydrophobic membrane filters sterilize the air used to form the hot-moldable plastic tube (parison). The air used to form the parison is known as the parison support air. The parison is subsequently blow-molded into the shape of an ampoule strip or a bottle.

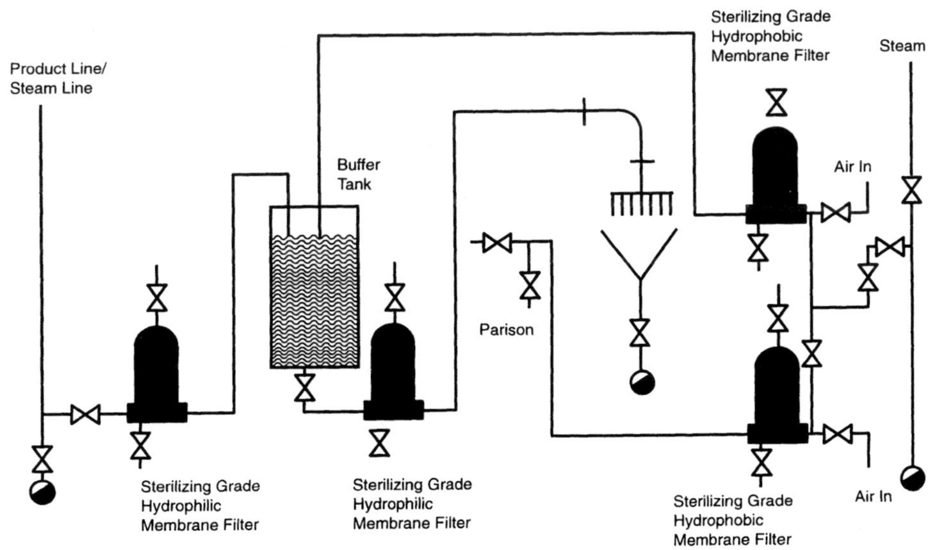

Figure 14 Air filtration applications in a blow–fill–seal operation.

Typical requirements for blow–fill–seal filters include that the filters be steam-sterilizable, integrity-testable, and the proper size to prevent restriction of gas flow. Hydrophobic membranes are used to prevent wetting out and to maintain high flow rates even in moist conditions.

4.4 Utilities

A number of peripheral unit operations can be required for a sterile process. The air filtration needs of these applications are discussed below.

Water-for-Injection Tank Vent

Sterilizing grade membrane filters can be used in vent applications in which the fluid in the tank is at an elevated temperature. One such application is the vent used to prevent contamination in a water-for-injection (WFI) tank. The water is at 80°C or higher. When a sterilizing grade air filter is used for this type of vent service, a steam-jacketed housing is typically used. It is only necessary to maintain the temperature of the filter cartridge at a temperature slightly above the dew point of the vapor. The steam introduced into the jacket should be at ambient pressure. Continuous operation of the jacket at a significantly higher steam pressure and temperature can reduce the service life of the filter due to accelerated aging of the hardware by oxidation.

Aging of the filters by oxidation depends on the status of the system. Oxidation does not occur when the cartridge is being steamed because there should be no air present in a properly operating steam-in-place system. If a cartridge is exposed to air at an elevated temperature, oxidation of the material in the filter, such as polypropylene hardware, will be accelerated. Oxidation will also occur when the filter is in a stagnant situation, i.e., there is no airflow through it. The flow of air through a filter can moderate the temperature environment, whereas under stagnant conditions the temperature of the filter will rise to the temperature of the housing. Stagnant conditions can exist when the tank is not being used or when it is empty. To prolong service life, when operating conditions permit, the steam jacket be turned off when there is no airflow through the filter for extended periods of time.

Hot Air

If an application involves hot air and a longer service life is desired, then high temperature filters can be used. High temperature filters can be used in continuous service at temperatures up to 120°C. These filters have a 0.2 μm microbial rating in liquid service and a particulate removal rating of 0.01 μm in gas service. The filter membrane is made of inherently hydrophobic PTFE, and the cage, core, and end caps are specifically designed for high temperature applications. For hot dry air, high temperature filter cartridges are expected to have a service life of up to 1 year at 100°C. However, change-out should be set for actual service conditions.

Steam Filtration

Process equipment and final filters are frequently sterilized by direct steam flow in situ during the normal line sterilizing cycle. This eliminates the need for making aseptic connections and risking recontamination. Filtered steam is required for this "sterilize in place" (SIP) treatment of filters, piping, vessels, and filling equipment.

Steam is also required for general equipment cleaning and sterilizing. The steam often contains significant amounts of pipe scale and other corrosion products. This particulate material should be removed in the interest of overall cleanliness and to avoid burdening the prefilters and final filters.

Particulate contamination in process steam is efficiently retained by porous stainless steel filters with an absolute gas rating of 1.2 μm. Porous stainless steel filter assemblies are typically sized at steam flow rates of 30–40 acfm per square foot of filter medium.

5 GENERAL CONSIDERATIONS FOR OPERATION (Haughney, 1995)

5.1 Filter Service Life

Filter cartridge change-out is usually based on actual experience, with a safety factor. Filters should be inspected on a monthly basis for oxidation. This should be supplemented by monitoring the pressure drop across the filters during operation to determine if the filters are plugging and routine integrity testing to confirm filter integrity during the service life of the filter. Alternatively, filter life studies, with an appropriate safety factor, could also be used to set a change-out schedule. Actual conditions for each application should be used during filter life studies.

5.2 Guidelines for Steam Sterilization of Sterilizing Grade Membrane Filters

Membrane filters can be sterilized by chemical sterilants (such as ethylene oxide, hydrogen peroxide in vapor form, propylene oxide, formaldehyde, and glutaraldehyde), radiant energy sterilization (such as gamma irradiation), or steam sterilization. The most common method of sterilization is steam sterilization, and it is the focus of further discussion regarding the sterilization of membrane filters used for air filtration.

Basic Procedures

Steam sterilization of a membrane filter can be accomplished either in an autoclave or in situ. In situ steam sterilization can be effectively accomplished by a variety of process arrangements. Below is an example of an effective procedure that can be employed for in situ steam sterilization (refer to Fig. 15). Steam sterilization is often the most critical portion of the process, and it is important that the procedures followed lead to sterilization of the system and do not damage the membrane filters.

1. Start with *all* valves closed.
2. Fully open valve C.
3. Fully open condensate drains I and D, housing drain J, and housing vent valve G.
4. Preset steam pressure to required steam pressure for the vent filter assembly. Then slowly open steam valve B. After condensate has been expelled from I and J, close both valves to crack.
5. Partially close vent valve G when steam flow is evident. Drain condensate from D. After condensate has been expelled, close D to crack.

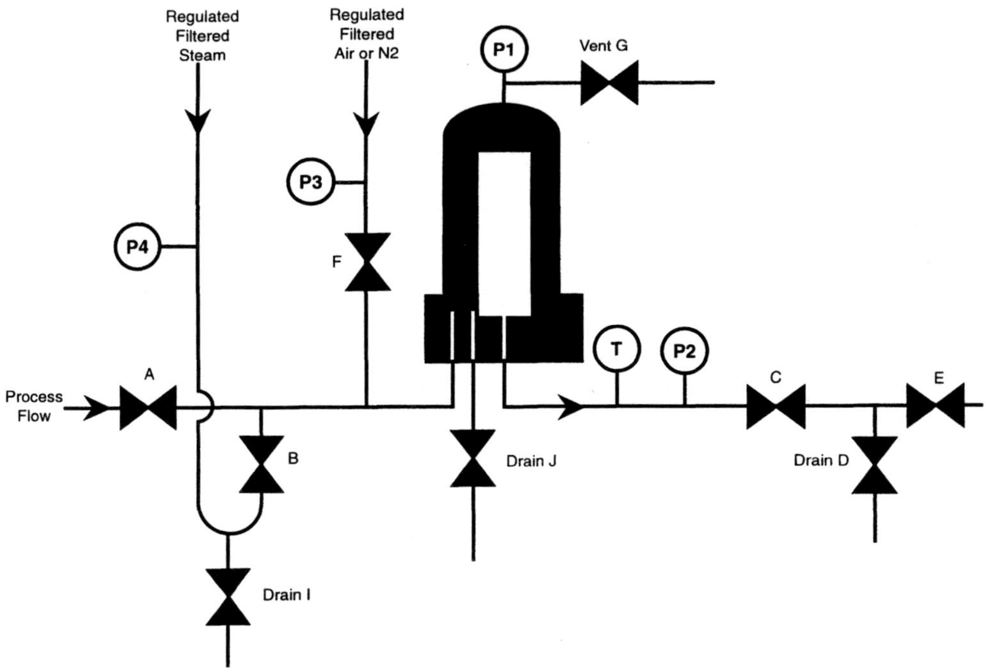

Figure 15 Steam sterilization arrangement (Haughney, 1995).

6. Permit steam to flow through the system for the required sterilization time, ensuring that no more than 5 psi pressure differential is developed across the filter.
7. Preset pressure of regulated air or nitrogen at 3 psi above the sterilization steam pressure. Close steam valve B, and immediately open air or nitrogen valve F when sterilization time is complete.
8. When sterilization time is complete, close B, drain valves D, J, and I, and vent valve G.
9. Steam may be flushed from the assembly to assist cooling by carefully opening vent valve G. Close valve G after venting.
10. Allow assembly to cool to ambient or to process temperature.
11. Close air or nitrogen valve F.
12. Relieve the gas pressure in the filter assembly via vent valve G. Filter assembly is now ready for use.

Sterilization of Filters and Downstream Equipment

In situ steam sterilization of filters and downstream equipment can be problematic. Sterilization of equipment assemblies requires very careful control and validation because the required steaming cycle is influenced by the equipment configuration, materials of construction, heat capacity, and volume of the downstream system. In addition, the vent filter must be steamed in the reverse direction.

It is always preferable to sterilize the filter and downstream components separately. However, if they are steamed simultaneously, appropriate vacuum relief safety devices must be fitted on downstream vessels that cannot withstand negative pressure without collapse.

Elimination of Reverse Pressurization Conditions During In Situ Steam Sterilization

At the conclusion of the sterilization cycle, it is recommended that an integrity test be conducted to ensure that the filter has not been damaged during the steaming procedure. Filter cartridges have occasionally been damaged at this stage. Analyses have shown that over 70% of such failures can be attributed to a reverse pressurization condition that developed during the cooling phase of the steam sterilization cycle. The possibility of the filter being damaged by exposure to reverse pressurization is increased during steam sterilization because the element is also subjected to elevated temperatures.

Reverse pressurization conditions can be avoided by following recommended procedures. During in situ steam sterilization, the steam is introduced into the filter housing in a procedure that displaces the air from the housing and then permits the steam to flow through the filter and exit through the downstream outlet of the system. At the conclusion of the in situ steam sterilization cycle, the steam valve is closed and air or nitrogen is applied to the system at approximately the same pressure as the steam. This procedure is the critical step in prevention of reverse pressurization damage.

The most common operator error at this point is to close the steam valve and not apply the specified air or nitrogen pressure. If the steam valve is shut and a noncondensable gas is not introduced, the housing is essentially an isolated system. Due to differential heat transfer during the cooling cycle, steam condenses to liquid water at different rates upstream and downstream of the filter. As a consequence, pressure differences of 5–15 psi across the wetted filter medium may develop. This condition may exist for only several minutes; however, this period is sufficient for permanent damage to be done to the filter. This situation can be completely avoided by maintaining the pressure through the introduction of a noncondensable gas (air or nitrogen) at the conclusion of the steaming cycle. This step eliminates the conditions for reverse pressurization.

Condensate Control

Condensate can form on filter membrane during the SIP (steam-in-place) procedure. The following guidelines should be followed to minimize the accumulation of condensate on either air or vent filters.

Plumbing

1. Figure 15 illustrates a recommended system configuration for steam sterilization. Recommended locations of drains are indicated (drains D, I, and J).
2. Pressure gauges and temperature sensors in the system should be checked on a routine basis for accuracy.
3. Steam traps should be checked periodically to make sure that they are working properly.
4. A temperature sensor should be installed on the downstream side of the filter, to verify that the steam is at the correct temperature.

5. Condensate traps should be located as close to the inlet of the filter housing as possible.
6. The filter cartridge should be positioned so that the open end is facing down to permit condensate to drain. The housing should be installed vertically to prevent condensate from accumulating on the upstream side of the filter.
7. Pressure gauges (accurate over the range of 0–45 psi) should be installed both up- and downstream of the filter housing, so that the pressure differential (ΔP) across the filter can be monitored. The pressure differential across the filter should not exceed 5 psid. A higher ΔP can cause damage to the filter when it is at elevated temperatures during the steam sterilization process. If a filter has been wetted with condensate and steam is introduced, the DP can rapidly exceed 5 psid.
8. It is recommended that the filter housing have a vent and a drain valve on the upstream side of the housing for the removal of condensate (Fig. 15: vent G and drain J). These valves should be partially open during steaming to prevent the accumulation of condensate.

Steam

1. Dry, saturated steam should be used to prevent excess condensate from entering the system. Superheated steam should *not* be used, because it could subject the filter to a high temperature and damage it.
2. The inlet pressure of the steam must be checked to verify that the required steam pressure is being delivered to the system, to ensure that the system is being properly sterilized.
3. Condensate should be drained from the steam line before introducing steam flow into the filter housing. This can be accomplished by ensuring that condensate drains in the upstream lines and in the housing are opened so that condensate is removed before steam flow is initiated through the filter.

Steam Cycle

During the steaming cycle, the drains and steam and steam traps must be partially opened to prevent a build-up of condensate.

Post-Steaming Procedure

A noncondensible gas, such as regulated air or nitrogen, must be introduced into the housing immediately after the steam valve is closed to prevent a vacuum from being formed on the upstream side of the filter. The gas pressure should be 3 psi higher that the steam pressure. This step is necessary to avoid reverse pressurization of the filter.

The upstream vent valve should be carefully opened when air is introduced after steaming. This will facilitate cooling by flushing the steam from the system. After venting, the valve may be closed.

Condensate can be removed from the membrane by continuing to apply a low air or nitrogen pressure after the steam has been removed from the system. The actual conditions should be validated for the application. This can be accomplished by weighing a dry filter prior to use. After the filter has been steamed and blown with air, it can be weighted to a constant weight to establish that it has been dried thoroughly. The constant weight should be within a gram of the dry filter weight. By using this procedure an amount of air required for drying a filter in a particular application can be established. As a starting point, 75 ft^3 of air per 10 in. filter is suggested.

Considerations for Exhaust Gas Filters

Condensate control in vent filter applications is dependent on the attention of the individual process operator. Many processes are operated according to experience and remove sufficient condensate to avoid filter blockage by condensate. This is evident from field reports. The following suggestions have been found to be useful for reduction of condensate accumulation on exhaust gas filters.

1. Condensation can be minimized in the vent filter housing by initiating steam flow through the vent housing only after the upstream vessel has developed some steam pressure. This will reduce the amount of wet steam entering the vent housing.
2. Water vapor can condense on a vent filter membrane during use if the fluid in the tank is water-based and the temperature of the filter is lower than the dew point of the fluid in the tank. A recommended procedure for avoiding the formation of condensate on the membrane is to maintain the filter assembly at a temperature slightly above the dew point of the liquid in the vessel. Formation of condensate can be prevented by fitting a heating section on the exhaust gas line upstream of the vent filter. The purpose of the heat exchanger is to ensure that the temperature of the exhaust gas at the filter is above the temperature of the exhaust gas at the fermentor exit. The effect of the heating unit is to lower the relative air humidity from 100% at the fermentor outlet to 20–50% downstream of the heating unit at the filter housing inlet. *Note*: The temperature of the filter should not exceed the vendor's recommendation for continuous service.
3. For filters that operate with backpressure in the head, condensate can be reduced on the exhaust filter if a pressure control valve is positioned at the fermentor exit upstream of the exhaust gas filter. The condensate will be reduced because the relative air humidity is lowered.
4. The amount of condensate that can accumulate in a filter is related to the exhaust gas flow velocity. At a higher flow velocity, the amount of condensate will increase. Thus, if there is any way in which the flow velocity of the exhaust gas can be reduced, the amount of condensate can be lowered. One possible solution would be to fit the exhaust gas line with a section of wider diameter piping.

6 CONCLUSIONS

This chapter has provided information on a variety of air filtration applications: fermentor inlet air, fermentor vent gas, vents on water-for-injection tanks, and vacuum break filters during lyophilization. In addition to a description of air filtration applications, guidelines were provided on the use of filters in these applications.

APPENDIX: SUMMARY OF ECONOMIC FORMULAS

Formulas are provided for various categories of cost savings associated with the use of Emflon II cartridges vs. fiberglass packed towers.

A.1 Contamination Cost Savings

Benefit 1. Reduced incidence of contaminated batches

Fermentation direct cost × product value multiplier × batches/year × Overall contamination rate × 0.5 contamination rate reduction factor

A.2 Energy Cost Savings

Benefit 2.1. Reduced pressure drop (see Fig. 9 for *K* factors)

Net energy savings = (K Factor$_{\text{Glass Tower}}$ − K Factor$_{\text{Emflon II}}$) × airflow (scfm) × energy rate ($/kWh) × equipment utilization rate

Benefit 2.2. Elimination of air heating

Net energy cost savings = Power rating of resistance tracing (kW) × energy cost savings rate ($/kWh) × aeration hours/year

Benefit 2 = benefits 2.1 + 2.2

A.3 Maintenance Costs Savings

Benefit 3. Reduced change-out costs.

Reduction in change-out costs (Annual change-out frequency × labor hours × labor hourly rate*) + (media cost/tower × annual change-out frequency)

*Including overhead

A.4 Equipment Productivity Savings (Reduction of Downtime)

Benefit 4.1. Unscheduled change-outs of glass wool tower

Hours saved = production hours/incident × incidents/year

Benefit 4.2. Extended sterilization cycle of glass wool media

Hours saved = production hours/cycle × frequency/year

Benefit 4.3. Cycle reduction due to increased aeration

Hours saved = fractional increase in aeration rate × peak aeration rate factor + production hours/year

Productivity factor = (Benefits 4.1 + 4.2 + 4.3)/(production hours/year)

Benefit 4 = fermentation direct cost × product value multiplier × batches/year × productivity factor

Total annual cost savings = sum of benefits (1 + 2 + 3 + 4)

A.5 Filter Costs

Annual cartridge cost = cost/module × No. of modules × change-outs/year

Annualized housing cost = (housing cost + installation cost)/depreciation period

Total annual filter costs = annual cartridge cost + annualized housing cost
Total annual conversion savings = total cost savings benefits − total annual filter costs

REFERENCES

ASTM. (1983). Standard Test Method for Determining Bacterial Retention of Membrane Filters Utilized for Liquid Filtration, ASTM Standard F838-83, American Society for Testing and Materials, Philadelphia.

Bruckshaw, N. B. (1973). *Filtr. Separ.*, May/June: 296.

Bruno, C. F., and L. A. Szabo. (1983). *Biotechnol. Bioeng.*, *25*:1223.

Conway, R. S. (1984a). *Biotechnol. Bioeng.*, *26*:844.

Conway, R. S. (1984b). Section criteria for fermentation air filters, in *Comprehensive Biotechnology* (C. Cooney, ed.) Academic, New York.

Fuchs, N. A. (1964). In *The Mechanics of Aerosols* (C. N. Davies, ed.), Macmillan, New York.

Haughney, H. (1995). Engineering considerations in sterile filtration processes, in K. E. Avis (ed.), *Sterile Pharmaceutical Products: Process Engineering Applications*, Interpharm Press, Buffalo Grove, IL, pp. 305–355.

Jaenchen, R., and R. Dellweg. (1989). Process Parameters for an Economic Use of Membrane filters in Fermentation Exhaust Gas Filtration, Publ. STR PUF 13, Pall Ultrafine Corp., East Hills, NY.

Martin, J. M., A. M. Trotter, P. Schubert, and H. Katz. (1994). Process filtration for biotechnology, in B. K. Lydersen, N. A. D'Elia, K. L. Nelson (eds.), *Bioprocess Engineering: Systems, Equipment, Facilities*, Wiley Interscience, New York, pp. 317–370.

Pall. (1989). The Sterilization of Fermentation Inlet Air; Economic Analysis of Pall Emflon® II Filter Cartridges vs. Glass Wool Packed Towers, Publ. STR PUF 11, Pall Ultrafine Corp., East Hills, NY.

Pall. (1994). Validation Guide for Pall Emflon® II Membrane Cartridges for Air and Gas Filtration, Publ. TR-870b, Pall Ultrafine Corp., East Hills, NY.

Perkowski, C. A. (1983). *Biotechnol. Bioeng.*, *25*,1215.

Porter, H. F. (1973). Gas–solid systems, *Perry's Chemical Engineers' Handbook*, 5th ed. (C. H. Chilton and R. H. Perry, eds.), McGraw-Hill, New York, Chap. 20.

Richards, J. W. (1968). *Introduction to Industrial Sterilization*, Academic, New York.

Stanbury, P. F., and A. Whitaker. (1984). *Principles of Fermentation Technology*, Pergamon, Oxford, UK.

Uberoi, T. (1992). Effectively select in-line filters, *Chem. Eng.*, March, p. 75.

Williamson, K., S. Tousi, and R. Hashemi. (1988). Recent developments in performance rating of gas/liquid coalescers, *Fluid/Particle Separ. J.*, *1*(2):111.

23

Sterility Testing with Membrane Filters

WAYNE P. OLSON
Oldevco, Beecher, Illinois

1 INTRODUCTION

This chapter is about sterility test practice as of 1996 and the near-term future of the test. For background see Olson [1]. The following terms are used herein.

Aseptic manufacturing. A system of manufacturing that removes or inactivates microbes in or on a product and thereafter excludes microbes from the product until the container in which the product is sealed is opened.

Barrier system. A system of rigid or flexible panels within a room. The barrier system is not fully enclosed and usually is constructed of optically clear plastic. Barriers tend to exclude humans, and microbes, from a system or product. The environment *inside* the barrier is maintained with HEPA-filtered air under positive pressure relative to the room outside the barrier.

Canister system. The Steritest canister system (Millipore Corp.) and the SteriSart (Sartorius) are self-contained membrane filter sterility test systems that operate under positive pressure from a peristaltic pump.

Dormant organism. An organism that is metabolically active and intact but unable to reproduce in certain conditions. Such an organism may be dysgenic, in which instance the genome is damaged. Dormancy may result from starvation or injury. A dysgenic condition may result from a genetic insult attributable to chemicals or extremes of physical conditions such as temperature.

First-order death. A survival curve shows, for example, 90% kill in the first increment of time, 90% of the survivors killed in the second increment of time, and so forth. A plot of $\log_{10}$ survivors versus time is approximately linear.

Isolator system. A fully enclosed housing or subroom that is not entered, topologically, by humans. The internal environment of the isolator and the surfaces of items in the isolator are sterilized with H_2O_2, or H_2O_2 + steam, or peracetic acid. Positive pressure is maintained inside the isolator with HEPA-filtered air; the air exits via a HEPA filter. Human manipulations inside the box are performed with long-arm gloves that are sealed to the isolator wall, or in a half or full suit attached to the isolator wall. Humans and the room environment are fully excluded from an isolator.

Manifold system. Manifolds for sterility testing are three- or six-place 47 or 50 mm diameter filter holders arranged on a single frame (usually of stainless steel) and operated under vacuum.

Overkill. A sterilization protocol that kills at least 6 logs of an organism that is resistant to the means of sterilization (e.g., *Bacillus stearothermophilus*, which is highly resistant to moist heat and also to H_2O_2).

Sterility assurance level (SAL). Probability of a unit being nonsterile. The pharmaceutical industry standard for terminally sterilized items is an SAL of 10^{-6}, usually established by validation following an overkill protocol. At this writing, the U.S. FDA guidelines for aseptically filled products is 10^{-3}.

Sterility test. A test, usually destructive, to establish that an item is free of viable microbes. The official sterility test used in the United States is the U.S. Pharmacopeial (USP) procedure (designated in the USP as <71> Sterility Tests). The USP test consists of verifying the sterility of 20 items from a lot (40 is proposed), preferably by the membrane method. Membrane-retained particles from half of the items are cultured in soybean casein digest (TSB) at 25°C, and half in fluid thioglycollate (FTM) at 32°C. Incubation times for TSB and FTM with membrane systems have been 7 days but will be lengthened to 14 days.

2 WHAT THE STERILITY TEST HAS BEEN AND WHAT IT IS NOW

The sterility test has been a means of determining whether the product in its final form is sterile. In the United States and some other countries, this meant that the contents of 20 final containers from a product batch are sampled into TSB and into FTM to ascertain whether the samples contain viable organisms. In the original form of the test, a small sample was recovered, aseptically, from each of a number of final containers and inoculated into TSB and into FTM. The media were incubated for 14 days at 25 and 32°C, respectively, and the appearance of turbidity was assumed to be the result of microbial growth. The growth would be streaked onto suitable nutrient agar plates to confirm the presence of organisms.

Problems existed with the testing of antibiotics. Although organisms resistant to a given antibiotic might be present in the final container, growth still would be suppressed in high concentrations of the drug. The membrane filter method was developed as a collaboration between the Sterility Test Branch of the U.S. FDA (this group no longer exists) and Millipore (Bedford, MA), so that any microbial contaminants in antibiotic solutions might be trapped on a membrane filter (MF) and subsequently rinsed free of the drug prior to MF immersion in growth medium. Membrane filter use for sterility testing became widespread, in part because the MF test is far more sensitive to small numbers of organisms than the direct inoculation process used previously.

In the 1960s and early 1970s, a pass in the sterility test was accepted widely within the pharmaceutical community as proof of the sterility of a lot of an injectable drug. Sterility test failures were commonplace, and retesting was done one or more times to provide a form of proof that contamination was not within the product but a result of the test procedure. The incompatibility of these views was not debated until major sterility issues with large volume parenterals surfaced in the 1970s [2].

In the early 1970s, putatively sterile large volume parenterals autoclaved in the final container (e.g., D5W) from major drug houses in the United States, United Kingdom, Sweden, and India were found to be contaminated with organisms introduced during the manufacturing process [2]. Later, Betadine solution (an iodine-containing antiseptic used during surgery) was found to be contaminated with an iodine-resistant pseudomonad introduced at the manufacturing site. Sterility failures in many lots of injectables galvanized the U.S. FDA and the British MCA to find the causes to ensure that repetitions were unlikely. The Clothier Report of MCA was a parliamentary investigation of such failures within a U.K. firm.

When the large numbers of sterility failures surfaced, with accompanying patient sepsis and some deaths, the quasi-collaborative relationship between the regulated industry and the regulators changed. In the early 1980s, product contamination and issues of probity arose with several U.S. generic houses. The relationship between the regulators and the regulated industry became strained and confrontational.

Within the same time frame, informal discussions among parenterals manufacturers (e.g., at Parenteral Drug Association meetings) related that media fills (fills of nonterminally sterilized bacteriological growth medium) showed contamination rates of one vial per 1000. At that time, retests of sterility test failures were commonplace and would result in a discrepancy statement (DS) in the lot record and quarantine of the lot until a retest was negative, presumably indicating that sterility test personnel had finally failed to contaminate the product. As many as five retests had been made in one company before a lot was rejected as contaminated. Two retests became standard, provided the organism isolated at the second test was different from the organism isolated the first time.

The reasons for the apparently cavalier attitude toward the sterility test (as of 1980) were that

1. The test was known to fail on occasion and was assumed to be at least as culpable as media fills, which had at that time a failure rate of about 0.1%.
2. It was understood then (as now) that the primary source of microbial contaminants is humans, and sterility test items (until recently) received considerably more human handling than a vial in a filling room.
3. Many manufacturing personnel assumed that a few nonpathogenic organisms in a putatively sterile item would do no harm to the patient. This attitude applied, in the main, to freeze-dried items and to cytotoxic drugs. (Late in the 1980s, the growing number of AIDS patients would make everyone more aware of immune-compromised patients, which often include the elderly.)

To the scientist, sterility is a statistical concept. Usually, under one set of conditions, organisms tend to die at a first-order rate. This is true whether the killing element is moist heat, dry heat, ethylene oxide, formaldehyde, glutaraldehyde, chlorine, ionizing radiation, or another agent. In law, and for compendial and regulatory purposes, a thing is sterile or it is not. Probabilities of kill are not considered. If a drug solution or a bandage is sold as a sterile product and it is not, the manufacturer is at fault. The law is concerned with the assignment of fault and with punishment. However, the only way in which a manufacturer of sterile solutions for injections or ophthalmic applications can be 100% positive that no items are nonsterile is to test everything that is produced. Sterility testing compromises the integrity of the final container. Testing all of the product leaves nothing to be sold and used.

Since 100% assurance of sterility is inconsistent with use of the product and with any approximation of reasonable business practice, and since the U.S. FDA is adamant that there will be no repetition of the sterility failures of the 1970s, practices are evolving that increase the SAL and aid in locating the source or sources of contamination. Sterility testing has no impact on the SAL but can play a major role in the detection of contaminants. The emerging view of the USP sterility test (1996) is:

1. The test is sensitive to contamination levels of 15% of the final containers or more (Table 1), but lower levels of contamination are unlikely to be detected if only 20 items are tested. Even if 100 samples from each lot were sacrificed for sterility tests, contamination levels of 0.1% would be detected in less than 10% of the lots produced. This alone disqualifies the USP sterility test as a useful quality control method. Although the test remains insensitive, the proposed number of items for test will be 40.
2. Since the test detects only a high frequency of contamination among putatively sterile articles, and since the use of isolators reduces the probability of a false positive to near nil, a failure must be viewed as proof of contamination.
3. The contaminating organism must be identified, at least as to genus and preferably as to species. An investigation must be undertaken to locate the source and correct the fault leading to the contamination.
4. Dysgenic organisms may not adapt to TSB or FTM swiftly enough to provide a positive growth reaction within 7 or even 14 days. Previously, a 7-day incubation was considered satisfactory for MF tests, but 14 days is now required, and evidence of this exists within the Australian, German, and U.S. pharmaceutical industries [3]. Some damaged organisms may be incapable of growth even after 14 days.

Table 1 Probability of Lot Rejection, Based on the Extent of Contamination and the Sample Size for Sterility Test

	Percent contamination				
N	0.1	1	5	10	15
20	0.02	0.18	0.65	0.89	0.96
50	0.05	0.39	0.92	0.99	
100	0.09	0.63			
200	0.18	0.87			
500	0.39				

Source: Modified from Ref. 1.

At this writing (1966):

Emphasis by the U.S. FDA, the USP, and the regulated industry is on manufacturing methods, and validation of those methods, to assure product sterility. The points of emphasis include

1. Clean room cleanliness as measured by particle counts
2. Microbiological evaluations of controlled environments
3. Personnel training
4. The design, construction, and maintenance of controlled environments
5. Sampling plans and sites
6. Alert and action levels
7. Airborne and surface sampling
8. Media and diluents used
9. Identification of environmental microbes
10. Media fills

The USP sterility test (half of each of 20 items for the TSB test, the other half of each for the FTM test as of the 1995 draft) is assumed to be a coarse evaluation of product sterility—an alarm of sorts.

Because it is more sensitive for the items actually sampled, the method of choice is the membrane filtration method [the direct transfer method (inoculation into medium) is to be used only where the membrane method is inappropriate].

A proposed change in <71> of the U.S. Pharmacopeia, published in the March/April 1995 issue of the *Pharmacopeial Forum*, is as follows: A sterility test failure, *when the testing is done in an isolator*, is considered proof of contamination, and a retest is not allowed. A retest with 40 items is allowed if sterility testing is done in a clean room.

The USP sterility test is evolving into a reliable test of aseptic practice in manufacturing; the test now is an ongoing check on the rigor of a manufacturer's cGMP compliance. I suggest that in major manufacturing operations in the near future a sterility test failure by any means will be considered presumptive proof of lot contamination.

Emphasis is placed on the membrane method for three reasons:

1. The MF method is far more sensitive to the presence of small numbers of organisms than direct inoculation because the entire contents of final containers can be sampled.
2. The organisms trapped on a membrane filter can be rinsed free of most growth inhibitors and toxic materials. With direct inoculation, the best that one can hope for is a significant dilution of the inhibitor.
3. The membrane method is the only practical means of testing the sterility of sterile-filtered bulks in the bulk tanks. The method of choice for bulk testing remains that of Gee et al. [4]. Where proper validations are done, it is possible to recycle into the next bulk the filtrate from the sterility tests.

3 TESTING OF STERILE BULKS

Most manufacturers of sterile items for injection perform a sterilizing grade filtration between the makeup tank and the sterile bulk tank. The sterilizing grade filter is usually in place when the bulk tank is autoclaved and may be in place but valved off during the latter part of the cycle if the sterile bulk tank is steamed in place. (If one passes all of the steam required for the sterilization of a bulk tank through the filter, pore collapse may occur.) Unless the product is highly labile, the sterile-filtered bulk is stored at 5–20°C for several days or until it can be sampled for sterility and composition prior to filling.

Usually, the sample is taken via a drop line to the bottom of the sterile tank, from which filling is done. Manufacturers are aware that any such sample is not truly representative of the bulk, although the sedimentation of particles greater in diameter than 3 μm may increase the probability of errant organisms in the sample if they are present.

Sampling of the sterile bulk requires several aseptic connections (i.e., the sterile pressure vessel or liter-sized evacuated vessel must be connected to the drop line of the sterile bulk tank; then the bulk sample must be transferred to the sterility test system; see Gee et al. [4] for some particulars). A preferable system incorporates the sterility test membrane filter for bulk testing directly into the sampling port of the sterile bulk tank. Where there is a lag between the sterilization process and filling, a sterile bulk must be sampled. In fact, early lines incorporating sterile filtration with filling of biologics also had a surge tank between the filter and the filling heads so that "bulk samples" could be taken. This was to accommodate the need of the FDA to see data on bulk sterility samples.

4 PERFORMANCE OF THE TESTS

4.1 Simple Aqueous Solutions and Membrane Filters

The Canister System

A Steritest canister system is shown in Fig. 1. The SteriSart canister system is similar. The sterile vented needle is placed into the item to be sampled. Through sterile tubing, a peristaltic pump impels the liquid into one of the canisters (each canister contains a sterile vent filter). The bottom of the canister is a 0.45 μm pore size membrane filter with a hydrophobic edge, supported by a porous plastic disk and a port with a removable plug. All of these components, including the needle that penetrates the elastomeric closure of the final container item, are supplied sterile. Downstream of the membrane filter and supports, when the plug is removed, a nonsterile connection is made to a vacuum bottle for the collection of the tested liquid. If the vacuum bottle and the tubing to it are clean and sterile, the system can be validated so that the collected liquid may be recycled to the next batch of product [4]. Half of the contents of each vial is filtered through each of the two canisters (three canisters in Europe, one of which contains Sabouraud's broth for yeasts, molds, and aciduric microbes). When all of the liquids have been filtered through the two (or three) canisters, the ports in the bottoms are closed (trapping some air beneath the wetted filters) and the two canisters are filled, one with TSB and the other with FTM.

The canister system, used in an isolator, is the most reliable in the avoidance of false positives. Chance microbial contamination is reduced by means of the canister, compared with the use of manifolded disk filters [5]. Any contaminant is streaked on nutrient agar to provide isolates for identification.

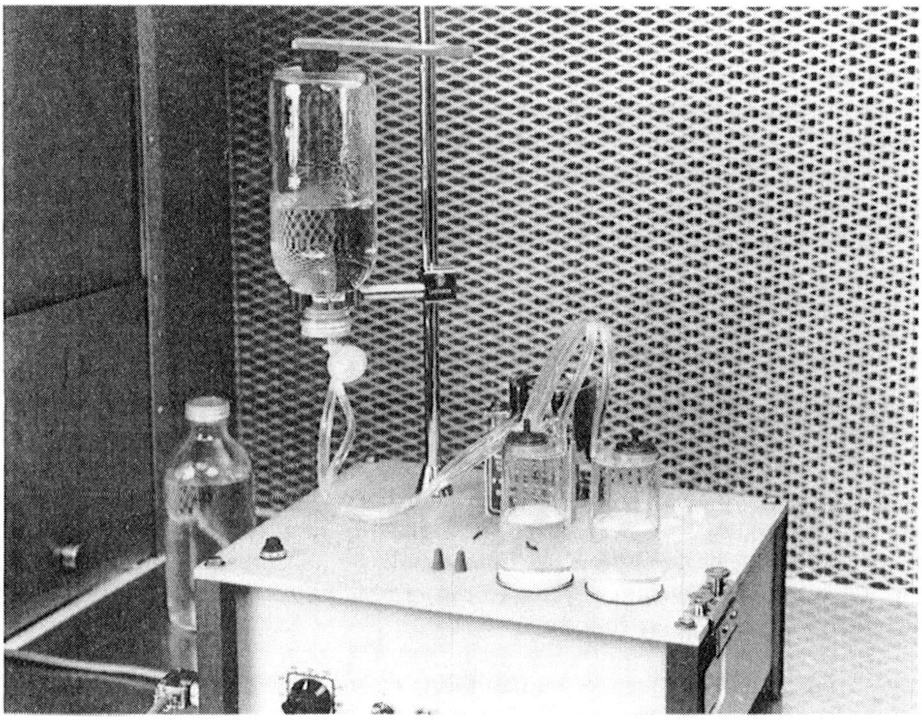

Figure 1 Steritest canister system with peristaltic pump drive. A final container is being sampled, and the feed is divided between the TSB and the FTM canisters. (Courtesy of Millipore Corp.)

The Manifold System

Stainless steel sterility test manifolds are outmoded and in declining use. The 0.45 μm pore size membrane filters, 47 or 50 mm in diameter and with a hydrophobic edge, are placed in the individual holders of a stainless steel manifold; each filter holder is usually capped with a clear plastic housing that has a removable lid for the addition of samples. This system is double-wrapped in autoclave paper and steam-autoclaved. The test manifold is carried into the sterility test clean room (by an appropriately gowned and gloved person) and placed in a biohazard hood (inside a clean room) that has previously been cleaned, disinfected, and turned on for at least 6 h prior to use (my preference). Immediately prior to placement of the manifold in the hood, the outer layer of autoclave paper (dirty, as a result of exposure to unclean air after removal from the autoclave) is removed and discarded. The manifold is connected to a vacuum source and is ready for use.

Usually, all of the contents of a number of final containers are passed through the smallest number of 47 mm filters as is consistent with filter clog and time constraints. Each of the filters is recovered with sterile forceps and cut in half with sterile scissors or a sterile guillotine. Half of the filter is incubated in a large tube of sterile TSB, and the other half in a large tube of sterile FTM. These are labeled and incubated at 20–25°C and 30–35°C, respectively, for 14 days. If either or both of the tubes become turbid, the turbidity is sampled with a sterile loop, streaked onto nutrient agar, and incubated under appropriate conditions (aerobic or anaerobic), and the organism(s) is/are identified.

The difficulties that can be encountered with such manifold systems, and the advantages of a closed system with paired glass holders for direct incubation, were described by Koppensteiner [6] and tested extensively by Hecker and Lukac [7]. The glass canister system is reusable and is in use where labor costs are sufficiently low that they do not dictate the use of disposables. A reusable canister system is shown in Fig. 2.

4.2 Liquids Containing Microbial Growth Inhibitors

Three diluting and rinsing fluids are designated in the USP, primarily for the rinse-down of the membrane filters after putatively sterile product containing growth inhibitors has been filtered through those membranes. The objective is to rinse away such materials before the TSB or FTM is added. For a solution or a suspension containing a penicillin or a cephalosporin, a quantity of β-lactamase sufficient to inactivate any residual activity on the filter should be added aseptically to fluid A and the filter rinsed with fluid A prior to the incubation of the filter with TSB or FTM. Fluid A is prepared as follows:

1. Add 1 g peptic digest of animal tissue to water to form 1 L solution.
2. Clarify by centrifugation or filtration.
3. Adjust pH to 7.1 ± 0.2.
4. Fill in 100 mL containers and steam autoclave.

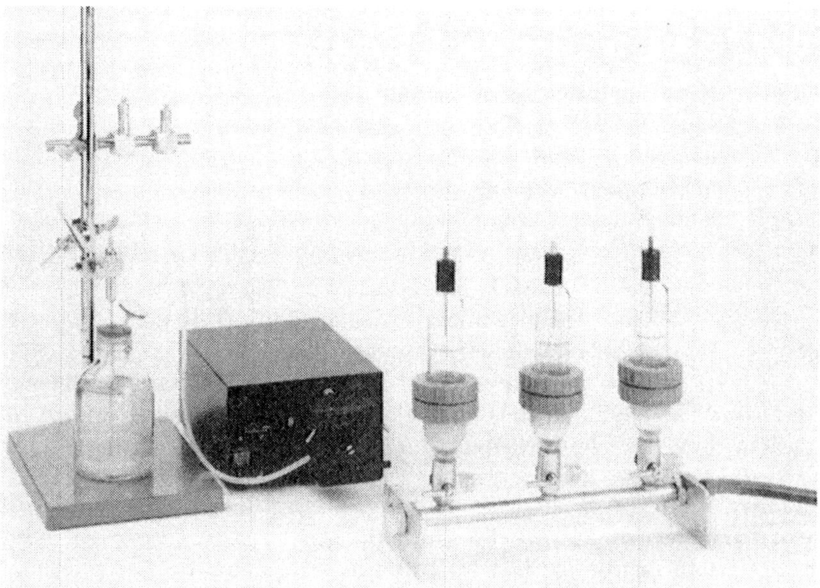

Figure 2 Reusable sterility test canister system. (Courtesy of Sartorius GmbH.)

4.3 Ointments and Oils

Most ointments and oils are soluble in isopropyl myristate (IPM), which, although not completely harmless to microbes, is less toxic than other membrane filter–compatible lipoid solvents. The amounts are no less than 100 mg from each of no fewer than 40 containers in no less than 100 mL of IPM. The IPM is sterile-filtered through a 200 nm pore size membrane filter; a water extract must have a pH of no less than 6.5. Warming the IPM to no more than 44°C reduces the viscosity and promotes the solubility of the ointment or oil under test without killing off most of the organisms, if present. Filtration through the sterility test membrane must be done promptly following dissolution, and the filter must not be allowed to run dry until all of the sample has been added.

Such filtrations can be done in the traditional manifold system, operating under vacuum only, but the clear plastic housing should be wrapped with a heat tape set to maintain a housing/oil temperature of about 40°C, since the filtrations are slow and become slower yet if the oil cools to ambient. Canister systems may function better than manifolds in such applications.

After the product has been filtered through the membrane filter but before exposure of the membrane to TSB or FTM, the membrane should be rinsed with 2 × 200 mL fluid D followed by 100 mL of fluid A. The small amount of Polysorbate 80 is sufficient to suspend and remove traces of oil. Fluid D is prepared as follows:

1. To 1 L fluid A add 1 mL Polysorbate 80.
2. Adjust the pH to 7.1 ± 0.2.
3. Dispense in 100 mL containers and steam autoclave.

If the oil or ointment is insoluble in IPM, it must be added directly to test media.

4.4 Emulsions

Phospholipid and other emulsions are used in total parenteral nutrition and for drug delivery. Such oil–water emulsions are filterable but must be intruded under positive pressure through the membrane filter (i.e., the lipid droplets must deform under pressure to penetrate the MF pores, and a proportion of the filter must become coated throughout with the lipid to facilitate lipid passage). Because the theoretical maximum pressure to be put on a sample in the manifold system is 1 atm (never achieved in practice), the canister system must be used. When the vent filter of a canister is plugged, the peristaltic pump is operating, and a vacuum is applied to the downstream side of the canister, an overpressure of more than 2 atm can be applied to an emulsion within the canister.

There is a period of 1 min or more during which no filtrate is observed in an overpressurized canister. Then the level of the emulsion commences to drop as filtrate is observed on the downstream side. During the quiescent period, the emulsion is intruding into the filter. Such testing has been validated and is in widespread use.

The addition of surface-active agents may make an emulsion more filterable but also may have a deleterious effect on the integrity of the microbial membrane. Glycerol and sucrose esters of fatty acids with substantial chain lengths are lytic [8] and are to be avoided. Tween 80 (10% w/v) appears to be more innocuous to organisms. Seemingly innocuous structures such as the glycerol and sucrose esters can be more lethal to vegetative organisms than the polyene antibiotics, and their use (unless properly validated) can *in*validate sterility test results [8]. Dimethylsulfoxide (DMSO) to 10% by volume has been used with emulsions [9], and an additive that mimics the effect of DMSO is required for conventional manifold systems that cannot be operated under positive pressure. Fluid K should be safer yet for microbes [1] and may make the emulsion filterable under negative pressure. This, too, must be validated. Fluid K is prepared as follows:

1. Dissolve 5 g peptic digest of animal tissue, 3 g beef extract, and 10 g Polysorbate 80 in water to 1 L.
2. Sterile filter the mixture, and adjust the pH to 6.9 ± 0.2.
3. Dispense in 100 mL containers and steam autoclave.

Another system (Septi-Chek), intended in part for use with lipid emulsions such as a total nutrition admixture (TNA), includes both a nutrient broth for growth of microbial contaminants and an agar slide [10]. Although the emulsion masks the turbidity of microbial growth, such growth on the slide within 24–72 h was obvious according to Murray and Sandrock [10]. What is needed is a comparison with the canister system operated under positive pressure for the extrusion of lipid emulsion through the membrane.

4.5 Nonfilterable Products

Direct Inoculation

Direct inoculation and manifolded membrane systems present multiple opportunities for contamination by sterility test personnel of the products under test, so this method is not preferred. An example would be a particulate drug or an oil that is insoluble in IPM. For this test, remove 1 mL (or, if the contents of final containers are less than 1 mL, the entire contents) from each container until one has 10 mL per medium. The 10 mL is added aseptically to 90 mL of TSB, and another 10 mL is added to 90 mL of FTM.

Incubation Period

The prevailing view has been that direct inoculation is less sensitive than the membrane filter sterility test, and where the bioburden is low and less than the entire contents of a final container is inoculated into growth medium, this is almost certainly true. The prevailing view also has been that incubation for 7 days is adequate for visible growth of membrane filter–collected organisms but that a 14 day incubation is necessary with directly inoculated media.

A German microbiologist [11] and an Australian group [12] have studied incubation times for membrane and direct inoculation sterility tests. Independently, they concluded (per Ref. 12) that the "membrane filtration method did not significantly enhance the efficiency of detection at seven days incubation." In both studies, a number of sterility tests were not positive until the 8th to 12th days. Therefore, unless more persuasive evidence to the contrary is published, the necessary conclusion is that the incubation time for the membrane filter sterility test must be increased to 14 days. At this writing (1996), the USP sterility test is being revised accordingly.

The reason for this may relate to the discussion of Tsuchido et al. [13]. They provided evidence of the kill of spores of *Bacillus subtilis* var. *niger* at temperatures well below 100°C in solutions of amphoteric surfactants (Tego compounds). However, they also point out that some of the spores are injured but capable of recovery. The portion of the discussion of Tsuchido et al. that relates to the recovery of organisms damaged during cleaning and sterilization is entirely consistent with the Australian [12] and German [11] studies that show occasional slow growth of contaminants during sterility testing.

4.6 Sterility Testing in Pharmacies

This text is about sterility testing in the pharmaceutical industry, but comments about ad hoc compounding of sterile items in the pharmacy, and testing of them, seem appropriate. Akers et al. [14] note that "pharmacists must perform end-product sterility testing on intravenous solutions to ensure their sterility." This is particularly true of the hospital pharmacy, which, in a decreasing number of locations, is a mini SVP/LVP manufacturing site.

4.7 The Sterility Test as an Analytical Method

In the absence of compelling evidence to the contrary, the U.S. FDA has held the view that multidose vials have some probability of contamination and that later administrations of drug may present a biohazard to the patient. However, multidose vials of lidocaine or heparin remain sterile, and when contaminated deliberately with *Staphylococcus aureus* at levels up to 10^8 CFU/mL the vials tend to become sterile over time. Two hundred emptied multidose vaccine vials (without preservative) showed no growth when sterility tested [15].

The results of Thompson and Thompson [14] are reminiscent of those of Gee et al. [16] wherein microbial die-off was shown as a possible result of the loss of critical cofactors (e.g., metals) from the microbes. Lidocaine, a hydrophobe, may disrupt the microbial membrane, killing the organisms; and the sulfate groups of heparin may sequester the iron and copper that microbes require for survival. However, the lidocaine results also may indicate that multiuse vials are far less of a microbial hazard than the FDA has supposed. Several additional studies along these lines would be most welcome and easily done.

5 MEDICAL DEVICES

A variety of devices presently are implanted into humans or are ex vivo but process blood and return it to the patient (e.g., artificial kidneys). They must be sterile at the time of implantation or use. Some of these are sterilized chemically (e.g., pig heart valves are immersed in 1% glutaraldehyde; the glutaraldehyde cross-links and inactivates immunizing antigens on the surfaces of the valves and, at the time of the addition, kills microbial contaminants).

Some devices are sterilized by ionizing radiation, in which case (provided proof of dosage is provided) sterility testing is not required. Implantable pumps may be steam-autoclaved or sterilized with ethylene oxide, depending on composition, and so forth. Where the device is produced in batches (e.g., artificial veins and arteries) and is sterilized by means other than ionizing radiation, sterility testing is usually done by complete immersion of one device (of a batch) in the growth medium, to a maximum of 1000 mL of medium. Immersion and examination for turbidity continue for 14 days. Although the sterility monitoring of devices is not a membrane method, it is included here for completeness.

The principal issue with the device sterility test is sensitivity. One device cannot be representative of a batch. If 5% of every batch of an implantable device are routinely contaminated, growth in a sterility test may not be detected in any of the lots produced over many years. Over 50% must be contaminated for a reasonable prospect of detecting poorly controlled manufacturing conditions.

Rinsing a device and passing the rinse fluid through a sterility test canister is not an adequate method. Bacteria and yeasts tend to form biofilms on surfaces. The organisms usually adhere to the adsorbing surface via secreted, highly porous oligo- and polysaccaride matrices that retain the organisms on the surfaces. See, for example, Ref. 17.

The sterility test has the inherent danger of inducing a false sense of security in the manufacturer, regulators, and users. The approach to device sterility that is most likely to ensure the desired result is intensive validation of process. The proof of the validity of this approach is the success of the industry with gamma-irradiated products that are not sterility tested. Devices sterilized by other validated means are likely to be as safe and not pose a risk to the patient.

6 ROBOTICS AND ISOLATORS

Robotic systems for sterility testing have been described [18], as have isolators [14]. As of mid-1987, Hoffmann-La Roche (Nutley, NJ) had been using robotic systems for two years [1], with no sterility test failures. The robotic systems have been in use since that time, and as of December 1994 the number of sterility test failures had been ''very, very small,'' according to a Hoffman-La Roche authority.

Consensus within the industry appears to be that isolators are the system of choice, and a walking tour of most modern pharmaceutical houses indicates that a large number of isolators have been put into service for sterility testing [19]. A sterility test isolator system is shown in Fig. 3.

The sterilization of most isolator interiors is by means of aerosolized H_2O_2 [14, 20] or chlorine dioxide (Alcide Corp., Norwalk, CT) [21] or peracetic acid [22]. Instructions for use, sterilization, and maintenance are provided by the manufacturers. The bioindicator spores are *Bacillus stearothermophilus* ATCC 12980 or equivalent for H_2O_2, *B. subtilis* var. *niger* for ClO_2, and *B. circulans* UC 9951 for peracetic acid. Provided the isolators are maintained and operated properly, false positives seem not to arise during sterility testing (see comment below). The current view of the U.S. Pharmacopeia is that viable microbes shown in a product in a properly operated isolator almost certainly indicate a contaminated product. For the revised USP sterility test, it is proposed that the recovery of a microbial contaminant from a final container in an isolator is definitive for lot rejection based on nonsterility.

Isolators are not perfect and beyond failure. A pinhole in a glove, partial masking of a portion of a final container from the lethal gas (e.g., hydrogen peroxide), a faulty seal on a port, and other occasional possibilities obtain for organisms to be present in an isolator during sterility testing. Therefore, in my view a second level of bacterial exclusion is appropriate (i.e., the SteriTest canisters). In and of themselves, the canisters are not proof against contamination but present a formidable barrier. Between the canisters and the isolator, the probability of false positives ap-

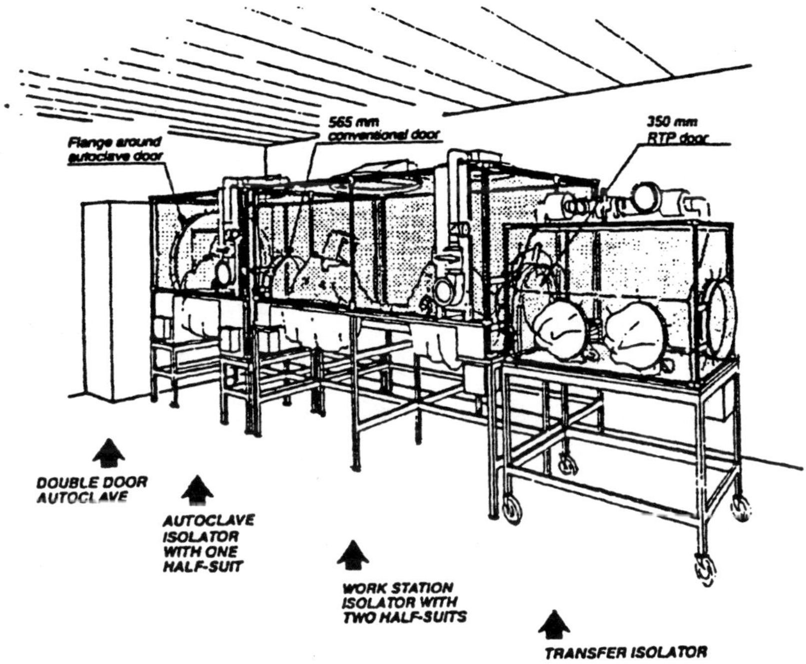

Figure 3 Sterility test isolator. (Courtesy of Isotech Designs, Montreal, Canada.)

proaches zero. Considering the economics of a false positive (lot failure), the costs are acceptable.

The monitoring of the air in isolators and overfilling lines in barrier systems (as well as in other locations) has been addressed best by Oxborrow [23]. My opinion has been that the use of settling plates (passive monitoring) is unacceptable and that any of the active sampling methods (centrifugal sampling, cascade impaction, liquid impingement) are preferable. Whyte's most recent arguments to the contrary [24] are persuasive but lack information on standard deviation. Airborne microbial counts monitored with settling plates and active samplers such as STA would be a most welcome addition to the literature assessed by pharmaceutical manufacturers.

Regardless of how the monitoring of air is done using published methods, the organisms must grow out overnight. The assumption has been that vegetative organisms trapped on a membrane filter in an air stream are desiccated and nonviable because they do not grow when placed on nutrient agar or other solid media. However, in light of the literature on dormant organisms [25], it is possible that air-dried organisms on filters are reproductively inactive on solid media but stain as viable cells (see Sec. 8). If that is the case, and if air stream–dried vegetative cells (trapped on a membrane filter) can be resuscitated with liquid medium, it follows that rapid aerosol monitoring can be done by a suitable stain of viable cells captured on a membrane filter. This study should be done because it would make possible the microbial evaluation of air within an hour or less of sampling rather than overnight. The method should also be less expensive and amenable to automation.

Very recent work [26] should revive interest in gelatin membranes, which appear to be as effective as the slit-to-agar (STA) sampler for the collection and enumeration of airborne bacteria. STA samplers as presently configured are not suitable for placement in isolators and under laminar flow lines; filters are more adaptable in this regard (in my opinion).

7 IDENTIFICATION OF ORGANISMS

For products terminally sterilized in the final container, a positive sterility test likely means contamination during testing, unless the sterilization cycle, or the closure of the final container, has failed. If the sterility test is not done in an isolator, a positive test may be due to a staphylococcus or other skin organism from sterility test personnel or people in filling or manufacturing. If the contaminant is random (i.e., one organism on a particle that has impinged into a single vial on the filling line) and from the surface of equipment, it may be a *Bacillus* sp. spore. Therefore, the identity of the organism provides critical clues as to the source.

My preference is to identify any such organism in an automated system such as the Microbial Identification System (MIS), a computer-interfaced gas chromatograph (GC) manufactured by Hewlett-Packard (Avondale, PA) and marketed by Microbial Identification Inc. (MIDI, Newark, DE). Units are presently being used within the U.S. pharmaceutical industry and in the U.S. FDA. These machines reliably identify the organisms according to fatty acid composition (Figs. 4 and 5). Although such devices are limited by the contents of their libraries, the libraries are updated periodically as a service of the vendor. For reliable identifications, the organisms must be grown under standardized conditions [27, 28]. A unique advantage of or-

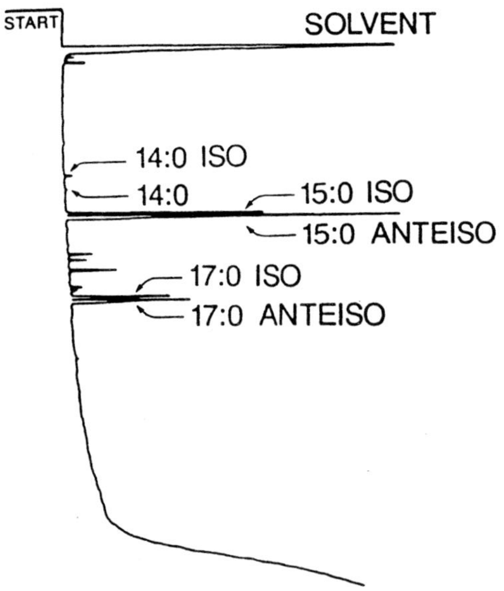

Figure 4 MIS gas chromatogram for *Bacillus subtilis* ATCC 6051. (From Ref. 27.)

HP 5998A: MICROBIAL IDENTIFICATION SYSTEM (Rev: 2.1) (Sw s/n: 2710A10107) (Hw s/n: 2612615

ID: 2 BACI SUBT ATCC 6051 Date of run: 16-OCT-
Bottle: 2 SAMPLE [AEROBE]

RT	Area	Ar/Ht	Respon	ECL	Name	%	Comment 1	Comment 2
1.569	38549000	0.077	. . .	7.014	SOLVENT PEAK	. . .	< min rt	
1.930	814	0.025	. . .	7.751	. . . .	. . .	< min rt	
2.140	1862	0.026	. . .	8.180	. . . .	. . .	< min rt	
6.561	1424	0.044	0.995	13.618	14:0 ISO	1.15	ECL deviates 0.000	Reference -0.003
7.074	696	0.042	0.983	13.999	14:0	0.55	ECL deviates -0.001	Reference -0.004
8.023	26247	0.040	0.967	14.623	15:0 ISO	20.54	ECL deviates 0.002	Reference 0.000
8.160	51544	0.041	0.965	14.713	15:0 ANTEISO	40.24	ECL deviates 0.002	Reference 0.000
9.627	3513	0.043	0.946	15.625	16:0 ISO	2.69	ECL deviates -0.001	Reference -0.002
9.844	2782	0.044	0.944	15.757	16:1 A	2.13	ECL deviates -0.000	
10.241	7036	0.044	0.941	15.998	16:0	5.36	ECL deviates -0.002	Reference -0.004
10.910	1904	0.045	0.936	16.389	17:1 ISO E	1.44	ECL deviates 0.002	
11.063	1418	0.049	0.935	16.478	Sum In Feature 5 . .	1.07	ECL deviates 0.002	17:1 ISO I/ANTEI B
11.323	14499	0.045	0.933	16.630	17:0 ISO	10.95	ECL deviates 0.001	Reference -0.002
11.481	17705	0.045	0.932	16.722	17:0 ANTEISO	13.35	ECL deviates 0.000	Reference -0.002
13.702	720	0.049	0.925	18.000	18:0	0.54	ECL deviates 0.000	Reference -0.006
*******	1418	. . .	. . .	. . .	SUMMED FEATURE 5 . .	1.07	17:1 ISO I/ANTEI B	17:1 ANTEISO B/i I

Solvent Ar	Total Area	Named Area	% Named	Total Amnt	Nbr Ref	ECL Deviation	Ref ECL Shift
38549000	129488	129488	100.00	123576	9	0.001	0.003

TSBA [Rev 2.0] Bacillus 0.602
B. subtilis 0.602

Figure 5 MIS printout, identifying an organism under test. (From Ref. 27.)

ganism identification by GC is that libraries for particular bacterial strains can be developed by the tester [29].

In most instances, strain identification would not be required of a parenterals manufacturer. However, since microbial contaminants in the final container will become increasingly rare, it would make good sense to freeze a sample for future reference. For example, if *Staphylococcus aureus* appears repeatedly, strain analysis may be the best means of determining who in manufacturing or in microbiological QC is consistently contaminating the product. This is not a matter of assigning blame but of correcting a fault.

8 DAMAGED ORGANISMS

An operating assumption of the USP, BP, and other sterility tests is that some organisms may not grow in the test media. The organisms of greatest concern to me and many others active in this area are not those species that tend not to replicate in TSB or FTM but those damaged by steam, sterilizing gases, or other agents, because they may be present as biofilms on the equipment (e.g., the moving belt that carries vials to the filling machine). Anderson et al. [30] examined the disinfection of PVC pipes (which are uncommon in pharmaceutical manufacturing, but their findings are nevertheless germane). *Pseudomonas aeruginosa* and *P. pickettii* embedded themselves into glycocalyces and resisted iodophors and phenolic disinfectants.

Organisms immersed in purified water or drinking water (and water for injection) tend, over a week or less, to lose their ability to replicate on solid media, but they remain viable. Recoverable plate counts on various solid media decline with time at 20–25°C for gram-negative and gram-positive genera (other than *Bacillus* and *Pseudomonas*) although the cells react with some dyes as do viable organisms [25]. Similar results have been obtained with monochloramine-damaged organisms in biofilms [31].

The exceptions (pseudomonads and genus *Bacillus*) noted by Byrd et al. [25] do not pose a detection problem. Pseudomonads grow to 10^6 CFU/mL in high purity water, and *Bacillus* species survive as spores; see the data in Gee et al. [16].

However, in the harsh conditions imposed by modern cleaning agents and steam-in-place operations, spores also are damaged, usually with lethal consequence but not always. Over an extended time, damaged or dormant organisms may resuscitate in liquid media [32], in which case they will be detected by the sterility test if it is protracted. The inference of the bulk of the literature is that where surfaces are examined, as with Rodac plates, damaged or dormant starved vegetative organisms may be inapparent. If there is an issue, in the main it is likely with the surfaces of manufacturing equipment and with medical devices. Discovery of such organisms must relate to the type of testing that is done and incubation time and conditions [3].

The phenomenon has been shown with e-beam-irradiated foodstuffs (parsley, deboned poultry meat, liquid egg white) under conditions that are clearly insufficient for sterilization by pharmaceutical industry standards but that are instructive. Viable counts with the AO technique on membrane filters were consistently higher by several orders of magnitude than aerobic plate counts [33].

Presumably, this phenomenon is not an issue with regard to the sterility of injectable products. For example, organisms that might dislodge from biofilms in WFI systems are likely to be killed in the tanks because WFI tanks are maintained at 60–80°C. Biofilms in drop lines, which most of the time are deadlegs, may be an issue (however, most firms steam out the entire WFI distribution system at least once per week and keep deadlegs very short, so that may not be an issue of consequence either).

Organisms on the surface of sterility test isolators or on filling line equipment in barrier systems are, we trust, killed and not merely damaged by vapor-phase hydrogen peroxide, peracetic acid, or chlorine dioxide. We know this where such systems are validated to a 6 log kill with the appropriate indicator organism. However, wherever surfaces or liquids are monitored as aerobic plate counts, the numbers of viable organisms can be severely underestimated. This may include the evaluation of the colony-forming units as standard plate counts in rinse water from pipes or tanks following cleaning and sterilization procedures.

Where plate counts are used to evaluate the cleaning and sterilization of equipment, I recommend supplementary studies with acridine orange on membrane-filtered liquid rinses or extracts.

9 VALIDATION

The sterility test system must be shown to be sensitive to as few as 100 viable organisms using the organisms listed in Table 2, and the results must be statistically significant. This is both a growth promotion test of the media and a test of one's methods. It is my recommendation (and a frequent practice in the industry) that the sensitivity of the test be shown for as few as 10 or so organisms. Therefore, one should validate a sterility test system at high and low levels of inoculum with the organisms listed in Table 2.

For valid test results, the organisms must be freshly harvested and their numbers estimated quickly. Growth of the aerobes is best done in TSB at 25°C with a harvest at 18–24 h and estimation of cell numbers by light scattering or another rapid method for which one has prepared a standard curve by logarithmic dilution and plating on or in nutrient agar. My preference is to centrifuge the cells and resuspend them in sterile PBS. To this end, a calibration curve of absorbance or other light measurement versus cell number as determined by plate count must be established well in advance of the sterility test validations. Barber [34] offers a practical outline of optical and Coulter-type methods. One wants to know the standard deviation that obtains in recovering 10 viable microbes from a freshly harvested cell suspension. Accordingly, the minimum number of replicates for the standard curve

Table 2 Test Microbes for the Validation of Growth Promotion

Medium	Microorganism[a]	Incubation *T* (°C)	Incubation O_2 or not
Fluid thioglycollate[b]	*Micrococcus luteus* ATCC 9341	30–35	Aerobic
	Candida albicans ATCC 10231	30–35	Aerobic
	Clostridium sporogenes ATCC 11437	30–35	Anaerobic
Soybean casein digest[c]	*Bacillus subtilis* ATCC 6633	20–25	Aerobic
	Candida albicans ATCC 10231	20–25	Aerobic
	Aspergillus niger ATCC 16404	20–25	Aerobic

[a]All microorganisms are available from the American Type Culture Collection, 12301 Parklawn Drive, Rockville, MD 20852. Note that the strict anaerobe *Bacteroides vulgatus* ATCC 8482 is not listed and that *Aspergillus niger* ATCC 16404 is included.
[b]Referred to in the text as FTM.
[c]Referred to in the text as TSB (trypticase soy broth).

should be 5, with 10 preferred. The validation containers should be incubated until obvious turbidity is demonstrated, or for 14 days.

10 PARAMETRIC RELEASE

Halls [2] has some useful comments on parametric release and notes that gamma-irradiated products have not been sterility tested for 20 years. He also makes the point that where a process is thoroughly understood, validated, and documented (e.g., steam sterilization) and the equipment is modern and fully controlled, parametric release should be an acceptable objective.

A thoroughly characterized and reliable process for the sterilization of product will be more reliable and useful than end product sterility testing, which, in my view, is antiquated and sufficiently insensitive as to be pointless in a properly run operation. The statistical pointlessness of the test when the contamination level is low has been known for around 50 years [35]. If 0.1% of a batch is contaminated, using 100 samples the probability of detecting the contamination using the USP sterility test is about 0.1.

I anticipate that contamination levels will drop below 0.01% in the near future when the use of barrier-associated filling systems becomes widespread. Even with 1000 samples, the probability of detecting the contamination using the USP sterility test is about 0.1. Where contamination levels are consistently low, the test is a waste of time, money, and skilled labor.

I suggest that the U.S. FDA, MCA, and other regulatory groups dangle a carrot (approval of parametric release) as a compelling incentive to the truly thorough characterization, validation, and documentation of the sterilization process. This is worth considering because the U.S. FDA is a magnificent watchdog, and, in the absence of that almost extrasensory canine conscience, the proposal would be most inappropriate. However, the sterility test should be continued as an end product evaluation of those items that do not have a satisfactory history of absence of sterility test failures.

REFERENCES

1. Olson, W. P. (1987). Sterility testing, in *Aseptic Drug Manufacturing, Technology for the 1990s* (W. P. Olson and M. J. Groves, eds.), Interpharm Press, Buffalo Grove, IL.
2. Halls, N. A. (1994). *Achieving Sterility in Medical and Pharmaceutical Products*, Marcel Dekker, New York.
3. Olson, W. P. (1996). The fourteen-day sterility test: How we got there [Letter to the Editor], *PDA J. Pharm. Sci. Technol.*, *50*(4):198.
4. Gee, L. A., J. M. G. H. Harvey, W. P. Olson, and M. L. Lee. (1985). Sterility test systems for product recovery, *J. Pharm. Sci.*, *74*:29–32.
5. Pickett, M., and W. Litsky. (1981). An effective alternative for testing antibiotic sterility, *Pharm. Technol.*, *5*(5):63–68.
6. Koppensteiner, G. (1976). A new test system for the proof of sterility of pharmaceuticals, *Drugs Made in Germany*, *19*:45–49.
7. Hecker, W., and J. Lukac. (1981). The sterility testing of small volume ampoules with a reusable holder for direct incubation, *CONCEPT Symposium* 12/8–9. English language translations are available from Sartorius GmbH, Gottingen, Germany.

8. Tsuchido, T., Y.-H. Ahn, and M. Takano. (1987). Lysis of *Bacillus subtilis* cells by glycerol and sucrose esters of fatty acids, *Appl. Environ. Microbiol.*, *53*:505–508.
9. Placencia, A. M., G. S. Oxborrow, and J. W. Danielson. (1982). *J. Pharm. Sci.*, *71*: 704–705.
10. Murray, P. R., and M. J. Sandrock. (1991). Sterility testing of a total nutrient admixture with a biphasic blood-culture system, *Am. J. Hosp. Pharm.*, *48*:2419–2421.
11. Besajew, C. (1992). Importance of incubation time in the test for sterility, *Pharmazeut. Ind.*, *54*:539–542.
12. Bathgate, H., D. Lazzari, H. Cameron, and D. McKay. (1993). The incubation period in sterility testing, *J. Parenter. Sci. Technol.*, *47*:254–257.
13. Tsuchido, T., K. Kanda, and I. Shibasaki. (1975). Enhancement of sporicidal activity of an amphoteric surfactant by heating, *J. Ferment. Technol.*, *53*:862–868.
14. Akers, J. E., J. P. Agalloco, and C. M. Kennedy. (1995). Experience in the design and use of isolator systems for sterility testing, *PDA J. Pharm. Sci. Technol.*, *49*:140–144.
15. Christensen, E. A., C. H. Mordhorst, and O. B. Jepsen. (1992). Assessment of risk of microbial contamination by use of multidose containers of injectable products, *J. Hosp. Infect.*, *20*:310–304.
16. Gee, L. A., R. Zeiner, and W. P. Olson. (1986). Membrane filter sterility test of antihemophilic factor, *Pharm. Res.*, *3*, 364–365.
17. Cormio, L., J. Vuopio-Varkile, A. Siitonen, M. Talja, and M. Ruutu. (1996). Bacterial adhesion and biofilm formation on various double-J stents *in vivo* and *in vitro*, *Scand. J. Urol. Nephrol.*, *30*:19–24.
18. d'Arbeloff, N. C., S. Rusmin, and D. Stack. (1991). Robotic applications in sterility testing, in *Sterile Pharmaceutical Manufacturing, Applications for the 1990s*, Vol. 2 (M. J. Groves, W. P. Olson, and M. H. Anisfeld, eds.), Interpharm, Buffalo Grove, IL.
19. Oles, P., B. St. Martin, J. Teillon, D. Meyer, and C. Picard. (1987). Isolator technology for manufacturing and quality control, in *Aseptic Pharmaceutical Manufacturing, Technology for the 1990s* (W. P. Olson and M. J. Groves, eds.), Interpharm Press, Buffalo Grove, IL.
20. Walker, N., and J. Wilkins. (1994). Case study: Evans Medical, Proceeding of the Barrier Isolation Technology Seminar, Int. Soc. Pharm. Eng., Philadelphia.
21. Jeng, D. K., and A. G. Woodworth. (1990). Chlorine dioxide gas sterilization under square-wave conditions, *Appl. Environ. Microbiol.*, *56*:514–519.
22. Davenport, S. M. (1989). Design and use of a novel peracetic acid sterilizer for absolute barrier sterility testing chambers, *J. Parenter. Sci. Technol.*, *43*:158–166.
23. Oxborrow, G. S. (1996). Quantitation of aerosolized organisms, in *Automated Microbial Identification and Quantitation* (W. P. Olson, ed.), Interpharm, Buffalo Grove, IL.
24. Whyte, W. (1996). In support of settle plates, *PDA J. Pharm. Sci. Technol.*, *50*(4): 201–204.
25. Byrd, J. J., H.-S. Xu, and R. R. Colwell. (1991). Viable but nonculturable bacteria in drinking water, *Appl. Environ. Microbiol.*, *57*:875–878.
26. Parks, S. R., A. M. Bennett, S. E. Speight, and J. E. Benbough. (1996). An assessment of the Sartorius MD8 microbiological air sampler, *J. Appl. Bacteriol.*, *80*:529–534.
27. Olson, W. P. (1992). Targeted drug delivery based on the mode of action of bacille Calmette-Guerin in bladder cancer, Ph.D. Dissertation, Univ. Illinois at Chicago.
28. Olson, W. P., M. J. Groves, and M. E. Klegerman. (1989). Fatty acids of *Mycobacterium bovis* BCG, *Mircobios*, *57*:151–155.
29. Smith, A. R. (1995). Cellular fatty acid analysis for classification and identification of bacteria, with emphasis on the genus *Bacillus*, in *Automated Microbial Identification and Quantitation* (W. P. Olson, ed.), Interpharm, Buffalo Grove, IL.
30. Anderson, R. L., B. W. Holland, J. K. Carr, W. W. Bond, and M. S. Favero. (1990). Effect of disinfectants on pseudomonads colonized on the interior surface of PVC pipes, *Am. J. Publ. Health*, *80*:17–21.

31. Stewart, P. S., T. Briebe, R. Srinivasan, C.-T. Chen, E. P. Yu, D. deBeer, and G. A. McFeters. (1994). Comparison of respiratory activity and culturability during monochloramine disinfection of binary population biofilms, *Appl. Environ. Microbiol.*, *60*: 1690–1692.
32. Magarinos, B., J. L. Romalde, J. L. Barja, and A. E. Toranzo. (1994). Evidence of a dormant but infective state of the fish pathogen *Pasteurella piscicida* in seawater and sediment, *Appl. Environ. Microbiol.*, *60*:180–186.
33. Copin, M.-P., D. Jehanno, and C. M., Bourgeois. (1993). Detection of irradiated deep-frozen foodstuffs by comparison of DEFT and APC counts, *J. Appl. Bacteriol.*, *75*: 254–258.
34. Barber, T. (1996). Optical methods for the estimation of microbial populations, in *Automated Microbial Identification and Quantitation* (W. P. Olson, ed.), Interpharm, Buffalo Grove, IL.
35. Knudsen, L. F. (1949). Sample size of parenteral solutions for sterility testing, *J. Am. Pharm. Assoc.*, *38*:332–337.

24

New Membrane-Based Technologies for the Pharmaceutical Industry

TONY ALEX and HOLLY HAUGHNEY
Pall Corporation, Port Washington, New York

1 INTRODUCTION

The intent of this chapter is to introduce new membrane filter technologies that can be employed in the pharmaceutical industry. Two of the technologies considered employ high shear devices for solid–liquid separations. The information on the high shear devices primarily is in reference to the DMF[1] dynamic membrane filter system and the PallSep[1] VMF vibrating membrane filter system. The DMF system's design employs a rotating disk to provide high shear; the PallSep VMF system uses vibration at the membrane surface for generation of high shear.

Another unique filtration application, the use of a single-pass membrane filter that can be backwashed (flow is reversed for contaminant removal) in solid–liquid separations, is also described.

2 HIGH SHEAR, SOLID–LIQUID MEMBRANE SEPARATION DEVICES

Both vibrating membrane technology (VMT) and the rotating disk membrane technology (RDMT) systems are membrane separation systems that operate with feed, bleed (retentate), and permeate (filtrate) streams. The difference between these devices and traditional crossflow devices such as cassette, spiral-wound, and tubular membrane configurations is that the retentate stream is not used for the generation of shear at the membrane surface. The retentate in the VMT and RDMT systems is

[1]DMF and PallSep VMF are trademarks of Pall Corporation.

used for fluid distribution across the membrane surface. The shear is created mechanically instead of by moving the fluid at a high crossflow, by vibration for VMT and rotating disk for RDMT. The shear rates for the RDMT (200,000–300,000 s^{-1}) and VMT (~100,000 s^{-1}) are considerably higher than for traditional crossflow devices, which can provide higher, more stable permeate flow rates and better product transmission.

Shear rate at the membrane surface for any membrane device will depend on fluid properties such as viscosity. For static crossflow devices, the shear rate is directly proportional to the fluid velocity and inversely proportional to the height of the channel. For both the VMT and RDMT systems the shear rate will have a radial profile across the membrane, with higher shear rates at the outer diameter, where the maximum membrane area is. The shear rate at the surface of the membrane in the VMT system is influenced by the amplitude and frequency of the oscillation. The angular velocity of the spinning disk influences the shear rate at the surface of the RDMT membrane.

The VMT and RDMT systems can be used in a variety of applications in pharmaceutical processing. These devices will outperform traditional crossflow membranes; however, if a traditional filtration method is able to meet both the economic and performance requirements for an application, then the high shear devices are probably not appropriate. High shear units can be considered if traditional techniques are not meeting performance requirements or too much membrane area is required for their use to be economical. RDMT or VMT can also be considered if a centrifuge or a system requiring a filter aid (such as a rotary vacuum filter) is used or being considered for an application. The VMT and RDMT systems can offer process benefits over these technologies also. A description of operation and some examples of performance for the VMT and RDMT separation systems are provided in the following sections. Comparisons of the performance with the more traditional technologies are also addressed.

3 VIBRATING MEMBRANE TECHNOLOGY SYSTEM

3.1 Description of System Operation

The vibrating membrane filter design effectively employs vibrational energy for better performance than traditional filtration-based separation processes. Flux (liters per square meter per hour), capacity (liters processed between cleaning cycles per square meter); and concentration factor achieved (ratio of feed volume to final retentate volume) are typically higher with the VMT system than with traditional crossflow systems.

Vibrating membrane filter systems use an oscillating disk filter stack vibrating at ≈60 Hz about a vertical axis. This type of design is described in a U.S. patent (Culkin, 1990). The filter stack moves back and forth with a vibrational frequency F (≈60 Hz) and vibrational peak-to-peak amplitude A (typically 0.5–1.0 in.). The oscillatory driving forces are provided by a torsion spring system. The oscillation, or vibration, is employed to provide a shear at the membrane surface that prevents fouling of the membrane. Figure 1 illustrates a full system setup; Figure 2 illustrates the mechanical components of the system.

The torsional spring–mass system consists of two masses connected by a torsion spring (Fig. 3). If one of the masses (mass A in Fig. 3) is rotated slightly in

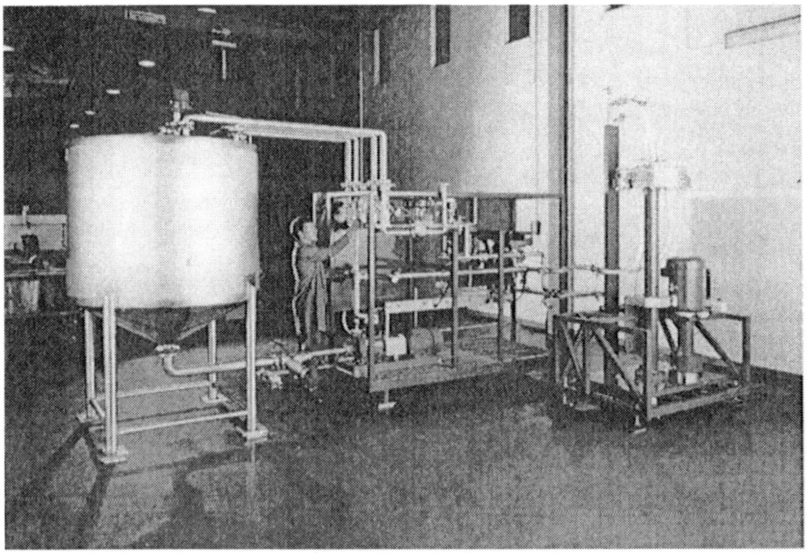

Figure 1 Full PallSep VMF system. (Courtesy of Pall Corporation.)

one direction, then the other mass will move in the opposite direction. This occurs because the torsion spring is "twisted" by the motion of the mass A. The twisted spring will exert a torque on mass B in the opposite direction. To create an oscillation of the masses, one of the masses is rotated back and forth with a specific amplitude, and this motion is translated through the torsion spring to the second mass. The motion is an angular simple harmonic motion.

For example, if the two masses have the same moment of inertia, then the amplitude of the motion and frequency of oscillation of each mass will be the same. One mass would, however, lag the other by a 180° phase. This oscillation of the masses requires that there exist a point on the spring where there is no torsional motion. For the above example, this point of no motion, or node, is at a location on the torsion bar that is equidistant from the two masses as depicted in Fig. 4.

The size, shape, and weight of the masses are important, because the equation of motion for this type of harmonic motion depends on the mass moment of inertia. A system such as this would be governed by the equation

$$\nu = \frac{1}{2\pi}\left[\kappa\left(\frac{1}{J_1} + \frac{1}{J_2}\right)\right]^{1/2} \tag{1}$$

where ν is the frequency of the oscillation, J_1 and J_2 are the mass moments of inertia of the masses, and κ is the torsional spring constant. The spring constant depends on the specific material properties and geometry of the torsion bar. The ratio of amplitudes of the two masses is inversely related to the ratio of their mass moment of inertia:

$$\frac{J_1}{J_2} = \frac{A_2}{A_1} \tag{2}$$

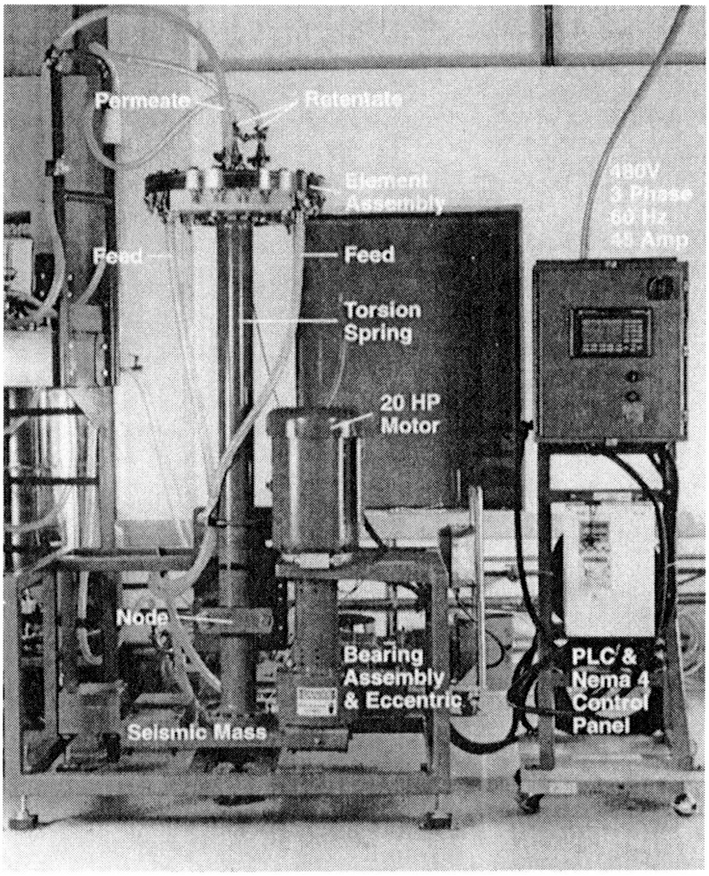

Figure 2 Mechanical components of the VMF system.

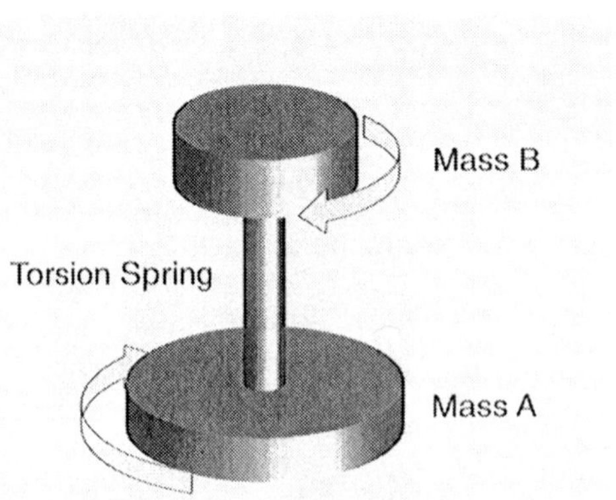

Figure 3 Torsion spring and mass design.

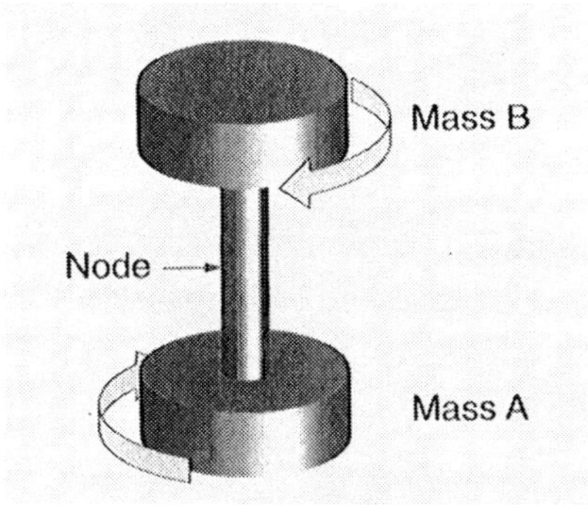

Mass A Moment of Inertia = Mass B Moment of Inertia

Figure 4 Torsion spring with masses that have equal mass moments of inertia.

In the case of the vibrating membrane filter unit torsion spring and mass design, the actual torsion spring and the two masses are indicated in Fig. 5. The mass at the bottom is the seismic mass, and the mass at the top of the torsion spring (or torsion bar) is the membrane assembly.

The goal of the design is to maximize the amplitude for the membrane element assembly to provide shear at the membrane surface. Thus, from Eq. (2), the seismic mass is designed to have a much larger moment of inertia than the membrane pack, so that the amplitude of the seismic mass is a minimum when the membrane assembly is at its operational amplitude.

To initiate and maintain the oscillatory motion, the spring must be excited. An alternating current (ac) motor controlled by a variable-frequency solid-state speed controller is used to produce the excitation in the following way. The ac motor spins an eccentric weight attached to the seismic mass. This weight is illustrated in Fig. 6; the weight is circular and has more mass on one side. The eccentricity of the mass causes a wobble, and the motion is translated to the seismic mass. The motion of the seismic mass increases as the ac motor speed increases. The objective is to keep the motion in the *xy* plane (back-and-forth motion of the seismic mass instead of an up-and-down motion). The design and supports for the seismic mass ensure that there is a maximum transfer of energy to the *xy* plane. The entire system rides on isolators to allow for free movement and prevent undesired motions. A U.S. patent describes the eccentric drive mechanism design (Culkin, 1991).

The energy from the movement of the seismic mass is translated through the torsion spring to the membrane pack. The membrane pack moves at a frequency 180° out of phase with the seismic mass. As the ac motor speed approaches the resonant frequency, the amplitude of the membrane pack reaches a useful maximum. A further increase in the ac motor speed once the membrane pack maximum amplitude is reached will cause a decrease in the membrane pack amplitude. Figure 7 illustrates the relationship between amplitude and frequency.

The vibrating membrane filter system is designed to operate below the maximum amplitude to reduce the stress to the torsion spring and to allow for a long spring life. The amplitude used is typically ¾ in., and the frequency is about 60 Hz.

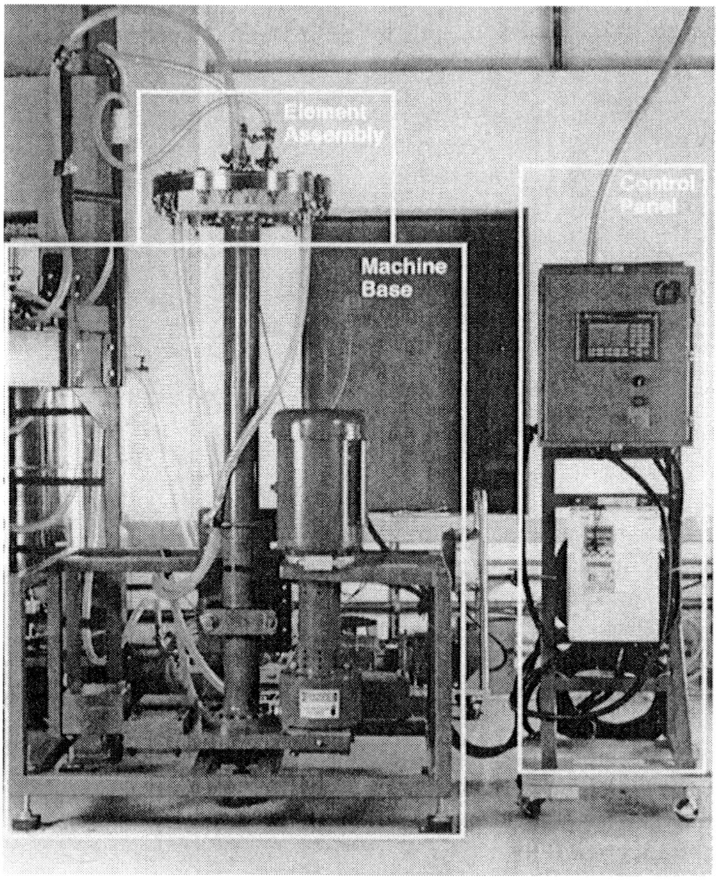

Figure 5 PallSep VMF unit torsion spring and masses.

3.2 Membrane Assembly

The filter pack is a set of circular disks with open channel spaces between them. The open channel is an essential feature that enables the fluid to remain stagnant; the introduction of any protuberance (for example, a screen for spacing) in the upstream fluid area would cause the bulk fluid to move, thus dampening this spring system.

The torsional vibration of the membrane filter pack with static fluid allows for the existence of a shear focused area at the membrane surface that retards the plugging of the membrane. Essentially all the shear is developed at the critical membrane/fluid interface. The membrane disks move back and forth while the bulk fluid is relatively stagnant. This is akin to the cup and saucer remaining on the table when the magician rapidly pulls the tablecloth from under it. Shear is developed at the interface of the moving membrane and the relatively stagnant fluid. Since all the vibrational energy is focused on the separation interface, very little energy is lost to the bulk fluid.

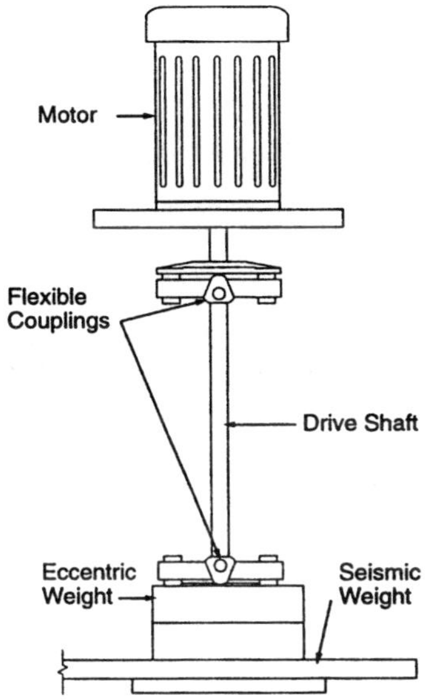

Figure 6 AC motor, eccentric mass, and seismic assembly.

Foulants are repelled at the membrane surface so that the desired material can penetrate the membrane at a high flow rate. The operation has feed, permeate, and retentate streams. The crossflow is not required for shear but is needed for fluid distribution. The flow pattern at the membrane surface is illustrated in Fig. 8.

The membrane assembly is essentially a set of flat disks separated by spacers at inner and outer locations. The entire disk pack is firmly mounted between two endplates that serve the functions of providing a pressure boundary, provide a site to attach the filter pack to the torsion bar, and provide for feed, permeate, and retentate piping connections. Each disk has membrane on both sides, so the space encapsulated by the two membranes defines the downstream side and the space provided by the interspersed spacers provides the upstream channel.

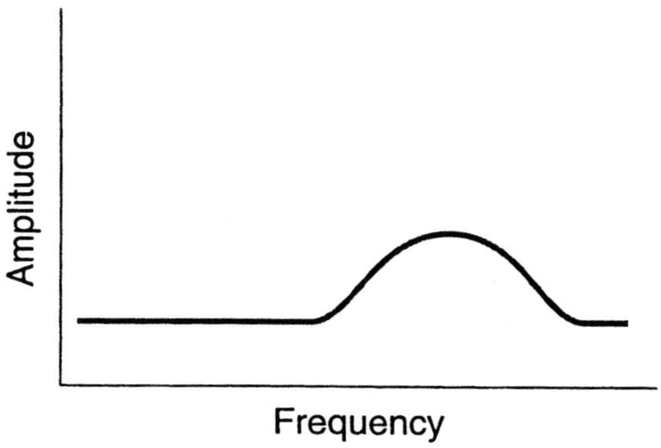

Figure 7 Amplitude–frequency relationship.

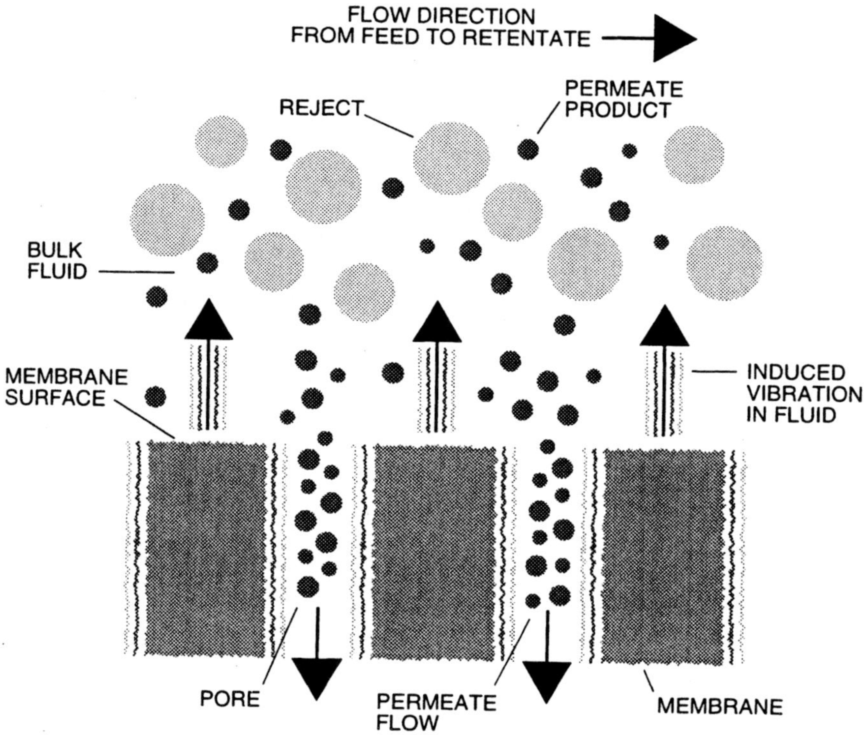

Figure 8 Flow pattern at membrane surface.

Standard membrane area in a membrane assembly is 40 m^2. However, the limitations to adding disks or membrane area are governed purely by the spring characteristics of the torsional spring system as defined by Eq. (1). Addition of more disks will cause J_1 to increase, causing the frequency (ν) to decrease. Hence by reducing the operational frequency (less shear) it would be possible to double the membrane area on a given spring system, or by increasing the spring constant it would be possible to double the membrane area.

Flow through the membrane assembly occurs when fluid is pumped to the feed ports on the bottom endplate. The feed is delivered to the first element through a feed distribution channel inside the bottom endplate of the membrane assembly. The feed is distributed to the membrane surface by distribution through feed openings on the outer diameter of each disk. There must be enough feed openings present to allow for a good distribution of flow across the membrane surface. The flow then moves radially inward toward the retentate openings located near the inner diameter of the disks. The fluid permeates the membrane and exits through the top end-plate permeate port. These are illustrated in Fig. 9.

The material rejected by the membrane is retained on the upstream side and becomes the retentate. The retentate flow and feed flow are directed up through the various disks of the element assembly. Ultimately flow is directed to the top of the membrane assembly, and concentrated material leaves the element assembly through the two retentate ports on the top endplate. Figure 10 shows a possible flow pattern

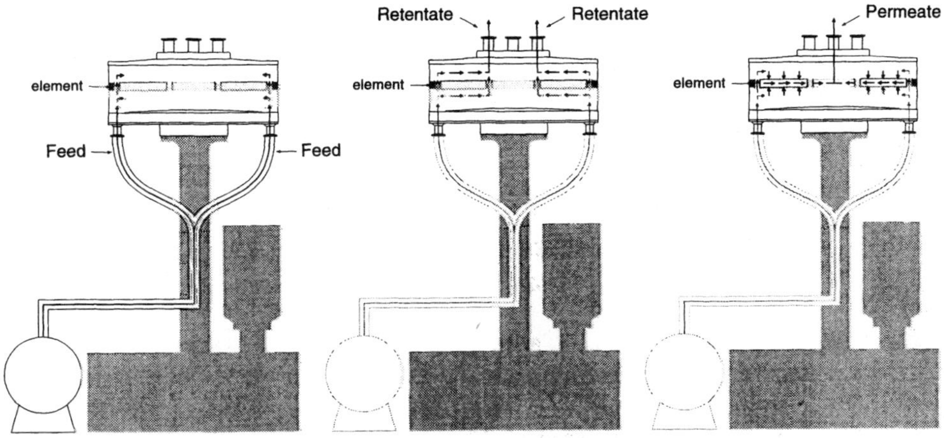

Figure 9 Illustration of flows in the membrane element assembly.

through the assembly. In this case all the disks are in parallel operation. It is possible to have a serial–parallel combination of the flow path.

Since the shear required for filtration is provided purely by the torsion spring assembly and is independent of the feed flow, independent control of system pressure and operational shear rate is possible. Decoupling the shear from the feed velocity has several benefits, the predominant one being that a large retentate-to-permeate ratio is not required for the proper operation of the system and thus a higher concentration can be achieved.

Moreover, since the shear rate is independent of feed velocity and the disks are open channel by design, upstream pressure drop (the pressure differential between the feed and retentate loops) is very low, usually on the order of a few pounds per square inch; thus fairly viscous fluids can be filtered. The device is an ideal concentrator.

Since the shear at the membrane surface is determined solely by the oscillation, it can be changed as desired without affecting the filter pack and the filtration process. Furthermore, due to the nature of the design there is the capability of generating shear an order of magnitude higher than that of conventional filtration devices.

The technology has the capability of using different types of membranes of the same geometry. It is possible to use this configuration to conduct microporous, ultrafiltration, and nanofiltration separations. The lack of solid rotating disks and a membrane pack designed with minimum hold-up volume permit a very high packing density.

The membrane material used for most pharmaceutical applications is a microporous PTFE. This nonstick material has been used for a variety of fluids, and in most cases the membrane provides stable fluxes over an extended time period with minimal cleaning (for example, a hot water flush between batches). The PTFE membrane has also demonstrated complete permeate flow recovery if there is a process interruption (stoppage of flow or vibration).

Energy draw for the system is predominantly determined by the shear generated, which is in turn primarily governed by two factors: vibrational frequency (F, Hz) and vibrational amplitude (A, in.). Typical energy draw is 0.03–0.15 kW/m^2

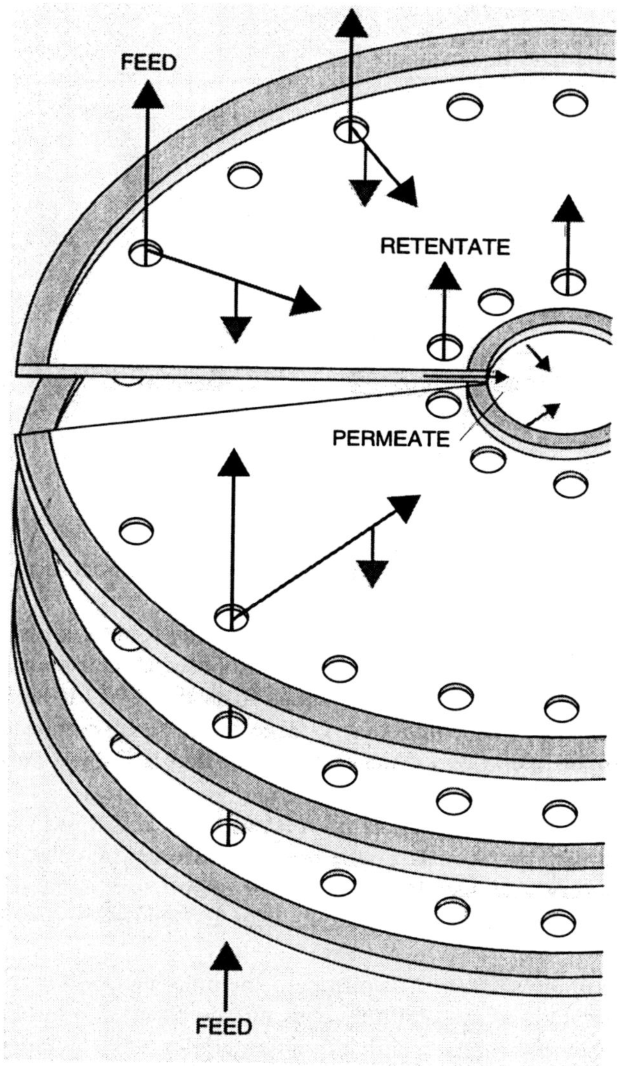

Figure 10 Flow pattern between the elements.

(0.004–0.019 hp/ft^2. A device of 40 m^2 membrane area usually draws less than 5 kW.

Low energy input requirements coupled with the high membrane area in the membrane filter pack makes this technology competitive for both low solids applications, which are typically handled by static crossflow systems, and high solids applications, which cannot be handled by static crossflow systems and are usually handled by centrifuges and filtration systems that use a filter aid precoat (rotary vacuum filters, for example).

3.3 Scale-Up for VMT System

Since the membrane assembly is constructed of a modular disk–spacer combination, the vibrating membrane filter system can be tested with one element or multiple elements. The single element can be used for feasibility testing, and multiple elements are intended for scaled-up pilot tests and actual processes. Testing indicates that scale-up is linear. A full-scale assembly is illustrated in Fig. 11. Another important point about the scale-up is that the optimization tests often required for traditional crossflow systems for the determination of the operating parameters (such as differential pressure, transmembrane pressure, and crossflow rate) are not required for VMT.

The general recommendation of vibrating membrane filter feasibility tests is that they be operated at the maximum allowable amplitude and the lowest possible pressure. As with all membrane-based technologies, there may be a need to optimize the membrane to meet the required effluent quality.

3.4 VMT Versus Traditional Crossflow Systems

To understand how the high shear devices compare with the traditional crossflow technologies, a comparison of the vibrating membrane filter and crossflow systems is given here.

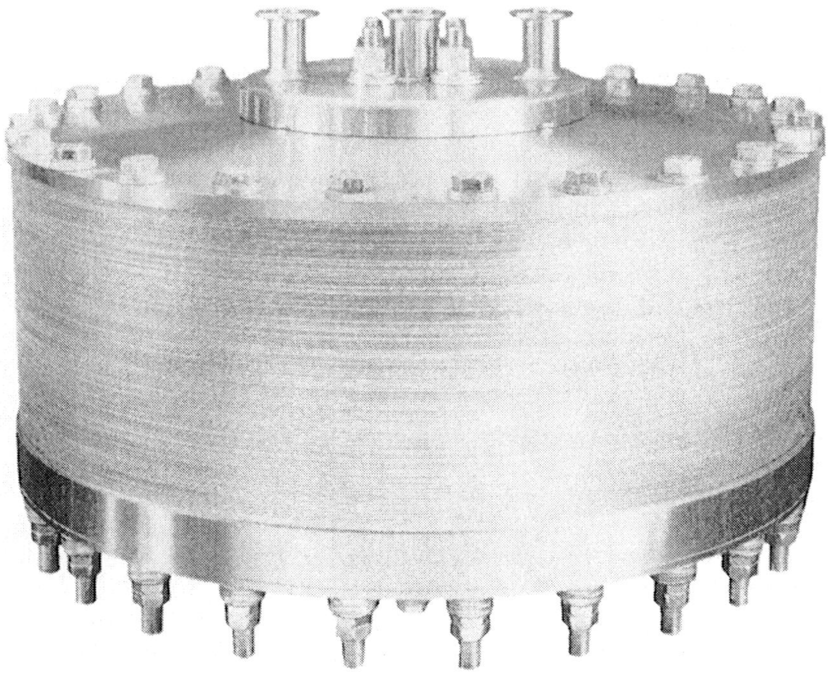

Figure 11 Full-scale element assembly. (Courtesy of Pall Corporation.)

A core difference between the technologies is the purpose of the crossflow. For the traditional static crossflow devices, such as a spiral wound filter shear is generated by the feed velocity, whereas for the VMT system (also for the RDMT system) the feed velocity is used to distribute the fluid on the upstream side of the membrane.

Since the shear in the VMT system is generated by mechanical means, the shear rate is independent of feed velocity and hence the pumping rate. A lower pumping rate will save energy costs and can improve product yield for cases in which the material can be damaged by the action of a high speed recirculation.

A high feed velocity for shear development means that a significant pressure gradient can develop between the inlet and the outlet (from feed to retentate). Such pressure gradients can affect the performance of the membrane and cause fouling. The vibrating membrane filter system can be operated in an essentially uniform transmembrane pressure (TMP) mode. This phenomenon is very valuable in microfiltration because differences in the TMP cause different parts of the membrane to experience different loadings, leading to premature fouling in some areas of the membrane. Premature fouling of the membrane can lead to severe difficulties in subsequent membrane regeneration.

Small gap sizes are required in spiral wound crossflow systems to achieve high velocity and thus a high shear. This is not the case in a VMT system. This independence of gap width promotes flexibility in choosing the appropriate gap width. This is particularly advantageous when the solids loading in the fluid is high.

Since the fluid velocity is not critical, the ratio of permeate to feed can be much better controlled in a vibrating membrane filter system than in a crossflow system. This improved control usually results in the ability to attain higher concentration factors. The energy consumed by the system is focused on the filtration regions and is not wasted in recirculating vast amounts of fluid as can be necessary in conventional crossflow systems.

The shear is developed at the membrane surface. Thus the upstream fluid is exposed to the high shear in a localized region only. This prevents the excessive damage that can be caused to shear-sensitive material during the high speed pumping of feed fluid that is required in conventional crossflow systems.

System footprint and holdup volume can be minimized with the vibrating membrane filter system. A small footprint for a system can be a benefit for applications in which space is limited. A low holdup volume can mean that more of the fluid can be recovered. Because of the design concept for the VMT system, a large amount of membrane can be packed into a small volume. The holdup volume is further reduced by the fact that a high flow recirculation loop is not necessary.

3.5 Application Examples for VMT System

Bioprocessing operations frequently involve the fermentation of bacterial, yeast, or fungal cells for the production of a specific product such as an antibiotic, vitamin, amino acid, flavor, or enzyme. The product may be extracellular (excreted from the cell) or intracellular (inside the cell). For extracellular products, the goal of the processing downstream of the fermentation tank is to separate the cells from the supernatant so that the product can be recovered and further purified. When the desired product is inside the cells, then the cells have to be lysed to set it free. The process goal is then to separate the product from the lysed material so that the product

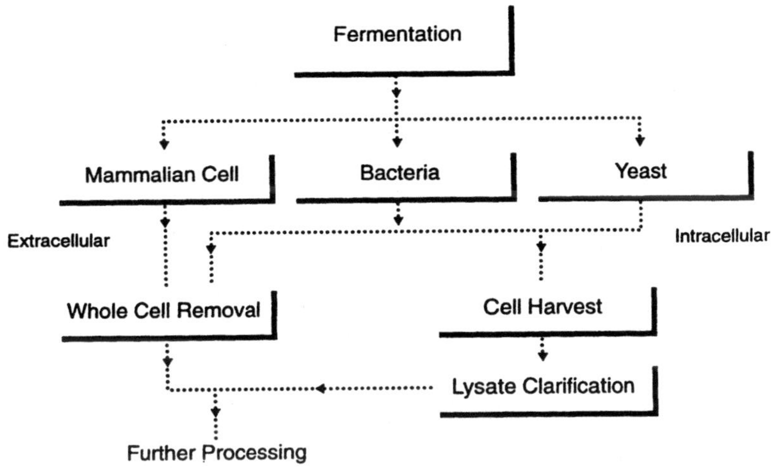

Figure 12 Pharmaceutical processes.

can be further purified. In some cases the cells are concentrated prior to lysis; in others the entire cell mass is subjected to the cell lysis conditions. The basic processes are schematically illustrated in Fig. 12.

Cell separation is a critical step in downstream processes after a fermentation; it is the initial clarification step for the process. As in any process that requires clarification and ultimately purification, it is preferable to remove as much of the contaminating materials as possible as early as possible in the process. Removal of the undesired material can have a significant impact on the further purification steps required for the product.

Another key point for a cell separation step is that the yield of the product should be optimized as much as possible. This can be accomplished by optimizing the cell concentration. A higher yield of the desired product in the broth filtrate after the cell concentration has been completed can be achieved by a diafiltration. For an extracellular product, diafiltration serves to "wash" out any product that remains in the concentrated cellular material. When the cells are the product (or contain the product), diafiltration is used to wash undesirable material off the cells.

Historically, rotary vacuum filtration (RVF) with a precoat (and other systems that require filter aid) and centrifuges have been used for many of the solid–liquid separation process steps required in pharmaceutical downstream processing. Recently, the industry has been evaluating and using membrane-based technologies in applications where RVFs and centrifuges were employed. The reasons a membrane-based technology, such as a VMT system, may be preferable to the RVF and to the centrifuge are described in the following section.

3.6 Membrane-Based Systems Versus RVFs and Other Systems That Require Filter Aid

Rotary vacuum filtration systems, pressure leaf systems, and belt filters are examples of solid–liquid separation systems that are usually operated with a filter aid. The filter aid can be body fed or recirculated to form a precoat on the filtration surface (for example, a cloth material).

There are many drawbacks to using a filter aid such as diatomaceous earth (DE). The use of filter aid requires a supply of the filter aid, since most filter aids are not indefinitely renewable. Thus, the cost of the filter aid and the costs of handling it and disposing of it are included in the operating cost. For some facilities, the cost and labor associated with the disposal of the filter aid can be considerable. For example, DE must be removed from the system (usually with water), and this slurry must then be handled as a waste. Landfills are a problem in some areas, and the slurry may require further treatment (water removal) before it can be moved.

A very important consideration when a filter aid is used is that the solid material collected with the filter aid cannot be separated from the filter aid. If this solid material has value and could be sold as product (for example, if there is nutritional value in solids, they can often be sold as animal feed), then the use of a filter aid is undesirable.

In many operations, the filter aid is used as a precoat, and a recirculation period is generally needed to establish the precoat and provide filtrate clarity. Membrane systems can provide the required clarity throughout the process.

Cleaning a filter aid based system after a process mission can be very labor-intensive, and there is direct operator contact with the DE and process fluid. Membrane systems provide a contained system.

Filter aid systems have the ability to provide a dry cake. Membrane-based systems usually require that the fluid be pumpable.

3.7 Membrane-Based Systems Versus Centrifuge Systems

There are many different types of centrifuge systems available for solid–liquid separations. The principle of operation is the use of centrifugal force (*g* force) to separate materials of different densities. Some examples include basket centrifuges, super (high *g* force) centrifuges, and solid bowl decanter and disk stack centrifuges. Centrifuges can retain solids for manual removal, periodically eject the solids, or continuously discharge them. Some types of centrifuges are capable of providing a dry cake (95–99% solids). The dryness will depend on the type of centrifuge and the process fluid. Centrifuges can provide a compact footprint, and some types are contained systems.

A centrifuge will provide only one level of separation, whereas with membrane-based technology different micrometer ratings will provide different effluent qualities as required for a specific application. Since membrane filters can provide a finer separation than the centrifuge, processing further downstream can be simplified.

Cleaning the system after a process mission, depending on the design of the centrifuge, can be very labor-intensive and can involve direct operator contact with the process fluid. Membrane systems provide a contained system.

Centrifuges generally have a high maintenance cost in comparison to membrane-based systems. However, even though there are some distinct advantages to the use of a membrane-based system such as a vibrating membrane filter system over the traditional equipment (RVFs or centrifuges), it may not be desirable to replace all of the existing equipment with VMT systems. The use of new membrane-based separations equipment is likely to be strongly considered for an expansion or a new process. It may prove to be judicious to use the membrane-based system in conjunction with the traditional equipment. For example, if a pressure leaf filter with a DE coat is currently being used to concentrate to a nonpumpable solid, then a VMT system could be used upstream of the pressure leaf filter to expand the capacity of the DE-based system. VMT systems require that the fluid be pumpable. This solution has the advantage of increased capacity with provision of the required high solids cake and a cleaner filtrate (at least for the fluid processed by the vibrating membrane filter system).

3.8 Applications of VMT Systems

There are a large number of potential applications for which a membrane-based system such as the vibrating membrane filter system could be used in place of existing technologies such as RVFs and centrifuges. Large-scale cell separations (on the order of 100,000 L fermentation broths) are one type of application for the VMT system.

Four examples of applications for a vibrating membrane filter system involving downstream processing are considered. These examples have been investigated and found to have both technical and economic relevance. They include two examples of cell separation where the desired product is an excreted product and two where the desired product is an intracellular product and the cells are concentrated and then lysed (Pall Corporation, 1997).

Example 1. Cell Separation for a Fungal Biomass with an Excreted Product

A vibrating membrane filter system can be used for cell separation of a fungal biomass and the product is excreted (extracellular). The current process employs a vacuum filter with a diatomaceous earth precoat. The fermentation medium components include materials such as fishmeal, peanut or soybean meal, corn steep liquor, beet molasses, lard oil or methyl oleate, glucose, methionine, and an antifoaming agent.

The basic goals of the process are to attain a maximum (90–95%) yield of product from the fermentor liquor with a minimized filtrate volume. The cells are concentrated, and since they are not contaminated with DE, disposal is more economical. Depending on the broth, it may be possible for the cells to be used as animal feed.

A summary of the application of the VMT for this process follows.

Total Process Volume. The total process filtrate volume was minimized as required. The VMT system is designed to concentrate to high solids levels. In this type of process, to maximize the yield of the product it is often necessary to diafilter the solids with water or buffer to maximize the product recovery. Since VMT is able to concentrate to a high solids level, the amount of fluid required for diafiltration is diminished. An example of the benefits of a higher concentration factor is presented in the Appendix.

Flow Rate. The flow rate was found to be on the order of 1000 L/h per machine.

Product Yield. The product yield was on the order of 95% or greater.

Clarity. Permeate clarity met requirements for the process.

Cleaning. Performance was recovered after the cleaning. Relatively mild cleaning treatments were found to be effective: water at 75°C and 0.02% caustic at ambient temperature.

Energy Usage. The energy required for the VMT system in this application is 0.0125 hp/ft^2 (0.009 kW/m^2) membrane area.

Antifoam Agent. No flux decline was observed due to the presence of antifoaming agent.

Example 2. Cell Separation for a Bacterial Biomass with an Excreted Product

For this example of a bacterial biomass cell separation, the current process uses a centrifuge followed by a vacuum filter with a diatomaceous earth precoat for further concentration. The broth material can be diluted for ease of separation. The VMT system would replace both unit operations. The fermentation broth can contain soybean oil, soybeans, corn flour, and calcium chloride plus an antifoaming agent. Sand can be present as a contaminant. The biomass is about 10–15% solids with 2–3% dry residuals.

The basic goal for the project is to attain a maximum (>90%) yield of the desired product. The cells are concentrated, and since they are not contaminated with DE, disposal is more economical. Depending on the broth, it may be possible for the cells to be used as animal feed.

A summary of the application of the VMT system for this process follows.

Total Process Volume. The total process permeate volume was minimized and was found to be less than the volume required in the current process. Essentially no dilution of the fermentation broth was needed. In this type of process, to maximize the yield of the product it is often necessary to diafilter the solids with water, or buffer, to maximize the product recovery. Since the VMT system is able to concentrate to a high solids level, the amount of fluid required for diafiltration is diminished.

Concentration Factor. The VMT system was able to provide a high concentration factor and is able to replace both the centrifuges and the RVFs in the process.

Permeate Clarity. For all experiments performed, the permeate appeared visually clear. Centrifuges and RVFs are unable to provide visual clarity. Downstream processing should be much improved with the membrane-filtered product.

Flux. The flow rate was on the order of 1000 L/h per machine.

Yield. A greater than 90% yield of the product was demonstrated. Transmission of the product was essentially 100%.

Cleaning. The membrane did not exhibit fouling; cleaning is expected to be straightforward for this process.

Energy Usage. The energy required for the VMT system in this application is 0.0125 hp/ft^2 (0.009 kW/m^2) membrane area.

Sand. Membrane abrasion due to the sand (abrasive material) was not observed.

Example 3. Cell Separation for a Bacterial Biomass with an Intracellular Product

This VMT system application is an example of a bacterial biomass (~1–3% solids) with the product inside the cells. The objective is to concentrate the biomass. The current process uses a centrifuge. The cell broth can be treated with the flocculent and decanted to make the separation easier. The fermentation medium is a synthetic tissue culture medium. A polypropylene glycol antifoaming agent is used.

The basic goals for the process are to attain a maximum yield (90–95%) of cells from the fermentor with minimized cell disruption.

A summary of the application of the VMT system for this process follows.

Total Process Volume. The total process permeate volume was minimized. In this type of process, in order to wash undesirable material off the cells, it is often necessary to diafilter the solids with water, or buffer, to clean the cells. Since the VMT system is able to concentrate to a high solids content, the amount of fluid required for diafiltration is diminished.

Concentration Factor. The VMT system was able to concentrate to a higher concentration factor than the current technology. The current technology can concentrate to about 8% solids; the VMT system demonstrated the ability to get to 16% solids by weight.

Flow Rate. The flow rate was found to be on the order of 1200 L/h per machine.

Product Yield. The cell yield was on the order of 95% or greater. The intracellular product activity was 100%. The product quality was judged to be better than the quality of the current process.

Flocculent and Decantation. It was not necessary to use flocculent with the VMT system; this would represent a simplification of the process.

Clarity. Permeate clarity was demonstrated to meet process requirements.

Cleaning. Performance was recovered after the cleaning. Relatively mild cleaning treatments were found to be effective. An enzymatic cleaner was used.

Energy Usage. The energy required for the VMT system in this application is 0.0125 hp/ft^2 (0.009 kW/m^2) membrane area.

Antifoaming Agent. No flux decline due to the presence of antifoam was observed.

Example 4. Cell Separation for a Bacterial Biomass with an Intracellular Product

This VMT system application is an example of a bacterial biomass (~7–9% solids by volume) with the product inside the cells. The objective is to concentrate the biomass. The current process uses a centrifuge. An organosilicate antifoaming agent is used.

The basic goal of the process is to attain a maximum (90–95%) yield of cells from the fermentor with minimized cell disruption and loss of cells in permeate.

A summary of the application of the VMT system for this process follows.

Diafiltration. In this type of process, in order to wash undesirable material off the cells it is often necessary to diafilter the solids with water, or buffer, to clean the cells. Since VMT is able to concentrate to a high solids content, the amount of fluid required for diafiltration is diminished. Diafiltration was demonstrated with the VMT system but is not possible with the centrifuge.

Flow Rate. The flow rate was found to be on the order of 1600 L/h per machine.

Product Yield. The cell yield was on the order of 95% or greater. No cells were found in the permeate. The centrifuge showed a 1–3% loss of product due to cell disruption in the filtrate.

Clarity. Permeate clarity was demonstrated to meet process requirements.

Cleaning. Performance was recovered after the cleaning. Relatively mild cleaning treatments were found to be effective. An enzymatic cleaner was used.

Energy Usage. The energy required for the VMT system in this application is 0.0125 hp/ft^2 (0.009 kW/m^2) membrane area.

Antifoaming Agent. Flux decline due to the presence of antifoaming agent was not observed.

Issues for Consideration

A concern for a membrane-based system in pharmaceutical processes is the issue of fouling. Fouling is a concern for a number of reasons. Membrane regeneration cycles can become extremely long and can interrupt process cycling; the flow through the membrane can diminish over time, leading to longer cycle times; and in some cases membrane fouling can mean that the desired product is not transmitted through the membrane, leading to a yield loss.

Foulants in the fermentation broth can include antifoaming agents, solid particles from the fermentation media (e.g., sand, undissolved salts), and proteinaceous material excreted from the cell in addition to the desired product. Lysates are usually more difficult to filter and can contain DNA and RNA, which are generally considered challenging materials for filtration.

The VMT system has been found to perform well under the various foulants.

Antifoaming Agents. Glycol- and silicone-based antifoaming agents have been used (about 1%) in material filtered by the VMT system. There has been no deleterious effect observed with either antifoaming agent.

Flux Stability. The expected permeate flow rate for a VMT system with a fermentation broth or lysate is on the order of 1000–2000 L/h per machine. The flows have been found to be stable with mild regeneration regimens.

Transmission or Yield. The transmission of the desired product has been found to meet requirements.

Abrasive Material. Abrasive materials such as sand have not been found to damage the membrane. (A general recommendation is to use a coarse prefilter to protect the pump in the system from abrasive materials.)

Vibrating membrane filter technology has been found to provide benefits over other technologies in cell separation applications and in concentration applications for fluids for which membrane technology has not been possible in the pharmaceutical industry.

4 ROTATING DISK MEMBRANE FILTER SYSTEM (Cole and Brantley, 1996)

The vibrating membrane filter system is able to generate shear at the membrane surface on the order of 100,000 s^{-1}. For most solid–liquid applications, this high shear will be adequate to provide the desired flow rates and product transmission. For cases in which a higher shear rate is necessary to perform at effective separation, there are devices that can produce shear rates in excess of 100,000 s^{-1}. These devices are classified as rotary shear devices.

An early design involves the use of concentric cylinders. A membrane can be placed on the surface of the center cylinder or on the inner surface of the outer cylinder. The center cylinder is rotated. The membrane is kept clean by the shear created by Taylor vortices (or eddies) formed in the gap between the concentric cylinders. This type of design is illustrated in Fig. 13. The technique has proven effective in terms of flow and transmission performance (Rebsamen and Ziegler, 1986; Holeschovsky and Cooney, 1991; Kroner and Nissinen, 1988; Murase, 1991); however, scale-up of the cylindrical design has been found to be impractical for high membrane areas.

4.1 Design and Operation of Rotating Disk Membrane Technology System

The stacked disk configuration has been used with the idea that it makes possible a more compact design in terms of membrane area. Figure 14 shows an RDMT system. The stainless steel rotors are rotated by a belt-coupled electric motor drive. The complete system is shown in Fig. 15. The system comprises all that is necessary to run the separation process, including heat exchangers, pumps, tanks, clean-in-place

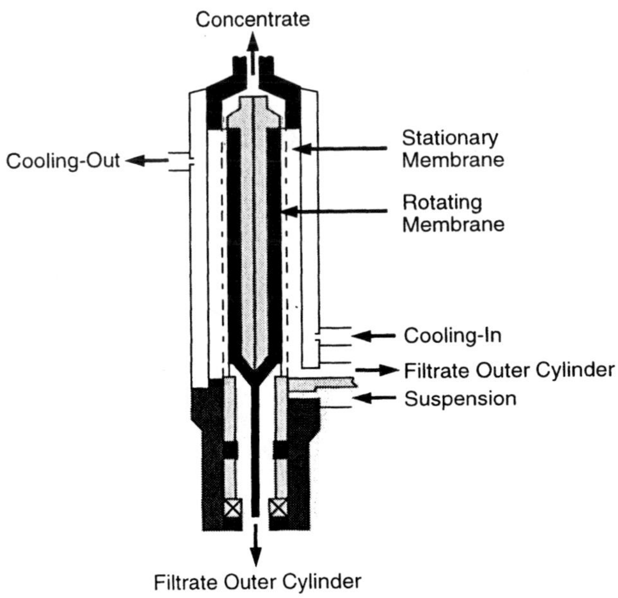

Figure 13 Rotating cylinder design (Cole and Brantley, 1996).

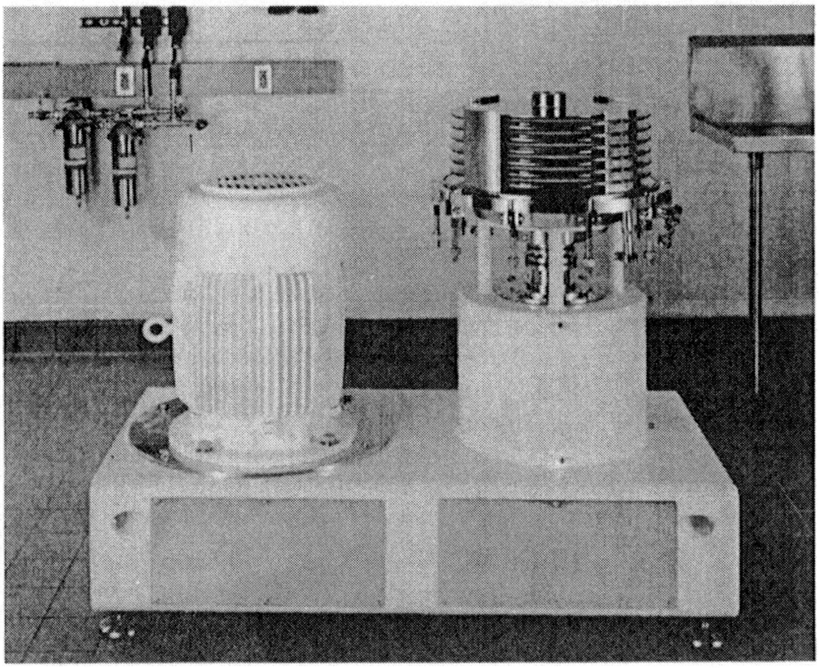

Figure 14 DMF unit. (Courtesy of Pall Corporation.)

capability, and steam-in-place capability. A full-scale unit is capable of processing 300–1500 L/h, the actual flow rate depending on the fluid.

The membrane elements are stacked between the rotors in 180° sectors. A sector is illustrated in Fig. 16. When assembled the two sectors form a membrane stack 16 in. in diameter. The membrane element consists of a plastic support disk with membrane bonded to both sides of the disk.

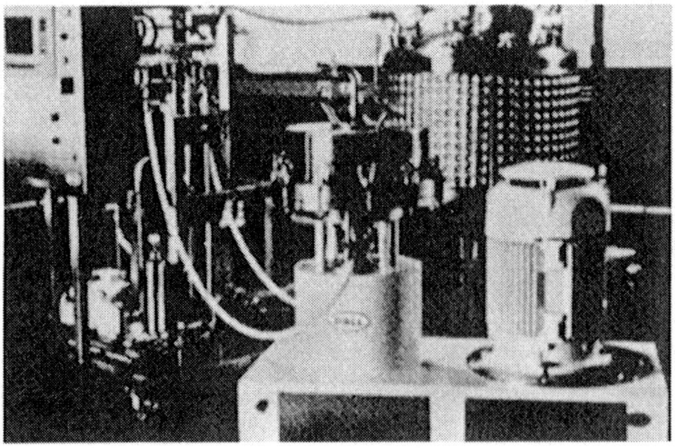

Figure 15 DMF system. (Courtesy of Pall Corporation.)

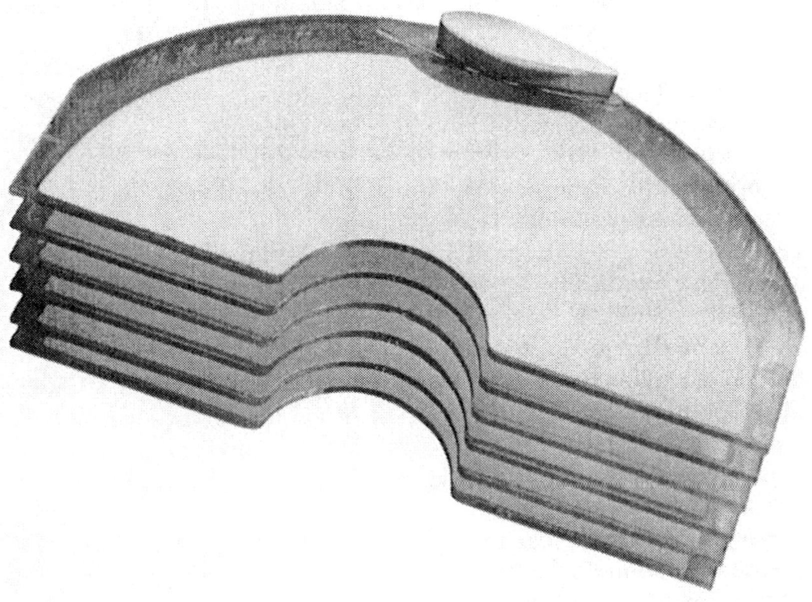

Figure 16 Sector of DMF membrane elements. (Courtesy of Pall Corporation.)

The stainless steel rotors are rotated at speeds of up to 1800 rpm. This high speed rotation causes high shear at the surface of the membrane. At the maximum rpm, the shear rate is estimated to be greater than 200,000 s^{-1}.

Figure 17 illustrates the flow pattern at the membrane surface. Shear is created in the gap between the solid rotating disk and the static membrane element. The competition between dynamic and viscous forces in the fluid results in rotation of

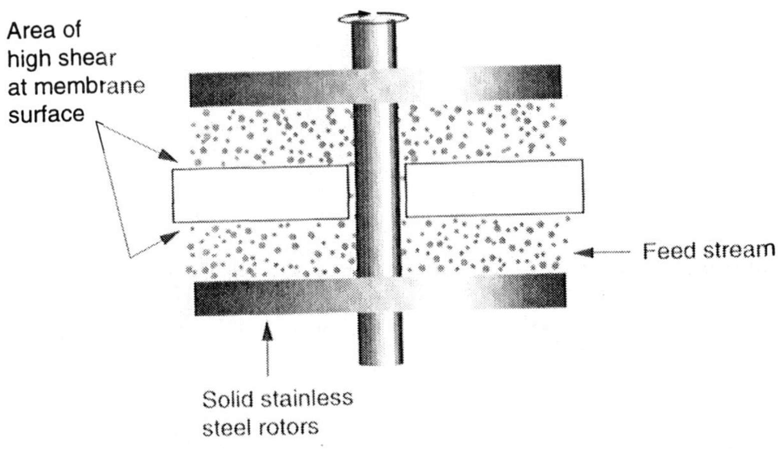

Figure 17 Flow pattern at membrane surface in DMF (Cole and Brantley, 1996).

the bulk of the liquid as a nearly rigid disk. There is significant shear in the boundary layer formed between the membrane surface and the bulk of the liquid.

Feed fluid is fed across the membrane for distribution (not for shear development). The feed is introduced into the top of the element housing assembly, and the retentate flow is directed to the center of the assembly and out the top of the housing. The flow pattern is illustrated in Fig. 18. Permeate flows through the membrane on both sides of the membrane element. The permeate flow is directed to the outside of the element and exits the assembly at the bottom.

For scaled-down tests, a 6 in. diameter dynamic membrane filter unit can be used. This unit is illustrated in Fig. 19, and the flow path is illustrated in Fig. 20.

The scaled-down device is intended for proof-of-concept testing. The membrane elements have membrane bonded on only one side of the plastic support disk. The fluid enters the assembly at the bottom of the rotating disk and is accelerated around the bottom of the disk to the upper surface of the membrane element, where it comes in contact with the membrane. The concentrate is directed to the center of the assembly, and the permeate to the outside. Both the permeate and retentate leave the unit through the top.

The differential pressure across the membrane (feed to permeate) requires a term for the pressure component due to rotation $[(1/8)(\rho r^2\Omega^2)]$. The pressure profile across the membrane is based on radial position. The appropriate equation for the 6 in. dynamic filter system is

$$\Delta P = P_{\text{feed}} + \frac{1}{8}(\rho r^2\Omega^2) - P_{\text{permeate}} \tag{3}$$

where

ΔP = differential pressure (dyn/cm^2)
P_{feed} = feed pressure (dyn/cm^2)
ρ = fluid density (g/cm^3)
r = radial position (cm)
Ω = angular velocity = rpm $\times$ $(2\pi/60)$
P_{permeate} = permeate pressure (dyn/cm^2)

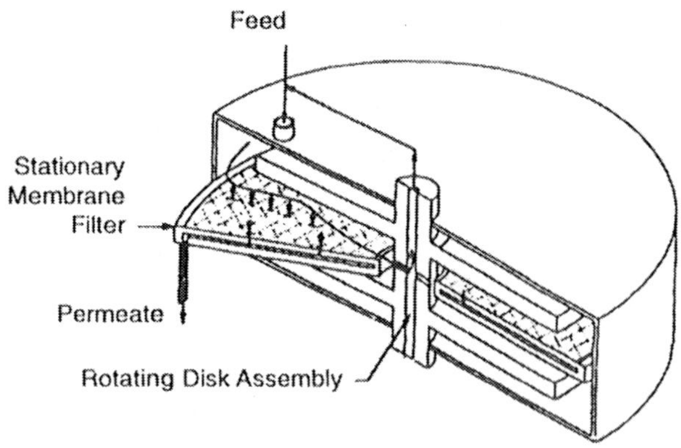

Figure 18 Flow pattern in DMF element assembly (Cole and Brantley, 1996).

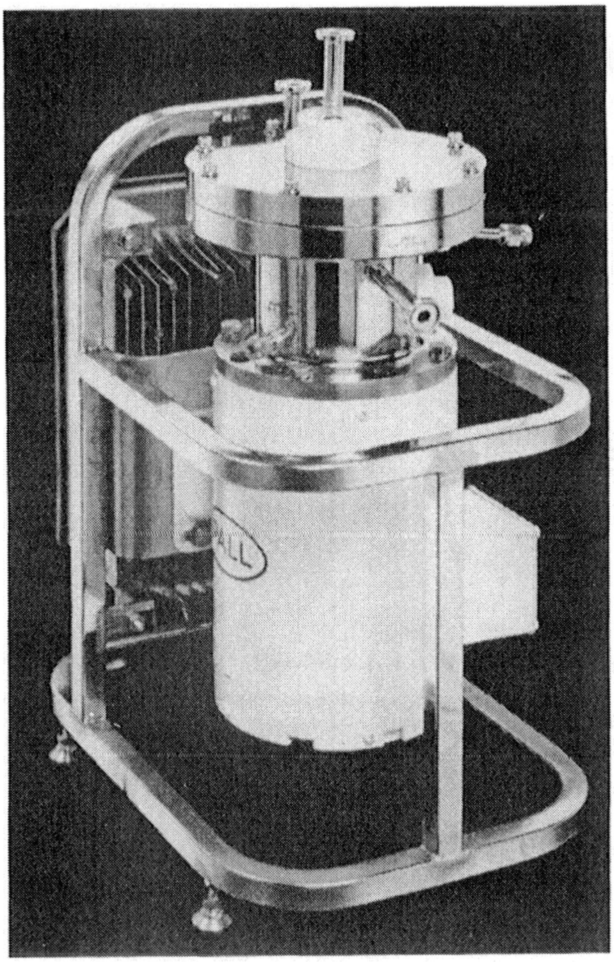

Figure 19 Scaled-down 6 in. DMF unit. (Courtesy of Pall Corporation.)

4.2 Performance Data

Comparison with Traditional Crossflow Devices

Lee et al. (1995) investigated the use of the RDMT, using the scaled-down design (Pall Corporation 6 in. DMF system), for an industrial recombinant yeast cell harvest. A summary of this investigation is presented here to highlight the performance of the dynamic membrane filter system in comparison with traditional cassette crossflow technology.

The strains used for the study were flocculating recombinant yeasts grown in a synthetic medium containing glucose, mineral salts, and glutamate. UCON LB625 antifoam (Union Carbide Corp, Danbury, CT) was used.

The product is intracellular, and one requirement for the operation is that the cell separation step be completed in less than 4 h because of the potential of product degradation. A 6× concentration factor followed by diafiltration is required to meet the yield requirements for the process.

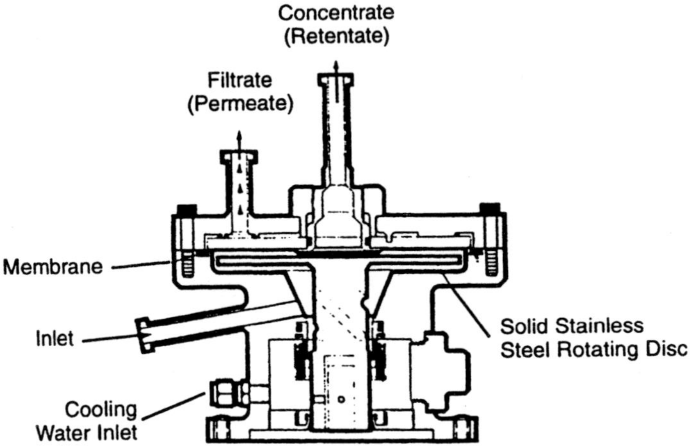

Figure 20 Six-inch DMF flow patterns (Cole and Brantley, 1996).

The cassette system tested exhibited a flux decline to <25 L/(m^2·h) with the recombinant yeast. If cassettes were used at the production scale, then the separation process time would be in excess of 8 h, which does not meet the <4 h requirement for the process. Also, a large filtration area would be needed.

The RDMT unit demonstrated average flux rates of >200 L/(m^2·h), and a sixfold concentration plus diafiltration could be achieved within 100 min—well within the 4 h maximum time.

Illustration of Operational Techniques for a Microporous Membrane

Lee et al. (1995) contains comparative data that illustrate an important point about the operation of a microporous membrane. A number of factors can lead to the plugging of a microporous membrane. These include relatively high differential pressures and high flow rates. Operation at a low pressure differential across the membrane (upstream to downstream differential) may lead to better long-term performance. Although there is an increase in flux with pressure, the flux tends to decline, and more frequent cleaning is required. Operation at a low pressure can result in a more stable condition, and fouling is likely to be reduced. Thus, cleaning requirements and reduced flux due to fouling may be less of an issue at lower differential pressures.

The other condition that can lead to premature fouling is excessive flow. During start-up, if permitted, the permeate flow rate can be very high. In traditional crossflow systems, this high start-up flux is followed by a sharp decline. If the start-up allows for a gradual increase in flow rate, the membrane will not be subjected to the initial fouling condition. Alternatively, the permeate flow rate can be controlled throughout the run.

During one experiment, the permeate flow rate was not controlled. At start-up the flow rate was very high [1600 L/(m^2 · h)] and then it decayed to about 100 L/(m^2 · h). The process time limit of 4 h for concentration and diafiltration could not be met because the sixfold concentration alone required 230 min.

In another experiment, the permeate flow rate was controlled and the sixfold concentration was accomplished in just over 3 h. With optimization, the use of a controlled permeate flow could meet the <4 h requirement.

Illustration of Protein Transmission (Cole and Brantley, 1996)

To illustrate the transmission performance of RDMT, the following data are presented for a scaled-down 6 in. diameter unit with microporous nylon membrane. The tests were performed with a 5% yeast suspension consisting of dry baker's yeast mixed with molasses and with ovalbumin and casein as protein transmission markers. Protein transmission was monitored by PAGE followed by Western blotting. Proteins were stained with amido black.

For a full-scale machine, the permeate flow rate would be on the order of 400 L/h. The results of the protein transmission assay are illustrated in Fig. 21. The figure shows that there is no difference between the feed, retentate, and permeate streams, indicating a transmission approaching 100%.

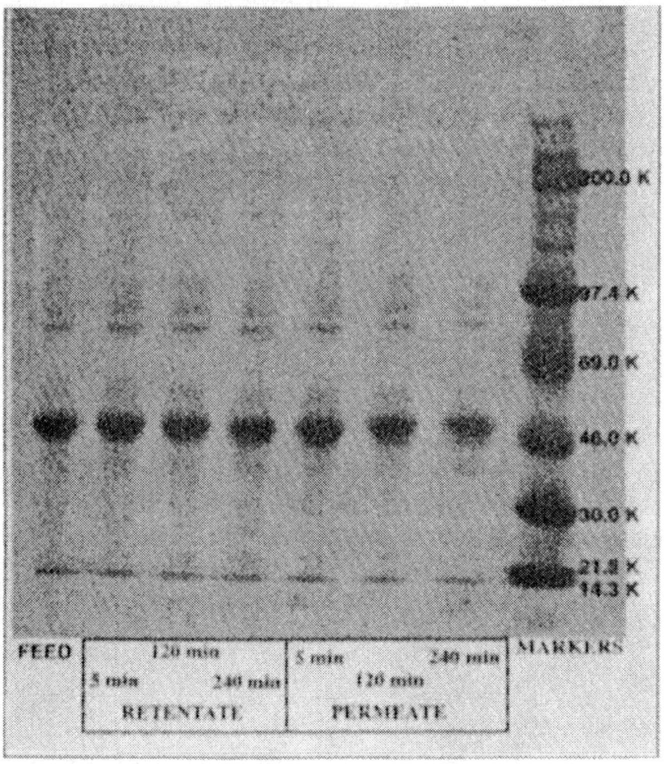

Figure 21 Protein transmission data (Cole and Brantley, 1996).

5 SOLID–LIQUID SEPARATION WITH A BACKWASHABLE SINGLE-PASS FILTER

5.1 Introduction

Production processes in the pharmaceutical industry can often involve the removal of solid particulate material such as activated carbon from the process stream. Activated carbon can be used to remove the color bodies in the process fluid downstream of a fermentation. The activated carbon can be added to a batch of the process fluid that requires decolorization. In some processes it is necessary to employ multiple decolorization steps. After the carbon has contacted the process fluid, it is necessary to remove the carbon from the fluid.

A backwash, or solid separations recovery, system using backwashable single-pass (or "dead end," in contrast to a crossflow filter assembly) filters can be used efficiently and economically for the removal of solid materials such as carbon from pharmaceutical process streams. The backwash technique involves the buildup of particulate contaminant material followed by initiating and cycling gas or liquid flow in the direction reverse to normal filtration flow through the filter element to remove the solid contaminants from the membrane. Various membrane materials can be employed; the filter element design must be robust enough to withstand pressure in both the forward and reverse directions.

The techniques used to perform a backwash operation are described in Sec. 5.2, and in Sec. 5.3 two test cases for the application of this technology in actual processes in the pharmaceutical industry are used to illustrate the economic benefits of the use of a backwashable polypropylene filter element.

5.2 Operation

A porous filter medium, either metallic or nonmetallic, with the appropriate pore size, will collect solids at or near the surface of the membrane. The solids will form a permeable cake. The cake is dislodged from the membrane at a predetermined pressure drop by initiating a reverse flow. The cake release is illustrated in Fig. 22.

The pressure drop is a function of cake thickness and cake compressibility. The dislodged solids are removed from the filter system. The solids can be returned to the process stream or to a storage or collection unit. The membrane filter is returned to flow in the forward direction. The pressure drop after a backwash (reverse-flow) cycle will remain essentially constant throughout backwash cycles. An example of the differential pressure versus time for a backwash operation is illustrated in Fig. 23.

For full-scale systems, multiple elements are installed in a filter vessel. The spacing of the filter elements is critical for proper cake formation and to prevent bridging between the cakes. The operation is automated so that the backwash cycles are controlled, and in multivessel installations the backwash cycles can be sequenced so that the flow is continuous. A full system design is illustrated in Fig. 24; an operating system is shown in Fig. 25.

There are two methods for the discharge of solids: the pressurized liquid method and the gas-assist method.

The pressurized liquid method can be used for an installation with multivessel systems, when process flow rates are high, or when a continuous uninterrupted flow

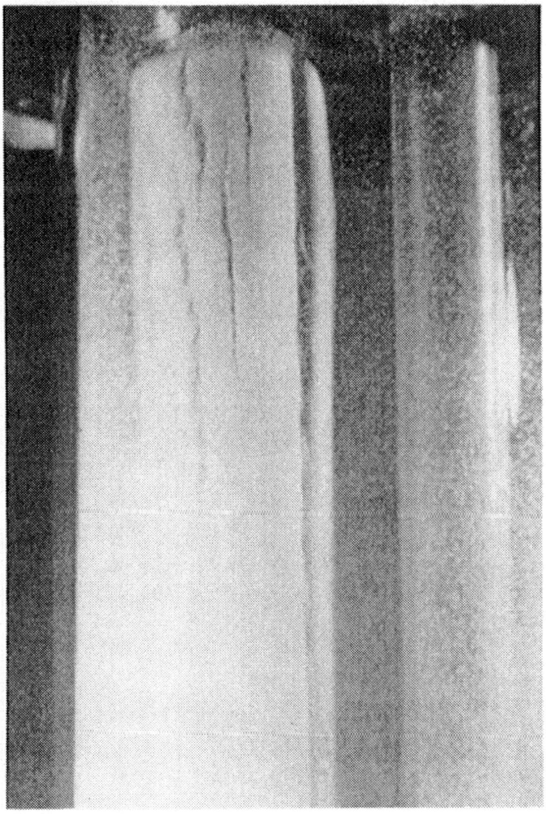

Figure 22 Backwash cake release.

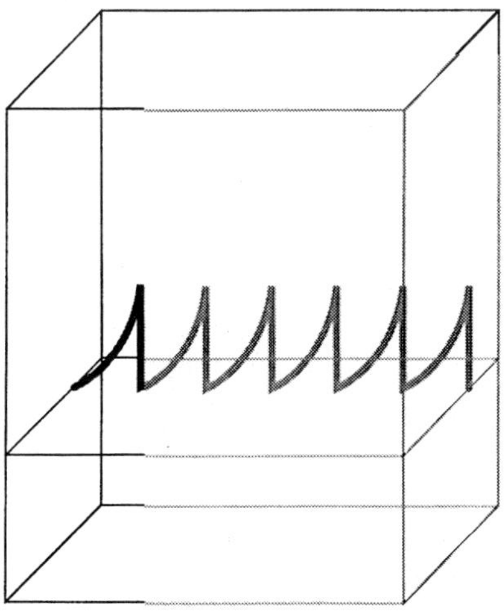

Figure 23 Differential pressure versus time for backwash operation.

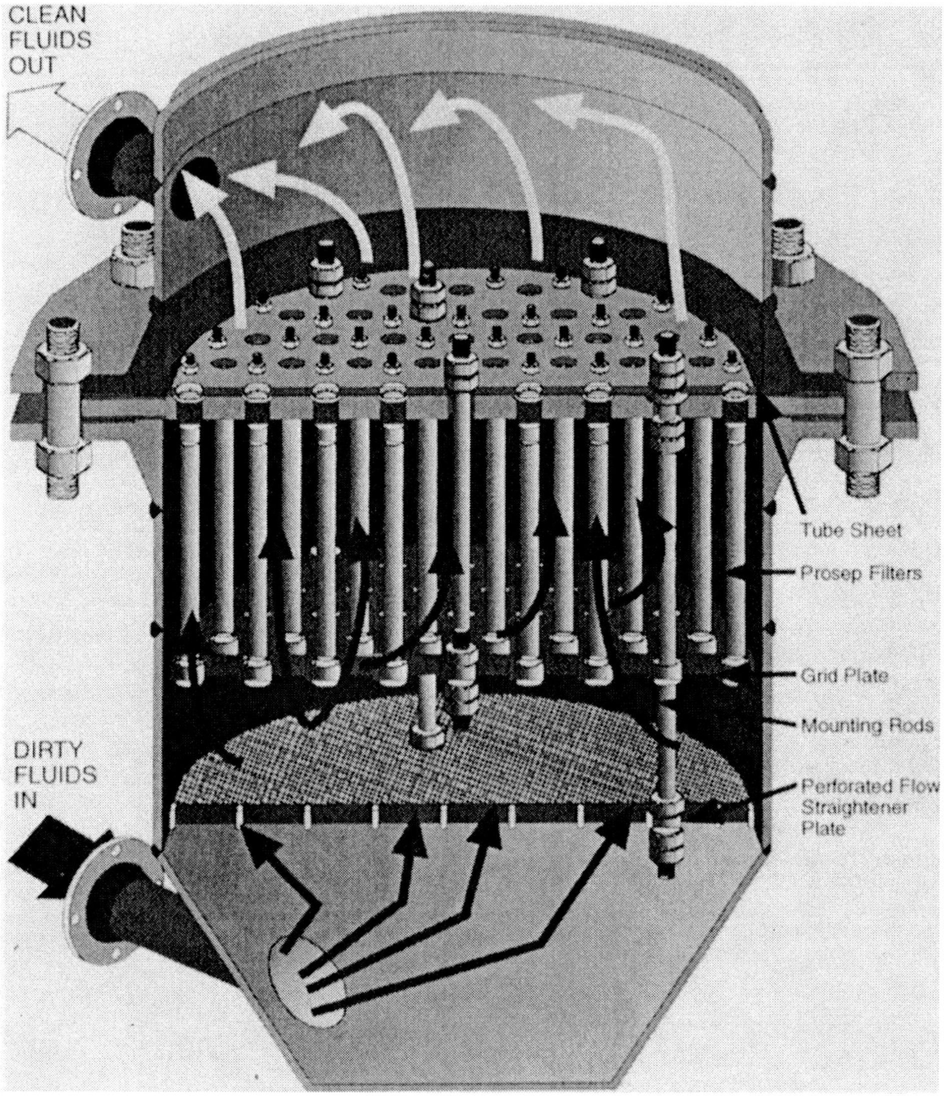

Figure 24 Full-scale backwash design.

is required. For backwash, one filter vessel is isolated and a reverse flow of low pressure liquid is initiated at a rate equal to or greater than the flow rate in the forward direction. The technique is illustrated in Fig. 26. The volume of liquid needed is approximately two vessel volumes. The liquid used to perform the backwash may be the filtrate or a buffer fluid. The use of filtrate for backwash fluid will minimize the loss of process fluid.

The gas-assist method can be employed when multivessel systems are installed, when process flow rates are high, or when a continuous flow is required. For the backwash, one vessel is isolated and the downstream side of the vessel is pressurized with a controlled quantity of filtered air or other suitable gas. The technique is

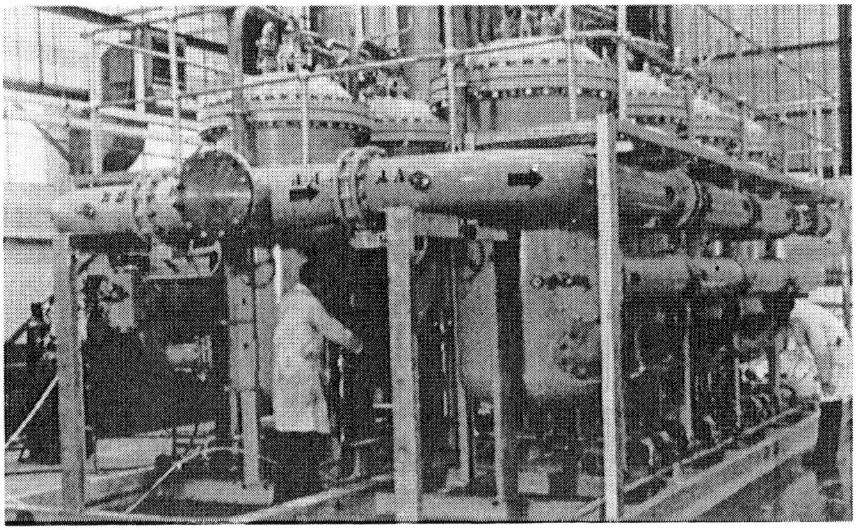

Figure 25 Full-scale operating backwash system.

illustrated in Fig. 27. The filter vessel drain port is opened rapidly. This causes a hydraulic pulse that acts to "bump" the collected solids from the filter surface. Flow in the forward direction is restored to the vessel after the backwash.

The solids removed from the filter may require further treatment. A further concentration of the solids may facilitate disposal or recovery. The slurry can be sent to a bag filter for recovery or further concentration.

The filtrate in the process may be valuable, and it may be desirable to minimize the filtrate losses in the operation. One technique that can be employed is the use of a scavenger filter near the center of the filter vessel. Scavenger filters are used to

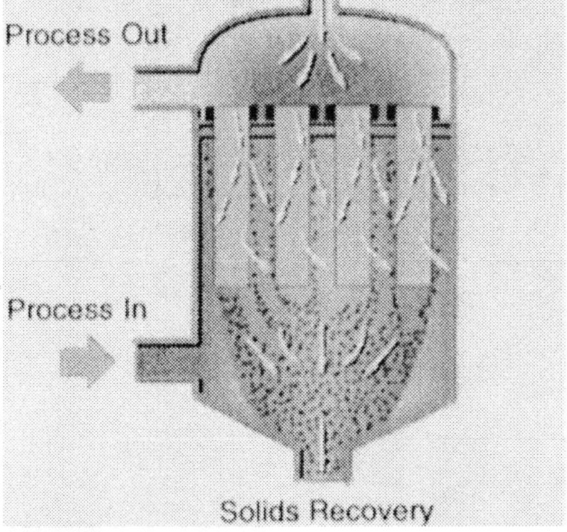

Figure 26 Pressurized liquid backwash.

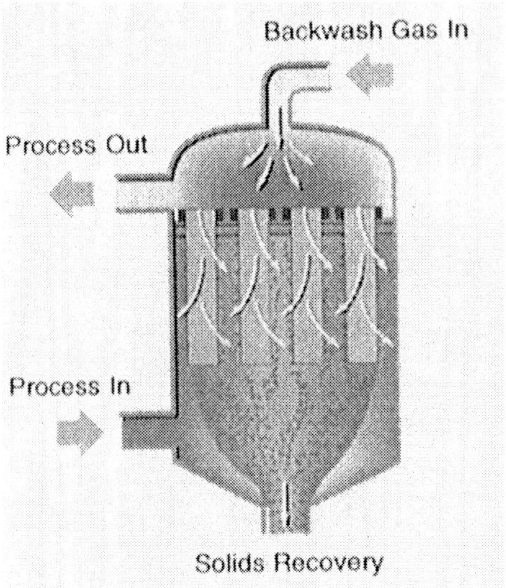

Figure 27 Gas-assisted backwash.

help drain the liquid just prior to the backwashing operation. The use of a scavenger filter is illustrated in Fig. 28.

Figure 29 illustrates a test stand developed for the evaluation and optimization of the use of the backwashing procedure as a filter reclamation process for backwashable filter elements. The test stand is portable and is designed for scaled-down tests. It can be used with a clear (transparent acrylic) filter housing, depending on the fluid compatibility, so that the filtration and backwash procedures can be observed. A variety of fittings can be used so that the backwashable filter test stand

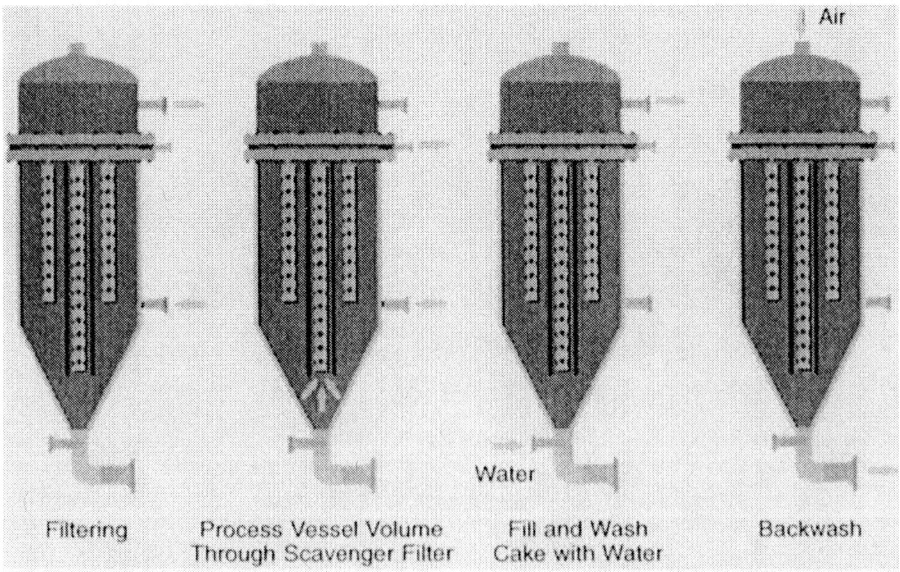

Figure 28 Scavenger filter design.

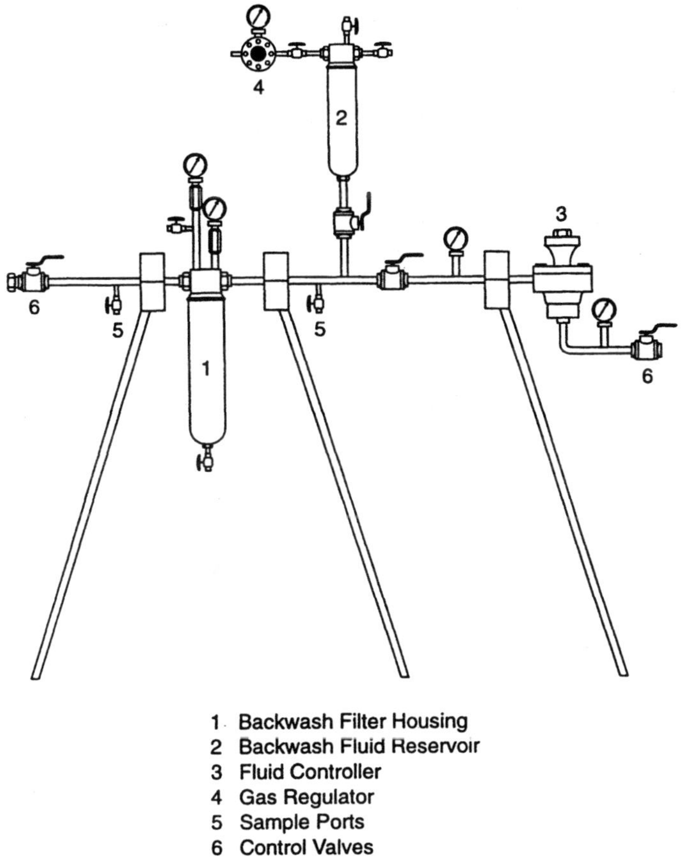

Figure 29 Scaled-down backwash test stand.

can be connected to the process stream, air or nitrogen gas stream, and, if required, a water supply for performance of a backwash.

During a typical evaluation, a backwashable element is used to filter a solution that contains a contaminant at a specified concentration. The filtration continues until a predetermined differential pressure is reached. The maximum differential pressure can depend on process requirements, cake thickness, and cake compressibility. The backwash procedure is then performed to remove the contaminant from the filter. Either a gas-assisted or a reverse-flow liquid backwash can be performed using the test stand. The liquid backwash can involve either a fluid that is compatible with the process fluid (such as water for water-based products) or the process fluid itself.

Multiple cycles are performed on the test material to determine information on the life of the filter in the application. The filter effluent can be analyzed to ensure that it meets the application requirements. For example, for a process that involves carbon removal, a gravimetric analysis or a turbidity measurement can be performed.

The backwash system design is flexible so that a variety of membrane types, metal and nonmetal, can be used for a backwash operation. The membrane elements need to have a pore size distribution such that particles are collected on the surface and do not penetrate into the depth of the medium. The elements must be designed to have strength and durability to withstand the cyclic loads that are applied during the reverse flow cycles. The filter surface must allow for an easy release of the cake on the surface of the membrane during the backwash.

The filter elements employed in a backwash operation may be used either with or without a filter aid precoat. The filter pore size rating can be selected for optimization of filtrate quality. Examples of filter elements that can be used are metal membrane filters and polypropylene (PP) depth filters.

Metal membrane filter medium is a thin, sintered matrix of fine stainless steel powder within a porous structure stainless steel woven wire mesh. The fine powder provides absolute filtration down to 2 μm. The woven wire mesh provides strength, but it is thin enough to permit the medium to be pleated into high area filter elements, which minimizes the resistance to flow. This product can be used in applications in which a precoat is desired.

Polypropylene (PP) filters have an outer (upstream) section in which the fiber diameter and pore size increase gradually to the filter element's outermost layer and an inner (downstream) section in which the pore diameter is constant. The variable-pore upstream section provides efficient prefiltration and is designed to provide long cycle times between backwash cycles. The filter element can be used with or without precoat. Solids concentrations in the feed stream can be up to 2500 ppm.

5.3 Test Cases

The following two example cases are provided to illustrate the evaluation of backwashable PP filters for pharmaceutical process applications (Haughney, 1993).

Case 1. The Removal of Activated Carbon from a Process Stream

The requirements for the application in which activated carbon was to be removed from a pharmaceutical process stream included a single-pass filtration system and a visually clear effluent. A liquid with a turbidity measurement in nephelometric turbidity units (NTU) of less than 1 is commonly considered to be visually clear. The backwashable PP filter element system was desired for the replacement of a filtration technology that involved the use of diatomaceous earth as a filtration aid. Diatomaceous earth, or any filter aid, was found to be unnecessary for the backwashable PP element tested in this application.

Process requirements for the application were a maximum differential pressure of 10 psid and a flow density of 1.1 gpm/ft^2.

Side-stream tests with a 12 μm ($\beta = 1000$ at 12 μm) backwashable PP element of 2 in. O.D. were performed as a slip stream. Additional testing with a 12 μm PP element was performed on a slurry of carbon and water. Gravimetric analysis was performed during the test. The carbon slurry was prepared in the same concentration as the carbon in the process solution.

The flow density during all of the testing was 1.1 gpm/ft^2. Cycles were terminated at a ΔP of 10 psid. At the end of a cycle, the element was subjected to two air-assisted backwashes at 30 psi. During the testing, on-line turbidity (NTU) was monitored. Gravimetric samples of the influent and effluent were taken. A total of six cycles were run. Full ΔP recovery after each cycle was obtained.

The results for six cycles are presented in Table 1. Average turbidity measurements are given for the beginning, middle, and late portion of each cycle. The in-

Table 1 Cycle Data for 12 μm Polypropylene Element Tested with Carbon and Water Slurry

Cycle number	Cycle duration (min)	Turbidity (NTU) Early	Middle	Late	Influent gravimetric analysis (g/L)
1	48	0.4	0.4	0.4	4.09
2	35	0.4	0.4	0.4	4.09
3	34	0.58	0.39	0.38	4.05
4	24	0.42	0.39	0.39	4.05
5	26	0.45	0.39	0.39	3.89
6	36	0.62	0.34	0.33	3.55

fluent gravimetric analyses are also presented. Table 2 presents effluent gravimetric analysis data for cycles 1 and 2. These analyses were performed over the entire cycle. Effluent gravimetric data for cycles 3–6 for analyses performed at given cycle times are presented in Table 3.

The average cycle length was 34 min. During the on-site testing, performed under the same conditions (terminal ΔP = 10 psid; flow density = 1.1 gpm/ft^2), cycle lengths were found to be quite similar.

The carbon and water slurry backwash tests indicate that high removal efficiencies are possible for carbon. For the worst case, the removal efficiency was 99.75%. The average removal efficiency for the six cycles was 99.92%. These removal efficiencies met the requirements for the application.

Case 2. The Removal of Active Raney Nickel Catalyst from a Process Stream

The requirement for this application was the removal of active Raney nickel catalyst from a process stream so that the effluent concentration of nickel is less than or equal to 3 ppm.

Active Raney nickel catalysts are pyrophoric. If allowed to dry in air, they smolder to red heat and provide a combustion source for exposed combustible materials. For this reason, an explosion-proof pump was used.

The process requirements were a maximum initial differential pressure equal to 2–5 psid and a maximum allowable pressure of 10–20 psi. The flow rate was 70–100 gpm, and a flow density of 0.2–0.3 gpm/ft^2 was desired for the application.

Table 2 Gravimetric Analyses Over Entire Cycle During Cycles 1 and 2 for 12 μm Polypropylene Element Tested with Carbon and Water Slurry

Cycle number	Gravimetric analysis (g/L)
1	0.0047
2	0.0100

Table 3 Gravimetric Analyses at Timed Intervals During Cycles 3–6 for 12 μm Polypropylene Element Tested with Carbon and Water Slurry

Cycle number	Effluent sample gravimetric analysis (g/L) taken at cycle time			
	2 min	12 min	22 min	34 min
3	0.0030	Not done	0.0025	0.0016
4	0.0003	<Detection limit[a]	0.0003	Not done
5	0.0016	<Detection limit[a]	<Detection limit[a]	Not done
6	<Detection limit[a]	<Detection limit[a]	<Detection limit[a]	Not done

[a]The detection limit is <0.0003 g/L.

A backwashable PP filter with an absolute rating of 12 μm with a 1.25 in. O.D. was tested for this application using the portable backwash test stand in a side-stream test. A 55 gal drum was used as the product supply. Twelve cycles were executed with a process stream that contained a given concentration of active Raney nickel at a flow density of 0.3 gpm/ft^2. The differential pressure for each cycle was less than 1 psid. The cycle duration was 15 min to simulate actual production batch cycle time. Samples taken from a downstream port during the testing were analyzed for nickel concentration and were found to meet the clarity requirements for the product. Filtered water was used as the backwash fluid. One backwash with 50 psig nitrogen gas between cycles was also performed. The data are presented in Table 4. The testing continued successfully for a total of 50 cycles.

Since filter feed can vary, PP grade selection and operating parameters can be adjusted according to ongoing in-plant experience for a wide range of operating conditions. PP elements (5 μm grade) were evaluated at full production scale and

Table 4 Cycle Data for 12 μm Polypropylene Element Tested with Active Raney Nickel Catalyst[a]

Cycle number	Cycle duration (min)	Flow density (gpm/ft^2)	Differential pressure (psid)
1	15	0.33	<1
2	15	0.33	<1
3	15	0.33	<1
4	15	0.33	<1
5	15	0.33	<1
6	15	0.33	<1
7	15	0.33	<1
8	15	0.33	<1
9	15	0.33	<1
10	15	0.33	<1
11	15	0.33	<1
12	15	0.33	<1

[a]Effluent was evaluated for each cycle and was found to be visually clear and to meet product requirements.

were found to meet the process requirements. A production unit with 300 ft^2 of area has run successfully for more than 770 cycles.

5.4 Advantages of Backwashable Filters

The following are some of the advantages of the use of backwashable PP filters in applications that involve the removal of solid materials from pharmaceutical process streams.

High removal efficiency. In both applications described above, the PP elements were able to provide visual clarity in the effluent immediately. Little or no recycling of the influent stream has been required in the use of backwashable PP filters. The benefit of a membrane-based technology is that the effluent quality can be set at a specified consistent level based on the membrane micrometer rating.

Low operating cost. The cycle life of PP filters for backwash applications is estimated to be as high as 100 cycles or greater for carbon and 1000 cycles for Raney nickel. Cost savings benefits that can be realized over technologies that require filter aid include

1. Cost savings associated with the reduction of labor requirements for cleaning the system
2. Equipment productivity savings (a recycle is not required to meet clarity requirements, for example)
3. Cost savings associated with filter aids as well as the waste treatment savings for filter aids

Containment. The system collects, washes, and discharges the contaminant without operator exposure.

Automation. A backwashable filtration system can be designed to collect solids and recover the product automatically or semiautomatically. Labor is reduced, and a consistent operation is possible.

Maintenance. There are no moving parts in a backwash system. This reduces the energy consumption, noise, and maintenance.

Holdup volume. A high volume backwash system can be designed in a compact footprint to minimize product holdup volume, backwash fluid volume floor space requirements, and installation facility costs.

APPENDIX: ESTABLISHMENT OF OPTIMAL PRODUCT RECOVERY SCHEME

The purpose of this discussion is to describe possible schemes for product recovery.

The VMT system is an excellent device for concentration. If a process requires diafiltration for a high product yield, then a concentration followed by continuous diafiltration will result in a lower volume of material, with a higher concentration, for further processing. The following calculations illustrate this point.

The mass balance for the desired product (for example, protein, enzyme, antibiotic) is

$$C_0V_0 = C_RV_R + C_PV_P$$

For a concentration operation the concentration of the desired product in the retentate is defined as

$$C_R = C_0(V_0/V_R)^s$$

For a continuous diafiltration operation the concentration of the desired product in the retentate is defined as

$$C_R = C_0 \exp[-V_D(1 - s)]$$

where

C_R = concentration of the desired product in the retentate stream
C_0 = concentration of the desired product in the feed tank (initial concentration)
V_0 = initial volume in the feed tank
V_R = volume of the retentate (concentrated material)
$s = 1 - C_P/C_R$
C_P = concentration of the desired product in the permeate
V_P = volume of the permeate
$V_D = V_P/V_0$

The transmission (C_P/C_R) is assumed to be 0.8.

The initial volume (V_0) is set at 100 L and the initial concentration (C_0) is set at 1 unit/L for this calculation. The desired result is a greater than 90% yield.

Option 1. Concentration Without Diafiltration

Conc. factor	C_R (units/L)	V_R (L)	C_RV_R (units)	C_PV_P (units)	V_P (L)	C_P (units/L)	Yield (%)
2×	1.14	50	57	43	50	0.86	43
3×	1.24	33	41	59	67	0.88	59
4×	1.32	25	33	67	75	0.89	67
5×	1.38	20	28	72	80	0.90	72
10×	1.58	10	16	84	90	0.93	84
20×	1.82	5	9	91	95	0.96	91

Option 2. Continuous Diafiltration

V_D	C_R (units/L)	V_R (L)	C_RV_R (units)	C_PV_P (units)	V_P (L)	C_P (units/L)	Yield (%)
1	0.44	100	44	56	100	0.56	56
2	0.21	100	21	79	200	0.39	79
3	0.09	100	9	91	300	0.30	91
4	0.04	100	4	96	400	0.24	96

Option 3. Twofold Concentration Followed by Continuous Diafiltration

Conc. factor	C_R (units/L)	V_R (L)	$C_R V_R$ (units)	$C_P V_P$ (units)	V_P (L)	C_P (units/L)	Yield (%)
2×	1.14	50	57	43	50	0.86	43

The initial volume for the diafiltration (V_0) is 50 L, and the initial concentration (C_0) is 1.14 units/L.

V_D	C_R (units/L)	V_R (L)	$C_R V_R$ (units)	$C_P V_P$ (units)	V_P (L)	C_P (units/L)	Yield (%)
1	0.51	50	26	31	50	0.62	74
2	0.23	50	11.5	45.5	100	0.45	88
3	0.10	50	5	52	150	0.35	95
Total for 2× concentration and three diavolumes:					200	0.47	95

Option 4. Threefold Concentration Followed by Continuous Diafiltration

Conc. factor	C_R (units/L)	V_R (L)	$C_R V_R$ (units)	$C_P V_P$ (units)	V_P (L)	C_P (units/L)	Yield (%)
3×	1.24	33	41	59	67	0.88	43

The initial volume for the diafiltration (V_0) is 33 L, and the initial concentration (C_0) is 1.24 units/L.

V_D	C_R (units/L)	V_R (L)	$C_R V_R$ (units)	$C_P V_P$ (units)	V_P (L)	C_P (units/L)	Yield (%)
1	0.56	33	18	23	33	0.70	82
2	0.23	33	8	33	66	0.50	92
Total for 3× concentration and two diavolumes:					133	0.69	92

Summary

The table below summarizes the operations that meet a 90% or greater yield. Initial volume = 100 L; initial concentration = 1 unit/L.

Option	Final permeate volume (L)	Final concentration of product in the permeate (units/L)	Yield of product (%)
20× concentration	95	0.96	91
3 diavolumes	300	0.30	91
4 diavolumes	400	0.24	96
2× concentration followed by 3 diavolumes	200	0.47	95
3× concentration followed by 2 diavolumes	133	0.69	92

The optimal option for processing appears to be a concentration followed by continuous diafiltration. The yield requirement is met, for this example, with a small final permeate volume. An even smaller volume would be possible if concentration alone were employed. However, a high concentration factor would be needed to meet the yield requirement.

If the high (20×) concentration factor is not desirable, then, assuming 80% transmission, a 92% yield could be attained with a 3× concentration followed by two diafiltration steps. For a 100 L batch, this would result in a final permeate volume of 133 L and 66 L for diafiltration.

To optimize a process, the actual permeate flow rates for the processing options would need to be established and considered in conjunction with the final permeate volume, final product concentration in the permeate, and overall product yield to establish the most economical processing option.

REFERENCES

Culkin, B. (1990). Device and method for filtering a colloidal suspension, 4,952,317, Aug 28.

Culkin, J. B. (1991). Eccentric drive mechanism, 5,014,564, May 14.

Cole, J., and J. Brantley. (1996). Dynamic membrane filtration in cell and protein production. *Biopharm.* 7(5):66–71.

Haughney, H. (1993). Removal of Solid Materials in Pharmaceutical Processes Through the Use of Pall Backwashable Prosep Filters, Pall Corporation, Port Washington, N.Y.

Holeschovsky, U. B., and C. L. Cooney. (1991). Quantitative description of ultrafiltration in a rotating filtration device. *AIChE J. 37*(8):1219.

Kroner, K. H., and V. Nissinen. (1988). Dynamic filtration of microbial suspensions using an axially rotating filter, *J. Membrane Sci. 36*:85.

Lee, S. S., A. Burt, G. Russotti, and B. Buckland. (1995). Microfiltration of recombinant yeast cells using a rotary disk dynamic filtration system. *Biotechnol. Bioeng. 48*(4):336.

Murase, T., E. Iritani, C. Pradistsuwana, K. Kano, K. Atsumi, and M. Shirato. (1991). High-rate microfiltration by use of a ceramic filter with rotating cylinders. *Kagaku Kogaku Ronbonshu 15*(3):630, and *Int. Chem. Engr. 31*(2):370.

Pall Corporation. *PallSep™ VMF™ Applications in Bioprocessing*. Port Washington, N.Y.

Rebsamen E., and H. Ziegler. (1986). Dynamic microfiltration and ultrafiltration in biotechnology. Proceedings World Filtration Congress IV (Ostend, B).

25

Prefiltration Technology

FORREST BADMINGTON
Millipore Corporation, Bedford, Massachusetts

1 INTRODUCTION

The term "prefiltration" is used to define the step or steps that may be taken to remove the larger insoluble contaminants from a process solution prior to final filtration. To be most effective, the prefiltration step is usually carried out within a short time prior to final filtration. The prefiltration step may include filtration, centrifugation, gravitational settling, precipitation, coagulation, or any other method that will reduce the particulate level prior to the final filtration step. This chapter focuses on those prefiltration steps in which a solution is passed through a filter medium incorporated into a cartridge design. The prefiltration step using filter cartridges may in some instances be a separate filter process; however, it is more often included within the final filter train.

In selecting the filter cartridges that will be used for aseptic processing in the pharmaceutical industry, much thought is given to selecting the final (sterilizing) filters to be used in the train. However, if you are required to produce a sterile effluent, your choices of types (micrometer sizes) of filter cartridges are limited to those membrane filters that meet the Health Industry Manufacturer Association's (HIMA's) and the Food and Drug Administration's (FDA's) regulatory guidelines defining a sterilizing grade filter. These filter cartridges will have retention ratings in the 0.1–0.2 μm range. Prefilter cartridges, on the other hand, will have retention ratings in the 0.2–10 μm range or higher.

Since the final sterilizing grade cartridges are the most expensive filters in the train, extending their capacity (useful lifetime) by choosing the best combination of prefiltration cartridges can substantially reduce the overall cost of the filtration train. However, with the number of types of prefilter cartridges available, choosing the best prefilter train offers a unique challenge. In this chapter I discuss filtration theory and practices related to the prefiltration process and define a series of steps that can

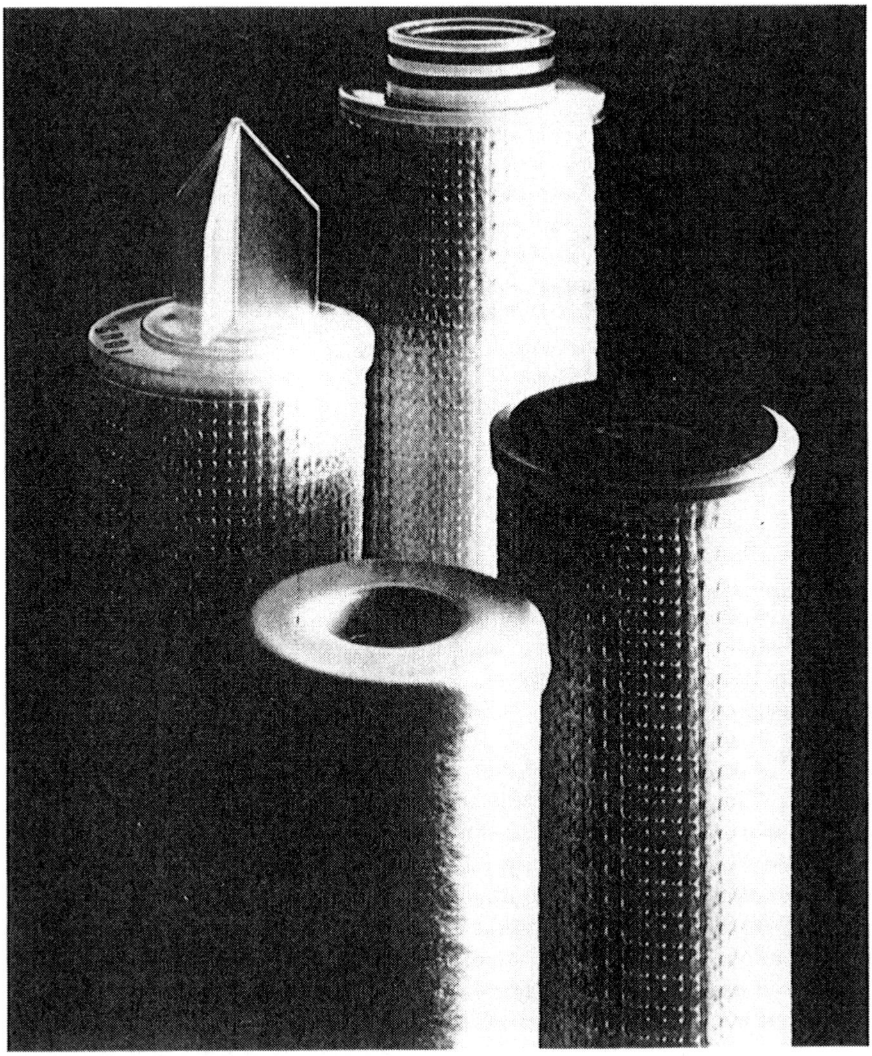

Figure 1 Depth prefilter cartridges with various sealing devices. (Courtesy of Millipore Corporation, Bedford, MA.)

be followed to select the most appropriate prefilter or combination of prefilters for specific applications.

2 PREFILTER CLASSIFICATIONS AND CHARACTERISTICS

2.1 Cartridges

A typical filtration system found in the pharmaceutical industry for aseptic processing of liquids consists of a series of filter cartridges. Each cartridge in this filter train is specifically chosen to protect and extend the life of the next cartridge. Prefilter cartridges are available in lengths from 1 to 40 in.; however, the 10, 20, and 30 in.

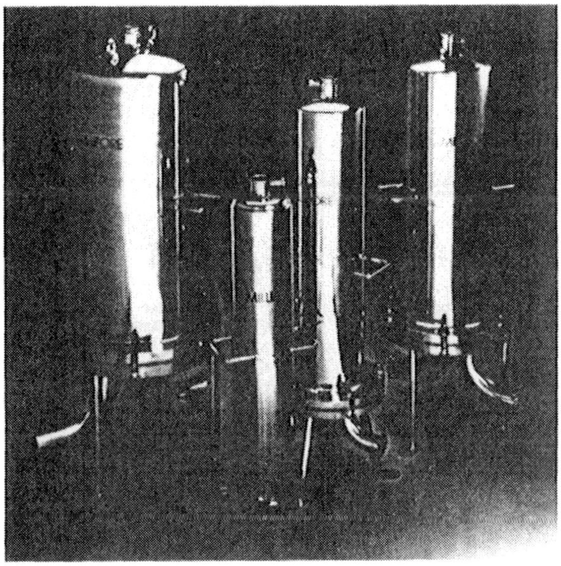

Figure 2 Typical multitube stainless steel housings used to filter large volumes of liquid. (Courtesy of Millipore Corporation, Bedford, MA.)

cartridges are the most commonly employed in standard process applications. For processing small to medium volumes of solution, single cartridges are placed into individual stainless steel housings. Cartridges are sealed into the housing using an O-ring or flat gasket seal, with process solution typically flowing from the outside of the cartridge into the central core (Fig. 1). For processing large volumes of solution (thousands of liters) multitube stainless housings such as those shown in Fig. 2 are employed. Prefilter cartridges used in pharmaceutical applications usually employ a double O-ring seal and interlocking tabs to lock the cartridge in place. Some filter cartridges are also equipped with a spear at the top of the cartridge to aid in centering and to prevent movement around the O-ring seal. For a detailed discussion of cartridge structure and design, see Chapter 16.

In relatively clean process solutions, the filter train may consist of only one prefilter and one final filter. More complex solutions, those that contain a large number of contaminants of various sizes, may require several different types of prefilters upstream of the final filter to effectively optimize the overall filtration process. The cartridge filters, placed upstream of the final filter, can be classified either by their position in the train (clarifying filter, prefilter) or by the structure and design of the filter medium (depth, surface, membrane) within the cartridge.

Classification by Position in Filter Train

Figure 3 shows filter cartridges identified by their position in the filter train. The clarifying filter cartridge would be the first filter cartridge in the train and the first filter to "see" process solution, the prefilter would be next, and then the final filter. In this case, the clarifying filter is the most open filter in the train and would remove the largest particles from the process solution and improve its overall clarity. Its main function is to extend the life of the prefilter. The prefilter in turn is used to extend

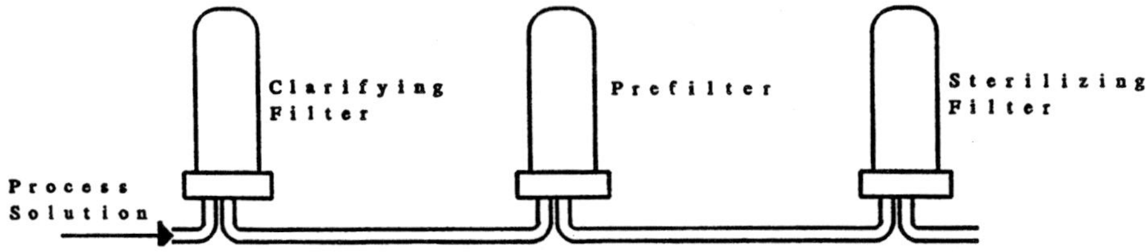

Clarifying Filter

1. Most open filter
2. Removes largest particles
3. Protects prefilter
4. May of may not be required
5. High capacity
6. Least costly
7. May be surface or depth filter
8. Nominal rating (based on hard particle retention)

Prefilter

1. Sized to protect final filter
2. Extends life of final filter
3. Protects final filter
4. Generally required
5. High capacity
6. More costly
7. May be surface or depth filter
8. Nominal rating (based on hard particle retention)

Final Filter

1. Least open filter
2. Removes smallest particles
3. Final filter (0.2 or 0.1 microns)
4. Required
5. Lower capacity
6. Most costly
7. Integrity testable
8. Absolute (based on microorganism retention)

Figure 3 Filter cartridges classified by their position in a filter train.

the life of the final filter. Generally filter trains contain a prefilter and a final filter; however, in the filtration of extremely dirty solutions or solutions with a large number of particles you may find that a clarifying filter is also needed. In these filter applications, the clarifying filter may be used to protect several prefilters in series.

Classification by Filter Structure

Filter cartridges are also characterized by the design or structure of the filter medium used in the cartridge. Under this classification, cartridges are referred to as depth, surface, or membrane filter cartridges.

Depth Filter

The depth filter consists of fibrous, granular, or sintered materials that produce a random porous structure. When fluid passes through a depth filter, particles become trapped in its tortuous network of flow channels. The construction of depth filter cartridges can vary. Most often the thick filter material (10–15 mm in depth) is wrapped or impregnated around a central core in the cartridge. In filter cartridges with a thin depth filter structure (3–5 mm in depth), the material may be placed into a pleated format (Fig. 4). A complete discussion of cartridge design is given in Chapter 3. The filtration material used in depth filter cartridges may consist of cotton, polypropylene, cellulose, acrylics, glass fiber, or any other polymeric material offering a porosity suitable for liquid flow. Due to the very open and random fibrous structure of depth filters it is difficult to characterize depth filter porosity in terms of a mean pore size distribution or rating. Depth filters are better characterized by their efficiency in removing hard particles of a specific size. Most filter manufacturers give depth filters nominal ratings, usually in the range of 90–99% retention efficiency of hard particles of a specified size. When referring to the porosity of depth filters, the term ‘‘percent void volume’’ (open space within the filter structure) is often mentioned. In general, filters have void volumes in the range of 30–80%; depth filters, due to their fibrous construction, are typically in the 30–40% range. Knowing the percent void volume of a depth prefilter is helpful in that, all other

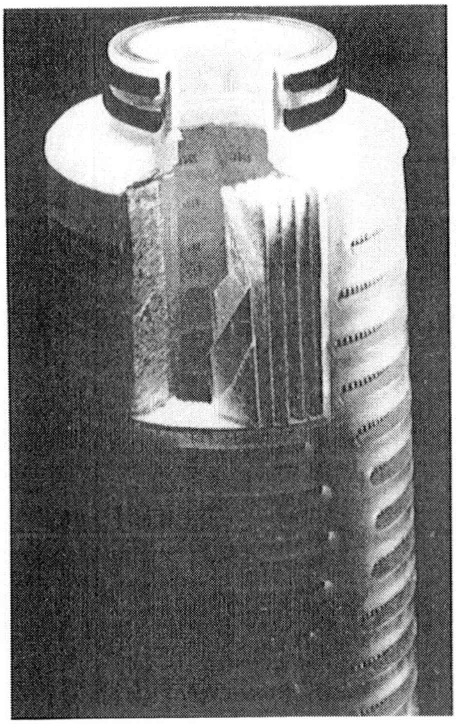

Figure 4 The pleated structure in a 10 in. filter cartridge. (Courtesy of Millipore Corporation, Bedford, MA.)

factors being equal, such as fiber length and diameter, the depth medium with the largest void volume will exhibit the highest capacity and lowest clean water pressure drop for a specified material thickness. This information can generally be obtained from the filter manufacturer. Scanning electron micrographs in Fig. 5 show the random porous structure of a glass fiber and a polypropylene depth filter. This type of structure would permeate the full depth of the filter material. A cutaway of a typical depth filter cartridge used in pharmaceutical filtration applications is shown in Fig. 6.

To increase the capacity of the depth filter, the thick filter matrix (3–20 mm) is constructed in a gradient density format. In this format, the filter material becomes progressively more retentive or tighter as the cartridge core is approached. The depth filter cartridge is generally used to remove the larger particles (0.5–100 μm) in the process solution.

With its thick filter matrix, the depth filter is an ideal format for adding a charge to the filter material. These charge-modified depth filters were first introduced in the mid-1970s to replace the use of asbestos filters in the pharmaceutical industry. The first charge-modified (CMS) depth filter (Zeta Plus) for pharmaceutical applications was introduced by AMF Incorporated, Cuno Division. Positively charged modified depth media have been used to reduce the endotoxin levels in water and pharmaceutical fluids (Hou and Zaniewski, 1990; Waterson, 1990; Wickert, 1991).

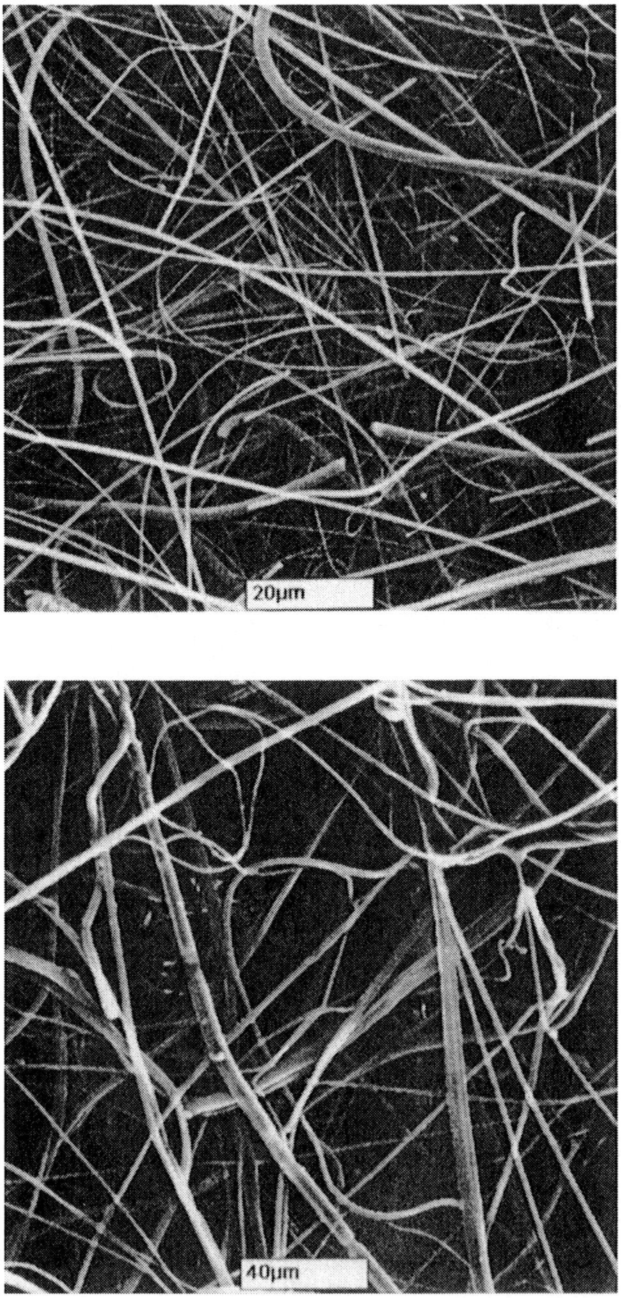

(a)

(b)

Figure 5 Scanning electron micrographs of the random porous structures found in (a) a glass fiber depth prefilter and (b) a polypropylene depth prefilter. (Courtesy of Millipore Corporation, Bedford, MA.)

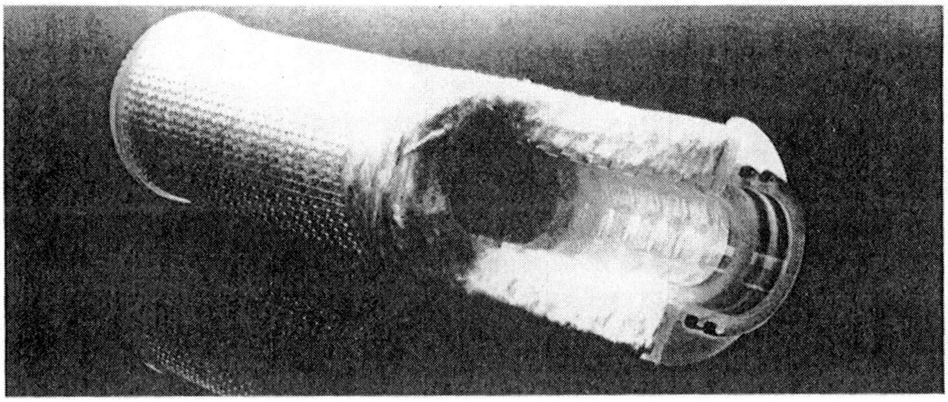

Figure 6 Cutaway view of an all-polypropylene depth prefilter cartridge. (Courtesy of Millipore Corporation, Bedford, MA.)

Prior to using any charge-modified medium it is important to evaluate your process solution with the materials for selective binding of low level product constituents.

Surface Filter

A surface filter is made up of multiple layers of media, usually glass or polymeric microfibers that are cast onto a paper or polyester support layer. As can be seen in Fig. 7, the surface filter has a much more uniform inner structure than the depth filter. When a fluid passes through a surface filter, particles larger than the spaces within the filter matrix are retained, primarily on the surface. In addition, smaller particles can be trapped within the filter matrix, giving a surface filter the properties of a depth filter as well.

Given the fact that some of the smaller particles are trapped within the structure of the surface filter, there is some conjecture in the industry as to the validity of using the surface and depth filter nomenclature or classification to describe these two types of prefilters. However, there are other distinct differences between the two. The surface filter usually has a higher retention efficiency rating than a depth filter and is used to remove the smaller particles (0.2–5.0 μm) in the process solution that would tend to plug the final sterilizing grade membrane filter. Because the filter material in a surface filter is thinner and tighter than the material in a depth cartridge, a large surface area is needed for flow, and surface filters are generally designed with a pleated structure (Fig. 4). For a further discussion of cartridge design, see Chapters 3 and 16. Surface filters are given nominal retention ratings of 99.0–99.99% retention efficiency based on a hard particle challenge.

Membrane Filter

Membrane filters, though acting similarly to surface filters in that most of the trapped material is on or near the surface of the filter, are in a unique class by themselves. The membrane filter can be thought of as a very thin (typically 0.1–0.2 mm), geometrically regular porous structure containing a number of layers of interconnecting cells. Membrane filters, generally thought of as final sterilizing grade filters, are used in many applications in the role of prefilter, especially in providing protection to a 0.1 or 0.2 μm sterilizing grade filter or to filters or devices that remove mycoplasma

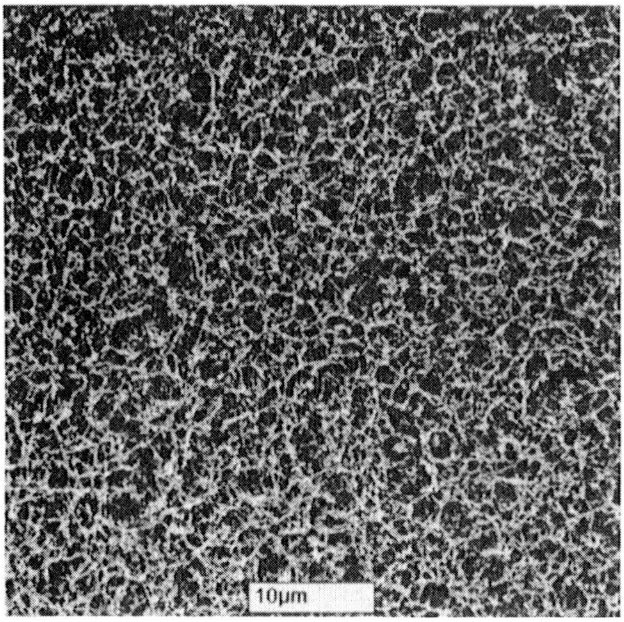

Figure 7 A scanning electron micrograph of the uniform structure found in a surface prefilter. (Courtesy of Millipore Corporation, Bedford, MA.)

and viruses. Membrane filters are cast from a variety of polymeric materials in a controlled manner that gives rise to a very uniform and consistent pore structure. Due to this consistency, membrane filters have been developed to retain 100% of certain microorganisms (Leahy and Sullivan, 1978; Tanny et al., 1979; Meltzer, 1983) and produce a sterile (free of microorganisms) effluent. These membrane filters have been traditionally termed "absolute" when referring to their retention efficiency. The absolute rating, however, applied to a 0.2 μm sterilizing membrane is specifically related to the complete removal of microorganisms by the size exclusion (sieving) mechanism and not based on a hard particle retention efficiency test. Membrane prefilters characterized by a hard particle challenge test, though sometimes referred to as absolute, should not be expected to retain 100% of the contaminant particles at their size removal rating. The membrane filter and its unique characteristics are described in detail in Chapter 12.

There can be quite a bit of overlap in the retention efficiency value and in the particle removal size rating assigned to each type (depth, surface, membrane) of cartridge prefilter. The chart shown in Fig. 8 lists the range of retention efficiencies and sizes of particles typically removed by the three types of prefilters.

To further improve the efficiency of a single-cartridge prefilter and in some cases to reduce the number of types of prefilter cartridges that may be needed in a filter train, cartridges are constructed with various combinations of membrane, surface, and depth media. In Fig. 9 a pleated cartridge is shown that is constructed with two layers of filtration material. The top layer, composed of borosilicate glass microfibers, acts as a depth filter, while the bottom layer of cellulose acts more like a surface filter. In some instances, a thick (10–15 mm) depth wrap material is placed

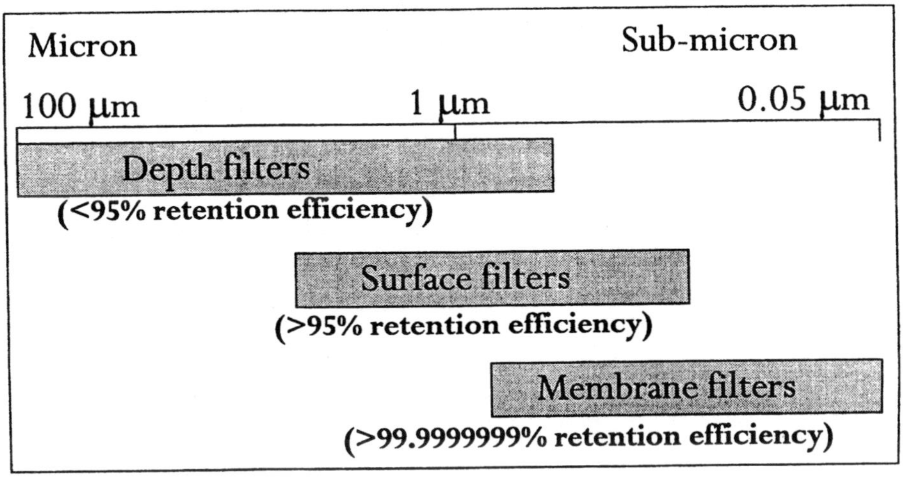

Figure 8 Chart showing the relative size removal and retention efficiencies of depth, surface, and membrane filters.

over a pleated surface filter to provide a true depth and surface structure in one cartridge (Fig. 10).

2.2 Bags

Bag filters have generally not seen much acceptance or use in the pharmaceutical industry. However, with the development of newly designed, stronger bag filters and better housing designs that will effectively hold and seal the bag into place under pressure and flux changes, the use of bag filters in this industry has been on the increase (Schrader, 1992). Bag filters are available in a variety of materials, including

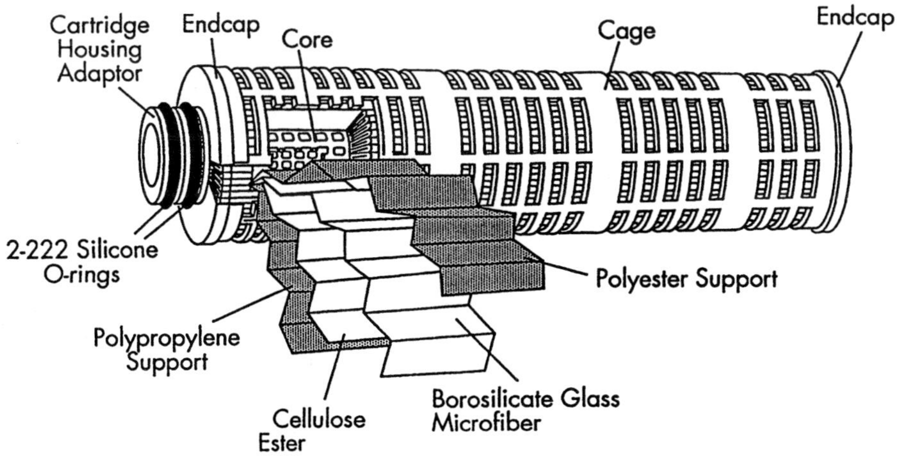

Figure 9 A cutaway view of a pleated prefilter cartridge containing a layer of glass fiber material over cellulose ester material. (Courtesy of Millipore Corporation, Bedford, MA.)

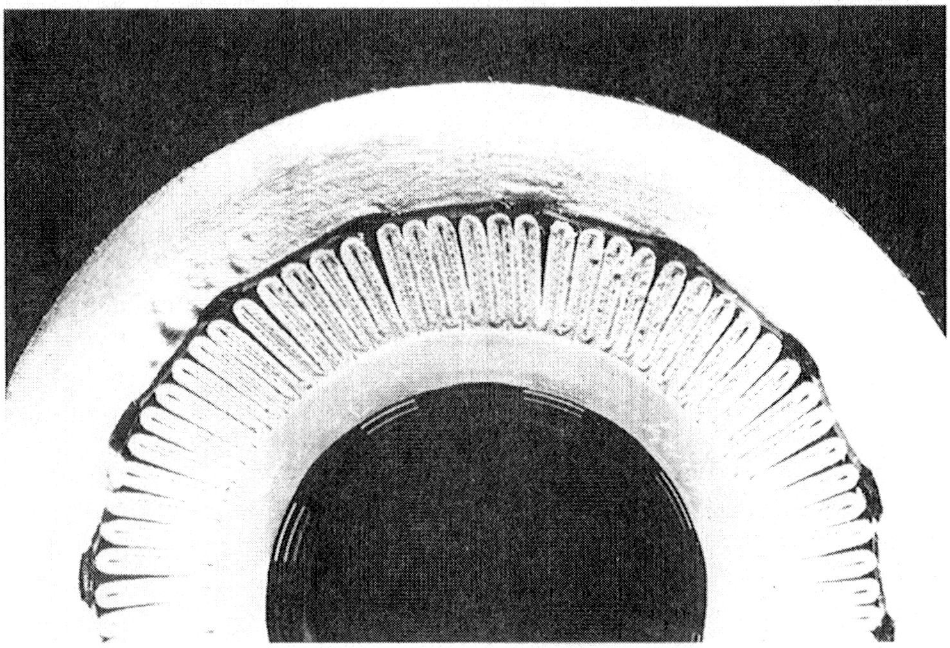

Figure 10 A cutaway view of a prefilter cartridge containing a gradient density depth filter material over pleated prefilter material. (Courtesy of Millipore Corporation, Bedford, MA.)

polypropylene, polyester, and nylon, and incorporate graded density depth filter media and pleated materials into their construction. They are supplied with retention efficiency ratings similar to those given for depth cartridges. Because of the high surface area available in the filter bag, it is most applicable for the filtration of high viscosity fluids. Bag filters with long sewn or thermally bonded seams are generally not good in filtrations where a high buildup of differential pressure is anticipated, in that the long seams in the bag supported by a stainless steel basket cannot take high pressure or dramatic pressure fluctuations. In general, bag filters are lower in cost than cartridges with the same effective filter area and would be the most suitable for noncritical process separations.

2.3 Pads

Filter media stacked in flat sheets or disks are generically referred to as pad filters. These pad filters can be classified as nonstructured depth filters and are often used in the very early stages of the pharmaceutical filtration process as a clarifying filter device. Pad filters are manufactured from a number of filter materials and come in a variety of sizes and shapes. During the filtration process they are usually placed into plate-and-frame holders or filter presses that will allow the process solution to flow through them. Pad filters offer the advantages that they are low in cost, are easily disposed of, and can be placed into configurations that afford effective depth filtration while maintaining a large effective filtration area. In many cases pad filters serve as the support material for various filter aids. One general disadvantage of the more brittle pad filters is that they may be difficult to seal tightly between the upstream and downstream sides of the filter medium and are therefore generally used to remove the largest contaminants upstream of the cartridge.

2.4 Filter Aids

Also classified as nonstructured prefiltration media are a series of materials known as filter aids. Filters aids are insoluble, inert materials of low bulk density that form a highly permeable cake with a low flow resistance. These materials are mainly used in two ways: as a precoat or as a "body feed." As a precoat the filter aid is added to a clean solution to make a slurry. The slurry is then processed through a filter to form a porous cake on the upstream side of the filter. This cake will become the filter medium for the process solution. As a "body feed" the filter aid is mixed directly with the process solution prior to the filtration step. The more common filter aids encountered in the pharmaceutical industry include diatomaceous earth, perlite, and cellulose. Diatomaceous earth (diatomite; called kieselguhr in Europe) is composed mainly of silica. The material originates from the fossilized skeletal remains of aquatic algae called diatoms. It is mined as a solid and separated into mixtures of various particle sizes for filtration use.

Perlite, which is mined from volcanic rock, is composed of alumina and sodium silicate. Perlite forms filter cakes with a pore size distribution significantly larger than that of the diatomaceous earth cakes. Cellulose fibers are sometimes used as filter aids, especially when high pH solutions are being filtered. However, the cellulose fibers have two disadvantages as a filter aid: They are more costly and more compressible than either diatomaceous earth or perlite.

A complete discussion of filter aids and their use in pharmaceutical applications is included in Chapter 1.

3 PARTICLE CAPTURE MECHANISMS

The key to selecting an optimized filtration system is to understand the particle–medium interactions in the filter matrix. To evaluate particle–medium interactions, we need to know the type of particle involved, the capture mechanism that is occurring, and the type of filter medium that is being challenged.

There are basically two types of particles: hard (nondeformable) particles and soft (deformable) particles. Typical hard particle contaminants encountered in pharmaceutical process solutions include dust, sand, metal fines, and diatomaceous earth. Typical soft contaminants include colloids, gels, bacteria, clays, and carbohydrates.

The capture mechanisms operating in liquid and gases have been extensively studied (Rubow, 1981; Rubow and Liu, 1986, Rubow et al., 1987). There are six basic capture mechanisms:

1. *Size exclusion or sieving* occurs when the particles are larger than the pores in the membrane.
2. *Adsorption or electrostatic deposition* occurs when there are attractive forces between the particles and the filter matrix.

3. *Inertial impaction* occurs when the inertia of the particles causes them to impact on the filter matrix. The inertia is developed as flow is diverted around the filter structure.
4. *Interception* occurs when the particle in the flow stream contacts the filter matrix.
5. *Diffusion* occurs when the small particles move in random or Brownian motion, which increases their probability of collision with the filter matrix.
6. *Gravitational settling* occurs when large particles settle out in slow-moving flow streams.

Depending on whether a gas or a liquid is being filtered, different capture mechanisms will predominate and directly influence the retention capabilities of the membrane filter. In gas filtration, the primary capture mechanisms are size exclusion, inertial capture, diffusion, and electrostatic deposition. The predominant capture mechanism depends on the particle size and the particle velocity. Small particles are retained by diffusion; larger particles, by inertial forces. Once a particle is retained on the filter's surface, it is difficult for that particle to become dislodged because of the electrostatic and intermolecular forces acting over the small distance between the particle and the filter surface. The open cell-like structure of a membrane filter causes a particle to be exposed to a large surface and to travel a very tortuous path through the filter. These effects magnify the retention mechanisms in gases, resulting in increased particle retention. The dominant capture mechanisms during liquid filtrations are size exclusion and adsorption. In prefiltration with depth filters, the two main capture mechanisms are entrapment and adsorption.

4 PREFILTER-PLUGGING MECHANISMS

In liquid filtration there have been several theoretical models presented for filter plugging (Hermans and Bredee, 1935, 1936; Grace, 1956; Hermia, 1982) over time. The caking model describes filter cake formation through particle buildup on the surface of the filter rather than inside the filter pores. Gradual pore blocking is characterized by gradual, controlled blocking of pores as a function of the amount of filtrate passing through the filter. Since contaminant particles are generally smaller than the pores, particles reaching the filter surface enter the pores and gradually build up on the inner walls until the pore is completely plugged. In complete blocking, a particle that reaches the filter surface completely blocks the pore. Intermediate blocking behavior falls between caking and gradual blocking; particles may either block the inner walls of pores or adhere to other particles on the surface.

The type of filter plugging encountered depends on the type of contaminant particles in the process solution and on the structure or micrometer rating of the filter medium. Hard (nondeformable) particles generally produce a filter cake, whereas soft (deformable) particles often lead to complete or gradual pore blocking. In real-world separations, solutions contain both types of particles; however, one type will usually predominate and give rise to one type of plugging mechanism. Biological solutions typically processed in the pharmaceutical industry contain mostly soft, deformable particles and typically block filters by a gradual or complete pore blocking mechanism. This works to our advantage in sizing systems (See Sec. 7.)

5 PREFILTER PERFORMANCE CRITERIA

Four key factors are critical in evaluating the overall performance of a prefilter cartridge: (1) percent retention efficiency (beta ratio), (2) capacity (throughput), (3) differential pressure drop versus flow rate, and (4) compatibility and extractables.

5.1 Percent Retention Efficiency

Percent retention efficiency is a measure of the ability of a cartridge to capture and retain particles. These particles are effectively removed from the solution as it passes through the filter. The percent retention efficiency on a cartridge prefilter is determined using the equation

$$\begin{aligned}&\%\ \text{Retention efficiency}\\&= \frac{(\text{No. of feed particles} - \text{No. of effluent particles})\ \text{size}\ X\ \text{and larger}}{\text{Number of feed particles size}\ X\ \text{and larger}} \times 100\end{aligned} \tag{1}$$

A term closely related to percent retention efficiency is beta ratio. The beta ratio term and concept, used more to define the retention of filters for industrial applications, was introduced by the Fluid Power Research Center (FPRC) at Oklahoma State University (OSU) in the late 1960s (Fitch, 1980). In 1973 the beta ratio concept was incorporated into a multipass method for evaluating the filtration performance of a fine hydraulic fluid power element issued by the American National Standards Institute (ANSI/B93.31) and the International Standards Organization (ISO 4572) issued in 1981. Beta ratio values are calculated from the equation

$$\text{Beta ratio}\ (\beta) = \frac{\text{number of feed particles of size}\ X\ \text{and larger}}{\text{number of effluent particles of size}\ X\ \text{and larger}} \tag{2}$$

As shown in Table 1, there is a direct relationship between beta ratio and percent retention efficiency, and either value can be derived from the other using Eqs. (3) and (4).

$$\%\ \text{Retention efficiency} = \frac{\beta - 1}{\beta} \times 100 \tag{3}$$

$$\text{Beta ratio}\ (\beta) = \frac{100}{100 - \%\ \text{retention efficiency}} \tag{4}$$

Table 1 Correlation of Percent Retention Efficiency and Beta Ratio

Beta ratio	Percent retention efficiency
1	0
2	50.0
10	90.0
100	99.0
1,000	99.9
10,000	99.99

Though the two methods developed by ANSI and ISO effectively measure the removal efficiency of the filter over its lifetime, they were specifically designed to measure cartridge efficiencies in hydraulic fluid under multipass (filter effluent returned to feed tank) flow conditions.

In 1988 the American Society for Testing and Materials (ASTM) issued a single-pass (effluent not sent back to feed tank), constant flow rate test method for determining filter efficiency in liquids (ASTM F795-88). This method provides a generalized diagram for a test system and an overall outline for the test procedure. The ASTM method, however, does not specify (1) a cartridge flow rate, (2) a cartridge pressure drop, (3) particle challenge type or concentration, or (4) test temperature. Varying any one of these factors can influence the retention efficiency results that are obtained. Most of the prefilter cartridge manufacturers and independent testing laboratories are currently using a version of the ASTM test procedure. Therefore, when using prefilter retention efficiency test data it is important to have the specific test method used to develop the data described in detail, especially if you are comparing prefilter cartridges from different manufacturers.

A number of particle contaminants have been used to measure the retention efficiency of filters. AC Fine Test Dust (ACFTD) is by far the most widely used particle contaminant for filter cartridge retention testing. It was originally used by the AC Spark Plug Division of General Motors to evaluate air filters in automobiles and was the main test particle used in the development of the ANSI/B93.31 and ISO 4572 test methods. It is a silica-based irregularly shaped hard particle with a wide particle size distribution in the range of 0.5–80 μm. A typical particle distribution by weight of ACFTD is listed in Table 2. ACFTD can no longer be obtained through the AC Division of General Motors but is now available at Powder Technologies Inc. (Burnsville, MN) as an SAE (Society of Automotive Engineers) standard test dust.

Latex beads and glass beads are other test contaminants used to evaluate the retention efficiency of filters. Both spherical latex (polystyrene) and spherical glass beads are very uniform in size and are available in a variety of specific particle sizes (Fig. 11). Beads offer the advantage that they can be used as a single-size monodispersed challenge contaminant of known size or as a mixture of known sizes. This allows filter retention efficiency testing to be done at specific sizes and will minimize particle sizing errors that may occur during the particle-counting steps with an unsized polydispersed particle challenge solution. The National Sanitation Foundation

Table 2 Particle Size Distribution in AC Fine Test Dust

Micrometer range	Percent by weight
0–5	39±3
5–10	18±3
10–20	16±3
20–40	18±3
40–80	9±3

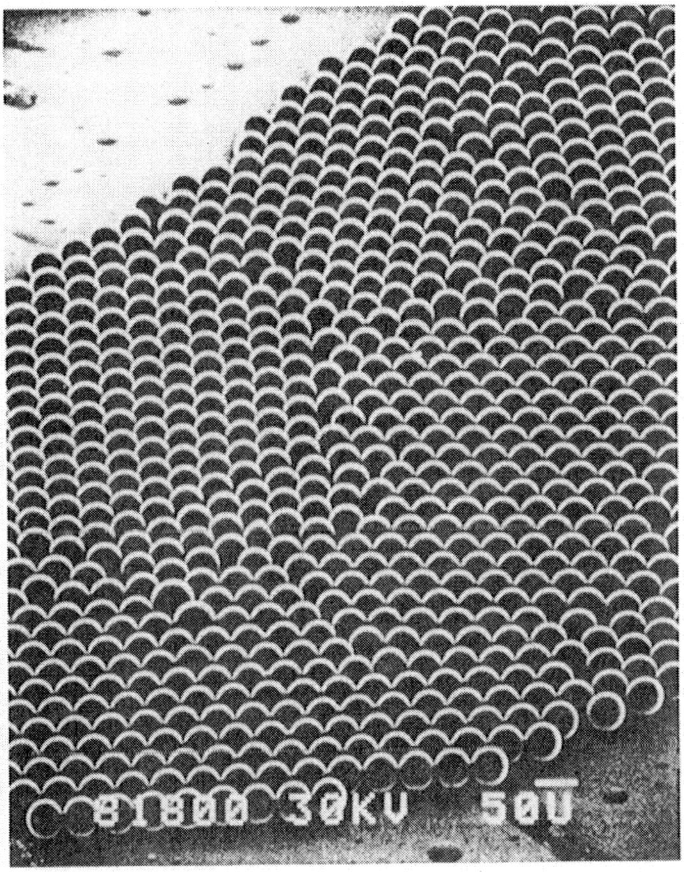

Figure 11 A scanning electron micrograph of spherical latex beads 44.1 μm in diameter. (Courtesy of Millipore Corporation, Bedford, MA.)

(NSF) recommends the use of latex beads (2.5–4.0 μm) as one of the acceptable test particles for certifying filter cartridges for cyst reduction in drinking water (NSF International, 1994). A fourth type of hard particle test contaminant, JIS Z-8901, is routinely used in Japan (JSA, 1989) for cartridge filter retention testing.

A schematic for a typical test system that would be used to measure the retention efficiency of prefilter cartridges is shown in Fig. 12. In this test system a solution of AC Fine Test Dust and latex beads are fed into a clean water feed stream flowing to a test cartridge. During the testing, recirculated cartridge effluent is cleaned with a 0.22 μm filter, and new ACFTD and latex beads are continuously added to this feed solution at a constant flow rate. This ensures that the particle level in the challenge solution remains constant. Sample ports upstream and downstream of the test cartridge provide on-line sampling to particle-counting sensors. The new particle-counting sensors used today can accurately determine particle levels within six to eight different size ranges simultaneously. The concentration of the test dust and latex beads in the feed solution is kept low (0.1 ppm) to allow for direct particle

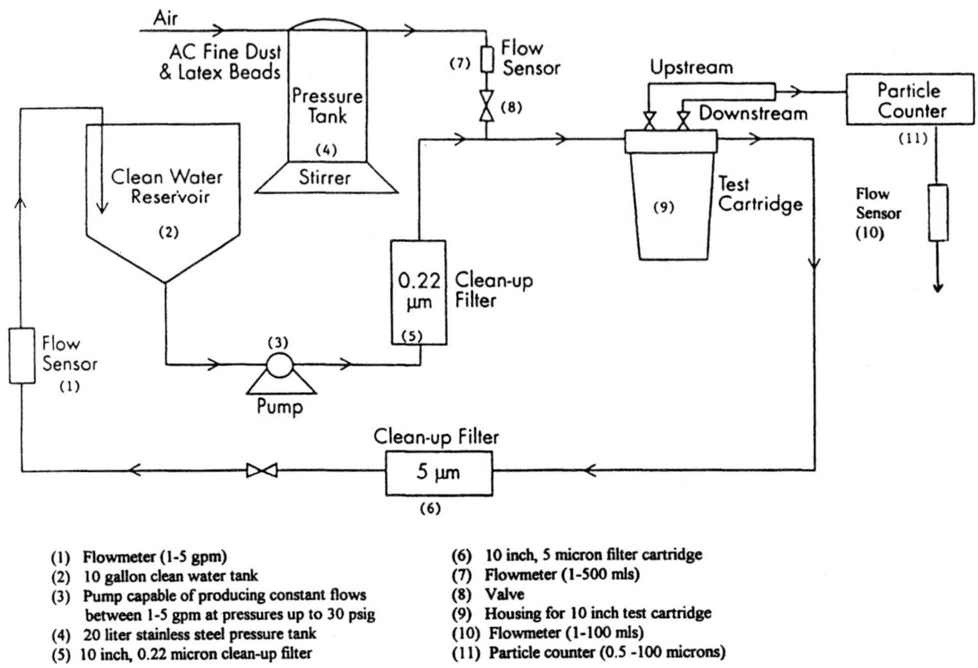

Figure 12 Schematic of a test system used to determine percent retention efficiency/beta ratio of prefilter cartridges. (1) Flowmeter (1–5 gpm); (2) 10 gal clean water tank; (3) pump capable of producing constant flows of 1–5 gpm at pressures up to 30 psig; (4) 20 L stainless steel pressure tank; (5) 10 in., 0.22 μm cleanup filter; (6) 10 in., 5 μm filter cartridge; (7) flowmeter (1–500 mL); (8) valve; (9) housing for 10 in. test cartridge; (10) flowmeter (1–100 mL); (11) particle counter (0.5–100 μm).

counting of the feed and effluent samples and so as not to build a filter cake or prematurely plug the cartridge. This test would provide an initial and reproducible retention efficiency rating for unused cartridges. Flow rates to the test cartridges would be maintained at the recommended usage levels for that type of cartridge. In most cases, flow rates in the range of 1–3 gpm are used when testing 10 in. prefilter cartridges. The percent retention efficiency or beta ratio data generated at various micrometer sizes are plotted and a retention curve is produced for each type of cartridge. Typical retention efficiency curves for a family of filter cartridges are shown in Fig. 13. Though the retention curves for individual prefilter cartridges are developed under a standard set of in-house test conditions with a standard hard particle contaminant, they allow us to make a direct comparison of initial cartridge retention efficiencies and are an invaluable tool for choosing the types of prefilters and/or clarifying filters that should be run during the initial screening trials with actual process solution. Remember that before final sizing recommendations are made, especially for large cartridge systems (greater than single 10 in. cartridges), a pilot run must be done with scaled-down cartridges at flow and processing conditions similar to those that will be employed during the full process runs.

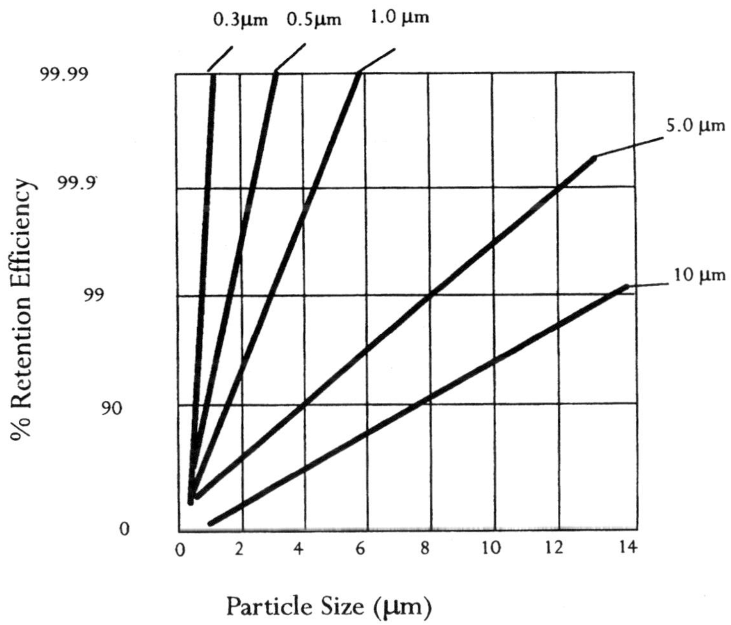

Figure 13 Retention efficiency curves for a series of depth prefilter cartridges.

Nominal Versus Absolute Retention Efficiency

Prefilters are given both nominal and absolute ratings. Absolute, in the classical definition, implies 100% removal, and this rating is generally reserved for sterilizing grade membrane filters.

Nominal ratings are given to filters that remove something less than 100% of the particles or contaminants at the filter rating. Unlike microorganisms, it is not possible to accurately measure the complete absence of very small particles or contaminants downstream of a filter with standard particle-counting equipment. The particle sensor is not capable of distinguishing the ever-present background (one to two particles) of particles smaller than 0.5 µm from the challenge particles used upstream of the filter.

Filter manufacturers have not standardized on the use of the two terms "nominal" and "absolute," nor have they agreed on the percent removal given to a filter cartridge with a nominal rating. Some filter manufacturers rate filters with 99.99% or 99.9% removal efficiency as absolute, whereas others give this filter a nominal rating. For a retention efficiency value to be meaningful it must include both a particle size and a percent retention value for the number of particles of that size.

5.2 Capacity (Throughput)

The dirt-holding capacity (throughput) of a filter can be defined as (1) the mass of contaminant held by the filter, (2) the volume of fluid fed to the filter, or (3) the mass of contaminant fed to the filter.

In practical applications, the capacity of a filter is a measure of the total volume of fluid that can be processed through the filter before a differential pressure develops across the filter that exceeds the limits of the filter system or when the flow through the filter is decreased to a rate that is unacceptable for the required processing conditions. In general, the capacity of a filter will vary dramatically depending on the types and particle size distribution of the contaminants being filtered. In some instances, prefilter cartridge capacity comparisons are made using in-house capacity data that have been generated with a synthetic solution. Generally these data are of no practical use, as the results are not directly related to the capacity data that are generated with real-world process solutions. Test trials to determine filter capacities or to compare filters can be done only with a representative sample from the actual process solution. Filter manufacturers will supply prefilter material cut into disks (47–90 mm) and depth filter cartridges in a 1–2 in. length for this testing. Section 7 in this chapter and Chapter 9 discuss this process in detail.

5.3 Flow Rate Versus Differential Pressure

One of the most important considerations when sizing a filtration system is the differential pressure drop that will be obtained across each filter. The maximum allowable pressure drop will control the minimum membrane area needed to do the job. The differential pressure across a filter is defined as the pressure upstream of the filter minus the pressure downstream of the filter at a specified flow rate. Filter manufacturers supply these data in the form of a pressure drop curve. The pressure drop curve shown in Fig. 14 gives the clean water pressure drop for a 10 in. filter cartridge at various flow rates and shows that there is a linear relationship between pressure drop and flow rate over the acceptable flow range for this cartridge filter. In most cartridge prefilters, the clean water pressure drop across the cartridge increases proportionally with flow rate (Johnston, 1992); therefore, in many instances pressure drop data are listed as the differential pressure (psid) at a specified flow rate, generally 1 gallon per minute (gpm).

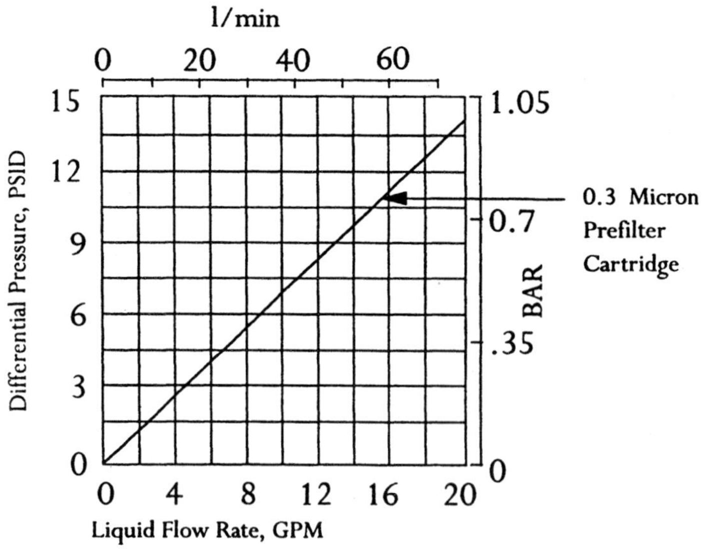

Figure 14 Pressure drop versus flow rate curve for a 10 in. 0.3 μm depth prefilter cartridge.

The pressure drop curve generated in Fig. 14 was generated with a clean water solution at 20°C (viscosity of 1.0 cP); however, a solution with a different viscosity would produce a different pressure drop across the filter. This is readily apparent when a cold water solution and a hot water solution are filtered under similar conditions. The cold water, having a higher viscosity than the hot water, would exhibit a higher pressure drop in the same cartridge at equivalent flows. For practical applications, the theory of pressure drop in prefilter cartridges can be simplified if two assumptions are made: (1) that the liquids being filtered are noncompressible and (2) that the fluids are Newtonian.

In Newtonian fluids the viscosity of the fluid is independent of shear. Pressure drop losses occur in two principal modes: laminar and turbulent. In laminar flow, pressure drop is proportional to velocity and viscosity. Because the characteristic dimension of surface and membrane filters is small, the liquid flow through the medium is generally always laminar. Therefore, the pressure drop across a filter cartridge with Newtonian solutions will increase linearly with an increase in viscosity (Johnston, 1990). For example, a filter with a pressure drop of 0.5 psid in water at 20°C (1.0 cP) would have a pressure drop of 5.0 psid in a solution with a viscosity of 10 cP. It is important to note that in the more open depth prefilter cartridges, where the clean water pressure drop is mainly due to turbulent flow, the pressure drop values at higher viscosities cannot be calculated directly from the clean water pressure drop data. For example, an open depth prefilter with a clean water pressure drop of 0.09 psid/gpm will have a pressure drop closer to 0.5 psid than to 0.9 psid when filtering a process solution with a viscosity of 10 cP. To size for pressure drop in these applications, obtain the filter manufacturer's viscosity–pressure drop–flow rate data for the specific filter cartridges in question.

Since water and most liquids are incompressible, the pressure differential across the filter will be independent of the absolute pressure of the system. This is not true for gases, however, and therefore filter manufacturers provide cartridge pressure drop versus flow rate curves for gases at various pressures.

5.4 Compatibility and Extractables

Extractables are defined as the total amount of material that is extracted from a filter during the time it is in contact with the process solution. An ideal, fully compatible filter material would be nonreactive with the process solution. It would neither adsorb nor remove any active ingredients from the process solution, nor would it impart any extractables back into the solution. Filter manufacturers have developed an excellent array of inert polymeric membrane filters that are compatible with the many solutions requiring filtration in the biopharmaceutical industry. Though compatible with the process solution, these membrane filters may have a small quantity (milligrams) of material extracted over time. Regulatory agencies require that filter manufacturers supply extractables data for their specific filter products. Generally, the quantity of extractable material is so small that it cannot be detected in an actual process solution even with the most precise and sophisticated analytical equipment. What is generally provided by the filter manufacturer is the quantity and type of material extracted using a clean solvent that is representative of the solvent found in the process solution (Stone et al., 1994, 1996). The filter manufacturer should also specify the exact test conditions used for the extraction, as described in Chapter 8.

Fiber Shedding

One area of concern directly related to extractables is that of cartridge fiber shedding. A fiber is defined by 21 CFR, part 210.3 (5) and Pharmaceutical GMPs (21 CFR, part 211) as any contaminant with a length at least three times greater than its width. 21 CFR, part 211.72 further states:

> Filters for liquid filtration used in the manufacture, processing or packaging of injectable drug products intended for human use shall not release fibers into such products. . . . If use of a non fiber releasing filter is necessary, an additional non-fiber releasing filter of 0.22 micron maximum mean porosity (0.45 micron if the manufacturing conditions so dictate) shall subsequently be used to reduce the content of particulates in the injectable drug product. Use of asbestos containing filter, with or without subsequent use of a specific non-fiber releasing filter, is permissible only upon submission of proof to the appropriate bureau of the Food and Drug Administration that use of a non-fiber releasing filter will, or is likely to, compromise the safety or effectiveness of the injectable drug product.

Some prefilter cartridges have a fiber-shedding claim; however, as stated in 21 CFR, section 211.72, clarifying and prefilter cartridges do not need to have a fiber-shedding claim as long as there is a non-fiber-releasing filter downstream. Many of the fibrous depth filters used as prefilters are constructed so as not to continuously release fibers into the product. The first requirement when more than one filter is used in a filtration train is to ensure that the final filter in line is a non-fiber-releasing filter of 0.22 μm (maximum mean porosity). It is preferable, where possible, to specify all filters in the filter train as non-fiber-releasing.

It is important to note that the German Federal Health Office has published standards for asbestos particulate limits in parenterals (BGA, 1993). This document states that the length of asbestos fibers is the decisive risk factor and has established three size categories:

1. Fibers exceeding 2.5 μm must be eliminated.
2. Fibers between 1 and 2.5 μm "may be found only in low concentrations." (The document further states that drug manufacturers should look for ways to remove fibers of this length, given that the current limits will be temporarily effective.)
3. Fibers not longer than 1 μm are not included in the quality assessment.

Considering these limitations for the final dosage form, it would be important to discuss any asbestos fiber related concerns with the prefilter cartridge manufacturer.

Protein Binding

In the first section of the extractables/compatibility discussion we mainly focused on the materials that would be extracted from the cartridge. It is also critical to know the extent to which the cartridge materials may remove any constituents from your product solution. When filters are used to process biotechnology products containing proteins that are extremely expensive or at a level where any loss is considered detrimental to the overall quality of the product, it is important to consider and evaluate what effects the membrane materials will have on the process solution. Because most polymeric microporous membrane filters have a large internal area accessible to proteins, there will be some nonspecific binding of proteins by the

Table 3 Protein Adsorption to Polymer Surfaces at a 1000 mg/L Protein Concentration

Membrane type	μg BSA bound/cm²	μg IgG bound/cm²
Hydrophilic polyvinylidene fluoride (PVDF)	3.4	3.8
Cellulose diacetate (CDA)	1.1	8.6
Mixed esters of cellulose acetate and cellulose nitrate	274	238

Source: Pitt (1987).

membrane. Certain polymer materials bind protein at higher rates than other materials. Filter manufacturers provide modified hydrophilic membranes specifically for protein applications. Since the level of binding is going to be dependent on the type of protein or peptide and its concentration in solution, it is recommended that an evaluation be done with a specific process solution and several filter materials before reaching a decision on one filter type. It is important to evaluate the entire filter train including any clarifying or any prefilters that the process solution will be in contact with during the filtration cycle. A number of papers have been published in this area (Pitt, 1987; Martin and Manteuffel, 1988; Van den Oetelaar et al., 1989; Sarry and Sucker 1992a, 1992b; Datar et al., 1992; Hu et al., 1993; Nema and Avis, 1993). Table 3 lists data on the nonspecific binding of bovine serum albumin (BSA) and sheep immunoglobulin G (IgG) with several commercial polymeric membranes. In addition to protein binding, it is important to monitor the adsorption of any other products or additives (preservatives) that may be in your process solution at low concentrations (Brose and Henricksen, 1994).

Shear Effects and Protein Degradation

In general, protein degradation, denaturation, or change in conformation is due more to the interaction of the protein (adsorption) with a specific polymer filter material than to the shear effects that are created as the protein solution is passed through a microporous membrane (Truskey et al., 1989). However, in one experimental study (Bowen and Gan, 1992) on the interaction of the enzyme yeast alcohol dehydrogenase (YADH) with microfiltration membranes, a loss in enzyme activity was attributed more to the shear effects occurring during the filtration than to a filter material interaction. Since many filtration applications require the use of pumps, these devices should also be evaluated as a potential contributor to shearing effects.

During the separation of mammalian cells from a protein product, shear may adversely affect the quality of the product passing through the filter. High flow rates and high differential pressures across the filter may cause cell lysis. This increase in cell debris may plug the downstream filter or contaminate the final product. It is recommended that these separations be run at low flow rates and low differential pressures and that the amount of cell lysis occurring during the filtration be continually monitored.

6 VALIDATION AND REGULATORY ISSUES

6.1 Regulatory Agencies

In the United States there are several key agencies involved in regulating aseptic filtration processing and providing requirements and test recommendations for validating filtration systems. They include the Food and Drug Administration (FDA), the Health Industry Manufacturers Association (HIMA), and the U.S. Pharmacopoeia (USP). The American Society for Testing and Materials (ASTM), though not a governmental regulatory agency, issues many test methods relating to the evaluation and testing of filter cartridges.

6.2 Prefilter Validation Requirements

Prefilter cartridges, unlike sterilizing grade filters, are not required to be integrity tested in the filter train. However, prefilter cartridges used in the final process filter train are required to meet the same stringent toxicity requirements as are listed

Table 4 Validation Responsibilities of Prefilter Supplier and Prefilter User

	Validation responsibility	
Parameter	Prefilter supplier	Prefilter user
Filter quality	Document all filter claims and manufacturing process.	Review data and audit manufacturer.
Filter consistency	Provide lot release data and document manufacturing process.	Show drug product consistency.
Structural integrity	Provide filter usage limits.	Validate for their process.
Extractables	Provide extractables data type and amount, pass USP oxidizables test.	Evaluate with their system and process solution.
Compatibility	Provide compatibility tables.	Evaluate with their solution.
Toxicity	Provide test data showing product meets USP Class VI plastics test and mouse safety test.	Document and verify information.
Adsorption	Provide known information.	Evaluate with their solution.
Product activity/stability	Provide known information.	Evaluate with their solution.
Endotoxins	Provide lot release data.	Evaluate filter and system.
Particles	Provide particle retention efficiency rating.	Product meets USP particulate standards for injectables.

for the sterilizing grade cartridges (CFR, 1990; FDA, 1987, 1994; USP, 1995). In the validation of prefilter cartridges, answers to the following questions need to be addressed:

1. Do all materials in the cartridge meet all toxicity and extractables/compatibility requirements?
2. What are the purpose and function of the prefilter?
3. What are its operating limitations?
4. Does the filter manufacturer supply all the necessary manufacturing and performance documentation on the cartridge?

Many filter cartridge manufacturers now include comprehensive validation guides with their prefilter products as well as their sterilizing grade products. These guides can greatly assist the prefilter user in addressing many of the validation questions, and it is therefore important to choose a filter supplier familiar with the regulatory agencies and their current requirements. The validation information that would be supplied by the prefilter manufacturer and the specific data that would be generated by the prefilter user are summarized in Table 4.

The United States Pharmacopeia (USP, 1995) issues a series of tests and requirements that should be met by all sterilizing grade membrane filter devices before they can be used to process solutions or drugs in the pharmaceutical industry. A specific test may be required as a one-time test, on an audit basis, or in limited testing for lot release. A summary of the USP tests directly applicable to prefilter cartridges is given in Table 5.

Table 5 USP 23 Tests for Specific Prefilter Cartridges Used in the Processing of Pharmaceutical Solutions

USP 23 test	Test description	Measurement criteria
⟨88⟩	Biological reactivity tests; in vivo Class VI plastics test	Extract from material when injected will not cause death or related systems in mice.
⟨88⟩	Biological reactivity tests; mouse safety test	Extract from filter device will not cause death or related systems in mice.
⟨788⟩	Particulate matter in injections	Filter device releases particles below current standard for process solution.
⟨85⟩	Bacterial endotoxins	Effluent from filter device below current endotoxin standard
⟨151⟩	Pyrogen test	Will not cause a pyrogenic response in a rabbit, or extract from filter is below current LAL standard.
Water for injection[a]	Oxidizables test	Passes the oxidizables substance test after a defined flush period.

[a]USP 23, pp. 1635, 1636.

7 PREFILTER SELECTION AND SIZING

7.1 Liquids

Filter Selection

Filtration systems for aseptic processing in liquid applications generally consist of a series of filter cartridges, with each cartridge in the series protecting and extending the life of the next filter cartridge.

Generally a great deal of thought and testing is devoted to the selection of the final (sterilizing grade) filter in the train. However, if you are required to produce a sterile effluent, your choice of the type (micrometer size) of filter cartridge is limited to those membrane filters and filter cartridges that meet the HIMA and FDA regulatory guidelines that define a sterilizing grade filter. Different polymeric materials are available for the various sterilizing grade filters, and those initially selected should be evaluated with your process solution for filter compatibility and/or product degradation or adsorption. Once you have chosen an appropriate final filter cartridge, the next task is to choose the most appropriate clarifying filters and/or prefilters to extend the life (capacity) of the final filter cartridge.

Filter Sizing

Choosing the appropriate prefilter combinations can be the key to filter train optimization and minimization of overall filtration costs. However, with the number of types of prefilter cartridges available, choosing the best prefilter train offers a unique challenge. To meet this challenge, two procedures are generally employed: (1) flow decay trials and (2) filterability trials.

Flow Decay Trials

Flow decay is the traditional method used to measure the flow rate and volume that will pass through a filter over a prescribed time period, generally until flow drops to 20% or 10% of the initial flow rate. Flow decay trials are run on small area filters, then scaled up to determine filter cartridge capacity. The effluent from the small area filter is then used to run a flow decay test on the next prefilter or the final filter in the filter train. By evaluating various prefilter media one can determine the best filter combination for protecting the final filter. The diagram in Fig. 15 shows the apparatus required to run the flow decay test.

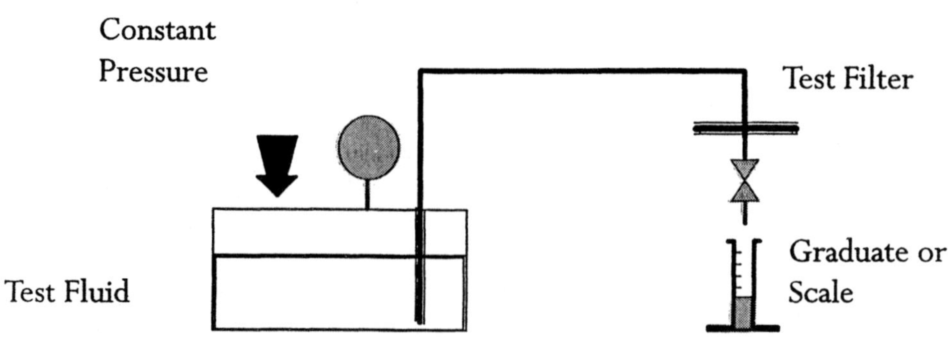

Figure 15 Flow decay test apparatus.

FLOW DECAY PROCEDURE. In the flow decay procedure, filter disks (generally 47 mm) are challenged with a representative sample of the process solution that will be used in the large-scale production runs. Tests are run at a constant upstream pressure until the flow rate to the disk declines to 10% or 20% of the initial flow rate. Final sterilizing grade filters (0.2 and 0.1 μm) and membrane-based prefilter materials are run at 20–30 psid or at the change-out differential pressure that the filter cartridge will experience in that application. The more open clarifying filters and depth prefilters are run at 5–10 psid. The filter with the highest retention in the train is run first in order to assess the effectiveness of various prefilter materials that will be tested to extend the life of this final filter. The total volume fed to each disk is recorded. The following formula is used to scale up the flow decay data on the disk to a cartridge:

$$\frac{\text{Cartridge filter area}}{\text{Disk filter area}} \times \text{volume fed to disk} = \text{volume cartridge will process}$$

Total Volume or Filterability Test

Filterability, an accelerated flow decay test based on the gradual pore-blocking mechanism, is used to predict the maximum volume that will pass through a filter over infinite time. The test was originally developed for filtration studies in the wine industry in the mid-1970s (Gaillard, 1976). However, it was not used routinely for general system sizing and prefilter optimization work in the pharmaceutical industry until the early 1990s (Badmington, 1992; Brose et al., 1994; Badmington et al., 1995; *Genetic Engineering News*, 1994). The filterability test is performed in exactly the same manner as the standard flow decay test but can be completed in 10–15 min. During this time the flow rate and cumulative volume through the filter disk or cartridge are recorded at 1 min increments. A straight-line plot of time (minutes) per unit volume (liters) versus time (minutes), modeled from the gradual pore-blocking mechanism, can be used to predict the total volume that will pass through a filter at an 80%, 90%, or complete (fully plugged, no flow) decline in the initial flow rate (Badmington et al., 1995). Usually at an 80–90% reduction in initial flow rate, a filter cartridge would be considered beyond its useful life. To calculate the volume of solution that will pass through the test filter as flow rate is reduced, the following equations are used:

$$V_{100\%} \text{ (V at 100\% flow loss)} = \text{1/slope of the straight-line plot} \tag{1}$$

$$V_{80\%} \text{ (}V\text{ at 80\% flow loss)} = 0.55 \times V_{100\%} \tag{2}$$

$$V_{90\%} \text{ (}V\text{ at 90\% flow loss)} = 0.68 \times V_{100\%} \tag{3}$$

The filterability test is very suitable for sizing in the pharmaceutical industry, as most biological solutions contain small deformable particles that will typically block filters by gradual pore blocking and therefore allow filterability data to predict the capacity of a filter. Filterability testing is extremely useful in sizing and optimizing filter trains in that it can dramatically reduce the time and the amount of process solution that will be required to test the capacity of a filter disk or cartridge compared to the traditional flow decay method.

Filterability Test Procedure

To perform a filterability test, filter disks (generally 47 mm in diameter) or depth cartridges (generally 1 or 2 in. in length) are challenged with a representative sample of the process solution. Tests are run at a constant upstream pressure for 10–15 min, with the cumulative volume through the filter being recorded at 1.0 min increments. The test apparatus shown in Fig. 15 for running flow decay tests can also be used for filterability trials. The upstream pressure used in the test should be very close to the pressure at which the cartridges would be considered plugged and changed out in the full-scale process run. For example, if the cartridge in the actual process filtration run was being changed out at a differential pressure across the cartridge of 10 psid, the filterability test would also be run at that pressure. The only exception to this rule would be in running the test on very open 1 or 2 in. depth prefilters. These filter cartridges should be run at 5 psid; otherwise initial flow rates and volumes collected in the first few minutes of the test would be too large to process effectively. In sizing a filter train, the filter with the highest retention in the train is run first. Therefore, in sizing a filter train that will produce a sterile effluent you would begin by testing the 0.2 μm sterilizing filter medium. This allows you to determine which prefilter materials will extend the life of this final filter.

To scale up the filterability data generated on disks or small cartridges use the following two formulas.

Disk Scale-Up to 10 in. Cartridge

$$\frac{\text{10 in. Cartridge filter area}}{\text{Disk filter area}} \times \text{volume fed to disk}$$

$$= \text{volume for a 10 in. cartridge}$$

Cartridge Scale-Up to 10 in. Cartridge

$$\frac{\text{Cartridge length (10 in.)}}{\text{Cartridge length in trial (1 or 2 in.)}} \times \text{volume fed to test cartridge}$$

$$= \text{volume for 10 in. cartridge}$$

The example listed in Table 6 illustrates the value of using the flow decay or filterability sizing approach to optimize a filter train. Based on the test data developed on 47 mm disks and then scaled up to 10 in. cartridge equivalents, filter train 3, containing two prefilters before the final filter, would offer a significant reduction in the filtration cost to process 1000 L of 5% calf serum compared to filter train 1 or 2.

As an additional benefit to filter train optimization, filterability testing can be used by production and quality control managers to monitor the batch-to-batch consistency of their process solution. In some instances, where the quality of process solutions may vary widely, a 10 min filterability test can easily predict if premature filter plugging can be expected in this process filtration step.

To be effective in sizing filter systems, it is important to

1. Understand your overall objectives.
2. Determine what is critical in your separation and answer the questions listed in Fig. 16 for your process solution characteristics and filtration conditions.
3. Record accurate data with your test solutions, and be sure that your test solution is representative of your final process solution.

Table 6 Filter Train Optimization to Process 1000 L of 5% Calf Serum[a]

	1.2 μm nominal cellulose prefilter	0.2 μm nominal cellulose prefilter	0.2 μm PVDF final filter	Total relative cost
Train 1 with final filter only				
Capacity on a 47 mm disk (liters) at 80% reduction in initial flow rate or $V_{80\%}$			0.26	
Disk capacity scaled to a 10 in. cartridge (liters)			130	
Number of 10 in. cartridges required to process 1000 L			8	100%
Train 2 with prefilter cartridge, then final filter				
Capacity on a 47 mm disk (liters) at 80% reduction in initial flow rate or $V_{80\%}$		0.46	3.3	
Disk data scaled to a 10 in. cartridge (L)		230	1600	
Number of 10 in. cartridges required to process 1000 L		5	1	44%
Train with two prefilter cartridges in series, then final filter.				
Capacity on a 47 mm disk (liters) at 80% reduction in initial flow rate or $V_{80\%}$	8.0	6.8	4.2	
Disk data scaled to a 10 in. cartridge (L)	4000	3400	2100	
Number of 10 in. cartridges required to process 1000 L	1	1	1	25%

[a]Data were generated in the laboratory on 47 mm filter disks. For the relative cost example, a prefilter cartridge was considered to be 50% of the cost of a final filter cartridge.
Source: Data from Badmington (1993).

4. Design a preliminary cartridge filter train based on your sizing data (Fig. 17).
5. In sizing large-scale filtrations (those requiring multiple cartridges or cartridges greater than 10 in. in length), perform a pilot-scale run with 2 or 4 in. cartridges before running the full-scale trial.
6. Rely on technical assistance and testing help from the filter manufacturers.

PROCESS SOLUTION:
Composition: ________________
Viscosity: ________________
Surface Tension: ________________
Particle Distribution: ________________
FILTRATION CONDITIONS:
Constant Pressure or Constant Flow Rate (circle one)
Sterilization of Filters: Steam in Place (SIP), Autoclave or Not Required (circle one)
Batch Size: ________________
Flow rate: ________________
Temperature: ________________
Initial Differential Pressure Requirements: ____________
Final Differential Pressure Requirements: ____________
Required Filtration Time: ________________

Figure 16 List of information needed for filter train sizing.

7.2 Gases

The aseptic guidelines of the U.S. Department of Health and Human Services (FDA, 1987) requires the use of sterilizing grade filters for critical contact gases. This would include the filter cartridges used on water-for-injection (WFI) tank vents, sterile product tank vents, bioreactor feed gas lines, lyophilizers, autoclaves, and biotechnology fermentation tank vents. Sterilizing grade gas filter cartridges must be integrity-testable, sterilizable, and non-fiber-releasing and be bacteria-retentive in dry and wet air. Ideally, they will have a lower pressure drop, both initially and throughout their

Filter Train Cartridge #	Type of Filter (clarifying, prefilter)	Micron Rating	Length (inches)	Number Required
#1				
#2				
#3				
Final Filter (Sterilizing)				

Figure 17 Summary of information on the filter cartridges needed in a filter train.

useful cycle, the ability to be repeatedly steam-sterilized, and the ability to withstand long-term exposure to high temperature air and be virus-retentive in dry and moist air (Keating et al., 1992). In many of these gas filtration applications such as tank vents, a prefilter is not generally required or used. However, in applications where in-house gases are fed to sterilizing grade filters, the addition of a highly retentive pleated prefilter cartridge directly upstream of the final filter should be considered. In high airflow applications, the prefilter would help prevent particle damage to the final filter.

Filter Selection and Sizing

In selecting prefilters for air filtration applications, the removal capacity of the filter device is generally not the critical performance parameter. Unlike water, air is compressible, and sizing of the air filters for initial flow rate versus pressure drop at various pressures becomes more complex. Filter manufacturers therefore supply airflow rate versus differential pressure drop curves for their filter cartridges at various pressures. Many filter manufacturers also have computer sizing programs available for specific products.

Prefilters used in the very early stages of the compressed air filtration sequence are generally required to remove oil and water droplets as well as particles. This is accomplished by the use of a coalescing filter. The coalescing filter usually contains a network of glass fibers that will trap dirt particles and water droplets. The water droplets that unite or "coalesce" at the side or bottom of the filter housing are separated from the filter matrix with a barrier that prevents liquid backflow. By continuously drawing off the liquid collected downstream of the antireentrainment barrier, large volumes of water can be effectively removed from the air stream. In some applications it may be necessary to install carbon adsorption filters downstream of the coalescing filters to remove oil vapors or organic odors that remain in the air.

It is very common to have a pleated cartridge filter between the coalescing filters and a final filter for sterilizing the air stream. This cartridge would contain a hydrophobic filter medium. All polypropylene pleated surface filter cartridges with nominal ratings between 0.5 and 1.0 μm are ideally suited for this application.

8 SPECIFIC APPLICATIONS

8.1 Antibiotic Processing Filtration

Antibiotic processing includes a variety of subprocessing steps. Common to most of the processes is the fermentation step. During fermentation, the metabolic process produces the desired antibiotic molecules, present in the antibiotic fluid or broth or retained in the cell. If the material is in the cell, the producing organism must be chemically induced to express the antibiotic molecule. This is largely accomplished by acidifying the broth. Subsequently, the task is to extract antibiotics from the media and bacteria. A level of 10% solids is considered common. The equipment used for the broth clarification step may vary from one antibiotic producer to another. However, it generally includes a combination of centrifugation and a filter aid separation. A dewatering centrifuge would be used to remove the larger particles from the broth. Most often a rotary drum filtration device consisting of a large drum rotating in a bath aspirates the broth by vacuum through a fine mesh stainless screen. A precoat of diatomaceous earth (DE) is built up on the surface of the drum to allow the broth particles to adhere to an open porous depth structure.

Once the large-scale removal has taken place, the solution is generally passed through a prefilter cartridge to prevent premature fouling in the subsequent purification steps of ion exchange and chromatography.

For antibiotic processing and for the general clarification of organic solvents, the surface filter offers two advantages over depth type prefilters. The large effective filtration area (EFA) in a pleated surface cartridge would (1) allow for higher initial flow rates per unit length of cartridge and (2) allow the hard particle contaminants found in the organic solvents to form a cake on the filter surface. As described earlier in Sec. 4, caking is an advantage when nondeformable hard particles are present, because the flow through the cartridge will continue at a reasonable rate as the differential pressure consistently rises across the cartridge. Filters used in this application must be compatible with aggressive organic solvents. Suitable filter and cartridge materials include polypropylene, nylon, glass fibers, Teflon, and polyvinylidene fluoride.

8.2 Cell Separation and Protein Clarification

In the protein clarification process, the protein solution is passed through the filter membrane while cells, larger molecules, and cell debris are retained. During the separation of protein products from large mammalian cells such as Chinese hamster ovary (CHO) cells or large particulate cell debris, both cartridge depth filters with nominal ratings in the 5–10 μm range and tangential flow filter (TFF) systems with microporous membranes are employed. Both systems bring advantages and disadvantages to this type of separation. TFF systems can be cleaned and reused. This will cut down filter costs, but extensive cleaning and validation protocols are required between runs. Prefilter cartridges, on the other hand, are used only once and thrown away. Because of this they result in a higher filter materials cost, but there is less cleaning and validation required between runs. Therefore, cleaning and validation support costs must be added to the costing equations. The selection of the best system can be made only after reviewing (1) the objective of the separation, (2) the characteristics of the process fluid, and (3) the overall processing costs.

During the next stage of the cell harvesting process, after the large cells have been removed by either a depth filter or a TFF system, a prefilter is generally required to extend the life of the sterilizing grade final filter cartridge or to protect a column that may be used in the final separation process.

8.3 Facilities Filtration

''Facilities filtration'' may include a variety of fluids, but it most commonly refers to the filtration processes for water, compressed air, and nitrogen. The filtration of these fluids and gases takes place either in the central distribution system or at the points of use.

In the central distribution system, cartridge filtration is only one of several operations. For water filtration, other operations typically include sand filtration, gravitational settling, ion exchange, and carbon bed filtration (chlorine removal). A central air filtration system includes an intake filter, compressor, receiver, dryer, and a coalescing filter (for oil removal).

Point-of-use filters for both water and air or nitrogen are typically 0.2 μm sterilizing grade filters. However, they may still need appropriate prefilter cartridges upstream to prevent costly oversizing and premature plugging of the final filters.

8.4 Large Volume Parenterals

Large volume parenterals (LVPs) are defined as those pharmaceutical products that are injected through the skin in doses greater than 100 mL and as high as 3–5 L. Batch sizes typically range from a low of a few hundred liters up to batches of 40,000 L. LVPs differ from other pharmaceutical products in that 0.45 μm filtration is used for particle removal prior to terminal heat sterilization. There has been a trend in the industry to filter these products at the 0.2 μm level prior to terminal sterilization, but this will require substantial prefiltration efforts, especially with high dextrose solutions.

Ingredients in typical LVPs are water, dextrose (5–50%), amino acids, salts, and occasionally viscous total parenteral nutrition (TPN) components. Final products include intravenous suspension bags and continuous ambulatory dialysis (CAPD) exchange solutions.

Depending on the type of LVP being processed, prefiltration cartridges may or may not be needed in this application. This can be determined during the initial filter train sizing trials. This is an appropriate application for small-scale sizing tests and may be appropriate for running an accelerated flow decay test prior to each run. (See discussion of filterability testing in Sec. 7.1.) For relatively clean solutions, it may be more advantageous to not use prefilter cartridges but to fill the need with extra final filters. This will give the needed flow rate capacity and keep the initial differential pressure across the filter train low. However, for the filtration of dextrose-containing solutions, choosing the correct prefiltration cartridges to extend the life of the final filters is critical.

Dextrose can vary substantially from lot to lot in the amount of insoluble material that is present, and therefore in some instances it is recommended that a second, parallel prefilter housing and cartridges be sanitized, installed in line, and ready to use if the first cartridges plug. With solutions that show variability, it may be helpful to run an accelerated flow decay test on the solution prior to beginning the filtration. From this quick test it can be determined if the filter train will adequately process the entire solution. (See Sec. 7.1.)

8.5 Small Volume Parenterals

Small volume parenterals (SVPs) include a wide variety of drug products, both traditional and bioengineered. They are typically in the 20–100 mL range and are packaged in small vials, prefilled syringes, ampoules, or lyophilized powders. Many of the SVPs are heat-sensitive and are packaged using aseptic (sterile filtration) processing. Filtration in SVP processing can be broken down into three basic areas: sterile filtration, prefiltration, and facilities filtration. The purpose of using a prefilter in this area is to prevent the final filter in the fill area from becoming plugged and building up a differential pressure that would reduce fill rates or cause a shutdown to replace the sterilizing grade final filters. Because each fluid is different, a prefiltration train must be designed and optimized for each fluid stream. Important characteristics of prefilters used in the SVP process include

High flow rates
Low extractables
Steam-sterilizability
High retention
Nonpyrogenic

Typically, raw materials used in SVP production are of high quality. Therefore, surface prefilters with high retention efficiencies are more useful than a less retentive depth filter.

8.6 Serum Filtration

A variety of human and animal sera are routinely processed via filtration, in many cases down to the 0.1 μm level to reduce mycoplasma. Filtration of serum can offer unique challenges, especially in the area of prefiltration. The length of time serum sits before filtration and the temperature of the filtration process will affect filter capacity. In the case of animal serum, the type of animal and its dietary intake will affect the amounts of lipids, triglycerides, and lipoproteins in the serum, which in turn affects filter capacity. With this large variability in the quality and condition of the serum to be filtered, a variety of prefilter cartridges and pretreatment methods are used in these applications. This is another area where the initial filter train sizing and optimization play a critical role. Due to the complexity and difficulty of serum filtrations, typical filter trains include multiple filter cartridges that combine the attributes of both depth and surface prefilters and clarifying cartridges. The prefilter media most suitable for this application include glass fibers (depth or surface filter), polypropylene (depth or surface filter), cellulose (surface filter), nylon (surface filter), and polyvinylidene fluoride (surface filter).

A typical filter train for processing human or mammalian serum is illustrated in Fig. 18. Raw serum being processed through this train would become a sterile serum product. In the filter train, a series of clarification and prefiltration cartridges

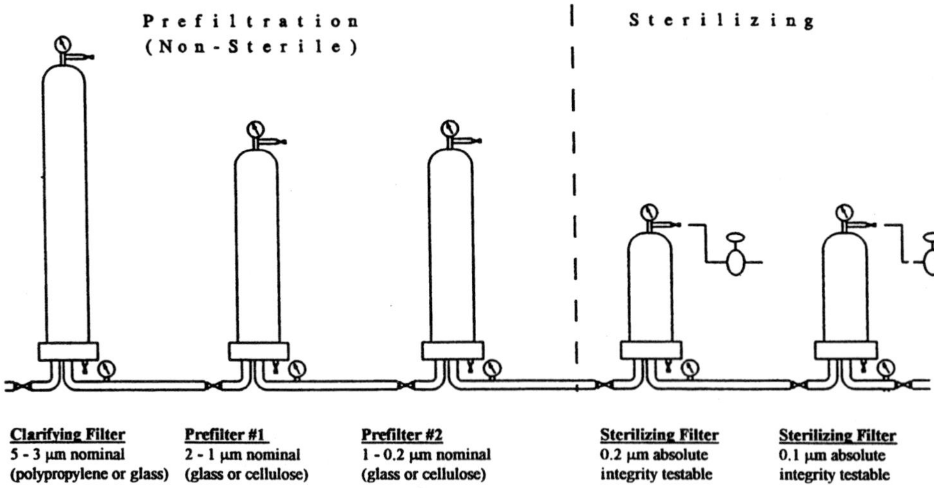

Figure 18 A typical filter train that may be used during the sterile filtration of serum.

are used to protect and extend the life of the final filters. Pressure gauges are placed both upstream and downstream of each housing to monitor the pressure increase across each filter cartridge. Valves are strategically located to vent all housings, and ports are placed on the sterilizing housings for integrity testing the filters inside. In serum filtrations, a 0.1 μm sterilizing grade filter is sometimes used as the final filter to increase the removal of any mycoplasma contamination that may be present in the serum. In these applications a standard 0.2 μm sterilizing grade filter often becomes the prefilter cartridge in the filter train. In filtrations where the sera may vary substantially in filterability from day to day, parallel prefilter systems could be incorporated into the train to allow changeover to new prefilters without stopping flow to the final filters. This could also be accomplished by placing a refrigerated holding tank and pump downstream of the first set of prefilters. The prefiltered serum in the holding tank would then be pumped to the set of prefilters directly upstream of the final sterilizing grade filters. This would also allow prefilters to be changed out in the middle of a run without stopping flow to the final bank of filter cartridges. It is important to size and optimize this application so that the final sterilizing grade filters do not plug.

ACKNOWLEDGMENTS

I wish to acknowledge the assistance given by Millipore in providing the product photographs and the time that was required to prepare this chapter. Thanks are also due to Robin De La Parra for providing the scanning electron micrographs and David Reader for assistance with the system flow diagrams.

REFERENCES

ASTM. (1988). Standard Practice for Determining the Performance of a Filter Medium Employing a Single Pass, Constant-Rate, Liquid Test, F795-88, *Annual Book of ASTM Standards*, American Society for Testing and Materials, West Conshohocken, PA.

Badmington, F. (1993). Reducing filtration costs through prefilter optimization, Poster Session, Parenteral Drug Association Annual Meeting, Orlando, FL.

Badmington, F., E. Honig, M. Payne, and R. Wilkins. (1995). V_{max} Testing for practical microfiltration train scale-up in biopharmaceutical processing, *Pharm. Technol., 19*(9): 64–76.

BGA. (1993). Promulgation Regarding Measures to Reduce the Asbestos Contamination of Parenteral Products, German Federal Health Office.

Bowen, R. W., and Q. Gan. (1992). Properties of microfiltration membranes: The effects of adsorption and shear on the recovery of an enzyme, *Biotechnol. Bioeng., 40*:491–497.

Brose, D. J., and G. Henricksen. (1994). A quantitative analysis of preservative adsorption on microfiltration membranes, *Pharm. Technol., 18*(3):65–72.

Brose, D. J., S. Cates, and F. A. Hutchison. (1994). Studies on the scale-up of microfiltration membrane devices, *J. Parenter. Sci. Technol., 48*(4):184–188.

CFR. (1990). Good Manufacturing Practices, U.S. 21 Code of Federal Regulations, Part 210-250.

FDA. (1987). Guideline on Sterile Drug Products Produced by Aseptic Processing, U.S. Dept. of Health and Human Services, Public Health Service, Food and Drug Administration.

FDA. (1994). Guideline for the Manufacture of In Vitro Diagnostic Products, U.S. Dept. of Health and Human Services, Public Health Service, Food and Drug Administration.

Datar, R., J. M. Martin, and R. L. Manteuffel. (1992). Dynamics of protein recovery from process filtration systems using microporous membrane filter cartridges, *J. Parenteral Sci. Technol.*, *46*(2):35–42.

Fitch, E. C. (1980). *An Encylopedia of Fluid Contamination Control*, Hemisphere Publishing Corp., Washington, D.C.

Gaillard, M. (1976). Etude sur les colloides glucidiques et la filterabilite des vins, Dissertation, Ecole Nationale D'Ingeniurs des Travaux Agricoles.

Genetic Engineering News. (1995). V_{max} Testing for optimizing filtration scale-up in bioprocess operations, February, p. 24.

Grace, H. P. (1956). Structure and performance of filter media. *AIChE J.*, *2*(3):307–336.

HIMA. (1982). Microbiological Evaluation of Filters for Sterilizing Liquids, HIMA Document No. 3, Vol. 4, Health Industry Manufacturers Association.

Hermans, P. H., and H. L. Bredee. (1935). *Rec. Trav. Chim. Pays-Bas*, *54*:680.

Hermans, P. H., and H. L. Bredee. (1936). Principles of the mathematical treatment of constant pressure filtration, *J. Soc. Chem. Ind., Trans. Commun.*, *55*:1–4.

Hermia, J. (1982). Constant pressure blocking filtration laws, application for power-law non-Newtonian fluids, *Trans. IChE*, *60*:183–187.

Hou, K. C., and R. Zaniewski. (1990). Depyrogenation by endotoxin removal with positively charged depth filter cartridge, *J. Parenter. Drug Assoc.*, *44*(4):204–209.

Hu, H., J. Camilleri, and W. Tamashiro. (1993). A new membrane for biopharmaceutical filtration, *Pharm. Technol.*, *17*(10):32–44.

JSA. (1989). *Dusts and Aerosols for Industrial Testing*, Japanese Standards Association, Tokyo, Japan.

Johnston, P. R. (1990). *Fundamentals of Fluid Filtration—A Technical Primer*, Tall Oaks Publishing, Littleton, CO.

Johnston, P. R. (1992). Fluid flow through filter media: A tutorial, *Pharm. Technol.*, *16*(9): 136–145.

Keating, P., R. Levy, M. Payne, S. Proulx, P. Rowe, and S. Pearl. (1992). Performance testing of membrane-based filters used in the filtration of industrial fermentation air, *Biopharm.*, *5*(1):36–41.

Leahy, T. J., and M. J. Sullivan. (1978). Validation of bacterial retention capabilities of membrane filters, *Pharm. Technol.*, *2*(9):65–75.

Martin, J. M., and R. L. Manteuffel. (1988). Protein recovery from effluents of microporous membrane filters, *Biopharm* *1*(10):20–27.

Meltzer, T. H. (1983). The absolute retention of *P. diminuta* by 0.2 μm-rated membrane filters, SVI Congress Nacional de Ciencias Farmaceuticas, Merida, Mexico.

Nema, S., and K. Avis. (1993). Loss of LDH activity during membrane filtration, *J. Parenter. Sci. Technol.*, *47*(1):16–21.

NSF Int. (1994). Drinking Water Treatment Units—Health Effects, Standard 53, NSF International, Ann Arbor, MI.

Pitt, A. (1987). The nonspecific binding of polymeric microporous membranes, *J. Parenter. Sci. Technol.*, *41*(3):110–113.

Rubow, K. L. (1981). Submicron aerosol filtration characteristics of membrane filters, Ph.D. Thesis, University of Minnesota, Minneapolis, MN.

Rubow, K. L., and B. Y. H. Liu. (1986). Characteristics of membrane filters for particle collection, *Fluid Filtration: Gas, Volume 1 ASTM STP 975* (R. R. Raber, ed.) American Society for Testing and Materials, Philadelphia, pp. 74–94.

Rubow, K. L., B. Y. H. Liu, and D. Grant. (1987). Characteristics of ultra-high efficiency membrane filters, Proceedings of the 33rd Annual Meeting of the Institute of Environmental Sciences, pp. 383–387.

Sarry, C., and H. Sucker. (1992a). Adsorption of proteins on microporous membrane filters: Part I, *Pharm. Technol.*, *16*(10):16–23.

Sarry, C., and H. Sucker. (1992b). Adsorption of proteins on microporous membrane filters: Part II, *Pharm. Technol., 16*(11):38–48.

Schrader, E. L. (1992). High efficiency bag filtration: Contaminant removal with engineered meltblown polypropylene composites. *Adv. Filtr. Separ. Technol., 6*:40–44.

Stone, T., V. Goel, and J. Leszczak. (1994). Methodology for the analysis of filter extractables: A model stream approach, *Pharm. Technol., 18*(10):116–130.

Stone, T., V. Goel, J. Leszczak, and S. Chrai. (1996). The model stream approach: Defining the worst-case conditions, *Pharm. Technol., 22*(2):34–51.

Tanny, G. B., D. K. Strong, W. G. Presswood, and T. H. Meltzer. (1979). The adsorptive retention of *Pseudomonas diminuta* by membrane filters, *J. Parenter. Drug Assoc., 33*(1): 40–51.

Truskey, G. A., R. Gabler, A. DeLeo, and T. Manter. (1989). The effect of membrane filtration upon protein conformation, *J. Parenter. Sci. Technol., 41*(6):180–193.

USP. (1995). USP 23 and National Formulary NF18, U.S. Pharmacopeial Convention, Rockville, MD.

Van den Oetelaar, Piet, J. M., I. M. Mentink, and J. B. Brinks. (1989). Loss of peptides and proteins upon sterile filtration due to adsorption to membrane filters, *Drug Dev. Ind. Pharm. 15*(1):97–101.

Waterson, R. M. (1990). Novel depth filtration technologies: Strategies for process development, *Pharm. Eng., 10*(5):22–29.

Wickert, K. (1991). Endotoxin control using charge modified filter media, *Pharm. Eng., 11*(4): 25–28.

26

The Filtration of Blood and Blood Fractions

WAYNE P. OLSON
Oldevco, Beecher, Illinois

1 INTRODUCTION

Human blood is infused into trauma patients when blood loss due to injury has been severe and is life-threatening. Some cells from whole blood or from bone marrow are isolated so that the regeneration of blood cells can resume following heroic chemotherapy or radiation treatment. Some plasma fractions that are human-sourced [e.g., antihemophilic factor (AHF, also called F-VIII)] are infused into patients periodically to correct specific genetic abnormalities. Human serum albumin (HSA) and immunoglobulins (IgGs) are used widely as therapeutic agents. Whole blood and components of whole blood are partially purified by filtration methods. This chapter is about some particulars of the methods used in these filtrations. Emphasis is on four areas:

1. Removal of aggregates from whole blood or packed erythrocytes
2. Purification of certain cells and platelets
3. Removal of bacteria and fungi from plasma fractions
4. Removal of viruses from plasma fractions

The reader will understand that this text is devoted to filtration but that other methods are also used to perform some of these steps (e.g., viral inactivation by means of heat or chemicals or both, in addition to viral removal by filtration). Many filtration-related methods exist that are not broached (e.g., blood oxygenation with an artificial lung).

2 SOME DEFINITIONS

A filter is a porous solid through which fluids can pass, leaving on or in the filter sterically hindered or adsorbed particles. *Filtration* is the act of passing a liquid or gas through that porous solid. *Microfiltration* relates to the removal of particles and microorganisms roughly in the range of 0.5–5 or 10 μm in diameter from suspension by means of a filter. *Ultrafiltration* is filtration through pores smaller than 0.05 μm (50 nm). *Dialysis* is the equilibration of small molecules across a membrane that prevents the passage of proteins and peptides, and *hemodialysis* is the dialysis of blood to remove the salts, urea, and some other materials of molecular weight (M_r) less than about 2000.

The *feed* is the fluid addressed to the filter, and the *filtrate* is the fluid downstream of the filter. Microfiltration is usually carried out in the *dead-end* mode, wherein all of the feed passes through to become filtrate. Ultrafiltration usually (but not always) is done in the *crossflow* or tangential flow mode (see Chapter 19). "Crossflow" is descriptive in that the feed flows in a narrow channel (in the neighborhood of 25 μm diameter) over the ultrafilter membrane (UF), and a proportion of the feed (5–95%, depending on plumbing on the filtrate side) passes through the filter to become filtrate. The feed that does not pass through the filter contains a concentrate of the excluded material and is usually recycled to the vat from which the feed is pumped. Viruses vary in size from about 100 nm down to about 20 nm. In this chapter, "matrix" refers to the polymer or ceramic of which an ultrafilter is constructed. Other definitions are given in the body of the text.

3 DEVICES AND PROCESSES

3.1 Filtration of Blood and Components at Bedside

Whole blood consists of cells and cell-like particles (erythrocytes or red blood cells; white cells or leukocytes; platelets) and plasma. Plasma is the liquid portion of whole blood, including fibrinogen and the various clotting factors. When plasma is processed in any way it is usually anticoagulated with ethylenediamine tetraacetic acid (EDTA, to complex Ca^{2+} and other cations necessary to clotting) or organic anticoagulants such as heparin, a sulfated polysaccharide that binds some clotting factors. Serum is plasma from which most of the fibrin and clotting factors have been removed.

Dialysis of Whole Blood

The best known mode of filtration of whole blood is *hemodialysis* and related phenomena. The whole blood is passed (as a relatively narrow film, cells and all) over membrane filters with nanometer-sized pores that retain most plasma proteins but permit the passage through the filter of water, salts, urea, and other solutes of low M_r. The bulk of the plasma proteins and all of the formed elements (cells and platelets) are retained on the upstream side of the dialysis filter. Outside of the dialysis tubing is the *dialysate* into which the salts, urea, and other solutes of low M_r diffuse, including some that are desirable (e.g., cytokines, which are intercellular signaling chemicals). The dialysate into which a substantial amount of molecular waste has diffused is said to be *spent*.

An Artificial Liver

The liver is the principal organ of detoxification. Liver failure, in the absence of a liver transplant from a donor, is fatal. Nose and coworkers at the Cleveland Clinic (Matsushita and Nose, 1986) created an experimental artificial liver intended to adsorb toxins from the blood of a patient. A schematic of the system is shown in Fig. 1.

The blood of the patient is anticoagulated with heparin and apheresed to separate formed elements from the plasma. The bulk of the plasma is exposed to sorbents (such as dextran-coated particles of charcoal) that adsorb toxic small molecules (aldehydes, free radicals, degraded hemoglobin, etc.) before the formed elements and plasma are recombined. The resin-adsorbed blood, immediately prior to reinfusion into the patient, is made recoagulable by the addition of protamine, which reverses the anticoagulant effect of heparin.

Artificial livers have not been particularly successful, in part because the multitude of detoxification functions of liver cells remain to be fully described. Also, most if not all of the liver functions are enzymatically mediated. Enzymes are capable of functioning at high rates for protracted periods. Adsorption, on the other hand, decreases in rate as the proportion of occupied adsorptive sites decreases.

Plasma Recovery

When a donor intends to present only plasma to the donor center, a process called *apheresis* is used. The filter over which the anticoagulated blood passes has pores large enough for all of the plasma proteins to pass through but retains the formed elements. Cell-free plasma is collected as filtrate, and the cells are returned to the donor. The pores of an apheresis filter are significantly larger (e.g., 0.1 μm diameter, in effect) than those of the filters used for hemodialysis to ensure the passage of plasma proteins.

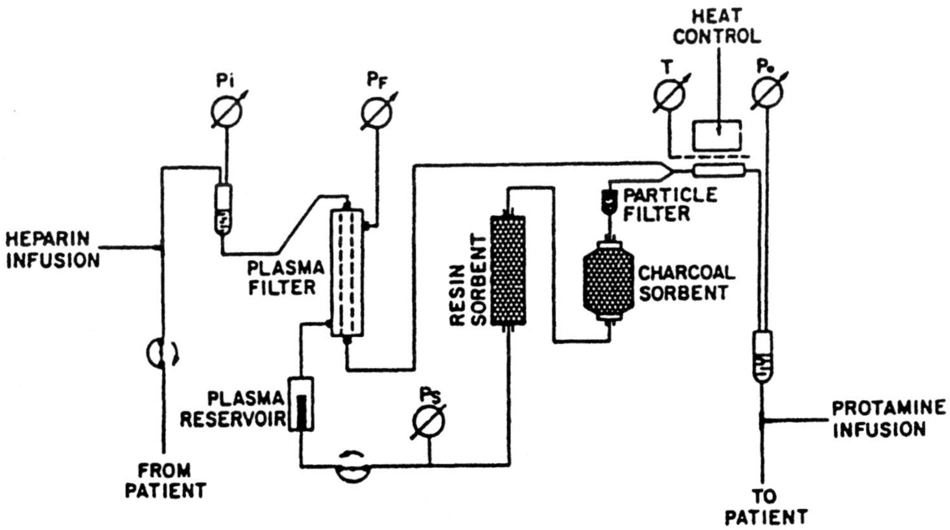

Figure 1 Artificial liver of the Cleveland Clinic.

Alternatively, anticoagulated whole blood is recovered into a bag, the cells and platelets are centrifuged to the bottom of the bag, the plasma proteins are expressed from the container, and the formed elements are returned to the donor. In this instance, when cells are returned with each donation, plasma donations can be made more frequently because the donor is less stressed.

Cell Recovery

Apheresis is also a first step in the purification of certain formed elements (e.g., platelets, erythrocytes, stem cells). The separation of cells from plasma (which can be done in several ways, including crossflow membrane filtration) also provides a cell concentrate that can be harvested for cell purification. In this instance a low-speed centrifugation of blood deposits the erythrocytes and leukocytes but only a proportion of the platelets, which then can be siphoned off, sedimented at higher *g*, resuspended in saline, and recentrifuged (i.e., washed). Platelets are small, anucleate elements that play a key role in clotting and are used widely in treating trauma patients. This can also be done as a crossflow filtration step, but for platelet recovery from small volumes, a centrifugal recovery and wash procedure seems simplest, cleanest, most efficient, and least expensive.

Leukocyte Removal

Leukocytes (white cells) include macrophages, T cells, and B cells, which are the primary cells involved in immune response to foreign bodies including parasites, bacteria, and viruses. Unfortunately, transplants (heart, kidneys, and other tissues) also engender an immune response that is mediated by these cells. As a result, the blood of transplant patients is often filtered through nonwoven filaments of chemically modified polyolefins to which leukocytes adsorb preferentially. The result is immune suppression of the patient at a time when the loss of those cells enhances the survival of the transplanted organ. Leukocyte removal from packed platelets is commonplace (Bowden et al., 1995).

Immune suppression also is done chemically. However, the use of chemotherapeutic agents to kill or maim these cells carries the inherent risk of destroying too much of the immune response (which also is the search-and-destroy system that kills tumors arising spontaneously in all people in addition to killing invading microbes). Rigorous chemotherapy can also kill the stem cells of the marrow that generate the formed elements of circulating blood, including red blood cells. The use of the leukocyte-removing filters reduces the need for chemotherapeutic suppression of immune function cells.

Leukocyte removal sometimes is done to recover antigen-presenting cells (such as macrophages) for the evaluation of T-cell response in patients who have been immunized.

Stem Cells

Stem cells are the progenitors of the panoply of blood cells. Heroic chemotherapy and radiation therapy destroy rapidly dividing cells (e.g., tumors) but also kill stem cells, which divide rapidly to produce formed elements (cells and platelets) of the blood. Stem cells can be recovered from the bone marrow and also (in lower concentration) from peripheral blood. Stem cells, purified and frozen with a cryopreservative, are thawed and returned to the patient following heroic therapy, in the hope that the purified stem cells contain no cancerous cells. They also are a frequent choice for gene therapy.

Stem cells are purified in this way. Mouse monoclonal antibodies (mMAbs) are prepared against the $CD34^+$ antigen (protein) that is unique to stem cells. The MAbs are immobilized on large dense beads or on the bottoms of small, sterile, optically clear plastic bottles. When these surfaces are brought into contact with the cell mixture recovered from the bone marrow or the cells or circulating peripheral blood, only those with the $CD34^+$ protein are immobilized by the MAbs (Olson, 1995).

Other cells are rinsed away. The desired cells remain. These cells are immobilized by small areas of the cell surface containing the $CD34^+$ protein. With agitation, these portions of the stem cell membrane tear away to release the cells free into suspension. This process is called immunoaffinity purification.

Removal of Clots from Whole Blood or Packed Red Cells, etc.

Some clotting occurs even in anticoagulated whole blood. Such clots, if infused into a patient, can occlude capillaries in the lung, eye, brain, liver, or other tissue; the potential exists to induce stroke. Such aggregates must be removed from whole blood packed erythrocytes. The simplest method is to pass the suspension through a filter that retains only large aggregates. The same type of filter is used to remove clots from the blood siphoned from the wound of a patient during surgery, with a view to recycling the blood and reducing the need for transfused material.

3.2 Industrial Filtration of Plasma and Plasma Fractions

Plasma

Whole plasma is quite viscous because it contains many proteins of high (M_r). For example, the M_r of immunoglobulin M (IgM) is about 900,000, indicating that this is a very large molecule. Plasma fibronectin is smaller in M_r (486,000) but is a linear molecule, so it contributes substantially to plasma viscosity, as does the F-VIII. Some fibrin clots tend to be present even in anticoagulated plasma, and these too contribute to plasma viscosity. However, in a well-run system, the plasma from which the proteins of high M_r have been removed is processed almost immediately and is seldom filtered. The exception is the handling of the high M_r proteins that precipitate from thawed fresh frozen plasma (cryoprecipitate).

Generation of the Cohn Fractions

The plasma proteins that are sterile-filtered in large volumes are fraction II (immunoglobulins or IgGs) and fraction V [human serum albumin (HSA)] (Cohn et al., 1946) as well as factor VIII and gamma globulins. The filtrations are described in some detail later in this narrative, but the generation of the fractions merits attention because proper (or improper) fractionation affects filterability and, more important, product quality and safety.

Cohn cold ethanol fractionation of proteins is possible because proteins have the following characteristics:

1. A protein tends to retain *in vitro* and *in vivo* function if it retains its characteristic (native) shape and cofactors (e.g., Ca^{2+}).

2. A protein in solution in the cold (+5 to −5°C) tends to retain its native shape.
3. A plasma protein is usually a monomer surrounded by bound water when it is in solution in its native shape.
4. The aqueous solubility of any protein is minimal at the pH at which the protein has no overall charge (the isoelectric point, p*I*).
5. Another molecule that complexes or otherwise binds water with a higher affinity than the binding of water by the protein will, at some concentration, strip some, perhaps most, of the water from a given protein.
6. A protein at its p*I* and with most of the bound water stripped away by a competing molecule such as ethanol tends to aggregate with others of its kind and precipitate from solution.

The special advantages of ethanol are the following:

1. Ethanol tends to desiccate and kill vegetative cells and inhibits the germination of bacterial and fungal spores; therefore Cohn fractions have few bacterial contaminants. However, many viruses are little affected by cold ethanol.
2. Because ethanol is a small molecule and volatile, it can be removed from a resuspension of the precipitated protein by dialysis through an ultrafilter or by placing the frozen ethanol-containing protein suspension in a vacuum so that the ethanol sublimes from the solid (frozen) state to the vapor phase.

The sequence of changes made in pH and ethanol concentration so as to precipitate the various Cohn fractions is shown in Fig. 2.

The ethanol and buffer constituents (for the alteration of pH) are added slowly with constant stirring. Acceleration of the additions results in local high concentrations of reagents, in which case many proteins precipitate instead of the few desired at a given stage of the process. However, if the additions are done slowly and the mixture is aged and stirred, the desired precipitate commences to form. The primary methods of precipitate recovery are centrifugation and filtration. Both methods merit comment.

Centrifugation

The centrifuge of choice is a continuous flow system, develops very high speeds, and can be cleaned easily and thoroughly. In most instances the centrifuge of choice is the Sharples Superspeed (Fig. 3). The rate of flow of suspensions through these refrigerated centrifuges is quite slow; hence units are often manifolded so that large volumes can be processed. The desired precipitate sediments on the wall of the bowl, which may be lined with plastic sheeting. The precipitate is subsequently scraped from the bowl and resuspended for further processing.

Not all of the precipitated proteins will resume their native shape when resuspended in solution; some will persist as denatured aggregates that are removed by filtration, most often through coarse, nonwoven filter of cellulose fibers. Other coarse filters are made of fine inorganic particles compressed between cellulosic pads. These filters are referred to as "depth" filters because, unlike membrane filters, which tend to retain particles on the filter surface, depth filters retain particles everywhere throughout the filter matrix.

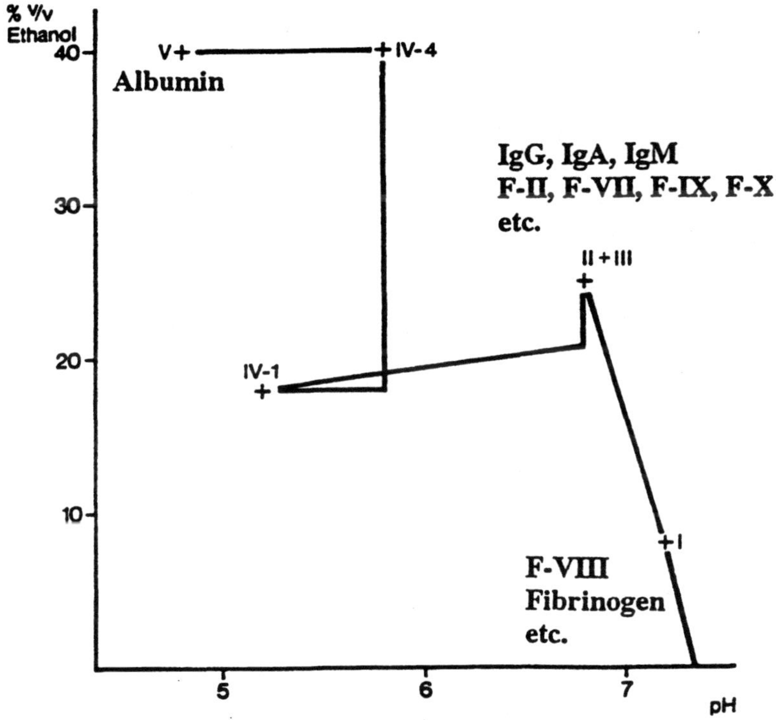

Figure 2 pH and ethanol concentration sequences to produce Cohn fractions of human plasma.

Depth Filtration for Cohn Fraction Recovery

Because filters are used even after centrifugation to recover a precipitate such as Cohn fraction II (IgG or gamma globulin), many blood fraction processors do not use centrifuges to collect each precipitated protein fraction. Rather, a fraction is recovered directly onto a depth filter, usually in the presence of a filter aid.

The concept is that if, for example, Cohn fraction II can be removed from suspension onto a depth filter, the particle-free filtrate, essentially IgG-free (the IgG is in the F-II precipitate), can be adjusted for precipitation of the next fraction. A rinse of the filter with the precipitating solution washes out residual non-IgG soluble proteins.

To recover the precipitated IgGs on the filter, an ethanol-free solution, passing slowly through the filter, resolubilizes and elutes the IgG as the ethanol is washed from the precipitate. The IgG is recovered downstream, in filtrate, as a dilute solution that is diafiltered (solvent exchange while being recirculated over an ultrafilter) and concentrated in an ultrafiltration (UF) system. The depth filters used in the collection of a precipitated fraction must be replaced for each filtration. In many facilities these filtration methods are the Cohn fraction recovery methods of choice.

The nonwoven depth filters most frequently are placed in plate-and-frame presses that contain many large filter sheets set up in parallel. That is to say, the feed is addressed to many of the sheets simultaneously. The sheets are supported by a stainless steel net, and the filtrate from each sheet is collected and repooled.

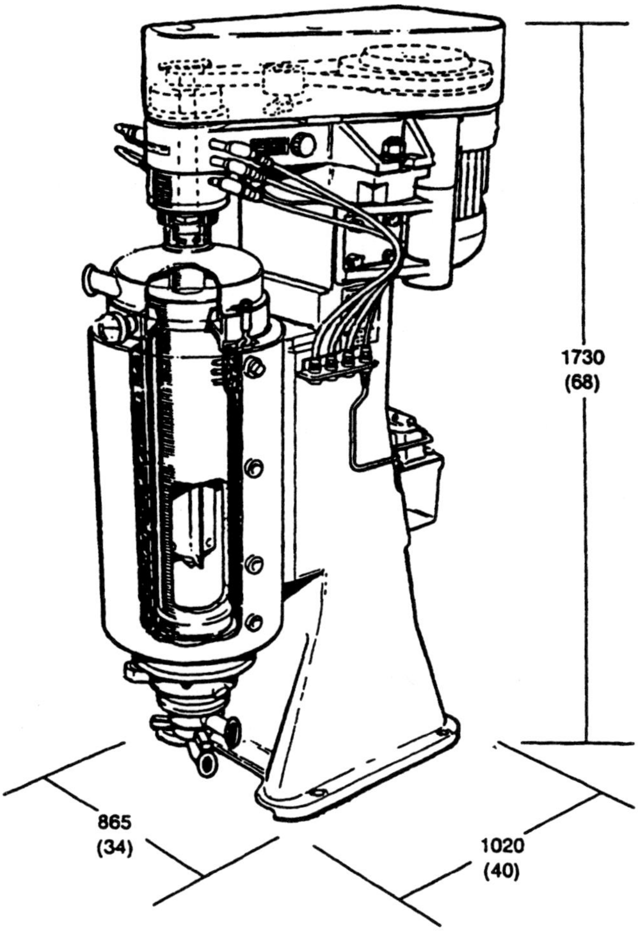

Figure 3 Sharples Superspeed centrifuge for the recovery of Cohn fractions from human plasma.

Advocates of positively charged filters argue that an advantage of the positively charged depth filter matrix is that it binds endotoxin (lipopolysaccharide, LPS) produced by gram-negative bacteria. This is partly true, for LPS has a negative charge imparted by phosphate groups, but the removal depends on several factors described in Chapter 10. Positively charged depth filters tend to be highly retentive because most particles are electronegative in aqueous suspension, but this also includes most plasma proteins. Therefore, positively charged depth filters are most effective in LPS removal in the absence of proteins. The positive charge may be provided by diethylaminoethyl (DEAE) or amino substituents that are weak anion exchangers (Fiore et al., 1980).

One philosophy is that the incoming frozen plasma used in Cohn fractionation ought not to have any significant levels of LPS unless the donation has been made by a septicemic person, in which case the donation should be rejected.

Plasma Fractions

Filtrations in General

Plasma has few medical applications at this time. However, when frozen plasma is thawed to −5 to 0°C (plasma is stored at −60 to −80°C), the high M_r proteins precipitate. This is the cryoprecipitate or cryo. The cryo contains some medically useful proteins (e.g., F-VIII), and the removal of the cryo leaves serum proteins (albumin, gamma globulins, other proteins of lower M_r) in solution. Serum is fairly stable, and its viscosity is not extremely high. F-VIII, whether from human blood or from genetically engineered animal cells in culture, is best purified by immunoaffinity methods (Olson, 1995).

If the cryo-free plasma is filtered, sterile muslin is used. As of the time of thaw, the bioburden is quite low, and any particles are residual platelets or fibrin clots. Fractionation is done with the addition of cold ethanol and adjustments in pH and conductivity, in the main at −5°C. Ethanol is sufficiently microbicidal that, together with the low temperature, the prospect of massive microbiological contamination is small during fractionation. Additions of ethanol and acetic acid or other pH adjustment solutions are made slowly with constant mixing to reduce local concentration effects so that the proteins that are intended to remain in solution at the indicated step do not precipitate. The resolubilization of proteins precipitated inadvertently is a lengthy process.

The end products of cold ethanol fractionation (Cohn et al., 1946) are relatively pure proteins, primarily normal human serum albumin (HSA, Cohn fraction V) and the immunoglobulins (Cohn fractions I, II, and III). The M_r of HSA is 68,000, the purity usually is about 97–98%; in trauma patients, substantial volumes of 5% and 25% solutions are administered intravenously to restore plasma volume and osmolarity.

Immunoglobulins are less pure, in part because they vary widely in charge (p*I* ranging from about 6 upward). Intravenous Ig preparations go through additional, non-Cohn steps such as chromatography for purification.

Sterilizing Grade Filtrations

A 5% HSA solution can be filtered successfully through any of the 0.2 μm-rated MFs available commercially, and provided the filter has been validated properly and nondestructively tested the filtration will remove all bacteria and fungi and particles that might cause capillary occlusion in the patient. The filters used are almost always in the form of a steam-sterilizable cartridge (Fig. 4) that is mounted in a stainless steel housing (Fig. 5) on a cleaned, steam-sterilized, vented tank into which the product (5% HSA in this instance) is pumped.

Five percent HSA adsorbs to surfaces but, depending on the surface charge of the filter, tends not to occlude filters rated at 0.2 μm. Even a highly adsorbing filter matrix like nylon 66, which adsorbs a significant amount of HSA on the 7000 cm^2 of filter area usually found in a 25 cm long cartridge filter, is suitable for HSA filtration because the amount of protein removed by filter adsorption is negligible relative to the batch volume and total protein. Our problem, though, is that due to the higher adsorption of nylon, fouling of the filter membrane is more likely. By way of contrast, hF-VIII in 1% HSA, filtered through a nylon 66 MF, is removed almost quantitatively. I speculate that a combination of hydrophobic and charge-

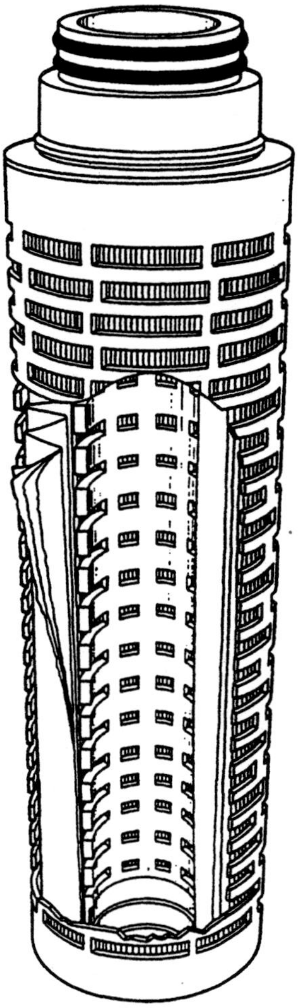

Figure 4 Pleated cartridge filter of about 2,000 cm^2 membrane filter area.

mediated events cause essentially irreversible unfolding of hF-VIII and adsorption of the molecule to the matrix.)

Cascade Filtration

One method for preliminary fractionation of plasma proteins that has not become widely used is cascade filtration, shown schematically in Fig. 6. Molecular microaggregates (e.g., fibrin clots) and immune complexes are removed from whole blood by filters with pore sizes ranging from 0.2 to 0.6 μm. Ultrafilters with pore sizes of 0.01–0.06 μm will tend to retain immunoglobulins (M_r 150,000 and higher) while allowing HSA (M_r 68,000) to pass through in the filtrate. Such strategies are actually applied in the diafiltration and concentration of IgG and HSA with ultrafilters, late rather than early in the process stream.

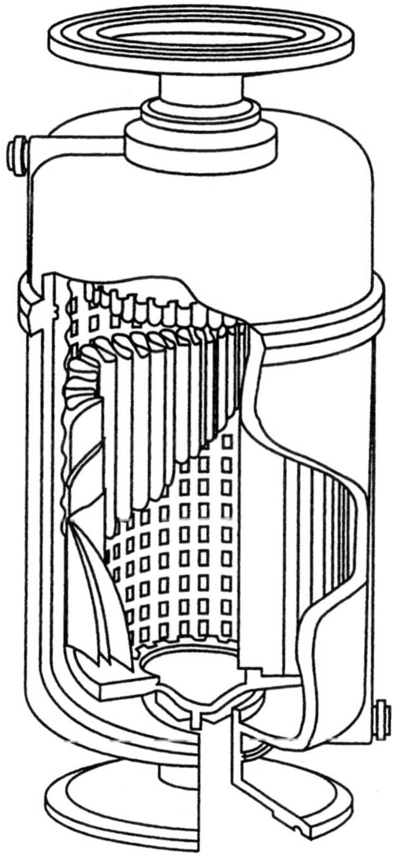

Figure 5 Pleated cartridge filter in a stainless steel housing.

Although cascade filtration works with fair efficiency, the worldwide standard method for plasma fractionation for over 50 years has been the Cohn cold ethanol method. Membrane methods like this are adjunct, not primary.

In several instances thus far in this chapter, adsorptive effects have been noted with depth and membrane filters. Such effects are important, often critical, in the purification of proteins and peptides, hence merit special consideration.

Rules of Thumb Regarding Protein Adsorption to Filters

Protein adsorption increases with

1. Charge on the filter (especially positive charges imparted by quarternary ligands, when the pH of the medium is at neutrality or higher) and charge density.
2. Hydrophobicity of the filter, especially as the salt-imparted conductivity of the solution increases.
3. Decreasing temperature when the solubility of the protein in the particular solution is near its limit.

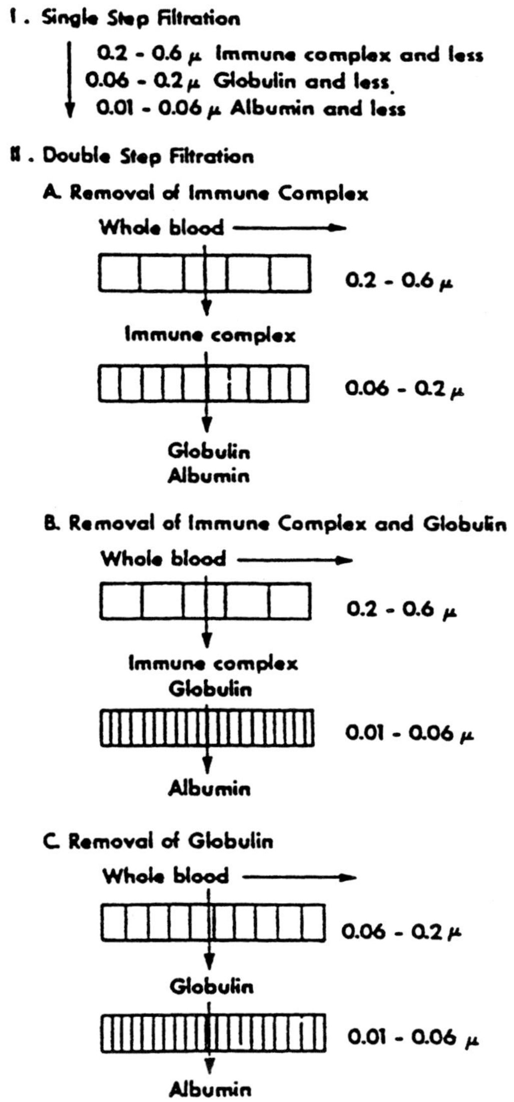

Figure 6 Schematic of cascade filtration.

Protein adsorption increases with

4. Protein M_r.
5. Average charge on the protein, relative to the matrix, at the pH of the suspending medium. Positively charged solutes at pH 7.0, for example most of the IgGs, will elute directly through a diethylaminoethyl-substituted filter matrix in a small volume of solvent but will be retained to varying degrees on a sulfated matrix at the same pH (many biochemists do not view this as a form of adsorption).
6. Increasing complexity of protein folding.

Minimal adsorption of proteins occurs when

7. The flux of the feed (face velocity, measured as milliliters of feed per square centimeter of filter area per minute, or cm/min) is small but continuous.
8. The internal filter surface area is minimal.
9. The filter surface is masked by polyols (e.g., oligosaccharides) with minimal free carboxyl groups.
10. Charge on the protein is the same as the charge on the filter.
11. Salts in solution are sufficient to mediate charge interactions between the protein and the filter but insufficient to cause the protein to precipitate.
12. Solutes of low M_r stabilize protein shape and folding (e.g., sodium caprylate added to HSA, whereby the alkyl moieties of the caprylate extend into the hydrophobic clefts of the HSA).

The points given above merit some explanation. The net charge on a protein is determined by groups that have the potential to lose a proton (e.g., carboxyl groups) or to gain a proton (e.g., amino groups). For example, carboxyl groups [R—C(O)OH] tend to be strongly electronegative when the proton is dissociated, which usually occurs in a protein at a pH above 4. The more strongly R attracts electrons, the more readily the proton will be dissociated and a negative charge established on the macromolecule. At approximately neutral pH (blood and plasma usually are at about 7.3–7.5), most plasma proteins have a negative charge.

However, even a highly negatively charged protein such as HSA (isoionic point or p*I* of 4, which is the pH at which intramolecular charges are balanced) has some positively charged amino acid residues on the surface of the molecule folded in the native state. Therefore, proximity of a lysine residue (positively charged) of HSA with a carboxyl residue on a filter may give rise to a transient binding, which may lead to a long-term binding. It is appropriate to note that adsorption of macromolecules or particles to surfaces tends to occur in two stages. The first is reversible and may last for seconds or minutes, depending on conditions. The second is an irreversible step with respect to molecular integrity and function.

Biologic Effects of Protein Adsorption

Proteins with significant hydrophobic zones internalize those areas as they fold into the native state; the exterior of such proteins (often globular) is largely hydrophilic. A plentitude of disulfide (R—S—S—R′) bridges between cysteine sulfhydryl residues maintains the shape of HSA. Fats (such as free fatty acids, e.g., sodium caprylate), held in place by hydrophobic interactions, stabilize hydrophobic zones in some lipid-binding proteins such as HSA. Since hydrophobic residues of amino acids tend to be internalized, hydrophobic interactions between a protein solute and the filter matrix usually involve unfolding of the protein, which often is tantamount to denaturation of the protein and loss of activity.

Gamma globulins have a Y shape, with the biologically active binding areas near the ends of the upright arms. The supporting tail, known as the Fc portion of an immunoglobulin, sometimes has a hydrophobic terminus that immobilizes the protein to the surface of a B cell. The biological binding arms are outstretched into solution. The IgG is bound to the surface of the B cell (a type of leukocyte) that produced it.

Gamma globulins have a strong tendency to adsorb, via Fc and by hydrophobic interaction, to plastics. [This effect was the basis of one of the early immunodiagnostic tests, which used plastic test tubes to which particular antibodies (Ab's) attach, strongly and essentially irreversibly but noncovalently. The target molecules in solution, to which a spike of known levels of radioactive target molecules have been added, is in turn bound by the immobilized Abs. From the radioactivity bound, one could determine the concentration of unlabeled target in the sample.]

One means of reducing the adsorption to plastic is the incorporation of a small amount of a poly(ethylene glycol) (PEG) of low M_r ($\approx$400). PEG is a flexible polyol with interspersed —CH_2— groups. The molecule can fold into accordion-like pleats, masking hydrophobic areas with an —OH exterior. The problem with this approach is that its effectiveness depends on PEG concentration and temperature, since PEG also can act as a precipitant at some critical concentration and set of conditions. The wisest arrangement minimizes the hydrophobic plastic surfaces that plasma proteins are exposed to during processing and avoids the addition of an unnecessary solute such as PEG.

Protein Adsorption and Sterilizing Grade Filtration

If excessive IgG adsorption is occurring with the filter in use, the filter material must be changed. The filters that are the least adsorptive to Ig's or any other proteins are those of unsubstituted cellulose acetate or polyol-covered polyvinylidene difluoride (PVDF). All nylon membranes, especially those of nylon 66, are powerfully adsorptive; these membrane materials are suitable for use only with HSA and some poorly adsorptive peptides that are filtered in high volumes from which adsorptive losses are negligible (Olson, 1987). Nevertheless, premature blocking can occur due to excessive fouling.

Proteins behave like particles. As proteins in solution approach a filter pore through which the solution is passing, some of the protein molecules do not quite make the turn into the pore and, like a racing car out of control at a sharp curve, impact into the filter matrix. This has been shown experimentally (Lindley et al., 1982). As far as resistance to flow is concerned, adsorption of macromolecular layers to the filter increases filter thickness. Also, with proteins of high M_r (e.g., hF-VIII), adsorption within the interior of the filter matrix causes a significant reduction in internal pore diameter and contributes dramatically to resistance to flow. For the given example (hF-VIII), adsorption of the protein from solution by the filter will

1. Remove a substantial proportion of the hF-VIII from the feed solution so that the concentration in the filtrate is dramatically less than in the feed.
2. Render the filtrate inoperable because internal and upstream surface adsorption will reduce the effective pore size and increase filter thickness so much that resistance to flow makes filter use impractical. Also, high losses of yield will be apparent.

Therefore, protein adsorption to sterilizing grade filters must be minimal and reproducible.

Protein Adsorption to Surfaces Other Than Filter Matrices

Immunoglobulins adsorb to glass, as do almost all proteins. Some of the adsorption may be attributed to hydrogen bonding between hydroxyls of the glass and carboxyl groups of the protein. It is possible, but not proven, that aluminum in the glass also imparts local high positive charges and promotes binding for it is known that aluminum can and does migrate within glass and leaches very slowly from the surface of glass into contained solutions over time (Quagliaro et al., 1988). The release of solutes from glassy polymers has been described mathematically (Peppas, 1982). Over the course of filtration, this is not a problem.

There are some circumstances in which irreversible binding of a protein to a filter is desirable. For example, if one wishes to immobilize an enzyme on a filter so that the enzyme can mediate a molecular conversion without contaminating the solution, covalent coupling of the enzyme to the filter is beneficial. A number of such molecular conversions are carried out in the manufacture of a variety of organic drugs. Pyruvate decarboxylase from the yeast *Candida utilis* converts benzaldehyde to L-phenylacetylcaronol, a key intermediate in the production of L-ephedrine (Shin, et al., 1996). A number of other examples are held proprietary. Although this technique is not applicable to the Cohn fractionation of plasma proteins, it merits mention because of its broad potential utility (e.g., modification of particular amino acid residues of a protein). The simplest means of coupling is the following. A filter matrix is substituted with a carboxylic acid. A water-soluble carbodiimide (WSCDI) is added to the carboxyl-substituted filter, and, after rinsing out the unreacted WSCDI at a pH no less than 6, the protein is added with mixing over time. Lysine amino groups of the protein react with the carboxyl groups on the filter to form peptide bonds that are quite stable. Sartorius (Göttingen) offers MA-series membranes (MA = membrane adsorbers) for bench-scale ion-exchange chromatography. The Sartorius literature indicates that the C15X product (weakly acidic cation exchanger) is carboxyl-substituted, and this should be suitable for the WSCDI-intermediated enzyme couplings. Some details on these methods can be found in (Olson, 1995).

Filtrations Other Than Microporous

The sterilizing grade filtrations with 0.2 μm pore size rated MFs are dead-ended, as are filtrations with depth matrices. The other major type of filtration is (UF) with skinned membranes that have pores of a size distribution in the nanometer range. Excellent reviews of ultrafiltration and all types of crossflow systems are given by Michaels et al. (1995) and in Chapter 16 of this volume.

Usually, the pore density of UF membranes does not approach that of the microporous filters, and for the skinned membranes operation in the dead-end mode rapidly results in filter clog due to the formation of a protein gel (polarization layer) on the upstream side. The gel layer on a dead-end mode ultrafilter converts the filter to a reverse osmosis function (only water passes through the gel into the filtrate, and then at low fluxes and under fairly extreme pressures).

The simplest cure, and one that is widespread, is crossflow (tangential flow), whereby the feed flows *across* the filter surface in a thin layer (as in hemodialysis) and a proportion of the feed is recycled on the upstream side. Forcing the feed into a thin channel above the filter results in considerable shear, which sweeps away particles and macromolecular solutes that otherwise would tend to form a polarization layer of protein gel plus particles on the surface. Because the channel above the UF membrane is usually 25 μm or less in depth, a coarse filtration of the UF crossflow feed (to remove particles greater than 20 μm in diameter) often is done with a nonwoven matrix of depth prefilters before the ultrafiltration is performed.

The amount of feed that passes through the ultrafilter is determined in part by the valving on the filtrate side. A high differential pressure from the upstream side is not necessary; the shear determines the continuity of flow.

Feed-and-Bleed Systems

One of the somewhat unconventional applications of ultrafiltration is feed-and-bleed, whereby UF systems are set up in series with constant feed and recovery of filtrate from each system. This approach is applied to the concentration of bovine and porcine plasma proteins in some applications by European food processors. Bleed is from each of the UF loops, which carry independent pumps. Booster pumps also are in place in the feed line between the UF loops. The emerging slurry has the consistency of a paste. To the best of my knowledge, such feed-and-bleed systems are not in use in pharmaceutical manufacturing.

Ranges in Pore Size and Configurational Variants

Ultrafilters usually are graded by the molecular weight range of the globular proteins that are excluded. Water and inorganic salts pass through freely. The exclusion curve (proportion of feed macromolecules retained, as a function of $\log_{10} M_r$) is almost always sigmoid in shape.

An ultrafilter rated at 10 kDa (M_r = 10,000) will usually retain over 98% of HSA (68 kDa) but will be poorly retentive of a small protein like insulin (5 kDa). The performance of an ultrafilter can also be measured as the retention of a well-described linear molecule. Dextran (polyglucose) fractions, or polyvinylpyrrolidone (PVP) or poly(ethylene glycol) (PEG) fractions may be substituted for proteins of known M_r in characterizing the ultrafilter. However, because the molecular weights of dextran or PVP or PEG fractions are far broader than those of specific proteins (tightly defined M_r, give or take a carboxyl group), the retention curve for an ultrafilter described with PVP will cover about two decades rather than one decade as when performance is measured with proteins.

The advantage of characterizing an ultrafilter with PVP or other nonprotein macromolecules is that small amounts of dextrans, PVP, and PEG are well tolerated as injections and can therefore be used in the characterization of an ultrafilter before the filter is used in the processing of an injectable drug. For example, solutions of dextrans formulated appropriately are approved as plasma expanders and in some circumstances used in place of HSA. Trace dextrans are recognized as safe by FDA, MCA, and other regulatory agencies. An ultrafilter can be characterized in terms of dextran rejection (retention), rinsed, and then used in the concentration or diafiltration (dialysis by means of a UF system) of plasma proteins intended for injections.

Ultrafiltration systems are produced and marketed as manifolded flat membranes, spiral-wound membranes, and hollow fibers. All presently are in use by various blood and/or plasma processors. Regeneration often is with 0.1 N NaOH. Many approaches to cleaning and validation have been validated [see Michaels et al. (1995) and this volume].

4 VIRUS REMOVAL BY FILTRATION

Human plasma often contains viruses that may be life-threatening such as hepatitis A, B, or C (HAV, HBV, HCV) or the human immunodeficiency virus (HIV-1). The detection of these viruses in individual plasma donations can be done by the polymerase chain reaction (PCR) (Mullis, 1987; Mullis et al., 1987). The current cost of a single PCR test makes this cost-prohibitive, however. Therefore, to ensure the general safety of blood-derived products, regulatory agencies throughout the world such as the Food and Drug Administration (FDA) in the United States and the Committee for Proprietary Medicinal Product (CPMP) in Europe have established guidelines for such plasma-derived products. These guidelines recommend minimal methods to determine the efficacy of the purification methods used in producing the blood-derived product in removing or inactivating any potential viruses in the bulk material. During the purification procedure there should be, according to these guidelines, at least two steps that remove or inactivate viruses, ideally using different physico-chemical means.

4.1 Viruses and Assays Used for Validation Studies for Viral Removal

To validate the efficacy of the UF system to remove or inactivate viruses, some means of quantifying the viruses is necessary. There are a variety of methods that could be employed to determine virus titers. Transmission electron microscopy is very tedious and inaccurate in quantifying virus titer and hence is unsuitable as an assay. Another possible method is to grow the viruses in cell culture containing ^{32}P, a hard beta emitter. However, the use of radioactive labels is normally avoided when possible, for obvious reasons, and does not result in absolute numbers.

Alternative methods applicable with any virus is the use of a monoclonal antibody (MAb) directed against the specific virus. The MAb can be radioiodinated or tritiated or labeled with any variety of beta or gamma emitters. A MAb can also be labeled with a fluorescent dye. Many such dyes are available, the best known being fluorescein isothiocyanate (FITC) and rhodamine B isothiocyanate (RBITC). These methods, however, cannot produce the accuracy of quantification that is required.

The most sensitive and useful method in quantifying virus titer is to use either a plaque assay or $TCID_{50}$ (tissue culture infectious dose) assay. The plaque assay is performed on a lawn of mammalian host cells that are lysed by the virus during their replication cycle. The plaques that are produced are counted, and there is a direct quantification of the viruses per volume. The $TCID_{50}$ assay is an indirect method of determining the titer of virus. The host cells are grown in multiple well plates, and a variety of concentrations of the virus-containing sample are inoculated onto the cells. It is then determined which concentration results in 50% of the wells being infected by the virus. These data can then be used in a variety of statistical formulas, such as the Spearman–Karber formula, to determine the actual titer of the virus. Either of these methods is acceptable to the regulatory authorities around the world.

According to the different regulatory guidelines, the viruses used in such a study should, when possible, be those viruses that are the potential contaminants of blood, such as HIV or HAV. When no practical assay is available for a specific virus in question, such as is the case (at the present time) with HBV and HCV, model viruses may be employed that closely resemble these viruses. In these examples the rabbitpox virus (as a model for HBV) and the bovine viral diarrhea virus (as a model for HCV) would be used.

In such a validation study using membrane filtration, a known amount of the virus will be spiked into the starting material prior to filtration. Following the filtration, the amount of virus will then be determined in both the retentate and the filtrate. This allows one to determine the distribution, e.g., mass balance, of the virus. In other words, the amount of the virus that is retained by the membrane, the amount that passes through the membrane, and the amount that is adsorbed on the membrane can be determined.

Once the mass balance has been determined, these values are used to calculate the reduction factor (RF) of the step being tested. This is calculated as follows.

$$\mathrm{RF} = \log_{10}\left[\frac{\text{(input virus titer/volume)} \times \text{input volume}}{\text{(output virus titer/volume)} \times \text{output volume}}\right]$$

For example,

$$\mathrm{RF} = \log_{10}\frac{(10^8\ \mathrm{IU/mL}) \times 10\ \mathrm{mL}}{(10^2\ \mathrm{IU/mL}) \times 20\ \mathrm{mL}} = 5.7$$

This example results in a reduction factor of 5.7 logs.

To achieve the greatest possible viral reduction, a variety of points must be taken into consideration. For example, the initial titer of the spiking virus must be the highest possible to ensure that the achievable reduction is not limited by the virus titer itself. Also, one must ensure that, when possible, the titrations are performed immediately and that samples are not frozen. Freezing and thawing the samples may result in a loss of titer due to inactivation of viruses by this additional step in the testing procedure.

4.2 Surrogate Viruses for Validation

Another approach to qualifying a filtration system for the removal of viruses it to use a harmless surrogate virion for which a simple quantitative assay is available. This may be useful in the initial phases of determining the efficacy of the membrane in removing viruses. This is due to the fact that the studies, as described above, although necessary for regulatory approval of the product in question, are too expensive to be carried out routinely for research purposes.

An example of a surrogate virus that could be used during the research phase of determining which membrane would be most effective in removing viruses is the coliphage MS2. Some information on this is provided in Bechtel *et al.* (1988).

4.3 Virus Removal During Microfiltration

There is little in the literature about the removal of virions from suspension with filters of rated pore sizes equal to or greater than 0.2 μm. I have removed MS2 from suspension with 10 kDa rated ultrafilters operating in the crossflow mode. However, dead-ended filtration through microfilters constructed of mixed esters of cellulose and rated at 0.2 and 0.45 μm also significantly reduced MS2 titers. Adsorptive removal of viruses is consistent with the studies of Tanny and Meltzer (1978) and Tanney et al. (1979).

Virus adsorption by a microporous filter is a function of the number of adsorptive sites, the composition of the adsorbing matrix, and the presence of solutes that promote or interfere with adsorption. Therefore, for proteinaceous solutions—exactly the type of solutions from which one wishes to remove viruses—virus removal by adsorption can be unreliable.

Adsorptive ligands can be immobilized on a support [e.g., the removal of hepatitis B virus (HBV) and other infectious virions from human plasma onto C_{18}-substituted materials]. The method works but is not sufficiently reliable for routine use in the manufacture of human injectables. The methods that are reliable and reproducible for the removal of viruses are size exclusion methods (e.g., UF), physical methods (e.g., heat, or solvent–detergent mixtures), or chemical methods (e.g., bisglutaraldehyde or hydrogen peroxide). In practice, combinations of methods must be used.

REFERENCES

Bechtel, M. K., A. Bagdasarian, W. P. Olson, and T. N. Estep. (1988). Viral removal or inactivation in hemoglobin solutions by ultrafiltration or detergent/solvent treatment, *Biomater. Artif. Cell Organs*, *16*(1-3):123–128.

Bowden, R. A., S. J. Slichter, M. Sayers, D. Weisdorf, M. Cays, G. Schoch, M. Banaji, R. Haake, K. Welk, L. Fisher, J. McCullough, and W. Miller. (1995). A comparison of filtered leukocyte-reduced and cytomegalovirus (CMV) seronegative blood products for the prevention of transfusion-associated CMV infection after marrow transplant, *Blood*, *86*:3598–3603.

Cohn, E. J., L. E. Strong, W. L. Hughes, D. J. Mulford, J. N. Ashworth, M. Melin, and H. L. Taylor. (1946). Preparation and properties of serum and plasma proteins. IV. A system for the separation into fractions of the protein and lipoprotein components of biological tissues and fluids, *J. Am. Chem. Soc.*, *68*:459–475.

Fiore, J. W., W. P. Olson, and S. L. Holst. (1980). Depth filtration, in *Methods of Plasma Protein Fractionation* (J. M. Curling, ed.), Academic, London, pp. 239–268.

Lindley, P. D., W. P. Olson, and M. R. Faith. (1982). Microporous membranes and crossflow filtration of macromolecules and proteins, in *Polymeric Separations Media* (A. R. Cooper, ed.), Plenum, New York, pp. 173–190.

Matsushita, M., and Y. Nose. (1986). Artificial liver, in *Evolution of Artificial Organs: A Festschrift to Dr. George E. Schreiner* (J. F. Maher, ed.), ISAO Press, Cleveland, OH, pp. 108–114.

Michaels, S. L., C. Antoniou, V. Goel, P. Keating, R. Kuriyel, A. S. Michaels, S. R. Pearl, G. de los Reyes, E. Rudolph, and M. Siwak. (1995). Tangential flow filtration, in Separations Technology: *Pharmaceutical and Biotechnology Applications*, W. P. Olson, (ed.), Interpharm, Buffalo Grove, IL, pp. 57–194.

Mullis, K. B. (1987). U.S. Patent 4,683,202.

Mullis, K. B., H. A. Erlich, N. Arnheim, G. T. Horn, R. K. Saiki, and S. J. Scharf. (1987). U.S. Patent 4,683,195.

Olson, W. P. (1987). Sterilization of small-volume parenterals and therapeutic proteins by filtration, in *Aseptic Pharmaceutical Manufacturing, Technology for the 1990s* (W. P. Olson and M. J. Groves, eds.), Interpharm, Buffalo Grove, IL, pp. 101–149.

Olson, W. P. (1995). Immunoaffinity purification of proteins for injection, and the issue of animal viruses, in *Separations Technology: Pharmaceutical and Biotechnology Applications* (W. P. Olson, ed.), Interpharm, Buffalo Grove, IL, pp. 391–425.

Peppas, N. A. (1982). Constant Solute Release Rates from Glassy Polymers, *Org. Coatings Appl. Polym. Sci. Proc. 46*:615–618.

Quagliaro, D.A., V. A. Geraci, R. E. Dwan, R. S. Kent, and W. P. Olson. (1988). Aluminum in albumin for injection, *J. Parenter. Sci. Technol., 42*:187–190.

Shin, H. S., and P. L. Rogers. (1996). Kinetic evaluation of biotransformation of benzaldehyde to L-phenylacetylcarbinol by immobilized pyruvate decarboxylase from *Candida utilis*. *Biotechnol. Bioeng., 49*:429–436.

Tanny, G. B. and T. H. Meltzer. (1978). The dominance of adsorptive effects in the filtrative sterilization of a flu vaccine, *J. Parenter. Drug. Assoc., 32*:258–267.

Tanny, G. B., D. K. Strong, W. G. Presswood, and T. H. Meltzer. (1979). The adsorptive retention of *Pseudomonas diminuta* by membrane filters, *J. Parenteral Drug Assoc., 33*:40–51.

SUGGESTED ADDITIONAL READING

Curling, J. M. (ed.) (1983). *Separation of Plasma Proteins*, Pharmacia Fine Chemicals AB, Uppsala, Sweden.

27

The Operation of the FDA: A Brief Summary

ANTHONY C. CELESTE
AAC Consulting Group, Inc., Bethesda, Maryland

1 INTRODUCTION

This chapter sets forth the general framework for the regulation of pharmaceuticals manufacturing by the U.S. Food and Drug Administration (FDA) under the federal Food, Drug and Cosmetic Act (FD&C Act) and its implementing regulations. The primary objective is to explain how agency operations affect manufacturers and other businesses in the pharmaceutical industry. Discussion of the following subjects, which are related to pre- and postmarket regulatory and/or enforcement activities, is based on the statute, regulations, FDA guidance, and industry practice and draws on my own expertise in the field.

FDA authority and industry oversight functions
Current good manufacturing practice requirements
Recall procedures
New drug application approval requirements
Adverse drug experience reporting requirements
Registration and listing

2 FDA OVERSIGHT

The FDA has broad authority under Section 704 of the FD&C Act to inspect pharmaceutical manufacturing establishments, including all equipment, finished and in-process materials, and containers. For prescription drugs, this authority extends to "all things" in an establishment bearing on whether there may be a violation of the FD&C Act including "records, files, papers, processes, controls, and facilities." The FDA typically conducts inspections prior to approval of a new marketing application, after a recall or for other causes, and on a periodic (biennial) or other basis without cause. Following an inspection, the investigator usually leaves a report of his or her observations known as an FDA-483. It is agency policy and a requirement for investigators that an FDA-483 be provided if the investigator observes deficiencies that, among other things, may result in a product becoming adulterated (in the case of pharmaceutical manufacturers, these would generally involve the current good manufacturing practice requirements described below). Few inspections of any magnitude will conclude without the issuance of an FDA-483. FDA-483's represent the individual views of investigators and are subject to review by the agency for a determination of whether the conditions in the establishment violate the law and warrant further action.

Although not required by law, it is customary industry practice for manufacturers to respond to an FDA-483 by explaining any corrective actions they have taken and attempting to resolve any misunderstandings that may have led to a particular observation. The FDA encourages prompt voluntary corrections and requests that responses include time frames for completing longer term actions. A response should address all of the listed observations and should speak to whatever systems may be affected as a result of the inspection and how the deviations, if indeed they are such, will be corrected.

Following inspections, investigators prepare reports officially referred to as Establishment Inspection reports (EIRs). In the normal course of the FDA review process, an FDA-483, the companion EIR, and a firm's response are reviewed at various management levels in the FDA district office. The report is first reviewed by the investigator's supervisor, who usually prepares a written summary of the more significant findings. If there appear to be serious violations or the firm has had past compliance problems, the supervisor may recommend that appropriate action of a regulatory nature be taken. The report is then referred by the district investigations branch to the compliance branch for further review. The totality of the evidence, including FDA-483's issued during previous inspections and any FDA sample results, is considered in view of agency guidelines and policies. District management then has at its disposal a number of options. Depending on the situation, managers can choose from a variety of regulatory options. These vary from a prompt reinspection through issuance of a warning letter to the recommendation of regulatory action to the Center for Drug Evaluation and Research. However, if a district determines, based on evaluation of the evidence and a firm's response, that no enforcement action is required, an EIR may be disposed of without any further action taking place.

The Center's Office of Compliance must make the initial decision on the appropriateness of a district recommendation for a regulatory action. The headquarters chain of command for regulatory action review and approval includes the FDA's offices of Regulatory Affairs and General Counsel. Ultimately, a decision is made by agency management as to the disposition of the recommendation. The agency has many enforcement tools at its disposal. These actions include administrative request to recall products, proceedings to withdraw product approval, seizure of a violative product in distribution channels, seizure of all raw materials and finished products at a facility, injunction to prevent continuing violations from occurring, and criminal prosecution to punish firms and individuals for previous violations of the law and to deter future violations. Depending on its assessment of the seriousness of the violation, the agency's action will vary. Sometimes more than one sanction is applied. Generally, higher levels of review take place when the agency is contemplating a criminal case or an action that would restrain a firm from doing business.

The sanctions available to the FDA for violations of the law are quite formidable. The differences between the criminal and civil sanctions are significant. Criminal cases, which involve the prosecution of responsible individuals as well as the business entity where appropriate, can result in time in jail as well as significant monetary fines. The civil sanctions used by the FDA usually involve action against a product or firm and can also result in significant monetary fines or expenses to bring the firm into compliance with the FDA's requirements. The most significant civil penalty that the agency can take is to enjoin a firm from continuing to operate. In this case the firm will essentially be closed until the court is satisfied that it can operate in compliance with all the FDA's requirements. The courts, naturally, rely on the FDA for this determination.

If agency management concludes that there is a serious violation, the initial action generally will be the issuance of a warning letter describing the violation and requesting that it be promptly corrected. In cases (including manufacturing violations) that meet predetermined criteria, the district office may issue a warning letter on its own initiative. The FDA may institute additional formal enforcement proceedings whether or not a satisfactory response to a warning letter is received. The letter is intended to stimulate the correction of the deficiencies identified during the inspection, whereas the civil and criminal actions are applied to meet other enforcement objectives. The FDA recommends product seizures, injunctions, and criminal prosecutions to the Justice Department, which is responsible for filing such cases in the U.S. district court where the violation occurred.

Although its enforcement powers are administered judiciously, the agency is not shy about using them when it deems that the situation warrants it. In recent years, the FDA has been particularly active in bringing action against those involved in drug manufacturing violations. For example, several pharmaceutical manufacturers (representing both the brand name and generic sides of the industry) are currently operating under court-ordered consent decrees that impose substantial restrictions on their operations. In cases of fraud, jail sentences and millions of dollars of fines have been levied against individuals and companies. In recent years the agency has regarded enforcement actions of this sort as a top priority and law enforcement generally as its principal mission.

3 MANUFACTURING REQUIREMENTS

Under Section 501(a)(2)(B) of the FD&C Act, a drug is deemed to be adulterated if it is not manufactured in accordance with current good manufacturing practice (CGMP). The FDA has promulgated regulations establishing minimum CGMP standards at 21 C.F.R. Parts 210 and 211. CGMP requirements are intended to provide assurance that drugs are manufactured under systems and procedures such that the products will have the quality, purity, safety, identity, and strength that they are labeled or purported to possess. The regulations cover finished dosage form products intended for human use. The FDA has not promulgated GMP regulations for the manufacture of bulk pharmaceuticals. However, the agency has stated and does use the CGMPs for finished pharmaceuticals as guidelines when conducting inspections of bulk manufacturing facilities.

The CGMP regulations are very general. They require manufacturers to establish programs to maintain drug quality, but they generally leave the content of those programs to the discretion of the manufacturers. Thus, in many areas there are a number of different ways in which a manufacturer may comply. The regulations require written standard operating procedures (SOPs) and production, control, and laboratory records (to which FDA has access under its inspection power). While the FDA has provided informal guidance on CGMP issues by making public its guidelines to investigators and other materials, manufacturers still retain substantial discretion in determining what is appropriate to satisfy CGMP standards. For example, the regulations require that manufacturing processes, analytical methods, and procedures be validated. They do not specify, however, how they should be validated. These procedures and others, such as how to sample and analyze a product, are left to the firm to decide. The appropriateness of the firm's decisions are reviewed by the FDA during the course of application review and establishment inspections.

The FDA, in an effort to establish uniformity in the conduct of CGMP inspections, has prepared a number of inspection guides that provide investigators with guidance as to what to look for during the inspection of certain types of pharmaceutical dosage form manufacturers. In addition, the FDA has also provided its investigators with guidance documents that are related to certain critical processes that are a part of all pharmaceutical operations. These include, for example, process validation, water systems, and quality control laboratories. While these documents are intended primarily to provide guidance to the field investigators, they also provide the industry with useful information on the agency's expectations in this ever-evolving area of current good manufacturing practices. These are also useful to the industry in the conduct of their own quality assurance and internal auditing programs.

By their nature, CGMP standards evolve over time. The law does not require, and the FDA does not expect, manufacturers to immediately replace all of their equipment with potentially improved technologies. Rather, manufacturers may properly keep older equipment and facilities in use, saving new methods and materials, as appropriate, for new plants or production lines. On the other side of this issue, the FDA allows companies to implement new and different manufacturing procedures and test methods provided they establish that these procedures and methods are equivalent to or better than their predecessors. Companies should use good judgment when applying the various FDA guidelines to their own unique processes and systems of control.

In addition to CGMP requirements, drugs generally must meet applicable standards established in the United States Pharmacopoeia (USP). The USP includes monographs for drug substances and drug products, which typically set forth requirements for drug purity, identity, and the like. The USP also includes standards for water quality and other matters pertaining to drug manufacturing. Although the USP requirements are distinct from CGMPs, compliance with the USP on a matter specifically covered by the compendium will usually be adequate to demonstrate compliance with CGMPs. Manufacturers also must comply with any additional specifications established in the approved new drug applications or abbreviated new drug applications for their products. The FDA expects and the regulations require drug manufacturers to adhere to all commitments made in approved applications. These include the names of all raw material suppliers, their specifications, the method of manufacture of the approved drug product, etc. Manufacturers wishing to make changes in application commitments must follow the FDA regulations set forth in 21 C.F.R. § 314.70.

4 RECALL STANDARDS

The FDA expects that from time to time even firms in compliance with CGMPs may experience product problems and deviations that would make a recall appropriate. Among other things, problems may occur as a result of employee error, changes to the manufacturing process, differences in raw materials, and other variations and anomalies. While the FDA does not have mandatory recall authority for pharmaceutical products, the agency has promulgated standards for voluntary recalls at 21 C.F.R. Part 7, Subpart C. Most responsible pharmaceutical manufacturers conform to these standards, under which manufacturers are expected to remove product from the market if it no longer meets its specifications and to notify and cooperate with the FDA. In addition, manufacturers are required to report to an FDA district office, through the "field alert" reporting system, the discovery of any mislabeling, contamination, or other adulteration of a marketed new drug product.

Under the recall standards, the FDA will classify a recall depending on the potential health hazard presented, and the recalling firm will determine which batches should be recalled and develop a strategy to remove them from the marketplace. A team of agency experts will classify the recall, with class I being the most serious and class III the least. Depending on the classification, the agency will expect the firm to take certain actions. For example, publicity in the form of a press release is usually associated with class I recalls. In addition, the recall classification will dictate the level of "effectiveness checks" and the level of communication to distribution channels. If a firm does not cooperate in conducting a recall, the agency may issue a public warning, then initiate a seizure or injunction to control the violative product.

The FDA evaluates both the seriousness of the violation that prompted the recall and the adequacy of the firm's actions. It will also usually follow up with an inspection of the firm to determine the root cause of the recall, review the action taken by the firm, and assess whether any other lots of the product may be affected. The inspection may result in the conclusion that serious control deficiencies at the facility caused the problem that resulted in the product recall. Under these circumstances, the recall could result in additional regulatory action being considered by the agency. The agency will follow the process described above when pursuing regulatory action as a result of a product recall.

5 APPROVAL REQUIREMENTS

A new drug cannot be marketed without prior approval by the FDA. For a drug that has never been marketed before, the manufacturer must file a full new drug application (NDA) with the FDA that includes data from tests in animals and humans demonstrating that the drug is safe and effective for its labeled indications. After an NDA has been approved and relevant patents and periods of market exclusivity have expired, other companies may obtain approval of the same compound through an abbreviated new drug application (ANDA). An ANDA must contain evidence that the drug product contains the same active ingredient as and is "bioequivalent" to the drug approved through an NDA. For topical drug products (including inhaled drugs), FDA regulations also require that the ANDA product generally must contain the same inactive ingredients as the NDA product (both qualitatively and quantitatively) unless the ANDA applicant can demonstrate that any differences will not affect the safety of the product [21 C.F.R. § 314.94(a)(9)(v)].

In addition, both NDAs and ANDAs must contain detailed information regarding the drug manufacturing process. The FDA will not approve an NDA or ANDA if it lacks assurance that the manufacturing methods, facilities, and controls are adequate to ensure the quality and purity of the drug product. The agency also can withdraw an approved NDA or ANDA if inadequacies develop after approval and are not corrected following notice. As part of the NDA and ANDA approval process, the FDA reviews the adequacy of the application and conducts an analysis on the finished product to check both the analytical method and the composition of the product. It then conducts an inspection of the facility to determine compliance with CGMPs and conformance to the commitments in the application and checks the data and information submitted in the application for accuracy.

6 ADVERSE EVENT REPORTING

Holders of approved NDAs and ANDAs must file reports of adverse drug experiences (ADEs) with the FDA under 21 C.F.R. § 314.80. The timing of these reports depends on the seriousness of the incident. The reports must be filed regardless of whether either the person making a report to the manufacturer or the manufacturer itself believes that there is a causal relationship between use of the drug and the adverse experience. The FDA maintains databases of ADEs submitted by manufacturers, and it releases this information under the Freedom of Information Act, subject to redaction of patient- and physician-identifying information. The regulations specifically provide that submission of an ADE report by a manufacturer or release of the report by the FDA "does not necessarily reflect a conclusion by the applicant or FDA that the report or information constitutes an admission that the drug caused or contributed to an adverse effect" [21 C.F.R. § 314.80(I)]. It is typical for there to be an increase in the number of reported ADEs following adverse publicity about a drug, such as would be occasioned by a class I recall that involved notice to consumers.

7 REGISTRATION AND PRODUCT LISTING REQUIREMENTS

The Food, Drug and Cosmetic Act requires that all persons, prior to engaging in the manufacture and/or processing of a drug, register with the FDA. This registration process has associated with it the listing of drugs that will be manufactured by the firm. This listing enables the FDA, through the National Drug Code Directory system, to provide a distinct identifying number to each drug marketed in the United States. The FDA regulations covering the drug registration and listing requirements are found in 21 C.F.R. Part 207.

These requirements for drug companies enable the FDA to determine the number of drug establishments and their location. The FDA uses this information to determine the size of the drug industry and the scope of products. This database also assists in the planning of inspection coverage, helps to locate violative products, and facilitates communications.

8 SUMMARY

The FDA conducts numerous and varied inspections of drug establishments during the course of a year. The primary emphasis over the last several years has been the preapproval inspection program. That program requires the FDA to make an affirmative decision on the status of a drug firm's CGMP compliance as well as its adherence to application commitments before an application (NDA, ANDA, AADA) is approved by the agency. The agency will withhold approval in any instance where a company may fall short of the agency's requirements. Detailed guidance documents in addition to those referenced above on the FDA's expectations during the conduct of these inspections, are available to the FDA and the industry. FDA officials have stated in a number of forums that they do not consider these guides binding on either the agency or the industry. They have articulated the position that if one follows the guidance provided in these documents, expectations are that the agency will find manufacturing practices to be acceptable.

In 1995, the FDA's Congressional Oversight Committee held hearings because of alleged agency retaliation against regulated persons who objected to agency decisions or refused to cooperate. It is the nature of the business for regulators and the regulated to disagree from time to time, and it is sometimes difficult for both parties to hide personal feelings in stressful situations. The FDA has had internal appeal and grievance investigation systems in place for many years and has worked diligently to ensure that its decisions are based on facts and good public policy. Businesses or individuals who wish to appeal a decision or question inaction by the agency on a matter should feel free to raise the issue to the next higher management level. Out of courtesy, the person who made an original decision should be informed that a matter is being appealed. The agency finds appeals that present facts in support of positions to be quite acceptable. Unsupported arguments or conjecture seldom add anything and indeed may cloud the important issues. If someone feels they have been treated unfairly by a major agency component and an appeal would be fruitless, they should contact the FDA Ombudsman.

28

Validation of the Counting Accuracy of Particle Counters with the New Particle Counting Model

JULIUS Z. KNAPP
Research & Development Associates, Inc., Somerset, New Jersey

1 INTRODUCTION

In Good Manufacturing Practices the pharmaceutical manufacturer has the ultimate responsibility for maintaining the quality of his products within the bounds established and published by the U.S. Pharmacopoeia (USP, 1995). The appearance of a definitive analysis of the counting errors in light extinction particle counters (Knapp, 1996; Knapp and Abramson, 1994, 1995; Knapp et al., 1994) can be used to eliminate a troubling inadequacy in the data available from them. This inadequacy has been the lack of a rigorous methodology to validate both the capability of a particle counting instrument and the operating conditions that will result in contaminating particle count data within a prescribed counting error. The result of this inadequacy has been contaminating particle assays with ambiguous, erroneous results that have been unreliable guides for parenteral manufacturing process controls.

Considering the importance of particle contamination to all concerned with the research, production, and quality assurance and the use of injectable products, a verbal description of the problem has been separated from the communication of mathematical details. Appendix 1 is an independent step-by-step counting validation procedure, and Appendix 2 contains a detailed development of the mathematics employed. The equation numbers in the body of the chapter are identical to those assigned in a continuous sequence with those of Appendix 2. Symbols and definitions are listed in Table 1.

Light extinction particle counters are well-behaved instruments fully capable of the workhorse task of making accurate, routine particle contamination measurements in injectable products. In principle, any particle counter instrument now in

Table 1 Glossary of Terms[a]

Symbol	Units	Definition
A	—	Arbitrary constant in curve-fitting equation
A_F	$cm^2 \times 10^{-6}$	Area of detector flow channel perpendicular to direction of sample stream
B_H	μm	Height of the scan beam
c	counts/mL	Detected counts per milliliter
c/n	—	Count efficiency ratio
$\bar{c}$	—	Particle count loss per milliliter due to the coincident count of multiples
$\bar{c}/n$	—	Count loss ratio
C^+	counts/mL	Total of coincident counts per milliliter
C_I	counts/mL	Initial, maximum, counts in a dilution experiment
C_0	counts/mL	Background counts, counts at infinite dilution
C'	counts/mL	Counts from the USP 23 specified −10% undercount concentration
C_{MAX}	counts/mL	Maximum count that a detector can record
$C(1)/N$	—	Single particle count ratio
$\bar{C}(1)/N$	—	Single particle count loss ratio
$\bar{C}_B(1)/n$	—	Bounded single particle count loss ratio
$C_B^+(1)/n$	—	Bounded multiple particle group count ratio
$C3$	—	Count limit for a particle size at a selected count error
D_P	μm	Diameter of test particle
D_{PE}	μm	Effective diameter of test particle including the analysis threshold selected
ε_C	—	Count error
f	—	Constant stepwise dilution factor
f_T	—	Total dilution factor between the concentration for a 1% undercount error to the noise-limited 1% overcount error
k	—	Arbitrary constant in curve-fitting equation
K^+	—	Ratio of all multiple event counts to single particle
n_T	—	Total number of particles in a suspension
N_E	—	Effective detector volumes per milliliter
N_{E3}	—	Effective detector volumes per milliliter for a selected particle size
N_I	—	The initial concentration of particles per milliliter in a dilution experiment
N'	—	USP 23 specified concentration of 10 μm particles at which there is a 10% undercount error for a detector
N''	—	Concentration of 10 μm particles for a 1% undercount error
N_3	—	Concentration for a selected count error
s	—	The sequential step number of a dilution experiment
S	—	The number of steps in a dilution experiment
V	mL	Unspecified volume
V_A	mL	Sample aliquot volume in a dilution experiment
V_{DE}	$cm \times 10^{-6}$	The effective volume of a detector including the effect of particle size
V_{DG}	$cm \times 10^{-6}$	The geometric volume of a detector based on its static dimensions
V_0	mL	The initial volume of a dilution experiment

[a]Asterisks indicate approximate values.

use, when operated within validated particle size and concentration contours, can deliver accurate counts of the number of single contaminating particles in a test volume. Accurate counts from particle counters are available within two error limits. The first limit to be encountered is at very low concentrations and is due to noise pulses. The count of noise pulses added to the count of particle pulses introduces a positive error into the count total recorded. With current instruments that are in good operating condition, a conservative 1% error limit is reached for the smaller particle ranges at a count of 100 particles/mL.

The second counting error limit for accurate particle counter counts is negative. The error results from a loss of counts. As particle concentration increases above the minimum set by noise pulses, an increasing loss of particle counts with concentration is observed. This loss of counts is due to the coincidental grouping of multiple particles in the sensitive volume of the detector. The grouped particle signal is aliased as a larger single particle. This count loss increases as the concentration of the particles being counted increases.

Operation within these two error limits results in reliable, replicable particle count data. Both positive and negative count error limits are specific to particle detector and particle counter designs and to the experimental use conditions. Operation within validated limits for noise and concentration, both within and below the USP 23 ⟨788⟩ control size range, will ensure single particle count accuracy without undercounts or the injection of false counts. These count limits vary with particle concentration and size and are determined by the capability of the counter. No test based on the counts of a suspension of a single particle size can characterize the complex particle size and concentration counting capability of a detector. In practice, selection of a counter with sufficient capability to provide the desired accuracy without constant dilution is an important consideration. When particle concentration exceeds the selected count accuracy contour, dilution and a repeat of the assay provides a practical solution.

The original concern of the USP was the effect of particle count loss due to coincidental particle group counts on the accuracy of the ⟨788⟩ SVI contaminating particle assay. Although the basic mechanism of the count loss due to the effect of particle concentration effect was identified correctly, the implications of this effect on the USP ⟨788⟩ SVI contaminating particle assay were not critically examined. As noted in this chapter, usable accuracy from a particle counter can result only when particle concentrations below and within the assay control range are related to the experimentally validated capability of the counter.

Accurate assessment of particle contamination quality in injectable products is an essential element in cost-effective parenteral manufacturing. For those operating in a single plant environment, the capability to test and validate particle counters with the equipment normally available in a pharmaceutical laboratory prior to their use is now at hand. In multiplant organizations, harmonization of particle contamination quality requires comparability of particle counter data. A simple, practical step to achieve control and comparability of these data is specification of a joint particle size/particle count contour based on the accuracy desired. This specification must be within the experimentally validated performance of the counters used. Selection and operation of particle counters within single particle count accuracy contours is the basis for secure particle counter data comparisons. Blind reliance on vendor specifications can now be replaced with assurance that GMPs have been satisfied. For those occasions when the selected particle size/particle count contour is exceeded, dilution of the test suspension and a repeated test can be employed. No methodology exists for the postmeasurement adjustment of invalid counts of random contaminating particle data.

From the initial FDA report (Munson, 1987) of ±50% membrane or microscopic particle assay variation by the same person on the same preparation with the same microscope setup, this assay method had limited value for control of parenteral manufacturing and enforcement value. The original membrane or microscopic assay results were comparable only when particle contamination was so gross that its error margin could be disregarded. The count accuracy data developed in the error sensitivity analysis of this chapter show that USP ⟨788⟩ particle counter assays of high concentration samples were also of limited value. The control of quality limits in achieving the lower levels of particle contamination that have been recorded can be attributed to the structuring of good manufacturing practices in the recent past. Reduction of particle contamination levels in many parenteral products has resulted from improvements in materials and manufacturing technology and is only casually related to the accuracy of the USP assays for contaminating particles measurement.

The FDA national symposium on the safety of large volume parenteral solutions in 1966 marked a turning point in particle contamination of injectable products. In the last ten years there has been no report of instant mortality associated with particle contamination in an injectable product. The 1966 national symposium developed practical, achievable particle contamination goals. Those goals are now a daily reality.

There have been many occasions when the utility of an advance in technology is so clearly visible that it is pressed into service immediately. Neat, all-encompassing, explanations of how the advance works and discovery of its limitations are eventually made and are dutifully documented in the scientific literature. The use of the Coulter, light extinction, and light scattering particle counters are prime examples of this phenomenon. This chapter analyzes count accuracy in light extinction particle counters; it does not deal with particle sizing problems.

The chapter is organized to provide the information that non-engineers and non-statisticians can use to evaluate the effect of particle coincidence error on the SVI particle data generated with light extinction particle counters. Two appendixes are provided.

Appendix 1 provides a step-by-step description of the experimental methods required to evaluate the capability of light extinction particle counters. With the results of Appendix 1, an operating contour of maximum concentration versus particle size is selected. This selection determines the single particle counting accuracy and the degree of ambiguity in the data from these counters.

Appendix 2 provides a detailed analysis of coincidence counting errors and ambiguities.

2 PARTICLE COUNTER APPLICATIONS

Light extinction particle counters offer the capability to register counts of suspended particles as the particles pass through a sensing zone. They operate as measurement transfer devices whose sizing accuracy is referred to the accuracy of the calibrating particles. The best sizing accuracy is obtained when two conditions are satisfied:

1. The counter is operated at a calibration point.
2. The refractive index ratio of spheres to the suspending liquid for which the instrument was calibrated are duplicated in the measurement.

Particle counter measurements replace tedious, eye-straining microscopic sizing and counting assays that require highly trained personnel with an automated device that can be operated by a technician. Counter data have shown good replicability; this convenience has tended to obscure the inherent limitations of the counts recorded. The methodology described in this chapter can add single particle counting accuracy to the list of benefits that these counters have made available.

Accurate count limits vary with particle size and concentration and are determined by the capability of the counter system in use. However, since all particle shapes are homogenized into "equivalent" spherical volumes by light extinction particle counters, they are not suitable for referee grade particle analysis. The "size" recorded for any nonspherical shape depends on its orientation as it passes through the scanning beam. The largest measurement errors occur for particles whose shapes vary most from the ideal sphere, for example, platelets and fibers.

In many research problems, the initial problem statement is deceptively simple. Complexity increases as the solution to the problem is approached. In the case of particle counting accuracy, the reverse has been the case. Accurate, comparable particle count data can become a commonplace laboratory occurrence. An overview of the "how" and "why" information needed to achieve accurate particle count data follows.

3 THE EFFECTIVE DETECTOR VOLUME

In every Poisson model of the counting process, the ratio of particles to detector volumes in the test volume is used to estimate the effect of the concentration-dependent coincidence error. However, the physical or geometric detector volume is affected by both the size of the measured particle and the selection of an analysis threshold. This interaction, shown in Fig. 1, illustrates the fact that the effective height of the detector, the dimension in the flow direction, varies with the diameter

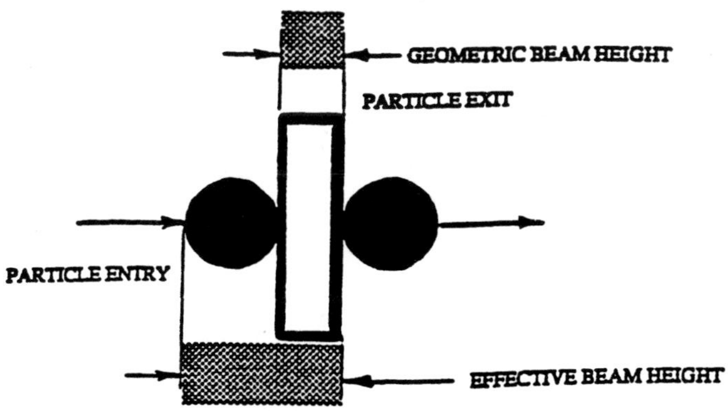

Figure 1 The particle signal starts when the particle edge is intercepted by the scan beam. It ends when the particle exits the scan beam. The effective height of the detector is the sum of the particle diameter and the scan beam width.

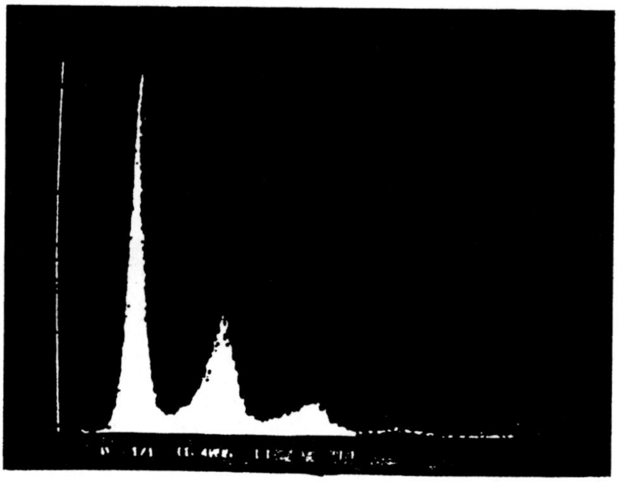

(a)

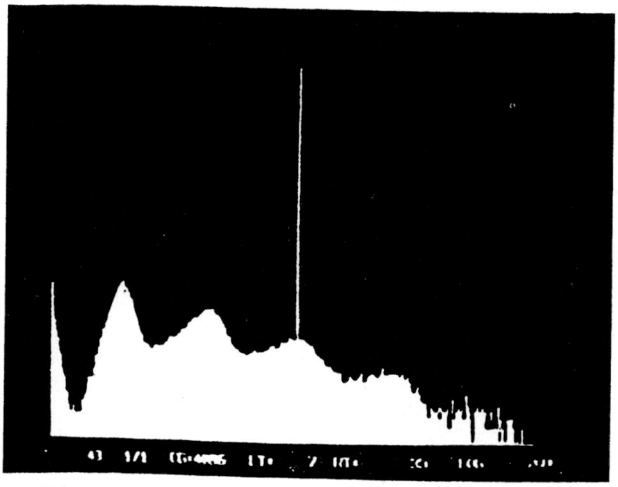

(b)

Figure 2 A pulse height analysis of the size and count of signals from a light extinction particle detector counting a high concentration of monosized particles. The horizontal axis is particle size; the vertical axis is particle concentration. Both records show the number of single particles counted and the occurrence of two, three, and four multiple coincident counting events. The particle size scale in both records is linear. (a) A linear analysis of particle concentration; (b) particle concentration in log form.

of the particle being measured. Since the effective detector height varies, the effective detector volume and thus the particle concentration also vary. The variable detector volume is defined as the effective detector volume. An important conclusion that can be drawn from this figure is that the concentration limit for particle counting accuracy decreases as particle size increases.

The pulse height analyzer photographs shown in Figs. 2a and 2b demonstrate the mechanism responsible for the loss of counts as particle concentration increases. These photographs were taken in the course of a dilution experiment with single-sized standard particles. In Fig. 2a is a linear display of particle counts versus particle size. In this photograph a series of five integral multiple particle sizes have been counted. The number of particles in the multiple particle groups counted diminishes rapidly with each successive peak. Since there are only single-sized standard particles in the sample counted, these pulse height analyzer photographs support the conclusion that, with increasing concentration, single and multiple particle groups are sized and counted. Figure 2b extends the dynamic range of observation by using a log count scale to display the fact that the number of particles in multiple occurrence particle groups is reduced as recorded size increases.

The physical or geometric detector volume is also affected by the selection of an analysis threshold as shown in the foreshortening of the measured particle size in Fig. 3. There is an interaction between the particle size chosen as an analysis threshold and the effective concentration. When the diameter of the particle size selected as the particle size analysis threshold is 10% or less of the diameter of the particle being counted, the effect is negligible. For accurate results with larger ratios, as Fig. 3 shows, the effective reduction in the area of the particle being measured must be considered. The effect of the analysis threshold is a reduction in the measured particle area by twice the threshold particle area.

Understanding the variation of the effective detector volume with the particle size being measured is an important step forward. Two constants are required to fully characterize the performance of a detector as particle size changes: (1) the physical or geometric detector volume and (2) the height of the scan beam employed. When these two constants are determined, the response of the counter to every particle size in its design range can be simply determined. Since there are two unknowns to be determined, two dilution experiments with two different standard precision particles can supply the set of simultaneous equations required for this determination. The

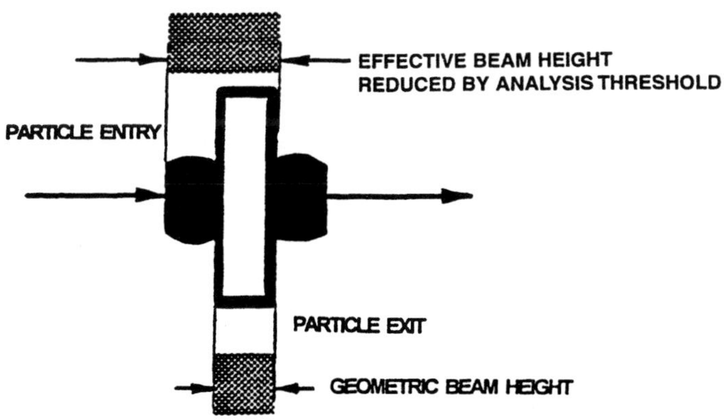

Figure 3 The reduction in particle width by the analysis threshold must be adjusted in the calculation of the number of detector volumes per milliliter. Raising the analysis threshold does not suppress coincidence count loss.

Table 2 Comparison of Specified and Experimental Values of the Beam height, B_H, and the Geometric or Physical Detector Volume, V_{DG}, for Two White Light and Two Laser Diode Particle Detectors[a]

Detector number	Light type	Geometric volume ($cm^3 \times 10^{-6}$)		Beam height (μM)	
		Specified	Expl	Specified	Expl
1	White	7.5	20.7	50	28.5
2	White	50.0	109.0	250	377.0
3	Laser	10.0	14.0	20	39.7
4	Laser	4.5	7.4	30	42.7

[a]Given the two experimental parameters B_H and V_{DG}, the effective detector volume, V_{DE}, can be calculated for any particle size within the range of a particle detector. N_E, the number of effective detector volumes per milliliter for a specific particle size, is then calculated as the reciprocal of V_{DE}.

availability of high accuracy standard particles with stable dimensions makes this determination possible.

The detector measurement data (Knapp and Abramson, 1994, 1995) listed in Table 2 show gross differences between commercial claims of detector performance and experimental results. The difference is attributable in part to the fact that the published dimensions were determined by static dimensional measurements. Basing the functional capability of a detector on static dimensional measurements, such as the design dimensions of the detector and the half-power points of the laser beam employed, ignores detector operating factors. Judging from a comparison of experimental results and vendor specifications, the use of static measurements to evaluate functional performance is as accurate as judging a horse race based on the weight of the horses at the starting line.

4 PARTICLE COUNTING ACCURACY WITH INCREASING CONCENTRATION

The relationship between the concentration of particles and the counts recorded from them is nonlinear. Accurate results are possible only in a concentration region that commences at the point where the positive count error due to background noise counts has diminished to acceptability and terminates where the negative count error due to coincidence is no longer acceptable.

Equation (1V) describes the relationship between the number of particles suspended per milliliter, n, and the number of particle signal counts recorded per milliliter, c.

$$\frac{c}{n} = \frac{\text{particle counts/mL}}{\text{single particles/mL}} = e^{-n/N_E} \tag{1V}$$

The ratio of counts recorded per milliliter to particles counted per milliliter is determined with an exponential measure of the particle concentration, the ratio of particles to effective detector volume. This count efficiency measure describes the relationship

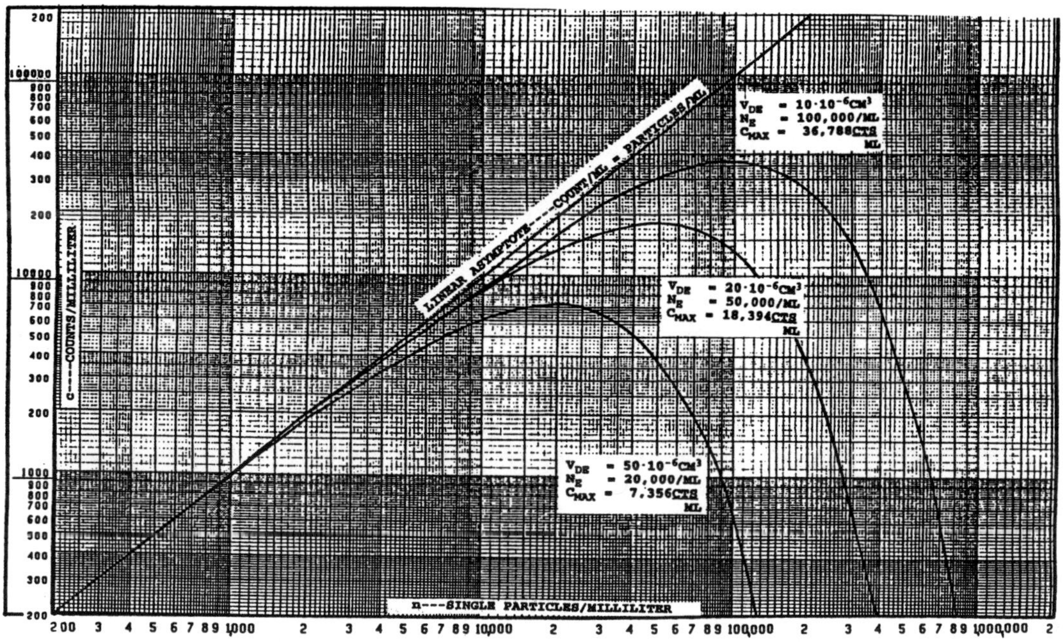

Figure 4 Counts per milliliter versus the concentration of particles per milliliter for detectors with effective detector volumes of 10×10^{-6}, 20×10^{-6}, and 50×10^{-6} cm^3 showing the increase of linear counting span and peak count capability as detector volume is decreased. The peak count for each detector occurs at N_E, the number of effective detector volumes per milliliter, $N_E = 1/V_{DE}$. The magnitude of each peak count is $0.3679N_E$.

between particle count and particle concentration for the class of all single particle counters. For the user this means that a maximum count limit at each particle size can be calculated within which a selected count accuracy can be maintained.

The three counting accuracy curves shown in Fig. 4 were published (Knapp and Abramson, 1994, 1995) to show the calculable relationship between the concentration of particles in a suspension and the recorded counts from them. The title block for each curve identifies three parameters: V_{DE}, the effective detector volume; N_E, the number of effective detector volumes in the test volume; and C_{max}, the maximum count that the detector can record.

The efficiency of the counting process and the extent of the linear counting range capability of a detector increased as detector volume decreased. The largest detector evaluated had the shortest linear span. Halving the effective detector volume doubled the linear count range, decreasing the effective detector volume to one-third tripled the linear count range, etc. All the recently designed detectors examined shared a common characteristic. The exponential characteristic for each detector was constant within experimental error for dilution experiments that ranged up to a ratio of approximately 20,000:1.

The occurrence of a maximum count was previously observed. What has been added here is the capability to calculate its magnitude, the concentration at which it occurs, and the count error at that concentration. The maximum count occurs at the concentration at which there is a ratio of one particle per effective detector volume.

The undercount error at that concentration is 63.2%. Some papers reported that the accurate count range of a detector increases as detector volume decreases. These curves support those observations with a calculated relationship between effective detector volume and the linear count range.

5 A UNIVERSAL COUNT ACCURACY CURVE FOR SINGLE PARTICLE COUNTERS

The count efficiency and count loss of all particle counters that count individual particle signals as a class are described graphically in Fig. 5. The curves of Fig. 5 were determined with Eq. (1V).

The parameter that relates the counts per milliliter recorded, c, to the concentration of particles per milliliter that have been counted, n, is N_E. N_E is a detector- and particle size–specific constant; it is determined by the physical volume of the detector, the height of the scan beam, and the size of the particle being measured. The counts recorded, c, can approach but never be exactly equal to n, the concentration of suspended particles. Good accuracy is available for routine, practical, qual-

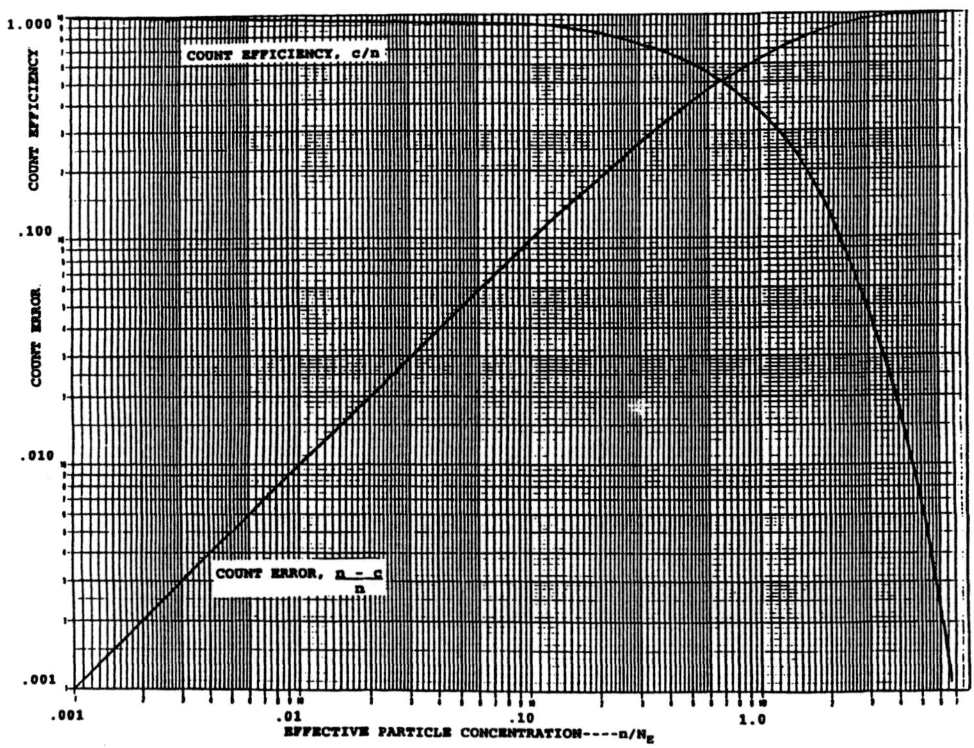

Figure 5 Universal count efficiency and count error curves for light extinction particle counters. The count efficiency, c/n, is the ratio of counts recorded per milliliter of suspended particles counted. The count error curve is labeled $(n - c)/n$ and is the count loss per milliliter of suspended particles counted. Both count efficiency and count loss are functions of the normalized effective particle concentration, n/N_E.

ity assurance particle contamination assays. A tabulation of scan beam heights and geometric detector volumes for particle sizes between 2 and 99 μm is listed for the four detectors shown in Table 2.

Figure 5 represents an advance in understanding and thus controlling particle measurements. It defines a calculable relationship between the concentration of particles and the counts recorded from them. It is, however, a limited advance. One experimental curve is required to describe the effect of concentration on the counts recorded for a single particle size in a specific detector.

With the normalized curves of Fig. 5, the limitations within which particle counters must be operated to achieve a selected counting error can be clearly visualized. At low concentration the error is seen to increase linearly as concentration increases. In fact, for concentrations up to 10% of N_E, the count error and the effective concentration are approximately equal. At the 10% concentration point the count error is 9.52%. As concentration is reduced, the undercount error more closely approaches the calculated effective concentration. At an effective concentration of 1%, the undercount error is 0.995%.

The conclusions reported were based on experimental data using electronic particle counters from three leading manufacturers. The data analyzed were obtained with both white light and laser diode based counters. The experimental conditions selected effectively eliminated any effect of sizing variability on the experimental data. The data recording range in the experiments reduced the effect of noise pulses on the counting experiment to 1% or less. Statistical variability of the counting data was minimized by using particle counts at each dilution step that ranged from 10,000 to over 300,000.

Figure 6 compares the impact of vertical and horizontal coincidence. The additive coincidence illustrated in frames 1 and 3 is described as vertical coincidence. The particle flow pattern illustrated in frames 1–4 are indicative of detector design and electronics that minimize or eliminate detector volume bridging incidents. The sequential frames 1 and 3 show the vertical or additive particle size coincidence error. The sensed particle signal is determined by the sum of the three uniform particles in frame 1 and the four particle signals of the coincidence occurrence group in frame 3 as the group passes through the scan beam. Frames 2 and 4 are completely blank, allowing time for the particle counter to reset its processing cycle to receive the next particle signal. The time required for counter reset using present solid-state electronics is a fraction of the full frame shown in the illustration.

The second coincidence mechanism is that due to random particle chains. In these random particle chains the signals are so closely spaced that the electronic reset signal that initiates the next sizing and counting cycle is suppressed. In a dilution experiment with uniform particles, the count from a horizontal coincidence particle chain can be of one particle or a vertical coincidental occurrence within the chain. The reset signal level, usually selected to be 10% below the level of the analysis threshold selected, is not reached due to the spacing of the particles in the fluid stream. The effect of the blockage of the reset signal is that each particle chain bridges together a number of detector volumes and produces a single count. In a random particle assay, the count can be from a vertical coincidence group or from the largest particle in a horizontal coincidence chain. Frames 5–8 in Fig. 6 represent a random particle chain in which the blockage of particle counter reset results in the recording of a single double occurrence count for all four frames.

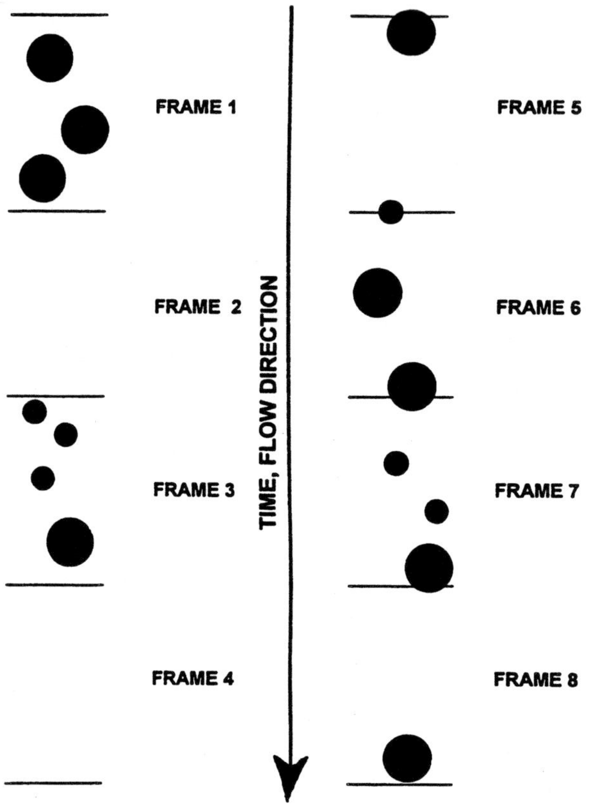

Figure 6 Frames 1 and 3 show vertical coincidence. A single particle is recorded in each frame whose size is equal to the sum of the cross sections of all particles present. Frames 5–8 show the effect of horizontal coincidence that results from the lack of counter reset between particle signals. One particle count is reported for the sequence of these four frames; its size is calculated as the equivalent of the sum of the cross sections of the two larger particles in frame 6.

The effective detector volume for the four interconnected frames is four times the basic effective volume detector. This change would be seen as a reduction to one-fourth of the expected linear measurement range and an increased count loss beyond that predicted by the particle-triggered Poisson model.

Technological progress has brought with it gain-bandwidth improvement in the instrumentation amplifiers used in particle counters. This improvement minimizes or eliminates the need to consider electronic coincidence. The term "electronic coincidence" was required when the bandwidth-limited pulse response of the amplifiers then available blocked the amplification of closely spaced signals. This type of blockage extended the detector volume with results similar to horizontal coincidence at lower concentrations. This limitation has been, happily, obsoleted with current solid-state amplifiers.

If horizontal coincidence were a factor in the dilution experiment data recorded, the exponential relationship of effective concentration to count efficiency could not have the constant characteristic that has been documented. The result of the bridging shown would be evidenced as a progressive change in the exponential relationship between concentration and count efficiency as the effective concentration increased. Although horizontal coincidence effects cannot be dismissed out of hand, they should not be a factor with present solid-state signal processing and currently available detectors. Accordingly, the balance of this chapter uses the particle-triggered Poisson model and the effective detector volume to evaluate the effect of vertical particle coincidence of particle counting accuracy. The tools with which to achieve replicable, accurate counts with light extinction particle counters are now available.

To summarize:

On the plus side, two normalized equations are now available with which the effect of concentration on particle count accuracy in all single particle counters can be analyzed. The first equation defines a dynamic relationship between the detector volume and the size of the particle being measured. The second equation describes the particle-triggered Poisson model. This new statistical model corresponds closely to the functioning of the actual counter. Horizontal and vertical coincidence have been investigated. The conclusion reached was that vertical coincidence was the major concern and, with present technology, may be the only coincidence error concern.

On the minus side, no distinction is made between single particle and multiple particle group counts. Resolving this problem is the next goal of this chapter.

6 INTENT AND REALIZATION OF COUNTING ACCURACY: PARTICLES COUNTED VERSUS COUNTS RECORDED

Before the results of particle count assays recorded by particle counters can be evaluated, the intent of these contaminating particle assays must be determined. Rereading of the new USP 23 ⟨788⟩ (1) as well as those in earlier USP revisions shows that the intent of these particle assays is to set acceptance limits for injectable products based on the number of single contaminating particles in a sample volume or in a container. The contamination limits for particles above 10 μm and above 25 μm were selected with both patient insult and perceived measurement reproducibility in mind.

Reviewing this measurement intention, count accuracy itself is a necessary but not sufficient analysis end point. The tools with which to realize the USP quality goal of evaluating the number of single particles counted can be formulated from the series that define the particle-triggered Poisson relationships.

7 COINCIDENCE ERROR REVISITED

All attempts to analyze the effect of coincidence error on particle counting accuracy use a model of the counting mechanism based on Poisson statistics. In these statistics, an infinite series of terms is used to model the response of a counter. A common characteristic of all Poisson series is that each term in the series represents an integral multiple of the signal for a single particle. The effect of particle signal coincidence is detected when multiples of the test particle size used in the test suspension are recorded. This type of additive coincidence signal can be observed and investigated with a pulse height analyzer as shown in the linear pulse height analyzer display of Fig. 2a or the equivalent data shown in a logarithmic display in Fig. 2b.

The initial application of the new particle-triggered Poisson model (Knapp et al., 1994; Knapp and Abramson, 1995) focused on an examination of the counts recorded from each of the particle size groups counted. The major concept introduced in the initial studies of counter performance was that of count efficiency, which was introduced in Eq. (7V). Count efficiency was defined as the ratio of the number of counts recorded to the number of single particles in suspension.

The next step forward began with an investigation of the complement to count efficiency, the loss of count efficiency. Using the second law of thermodynamics, the sum of the count efficiency and count loss is shown to be equal to 1 in Eq. (2V) and Eq. (2) its algebraic equivalent, these are efficiency balance equations. The relationship that they define is essential in the analysis of count loss due to particle signal coincidence.

$$1 = \text{count efficiency} + \text{count loss} \tag{2V}$$

$$1 = \frac{c}{n} + \frac{\bar{c}}{n} \tag{2}$$

Equation (2) uses c/n for count efficiency and $\bar{c}/n$ (c not on n) for the count loss symbol. The use of the particle-triggered Poisson model in combination with count efficiency and count loss accurately describe the single particle counting capability of all light extinction particle counters. This description is implemented with constants and relationships that can be validated experimentally in modestly equipped pharmaceutical laboratories. The single particle count capability of light extinction particle counters is developed by expressing the count efficiency ratio as the sum of the single particle count efficiency ratio and the count efficiency ratio of all multiple particle occurrence groups. The single particle count efficiency ratio is available in the particle-triggered Poisson series. This series, whose applicability was validated in Knapp and Abramson (1994), is written as a sum of the count efficiency ratios of all particle occurrence count groups. A verbal restatement of Eq. (9) of that paper is

(Overall count efficiency) = (count efficiency of single particle groups)
+ (count efficiency of two-particle groups)
+ (count efficiency of three-particle groups) + ··· (3V)

The Poisson series of Eq. (3V) is expressed symbolically in Eq. (3). The ratio of counts to single particles in suspension is c/n, the overall count efficiency. Each individual term on the left is the count efficiency of a group count commencing with $C(1)/n$, the single particle group term. The remaining terms are in order of the multiplicity of the number of particles in the group.

$$\frac{c}{n} = \frac{C(1)}{n} + \frac{C(2)}{n} + \frac{C(3)}{n} + \frac{C(4)}{n} + \cdots \tag{3}$$

Expressing this Poisson series algebraically entirely in terms of the count efficiency is accomplished in the equation

$$\frac{c}{n} = \left(\frac{c}{n}\right)^2 + \left(\frac{c}{n}\right)^2\left(1 - \frac{c}{n}\right) + \left(\frac{c}{n}\right)^2\left(1 - \frac{c}{n}\right)^2 + \cdots \tag{3A}$$

There is a term-by-term correspondence between Eqs. (9V), (4A), and (9). Using this correspondence, $C(1)/n$, $C(2)/n$, $C(3)/n$ and $C(4)/n$, the count efficiency of single, double, triple, and quadruple occurrence groups, can be written by inspection. Equation (10V) expresses the single particle group count efficiency as the square of the raw count efficiency. Equation (4) restates Eq. (4V) algebraically.

$$\begin{pmatrix}\text{Count efficiency}\\ \text{ratio of}\\ \text{single particle groups}\end{pmatrix} = \begin{pmatrix}\text{Overall}\\ \text{count efficiency}\\ \text{ratio}\end{pmatrix}^2 \tag{4V}$$

$$\frac{C(1)}{n} = \left(\frac{c}{n}\right)^2 \tag{4}$$

The overall count efficiency ratio can also be written as the sum of single particle group count efficiency and multiparticle group count efficiency as in Eq. (5V). The equivalent symbolic relationship is shown in Eq. (5).

$$\begin{pmatrix}\text{Overall}\\ \text{count}\\ \text{efficiency}\end{pmatrix} = \begin{pmatrix}\text{count}\\ \text{efficiency of}\\ \text{single particle}\\ \text{groups}\end{pmatrix} + \begin{pmatrix}\text{count}\\ \text{efficiency of}\\ \text{multiparticle}\\ \text{groups}\end{pmatrix} \tag{5V}$$

$$\frac{c}{n} = \frac{C(1)}{n} + \frac{C^+}{n} \tag{5}$$

The effect of multiparticle groups on any experimental particle size distribution can be estimated with C^+/n, the count efficiency of multiparticle groups. The subtraction of the count efficiency ratio of single particle groups from the overall count efficiency ratio results in the count efficiency ratio of all multiple count groups. The results are shown in Eqs. (6V), (6), and (6A).

$$\begin{pmatrix}\text{Count efficiency}\\ \text{of multiple particle}\\ \text{groups}\end{pmatrix} = \begin{pmatrix}\text{overall count}\\ \text{efficiency}\end{pmatrix} - \begin{pmatrix}\text{count efficiency}\\ \text{of single}\\ \text{particle groups}\end{pmatrix} \tag{6V}$$

$$\frac{C^+}{n} = \frac{c}{n} - \frac{C(1)}{n} \tag{6}$$

$$\frac{C^+}{n} = \left(\frac{n}{n}\right)\left(1 - \frac{c}{n}\right) \tag{6A}$$

Substituting for the count efficiency, c/n, its equivalent in Eq. (5) into the efficiency balance equations, Eq. (4), results in the verbal count efficiency balance equation, Eq. (7V) and its symbolic equivalent, Eq. (7).

$$\begin{pmatrix}\text{Single}\\ \text{particle group}\\ \text{count}\\ \text{efficiency}\end{pmatrix} + \begin{pmatrix}\text{multiple}\\ \text{particle group}\\ \text{count}\\ \text{efficiency}\end{pmatrix} + \text{count loss} = 1 \tag{7V}$$

$$\frac{C(1)}{n} + \frac{C^+}{n} + \frac{\bar{c}}{n} = 1 \tag{7}$$

The count efficiency balance equations (7) and (7V) supply a new tool to the study of coincidence errors. They show that single particle count loss has two sources: the count of particle clusters and the loss of counts within the particle clusters that were not recorded.

The raw count efficiency balance of Eq. (2) is also applicable to the count efficiency of single particles. Solving this equation provides a convenient expression for the single particle count loss as in Eq. 8.

$$\begin{pmatrix}\text{Count loss}\\ \text{of single particles}\end{pmatrix} = 1 - \begin{pmatrix}\text{Count efficiency}\\ \text{of single particles}\end{pmatrix} \tag{8V}$$

$$\frac{\bar{C}(1)}{n} = 1 - \frac{C(1)}{n} \tag{8}$$

This completes an introductory survey of the tools with which to analyze the accuracy of single particle counts and the effect of coincidence on the counts recorded by light extinction particle counters. A more complete examination of this important topic is contained in Appendix 2. A summary of useful equations with which to analyze coincident interactions is listed in Table 3.

Table 3 Count Efficiency Analysis Tools

Eq. (1)	$\frac{c}{n} = e^{-n/N_E}$	Raw count efficiency
Eq. (2A)	$\frac{\bar{c}}{n} = 1 - \frac{c}{n}$	Raw count loss ratio
Eq. (9)	$\frac{C(1)}{n} = e^{-2n/N_E}$	Single particle count efficiency
Eq. (4)	$\frac{C(1)}{n} = \left(\frac{c}{n}\right)^2$	Single particle count efficiency
Eq. (8A)	$\frac{\bar{C}(1)}{n} = 1 - \left(\frac{c}{n}\right)^2$	Single particle loss ratio
Eq. (6)	$\frac{C^+}{n} = \left(\frac{c}{n}\right)\left(1 - \frac{c}{n}\right)$	Count ratio of all multiple occurrences
Eq. (11)	$\frac{C(2)}{n} = \left(\frac{c}{n}\right)^2\left(1 - \frac{c}{n}\right)$	Count ratio of double multiple occurrences
Eq. (12)	$\frac{C(3)}{n} = \left(\frac{c}{n}\right)^2\left(1 - \frac{c}{n}\right)^2$	Count ratio of triple multiple occurrences
Eq. (13)	$\frac{C^+(3)}{n} = \left(\frac{c}{n}\right)\left(1 - \frac{c}{n}\right)^2$	Count ratio of triple and higher multiple occurrences
Eq. (14)	$\frac{C(4)}{n} = \left(\frac{c}{n}\right)^2\left(1 - \frac{c}{n}\right)^3$	Count ratio of quadruple multiple occurrences
Eq. (2)	$\frac{c}{n} + \frac{\bar{c}}{n} = 1$	Efficiency balance equation
Eq. (7)	$\frac{C(1)}{n} + \frac{C^+}{n} + \frac{\bar{c}}{n} = 1$	Count efficiency balance equation

8 CONTAMINATING PARTICLES: SINGLE PARTICLE COUNTS VERSUS PARTICLES COUNTED

The universal count efficiency and count error curves shown in Fig. 4 represent a significant but not final step toward achieving a description of single-particle count efficiency and count error response. Equation (1), on which Fig. 4 is based, does not differentiate between counts of single particles and counts of coincident particle groups. In retrospect, the graphical legends in Figs. 4 and 5 must be changed to reflect the fact that these are raw count curves.

The relationship between the number of single particle counts, $C(1)$, recorded by a light extinction particle counter and the number of single particles in suspension, n, is also exponential:

$$\frac{C(1)}{n} = \frac{\text{single particle counts/mL}}{\text{single particles/mL}} = e^{-2n/N_E} \tag{9V}$$

The exponent in Eq. (1) that related counts to suspended particles counted was n/N_E. In Eq. (9) the exponent relating single particle counts to the number of single suspended particles counted is $-2n/N_E$. The exponential term is the square of the term in the raw count relationship. The exponent $-2n/N_E$ can be written as $-n/(N_E/2)$, showing that the linear count region for single particle counts is shorter than that for raw counts. The exponential curves of single particle counts versus concentration and the corresponding error curve are graphed in Fig. 7.

Figure 7 is a normalized, universal description of all single particle count efficiency and single-particle count error curves. The universal curves in this figure are based on the particle-triggered Poisson model and the effective detector volume. This figure provides the capability to define single particle count accuracy and count error for USP ⟨788⟩ contaminating particle assays. It provides the information required to operate light extinction particle counters within selected accuracy limits. The selected count accuracy limits are defined by a concentration and particle size contour.

As in the earlier universal curve of raw counts versus effective concentration, the occurrence of a maximum count is observed. The maximum single particle count occurs at one-half the concentration at which the raw count maximum appeared. The concentration at which the maximum single particle count occurs is half that for the raw count curve. The single particle maximum count occurs at a ratio of one-half particle per effective detector volume. The undercount error at that concentration is 63.2%. The concentration capability of a detector for single particle counts is half of the raw particle count capability.

9 APPLICATION TO THE USP ⟨788⟩ CONTAMINATING PARTICLE ASSAY

This section provides an overview of the problems addressed. A more complete treatment follows in Appendix 2.

USP 23, p. 1814, Test Apparatus, Sensor Concentration Limits, defines the limiting concentration that can be assayed as that at which the coincident counts amount to 10% of the single 10 μm particles present. This concentration-related

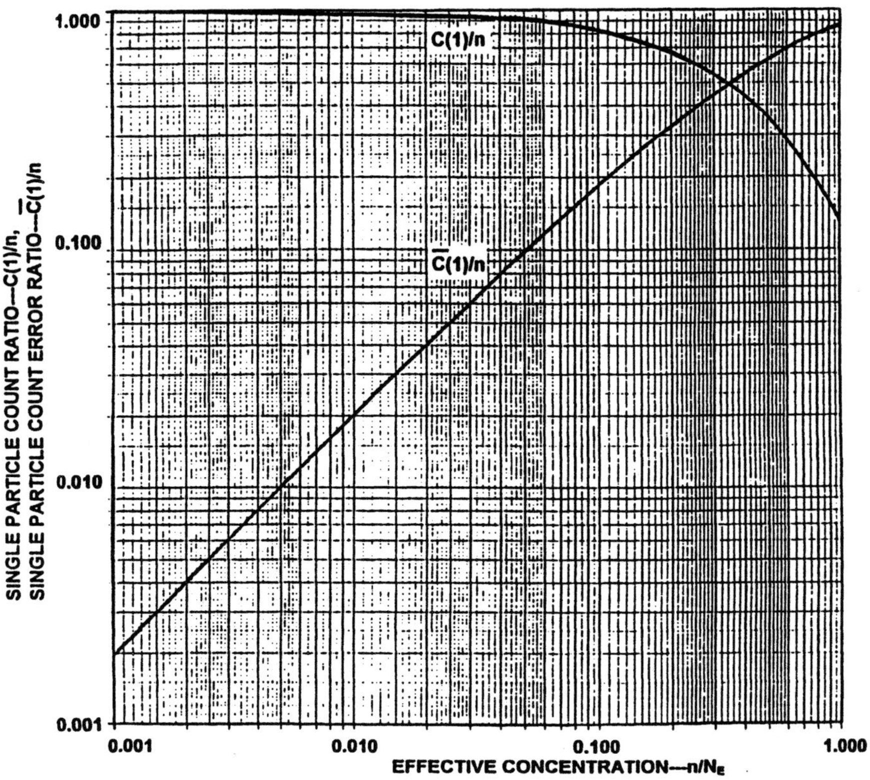

Figure 7 The universal single-particle count efficiency, $C(1)/n$, and count error curves, $\bar{C}(1)/n$, versus the effective concentration measure, n/N_E, for light extinction particle counters. Both measures are per milliliter of suspended particles counted. Implementation of the intent of USP ⟨788⟩ to assay particle contamination in a count of single particles can now be accurately realized.

specification has not been measured directly. Its determination rests on an undefined model-based calculation. The particle counting accuracy that results is examined in detail below.

A comparison of the effect of the choice of a counter model and choice of a concentration measure on the resulting assay count accuracy (Knapp et al., 1994; Lieberman, 1975) was recently made using the No. 3 detector listed in Table 2. In these analyses the multiple particle group count efficiency ratio was equated to 0.10 of the count efficiency ratio.

An alternative, more rigorous analysis follows based on the count ratio balance equation. The primary data are those of count efficiency and relative particle concentration. The relative particle concentration is the ratio of particles per detector volume: n/N_G for the Jaenicke geometric model and n/N_E for the particle-triggered model using the effective concentration measure.

The count efficiency that results from a 10% multiple occurrence rate for both of the published Poisson models is calculated. The calculated count efficiency is particle size–free. To calculate the concentration of particles at which the 10% coincidence rate occurs, detector parameters and particle dimensions are required. Assuming a specific detector No. 3 in Table 2, the coincidence error for the 10% multiple occurrence concentration is then calculated for both models.

10 JAENICKE GEOMETRIC MODEL CALCULATIONS

The static, geometric concentration measure, n/N_G, at which there is a 10% multiple occurrence count ratio involves the digital solution of exponential equations. The details are listed in Appendix 2. The relative concentration for the Jaenicke geometric model, n/N_G, at which there is a 10% multiple occurrence rate is calculated to be 0.85145 with Eq. (24). This relative concentration is then used to determine the count efficiency ratio for single particle counts with Eq. (27). The single particle count efficiency ratio is 42.7%. The corresponding single particle loss ratio is 57.3%. To calculate the particle concentration for this condition, the No. 3 detector in Table 2 was assumed. The particle concentration was estimated with Eq. (20) to be 60,818 particles/mL.

11 PARTICLE-TRIGGERED MODEL WITH EFFECTIVE CONCENTRATION MEASURE

Equation (6V) relates the count efficiency of multiple particle groups to the overall count efficiency and the count loss.

$$\begin{pmatrix}\text{Count efficiency}\\ \text{of multiple particle}\\ \text{groups}\end{pmatrix} = \begin{pmatrix}\text{overall count}\\ \text{efficiency}\end{pmatrix} - \begin{pmatrix}\text{count efficiency}\\ \text{of single particle}\\ \text{groups}\end{pmatrix} \qquad (6V)$$

Substituting for the count efficiency ratio of multiple particle groups the USP 23 specification of 0.10 results in a quadratic expression. Solving for the count efficiency results in two roots to the equation, 0.8873 and 0.11276. The count efficiency for the particle-triggered model exhibits a peak count and then a decay of counting capability. Only the count efficiency solution before the peak is of interest. Substituting 0.8873 in Eq. (4) and squaring, as indicated, results in a single particle count efficiency equal to 0.7873. The resulting single particle count loss at this concentration is 21.3%. This is the smallest count error that will result in this assay. The count error for all larger particles will be greater.

$$\begin{pmatrix}\text{Count efficiency}\\ \text{ratio of}\\ \text{single particle groups}\end{pmatrix} = \begin{pmatrix}\text{overall}\\ \text{count efficiency}\\ \text{ratio}\end{pmatrix}^2 \qquad (4V)$$

12 THE PARTICLE-TRIGGERED POISSON MODEL EVALUATION OF THE SINGLE PARTICLE COUNT LOSS FOR THE JAENICKE GEOMETRIC MODEL CONCENTRATION ESTIMATED AT A 10% MULTIPLE OCCURRENCE RATE

The Jaenicke geometric model calculation showed a concentration of 60,818 10 μm particles/mL for a 10% multiple coincident occurrence rate. Using the No. 3 detector data in Table 2, N_E for 10 μm particles is 57,057. The particle triggered model count efficiency for single particle counts is calculated with the equation

$$\frac{C(1)}{n} = \left[\frac{\text{Single particle counts/mL}}{\text{Single particles/mL}}\right] = e^{-2n/N_E} = e^{-2.60,818/57,057} = 0.1186 \qquad \text{(9A)}$$

Substituting 60,818 particles/mL for n and 57,057 for N_E results in a single particle count efficiency at this concentration of 11.86%. The single particle count loss is therefore 88.14%, approximately twice the error calculated with the Jaenicke geometric model. These results are worse than those from the original evaluation.

13 CONVERSION OF USP 23 ⟨788⟩ COUNTER ACCURACY SPECIFICATION FOR ACCESS TO PARTICLE-TRIGGERED MODEL ANALYSIS

N' and N'_E are, respectively, the concentration and number of effective particle volumes for milliliter that satisfy the USP 23 ⟨788⟩ coincidence ratio specification for single particle counts. N'_E, the number of detector volumes per milliliter for 10% coincidence ratio error, is calculated with Eq. (10). A summary of all symbols used is listed in Table 1.

$$N'_E \text{ (USP 10 μm minimum)} = 8.363\, N' \qquad (10)$$

Table 4 The Effect of Count Efficiency Variation from 0.99 to 0.70 on the Single Particle Group Count Efficiency and Single Particle Group Count Loss Using the Particle-Triggered Poisson Model with the Effective Particle Concentration Measure[a]

Raw count efficiency, c/n	Single particle count efficiency, $C(1)/n$	Single particle count loss, $\bar{C}(1)/n$
0.99	0.98	0.02
0.9747[b]	0.95[b]	0.05[b]
0.95	0.90	0.10
0.8873[c]	0.7873[c]	0.2127[c]
0.85	0.72	0.28
0.80	0.64	0.36
0.75	0.56	0.44
0.70	0.49	0.51

[a]A single particle count efficiency of 0.7873 for 10 μm particles satisfies the USP ⟨788⟩ SVI 10% coincidence count loss specification. The single particle count efficiency for all larger particle sizes decreases as particle size increases.
[b]Single particle count error 5.00% (at 0.9747 single particle group count efficiency).
[c]Single particle count error 21.3% (at USP 23 SVI 10% multiple group coincidence).

The 16.679 conversion constant determines the minimum N_E that will result in a 10% coincidence rate for 10 μm particles when the concentration that results from application of the USP 23 ⟨788⟩ SVI coincidence limit test is used.

The minimum N_E, N'_E, for a 10% C^+/n for 4000 10 μm particles per milliliter calculated for a single particle count loss is shown to be 33,452 in the equation

$$N'_E(10\ \mu m) = 8.363 \times 4000 = 33{,}452 \tag{10A}$$

Operating at the USP concentration limit for 10 μm particles results in a single particle count loss of 21.3%. The single particle count loss for all larger particles at this concentration will be greater. The use of the raw count efficiency relationship, Eq. (1V), with minimum N'_E to determine single particle count loss results in an underestimate of 53%. The result is an undercount of 11.27%, compared to the 21.3% single particle count loss that actually occurs.

The conversion constant in Eq. (11) transforms the USP 23 ⟨788⟩ SVI coincidence ratio specification into a measurable and calculable validation procedure. This procedure can be accomplished by even a modestly equipped pharmaceutical laboratory. Major considerations in the use of this conversion constant for a concentration of 10 μm particles is that its accuracy relies on the results of unspecified measurement methods. Although a relationship between the USP 23 ⟨788⟩ SVI coincidence rate specification and the particle-triggered Poisson model has been established, the effect of this specification should be considered before it is used for selection of concentration limits. The final result of operating at a concentration limit resulting from the USP 23 ⟨788⟩ SVI coincidence specification is operation with a 21.3% single particle group undercount for 10 μm particles, the smallest particle size specified in the assay. The counting error increases as particle size is increased.

See Appendix 2 for a detailed examination of this conversion factor.

A methodical examination of single particle count ratio error versus the count efficiency of operation is shown in Table 4. The data in this table show that a count efficiency of 0.9747 is required to achieve a 5% single particle error rate. A raw count efficiency of 0.95 for 10 μm particles that satisfies the USP ⟨788⟩ SVI 10% coincidence count loss specification results in a single particle count loss of $(1 - 0.95^2)$, which is equal to a 9.75% single particle count loss. Also see Table 5.

The single particle count balance expressed in Eqs. (7) and (7V) provides the means to resolve counts of single particles from the total counts recorded. In Fig. 7 the count loss ratio from multiple particle group occurrences and the count loss ratio due to the uncounted particles within each cluster are included. The total coincidence count loss is the sum of both loss ratios. Within a 20% total error limit, the contributions of both loss ratios are seen to be approximately equal. Neglecting the count loss contribution of either coincidence component results in a 50% underestimation of the single particle count error.

14 CONTAMINATING PARTICLES: COUNTS RECORDED VERSUS NUMBER OF PARTICLES COUNTED

The intent of USP ⟨788⟩ is to consider contamination measurements evaluated by counts of single particles. The universal count efficiency and count error curves

Table 5 Variation of N_E, the Experimental Detector and Particle Size Specific Constant, as Particle Size Varies from 2 to 99 μm

Particle size (μM)	Experimental N_E Geometric detector volume[a] (cm^3 × 10^{-6}) 7.5 (W)	50 (W)	10 (L)	4.5 (L)
2	45,141	9,126	68,003	129,089
5	41,099	9,054	63,439	120,970
5.773	29,815	9,036	62,360	119,041
7.071	38,706	9,005	60,630	115,936
10.0	35,761	8,937	57,057	109,493
15.0	31,651	8,823	51,841	100,000
17.678	30,859	8,763	49,422	95,569
20.0	28,388	8,712	47,499	92,030
25	25,735	8,604	43,829	85,233
30.0	23,535	8,498	40,685	79,371
40.0	20,099	8,294	35,580	69,774
50.0	17,539	8,100	31,613	62,247
60.0	15,557	7,915	28,442	56,186
70.0	13,978	7,738	25,850	51,200
80.0	12,690	7,568	23,690	47,027
99.0	10,799	7,266	20,445	40,722

[a]Values from commercial literature. (W) and (L) following the specified detector volume refer to the employment of a white or laser excitation source.
[b]N_E in effective detector volumes per milliliter.

shown in Fig. 3 represent a significant but not final step toward achieving a similar description of single particle count efficiency and count error response. In retrospect, the graphical legends in Figs. 3 and 4 must be changed to reflect the fact that these are raw count curves.

The universal single particle count efficiency and count error curves in Fig. 5 provide the capability required for USP ⟨788⟩ to define single particle count accuracy and count error. To satisfy the USP contamination measurement intent, the count balance relationship based on vertical single particle coincidence count errors is employed. These universal curves, employing the effective particle concentration measure n/N_E, apply to all single particle counters.

As in the earlier universal curve of raw counts versus effective concentration, the occurrence of a maximum count is observed. The maximum count occurs at the concentration at which there is a ratio of one-half particle per effective detector volume. The undercount error at that concentration is 63.2%. These curves provide the information required to operate light extinction particle counters within selected accuracy limits. The selected count accuracy limits are defined by a concentration and particle size contour. Comparing these results to those obtained for the raw count maximum, the concentration for the peak count is half of that for the raw counts. The concentration at which this single particle count peak occurs is half of that calculated for the raw count curve.

15 COINCIDENT OCCURRENCES AND THE USP ⟨788⟩ PARTICLE ASSAY

The effect of coincident occurrences on the count accuracy of the USP ⟨788⟩ contaminating particle assay is determined by both particle concentration and particle size. The coincident occurrences that can affect the USP ⟨788⟩ particle assay count accuracy originate within the 10–25 μm control region and from the steeply rising concentration of particles immediately below the 10 μm control threshold. The maximum coincidence errors in the USP ⟨788⟩ particle assay can result from both the maximum acceptable particle concentrations defined in the assay and the uncontrolled particle concentrations immediately below the 10 μm lower boundary.

The number of multiple occurrences at each particle size that can occur with concentration and their effect on the USP ⟨788⟩ assay counts recorded are summarized in Table 6. This table shows that the coincidence effect of sub-10 μm particles is injection of false counts within the assay limits. For particles ranging in size from 10 to 12.5 μm, the predominant coincidence effect is an undercount error. For particles from 12.5 to 17.6777 μm, both false counts and undercounts can result based on the concentration of particles counted. From 17.6777 to 25 μm, the predominant (and potentially more serious effect) is the generation of false counts of particles greater than 25 μm in diameter.

To examine the effect of coincidence error with realizable, measured particle distributions, the effect of coincidence on two particle sizes was calculated. The

Table 6 The Effect of Multiple Occurrences on the USP ⟨788⟩ Contaminating Particle Assay from Below and from Within the Controlled Particle Size Range

Particle area	Particle diameter (μm)	Multiple coincident occurrences, *n*	Effect
10 μm/3	5.7735	3	False counts >10 μm, $n > 3$
10 μm/2	7.0711	2	False counts >10 μm, $n > 2$
			Start USP limit zone >10 μm
25 μm/6.25	10.0000	6	
25 μm/5	11.1803	5	Undercounts $10\ \mu m < D_P < 25\ \mu m$
25 μm/4	12.5000	4	False counts > 25 μm, $n > 4$
25 μm/3	14.4338	3	False counts > 25 μm, $n > 3$
25 μm/2	17.6777	2	False counts > 25 μm, $n > 2$
			End USP limit zone < 25 μm
			Start USP limit zone > 25 μm

Note: Multiple coincident occurrences are calculated in integral digital increments in any Poisson model of the counting process.

measured particle distribution for both particle sizes was assumed to be 5%. The $n = 4$ entry for the asterisked 11.5 μm particle size shows that up to a 4× coincident occurrence the resulting false multiple particle count will remain under 25 μm, thus producing undercounts. The asterisked 21.7391 μm particle size, with a similar distribution, indicates that in the absence of coincidence error a $+3\sigma$ retention of single particle counts will remain within the 25 μm control limit. Double coincidence occurrence with this particle size will result in a 30.744 μm particle size peak.

16 SENSITIVITY ANALYSIS OF COINCIDENT PARTICLE INTERACTIONS

The effect of the coincidence-magnified particle signals on particle contamination assays has been obscured by the focus on undercount error. Figure 8 summarizes the eight major coincidence effects that can occur in the USP ⟨788⟩ assay as a result of the particle concentration being measured.

Analysis of the interaction problem begins by dividing the particle sizes that should be considered into five zones. The geometric mean particle size in each zone, shown in parentheses, will be used for performance comparisons. Zone I is the particle size group that generates from one-third to one-half of the signal from 10 μm particles. It is the source of false counts greater than 10 μm from triple and higher coincident occurrences.

The particle size group in zone II commences with particles whose signals range from one-half to the entire signal from the 10 μm particle size. All coincident occurrences in this zone will register false USP particle assay counts.

The zone III particle size group ranges from 10 μm particles to a size that produces less than half the signal of a 25 μm particle. Depending on the particle size and the capability of the detector undercounts, false USP ⟨788⟩ SVI assay counts greater than 25 μm and undercounts can both originate in this zone. The undercounts

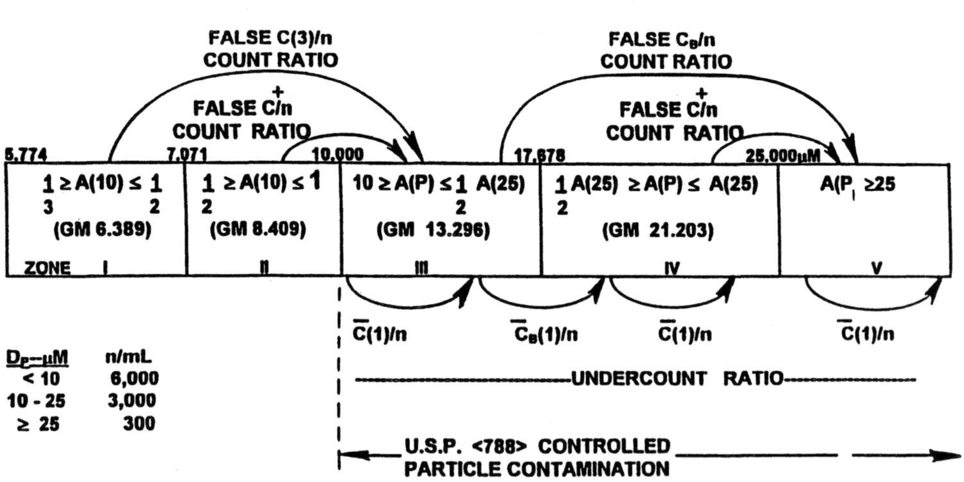

Figure 8 A structured sensitivity analysis of a light extinction particle detector to coincidence errors in the USP ⟨788⟩ SVI contaminating particle assay. All symbols refer to counts of single particle groups rather than to raw counts. GM = geometric mean.

are caused by the count loss due to horizontal coincidence plus that due to the count loss from multiple occurrence events. Accordingly, zone III is shown as the origin of three undercount loops and a false count interaction loop. The false count loop shows the possibility of false counts greater than 25 μm originating in zone III.

Zone IV commences with particles whose signal is at least half that of a 25 μm particle. Any multiple coincident occurrence in this zone will create false counts in zone V. Zone V begins at the 25 μm particle size and extends up to the visible particle zone. The count loss in zones IV and V consists of both horizontal and vertical multiple occurrences; their effect is shown as self-loops.

To demonstrate the use of this loop analysis, two detectors in current use were selected. The first is a new, well-designed detector with laser excitation. It has high concentration counting accuracy and a low pressure drop across the detector flow path. The low pressure drop design minimizes the possibility of cavitation-induced false background counts. The second was an older, well-regarded white light detector.

A comparison of the assay results of the same 2 mL SVI container with both of these detectors follows. This comparison supports the lack of comparability for particle counter data that has become common experience.

17 SVI CHALLENGE OF SENSITIVITY ANALYSIS

The assumed particle contamination in the 2 mL container is based on the new USP 23 SVI limits. Any example based on USP 22 SVI limits is too extreme to be useful. The contaminating particle concentration is set at the upper USP 23 SVI limit of 6000 particles per container or 3000 particles/mL of a size 10 μm or greater. This limit includes a maximum of 600 particles 25 μm or larger. For this example a concentration of 6000 particles/mL is assumed in the two unspecified zones below the 10 μm control threshold. In each zone, coincidence calculations use the geometric mean particle size. The effect of the coincidence error as a percent of the USP acceptance level is shown adjacent to the loop affected.

18 NEW LASER DETECTOR SENSITIVITY ANALYSIS

Figure 9 shows the calculated sensitivity of the new laser detector to particle counting interference in the USP ⟨788⟩ SVI particle assay. The experimental geometric detector volume and scan beam height were evaluated with the protocol included in Knapp and Abramson (1994) and are listed in the legend for this figure. The effects of the coincident interactions on the assay results are noted on each loop. The selection of the geometric mean particle size, 13.296 μm, in zone III for this example eliminates the need for a self-loop in the 10.0–12.5 μm span.

The loop from zone I to zone III is a false count loop for triple or higher coincident occurrences. At the assumed 6000 particles/mL particle contamination level this loop contributes 58.9 false counts per container greater than 10 μm, or approximately 1.0% of the allowable total. These false counts can be considered a minor annoyance. The zone II–III loop contributes 852.1 false counts ≥10 μm, 14.2% of the allowable total based on the same 6000 particles/mL concentration in the unspecified half to full 10 μm size group. Zone III, with particles ranging from 10 μm to those with half the area of a 25 μm particle, is seen to be a source of both false counts ≥25 μm and undercounts. The undercounts are due to horizontal

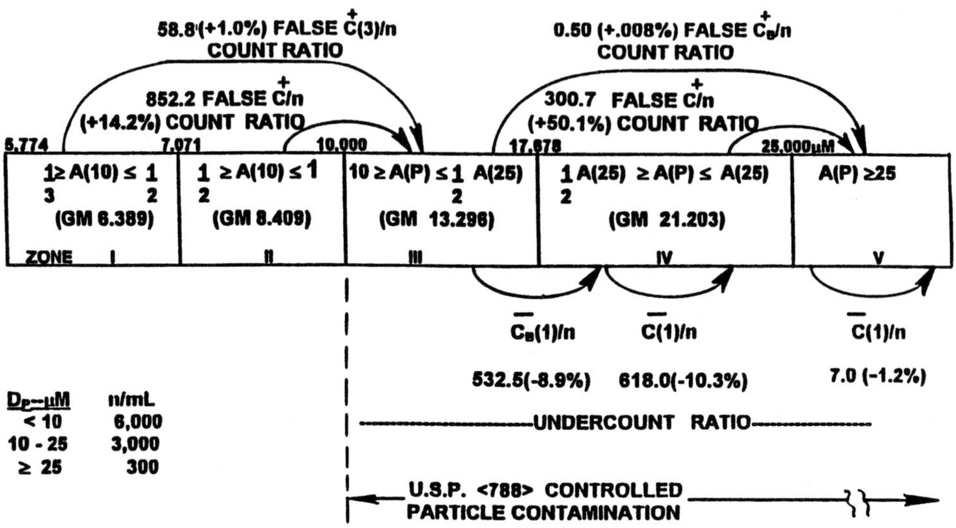

Figure 9 Sensitivity analysis of a new laser-sourced detector to coincidence errors in the USP ⟨788⟩ SVI contaminating particle assay of a 2 mL container. The experimental detector parameters are geometric detector volume V_{DG} = 10.2 cm^3 × 10^{-6}; beam height B_H = 27.3 μm. All symbols refer to counts of single particle groups rather than to raw counts. GM = geometric mean.

coincidence count loss and the portion of vertical coincidence count loss that remains within the 10–25 μm particle size span. The response of this laser-source detector includes 523.3 undercounts, 8.9% of the allowable 6000 per container within the 10–25 μm span and 0.50 false count ≥25 μm, 0.08% of the 600 particles per container that are the acceptable limit.

In zone IV all coincident occurrences result in false counts >25 μm. Counting 3000 particles/mL in this 2 mL container, this detector records 252.9 false counts >25 μm per 2 mL container, 42.1% of the 600 particle limit.

The count of 600 25 μm particles by this detector is accomplished with distinction. The new laser source detector responds with an undercount of 7 particles, 1.2% of the acceptable total.

The assay of this 2 mL SVI container with the older, well regarded white light detector is shown in the sensitivity analysis of Fig. 11 in Sec. 20.

19 OLDER WHITE LIGHT DETECTOR SENSITIVITY ANALYSIS

The sensitivity to coincidence interference of the USP ⟨788⟩ assay data evaluated by the white light detector is tested in Fig. 10. The measured detector constants (Knapp and Abramson, 1994) for the older white light detector are shown in the legend for this figure. There is an approximate doubling in each false count or undercount category that was tabulated for the new laser source detector. The false count contribution from the zone I–III loop is again negligible. It is 205 counts, 3.4% of the allowable total. The false counts in the zone II–III loop amount to 25.3% of the allowable counts ≥10 μm, an error that cannot be lightly disregarded. The under-

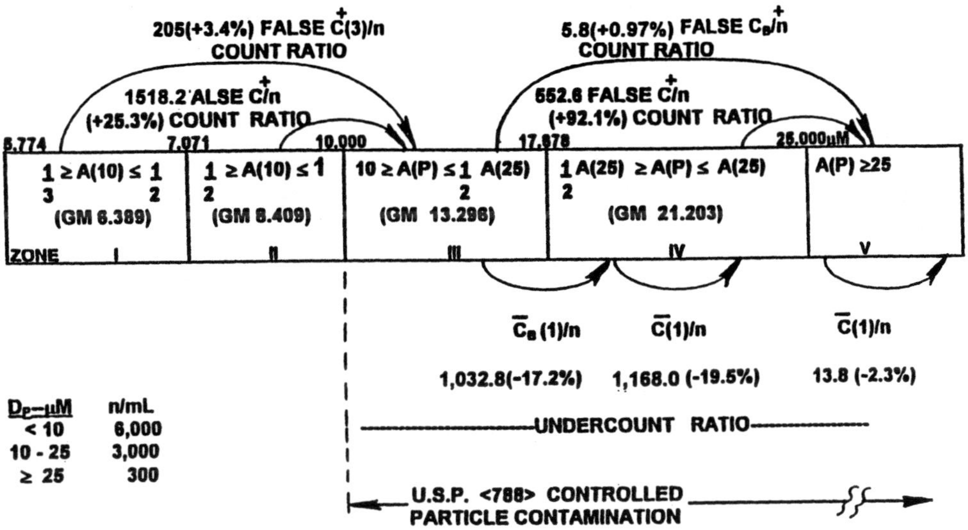

Figure 10 Sensitivity analysis of an older white light detector to coincidence errors in the USP ⟨788⟩ SVI contaminating particle assay of a 2 mL container. The experimental detector parameters are geometric detector volume $V_{DG} = 20.7\ \text{cm}^3 \times 10^{-6}$; beam height $B_H = 28.5$ μm. All symbols refer to counts of single particle groups rather than to raw counts. GM = geometric mean.

count shown in the zone III–IV loop is 1518 counts, 25.3% of the allowable total ≥10 μm. There is a negligible false count contribution in the zone III–V loop of 3.6 counts, 0.06% of the maximum allowable particle count ≥25 μm.

The zone IV–V loop contributes 552.6 false counts ≥25 μm, 92.1% of the allowable 600 particle per container maximum. The 13.8 undercounts calculated for a concentration of 600 25 μm particles, 2.3% of the allowable total, brings an important note of optimism that count accuracy is possible.

20 SENSITIVITY ANALYSIS RESULTS

Zone I

The injection of false counts into the USP ⟨788⟩ SVI particle assay from particles whose light extinction signal is between one-half and one-third of the 10 μm lower control boundary ranges from 3.4% for the older white light detector down to 1% for the laser-sourced detector for the numerical values selected. These false counts do not inject serious errors.

Zone II

False counts from this zone, from particles whose signals lie between one-half and just below the 10 μm particle signal range from +25.3% for the older white light detector down to +14.2% for the newer laser-sourced detector. This and the zone I count error are removable errors. Specification of control limits for this presently unspecified particle size region can control this error.

Zone III

Particle signals in this region range from 10 μm to just less than half the signal of a 25 μm particle. For the present SVI control limits, false counts greater than 25 μm from either detector lie below 0.10% and can be neglected. Single-particle undercounts range from 17.2% for the older white light detector down to 8.9% for the newer laser-sourced detector. These errors can be controlled with sample dilution for both detectors.

Zone IV

This region commences with particle signals that are one-half that of a 25 μm particle and ends with particles just below the 25 μm particle size limit. This region is seen to be the source of both undercounts and false counts greater than 25 μm. The undercounts, calculated on the basis of 3000 particles/mL, range from 19.5% for the older white light detector down to 10.3% for the newer laser-sourced detector. The effect of false counts greater than 25 μm from this particle size region, for both detectors, is the most significant count error in the contaminating particle assay. The false count error of particles greater than 25 μm for the older white light detector is +92.1%; for the laser-sourced detector this error is reduced to 42.1%. Both types of count errors are correctable without the advent of new technology. Both types of count errors can be corrected by sample dilution.

Zone V

The single particle undercount errors in this zone, 2.3% for the older white light detector and 1.2% for the newer laser-sourced detector, are indicators that the technology in presently available counters can deliver the replicability and count accuracy that are essential to any assay.

21 SINGLE PARTICLE COUNT ACCURACY CONTOURS FOR THE LASER-SOURCED DETECTOR

The possibility of usably accurate count results with a commercially available instrument is examined in Fig. 11. The peak count/accuracy contours shown in this figure are for the laser detector whose characteristics were used in the preceding example. The scan beam height and geometric detector volume were evaluated with the protocol described in Knapp and Abramson (1994, 1995) and Knapp et al. (1994). The dilution experiments were calculated with 9.87 and 25.7 μm particles corrected for a 3 μm analysis threshold.

The count accuracy contours for 7.5–25 μm particles is proof that practical count accuracy performance is available. The four contours range from a high of 98% accuracy through 95%, 90%, and 85% single particle count accuracy contours.

To limit single particle counting error to 2%, the maximum count ranges from a high of 793 counts/mL at 7.5 μm to a low of 523 counts/mL, or 1046 per container, for 25 μm particles. This limit is sufficient for many marketed injectable products. To maintain 5% single particle count accuracy, the count limit ranges from 1977 counts/mL at 7.5 μm to a low of 1321 counts/mL, 2642 per container at 25 μm, a contamination range that should encompass most injectable products. Count accuracy limits of 90% and 85% are also shown in this graph.

The experimental results shown here are based on experimental data from a single Particle Measurement Systems, Inc. particle counter. Similar results have been

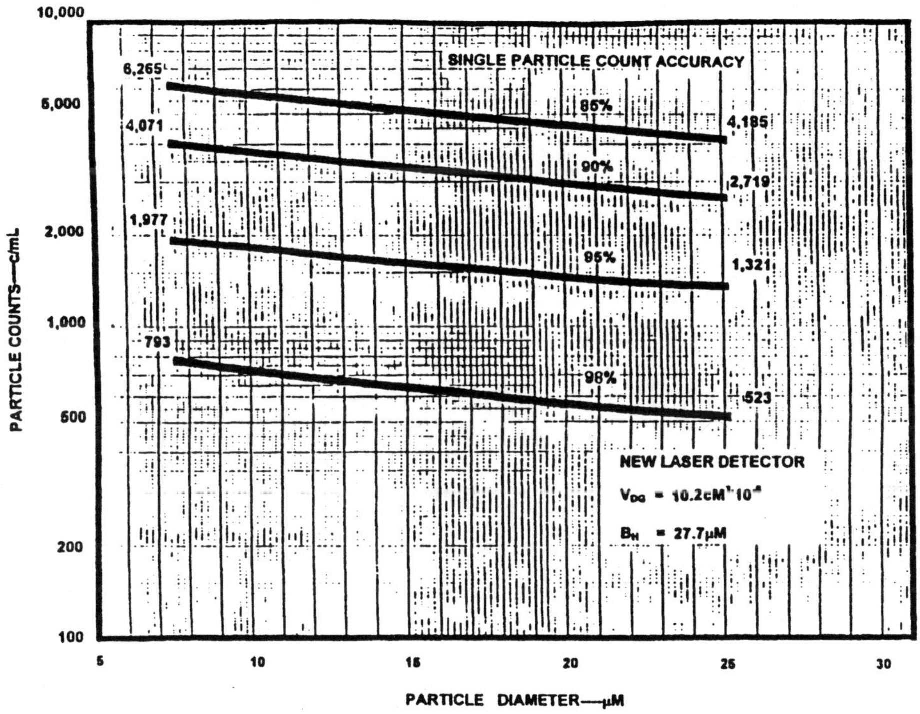

Figure 11 Single particle count accuracy contours for a recent laser-sourced particle detector. The equivalent capability of this detector is commercially available from several manufacturers. The counting accuracy contours shown here demonstrate that accuracy of light extinction particle counter assays is now achievable.

obtained with a HIAC/Royco laser-sourced particle counter and should be available from Clime Co. Instruments. The response characteristics reported are not a brief for a particular instrument. They are a demonstration that count accuracy is possible when the peak count is controlled during an assay. These count accuracy curves also demonstrate that the evaluation of particle counter accuracy is within the reach of even modestly equipped laboratories.

22 CAPABILITY OF SINGLE PARTICLE COUNTERS

The error sensitivity results have shown that the need to obtain clear, unambiguous contaminating particle assay results for the control of parenteral production imposes stricter concentration limits than those listed in the USP 23 ⟨788⟩ specifications. The single particle count efficiency has been shown to be equal to the raw count efficiency squared, $(c/n)^2$. The most probable source of false counts has been shown to be the count efficiency ratio of all multiple occurrences, $C^+/n = (c/n)(1 - c/n)$. Achievable accuracy with laser-sourced counters, based on the selection of a 5% multiple occurrence ratio, is a single particle undercount error of 2.5%. Even the selection of these concentration limits does not ensure useful assay results without interpretation in all cases. A concentration of 300 particles/mL less than 25 μm and greater than 17.678 μm in diameter at the selected concentration limit will result in a false count of 15 particles greater than 25 μm in size. If this concentration increases to 3000 particles/mL, an acceptable level for a 2 mL fill volume, each milliliter would contribute 150 false coincident group counts greater than 25 μm, for a total of 300 counts against the allowable total of 600 particles greater than 25 μm.

Single particle counters are well-behaved instruments fully capable of the workhorse task of making accurate, routine particle contamination measurements in injectable products. In principle, any particle counter instrument now in use can deliver accurate particle counting data when operated within defined maximum count limits. These limits vary with particle size determined by the capability of the counter system in use. In practice, selection of a counter with the concentration capability to provide the desired accuracy without the burden of constant dilution is an important consideration. For concentrations that exceed the selected count accuracy contour, dilution and a repeat of the assay provide a practical solution. There is no methodology that can correct erroneous count data from random particulates.

Since all particle shapes are homogenized into "equivalent" spherical volumes, these counters are not suitable for referee grade particle analysis. The size recorded for any nonspherical shape depends on its orientation as it passes through the scanning beam. The largest measurement errors are for platelets and fibers.

A problem that must be faced is that these counters are not specified in a manner that is helpful to the user who needs counting accuracy. For the measurement of concentrations that do not exceed some hundreds of particles 5–100 μm in size per milliliter, the lack of adequate specifications may be more of an annoyance than a crisis problem. For those who must correlate their analyses over time or with other locations or occasionally make accurate measurements that approach the USP ⟨788⟩ SVI limits, the step-by-step coincidence effect evaluation procedure detailed in Appendix 1 is recommended. The end user requires two pieces of information that have been determined in a validation demonstration to ensure that the data being collected are meaningful. The information required is the functionally measured geometric volume of the detector, V_{DG}, and the functionally measured height of the scan beam, B_H. Functional measurement requires that these determinations be made from particle counting data. With these two pieces of information in hand, a count accuracy contour for the entire range of measured particles can be selected that can control both assay undercounts and false counts. With these errors controlled, particle counting assays can become truly independent of instrument and measurement laboratory.

The physical world does not recognize the lower boundary established by the U.S. Pharmacopoeia for these contaminating particle measurements. An exponentially increasing population of contaminating particles has been described as particle size decreases. Monitoring data in the 5–10 μm particle size range provides insurance against this potential measurement interference. When an interference is determined, dilution or particle size separation prior to measurement can preserve counting accuracy.

The intent of the USP 23 particle contamination quality standards has never been in doubt. It has been to evaluate particle contamination in injectable fluids by counts of single particles in two size ranges: single particles greater than 10 μm and a much smaller number larger than 25 μm. In this chapter a count efficiency balance equation has been used to distinguish group count accuracy from single particle count accuracy. The application of a maximum particle count contour for the range of contaminating particle sizes that must be controlled makes possible a new era in accurate particle assays. The control of particle concentration before final measurement makes possible the correlation of assays rather than the present rough comparisons that are now possible.

ACKNOWLEDGMENT

Sincere thanks are tendered to Mr. A. Lieberman of Particle Measurement Systems, Inc., for his substantial part in shaping the Coincidence Effect Evaluation Procedure and to my colleague Dr. Lee R. Abramson, for his continued help with the statistical concepts described.

REFERENCES

Jaenicke, R. (1972). The optical particle counter: Cross-sensitivity and coincidence, *Aerosol Sci.*, *30*:95–111.

Knapp, J. Z., (ed). (1996). *Liquid and Surface Borne Particle Measurement Handbook*, Marcel Dekker, New York.

Knapp, J. Z., and L. R. Abramson. (1994). A new coincidence model for single particle counters, Part I: Theory and experimental verification, *J. Pharm. Sci Technol.*, *48*(3): 110–134.

Knapp, J. Z., and L. R. Abramson. (1995). A new coincidence model for single particle counters, Part III: Realization of single particle counting accuracy, *J. Pharm. Sci. Technol.*, *50*(2):99–122.

Knapp, J. Z., A. Lieberman, and L. R. Abramson. (1994). A new coincidence model for single particle counters, Part II: Advances and applications, *J. Pharm. Sci. Technol.*, *48*(5): 255–292.

Lieberman, A. (1975). Flow rate and concentration effects in automatic particle counters, presented at National Conference on Fluid Power, Chicago, IL.

Munson, T. E. (1987). F.D.A. perspectives on particulate matter testing in small volume injections, Proc. Int. Conf. on Liquid Borne Particle Inspection and Metrology, May 11–13, p. 827.

USP. (1995). United States Pharmacopoeia, 23 U.S. Pharmacopeial Convention, Inc., Rockville, MD.

APPENDIX 1: COINCIDENCE EFFECT EVALUATION PROCEDURE

A1.1 Scope

This procedure defines the effect of concentration on the coincidence errors of single particle counters. These errors include both undercounts and false counts that can affect USP 23 ⟨788⟩ particle assay results. It is particularly applicable to an optical liquid-borne particle counter (optical particle counter). The procedure is designed for volumetric optical particle counters used for contamination testing of small volume parenterals as described in USP 23 ⟨788⟩. With world pharmaceutical standards in mind, the subvisible particle size control range is from approximately 2 μm to those particles with diameters in excess of 100 μm. The upper concentration limit for this procedure ranges up to 6000 particles per milliliter for the 1 mL container, the smallest SVI container in widespread use. Coincidence count loss determination for particles at the maximum sensitivity of the optical particle counter is not part of this procedure. Operation within defined count limits over the operating range of the optical particle counter is the basis for accurate count determinations.

A1.2 Limitations

Particle counting errors occur when the optical particle counter reports more or fewer particles than are actually present in the suspension. The errors can result from incorrect optical particle counter design or construction, from incorrect optical particle counter operation, or from incorrect sample handling procedures. Accurate determination of the count efficiency, the ratio of counts to single particles that have been counted, for optical particle counter's must commence with the recognition that the relationship between the number of single particle counted and the resultant count is exponential. The high concentration operating limit is reached when the undercount loss exceeds the acceptable measurement error. The ratio of counts per milliliter to particles per milliliter at low particle concentrations approaches but never becomes an ideal linear relationship.

With some optical particle counter's, some background electronic noise pulses are large enough to be recorded as counts at the smallest particle size threshold of the counter. As the particle size analysis threshold is increased, the number of noise pulses/mL recorded decrease. These noise pulses will most affect the accuracy of the low concentration, lower size range measurements. The effect on counting accuracy of noise pulses is usually negligible in higher particle concentrations and for larger particle sizes. The low concentration operating limit is reached when the positive count error introduced by noise pulses exceeds the acceptable measurement error. Special care must be exercised to obtain accurate results.

A1.3 Definition of Terms and Symbols Specific to This Procedure

3.1. Coincidence. Signal coincidence describes the mechanism that reduces the count of particles present in a suspension by counting random groups of particles as single, larger, counting events. Coincidence reduces the total number of particles counted and distorts the distribution of particles being measured toward larger sizes.

3.2. Effective Detector Volume. In all presently available particle counters used for the evaluation of particle contamination in pharmaceutical products, the diameter of the particle measured is a non-negligible fraction of the scan beam height. For this case, the effective detector volume is larger than the physical or geometric detector volume of the detector. The effective height of the detector is the sum of the scan beam height and the diameter of the particle being measured. The effective detector volume is the product of the effective height of the scan beam and the flow cross section.

3.3. Measurement Units. All parameters are defined per milliliter of test volume.

3.4. Effective Particle Concentration. The effective particle concentration is measured as the ratio of particles per milliliter, n, to the number of effective detector volumes per milliliter, N_E.

3.5. Other Symbols Employed:

- f = Stepwise dilution factor.
- f_T = Total dilution factor between the −1% undercount concentration and the +1% noise-limited count.
- N' = The concentration at which a −10% count error occurs when 10 μm particles are counted by a detector.
- N'' = Concentration of 10 μm particles at which a 1% undercount error occurs.
- N_I = Initial particle concentration in a dilution experiment.
- s = The sequential step number of a dilution experiment.

S = The number of steps in a dilution experiment. Note: An asterisked quantity indicates an approximate value.

A1.4 Summary of Procedure to Determine Counting Accuracy

4.1. Sensor calibration, carried out at the manufacturers recommended flow rate, must precede the count accuracy procedure.

4.2. The background count C_0 of the filtered, surfactant treated, clean water that is used as a diluent is determined. The dilutent shall contain no more than 1 particle/mL >10 μm. This is the count at infinite dilution. The volume of diluent for this determination shall be no less than 500 mL.

4.3. The choice of experimental parameters provides four data points in the low count error concentration range. These four data points with C_0, the background count, contribute to the extrapolated determination of the initial concentration, N_I. At each dilution point, six 10 mL aliquots are taken. The first aliquot is discarded and the data of the five remaining aliquots are averaged. The accurate determination of the concentration of particles per milliliter at each dilution step rests on the accuracy with which the initial suspension is determined and the stepwise dilutions are performed.

4.4 The initial concentration of particles in the undiluted master suspension is selected to have a ratio of approximately 0.60 particles per detector volume. Accurate experimental determination of N_E, the number of effective detector volumes per milliliter is calculated from the initial dilution steps. At these initial steps particle concentration is high and high undercount error is observed.

4.5 The determination of N_I is performed by extrapolation from the data recorded between a concentration ratio of $0.01N_E$ and the concentration where the background noise count, C_0 /mL is 1% of recorded counts. A nominal value for this limit is 100 counts/mL. Accuracy in the determination of N_E rests upon the accuracy with which the concentration of the initial particle suspension is determined and the accuracy of the dilution sequence employed.

A1.5 Significance

Optical particle counters are calibrated with suspensions of well defined particles of known concentration and sizes. However, optical particle counters are used with liquids whose contamination level is not known. If the concentration of particulates exceeds the accurate counting limit of the detector or if the flow rate through the optical particle counter is not within the specified range then control of the coincidence undercount error limit will be degraded. Errors in reported particle size range and/or concentration will occur with no indication of the extent of error. No correction after measurement is possible because of the random nature of the particles being measured. This procedure will aid in defining the operating range of the optical particle counter where acceptable counting and sizing accuracy can be expected.

A1.6 Interferences

6.1 Improperly cleaned containers used to prepare dilutions and to contain samples will release artifact particles that will result in counting and analysis errors.

6.2 Inadequately dispersed samples during any measurements will result in wide variations in particle concentration and thus wide variations in data from sequential aliquots. Depending upon the nature of the suspension being counted, particle sedimentation and fluid dynamic forces during sample flow may also cause counting errors. For this reason, this procedure requires continuous stirring of the sample during handling and measurement. The stirring must be at a sufficient speed to suspend the particles being counted but must be maintained below cavitation level.

6.3 The creation of cavitation in the test suspension invalidates all measurements.

A1.7 Apparatus and Materials

7.1 A balance with load capability of at least 1 kg and 0.1 g accuracy or a volumetric delivery system that can maintain 1% aliquot accuracy is required.

7.2 Sample containers from which samples will be fed to the optical particle counters should be approximately 250 mL; for aliquot addition approximately 100 mL containers, with covers, shall be used. The use of narrow-mouth containers minimizes the entry of airborne particulates. New sample containers are desirable because their surface will be free from crazing and thus be easier to clean.

7.3 An external field driven magnetic stirrer with Teflon coated stirring bars shall be used.

7.4 The optical particle counters system shall include a liquid feeder with flow rate control and volumetric measurement.

7.5 Standard latex particles with nominal size of 10 μm and relative standard deviation no greater than 5% shall be used.

7.6 Nonionic surfactant shall be used for diluting latex particle suspensions. Triton X-100 (Rohm & Haas), Tween 20 (Atlas Chemical Co.) or equivalent materials have been found satisfactory.

7.7 Prepare a mixture of approximately 2 L of clean water with 0.01% surfactant. Filter the mixture through a 47 mm diameter filter with a pore size less than 0.50 mm. Test the mixture for particle contamination. The mixture is acceptable for use if it contains no more than 1 particle/mL >10 μm.

A1.8 Calibration

8.1 Verify that the calibration of the optical particle counters is current and is in accordance with ASTM F658 for particle sizing accuracy. Verify that the flow rate used during sizing calibration is set within the manufacturers recommended range. This flow rate shall be used for all subsequent measurements.

A1.9 Coincidence Count Effect Protocol Parameters

9.1 Using the instrument manufacturer's specification of the concentration, N', at which there is a 10% occurrence of coincidence, calculate N_E.

$$N_E = 8.363N'$$

9.2 To optimize extrapolation accuracy in the calculation of N_I a low counting error span with equal and opposite error end points is selected. The maximum particle concentration data point used is limited to the concentration, N'', for a 1% undercount error. Calculate the nominal 1% undercount concentration, N'' as $0.01N_E$.

$$N'' = 0.01N_E$$

9.3 Approximately 12 dilution steps between $0.01N_E$ provide adequate dilution data for the high concentration end. The approximate dilution factor is determined from the ratio of N'', which is equal to $0.01N_E$ to $5.0N'$, which is equal to $0.6N_E$.

$$f^* = \left[\frac{0.01N_E}{0.6N_E}\right]^{1/12} = (0.01666)^{1/12} = 0.7109$$

Round f^* to $f = 0.70$ and maintain the rounded dilution factor f, calculated in 9.5 throughout the entire dilution sequence. *Note*: Increasing f will provide more detailed dilution data when required.

9.4 The lowest concentration data point for the extrapolation is determined by the concentration at which 1 count/mL will result in a +1% noise pulse count error. This choice results in a low concentration end point of 100 counts/mL. Estimate the noise limited concentration of 100 counts/mL, N_{NI} in terms of N_E. An order of magnitude estimate of current N_E values is 100,000.

$$\frac{N_N}{N_E} = \frac{100}{100{,}000}$$

$$N_N = 0.001N_E$$

9.5 Three dilution steps between $N'' = 0.01N_E$ and $N_N = 0.001N_E$ counts/mL, when anchored by the data point at infinite dilution C_0, usually provide adequate data for an accurate extrapolation of N_I. The number of dilution steps, d, is calculated.

$$d^{0.7} = \left[\frac{N''}{N_N}\right] = \left[\frac{0.01N_E}{0.001N_E}\right] = 0.1$$

$$d = 3.29$$

9.6 Calculate the approximate value of the initial particle suspension N_I^* from N', the counter manufacturer calculated concentration for 10% 10 μm coincidence occurrence as required for compliance with USP23.

$$N_{I^*} = 0.6N_E = 0.6(8.363N') = 5.0178N' \approx 5.0N'$$

9.7 Calculate the initial counts/mL, C_I, resulting from a concentration of N_I particles/mL using the particle triggered Poisson model conversion factor calculated in 9.1 and readjust the suspension if required.

$$C_I = N_I e^{-N_I/N_E}$$

9.8 Select the aliquot volume V_A. The aliquot volume is selected to be large enough to provide separation from the preceding particle concentration and to provide an accurate sampling of the suspended particles. The aliquot volume selected should provide an acceptable 95% confidence interval for the smallest count planned. Six 10 mL aliquot volumes have been found to yield accurate results. The first 10 mL aliquot is discarded and the average of the counts for the remaining 50 mL is recorded.

9.9 Select the sample volume, V_0

$$f = 1 - V_A/V_0$$

Note: Use of a 60 mL volume balance after sampling avoids possible cavitation from the stirring bar.

A1.10 Coincidence Count Loss Protocol

10.1 Validate cleanliness of the containers to be used by rinsing sample components with clean diluent and passing a series of 10 mL samples through the optical particle counter. Discard the data from the first sample and verify that the average is ≤1 particle/mL ≥ 10 μm.

10.2 Tare the selected clean container with the stirring bar and cover until used.

10.3 Prepare the master suspension of the 10 μm standard PSL particles at a concentration of N_I particles per milliliter as calculated in 9.6 by adjusting counts per milliliter to the value calculated in 9.7. Adjust the master suspension within ±5% of the calculated counts per milliliter for the N_I desired.

10.4 Set the optical particle counter data system within the dynamic range of the instrument to record data in the cumulative mode. Set particle size thresholds including 2, 5, 10, 25, and 50 μm. Smaller and larger size thresholds can also be used. At no time should the smallest size threshold be set so that the particle count for the diluent indicates more than 1 particle per milliliter greater than 10 μm. *Note*: Selection of a threshold value affects the concentration error. The count data required is the differential count above 7.5 μm to ensure inclusion of the full tail of the distribution. The sequential dilution experiment is continued from the initial concentration until the background noise count, C_0/mL, is 1% of recorded counts. A nominal value for this limit is 100 counts per milliliter.

This analysis selection is made to ensure inclusion of the lower tail of the 10 mm particle distribution. When the analysis threshold is greater than 10% of the measured particle, the particle diameter D_{PE} is less than D_P.

$$D_{PE} = (D_P^2 - 2D_T^2)$$

10.5 Place the sample container in the optical particle counter feeder assembly. Set the stirring speed so that a 5 mm vortex is seen at the liquid surface but no air is drawn into the liquid. Set the optical particle counter sampler to pass liquid to the optical particle counter at the flow rate for which the optical particle counter was calibrated. Pass six 10 mL sample aliquots through the optical particle counter sensor and record the data from the last five samples. Select 10 μm as the lower particle size threshold that will include 99.9% of the 15 μm particle population. Calculate the average particle size dispersed, and mix the suspension for 1 min before taking an aliquot.

10.6 Sample the reestablished test volume using six 10 mL aliquots. The remaining volume is $V_0 - 60$ mL.

10.7 For dilution experiments using gravimetric volume determinations, transfer 60 mL of the prepared clean diluent in a clean tared container to the test volume after the completion of the counter sampling cycle. Cover the container with clean aluminum foil until use. Weigh the container after the transfer of the 60 mL and adjust the total liquid volume transferred. Calculate all concentration factors from the recorded gravimetric data of the sample container only. To ensure that the suspension has been uniformly dispersed, mix the suspension for 1 min before taking an aliquot.

Note: For samples that include 1 mL tare volumes, decrease the test aliquot to 9 mL.

10.8 For volumetrically controlled experiments, add six 10 mL precision syringes of surfactant-treated clean water to return to an approximate volume of V_0 mL. Record the test volume to 0.1 mL. This dilution corresponds to a ratio of d as determined by weight of the total sample plus diluent. To ensure that the suspension has been uniformly dispersed, mix the suspension for 1 min before taking an aliquot.

10.9 Carry out the procedures of steps 10.8 and 10.9 or 10.10 until the concentration is approximately 100 counts/mL, recording indicated average concentration >10 mm after each dilution.

A1.11 Count Accuracy Data Analysis

11.1 Review the data. Prepare a data table showing the sequence of dilution steps, the dilution factor and the average counts/mL at each step. Use either 11.2 or 11.3 to select and edit the linear data points for the determination of N_I.

11.2 From the data table make a log-log graph of the number of counts versus dilution factor. Select the log-log plot data points for numeric analysis that lie on a unit slope line and that appear to be in the linear count region. Edit erroneous data points.

11.3 Test the linear count data points using C_0 and each point in turn in the linear count region. c is the cumulative particle count >10 μm, f is the dilution factor for the recorded count, and N_I is the initial particle concentration. Edit erroneous data points.

$$c = C_0 + fN_I$$

11.4 Prepare a data table of the selected linear response data and use a linear regression analysis to include the C_0 data anchor point.

11.5 Select the linear regression solution using those data points in the calculation that result in the minimum zero offset to select the optimum value for the initial concentration of particles, N_I.

11.6 For each dilution data point calculate the concentration of single particles in suspension as the product of the initial concentration and the corresponding dilution factor, $n = N_I f^S$.

11.7 Determine the count error for each dilution data point.

$$\varepsilon_c = (n - c)/n$$

11.8 Determine the experimental value of N_E, the number of effective detector volumes/mL. Use data points that depart from the linear dilution equation by at least 30% to assure accuracy.

$$N_E = -\frac{n}{\ln(c/n)}$$

11.9 Calculate N', the model-based single particle concentration for a 10% coincidence count limit with the experimentally determined value of N_E.

$$N' = \frac{N_E \ln 0.7833}{2}$$

11.10 Calculate C', the model-based count at which there is a 10% coincidence count limit undercount error.

$$C' = 0.7833N'$$

A1.12 Determination of Geometric Detector Volume and Effective Beam Height

12.1 To determine the coincidence count loss for the full particle size design range of a detector, V_{DG} and B_H for the detector must be evaluated. B_H is evaluated following two determinations of N_E, the number of effective detector volumes for two particle sizes, N_{E1} and N_{E2}.

$$B_H = \frac{(N_{E2}/N_{E1})(D_{P2} - D_{P1})}{1 - N_{E2}/N_{E1}}$$

12.2 Using the calculated value of B_H from 12.1, calculate V_{DG}, the geometric detector volume using paired values of V_{DE} and D_P.

$$V_{DG} = \frac{V_{DE}}{(1 + DP/BE)}$$

A1.13 Calculation of a Selected Count Accuracy Contour for a Range of Particle Sizes

13.1 Calculate V_{DE3}, the effective detector volume for the selected particle size.

$$V_{DE3} = V_{DG}(1 + D_P/B_H)$$

13.2 Calculate N_{E3}, the number of effective detector volumes per milliliter for the selected arbitrary particle as the reciprocal of V_{DE3}.

$$N_{E3} = 1/V_{DE3}$$

13.3 Calculate N_3, the concentration limit for the selected particle size and count error.

$$N_3 = N_{E3} \ln(c/n)$$

13.4 Calculate the particle count that results from an N_3 concentration. The count efficiency is 1 minus the count error.

$$C_3 = N_3(1 - \varepsilon_C)$$

13.5 Calculate the count error contours for the counters designed particle size range.

13.6 Plot the calculated count accuracy contour. To operate with the selected count accuracy, maintain peak counts within the count accuracy contour selected.

APPENDIX 2: TECHNICAL DETAILS

A2.1 The Effective Concentration Measure

One equation is required to determine the concentration effects on counting accuracy for each particle size. To have this count–concentration relationship available for the range of particle sizes within the capacity of a detector, a relationship between particle size and N_E is essential. This relationship is

$$V_{DE} = \dot{V}_{DG}\left(1 + \frac{D_P}{\dot{B}_H}\right) \tag{15}$$

where

$\dot{B}_H$ = scan beam height
D_P = particle diameter
V_{DE} = effective detector volume = $1/N_E$
$\dot{V}_{DG}$ = geometric detector volume

The dots designate unknown terms.

Equation (15) has two unknowns: V_{DG}, the functionally measured geometric detector volume, and B_H, the functionally measured scan beam height. Both the geometric detector volume and the scan beam height, in manufacturer's specifications and in prior publications, have been determined by static measurements. Static measurements cannot fully gauge the dynamic interaction of a particle with the variability of flow within the detector and with the variation of the scan beam scatter as it passes through the detection zone. The two unknown constants in Eq. (15) are determined with simultaneous equations using data from two dilution experiments with different particle sizes.

A2.2 The Effect of the Analysis Threshold

When the analysis threshold reduces the sensed area of the particle, the experimental results have been determined for the effective particle diameter, D_{PE}, not the actual particle diameter.

The relationship of the effective particle diameter to the experimental determination of coincident count loss is discussed below.

When the particle size analysis threshold selected is no more than one-tenth of the calibrating particle diameter, it will affect the experimental results by 1% or less and can be ignored. The selected threshold reduces the sensed particle diameter as shown in Eq. (2). D_P is the diameter of the calibrating particle, D_T is the diameter of the particle selected as an analysis threshold, and D_{PE} is the effective reduced particle diameter, which controls the count loss due to increasing concentration.

$$D_{PE} = (D_P^2 - 2D_T^2)^{1/2} \tag{16}$$

The effect of a 5 μm analysis threshold on a 15 μm particle is examined in Eq. (16A).

$$D_{PE} = [(15)^2 - 2(5)^2]^{1/2} = 13.23\ \mu\text{m} \tag{16A}$$

The effect of a 5 μm analysis threshold on a 19.5 μm particle is examined in Eq. (2B).

$$D_{PE} = [(19.5)^2 - 2(5)^2]^{1/2} = 18.17\ \mu\text{m} \tag{16B}$$

The choice of a detection threshold will affect concentration test results by reducing the detected size of particles. If the reduction in particle width caused by an elevated analysis level is not considered, results based on the nominal size of the calibrated particles will be in error. A constant high analysis threshold will result in an increasingly oversized determination of N_E as the test particle diameter is reduced. An uncorrected computation based on dilution experiment counting data of 15, 19.5, and 25 μm particles with a 5 μm threshold will result in an oversizing of N_E by 16.7%, 6.8%, and 4%, respectively. This oversizing of N_E will result in underestimates of the coincidence effect counting errors for the detector.

A2.3 The Basic Particle-Triggered Poisson Model

The validated relationship between particle counts and the number of particles counted introduced in Knapp and Abramson (1994) for single particle light extinction counters described the use of the particle-triggered Poisson model for particle counting events. (Table 1 provides a summary of the symbols used.) The total for the Poisson series shown in Eq. (17) is 1. It sums the occurrence probability of single, double, triple, and higher multiple occurrence particle groups.

$$1 = e^{-n/N_E} + e^{-n/N_E}(1 - e^{-n/N_E}) + e^{-n/N_E}(1 - e^{-n/N_E})^2 + e^{-n/N_E}(1 - e^{-n/N_E})^3 + \cdots \tag{17}$$

Denoting the ratio of the total number of counts to the total number of single particles by c/n and multiplying each term in Eq. (3) by c/n results in a Poisson series in count efficiency:

$$\frac{c}{n} = \frac{ce^{-n/N_E}}{n} + \frac{ce^{-n/N_E}}{n}(1 - e^{-n/N_E}) + \frac{ce^{-n/N_E}}{n}(1 - e^{-n/N_E})^2 + \frac{ce^{-n/N_E}}{n}(1 - e^{-n/N_E})^3 + \cdots \tag{17A}$$

Each term on the right-hand side is the probability of an individual counting occurrence ratio. One common characteristic in all these terms is that each represents the probability of a count occurrence ratio group that is an integral multiple of the single particle ratio group. This type of additive coincidence signal is called vertical coincidence. (The use of faster electronics eliminated horizontal coincidence.)

Equation (17B) is the symbolic equivalent of Eq. (17A). In Eq. (17B), the count ratios are separated into multiplicity occurrence groups.

$$\frac{c}{n} = \frac{C(1)}{n} + \frac{C(2)}{n} + \frac{C(3)}{n} + \cdots \tag{17B}$$

To determined the number of single monosized particles in the total count, each count multiplicity term is multiplied by the multiplicity of particles in that count. This relationship is expressed as

$$n = C(1) + 2C(2) + 3C(3) + 4C(4) + \cdots \tag{18}$$

Dividing each term of Eq. (18) by n results in Eq. (19), which expresses the number of single particles in each counting event as a fraction of the total number of single particles in the sample that have been counted.

$$1 = \frac{C(1)}{n} + \frac{2C(2)}{n} + \frac{3C(3)}{n} + \frac{4C(4)}{n} + \cdots \tag{19}$$

Substituting each group of counted occurrences from Eq. (17) into Eq. (19) results in (19A).

$$n = ce^{-n/N_E}[1 + 2(1 - e^{-n/N_E}) + 3(1 - e^{-n/N_E})^2 + 4(1 - e^{-n/N_E}) + \cdots] \tag{19A}$$

Since the bracketed term in Eq. (5A) is equal to e^{2n/N_E},

$$n = ce^{n/N_E} \tag{20}$$

Equation (6) relates counts to particles. Solving for the desired effective counting efficiency, c/n, the ratio of raw counts to the number of particles counted for the particle-triggered Poisson model is

$$\frac{c}{n} = e^{-n/N_E} \tag{1}$$

Experimental verification of Eq. (7) commences with rewriting the equation as

$$\ln(c/n) = \frac{-n}{N_E} \tag{21}$$

Using Eq. (1) the particle-triggered Poisson series in Eq. (17A) is rewritten in count efficiency terms as

$$\frac{c}{n} = \left(\frac{c}{n}\right)^2 + \left(\frac{c}{n}\right)^2\left(1 - \frac{c}{n}\right) + \left(\frac{c}{n}\right)^2\left(1 - \frac{c}{n}\right)^2 + \cdots \tag{22}$$

There is a term-by-term correspondence between Eqs. (17A), (17B), and (22). Using this correspondence, $C(1)/n$, $C2/n$, $C3/n$, and $C(4)/n$, the count efficiency of single, double, triple, and quadruple occurrence groups, are written by inspection in Eqs. (11)–(14). Note that the single particle group count efficiency is the square of the raw count efficiency.

$$\frac{C(1)}{n} = \left(\frac{c}{n}\right)^2 \tag{4}$$

$$\frac{C(2)}{n} = \left(\frac{c}{n}\right)^2\left(1 - \frac{c}{n}\right) \tag{11}$$

$$\frac{C(3)}{n} = \left(\frac{c}{n}\right)^2\left(1 - \frac{c}{n}\right)^2 \tag{12}$$

$$\frac{C(4)}{n} = \left(\frac{c}{n}\right)^2\left(1 - \frac{c}{n}\right)^3 \tag{14}$$

The first term in Eq. (17A) is an exponential expression for single particle count efficiency, $C(1)/n$. Substituting e^{-n/N_E} from Eq. (1) for its equivalent c/n results in the equation

$$\frac{C(1)}{n} = e^{-2n/N_E} \tag{9}$$

The logarithmic form of Eq. (9) is

$$\ln\left[\frac{C(1)}{n}\right] = \frac{-2n}{N_E} \tag{9B}$$

Using these relationships, the count efficiency of all multiple group occurrences is determined by subtracting from the count efficiency, c/n, the single particle count efficiency as in Eq. (6).

$$\frac{C^+}{n} = \frac{c}{n} - \frac{C(1)}{n} \tag{6}$$

which is equivalent to

$$\frac{C^+}{n} = \left(\frac{c}{n}\right)\left(1 - \frac{c}{n}\right) \tag{6A}$$

In the analysis of the effect of coincidence error, the group count efficiency for triple and higher multiple group occurrences is useful. It is determined by subtracting from the count efficiency, c/n, the sum of single and double particle group count efficiencies. The result, after simplification, is

$$\frac{C^+(3)}{n} = \left(\frac{c}{n}\right)\left(1 - \frac{c}{n}\right)^2 \tag{13}$$

Equation (17B) the particle-triggered Poisson equation expressed in count efficiency terms, can also be expressed as a sum of single particle group count efficiency and the sum of multiple group count efficiency, as shown in Eq. (5). The algebraic equivalent of Eq. (5) is Eq. (22A).

$$\frac{c}{n} = \frac{C(1)}{n} + \frac{C^+}{n} \tag{5}$$

$$\frac{c}{n} = \left(\frac{c}{n}\right)^2 + \left(\frac{c}{n}\right)\left(1 - \frac{c}{n}\right) \tag{22A}$$

Using the second law of thermodynamics, the sum of the count efficiency and count loss is shown to be equal to 1 in Eq. (2), an efficiency balance equation. This relationship is an essential step in the analysis of count loss due to particle signal coincidence.

$$1 = \frac{c}{n} + \frac{\bar{c}}{n} \tag{2}$$

Solving Eq. (2) for $\bar{c}/n$ as 1 minus the count efficiency is shown in Eq. (2A). The count loss ratio, $\bar{c}/n$ (c-not on n) for the class of all single particle light extinction particle counters is defined in this equation. Incorporation of the effect of the count loss ratio will be seen to be essential to resolving the count accuracy problem at high concentration ratios.

$$\frac{\bar{c}}{n} = 1 - e^{-n/N_E} = 1 - \frac{c}{n} \tag{2A}$$

Substituting for c/n in Eq. (2), the efficiency balance equation, its equivalent value in Eq. (5), the sum of $C(1)/n$ and C^+/n results in a general count efficiency balance equation, expressed symbolically as

$$1 = \frac{C(1)}{n} + \frac{C^+}{n} + \frac{\bar{c}}{n} \tag{7}$$

Equation (7) states that the sum of single particle counts plus the sum of multiple group particle counts plus the loss of the single particle counts lost within the multiple particle group counts is unity. This general count balance equation is applicable to both Poisson counting models described in the literature. It summarizes the essential information required to understand and analyze the coincidence error that occurs in particle counting.

The loss of single particle group counts is another application of the efficiency balance relationship developed in Eq. (15). Applying the second law of thermodynamics to the single particle group count efficiency, the sum of the single particle group count efficiency and count loss is equal to 1:

$$1 = \frac{C(1)}{n} + \frac{\bar{C}(1)}{n} \tag{23}$$

Solving Eq. (16) for the single particle count loss gives

$$\frac{\bar{C}(1)}{n} = 1 - \frac{C(1)}{n} \tag{23A}$$

The simple and powerful relationships listed in this section describe the concepts that reduce the problems surrounding the accuracy of particle counting to a manageable laboratory routine.

A2.4 Application to the USP23 ⟨788⟩ SVI Contaminating Particle Assay

The USP23 ⟨788⟩ specification for a concentration limit for electronic counters on p. 1814 under Sensor Concentration Limits is that count level at which coincidence counts due to the presence of two or more particles in the sensor view volume comprise less than 10% of the counts collected for single 10 μm particles.

In Knapp et al. (1994), a constant was calculated to facilitate use of the count efficiency relationships from vendor-specified coincidence data for the USP ⟨788⟩ 10 μm SVI working standard of 4000 particles/mL. Multiplication by this constant resulted in the value of N_E for the detector. The constant was based on the use of raw counts and the assumption that the coincidence occurrence count rate could be equated to 10% of the single particle count ratio.

The following more rigorous development commences with a count efficiency equation for total coincident ratio occurrences based on single particle counts. This development restricts even further the particle concentration for a selected single particle count accuracy.

The analysis uses symbolic Eq. (6), which shows that the count efficiency ratio of multiple particle groups is equal to the raw count efficiency less the count of single particle groups. This symbolic equation applies to both Poisson models; the specific algebraic equations will, of course, differ. The analysis is begun by setting the multiple particle occurrence count ratio to the USP 10% maximum acceptable limit in each detector model and then solving for either the count efficiency or the relative concentration, the ratio of particles per detector volume, for that model. The resulting data provide the basis for determining the particle concentration for the 10% multiple group coincident occurrence ratio.

A2.5 Jaenicke Geometric Poisson Model with Static Concentration Measure: Single and Raw Particle Count Loss at 10% Coincidence

Equation (24) is an algebraic application of symbolic Eq. (6) for the count efficiency of multiple particle groups for the Jaenicke Poisson model.

$$\frac{C^+}{n} = \frac{1 - e^{-n/N_G} - (n/N_G)e^{-n/N_G}}{n/N_G} \tag{24}$$

Putting the multiple occurrence count ratio in Eq. (24) equal to 0.10 and solving numerically for n/N_G, the relative particle concentration, results in the equation

$$\frac{n}{N_G} = 0.85145 \tag{25}$$

Equation (26) expresses the count efficiency for single particle counts in this Jaenicke Poisson model.

$$\frac{C(1)}{n} = e^{-n/N_G} \tag{26}$$

Substituting the relative concentration calculated in Eq. (25) into Eq. (26) results in Eq. (27), the single particle group count efficiency corrected to four significant figures.

$$\frac{C(1)}{n} = e^{-0.85145} = 0.4268 \tag{27}$$

The calculated Jaenicke geometric single particle count efficiency for a 10% multiple occurrence rate is 42.7%; the single particle count error rate calculated with the Jaenicke geometric model for this condition is 57.3%.

The effect of these efficiency ratios is illustrated with the No. 3 detector of Table 2, the geometric detector volume is 14×10^{-6} cm^3. N_G, the number of detector volumes per milliliter, equals $1/V_{DG}$ and is 71,429. The Jaenicke geometric model particle concentration is 60,818 particles/mL as shown by the equation

$$\frac{n}{N_G} = \frac{n}{71{,}429} = 0.85145, \qquad n = 60{,}818 \text{ particles/mL} \tag{28}$$

When only raw counts are considered, the raw count efficiency for the Jaenicke geometric model is expressed as

$$\frac{c}{n} = \frac{1 - e^{-n/N_G}}{n/N_G} \tag{29}$$

Substituting the calculated relative particle concentration, $n/N_G = 0.85145$, into Eq. (29) results in

$$\frac{c}{n} = \frac{1 - e^{-0.85145}}{0.85145} = 0.6732 \tag{29A}$$

The raw count efficiency for the 10% coincident count ratio limit is 67.3%; the corresponding count loss rate is 32.7%, significantly less than the 57.3% count loss that results when single particles are the basis of the computation.

A2.6 Particle-Triggered Poisson Model with the Effective Concentration Measure: Single Particle Group Count Loss at 10% Coincidence

In Eq. (6B) the 0.10 occurrence ratio for all multiple occurrences is substituted into the algebraic equivalent of the symbolic equation for C^+/n, the multiple occurrence count efficiency for the particle-triggered Poisson model. This substitution results in a quadratic equation in count efficiency, c/n.

$$\frac{C^+}{n} = 0.10 = \frac{c}{n} - \left(\frac{c}{n}\right)^2 \tag{6B}$$

Solving Eq. (6B) with the quadratic formula results in two roots, count efficiencies of 0.8873 and 0.1127. The particle-triggered model count efficiency is a peaked function. The count efficiency value of interest is the one that occurs before the peak count is reached, as shown in the equation

$$\frac{c}{n}\left(\frac{C^+}{n} = 0.10\right) = 0.8873 \tag{6C}$$

Equation (4) expresses the single particle count efficiency as the square of the raw count efficiency for the particle-triggered model. Substituting the result of Eq. (6C) into Eq. (4) and simplifying the results gives Eq. (30).

$$\frac{C(1)}{n} = \left(\frac{c}{n}\right)^2 \tag{4}$$

$$\frac{C(1)}{n} = (0.8873)^2 = 0.7873 \tag{30}$$

Equation (8) expresses the single particle count loss as 1 minus the single particle count efficiency, or 21.3%. By comparison, the earlier work based on an assumed 90% single particle count efficiency resulted in a single particle count error of 19%.

$$\frac{\bar{C}(1)}{n} = 1 - \frac{C(1)}{n} = 1 - 0.7873 = 0.2126 \tag{8B}$$

The calculations to this point are independent of particle size. To relate the calculated single particle count efficiency to the count of a selected particle size, the basic parameters for a specific detector are required. The parameters are N_E, the number of effective detector volumes per milliliter, and B_H, the effective height of the scan beam. Using detector No. 3 of Table 2, as in the previous calculation, N_E for 10 μm particles is 57,057 detector volumes per milliliter. Substituting the single particle count efficiency and the selected value of N_E into Eq. (9A) results in

$$\ln(0.7873) = -\frac{2n}{57{,}057}, \qquad n = 13{,}645 \text{ particles/mL} \tag{31}$$

Limiting the particle concentration measured to 13,645 particles/mL limits single particle count loss to 21.3% as calculated with Eq. (8B).

A2.7 The Particle-Triggered Model Single Particle Group Count Loss for the Jaenicke Geometric Model at a 10% Coincidence Rate

The N_E for 10 μm particles for detector No. 3 from Table 2 is 57,057. Substituting $n = 56{,}565$, the concentration at a 10% single particle occurrence rate determined with the Jaenicke geometric model, and the $57{,}057 N_E$ for 10 μm particles for detector No. 3 into Eq. (9) determines the single particle count efficiency at the concentration calculated with the Jaenicke Poisson model:

$$\frac{C(1)}{n} = e^{-2(60{,}818)/57{,}057} = 0.1186 \tag{32}$$

The single particle count efficiency using the concentration calculated with the Jaenicke geometric model is 11.9%: the corresponding single particle count loss is 88.1%. The Jaenicke geometric model results are not representative of particle counter performance.

A2.8 Minimum N_E to Satisfy USP 23 Multiple Occurrence Specification: Raw Counts Versus Single Particle Counts

The minimum N_E, N'_E (single particle), that can be used to satisfy the USP ⟨788⟩ SVI specification for single particle counts at a concentration of 4000 particles/mL is calculated by substituting $C(1)/n = 0.7873$ into Eq. (9) as shown in Eq. (33).

$$\ln(0.7873) = -2 \times 4000/N_E$$

$$N'_E \text{ (single particle group data)} = 33{,}452 \tag{33}$$

The results of Eq. (33) show that a minimum N_E' of 33,452 is required to accurately satisfy the USP coincidence specification of 10% coincidence occurrence for counts of single 10 μm particles at a concentration of 4000 particles/mL. Use of this specified concentration results in a 21.3% single particle group count loss.

When raw particle count data are used to calculate the particle concentration for the USP coincidence limit test, a 53% underestimate of the count loss results. N_E' for 10 μm particles remains unaltered at 33,452. The numerator of the effective concentration ratio, n/N_E', for raw counts is ½ that of single particle counts. The result is a raw count loss of 11.27% versus the 21.3% loss of single particle counts as shown in Eq. (1B).

$$\frac{c}{n} = e^{-4,000/33,452} = 0.8873 \tag{1B}$$

$$\frac{\bar{c}}{n} = 0.1127 = 11.27\% \tag{34}$$

A2.9 Conversion Constant from USP 23 SVI 10% Total Coincidence Specification for 10 μm Particles to N_E Detector Volumes per Milliliter for These Particles

When the concentration for the USP 23 ⟨788⟩ SVI 10% coincidence error is accurately known, the determination of N_E at 10 μm for the detector involves only multiplication by a conversion constant. The present USP 23 ⟨788⟩ SVI count accuracy limit specification does not differentiate between raw counts and single particle counts. Accordingly, both are treated in the following section.

For single particle counts, 0.7873 is substituted for $C(1)/n$ in Eq. (9C):

$$N_E = \frac{-2n}{\ln(C(1)/n)} = \frac{-2n}{\ln 0.7873} = +4.1815(2n) = 8.3631n \tag{9C}$$

The total conversion constant is 8.3631. A major consideration in the use of this conversion factor is that the accuracy of the calculated result depends on the vendor's unspecified experimental methods.

N_E is a basic parameter of detector performance and is unchanged for use with either raw counts or single particle counts. What does change is the numerator of the effective concentration ratio and thus the value of the exponent that determines the count efficiency. For raw count efficiency, this ratio is n/N_E; for single particle counts this ratio is $2n/N_E$. Comparing these ratios, the effective concentration for single particle counts is twice that for raw particle counts resulting in the lower count efficiences for single particle counts that have been experienced.

The N_E required to comply with the USP ⟨788⟩ SVI concentration limit using the raw count equation, Eq. (7), results in twice the concentration calculated with the single particle count conversion constant.

Although this conversion constant has been developed, accurate results from its use depend on the accurate determination of the concentration for the USP 23 10% coincidence limit point. Given the required accuracy in the evaluation of the specified concentration, the final result of operating at these conditions for contaminating particle assays is data that are ambiguous and unreliable.

A2.10 Counts and Single Particle Group Counts

Each term in Eq. (3A) represents the occurrence probability of a multiple particle group as shown in the symbolic equivalent statement of Eq. (3). This 1:1 relationship between the algebraic series and the logical equivalent statement can be used to determine the efficiency ratio of selected groups. The first term $(c/n)^2$ is the efficiency ratio of the number of particles that have been counted as individual occurrences. The count efficiency of single particle group counts is expressed as

$$\frac{C(1)}{n} = e^{-2n/N_E} \tag{9}$$

The ratio of Eq. (9A) to Eq. (1) provides the ratio of single particle counts to all counts:

$$\frac{C(1)}{c} = e^{-n/N_E} \tag{35}$$

Equation (35) shows that raw counts are exponentially related to single particle group counts. The use of a count limit specification for single particle counts using raw count values will result in an erroneous determination.

A2.11 Boundary Effects, Undercounts, and False Counts

The computation of the single particle group count efficiency, Eq. (10), and the count efficiency of all multiple occurrence counts, Eq. (14A), assumes an effectively infinite measurement span. When boundaries are introduced as in the USP ⟨788⟩ contaminating particle assay, their effect on the computation of undercounts and false counts must be considered when single particle count loss is to be accurately calculated.

The effect on single particle count loss of coincident occurrences within a boundary is determined by the coincidence occurrence multiple that can be contained within the selected boundary. Considering ideal particle samples and ideal counters, the ratio of multiple occurrences that can be contained within the 10–25 μm particle size boundaries of the USP (788⟩ particle assays is determined by the size of the particle as shown in Table 2.

As an example, the bounded single particle undercount ratio, $\bar{C}_B(1)/n$, and C_B^+/n, the bounded false count ratio for the 13.296 μm geometric mean particle size in zone III of the sensitivity analysis will be analyzed. Consulting Table 2 shows that double and triple occurrences for this particle size can be contained in the USP defined contamination span. The total number of single particle counts lost within the 25 μm boundary is the sum of the horizontal coincidence count loss and the loss in counts due to the single count for each particle grouping in vertical multiple occurrence events. This count loss is equal to one count for each double occurrence event and two counts for each triple occurrence event. Equation (36) is the symbolic sum of these losses.

$$\frac{\bar{C}_B(1)}{n} = \frac{\bar{c}}{n} + \frac{C(2)}{n} + \frac{2C(3)}{n} \tag{36}$$

Substituting for the symbolic terms in Eq. (36) their algebraic equivalents from Eqs. (2A), (11), and (12) results in

$$\frac{\bar{C}_B(1)}{n} = \left(1 - \frac{c}{n}\right) + \left(\frac{c}{n}\right)^2 \left(1 - \frac{c}{n}\right) + 2\left(\frac{c}{n}\right)^2 \left(1 - \frac{c}{n}\right)^2 \tag{37}$$

For simpler manipulation, Eq. (31) is rearranged as

$$\frac{\bar{C}_B(1)}{n} = \left(1 - \frac{c}{n}\right)\left[1 + \left(\frac{c}{n}\right)^2 \left(3 - 2\frac{c}{n}\right)\right] \tag{37A}$$

The single, double, and triple occurrence particle counts of the 13.296 μm particles were seen to remain below the 25 μm boundary. Each false count, C_B^+/n, will therefore originate in a multiple occurrence event greater than 4. The bounded false count ratio is determined by subtracting from the multiple group count efficiency the count efficiency of double and triple coincident occurrences. Equation (38) is the resulting symbolic equation; the algebraic equation, Eq. (39) then follows and is simplified in Eq. (39A).

$$\frac{C_B^+(1)}{n} = \frac{C^+}{n} - \left(\frac{C(2)}{n} + \frac{C(3)}{n}\right) \tag{38}$$

$$\frac{C_B^+(1)}{n} = \left(\frac{c}{n}\right)\left(1 - \frac{c}{n}\right) - \left(\frac{c}{n}\right)^2\left(1 - \frac{c}{n}\right) - \left(\frac{c}{n}\right)^2\left(1 - \frac{c}{n}\right)^2 \tag{39}$$

$$\frac{C_B^+(1)}{n} = \left(\frac{c}{n}\right)\left(1 - \frac{c}{n}\right)^3 \tag{39A}$$

A2.12 Maximum Raw Particle Count Capability of the Particle-Triggered Poisson Model and the Concentration at Which it Occurs

Solving Eq. (1) for c as shown in Eq. (1A) facilitates determination of the concentration capability of a detector as shown in Fig. 3.

$$c = ne^{-n/N_E} \tag{1A}$$

Differentiating Eq. (1A) with respect to n yields C_{MAX}, the peak of the particle count versus concentration curve as shown in Eq. (40). The number of single particles in suspension at the peak count is given in Eq. (40A),

$$C_{MAX} = N_E e^{-1} = 0.3679 N_E \tag{40}$$

$$n(C_{MAX}) = N_E \tag{40A}$$

In Fig. 3, Eq. (1A) has been used to demonstrate the effect on counting capability of detector volume as particle concentration increases. Equations (40) and (40A) have been used to calculate the peak count capability and the concentration at which it occurs.

A2.13 Maximum Single Particle Count Capability of the Particle-Triggered Poisson Model and the Concentration at Which it Occurs

The determination of universal curves of counting accuracy and counting error for all single particle counters was a major but not final step to understanding and controlling the counting error of particle counters. The next step is to differentiate Eq. (9) with respect to n to yield $C(1)_{MAX}$. The simplified results, shown in Eq. (41) are used to calculate the peak number of single particles in suspension, $C(1)_{MAX}$. Equation (41A) determines the concentration, $n(C_{MAX})$, at which the peak of the single particle group count versus particle concentration curve is located.

$$C(1)_{MAX} = N_E \frac{e^{-1}}{2} = \frac{0.3679 N_E}{2} = 0.1839 N_E \tag{41}$$

$$n[C(1)_{MAX}] = \frac{N_E}{2} \tag{41A}$$

Equation (41) states that the maximum number of single particle group counts reported by a counter will be 18.39% of the number of effective detector volumes per milliliter for the detector. Equation (41A) locates this maximum single particle group count at a concentration of $N_E/2$ particles per milliliter.

Comparing the peak raw count and single particle peak count and the concentration at which they occur is accomplished by comparing Eqs. (40) and (40A) with Eqs. (41) and (41A). The single particle peak count is half that of the raw count maximum. The single particle count maximum occurs at half the concentration at which the raw count maximum appeared.

These relationships provide the means with which to evaluate the effectiveness of the minimum acceptable light extinction count accuracy specification defined in USP 23 ⟨788⟩ for 10 μm particles.

A2.14 Estimation of Counting Errors with Detector Parameters

The raw count error for this Poisson model is calculated with Eq. (21). At small n/N_E ratios, the count error is approximated with Eq. (21A).

$$\varepsilon_C = (1 - e^{-n/N_E}) \tag{42}$$

$$\varepsilon_C = 1 - n/N_E \tag{42A}$$

The single particle count error is calculated with Eq. (43). At small n/N_E ratios, the count error is approximated with Eq. (43A).

$$\varepsilon_C = (1 - e^{-2n/N_E}) \tag{43}$$

$$\varepsilon_C = 1 - 2n/N_E \tag{43A}$$

A2.15 Primary Verification of Particle Counting Accuracy

Primary verification of particle counter counting accuracy is obtained with the standard membrane microscopic assay at low concentration obtainable in the terminal steps of the dilution experiment. This verification is performed by counting a suitable low concentration of single particles and then diluting the counted particle concentration for accurate membrane microscopic assay results. A description of the procedure follows.

A particle suspension is counted at a concentration at which neither the positive noise error pulses nor the negative undercount error for single particles can contribute an error greater than 1%. This requirement is conservatively equivalent to the choice of a concentration greater than 100 particles/mL and less than the concentration at which the count efficiency (the ratio of single particle counts to the number of single particles in solution) is equal to 0.99 as shown by the substitution in Eq. (9).

$$\frac{C(1)}{n} = 0.99 = e^{-2n/N_E} \tag{9D}$$

The solution for the relative concentration, n/N_E, is

$$\frac{n}{N_E} = \frac{0.01005}{2} = 0.005025 \tag{44}$$

Substituting the solution of Eq. (44) for n in Eq. (45) results in the concentration per milliliter at which there is a 1% single particle undercount error.

$$n(\varepsilon_n = 1\%) = 0.005025N_E \tag{45}$$

The dilution required to adjust the particle concentration to an appropriately low level suitable for microscopic verification, say 50 ± 25 particles/mL, can then be calculated, prepared, and finally verified with a standard membrane microscope assay. This determination is repeated to achieve the desired statistical confidence interval. Equation (44) is also the dilution ratio required for the 1% single particle count error when the particle concentration is N_E particles/mL. When the initial concentration is K times N_E, the dilution factor is adjusted as shown in Eq. (46).

$$\frac{n}{KN_E} = \frac{0.005025}{K} \tag{46}$$

This describes an experimentally validated method of responding to the count accuracy specification included in USP 23. The effect on assay accuracy of particle interaction from below the 10 μm particle control region and from within the 10–25 μm particle control band analyzed in Knapp and Abramson (1995) merit serious consideration.

A2.16 Population Estimate for a Sub-10 μm USP ⟨788⟩ False Count Test

The highest probability multiple coincidence event is that of the double. To test the false count contribution of sub-10 μm particles on the USP ⟨788⟩ SVI particle assay, a population of these 10 μm particles will be defined. The particle size is selected to have half the area of a 10 μm particle; its diameter is therefore 7.071 μm. The concentration of these 7.071 μm particles is determined by fitting an exponential equation to a two-point particle distribution defined by the SVI acceptance criteria of USP ⟨788⟩.

An exponential equation with two unknowns can be fitted to USP ⟨788⟩ SVI acceptance limit criteria for both revisions 22 and 23. Following the calculated fit, both equations are used to estimate a concentration of 7.071 μm particles/mL with which to test for the injection of false counts into the SVI ⟨788⟩ assay.

Although the contamination quality standard is based on the number of particles per container, count accuracy criteria are calculated per milliliter. The exponential relationship is

$$n = Ae^{-kD_P} \tag{47}$$

where

n = concentration, particles/mL
D_P = particle diameter, μm
A, k = arbitrary constants

In each of the ⟨788⟩ distributions selected, the maximum acceptable value for 25 μm is used and the balance of the test group is assumed at 10 μm. For USP 23 the resulting two-point particle distribution is 5400 particles per container at 10 μm and 600 at 25 μm. This pair of values satisfies the proposed SVI maximum limits of 6000 particles > 10 μm and not to exceed 600 particles of over 25 μm. Considering the broadly used 2 mL container as the highest particle concentrations that should be of concern, the corresponding concentrations in particles per milliliter will be 2700 particles/mL for 10 μm particles and 300 particles/mL for 25 μm particles.

With two unknowns, a pair of equations are required for solution:

$$2700 = Ae^{-10k} \tag{48}$$

$$300 = Ae^{-25k} \tag{49}$$

The joint solution of these two equations for the arbitrary constants results in $A = 11{,}682.3$, $k = 0.146482$. The population of 7.071 μm particles/mL is estimated with the equation

$$n = 11{,}682.3e^{-7.071\times 0.146482} \tag{50}$$

or

$$n = 4146.4 \text{ particles/mL}$$

The corresponding total of 7.071 μm particles in the 2 mL container is twice the value calculated with Eq. (43), or 8293.2 particles per container.

As in the case of the USP 23 ⟨788⟩ SVI assay, in the selection of a test group for USP 22, the maximum acceptable value for 25 μm is used, and the balance of the test group is assumed at 10 μm. The resulting two-point particle distribution is 9000 particles per container at 10 μm and 1000 at 25 μm. This pair of values satisfies the SVI maximum limits of 10,000 particles > 10 μm of which no more than 1000 shall exceed 600 particles > 25 μm. Again considering the broadly used 2 mL container as having the highest particle concentrations that should be of concern, the corresponding concentrations in particles per milliliter will be 4500 particles/mL for 10 μm particles and 500 particles/mL for 25 μm particles.

When USP 22 ⟨788⟩ limits are used to calculate a 7.071 μm particle population, the following equations are used.

$$4500 = Ae^{-10k} \tag{51}$$

$$500 = Ae^{-25k} \tag{52}$$

Since the ratio of the concentrations selected is the same for both cases, 2700/300 = 4500/500 = 9, the arbitrary constant k is the same for each: k = 0.146482. Substituting this value of k into Eq. (25D) and solving for A gives A = 38,940.9. The estimated concentration of 7.071 μm particles is then calculated with Eq. (46):

$$A = \frac{4500}{e^{-10\times0.146482}} = 19{,}470.4 \text{ particles/mL} \tag{53}$$

For USP 22, the arbitrary constants k and A are respectively 0.146482 and 19,4760.4. The concentration of 7.071 μm particles is calculated as

$$n = 19{,}470.4e^{-7.071\times0.146482} = 6911.1 \text{ particles/mL} \tag{54}$$

The concentration of these interfering particles is 13,822 particles per container. It must be stressed that the intent of this discussion is to demonstrate ⟨788⟩ assay sensitivity to sub-10 μm particles with a numerical example. It is not intended to propose an analytical description of the distribution of random particulates in parenteral products.

With constants A and k determined for USP 22 and 23, the calculation of an interfering population of 5.773 μm particles/mL is a 2 mL container yields respective values of 8358 and 5015 particles/mL.

29

Validation of Filtrative Sterilizations

MAIK W. JORNITZ
Sartorius AG, Göttingen, Germany

THEODORE H. MELTZER
Capitola Consulting Company, Bethesda, Maryland

1 INTRODUCTION

In its Guideline on General Principles of Process Validation, the Food and Drug Administration (FDA) makes plain that the validation of sterile processes is required of the manufacturers of sterile products. The testing of final products alone cannot suffice for this purpose if only because no practical sampling plan can provide complete assurance regarding untested units [1].

In its continuing development, filter validation has evolved from the concept that particles such as organisms are filtratively separated from their suspensions by sieve retention solely because they are too large to negotiate the pore passageways. It is now commonly accepted that organisms are retained by filters because of adsorptive sequestration mechanisms in addition to sieve retention. The adsorptive effects make it possible for filters to remove particles that are smaller than the filter pores. Nevertheless, certain current validation practices still derive from the earlier assumption that filtrative sterilizations are based solely on the sieve retention mechanism. It is from these origins that the 1×10^7 CFU/cm^2 challenge arises, that establishing the exact organism size becomes of concern, and that the pore size rating, often erroneous and even misleading, is of interest [2].

To be sure, where sieve retention is operative, filter efficiency is complete and invariant, an axiomatic expression of solid geometry. The particle is too large to penetrate the pore regardless of the filter conditions or the composition of the suspending fluid. Adsorptive influences, on the other hand, are responsive to these factors. In any given sterilizing filtration it is not possible to sort out the mechanisms at work. The filter adequate to the required performance under one set of filtration conditions may prove deficient in another. Hence the stipulation of "worst-case conditions." Hence also the need for filter validation, to demonstrate that the vagaries of the adsorptive effect do not introduce uncertainties into the very filtration of interest under the most severe filtration conditions being used specifically for the product being filtered, those least likely to promote organism retention by the filter.

2 CURRENT APPROACHES

The FDA view is that the most reliable way to conduct filter validations is to challenge the sterilizing filter in the specific drug preparation of interest, in a manner consonant with production conditions, with a suspension of properly sized *Brevundimonas diminuta*, (formerly called *Pseudomonas diminuta*) [3] sufficient to provide 1×10^7 CFU per square centimeter of available filter surface. A sterile filtrate is expected. This provides an opportunity to assess the effect of the particular drug on the filter, in terms of altering the pore size, and on the organism, in terms of modifying its size.

In actual practice, the microbiological assay of the total filtrate is usually performed using the recovery method. However, the assay method to be used is not specific. Regardless of how it is performed, its purpose is to search for viable organisms in the filtrate.

A problem arises when the specific product is inhibitory to the organisms, for the current microbiological assay requires the detection of *viable* organisms. The counting also of dead organisms, as could be accomplished with the epifluorescence technique [4], would not be useful because they may have been present in the filter and/or the filter assembly, their demise occasioned by the sterilization of the filter prior to its use. The presence of dead *B. diminuta* could be detected, however, by the use of RNA typing techniques [5], if desired.

It might be thought that the killing or inhibiting of the model organisms (e.g., *B. diminuta*) by the suspending medium would render moot the validation of the filter to achieve sterilization. The concern, however, is with the possible presence of organisms native to the preparation that may conceivably not be killed by the inhibitory agent. Attempts are then made to use the product minus its antagonistic component(s), a so-called placebo solution. The inhibitory agents are omitted from the formulation, the requisite organism challenge is added, and the filtration is performed under worst-case conditions. Microbiological assessment then follows.

Another useful approach is possible. In a viability test, the organism kill rate may be determined at different time intervals starting with a known organism concentration. This may permit the addition of so high a concentration of organisms as to ensure the survival of the requisite number, 1×10^7 per square centimeter of filter area, sufficient for the duration of the test.

The drug preparation is considered nonbactericidal if over the exposure time the organism count is not diminished by more than one log. The quantity of organism suspension directly inoculated into the drug should be minimized, below 10% of the total volume if possible, to lessen its adulterating effect.

Where biocidal or inhibitory ingredients are not minor in content, however, recourse is had to a third direction. The filter is exposed to the specific preparation, inhibitory though it be. This provides opportunities for any tendency toward filter incompatibility to alter the pore sizes of the filter. (Compatibility assessment techniques are beyond the scope of this writing. Reference can be made to Lukaszewicz and Meltzer [6] or to Chapter 8 in this book.) The filter is then washed as copiously as necessary to flush out the inhibitory agent. (It should be noted that this is sometimes accomplished only imperfectly.) The filter, free of inhibitory agent but with its pore structure perhaps altered by contact with the test preparation, is then challenged with the proper suspension of organisms. This allows the effect of the drug on the organism size to be assessed. The challenge is to be done under "worst-case or process" conditions. Often, however, these conditions are defined only in terms of the filtration modality employed in the production mode. Often the organism-suspending medium is seen as being unimportant—even water is sometimes used; but the attributes of the suspending liquid also may contribute to the worst-case conditions. Additionally, it too must be assessed for its effects on the size of the organisms. Bacterial suspensions in liquids other than actual product may also not reveal adsorptive capture involvements.

When filters are challenged with product formulations absent their inhibitory compounds (for the challenge organism), the product parameters should be viewed carefully. If changes in the product properties occur as a result of the removal of inhibitory compounds—i.e., changes in osmolarity, surface tension, or pH—then such changes should be compensated for by adjusting the properties of the product to its original nature. This may be done by adding suitable substances that are otherwise nonhibitory to the challenge organism, e.g., glycerol to increase viscosity.

The effect of the specific drug preparation on the filter is investigated by exposing the filter to its action under actual processing conditions, e.g., transfilter pressure, time, temperature, and flow rate. Either a recirculatory mode or a single-pass style of drug flow may be used.

Depending on the bactericidal power of the drug preparation and the viability of the test organism over the exposure time, different techniques may be used to achieve the desired total organism challenge over the duration of the filtration as in production.

As stated, so high a total initial organism concentration may be inoculated that at the experimentally defined kill rate 1×10^7 CFU/cm^2 some organisms remain viable throughout the production cycle. Alternatively, the desired total organism density can be achieved by metering in incremental quantities of the organism suspension over the course of the filtration.

Other approaches are also possible, including the omission of the bactericidal ingredient or modification of, e.g., the temperature or the filtration duration, if that should be the cause of the organism kill. These techniques, however, suffer from a lack of identity with the specific drug preparation or the actual filtration conditions governing in production.

The subject of surrogate solutions or placebos to be used in place of the specific, but cidal, drug preparations arises from these considerations.

3 PORE SIZE CONSIDERATIONS

The pore size is of direct concern in the sieve retention mechanism in its relevance to the size of organisms expected to be retained by the filter. The size of the pore relative to smaller particles also influences adsorptive particle arrests, particularly in conjunction with appropriate rates of flow, viscosity, etc., as discussed in Chapter 10.

Originally, the microporous sterilizing filter was assigned a pore size rating of 0.45 μm. It was found, however, that a certain organism, then called *Pseudomonas diminuta* but now reclassified as *Brevundimonas diminuta*, could penetrate such membranes where protein was present in the suspending medium [7]. The pore size of sterilizing filters was halved to retain these organisms, and the 0.2 or 0.22 μm microporous membrane became the standard designation of sterilizing filters.

Unfortunately, there is no filtration industry standard for rating microporous membrane filters. Indeed, one widely used 0.2 μm rated membrane, successful in its application to filtrative sterilizations, is stated by its manufacturer to be deserving of a 0.46 μm rating on the basis of its retention of latex spheres of appropriate sizes [8]. To avoid the complications presented by the nonstandard ratings, a functional definition of the sterilizing filter was based on its ability to retain 1×10^7 CFU of *B. diminuta*, grown in a specified way to limit and delineate the organism size, per square centimeter of membrane surface under stipulated applied differential pressures or given rates of flow [9]. Filter manufacturers thereby became entitled to call their membrane product a sterilizing filter if it met this defined operational performance. Presumably, this functional definition finessed the need to define pore sizes dimensionally or to elucidate the captive mechanisms involved.

Although filter manufacturers possessed a standard for conferring the appellation "sterilizing filter," a membrane thus labeled does not necessarily produce sterile filtrate under all circumstances. This happens mainly when organisms smaller than the above-mentioned challenge organisms are present. In this case, filter types of smaller pore sizes need to be used if the absoluteness of sieve retention is sought.

4 PORE SIZE DESIGNATIONS

Initially, the bubble point integrity test was seen to serve as a numerical measurement of the set of largest pores present in a filter. These are significant because their dimension would provide passageways least likely to be sieve-retentive. It soon became evident that the integrity tests did not supply sufficiently precise measures of the pore diameters [10].

The bubble point measurement, and subsequently the other integrity tests that were developed (see Chapter 11) perform a most important function. They provide a nondestructive test whereby the individual filters being used in a sterilization exercise can be assayed to see whether they accord with the filter manufacturer's correlation of organism challenge levels with given integrity test values. A proper integrity test value affirms that the filter being used conforms to the filter manufacturer's experimentally determined correlation with the successful 1×10^7 CFU/cm^2 challenge in his qualifying testing mode, that he is justified in labeling the filters a "sterilizing grade" membrane. It does not ensure, however, that the filter's use will invariably yield sterile filtrate under any and all use conditions. That, indeed, is the purpose of the filter validation function. It is a consequence of the organism retention mechanisms that are operative in a given filtration. These, described in Chapter 10, reflect the conditions governing the filtration and the composition of the organism-suspending fluid.

5 PORE NUMBERS AND DISTRIBUTIONS

The early assumption (unwarranted) that sterilizing grade filters removed organisms solely by the sieve retention mechanism, however simplistic, had to accommodate a number of considerations: elucidation of the number of pores per given filter area, the phenomenon of pore size distribution, and the dimensional significance of the pore size rating. Almost instinctively, the user of a 0.2 or 0.22 μm rated membrane, the common numerical designation of the sterilizing filter, believes the numerical value to be the expression of the minimum size particle the filter will retain by sieving. But that is not so. With very few exceptions, the pore size designation is not based on the sieve retention of particles of specific sizes. Pore size ratings are assigned on the basis of any of a number of measuring techniques [11]. This is one reason why sterilizing membranes came to be qualified by the HIMA convention of retaining 1×10^7 CFU *B. diminuta* organisms per square centimeter of membrane surface, and not by the numerical matching of assigned pore sizes to the particle size whose retention is desired.

Almost nothing is known about the sizes and shapes of the restrictive pores of a filter. An inquiry into the matter based on pore-formation physics has received only scant attention [12,13]. The governing attitude is that the actual sizes and shapes of the pores need not be elucidated, that, academic interests aside, the operational performance of the filter is, in the final analysis, all that counts. It is known, however, that the pores of a microporous membrane are represented by a pore size distribution. Presumably, the bubble point integrity test measures the set of largest pores. Nevertheless, the largest pores may be so few in number as not to find expression even in integrity test measurements, sensitive though they be. One would wish, therefore, to challenge the filter with enough organisms to encounter even the very few largest pores that may be present. This introduces the concept of challenge density.

For any given filter the number of restrictive pores that are present is unknown. Arithmetical calculations taking into account a given expanse of filter area, its total porosity, and the 0.2 μm dimension of the sterilizing pore have yielded numbers similar to $1 \times 10^7/cm^2$ or thereabouts. It becomes convenient to have a number with which to perform calculations, but the calculated number is meaningless. The total porosity is not easy to measure with accuracy. Furthermore, the total porosity is not neatly divided into metering or restrictive pores. Much of the space is vestibular, consisting of large entryways leading to the restrictive pores whose numbers are only being guessed at [13]. The number of restrictive pores cannot be determined directly from the number of organisms retained because single organism arrests at single choke pores cannot be assumed.

It is from such findings, however, that it is concluded that even 0.45 μm rated membranes can retain 1×10^4 or 1×10^5 CFU challenge levels of *B. diminuta*. However true for such membranes as may have been investigated, the conclusion cannot be justifiably extended to all other similarly rated filters, there being no standardization of pore size ratings. Moreover, there have been no reported investigations of the coacervation technique whereby microporous membranes are manufactured to show that the variations of the process used by different manufacturers yield the same pore architecture, particularly in the uninvestigated area of pore size distributions.

In the belief that each and every pore should be challenged by an organism, 1×10^7 CFU are conventionally used per square centimeter of available filter surface. Indeed, this very challenge number has become enshrined in the filter validation protocol irrespective of the bioburden level determined to be present in the drug preparation whose filtrative validation is being sought, which usually is found to be lower. This challenge density was arrived at by a HIMA group whose most notable accomplishment may have been a consensus agreement by an assemblage of filter manufacturers and users previously known for their competitive rivalry. The number arrived at was, however, a product of the belief current at the time regarding the number of 0.2 μm pores present in a sterilizing membrane. The number was stipulated at 1×10^7. Clearly, the number lacked precision. Therefore, the exact expression used was "a minimum of 1×10^7 CFU." At least one filter company sees a virtue in testing to a higher challenge level, finding that their 0.2 μm rated membrane is not covered by a monolayer of *B. diminuta* at the 1×10^7 CFU level [14]. But it is this very membrane that the same manufacturer discloses to be 0.46 μm in pore size rating on the basis of latex particle retention [2,8]. Therefore, even if this finding were correct, it could not suitably be extended to the more conventionally labeled 0.2 and 0.22 rated filters.

There may be reason to test at challenge densities greater than 1×10^7 CFU/cm^2 of filter surface. It is, however, incorrect to impute an inability to retain higher challenges to those sterilizing filters whose testing is performed at the 1×10^7 level.

The 1×10^7 CFU/cm^2 challenge density is an exaggeration of the number of restrictive pores. Ironically, the greater the challenge density beyond that needed to confront each individual pore, the easier the retention of the challenging organisms, if only as an expression of pore bridging and cake formation. Additionally, there is evidence from silica particle retention studies that more dilute challenge confrontations, albeit to the same total challenge density, are the more difficult ones for filters to retain [15,16]. While it may be convenient to designate a total of 1×10^7 CFU/cm^2 challenges as suitable for filter validation work, it would be more revealing and significant to base challenge levels and dilution levels on actual bioburden studies relative to the actual drug preparation whose filtrative validation is being investigated.

Interestingly, even if the sterilizing filter contained 1×10^7 restrictive pores per square centimeter, challenging with a like number of organisms would not, on the basis of probability, result in a one-on-one confrontation. Statistical considerations would result in 15% of the pores receiving multiple challenges, while approximately a like number would remain uncontested [17].

6 ORGANISM SIZING

The organism size–pore size relationship productive of filtrative sterilizations obviously requires some precise sizing of the organisms as well as of the pores. It is known that the cultivation medium can have a profound effect on both cell size and cell arrangement.

Leahy and Sullivan [18] relied on saline lactose broth as the cultivation medium for *B. diminuta* challenge organisms. Its formulation consists of 7.6 g sodium chloride, 30.0 mL lactose broth [1.3 g dehydrated lactose broth (BBL) per 100 mL distilled water], and 970 mL distilled water. Scanning electron micrographs of the resulting cultures reveal organisms that are coccobacillary in appearance and are present as single cells. Their aspect ratios are 1.0–2.5. Following the incubation stage the broth culture is filtered through 0.45 μm rated filters but are retained by 0.22 (0.2) μm rated membranes.

Fennington and Howard [19] used a growth medium consisting of 7 g trypticase, 2.5 g of yeast extract, 0.5 g sodium chloride, and 2 mmol magnesium sulfate per liter. The cultivated cells were stored as frozen cell pastes after suitable manipulations and treatments and reconstituted from the cell paste. The cell size was confirmed by scanning electron microscopy (SEM) as having widths of 0.32–0.35 μm and lengths of 0.82–0.96 μm. These dimensions are consistent with previously reported cell sizes of 0.3–0.4 × 0.6–1.0 μm for *B. diminuta* [18]. The passage of the organisms through 0.45 μm rated membranes, after a titer reduction of four logs, followed by their retention by 0.2 μm rated membranes serves microfiltratively to define the correctness of the organism sizes.

Some investigators fear that organism suspensions reconstituted from pastes may result in at least partial organism agglomeration. Those of Fennington and Howard [19] were free of such defects, as indicated by SEM, plate count, and direct microscopic count measurements.

It is *B. diminuta* organisms thus suitably prepared to proper size by techniques such as the foregoing that are used in the challenge work central to the filter validation exercise. Still to be considered are the effects of the filtration conditions and of the attributes of the specific drug solutions on the organism–pore size relationship and on the adsorption of organisms by the filter within the context of worst-case conditions.

7 SIEVE RETENTION

The principle of sieve retention is simple. Unless the particle or pore becomes distorted, a particle larger than the pore cannot pass through the pore aperture. Hence, the emphasis is on the size of the pores and the relative size of the organisms. The number of challenging particles makes no difference; the applied differential pressure, short of its effect on deformation, is without influence. The nature of the particle-suspending medium, provided it is not incompatible with either the filter or the particle, has no effect; nor do the various filtration conditions of temperature, viscosity, osmolarity, ionic strength, pH, etc. Where the smallest particle of the particle size distribution is larger than the largest pore of the pore size distribution, the filter is absolute in its retention, but only then.

However, even subtle incompatibilities between the microporous membrane and the contacting fluid can alter the pore size dispositions. Pore enlargement may endanger the sieve retention of the organisms. Plasticization of the polymeric microporous membrane, a manifestation of liquid–solid incompatibility, results in a diminution of its solid-state viscosity. In consequence, polymeric intersegmental movement becomes possible. Swelling, and the release of stresses inevitably built in during the membrane casting process will result. In the complex of antagonistic swelling and shrinking forces, individual pores may become larger. Significant pore enlargements should be detectable by bubble point integrity test measurements [6].

The surety of the sieve retention of *B. diminuta* by sterilizing filters can also be imperiled by shrinkage of the organism size. Ionic strengths and osmolarities can affect the sizes of organisms.

7.1 Osmolarity

Size changes in an organism can result from responses to osmolarity differences. Osmolarities of about 150–500 mosM result in a shrinking of bacterial cell size [20–23]. This is a consequence of the movement of water from within the bacterial cell across its semipermeable membrane in response to the higher saline gradient of the suspending medium. Levy et al. [24,25] reference numerous examples of such occurrences. These authors cite work [26] wherein cells cultured in 150 mosM sodium chloride medium exhibited a decrease of 15 or 21%, respectively, when osmotically shocked to 300 or 500 mosM. High osmolarity would therefore constitute a worst-case condition in that it would tend to reduce the likelihood of sieve retentions.

7.2 Ionic Strength

High osmolarities are produced by high ionic strengths. Where the ionic components of the solution cannot permeate the bacterial membrane, their effect, through the Donnan equilibrium, is to draw water out of the cell, thus reducing its size. This threat to the sieve retention of organisms makes high ionic strength a worst-case situation.

The influence of high ionic strengths in reducing the negative charges on filter surfaces, along with its concomitant effect on adsorptive sequestrations, is discussed shortly. In this situation, low ionic strengths present a worst-case scenario.

7.3 Assimilable Organic Carbon

The availability of assimilable organic carbon is a key determinant of both cell size [27,28] and cell surface interactions [29,30]. As nutrient levels decrease, cells increase their cell surface/volume ratio and export hydrophobic proteins to the cell wall exterior. The net effect of these two actions is to miniaturize cell size and increase hydrophobic interactions with substrata, respectively.

Several workers have shown that nutrient-limiting environments promote the attachment of bacteria to surfaces [31,32]. For example, Davies and McFeters [33] found that planktonic (free-floating) bacterial growth on low nutrient minimal media resulted in a significant reduction in bacterial size in a simulated drinking water environment. Predictions of whether a given organism will adhere to a particular surface are highly dependent on the nature of the suspending milieu and the physiological status of the bacterial community present. Bacterial metabolism and cell surface structures are influenced by the physicochemical characteristics (e.g., surface charge, functional groups, stearic factors) of the substratum (Fig. 1).

A low assimilable carbon level, in tending to reduce cell size, would offer a worst-case situation. However, by promoting organism attachments to surfaces, it

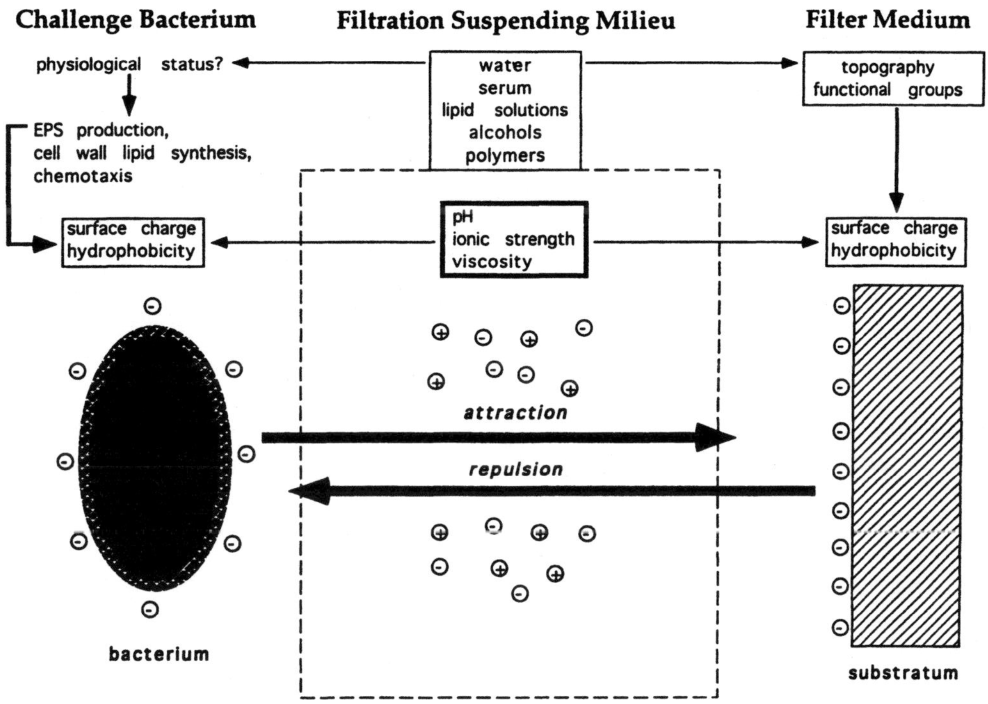

Figure 1 Influence of bacterial physiology and characteristics of substratum on adherence. (From Ref. 60.)

would present an opposite effect. Because of the importance to the validation effort of the sieve retention mechanism, the tendency here is to regard low assimilable carbon levels as a worst case.

8 ADSORPTIVE SEQUESTRATION

That adsorptive influences serve to retain organisms on filter surfaces has been long known [34]. Recognition of the fact by the practitioners of pharmaceutical filtration was, however, delayed. There was an adherence to the comforting concept of sterilizing membranes being inherently "absolute," that is, dependent on sieve retention. That view is not without its adherents even today. Those who share this view possibly tend to regard the FDA's insistence on filter validation as an unnecessary exercise.

8.1 Charge-Related Adsorption

The adsorption of bacteria to polymeric membrane surfaces derives from van der Waals forces, the secondary valence effects resulting from the unequal sharing of electrons by the atoms constituting the molecular species involved. The electric charges are partial, weak in character, and operative over only short distances. They are seldom, if ever, full blown in ionic nature. Nevertheless, they are charge-related and are responsive to modification by the addition of other charged entities such as hydronium ions (i.e., changes in pH), particularly multivalent cations derived from soluble salts.

The special case of hydrogen bonding may also find expression in adsorptive sequestration. In this instance, a hydrogen atom bearing a partial positive charge because it was deprived of its equal share of bonding electrons by an adjoining atom (e.g., part of a bacterium surface), may become charge-bonded to an oxygen or nitrogen atom constituting part of another molecular structure (e.g., part of a polymeric filter surface). The oxygen or nitrogen atom involved comes to bear a partial negative charge, the result of its possessing more than its equitable share of the electrons involved in its covalent bonding within the molecule.

8.2 Hydrophobic Adsorption

Whatever the origins of the charge governing adsorption, their nature is widely comprehended. It is generally appreciated that bacterial adsorption can result from electrical attractions between unlike-charged atoms. What is less widely understood is that bacterial adsorption onto filter surfaces may be the result of hydrophobic adsorption, a phenomenon completely independent of charge considerations [35].

Molecules of like cohesive energy densities tend to associate with one another. The cohesive energy density (CED) is a summation of the bonding characteristic that constitutes a molecule [36]. The alchemists described the phenomenon as "like dissolves like." There is a hierarchy of wetting, plasticizing, swelling, and dissolving that mirrors an increasing similarity in the CEDs of molecules. Molecules of unlike CED segregate from one another. Molecules of like CED tend to intermingle. Thus, polar water does not wet nonpolar polyethylene surfaces, but nonpolar hydrocarbons do. Nonpolar areas on bacterial surfaces, in like fashion, adhere to (wet) nonpolar areas on polymeric membrane surfaces. A consequence of hydrophobic adsorptions is a minimization of the free surface energy of the system. Hydrophobic adsorption results is a lessening in the extent of hydrophobic surfaces exposed to a hydrophilic liquid medium.

For whatever reason, hydrophobic adsorption is not as widely appreciated as its charge-induced counterparts. Thus, the literature contains disclaimers of organism adsorption by filters on the basis that the results are not responsive to pH changes or to the presence of multivalent cations. Hydrophobic adsorption, not being charge-governed, would be impervious to such influences. It would, however, be affected by the presence of surfactants, particularly nonionic ones [37,38]. There is reason to believe that most bacterial sequestrations by polymeric membranes are hydrophobic in character.

8.3 Surface Charge and Ionic Strength

The theory of colloid stabilization [39] as applied by Marshall et al. [32] holds that the separation between bacteria and adsorbents in an electrolyte solution is dependent on a balance between attractive and repulsive forces. The repulsive forces, mediated by like charges on the bacterial and substratum surfaces, are balanced by attractive forces, which include the hydrophobic effect and hydrogen bonding. This relationship can be described by the equation

$$V_t = V_r + V_a$$

where

V_t = total energy of interaction
V_r = energy of repulsion
V_a = energy of attraction

Bacterial adhesion to filter surfaces is often consonant with colloidal phenomena. Most particles, both bacteria and filter surfaces, are negatively charged. This is often a function of carboxylate groups that are associated with various organic compounds, usually a result of some degree of oxidation. In any case, this results in mutual repulsions of their double layers. Even were the charges of opposite types, there might be no attraction because the van der Waals forces act over only very small distances. The presence of higher ionic concentrations serves, however, to reduce the double layers, thus diminishing the distances between the charged particles and the surface. This being so, where appropriate attractive forces can manifest themselves, they do. Between like-charged surfaces, mutual repulsion still governs. However, as ionic strengths increase, the distances shrink to the point where hydrophobic, surface energy minimizing forces (not charge-related, but also operative only at short ranges) assert their influences and permit hydrophobic adsorption to occur. Indeed, as stated, for hydrophobic retentions, low ionic strengths serve as worst-case conditions in that they minimize organism arrests.

Ionic strength is a major determinant of cell surface charge and, by extension, the association of bacteria with charged surfaces. Fletcher [40] showed, for example, that the adhesion of *Pseudomonas fluorescens* to glass substrata was favored under conditions of increased ionic strength (addition of NaCl). A number of workers have reviewed the importance of cell surface charge on bacterial sorption to various surfaces [32,41–44].

The extent and direction of this influence depends on the magnitude of the ionic strength. It is for reasons such as this that different preparations, each containing the $1 \times 10^7/\text{cm}^2$ challenge of *B. diminuta*, may yield different degrees of retention with the same sterilizing filter. This is also why there is an insistence that the efficacy of the sterilizing filter be demonstrated under the circumstances of severest use, under worst-case conditions.

9 PRODUCT-SPECIFIC ATTRIBUTES

Ionic strength is just one of the product-specific attributes that may influence organism retention by filters through the adsorptive mechanism. Other compositional attributes under worst-case conditions, considered below, include pH, osmolarity, viscosity, and surface tension, particularly as related to the influence of surfactants.

The effects of osmolarity and assimilable organic carbon levels on organism size and, through those agencies, on the reliability of the sieve retention mechanism have already been remarked on.

9.1 pH Effects

pH measurements reflect the concentrations of hydrogen ions (hydronium ions, H_3O^+) and hydroxyl ions present in the solution. The influences of such charged entities on the surface charges represented by the double layers of polymeric membrane surfaces are similar in kind to those exercised by other like-charged ions. The effects on double layer distances and on hydrophobic adsorption can be expected to be similar. Nevertheless, as Levy et al. [24,25] indicate, it is difficult to predict the effects of pH on organism adsorption. At the pH level at which the polymeric filter has a negative charge, it is unsuited for bonding to negatively charged organisms. However, proteinaceous constituents of the bacterial cell surface may possess positive charges. Adsorptions may result. Levy et al. [24,25] state that nitrocellulose filters exhibit a positive charge below pH 4. Values of pH above this level would therefore increasingly constitute a "worst case" in terms of repelling negatively charged organisms, additionally frustrating their adsorption.

Levy [45] and Leahy [46] reported that varying the pH does not affect the organism retention by given mixed esters of cellulose membranes. Leahy and Sullivan [18] show, however, that the degrees of retention by these filters do vary with differential pressure, an indication that adsorptive influences are involved. Furthermore, nonionic surfactants do affect particle retention [37,38]. The implications are that hydrophobic adsorptions, not charge-related attractions, are at work. As stated, most organism adsorptions to polymeric filters are believed to be hydrophobic in nature.

The literature indicates that pH influences cell surface charges and hence the cell's adhesion to surfaces as well as the binding capacity of the cell surface. Additionally, pH importantly governs extracellular polymer stability. The chief consideration of pH may be the negative effects of pH values below 6 on organism survival. The optimal range for challenge organism viability is probably $6.5 \leq \text{pH} \leq 7.5$. Since the validation study requires the presence and detectability of live organisms (bacteria), surrogate solutions should be within that pH range.

9.2 Surface Tension

Surface tension that is the result of the presence of surfactants in a solution is an attribute to be considered. The adsorption of surfactant by both filter and organisms creates mutual repulsions [37]. Ridgway explains this as being due to the hydrophobic adsorption of surfactant to both surfaces, leaving the relatively polar moieties of these molecules to face and repel one another (Fig. 2). As a result, surfactants, even in concentrations of less than 0.05%, serve to prevent organism adsorption. Tolliver and Schroeder [38] demonstrate the effect of such a concentration of a nonionic surfactant on influencing the organism retention by membranes of different polymeric compositions (Table 1). The surfactant preempts the surfaces present by hydrophobic adsorption, competitively preventing organism–filter interfacing. Nonionic surfactants are the operative entities. Cationic and anionic surfactants are not as effective. The presence of nonionic surfactants, therefore, contributes to a worst-case situation.

The presence of surface-active agents, as stated, disrupts hydrophobic-type interactions between challenge organisms and filter media. Indeed, surfactants are useful in removing fouling organisms from membrane media [47] and other surfaces. They should be expected to influence organism retention by adsorption.

Lytle and Roustson [48] examined the influence of a buffered saline solution containing surfactants, serum, or culture broth on viral retention by nitrocellulose and cationic polysulfone membranes. They found that various challenge viruses could be bound by hydrophobic and electrostatic interactions and that the nonionic

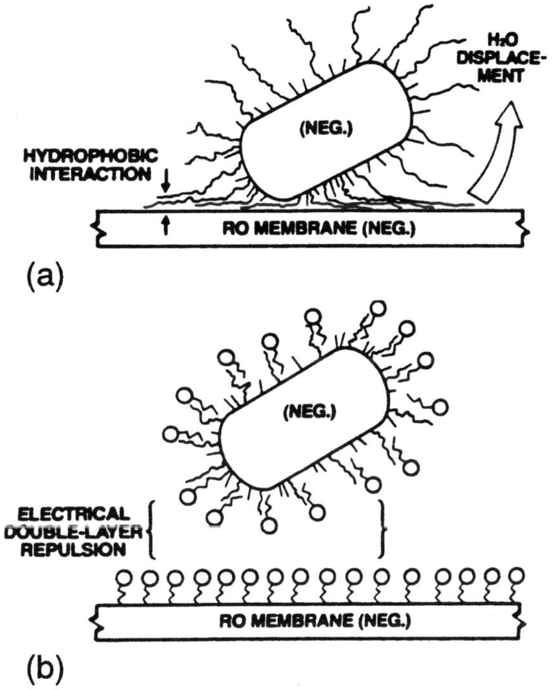

Figure 2 Diagrammatic illustration of surfactant activity. (a) Displacement of a structured layer of absorbed water by approaching surfaces increases system entropy, which drives the reaction forward. (b) In the presence of a surfactant, hydrophobic sites on the cell and reverse osmosis membrane are masked by detergent molecules, thereby precluding a hydrophobic interaction. (From Ref. 47.)

detergents Triton X-100 and Tween 80 minimized adsorptive capture by either type of interaction. Similar findings were reported for a 5% serum addition. Interestingly, neither sodium dodecyl sulfate (an anionic detergent) nor fluorochemical surfactants (cationic) were effective in this regard. It is likely that these findings could be ex-

Table 1 Percent Retention of 0.198 μm Latex Particles by Various 0.2 μm Rated Membranes Using Turbidity Measurements

Filter type	In water	In 0.05% Triton X-100
Polycarbonate	100.0	100.0
Asymmetric polysulfone	100.0	100.0
Polyvinylidene fluoride	74.8	19.2
Nylon 66	82.1	1.0
Cellulose esters	89.4	25.1

Source: Ref. 38.

tended to the minimization of adsorptive bacterial capture using the same membranes.

9.3 Viscosity

It has been commonly supposed that higher viscosities would militate against adsorptive organism retention by making it more difficult for microbes, suspended midstream, to reach pore walls under the impetus of Brownian motion before the flow conveys them through the filter. The key consideration is the rate of flow. At any viscosity, given a Hookean response by the liquid, flow rate varies directly with differential pressure. The rates involved in adsorptive attachments are unknown. If they are not instantaneous, it can be postulated that the bacterium, regardless of its proximity to the pore wall, could be ejected through the pore passageway before adsorption could occur.

Perhaps viscosity is not among the significant attributes to consider given the findings of Aranha and Meeker [49], namely, that the filtrative removal of challenging organisms was not affected by testing in 80% glycerol, a medium of 75 cP viscosity at 25°C and 16 cP at 42°C. These investigators found that 80% glycerol did not effect a significant loss in challenge organism viability. Viable *B. diminuta* were not recovered from the test filtrates.

In any case, product-specific attributes and their influence in respect to organism retention need to be evaluated before the challenge test is performed. This is commonly done with a viability test to investigate the survival of the organism or possible damage to the organism. Challenge tests performed without an initial viability test are meaningless, due to the fact that one does not know what viable titer is actually challenging. Filter validation work should include and document the outcome of a viability test.

10 FILTRATION CONDITIONS

In addition to the particular attributes of the specific organism-suspending medium, the operational conditions governing the filtration define the extent of adsorptive retention achieved by a given filter. Temperature and its effects on viscosity, applied differential pressure, and duration of the filtration, all interrelated factors, exert their influence.

10.1 Temperature

Temperature has several effects that require consideration. Viscosity varies directly with temperature. One of the consequences is that at a given differential pressure a fluid will flow faster at more elevated temperatures. This, in turn, will govern the duration of the filtration. In this sense, higher temperatures become the equivalent of higher differential pressures. Leahy and Sullivan [18] showed that organism retention by membrane filters could decrease at elevated transmembrane pressures. This occurs for ''nonsterilizing'' filters presumably because of the reduced intervals for adsorptive removal as occasioned by shorter residence times of the fluid within the filter. Therefore, elevated temperatures would define the worst-case condition. For ''sterilizing'' filters, the sieve retention mechanism is operative, in the Leahy and Sullivan work, regardless of the differential pressures investigated, namely, 50 psi.

Table 2 Rate of Kill by Heat of *Pseudomonas pickettii* in 0.9% Sodium Chloride Solution

Temperature	*D* value[a]
50°C (122°F)	26.0
55°C (131°F)	1.9
60°C (140°F)	0.7

[a]*D* value = time required for 90% kill or 10 log reduction.
Source: Ref. 50.

Higher temperatures in conjunction with some particular ingredients may also have untoward effects on filter compatibilities. This can be assessed through application of filter integrity testing to detect changes in values.

The influence of temperature on microbial growth and reproduction requires consideration (Table 2). Organism growth and survival temperatures between 35 and 40°C are suitable. Aranha and Meeker [49] found that a 3 h exposure to 42°C (in glycerol) resulted in significant losses in *B. diminuta* viability. As Levy et al. [24,25] state, "It may be reasonable to hypothesize that bacteria, such as *B. diminuta*, would reproduce more effectively at 35°C than at 20°C. This could produce a higher effective challenge over a longer duration."

It is assumed on the basis of the above considerations that higher temperatures, but not exceeding 40°C (for *B. diminuta*), define a worst-case situation.

10.2 Flow Rate, Differential Pressure, Processing Time

Higher differential pressures produce higher flow rates and therefore shorter processing times. However measured, these interconnecting phenomena, by minimizing opportunities for adsorptive sequestration by way of decreasing contact times, become defined as worst-case conditions. It should be pointed out, however, that longer filtration time promotes opportunities for organism proliferation and therefore could constitute a more severe challenge [17,49].

Tanny et al. [51] show that for a filter dependent upon adsorptive captures to achieve solution sterilization, lower applied differential pressures are more effective (see Table 3). Leahy and Sullivan [18] find the same effect (Table 4).

11 ORGANISM CHALLENGE LEVEL

In addition to the suspending solution's compositional attributes and the physical and hydraulic factors mentioned, the organism challenge level itself influences the extent of adsorptive sequestration [52,53]. As shown in Fig. 3, the larger the pore size and the greater the challenge level, the more likely are the organisms confronting the filter to escape adsorptive arrest. This factor would seem not to be important in the validation exercise, given its standardization by the FDA at the 1×10^7 CFU/cm^2 level. However, the organism dilution level comprising the total challenge has been neither defined nor investigated.

Table 3 Capture Efficiencies of 0.45 μm Cellulose Triacetate Membranes at Various Pressures. Challenge Concentration 1×10^5 Organisms/mL or $2 \times 10^7/cm^2$ Filter Area

Operating pressure (psi)	Organisms per 100 mL 500 mL	1000 mL	1500 mL	2000 mL	Number of organisms in filtrate/mL	Capture efficiency E
5	0	0	0	0	0	0.99995_0
5	4	12	7200	7200		
5	0	0	0	0		
15	0	13	19	39	10–20	0.9999_0
15	3	2	0	7200		
15	6	15	12	11		
30	93	91	61	66	50–100	0.999_5
30	38	34	39	52		
30	7200	7200	7200	7200		

Source: Ref. 51.

It has largely been assumed that the more massive organism challenges pose the worst-case conditions. Most filter validations therefore emulate the qualification procedures whereby the filter manufacturers confront the filter being tested with a high concentration of organisms. This also serves the practical purpose of minimizing the total volume of liquid being filtered. Convenience and even practicality notwithstanding, there is reason to believe that a diluted organism suspension whose total challenges add to 1×10^7 organisms per square centimeter of filter surface constitutes the worst-case condition, the very opposite of the filtrative exercise often practiced.

Roberts et al. [15] and Grant and Zahka [16], found that confronting microporous membranes with relatively dilute suspensions of monosized cross-linked polystyrene spheres resulted initially in their complete retention followed by a decrease in their arrests. With further filtration, some restitution of better retention resulted. The latter can be explained by the incipient development of a filter cake and its contribution to particle capture. However, given pore size distributions and the

Table 4 Effect of Pressure on the Passage of *P. diminuta* Through Membranes of Various Pore Sizes

Filter type	Pore size (μm)	β ratio 0.5 psid	5 psid	50 psid
GS	0.22	$>10^{10}$	$>10^{10}$	$>10^{10}$
HA	0.45	10^8	10^7	10^6
DA	0.65	10^4	10^4	10^3
AA	0.80	10^2	10	10

Source: Ref. 18.

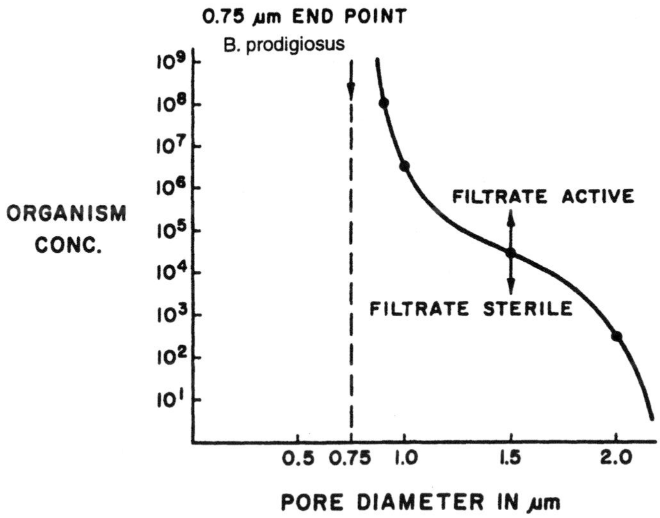

Figure 3 Pore diameter versus *Bacillus prodigiosus* concentration. Whether the effluent is sterile or active is a result of these parameters. (From Ref. 53.)

greater tendency for fluid to flow through larger pores, the first particles might have been expected to find the larger pores and pass through them without capture. The observed phenomena can be rationalized as follows. The hydrodynamic flow bearing the particles does seek the larger pores. These, however, are so few in number as to escape substantial challenge because the liquid flow reflects the presence of far more numerous smaller pores. It is the retaining action of these small pores that makes for the initial complete retention. As the smaller pores become blocked by the particles they retain, they are removed from further filter action. The relatively fewer large pores become increasingly important, progressively representing a larger proportion of the operative pores. Particles are increasingly borne to these larger pores with heightened possibilities of escaping capture. Interestingly, more massive initial challenges of filters do not reveal declines in the perfection of the particle retention. This may be due to particle agglomerations forming large particles capable of blocking the larger pores, to the bridging of large pores, or to a shortening of the time needed to form a filter cake.

Irrespective of the correctness of the above rationalization, a less dense challenge, not a more concentrated challenge, may constitute worst-case conditions. If so, what actual dilution of organisms is appropriate to filter validation? The answer should mirror the actual bioburden typical of the drug preparation being filtered. Since this may differ from lot to lot, historical data should be developed. Bioburden characterizations of the drug preparations are therefore an integral part of the filter validation requirement to establish the appropriate log reduction. Although required, these determinations are not always performed. Nevertheless, most filter vendors conduct the product bacterial challenge test by the incremental addition of the bacterial suspension to the recirculated product or placebo. A full range of challenge levels, up to the level of 1×10^7, is thus introduced.

12 TESTING: METHOD AND SCALE

12.1 The Test Method

The organism suspension challenging the filter whose sterilizing performance is being validated is led into the housing containing the filter. The effluent is then passed through the reference filter whose function is to retain any organisms that were not removed by the filter being tested. The presence of organisms, if any, on the reference filter is then ascertained.

12.2 The Scale of the Test

The scale on which the validation exercise is performed requires thought. The more closely the test resembles actual production conditions, the more dependable and significant its revelations. However, the greater the volume of test liquid involved, the less practical the operational transactions. Convenience is not the only consideration. Contamination of the test results and the finding of false positives occasioned by more extensive and prolonged manipulations must be considered. Additionally, some products are considerably more costly to validate. The greater the volume or volumes required for the validation work, the more considerable the cost factor. For this reason, at least two different approaches seek to make the exercise practical. In the first, rather than a filter device, a section of the membrane filter, usually a 47 mm disc, is used. An actual filter device is more complicated, and its filter action may be different, perhaps even significantly so; however, the use of a small section of membrane makes it possible to test the entire volume of the filtrate, a necessity where sterility is to be ensured. Assaying aliquot portions of the filtrate to demonstrate their sterility leaves unanswered the question of the sterility of the untested remainder. Therefore, the *total* filtrate must be assayed, sterility being an absolute condition. In this approach, efforts are made to keep the volume, surface, and time relationships as similar as possible to those existing in an actual production run. Unfortunately, the flaw in this approach occurs when there is an increase in scale, such as going from beaker to pilot plant to full-scale operation, which may involve very different rates and interactions and may yield different results. Therefore, there are those who champion filter validations using actual filter devices. These can even be 10 in. filter elements, which can cause the above-mentioned complications. For this reason some filter manufacturers use small-scale pleated filter units that are equal in material choice and construction to the larger filter elements.

12.3 Hydraulic Shock

One reason for basing the validation test on a pleated filter device rather than on flat membrane discs of whatever size is that flexing of the side seams and of filter pleats, as well as the stressing of the points of bonding of filter to end cap, is occasioned by the pumping action that takes place. Indeed, the hydraulic stressing of the filters could conceivably lead to failure and requires assessment as part of the filter validation effort. At the very least, repetitive pulsing studies on the filter should be carried out.

A first approach could use a small pleated device, possibly a capsule, flexed for the number of times it, or a cartridge, would receive pumping impulses during its service life. Even here, assumptions are made. Pleat lengths will differ between the actual cartridge filter and the smaller prototype being tested. The stresses and their effects will not be the same. Some filter vendors implement pulsation test procedures to investigate the performance of their filters under hydraulic shock conditions. The results of such tests are usually described and documented in the product qualification documentation available from the vendor.

13 RECOVERY METHOD

The ultimate decision on whether the filter being validated has completely retained its organism challenge is commonly made by using the recovery method. The liquid filtered through the membrane is passed through a collection membrane intended to capture any organisms that were not arrested by the filter being assayed. The collection filter with its retained microbes, if any, is placed on nutrient and incubated. After a suitable interval, the colonies formed by the organisms are counted under a microscope.

Traditionally, a 0.45 μm rated membrane is used for this purpose. It might be thought that a 0.2 μm rated collection filter would be more likely to ensure the trapping of organisms; however, Sladek et al. [54] demonstrated that, for whatever reason, larger populations of organisms are recovered using 0.45 μm rated membranes. This experimental observation is confirmed by Bordner [55] on the basis of extensive studies on microbiological assays of water. Periodically, efforts are made to use a 0.2 μm rated membrane in recovery contexts. Claims of superiority for 0.2 μm filters have thus far not been convincing [56]. To be sure, the 0.2 μm rated filter may be more retentive, but fewer of the retained organisms may survive to be tallied than when a 0.45 μm rated filter is used. The 0.2 μm rated filter is used in the sterility procedure wherein the filter and its retained organisms are directly transferred into nutrient broth for incubation and for turbidity detection of microbial growth. This sterility test method, however, lacks the possibilities of quantitation and speciation sought by some from the recovery method.

Groves [57] centers on the problem involved in the recovery method. He asks, "Why should a second filter collect particles that have already passed through a first filter?" Inherent in his question is the knowledge that the referenced filter expected to retain the organisms is 0.45 μm rated. These microbes have just negotiated a 0.2 μm rated membrane. An exclusive reliance on the sieve retention mechanism underlies the logic of Groves' question. The use of the 0.45 μm rated membrane in the recovery method has rested on the experience of Sladek et al. [54]. Interestingly, the recovery method was designed for microbiological water assays. Sterility is usually not a concern in drinking or recreational water examinations. The 0.45 μm membrane was not expected to contribute quantitative colony counts, but rather larger numbers, perhaps more meaningful to compare, than the 0.2 μm rated filter.

Levy [58], in reply to Groves, states that the 0.45 μm rated reference filters "do not allow any *Pseudomonas diminuta* to pass through until concentrations > 1000 colony-forming units have challenged this filter." This is perhaps the key issue. Has this filter action itself been validated? The complexity of filter validation is shown by the need for the recovery method itself to be validated as yielding absolute retentions. The work of Leahy and Sullivan [18] demonstrates that the 0.45 μm rated mixed esters of cellulose membrane can completely retain 1×10^4–1×10^5 CFU of *B. diminuta* before organism passage commences. Carter [59] validates that the

0.45 μm rated polyvinylidene fluoride membrane is also suitable as a reference filter in the recovery method. It is often assumed that other 0.45 μm rated membranes available in the market perform similarly. Some filter manufacturers advise that their 0.2 μm rated membrane be used for recovery purposes.

14 STERILITY TESTING

Validation procedures are classically divided into four steps: design qualification (DQ), installation qualification (IQ), operational qualification (OQ), and performance qualification (PQ). In the last step, the properly designed, installed, and operationally tested purification units are tested in an ongoing production mode to determine how the entire integrated process performs. Munson [60] considers the present filter validation status as possibly lacking the PQ stage. He suggests as a suitable PQ the filtering of the effluent from the sterilizing filter by passing it through a tighter reference filter—possibly using a 0.2 μm rated membrane followed by a 0.1 μm rated filter. The residence filter is to be examined for retained organisms by a sterility test, by being incubated while immersed in nutrient. The sterility testing method, the use of a reference filter tight enough unequivocally to retain organisms that may penetrate the test filter followed by immersion in growth medium, offers an alternative to the recovery method.

15 DIRECT TRANSFER METHOD

Attempts, anecdotally reported, have been made to validate the recovery method by subjecting the entire effluent from the reference membrane to the direct transfer sterility-type assay. One filter company mixed 100–200 mL portions with concentrated tripicase soy broth and incubated the mixture at 30°C for 7 and 14 days. No organism growth resulted. Larger volumes can be handled as multiples of such portions albeit at the risk of encouraging false positives. Efforts, again anecdotally reported, have been made to substitute the direct transfer method for the recovery method. One filter company, after challenging the filter being validated by a suspension of *Pseudomonas diminuta* in growth medium, incubated the entire 20–25 L effluent in a 30 L container. The inconvenience of handling so large a volume was finessed by a filter user who challenged a 10 in. cartridge filter being validated with a 1 L suspension of organisms and recirculated the effluent by pumping, to mimic the requisite larger volume. In the presence/absence direct transfer method of sterility testing, the development of turbidity, subject to the elimination of false positives, would be taken as evidence of lack of sterility.

The solution volume used is not so critical in examining those aspects of filter validation—pH, viscosity, flow rates, pressure, temperature, hydraulic shock, and compatibility—that do not involve demonstrating sterility, the complete absence of organisms. Here smaller portions can be used based on the simple ratio of volume to filter surface, as established by the area of the test filter. Alternatively, a small portion of a solution can be recirculated repetitively through a given filter to simulate exposure to a larger volume or for a longer time. This is also of use where an expensive drug is involved.

16 FURTHER VALIDATION ASPECTS

Besides the validation of the filter in terms of its retentive capabilities with the actual drug product, other validation features need to be considered. These elements do not have to be applied in every instance but are commonly needed for proper documentation and understanding of the process. Such validation aspects are, for example, product integrity test values, particulate counting, chemical compatibility testing, and adsorption and extractable studies, just to name a few. Some of these evaluations are done during the product stability test phase; nevertheless, other tests are also performed by the user or by the filter vendor in close conjunction with the user.

16.1 Product Integrity Testing

The filter integrity test is a nondestructive test to evaluate whether the filter unit is integral or contains a flaw. The tests most commonly used are the diffusive flow, pressure-hold, and bubble point procedures. Due to the physics of the tests, all can be influenced by the properties of the product; for example, a reduced surface tension will create a lower bubble point value. To avoid any such influences on the water integrity test values given by the filter vendor, water can be flushed through the filter when the integrity test is performed after product filtration. Nevertheless, it is often difficult to remove all product residues from the filter matrix; furthermore, surface-active substances are extremely difficult to flush out. For these reasons an excessive amount of water may be needed to achieve a reliable integrity test result. In some cases, when protein solutions are filtered, the fouling of proteins on the membrane influences the integrity test value. In these instances one can flush the filter with solvents before performing the integrity test.

To avoid any of the above-mentioned lengthy and costly proceedings, filter vendors offer to evaluate the product integrity test limits for their specific filter units. A correlation between the water test limit and the product is established. This is usually performed with a minimum of three different filter lots and, in the case of variable product specifications, also with three lots of product. A helpful tool to evaluate the product integrity test limits is the multipoint diffusion test. It tests the filter element at several different test pressures and yields a graph from a low diffusion level to the bubble point itself [61]. The graph shows whether the product bubble point value shifted from the water value as expected or whether the slope of the graph shifted, as if due to a fault. Multipoint diffusion testing offers enhanced reliability in evaluating product integrity test limits.

16.2 Particulate and Chemical Compatibility Tests

Most filter vendors test their filters for particulates to fulfill USP 23 requirements. These tests are performed in the product qualification stage of the filter product validation. Usually the test is performed using high purity water. The test results are documented in the validation or product qualification guides. This is also done for the chemical compatibility, which is listed for a variety of chemicals. Compatibility tests are performed over a 7-day period. After this period the filter elements are checked in terms of their performance and integrity. Despite the tests performed at the filter vendor's facility, particulates and chemical compatibility testing by the filter user is still needed in certain instances, as when the product/filter behavior is unknown or thought to cause problems. Particulates should specifically be assessed for when the actual product is a small-volume parenteral; chemical compatibility should be tested when the solvent used for the products is known or suspected to cause problems or interactions.

16.3 Extractables Testing

As with particulates, especially with chemical compatibility testing, extractables testing is important to gain knowledge of product–filter interactions or to learn whether the filter releases substances that could influence the product quality. The initial extractables testing is repeated during the product qualification stage and is documented in the vendors' guidelines. Often, only gravimetric measurements are performed. However, these are quantitative only for nonvolatile residues and do not reveal chemical identities. More modern techniques, described in Chapter 8, are required. These are more precise and revealing. Their methodologies and results have general application to product extractables testing. Usually these are necessary only when it is known that a product–filter interaction is possible or that the process conditions, e.g., elevated temperatures or long contact times, promote the chance of extractables release. In any case, these more sophisticated extractable studies offered by the individual filter vendor are available to the filter users.

17 ORGANISM-SUSPENDING PLACEBO

As discussed, the surest demonstration of filter validation requires the use of product-specific media under the conditions defined as worst-case or praxis for that particular filtration operation. Such preparations can contain ingredients that are inhibitory to organism growth in quantities too large to be removed without substantially changing the nature of the drug. In such cases, as stated, the filter is equilibrated with the product, which is then removed by washing. The filter is then challenged with the standard suspension of *B. diminuta*. Often, no special attention is paid to the organism-suspending fluid; even water is sometimes used. Challenge suspensions in saline lactose have been accepted by the regulatory authorities.

The rationale for exposing the filter to the drug and then washing out the inhibitory (and other) ingredients is that the filter's contact with the specific drug preparation may engender pore enlargement where incompatibilities exist. The larger pores will become manifest by passing more organisms. If such failures at organism containment do not occur, validation of the filter is assumed. The emphasis is on sieve retention, but unfortunately not sufficiently so. The influence of the drug product on organism size and the adsorptive influences arising from the product attributes and the "worst-case conditions" will not be known. A suitable placebo or surrogate solution is required for this purpose [62]. A proper assessment of the product-exposed and washed filter requires a confrontation with organisms in a vehicle whose attributes match those of the drug product of specific interest as closely as possible. Water or some other innocuous liquid does not suffice. Although it is true that FDA inspectors may accept organisms-in-water or organisms-in-saline lactose challenges, if these lead to perverse consequences, the drug preparer, not the FDA, will be held liable. The goal is for the surrogate solution to be imitative of the specific drug preparation in its attributes.

18 DEVISING SURROGATE SOLUTIONS

A more ambitious goal might also be attempted: an effort to define more universal surrogate solutions to substitute for the product-specific media that are now required. However, all too few studies have been directed specifically to the elucidation of particular solution attribute effects on organism retention by membrane filters. Comprehension of the several processing and solution attributes governing filtration validations are imperfectly understood. Their quantitation and the assessment of their interactions can, at best, be only approximated [62]. Under these circumstances, specific guidance is not presently feasible. Nevertheless, knowing the directions of the influences of the several attributes and filter conditions on adsorptive effects and on organism and pore sizes can permit beginnings of tests even in that direction, subject to eventual refinements.

One purpose of this chapter is to examine the attributes generally considered as defining worst-case conditions with a view to devising proper surrogate solutions. The desired suspending medium would expose the organisms to virtual product conditions and would militate against their retention by adsorption. Additionally, it would investigate the solution's influence on the challenge organisms, including their viability. This would ensure that the sterilizing action of the filter being tested is solely the consequence of sieve retention, its dependability ascertained by assessment of the solution's influence on the size of the organisms and pores.

Surrogate solutions can be postulated as organism-suspending media that would minimize, if not eliminate, adsorptive retention. Such a solution could be high in viscosity. It would be low in surface tension, as caused by the presence of a nonionic surfactant. Its pH would reflect the charge optimization appropriate to the particular filter being validated, as defined by the filter manufacturer. As has been discussed, both high and low ionic strengths can operate to create worst-case conditions, high ionic strengths operating to diminish organism size. Osmolarities, likewise, pose worst cases in both their low and high values. The high osmolarities, when the solutes are not transferable into the microbe, tend to shrink the organisms. The construction of the placebo would imitate the specific drug of interest in the choice of the high or low alternative concentrations.

This surrogate solution would be employed at an appropriate processing temperature, preferably in the range of 35–40°C, to avoid evaluation of the complicating influences of temperature on organism proliferation, viscosity, and adsorptive bonding. The organism challenge would be performed at high differential pressures for a duration of time relevant to the processing practice. The presence of protein in the surrogate solution could be explored for its interference with organism adsorption to the filter, as has been alleged. Above all, however, it would be necessary to make certain that the requisite organism concentration could survive in the synthesized placebo. Where helpful to this end, low concentrations of assimilable carbon sources could be employed as nutrients.

19 GROUPING OF PRODUCTS

The requirement that a filter be validated for use with each specific drug product can pose an impractical and costly burden on the manufacturers of multiple drug products. It can also be an unnecessary tax in cases where drug products may not differ appreciably from one another. Efforts are therefore made to group drugs in terms of similarity of composition, properties, and/or filtration conditions to minimize the number requiring individual validation. However, attempts at grouping products suitable for a single validation encounter the same problems as those involved in devising surrogate solutions, namely, the quantitation and balancing of the several conflicting and/or reinforcing product attributes and operational filtration conditions simultaneously influencing the overall result.

An early effort at grouping, impressive in its reach, was undertaken to construct an envelope of acceptable limits for drug attributes and filtration conditions as defined by successful validations. Drugs not yet validated would not require testing, provided their attributes and filtration parameters fell within the acceptance envelope [24,25]. This effort was considered too broad in scope to be justifiable, particularly in that the interactions of the various influences were unknown and unquantified and therefore incapable of being properly balanced.

A narrower scope, called bracketing, could be acceptable. An unvalidated drug preparation whose attributes were between those of two drugs that had been successfully validated might not require individual testing provided that the limiting experiences were only narrowly separated. The judgment on "narrow" would have to be that of the FDA. It would likely be made on the basis of some quantitative measure, e.g., by considering the percentage of difference between the not-yet-validated drug and the validated drugs. Judgments would be made on a case-by-case basis, not by a set formula.

Two types of groupings seem beyond reasonable challenge. A series of preparations differing only in the concentration of an active ingredient, e.g., 0.1% vs. 20%, all filtered under the same filtration conditions. Validation of the low, high, and possibly the middle concentrations would suffice. Again, a series of, say, 20 products differing only in the attribute of, say, viscosity could require the validation of only the low, high, and middle viscosity preparations. In general, single-parameter variations, whether of drug attribute or operational filtration condition, would seem to justify a grouping arrangement.

Whatever the attempt at grouping, the FDA must be informed of its rationale and history. The rationale is to be based on scientific principles. A successful history would sanction the rationale. Without a successful history, any effort at grouping will remain suspect. As has been observed in other human endeavors, nothing succeeds like success. Given the complexity of the situation, it remains certain that FDA judgments regarding the practice of grouping will be on a case-by-case basis.

20 RESPONSIBILITY FOR VALIDATION

That the drug processor has the ultimate responsibility of performing the filter validation is understood. On occasion this obligation may perhaps have been acknowledged somewhat perfunctorily, strong reliance, sometimes too strong, having been placed on filter vendors. The concurrence of the drug manufacturer in a validation plan discussed with a filter vendor, while appearing collegial, may have been only cursory, it being expected that the filter manufacturer was likely to possess the knowledge and experience necessary to the validation. Decisions concerning the filter validation protocol can indeed be mutually agreed upon between the drug preparer and the filter manufacturer when the latter performs the exercise for the former. The responsible discharge of the drug preparer's obligation requires, however, that he knowledgeably comprehend and endorse what the filter manufacturers may suggest be done. The decision making can be a shared enterprise; the responsibility, however, remains exclusively that of the drug manufacturer.

While the drug preparer has the responsibility for the filter validation activity, whether performed by him or by others on his behalf, the exercise must conform to the views and requirements of the FDA. Unfortunately, this necessary and prudent oversight function can have a chilling effect on those called upon to define the validation protocol. The result may be a tendency to wait for the FDA to state exactly what should be done. That is neither the agency's intention nor its function. Indeed, following FDA suggestions and even guidelines confers no immunity from untoward consequences should they occur. How to validate, precisely what to do and when, is the decision of the drug manufacturer alone. The filter vendor cannot be knowledgeable for him. The drug manufacturer must be aware of what is involved.

The practice of certification by vendors is beyond the scope of this chapter. To the extent, however, that certification of an event by a filter vendor is seen as relieving the drug preparer of his responsibilities to ascertain and evaluate an action or performance, it is judged unacceptable. Certification may serve as an assurance to its receiver. It does not, however, negate or transfer responsibilities.

It is hoped that the foregoing discussion will help guide the biopharmaceutical industry to an increasingly meaningful performance of filter validations, to the attainment of a mutually appreciated responsibility and goal.

REFERENCES

1. FDA, Guideline on General Principles of Process Validation, Center for Drugs and Biologicals and Office of Regulatory Affairs, Washington, DC, September 1985.
2. H. C. Mouwen and T. H. Meltzer, Sterilizing filters: Pore-size distributions and the $1 \times 10^7/cm^2$ challenge, *Pharm Tech.*, *16*(7):28–32 (1992).
3. P. Segers, M. Vacanneyt, B. Pot, U. Torck, B. Hoste, D. Dewettinck, E. Falsen, K. Kersters, and P. DeVos, Classification of *Pseudomonas diminuta* Leifson and Hugh 1954 and *Pseudomonas vesicularis* Busing, Doll and Freytag 1953 in *Brevundomonas* gen. nov. as *Brevundimonas diminuta* comb. nov. and *Brevundimonas vesicularis* comb. nov., respectively, *Int. J. Syst. Bacteriol.*, *44*:499–510 (1994).
4. American Society for Testing and Materials, Enumeration of aquatic bacteria by epifluorescence microscopy counting procedure, in *Water*, Vol 11.02, D-4455 85, Philadelphia, PA, 1985, pp. 632–635.
5. M. A. Innis, PCR protocols, *A Guide to Methods and Applications*, Academic, San Diego, CA, 1990.
6. R. C. Lukaszewicz and T. H. Meltzer, On the structural compatibilities of membrane filters, *J. Parenter. Drug Assoc.*, *34*:463–472 (1980).
7. F. W. Bowman, M. P. Calhoun, and M. White, Microbiological methods for quality control of membrane filters, *J. Pharm Sci.*, *56*(2):453–459 (1967).
8. V. Krygier, Rating of fine membrane filters used in the semiconductor industry, Fifth Annual Semiconductor Pure Water Conference, Jan. 16–17, San Francisco, CA, 1986, pp. 232–251.
9. HIMA Document No. 3, Vol. 4, *Microbiological Evaluation of Filters for Sterilizing Liquids*, Health Industry Manufacturing Association, Washington, DC, 1982.

10. P. R. Johnston, R. C. Lukaszewicz, and T. H. Meltzer, Certain imprecisions in the bubble point measurement, *J. Parenter. Sci. Tech.*, *35*(1):36–39 (1981).
11. T. H. Meltzer, *Filtration in the Pharmaceutical Industry*, Marcel Dekker, New York, 1987, Chap. 3.
12. T. H. Meltzer, The pore structures of microporous filters, *Ultrapure Water*, *5*(5):49–55 (1988).
13. R. E. Williams and T. H. Meltzer, Membrane structure, the bubble point and particle retention: A new theory, *Pharm. Tech.*, *7*(5):36–42 (1983).
14. M. Osumi, N. Yamada, and M. Toya, Bacterial retention mechanisms of membrane filters, *PDA J. Pharm. Sci. Technol.*, *50*(1):30–34 (1996).
15. K. L. Roberts, D. J. Velasquez, and D. M. Stofer, Challenging the membrane filter ratings, *Semicond. Int.*, *13*(11):80–84 (1990).
16. D. C. Grant and J. G. Zahka, Sieving capture of particles by microporous membrane filters from clean liquids, *Swiss Contam. Control*, *3*(4a):160–164 (1990).
17. J. M. Juran (ed.), *Quality Control Handbook*, 3rd ed., McGraw-Hill, New York, 1974, pp. 22–29; App. 2, p. 2.
18. T. J. Leahy and M. J. Sullivan, Validation of bacterial retention capabilities by membrane filters, *Pharm. Technol.*, *2*:65–75 (1978).
19. G. J. Fennington and G. Howard, Jr., Preparation and evaluation of bacterial stock for filter validation, *PDA J. Pharm. Sci. Technol.* *51*(4):153–155 (1997).
20. W. G. Characklis, Microbial biofouling control, in *Biofilms* (W. G. Characklis and K. C. Marshall, eds.), Wiley, New York, 1990, pp. 585–683.
21. P. J. Herald and E. A. Zottola, Attachment of *Listeria monocytogenes* and *Yersinia enterocolitica* to stainless steel at various temperatures and pH values, *J. Food Protect.* (abstr.). *50*:894 (1987).
22. G. K. Richards, R. F. Gagnon, G. Obst, and G. B. Kostiner, The effect of peritoneal dialysis solutions on rifampin action against *Staphylococcus epidermidis* in the fluid and biofilm phases of growth, *Periton. Dial. Int.*, *9*:183–186 (1993).
23. A. W. Hoadley, Effects of injury on the recovery of bacteria on membrane filters, in *Membrane Filtration: Application, Techniques, and Problems* (B. J. Dutka, ed.), Marcel Dekker, New York, 1981, pp. 413–450.
24. R. V. Levy, K. S. Souza, and C. B. Neville, The matrix approach: Microbial retention testing of sterilizing-grade filters with final parenteral products, Part I, *Pharm. Technol.*, *14*:160–173 (1990).
25. R. V. Levy, K. S. Souza, D. L. Hyde, S. M. Gambale, and C. B. Neville, The matrix approach: Microbial retention testing of sterilizing-grade filters with final parenteral products, Part II, *Pharm. Technol.*, *15*:58–68 (1991).
26. W. W. Baldwin, R. Myer, T. Kung, E. Anderson, and A. L. Koch, Growth and buoyant density of *Escherichia coli* at very low osmolarities, *J. Bacteriol.*, *177*:235–237 (1995).
27. R. Y. Morita, Starvation and miniaturization of heterotrophs, with special emphasis on maintenance of the starved viable state, in *Bacteria in the Natural Environments: The Effect of Nutrient Conditions* (M. Fletcher and G. Floodgate, eds.), Soc. Gen. Microbiol., London, 1985, pp. 111–130.
28. T. Nystron, R. M. Olsson, and S. Kjelleberg, Survival, stress resistance, and alterations in protein expression in the marine *Vibrio* sp. strain s14 during starvation for different individual nurients, *Appl. Environ. Microbiol.*, *58*:55–65 (1992).
29. B. Dahlback, M. Hermannsson, S. Kjelleberg, and B. Norkrans, The hydrophobicity of bacteria—An important factor in the initial adhesion at the air–water interface, *Arch. Microbiol.*, *128*:267–270 (1981).
30. M. Wrangstadh, P. L. Conway, and S. Kjelleberg, The production and release of an extracellular polysaccharide during starvation of a marine *Pseudomonas* sp. and the effect thereof on adhesion, *Arch. Microbiol.*, *145*:220–227 (1986).

31. M. W. Mittelman and D. C. White, The role of biofilms in contamination of process fluids by biological particulates, in *Particles in Gases and Liquids* (K. L. Mittal, ed.), Plenum, New York, 1990, pp. 35–50.
32. K. C. Marshall, R. Stout, and R. Mitchell, Mechanisms of the initial events in the sorption of marine bacteria to surfaces, *J. Gen. Microbiol.*, *68*:337–348 (1971).
33. D. G. Davies and G. A. McFeters, Growth and comparative physiology of *Klebsiella oxytocia* attached to GAC particles in liquid media, *Microb. Ecol.*, *15*:165–175 (1988).
34. T. H. Meltzer, *Filtration in the Pharmaceutical Industry*, Marcel Dekker, New York, 1987, Chap. 8.
35. C. Tanford, *The Hydrophobic Effect*, 2nd ed., Wiley, New York, 1980.
36. A. V. Tobolski, *Properties and Structure of Polymers*, Wiley, New York, 1960, pp. 64–66.
37. H. F. Ridgway, Microbial fouling of reverse osmosis membranes: Genesis and control, in *Biological Fouling of Industrial Water Systems: A Problem Solving Approach* (M. W. Mittelman and G. G. Geesey, eds.), Water Micro Associates, Long Beach, CA, 1987, pp. 133–198.
38. D. L. Tolliver and H. G. Schroeder, Particle control in semiconductor process stream, *Microcontamination*, *1*(1):34–43, 78 (1983).
39. B. V. Derjaguin and L. Landau, Theory of the stability of strongly charged lyophobic soils of the adhesion of strongly charged particles in solutions of electrolytes, *Acta Physicochim.*, *14*:633–662 (1941).
40. M. Fletcher, Attachment of *Pseudomonas fluorescens* to glass and influence of electrolytes on bacterium–substratum separation distance, *J. Bacteriol.*, *170*:2027–2030 (1988).
41. M. C. M. van Loosdrecht and A. J. B. Zehnder, Energetics of bacterial adhesion, *Experientia*, *46*:817–822 (1990).
42. J. Sjollema, H. J. Busscher, and A. H. Weerkamp, Experimental approaches for studying adhesion of microorganisms to solid substrata: Applications and mass transport, *J. Microbiol. Methods*, *9*:79–90 (1989).
43. G. Reid, A. E. Khoury, C. A. Preston, and J. W. Costerton, Influence of dextrose dialysis solutions on adhesion of *Staphylococcus aureus* and *Pseudomonas aeruginosa* to three catheter surfaces, *Am. J. Nephrol.*, *14*:37–40 (1994).
44. H. J. Busscher and A. H. Weerkamp, Specific and non-specific interactions in bacterial adhesion to solid substrata, *FEMS Microbiol. Rev.*, *46*:165–173 (1987).
45. R. V. Levy, The effect of pH, viscosity, and additives on the bacterial retention of membrane filters challenged with *Pseudomonas diminuta*, in *Fluid Filtration: Liquid*, Vol. II, ASTM, Washington, DC, 1987.
46. T. J. Leahy, Validation of bacterial retention by membrane filters: A proposed approach for determining sterility assurance, Ph.D. dissertation, University of Massachusetts, Amherst, MA, 1983.
47. H. F. Ridgway, D. M. Rogers, and D. G. Argo, Proceedings of the Semiconductor Pure Water Conference, San Francisco, CA, 1986, pp. 133–164.
48. C. D. Lytle and L. B. Roustson, Minimized virus binding for tests of barrier materials, *Appl. Environ. Microbiol.*, *61*:643–649 (1995).
49. H. Aranha and J. Meeker, Microbial retention characteristics of 0.2-microns-rated nylon membrane filters during filtration of high viscosity fluids at high differential pressure and varied temperatures, *J. Pharm. Sci. Technol.*, *49*:67–70 (1995).
50. R. L. Anderson, L. A. Bland, M. S. Favero, M. M. McNeil, B. J. Davis, D. C. Mackel, and R. R. Gravell, *Appl. Environ. Microbiol.*, *50*(6):1343–1348 (1985).
51. G. B. Tanny, D. K. Strong, W. G. Presswood, and T. H. Meltzer, Adsorptive retention of *Pseudomonas diminuta* by membrane filters, *J. Parenter. Drug Assoc.*, *33*:40–51 (1979).

52. S. F. Emory, Y. Koga, N. Azuma, and K. Matsumoto, The effects of surfactant types and latex-particle feed concentration on membrane retention, *Ultrapure Water*, *10*(2): 41–44 (1993).
53. W. J. Elford, The principle of ultrafiltration as applied in biological studies, *Proc. Roy. Soc.* (*Lond.*), *12B*:384–406 (1933).
54. F. J. Sladek, R. V. Suslavich, B. I. John, and F. W. Dawson, Optimum membrane structures for growth of coliform and fecal coliform organisms, *Appl. Microbiol.*, *30*:685–689 (1975).
55. R. H. Bordner, Environmental Protection Agency, private communications.
56. J. L. Clancy and L. Cimini, Methods for the improved recovery of high purity water bacteria, Ultrapure water Expo '91-East Conference on High-Purity Water, Proceedings, Philadelphia, PA (April 29–May 1, 1991).
57. M. J. Groves, Letter to the Editor, *Pharm. Tech.*, *15*(1):18 (1991).
58. R. V. Levy, Letter to the Editor, *Pharm. Tech.*, *15*(1):18, 20 (1991).
59. J. Carter, Evaluation of recovery filters for use in bacterial retention testing of sterilizing-grade filters, *PDA J. Pharm. Sci. Technol.*, *50*(3):147–154 (1986).
60. T. Munson, Private communication, 1996.
61. P. J. Waibel, M. W. Jornitz, and T. H. Meltzer, Diffusive airflow integrity testing, *PDA J. Pharm. Sci. Technol.*, Nov./Dec.: 311–316 (1996).
62. T. H. Meltzer, M. W. Jornitz, and M. W. Mittelman, Surrogate solution attributes and use conditions: Effects on bacterial cell size and surface charge relevant to filter validation studies, PDA Second Asian Symposium, Feb. 17–19, 1997, Osaka, Japan.
63. M. W. Mittelman, M. W. Jornitz, and T. H. Meltzer, Bacterial cell size and surface charge characteristics relevant to filter validation studies, *PDA J. Pharm. Sci. Technol.*, 1997 (Accepted by PDA Journal of Pharmaceutical Sci. & Technol.).

Index

ISBN 0-8247-9896-1

EAN

9 780824 798963

90000>